Staphylococci in Human Disease

Staphylococci in Human Disease

EDITED BY

KENT B. CROSSLEY, MD
Professor of Medicine
University of Minnesota Medical School
Associate Chief of Staff for Education
Minneapolis Veterans Affairs Medical Center
Minneapolis, Minnesota, USA

KIMBERLY K. JEFFERSON, PHD
Assistant Professor of Microbiology and Immunology
Virginia Commonwealth University School of Medicine
Richmond, Virginia, USA

GORDON L. ARCHER, MD
Professor of Microbiology and Immunology
Senior Associate Dean for Research
Virginia Commonwealth University School of Medicine
Richmond, Virginia, USA

VANCE G. FOWLER JR, MD, MHS
Associate Professor of Medicine
Division of Infectious Diseases
Duke University Medical Center
Durham, North Carolina, USA

SECOND EDITION

WILEY-BLACKWELL
A John Wiley & Sons, Ltd., Publication

This edition first published 2009, © 2009 by Blackwell Publishing Ltd

Blackwell Publishing was acquired by John Wiley & Sons in February 2007.
Blackwell's publishing program has been merged with Wiley's global Scientific,
Technical and Medical business to form Wiley-Blackwell.

Registered office: John Wiley & Sons Ltd, The Atrium, Southern Gate, Chichester, West Sussex,
PO19 8SQ, UK

Editorial offices: 9600 Garsington Road, Oxford, OX4 2DQ, UK
The Atrium, Southern Gate, Chichester, West Sussex, PO19 8SQ, UK
111 River Street, Hoboken, NJ 07030-5774, USA

For details of our global editorial offices, for customer services and for information about how to apply for permission to reuse the copyright material in this book please see our website at www.wiley.com/wiley-blackwell

Library of Congress Cataloging-in-Publication Data
Staphylococci in human disease / edited by Kent B. Crossley . . . [*et al.*]. – 2nd ed.
p. ; cm.
Includes bibliographical references and index.
ISBN: 978-1-4051-6332-3
1. Staphylococcal infections. I. Crossley, Kent B.
[DNLM: 1. Staphylococcus–pathogenicity. 2. Staphylococcal Infections.
QW 142.5.C6 S7935 2010]
QR201.S68S84 2010
616.9′297–dc22

2009004429

A catalogue record for this book is available from the British Library.

Set in 9.25/12pt Palatino by Graphicraft Limited, Hong Kong
Printed in and bound in Singapore by Fabulous Printers Pte Ltd

1 2009

Contents

Contributors

Deverick J. Anderson, MD, MPH
Assistant Professor of Medicine
Duke University Medical Center
Associate Hospital Epidemiologist
Chair, Antibiotic Evaluation Committee
DU Box 3605
Durham, NC 27710, USA

Elie F. Berbari, MD
Associate Professor of Medicine
Mayo Clinic College of Medicine
200 First St SW
Rochester, MN 55902, USA

Brigitte Berger-Bächi, PhD
Institute of Medical Microbiology
University of Zürich
8006 Zürich, Switzerland

Gregory A. Bohach, PhD
Director, Experimental Station; Associate Dean, College of Agricultural and Life Sciences; Professor, Department of Microbiology, Molecular Biology, and Biochemistry
University of Idaho
PO Box 442331
Moscow, ID 83844-0001, USA

Helen W. Boucher, MD FACP
Director, Infectious Diseases Fellowship Program
Assistant Professor of Medicine
Division of Geographic Medicine and Infectious Diseases
Tufts Medical Center
800 Washington Street, Box 238
Boston, MA 02111, USA

John M. Boyce, MD
Chief, Infectious Diseases Section
Hospital of Saint Raphael;
Clinical Professor of Medicine
Yale University School of Medicine
1450 Chapel Street
New Haven, CT 06511, USA

Henry F. Chambers, MD
Professor of Medicine
University of California San Francisco;
Chief, Division of Infectious Diseases
San Francisco General Hospital
San Francisco, California, 94110, USA

Liang Chen, PhD
Public Health Research Institute Tuberculosis Center
University of Medicine and Dentistry of New Jersey
225 Warren Street
Newark, NJ 07103, USA

G. Ralph Corey, MD
Division of Infectious Diseases
Duke Clinical Research Institute
Duke University Medical Center
Durham, North Carolina, 27715, USA

Sara E. Cosgrove, MD
Assistant Professor of Medicine
Division of Infectious Diseases
Johns Hopkins University School of Medicine
Baltimore, Maryland, 21287, USA

Lisa E. Davidson, MD
Assistant Professor of Medicine
Division of Geographic Medicine and Infectious Diseases
Tufts Medical Center
800 Washington Street, Box 238
Boston, MA 02111, USA

Aaron DeVries, MD, MPH
Adjunct Assistant Professor of Medicine
University of Minnesota School of Medicine;
Medical Epidemiologist
Infectious Disease Epidemiology, Prevention, and Control Section Minnesota Department of Health
Acute Disease Investigation and Control Section
625 Robert Street North
PO Box 64975
St. Paul, MN 55164-0975, USA

Odette C. El Helou, MD
Instructor in Medicine
Mayo Clinic College of Medicine
200 First St SW
Rochester, MN 55902, USA

Miriam Ender
PhD student
Institute of Medical Microbiology
University of Zürich
8006 Zürich, Switzerland

Jerome Etienne, MD, PhD
INSERM U851;
Centre National de Référence des Staphylocoques
Faculté de Médecine Laennec
Université Lyon 1
Lyon, F-69008 France

Tristan Ferry, MD, PhD
INSERM U851;
Centre National de Référence des Staphylocoques
Faculté de Médecine Laennec
Université Lyon 1
Lyon, F-69008 France

Paul D. Fey, PhD
Associate Professor
Departments of Pathology and Microbiology and Internal Medicine
University of Nebraska Medical Center
Omaha, NE 68198-4031, USA

Linda A. Ficker, BSc, FRCS, FRCOphth
Consultant Ophthalmic Surgeon
Moorfields Eye Hospital NHS Foundation Trust
London, UK
162 City Road
London EC1V 2PD

Betty A. Forbes, PhD, D(ABMM), F(AAM)
Department of Pathology
Virginia Commonwealth University School of Medicine
PO Box 980662
Richmond, VA 23298, USA

Timothy J. Foster, PhD
Microbiology Department
Moyne Institute of Preventive Medicine
Trinity College
Dublin 2, Ireland

S. Gatermann, MD, PhD
Abt. Med. Microbiologie
Ruhr-Universitaet Bochum
44801 Bochum, Germany

Steven R. Gill, PhD
Infectious Disease and Genomics
Departments of Oral Biology/Microbiology and Immunology
Center of Excellence in Bioinformatics and Life Sciences
University of Buffalo
701 Ellicott Street
Buffalo, NY 14203, USA

Rachel J. Gorwitz, MD, MPH
Division of Healthcare Quality Promotion
National Center for Preparedness, Detection, and Control of Infectious Diseases
Centers for Disease Control and Prevention
MS A35
1600 Clifton Rd NE
Atlanta, GA 30333, USA

Hattie D. Gresham, PhD
Research Microbiologist and Professor
New Mexico Veterans Affairs Health Care System
University of New Mexico
Albuquerque, NM 87131, USA

Nada Harik, MD
Department of Pediatrics
Section of Infectious Diseases
Arkansas Children's Hospital
800 Marshall Street
Little Rock, AR 72202, USA

Mark E. Hart, PhD
National Center for Toxicological Research
Division of Microbiology
3900 NCTR RD
Jefferson, AR 72079, USA

Loreen A. Herwaldt, MD
Professor
University of Iowa Carver College of Medicine
University of Iowa College of Public Health;
Hospital Epidemiologist
University of Iowa Hospitals and Clinics
200 Hawkins Drive
Iowa City, IA 52242-1081, USA

Roni Heusser
PhD student
Institute of Medical Microbiology
University of Zürich
8006 Zürich, Switzerland

Keiichi Hiramatsu, MD, PhD
Department of Bacteriology
Department of Infection Control Science
Juntendo University
2-1-1 Hongo, Bunkyo-ku, Tokyo, Japan 113-8421

David C. Hooper, MD
Professor of Medicine
Harvard Medical School;
Chief, Infection Control Unit
Division of Infectious Diseases
Massachusetts General Hospital
55 Fruit Street
Boston, MA 02114-2696, USA

Judith Hübscher
PhD student
Institute of Medical Microbiology
University of Zürich
8006 Zürich, Switzerland

John A. Jernigan, MD, MS
Deputy Branch Chief, Prevention and Response Branch
Division of Healthcare Quality Promotion
National Center for Preparedness, Detection, and Control of Infectious Diseases
Centers for Disease Control and Prevention
MS A35
1600 Clifton Rd NE
Atlanta, GA 30333, USA

Joseph John, MD
Associate Chief of Staff for Education
Ralph H. Johnson Veterans Affairs Medical Center;
Clinical Professor of Medicine
Professor of Microbiology and Immunology
Medical University of South Carolina
109 Bee Street
Charleston, SC 29401-5703, USA

Zeina A. Kanafani, MD, MS, CIC
Assistant Professor of Medicine
Division of Infectious Diseases
American University of Beirut Medical Center
Cairo Street PO Box 11-0236; Riad El Solh 1107 2020
Beirut, Lebanon

Keith S. Kaye, MD, MPH
Professor of Medicine
Wayne State University and Detroit Medical Center
Corporate Director, Infection Prevention,
Epidemiology and Antimicrobial Stewardship
University Health Center, 4021 Saint Antoine,
Suite 2B, Box 331, Detroit, MI 48201, USA

Marin H. Kollef, MD
Washington University School of Medicine
Campus Box 8052
680S Euclid Avenue
St Louis, MO 63110, USA

Barry N. Kreiswirth, PhD
Public Health Research Institute Tuberculosis Center
University of Medicine and Dentistry of New Jersey
225 Warren Street
Newark, NJ 07103, USA

Chia Y. Lee, PhD
Department of Microbiology and Immunology
University of Arkansas for Medical Sciences
4301 W. Markham, Mail Slot 511
Little Rock, AR 72205, USA

Jean C. Lee, PhD
Associate Professor
Channing Laboratory
Department of Medicine
Brigham and Women's Hospital and Harvard Medical School
181 Longwood Avenue
Boston, MA 02115, USA

Mark Loeb, MD, FRCPC, MSc
Departments of Pathology and Molecular Medicine
Clinical Epidemiology and Biostatistics
McMaster University
Michael G. DeGroote Centre for Learning Room 3203
1200 Main Street West
Hamilton, Ontario, Canada L8N 3Z5

Barun Mathema, MPH
Public Health Research Institute Tuberculosis Center
University of Medicine and Dentistry of New Jersey
225 Warren Street
Newark, NJ 07103, USA

Nadine McCallum, PhD
Institute of Medical Microbiology
University of Zürich
8006 Zürich, Switzerland

John K. McCormick, PhD
Associate Professor
Department of Microbiology and Immunology
University of Western Ontario
DSB3014, 1151 Richmond St.
London, Ontario, Canada N6A 5C1

José R. Mediavilla, BS
Public Health Research Institute Tuberculosis Center
University of Medicine and Dentistry of New Jersey
225 Warren Street
Newark, NJ 07103, USA

Esteban C. Nannini, MD
Division of Infectious Diseases, Sanatorio Parque;
Facultad de Ciencias Médicas
Rosario, Argentina

Douglas H. Ohlendorf, PhD
Department of Biochemistry, Molecular Biology, and Biophysics
University of Minnesota
321 Church St SE
5-118 NHH
Minneapolis, MN 55455-0250, USA

Douglas R. Osmon, MD, MPH
Associate Professor of Medicine
Mayo Clinic College of Medicine
200 First St SW
Rochester, MN 55902, USA

Richard A. Proctor, MD
Professor Emeritus of Medical Microbiology/Immunology and Medicine
5301 Microbial Sciences Building
University of Wisconsin School of Medicine and Public Health
1550 Linden Dr.
Madison, WI 53706, USA

Kathie L. Rogers, PhD
Department of Pathology and Microbiology
University of Nebraska Medical Center
Omaha, NE 68198-4031, USA

Karen L. Roos, MD
John and Nancy Nelson Professor of Neurology
Indiana University School of Medicine
550 North University Boulevard, Suite 4411
Indianapolis, IN 46202-5124, USA

Ethan Rubinstein, MD, LLb
Sellers Professor of Medicine
Section of Infectious Diseases
Faculty of Medicine
University of Manitoba
543-730 William Ave
501 Basic Medical Sciences Building
Winnipeg, Manitoba, Canada R3E 0W3

Mark E. Rupp, MD
Professor and Hospital Epidemiologist
Department of Internal Medicine
University of Nebraska Medical Center
Omaha, NE 68198-4031, USA

Adam C. Schaffer, MD
Instructor
Department of Medicine
Harvard Medical School
Brigham and Women's Hospital
PBB-B-422, 75 Francis Street
Boston, MA 02115, USA

Patrick M. Schlievert, PhD
Department of Microbiology
University of Minnesota
420 Delaware St SE
Minneapolis, MN 55455-0341, USA

Bettina Schulthess
PhD Student
Institute of Medical Microbiology
University of Zürich
8006 Zürich, Switzerland

Brian S. Schwartz, MD
Assistant Professor of Medicine
Division of Infectious Diseases
University of California San Francisco
513 Parnassus Avenue Room S380
San Francisco, California 94143, USA

Kati Seidl
PhD student
Institute of Medical Microbiology
University of Zürich
8006 Zürich, Switzerland

Maria Magdalena Senn, PhD
Institute of Medical Microbiology
University of Zürich
8006 Zürich, Switzerland

Robert J. Sherertz, MD
Professor of Medicine and Infectious Diseases
Wake Forest University School of Medicine
Section on Infectious Diseases,
Medical Center Blvd
Winston-Salem, NC 27157, USA

Andrew E. Simor, MD, FRCPC, FACP
Department of Microbiology and Division of Infectious Diseases
Sunnybrook Health Sciences Centre
University of Toronto
B103-2075 Bayview Avenue
Toronto, Ontario, Canada M4N 3M5

Mark S. Smeltzer, PhD
Department of Microbiology and Immunology
University of Arkansas for Medical Sciences
4301 W. Markham, Mail Slot 511
Little Rock, AR 72205, USA

Greg A. Somerville, PhD
Assistant Professor
Department of Veterinary and Biomedical Sciences
University of Nebraska
Fair St. and East Campus Loop
Lincoln, NE 68583-0905, USA

Jacob Strahilevitz, MD
Department of Clinical Microbiology and Infectious Diseases
Hadassah Medical Center
Hebrew University
Jerusalem 91120, Israel

Martin E. Stryjewski, MD, MHS
Assistant Professor of Medicine
Department of Medicine and Division of Infectious Diseases
Centro de Educación Médica e Investigaciones Clínicas "Norberto Quirno"
Buenos Aires, Argentina;
Division of Infectious Diseases
Duke Clinical Research Institute
Durham, North Carolina 27705, USA

Patricia Stutzmann Meier, MD, PhD
Institute of Medical Microbiology
University of Zürich
8006 Zürich, Switzerland

Karl M. Thompson, PhD
Postdoctoral Fellow in Research
Department of Microbiology and Immunology
Virginia Commonwealth University
PO Box 980678
Richmond, VA 23298, USA

Henri A. Verbrugh, MD, PhD
Professor of Clinical Microbiology and Antimicrobial Therapy
Department of Medical Microbiology and Infectious Diseases
Erasmus University Medical Center
3015 CE Rotterdam, The Netherlands

Mark H. Wilcox, MD, FRCPath
Professor of Medical Microbiology
Leeds Teaching Hospitals and University of Leeds
Leeds General Infirmary
The Old Medical School
Thoresby Place
Leeds, LS1 3EX, UK

Hidetaka Yanagi, MD
Tokai University School of Medicine
Division of General Internal Medicine
143 Shimokasuya,
Isehara, Kanagawa, 259–1143 Japan

Preface to the Second Edition

In the preface to the original edition of this book, written over a decade ago, we noted that there were three reasons to plan and edit a book about staphylococci and staphylococcal infection. These same reasons are even more important today than they were in 1997.

Firstly, the significance of staphylococcal infection has continued to increase. When the original edition was published, methicillin-resistant staphylococci were relatively uncommon. That has changed dramatically in the last decade. In 2005, 19 000 deaths in the USA resulted from methicillin-resistant *Staphylococcus aureus* (MRSA) infection. This number exceeded both HIV-AIDS and homicide as causes of mortality. Community-acquired MRSA infections, almost unknown in 1997, have become a substantial problem in subsequent years. Nothing we have read suggests to us that mortality from staphylococcal infection is lower than it was in 1997 or that newer antistaphylococcal antibiotics are likely to result in more favorable outcomes. Staphylococci remain the most important cause of nosocomial infections in the USA and MRSA has become the most common cause of skin and soft tissue infection in the community.

Secondly, the volume of information about staphylococci and staphylococcal infection has grown at a rapid rate. In 1997, there were 2283 papers indexed by the National Library of Medicine under the headings "staphylococci" or "staphylococcal infection." In 2008, there were 12 330 papers in these categories. This extraordinary amount of information demands assessment by skilled and critical authors and editors. We have an outstanding group of authors who have carefully sifted through this information and provided succinct evaluations of their part of this enormous collection of literature.

Finally, no other book like this has been published since our first edition. The books about staphylococci that have been published in the last decade have focused on laboratory science or have been symposia proceedings.

Our goal here – as with the first edition – is to provide a comprehensive review of both basic and clinical science about staphylococci. This volume should be of value to both researchers and clinicians. We hope you find it useful.

Kent B. Crossley
Kimberly K. Jefferson
Gordon L. Archer
Vance G. Fowler, Jr.
September 2009

Section I
The Organisms

Biology and Taxonomy

Chapter 1 The Biology of Staphylococci

Greg A. Somerville[1] *and Richard A. Proctor*[2]
[1] Department of Veterinary and Biomedical Sciences, University of Nebraska, Lincoln, Nebraska, USA
[2] University of Wisconsin School of Medicine and Public Health, Madison, Wisconsin, USA

Historical perspective of the isolation and characterization of the staphylococci

The staphylococci make up the family of Gram-positive cocci, Staphylococcaceae, which is in the order Bacillales. The term "staphylococcus" was synthesized from the Greek word *staphyle*, meaning bunch of grapes, for their ability to form microscopic grape-like clusters, and the term "coccus," meaning grain or berry. *Staphylococcus aureus* was one of the first bacterial pathogens identified, and causes a very broad range of infections including impetigo, folliculitis, superficial and deep skin abscesses, wound infections, osteomyelitis, suppurative arthritis, pneumonia, pleural emphysema, meningitis, septicemia and endocarditis, toxic shock syndrome, scalded skin syndrome, and food poisoning [1].

Koch first differentiated Gram-positive cocci in 1878 and recognized that different diseases such as abscesses correlated with the presence of clusters of Gram-positive cocci. Shortly thereafter, in 1884, Rosenbach differentiated species of staphylococci on the basis of colonial pigmentation, whereby the most pathogenic species formed a golden pigment and less pathogenic staphylococci formed white colonies called *S. albus*, now *S. epidermidis*. Also included in the *S. albus* strains were many other coagulase-negative staphylococci that fail to form pigment. Alexander Ogston, in 1880, found "a cluster forming coccus was the cause of certain pyogenous abscesses in man." When Ogston injected the pus from humans containing staphylococci into mice, it produced abscesses; however, when the pus was heated or treated with phenol, it failed to produce abscesses. In 1882, Ogston named the organism staphylococcus. Pasteur had reached similar conclusions at approximately the same time. Coagulase testing later provided a more certain classification of staphylococci than pigment production, wherein a positive coagulase test, which confirmed the identity of *S. aureus*, correlated much better with pathogenicity.

Another common human pathogen is *S. saprophyticus*, which produces urinary tract infections in young women [2]. *Staphylococcus haemolyticus* is somewhat less common, but is important because it can be highly antibiotic resistant even to glycopeptides and linezolid [3]. Many other coagulase-negative strains (41 species identified at present) such as *S. schleiferi* and *S. lugdunesis* have been described, and they can produce a variety of nosocomial infections (reviewed by von Eiff *et al.* [4,5]).

Morphology

Staphylococci have a diameter of 0.7–1.2 μm and a Gram-positive cell wall (Figure 1.1). Division planes occur at right angles and the cocci separate slowly, hence tetrads are frequently found. Clustering of cocci is promoted by growth on solid medium. On occasion, the clusters may be asymmetrical.

Microbiological differentiation of staphylococci

Growth under various conditions

Staphylococci are facultative anaerobes that grow most rapidly under aerobic conditions and in the presence of CO_2. Colonies of *S. aureus* are β-hemolytic due to the production of several hemolysins: α-toxin, β-toxin, γ-toxin, and δ-toxin. Some *S. epidermidis* strains are β-hemolytic due to the production of δ-toxin [6]. Pigmentation is more pronounced after 24 hours and when held at room temperature, or in media enriched with acetate or glycerol monophosphate [7,8]. The pigments are carotenoids, whose biosynthetic pathway has recently been identified in *S. aureus* [9]. Pigment is not produced under anaerobic

Staphylococci in Human Disease, 2nd edition. Edited by Kent B. Crossley, Kimberly K. Jefferson, Gordon Archer, Vance G. Fowler, Jr.

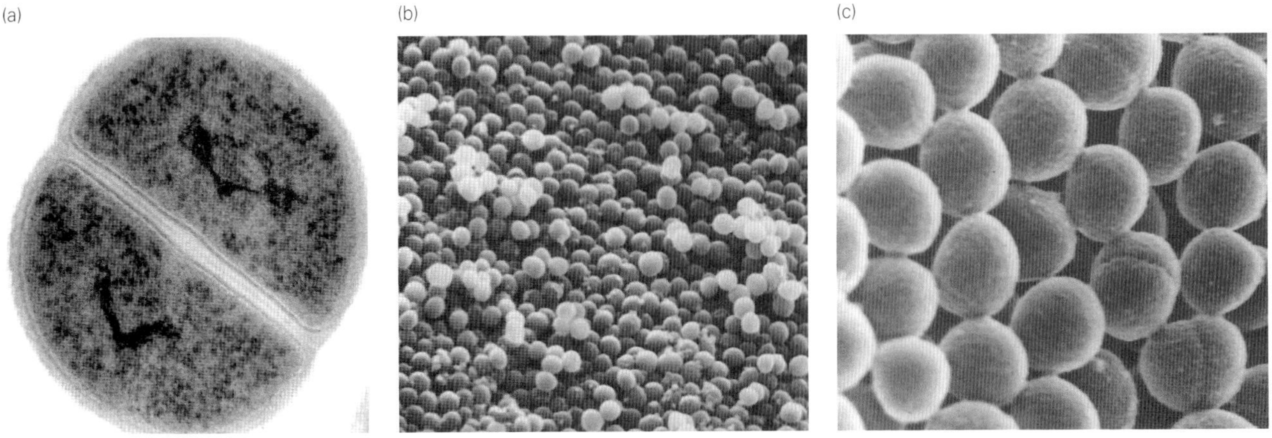

Figure 1.1 (a) Transmission electron microscopy at 126 700× magnification of *S. aureus* cells displaying cell separation by a cross-wall surrounding a highly contrasting splitting system. Scanning electron microscopy of *S. aureus* cells at (b) low (6700×) and (c) high (35 000×) magnification. Reproduced with permission from Kahl BC, Belling G, Reichelt R, Herrmann M, Proctor RA, Peters G. Thymidine-dependent small-colony variants of Staphylococcus aureus exhibit gross morphological and ultrastructural changes consistent with impaired cell separation. *J Clin Microbiol* 2003;41(1):410–3.

conditions or by small colony variants [10]. The formation of pigments is dependent on the stress sigma factor, σ^B [11]. A few *S. aureus* strains produce abundant exopolysaccharide (e.g., Smith strain, which produces a mucoid colony); however, most strains produce only a microcapsule and the colonies appear non-mucoid [12]. When encountered in clinical strains, the most frequent *S. aureus* serotypes are capsule types 5 and 8 [12]. In contrast to *S. aureus*, most clinical *S. epidermidis* isolates produce more exopolysaccharide.

Staphylococci can grow in a wide pH range (4.8–9.4), resist drying, and can survive at temperature extremes as high as 60°C for 30 min. In addition, *S. aureus* grows in high-salt medium due to the production of osmoprotectants [13], and can tolerate 7.5–10% NaCl. The ability of *S. aureus* to ferment mannitol is the basis for differentiating it from *S. epidermidis* and *S. saprophyticus*. When grown on mannitol salt agar, fermentation of mannitol produces a yellow zone around the colony. In addition to mannitol, *S. aureus* can metabolize glucose, xylose, lactose, sucrose, maltose, and glycerol. Further differentiation of staphylococci can be achieved by growth in the presence of novobiocin. *Staphylococcus saprophyticus* [14] and *S. xylosus* [5] are intrinsically resistant to novobiocin because their version of the DNA gyrase B enzyme does not bind novobiocin whereas other coagulase-negative staphylococci such as *S. epidermidis*, *S. haemolyticus*, *S. hominis*, *S. lugdunensis*, and *S. schleiferi* are novobiocin susceptible [5].

Special media

Several nonroutine agars are used to study *S. aureus* enzymes. Lipases produce clearing on egg yolk agar, especially when grown under anaerobic conditions [15]. *Staphylococcus aureus* protease activity can be monitored on casein agar plates, where protease-positive strains produce clearing of the agar [16]. When V8 protease (encoded by *sspA*) is present, it produces a zone of white precipitates around the colony [16]. Finally, tellurite is often added to growth media for the selection of *Corynebacterium diphtheriae* in pharyngeal specimens; *S. aureus* may be found in the pharyngeal specimens and can grow in the presence of tellurite, producing gray-black colonies that allow it to be confused with *C. diphtheriae*.

Other methods for differentiation of staphylococci

Staphylococci can be differentiated from micrococcus species based on their susceptibility to lysis by lysostaphin [17]. Lysostaphin is a metalloendopeptidase that targets the pentaglycine bridge of peptidoglycan [18].

Phenol soluble modulins have been associated with more severe staphylococcal infections and require specialized chromatography and mass spectrometry for identification and quantification [19].

While polymerase chain reaction (PCR) testing is not yet routine practice, its use is becoming more widely available in clinical as well as research laboratories. One of the most reliable PCR tests for *S. aureus* [20] detects the presence of the thermonuclease gene *nuc* [20–22]. PCR can also be used to test for the presence of genes encoding Panton-Valentine leukocidin (PVL), which is indicative of strains of community-acquired methicillin-resistant *S. aureus* (CA-MRSA) [23].

Colonization with staphylococci

Nasal carriage of *S. aureus* is persistently present in 30% of people and transiently found in 70% of people; conversely, 30% of people resist nasal colonization [4,24]. A higher incidence rate of nasal carriage of CA-MRSA has also been associated with individuals having frequent contact with cats, dogs, pigs, and horses, suggesting that animals can be vectors in the spread of CA-MRSA [25–28]. *Staphylococcus aureus* reportedly adheres to nasal mucosa through several surface protein adhesins, including SasG, clumping factor, and fibronectin-binding protein [29–32]. Indeed, the staphylococci have a large array of surface proteins and carbohydrates that enable binding to a broad range of host tissues, including platelets, epithelial cells, endothelial cells, and host intercellular matrix proteins [33]. More detailed information concerning staphylococcal adherence to host tissues is covered in Chapter 7.

CA-MRSA demonstrate distinctive patterns of colonization, as they may be found solely in the throat or on the skin but are culture negative in the nares [34,35]. For this reason, testing individuals for colonization by nasal culture alone may not be sufficient for detection of CA-MRSA colonization.

Several recent studies suggest that streptococci may compete with CA-MRSA for colonization of mucosal surfaces. In a study by Chen *et al.* [36], it was observed that 17% of pregnant women were found to be vaginally colonized with *S. aureus* but only 0.5% were colonized by MRSA. Colonization of the vagina with *S. aureus* was associated with an 11-fold increased risk of postpartum fever. Interestingly, patients vaginally colonized with CA-MRSA were 12.5 times less likely to carry group B streptococci. In contrast, when methicillin-sensitive *S. aureus* (MSSA)-colonized patients were compared with patients who were not *S. aureus* colonized, the MSSA patients were 4.5 times more likely to carry group B streptococci [37]. These data suggest that group B streptococci are especially important for competing with CA-MRSA for colonization of vaginal mucosa. Similarly, on the oropharyngeal mucosal surfaces, *Streptococcus pneumoniae* may be important for preventing oral colonization by CA-MRSA. Children carrying *Streptococcus pneumoniae* are less likely to carry *S. aureus* [38], and pneumococcal vaccination increases *S. aureus* colonization [39,40]. While the heptavalent conjugate vaccine was not licensed for use in children in the USA until 2000 and in Europe until 2001, the first report of oral colonization by CA-MRSA was in 1998 [41]. Nevertheless, vaccination and subsequent eradication of competing bacterial species may be contributing to the rapid spread of CA-MRSA. *Streptococcus pneumoniae* can produce hydrogen peroxide at concentrations capable of killing *S. aureus* [39], but this does not appear to be a major determinant of the patterns of co-colonization [42]. When looking specifically at CA-MRSA colonization, the rate of *S. aureus* colonization is increased in patients receiving the pneumococcal vaccine, but there is no particular increase in CA-MRSA strains [43]. Thus, streptococci on mucosal surfaces compete with *S. aureus*, but this is only one potential factor contributing to the current CA-MRSA outbreak.

Staphylococcus epidermidis resides more permanently on the skin because it is better able to tolerate the acidic pH, lipids, and salt found on skin [44] than is *S. aureus*, which can only persist on the skin for several hours. Recently, USA300, a CA-MRSA strain responsible for a rapidly spreading epidemic of skin and soft tissue infections, was found more frequently on the skin in the absence of nares colonization relative to other strains of *S. aureus* [34,35], suggesting that USA300 strains are particularly well adapted to persist on the skin. Whether skin colonization is permanent or transient, this colonization creates a major problem in hospitals because hands are an excellent means of transmitting MRSA, thus creating a major threat to patient welfare [45].

In addition to the two predominant staphylococcal human pathogens, several other staphylococci are capable of causing disease in humans and animals. *Staphylococcus saprophyticus* is able to colonize the urinary tract and cause infections, showing lower levels of colonization when higher concentrations of Tamm–Horsfall protein are present [46]. Coagulase-negative staphylococci are frequently found on the skin and mucous membranes [5], binding to tissues via teichoic acids, hemagglutinin, fibronectin, and autolysins [47,48]. *Staphylococcus anaerobius* is a pathogen of sheep that causes skin abscess, but only rarely has it produced abscesses or sepsis in humans [49].

Cell structure

The staphylococcal cell envelope is a complex structure that consists of a cell membrane composed of lipids and proteins, a cell wall made from peptidoglycan and teichoic acids, and polysaccharides. As with all cell membranes, its integrity is crucial for maintaining a boundary between the external environment and the cytoplasm. The membrane also contains a large number of proteins that transport solutes across chemical gradients, expending ATP or membrane potential. The electron transport machinery (NADH oxidase, cytochromes, and F_0F_1-ATPase) is also localized to the cell membrane, producing ATP and establishing the electrochemical gradient across the membrane that powers a multitude of activities. The cell wall contains the high osmotic pressure of the cytoplasm of staphylococci.

Membrane

The bacterial membrane is a lipid bilayer where the inner and outer leaflets contain asymmetrically placed lipids [50]. While the basic lipid components of the staphylococcal membrane were defined several decades ago [51] and found to change during different phases of growth [52], the ability of the membrane to respond to environmental, host defense-related, and antimicrobial challenges has only recently been appreciated.

The membrane phospholipids of *S. aureus* include phosphatidylglycerol, lysyl-phosphatidylglycerol, phosphatidic acid, cardiolipin, and traces of phosphatidylethanolamine and phosphatidylglucose [51–53]. These phospholipids, together with the carotenoids, menaquinone, and the glucolipids (monoglucosyldiglyceride and diglucosyldiglyceride), make up the major components of the staphylococcal membrane [52]. The phospholipids total about 60 μmol, the carotenoids 0.1 μmol, the vitamin K_2 isoprenologues 0.2 μmol, and the glucolipids 10 μmol per gram dry weight in exponentially growing cells [52]. *Staphylococcus aureus* accumulates cardiolipin and loses phosphatidylglycerol during the stationary phase of growth. The minor lipids, phosphatidylethanolamine and phosphatidylglucose, also accumulate, whereas the lysyl-phosphatidylglycerol content of the membrane remains constant during the stationary phase [51].

Because optimal membrane fluidity must be maintained for cell function, staphylococci must adapt to changes in environmental conditions by altering their membrane fluidity [54,55]. Adjustments in membrane fluidity, effected by changes in lipid composition, must occur in response to variations in temperature, pressure, ion concentrations, pH, nutrient availability, and xenobiotics. In many bacterial species membrane fluidity is greatly increased by introducing unsaturated fatty acids into the lipid bilayer, which disrupts packing of the lipids. However, this strategy is not utilized by *S. aureus*, which employs anteiso-branching of the fatty acids to increase fluidity in response to conditions such as high salt concentrations [44], and increases iso-branched fatty acids and carotenoids to decrease fluidity. The production of branched-chain fatty acids is regulated in part by the two-component regulatory system YycFG [56].

Some examples of changes in membrane lipids in response to environmental challenges are described here. Cardiolipin content in the membrane increases when *S. aureus* is challenged with cell wall-active antibiotics [57]. Cardiolipin is synthesized from two phosphatidylglycerol molecules [51], and it helps to place a cap on the extracellular face of the membrane to prevent protons from slipping through the bilayer [58]. Cardiolipin concentrates around the F_0F_1-ATPase, which may help to direct protons into this ATP-forming complex [58,59]. The carotenoid pigments of *S. aureus* are optimally produced when the bacteria are held at room temperature rather than 37°C [60]. In *S. aureus*, these pigments are triterpenoid carotenoids possessing a C_{30} chain, whereas most other bacterial carotenoids are C_{40} [61,62]. These pigments have multiple functions, including protection from ultraviolet light [63], resistance to detergents [54,64], stabilization of more fluid membranes [54,64,65], increased tolerance to thermal challenge [66], and protection from oxidant challenge [67]. The apparently contradictory responses, i.e., increased production of carotenoids at room temperature, yet increased protection from thermal stress probably relates to their role in stabilizing the membrane. Under cold conditions, carotenoids stabilize the membrane that has become much more fluid due to changes in lipid composition. In contrast, heating disorganizes the membrane, so stabilization will again be advantageous. Carotenoid pigment biosynthesis is part of the σ^B regulon [63], and it probably accounts for many of the protective stress responses that are induced by σ^B. The function of carotenoids and membrane fluidity extends beyond stress survival; decreased pigmentation is also associated with increased toxic shock syndrome toxin-1 production [68].

Altering the chemical composition of the membrane not only changes membrane fluidity but also the surface charge of the membrane. For example, addition of L-lysine to phosphatidylglycerol can confer a positive surface charge, e.g., lysyl-dipalmitoylphosphatidylglycerol (lysyl-DPPG) [69]. Similarly, modifying teichoic acid by adding D-alanine can decrease negative charge [69]. Each of these changes decreases the negative charge on the surface of the bacteria, which reduces the ability of cationic peptides and positively charged antimicrobial agents such as gentamicin and calcium carrying daptomycin to bind to *S. aureus*, making it more resistant to these challenges [70].

For bacteria to maintain the chemical (ΔpH) and electrical (ΔΨ) components of the proton motive force, the membrane of bacteria must act as a barrier to the movement of hydrogen ions [71]. Therefore, increased membrane fluidity, as caused by warmer temperatures, decreases packing of the lipids in the membrane [72], which allows protons to flow through the disordered lipids of the membrane [73–75]. Cardiolipin acts as a barrier to proton flux across the membrane and it often surrounds the F_0F_1-ATPase, which enhances ATP production since protons do not leak back into the cytoplasm without producing ATP [76,77].

Cell wall

Peptidoglycan: structure, synthesis, autolysis, and cell division

Peptidoglycan, also called murein, is a large macromolecule that is cross-linked into a three-dimensional structure forming a rigid cell wall. It is composed of alternating β-1,4-linked amino sugars composed of *N*-acetylglucosamine (GlcNAc) and *N*-acetylmuramic acid (MurNAc) that are cross-linked by short peptide chains usually composed of tetrapeptides of L-alanine, D-isoglutamine, L-lysine, and D-alanine [78,79]. These short peptides are linked via an amide bond to the D-lactyl moiety of MurNAc [80–82]. The peptides are then cross-linked in a second dimension by interpeptide bridges consisting of penta- or hexa-glycine peptides extending from the carboxy-terminal D-alanine to the ε-amino group of the L-lysine in position 3 of the adjacent peptide. The glycan strands and the cross-linked peptides create a three-dimensional macromolecule with various cross-links that give the cell wall rigid structure [82,83]. The biosynthetic pathway is shown in Figure 1.2.

Peptidoglycan biosynthesis occurs in five stages. The first stage involves the biosynthesis of MurNAc and the addition of a pentapeptide to the MurNAc, which uses

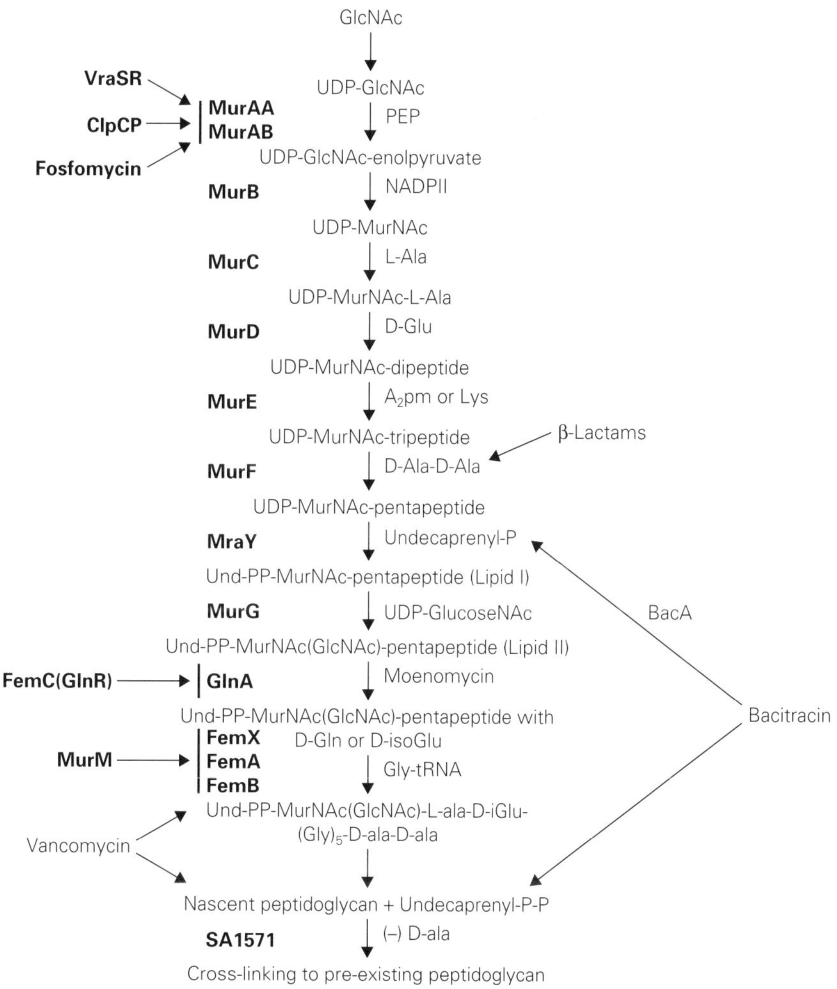

Figure 1.2 The biochemical pathway leading to peptidoglycan synthesis. Enzymes that catalyze each step are shown in bold. Antimicrobial agents that inhibit different steps are indicated.

the enzymes MurAA, MurAB, MurB, MurC, MurD, MurE, and MurF. In the second stage, an undecaprenyl acyl chain is added by MraY forming Lipid I, as the macromolecule is localized to the membrane. Next, GlcNAc is added by MurG to form the disaccharide MurNAc-GlcNAc, called lipid II. In the fourth stage, a pentaglycine peptide is added to the ε-amino group of the L-lysine by FemX, FemA, and FemB [84]. The fifth step involves release of the undecaprenyl group, movement of the nascent peptidoglycan to the outside of the cell, removal of the terminal D-alanine, and cross-linking to the preexisting peptidoglycan via penicillin-binding proteins (PBPs). Variations can occur in the initial tetrapeptide attached to the MurNAc such that the isoglutamate residue can be a glutamine or a meso-2,6-diaminopimeloyl (DAP). Of note, DAP is added with very low efficiency and does not allow the Fem factors to work properly. This results in increased susceptibility of MRSA strains to methicillin.

Lipids I and II

Lipid I (undecaprenylphosphate-MurNAc-pentapeptide) is formed in the first lipid-linked step of cell wall synthesis by MraY, which transfers the soluble UDP-MurNAc-pentapeptide to the lipid carrier undecaprenylphosphate (C55-P). The translocase MurG subsequently links UDP-activated *N*-acetylglucosamine (UDP-GlcNAc) to the muramoyl moiety of lipid I, thus yielding lipid II (undecaprenylphosphate-GlcNAc-MurNAc-pentapeptide) [85]. Recently, farnesol has been reported to increase β-lactam susceptibility of MRSA by inhibition of cell wall biosynthesis through reduction of free C55 lipid carrier with subsequent retardation of murein monomer precursor transport across the cell membrane [86] but it had no effect on PBP2′, which is the altered PBP in MRSA. In addition, it completely suppressed staphyloxanthin production [86]. The D-glutamyl residue in lipid II is converted to D-iso-Glu or D-Gln by GlnA (FemC), which is also needed for methicillin resistance [87].

Pentaglycine bridge

The pentaglycine bridge is synthesized by three enzymes, FemX (*fmhB*), FemA, and FemB, that add the first, second and third, and fourth and fifth glycines, respectively [88]. The pentaglycine interpeptide bridge links the ε-amino group of the L-lysine of one peptidoglycan chain to the D-alanine in position 4 of a neighboring chain [88].

Penicillin-binding proteins

PBPs are DD-transpeptidases that catalyze the last step of peptidoglycan biosynthesis [89]. This occurs on the external surface of the cytoplasmic membrane [89]. PBPs catalyze both the transglycosylation and the transpeptidation reactions required for assembly from the disaccharide oligopeptide precursors, leading to incorporation of the lipid-linked peptidoglycan precursors into the growing cell wall. PBPs probably function in multienzyme complexes that combine peptidoglycan synthetases and hydrolases into a macromolecular peptidoglycan synthesizing complex [90,91]. *S. aureus* has only one mode of cell wall synthesis, which takes place at the septum [92].

The PBPs of *S. aureus* are of particular importance because MRSA strains have acquired resistance to all β-lactam antibiotics due to a modified PBP2 called PBP2a (see Chapter 8 for a more detailed discussion), which is capable of transpeptidation even in the presence of high concentrations of antibiotic because of its low affinity for β-lactam antibiotics [93,94]. Nevertheless, PBP2 is also required for the full expression of methicillin resistance [95]. In the presence of high concentrations of methicillin, PBP2a is responsible for the transpeptidation of peptidoglycan, but the transglycosylase function of PBP2 is still required for the expression of resistance, suggesting cooperation between these PBPs [96,97]. The β-lactam antibiotics bind and inactivate the transpeptidase domain of PBPs in an irreversible manner [98] by preventing the acylated protein from binding to its substrate, the D-Ala-D-Ala terminus of peptidoglycan muropeptides. PBP2 is normally localized at the division septum, the primary location of cell wall synthesis in *S. aureus*; however, oxacillin causes PBP2 to become dispersed over the entire surface of the cell [92].

Once the cell wall has been formed, it must be broken to allow cell division. The cell division plane is formed by FtsZ, a protein that directs autolysins to a localized site in the cell wall as well as PBP2 for new cell wall formation [95]. Atl in *S. aureus* and AtlE in *S. epidermidis* are the major autolysins in these organisms and possess both amidase activity (targets the amide bond between MurNAc and L-alanine) and glucosaminidase activities [99]. How these activities are regulated in staphylococci is an area of active research.

Teichoic acids

Low guanosine plus cytosine (GC) organisms like staphylococci produce lipoglycans with phosphodiester bonds in repeating units called teichoic acids [100]. Teichoic acids are polyanionic molecules [80,100,101] that can be subdivided into wall teichoic acids (WTAs), which are covalently linked to the peptidoglycan, and lipoteichoic acids (LTAs), which are anchored in the outer leaflet of the cytoplasmic membrane via a glycolipid [100,101]. Both LTAs and WTAs extend to the bacterial surface and alter the surface properties of the organisms. Most staphylococci produce both types of teichoic acids (Figure 1.3).

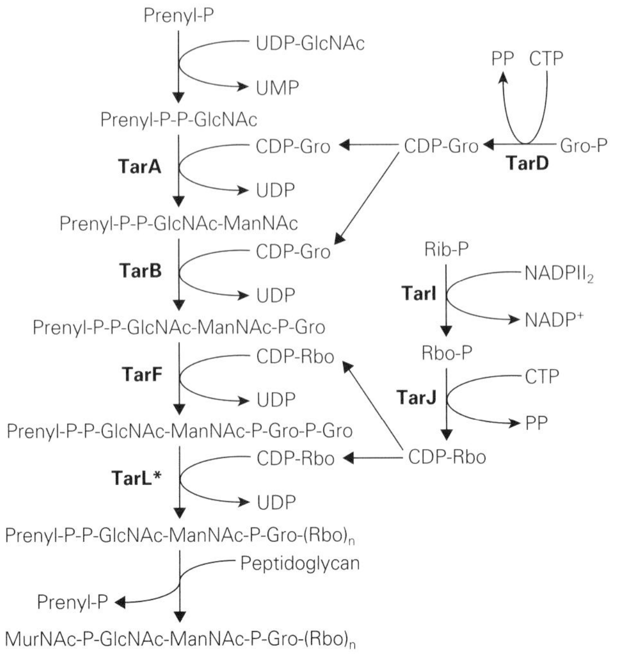

Figure 1.3 The biochemical pathway leading to teichoic acid synthesis. Enzymes that catalyze each step are shown in bold. * Details of the last step are still under investigation, but *S. aureus* appears to lack TarK and use TarL instead.

WTA mutants have been generated [32,102,103]; however, LTA mutations have proven to be lethal [104]. One reason why mutations in LTA may be lethal is that LTA affects cell division [104] and autolysin activity [105].

In staphylococci and many bacilli, LTA is composed of poly(glycerolphosphate) ([Gro-P]$_n$) attached to the glycolipid anchor β-D-Glcp^{II}-(1→6)-β-D-Glcp^{I}-(1→3)-diacylglycerol (DGlcDAG) [106]. Recently, several genes in the biosynthetic pathway of LTA have been identified. YpfP is a glycolipid synthase that mediates DGlcDAG in *S. aureus* [107]. Translocation of DGlcDAG from the inner to the outer leaflet is probably accomplished by LtaA [104]. The LTA is polymerized by LtaS [108]. A deletion in YpfP markedly reduced LTA content in *S. aureus*, but there was no change in WTA content [109].

LTA has a function in the regulation of autolysin activity, surface hydrophobicity, and biofilm formation [107]. (–)-Epicatechin gallate (ECg), a component of green tea, sensitizes MRSA to β-lactam antibiotics, promotes staphylococcal cell aggregation, and increases cell wall thickness by reducing peptidoglycan cross-linking [110]. ECg promotes LTA release from the cytoplasmic membrane, but it does not alter PBP2a expression, even though it reduces Triton X-100 autolysis, suggesting that ECg effects focus on loss of the LTA-inhibitory activity against the autolysin.

Exopolysaccharides

Biosynthesis and regulation of polysaccharide intercellular adhesin

In *S. epidermidis*, and to a lesser degree in *S. aureus*, the synthesis of polysaccharide intercellular adhesin (PIA) is an important process for medical device-associated infections [111,112], is required for the maturation of biofilms (for further review see Chapter 5) [113], and is important for evasion of the host innate immune system [114,115]. PIA is a β-(1,6)-linked GlcNAc polymer [116] of at least 130 residues [117] whose synthesis requires the enzymes encoded within the intercellular adhesin (*ica*) operon (*icaADBC*) [113]. IcaA and IcaD are thought to form a heterodimeric, cell membrane-associated, UDP-GlcNAc transferase [118]. IcaC is a membrane-associated protein hypothesized to be involved in the formation of long polymers and the subsequent export of the growing PIA chain [118]. IcaB catalyzes the deacetylation of poly-GlcNAc [114]. Of importance in the synthesis of PIA is the availability of GlcNAc.

Regulation of the *icaADBC* operon is complex, involving at least two DNA-binding proteins (IcaR and SarA), the alternative sigma factor σ^B, and the *luxS* quorum-sensing system. IcaR is a transcriptional repressor that binds immediately 5′ to the *icaA* transcriptional start site of the *ica* operon [119,120]. SarA is a positive regulator of *ica* transcription that binds to the *icaA* promoter region [121,122]. σ^B affects PIA synthesis indirectly by regulating the expression of *icaR* [123–125]. The *luxS* quorum-sensing system negatively regulates PIA synthesis and biofilm formation; however, the mechanism of regulation remains to be determined [126]. In addition to these regulatory elements, staphylococci regulate the synthesis of PIA and the formation of biofilms in response to nutrient availability, oxygen tension, and a variety of stress factors [127–131]. Interestingly, many of the same environmental and stress factors that affect PIA synthesis also alter tricarboxylic acid (TCA) cycle activity, leading to the hypothesis that PIA synthesis is linked to TCA cycle activity and that regulatory proteins capable of responding to TCA cycle-associated signals control this process [132].

Capsule biosynthesis and regulation

As stated earlier in this chapter, the most commonly encountered *S. aureus* capsule types are 5 and 8 [12]. Both capsule types 5 and 8 are polymers of *N*-acetyl-D-fucosamine, *N*-acetyl-L-fucosamine and *N*-acetyl-D-mannosaminuronic acid (discussed in a later chapter of this book). The biosynthetic precursor of the three capsule sugars is UDP-GlcNAc, the same amino sugar used in synthesizing PIA. GlcNAc is synthesized from the glycolytic intermediate fructose 6-phosphate, and in a rich medium containing glucose abundant levels of fructose 6-phosphate will be generated by the glycolytic (Embden–Meyerhof–Parnas) pathway; however, capsule is most abundantly synthesized in the postexponential phase of growth when glucose is growth limiting [133]. In the absence of glucose, fructose 6-phosphate can be synthesized by gluconeogenesis from the TCA cycle intermediate oxaloacetate. The first step of gluconeogenesis is ATP-dependent decarboxylation and phosphorylation of oxaloacetate by phosphoenolpyruvate carboxykinase (*pckA*) to generate phosphoenolpyruvate (PEP) [134]. Gluconeogenesis can then generate fructose 6-phosphate from PEP, which can be used for UDP-activated GlcNAc biosynthesis. Support for the idea that postexponential capsule biosynthesis requires TCA cycle activity and phosphoenolpyruvate carboxykinase can be found in the observation that capsule is made during aerobic growth [135]. In addition, inactivation of phosphoenolpyruvate carboxykinase (*pckA*), the TCA cycle (*citB*, *citC*, *citG*, or *odhA*), or GlcNAc biosynthesis (*glm*M) reduces killing in a *Caenorhabditis elegans* killing assay to the same extent as do mutations in capsule genes [136]. These data suggest that regulators of TCA cycle activity, such as CodY, are likely to regulate capsule biosynthesis.

Metabolism

Amino acid requirements for staphylococcal growth

Numerous phenotypic studies of *S. aureus* have attempted to determine the amino acid requirements for growth [137–142]. These studied revealed that *S. aureus* required between three and twelve amino acids for growth, with proline, arginine, valine, and cysteine being most frequently required; hence, these studies concluded that *S. aureus* frequently possessed multiple amino acid auxotrophies. Interestingly, it was also observed that these auxotrophies would revert to a prototrophic state at a high frequency, suggesting the auxotrophies were not due to the absence, or genetic inactivation, of biosynthetic pathways [137,143]. This suggestion was subsequently confirmed by whole-genome sequencing of *S. aureus*, where it was determined that biosynthetic pathways exist for all amino acids [144–149]. If the amino acid auxotrophies are not due to inactive or absent biosynthetic pathways, then the two more likely explanations are feedback inhibition of the biosynthetic enzymes or repression of enzyme synthesis. Although the former possibility is the more transient phenomenon, both possibilities should be quickly reversed by growth in culture medium lacking the inhibitor/amino acid; however, it was observed that reversal of *S. aureus* auxotrophies could require several passages of the bacteria in medium lacking the specific amino acid [137,143]. These observations imply that metabolic regulation in staphylococci can be unconventional, or at least divergent from that of *Escherichia coli* and *Bacillus subtilis*, and that we need to look elsewhere for the cause of the amino acid auxotrophies. One possibility is that feedback inhibition or repression of

Table 1.1 Metabolic pathways and biosynthetic intermediates.

Embden–Meyerhof–Parnas	Pentose phosphate pathway	Tricarboxylic acid cycle
Glucose 6-phosphate	Ribose 5-phosphate	Oxaloacetate
Fructose 6-phosphate	Sedoheptulose 7-phosphate	α-Ketoglutarate
Dihydroxyacetone phosphate	Erythrose 4-phosphate	Succinate
Glyceraldehyde 3-phosphate		
Phosphoenolpyruvate		
Pyruvate		
Acetyl-Coenzyme A		

enzyme synthesis could occur at an earlier step in amino acid biosynthesis; specifically, decreasing the availability of amino acid biosynthetic precursors.

Bacteria live in environments subject to rapid changes in the availability of the nutrients necessary to provide energy and biosynthetic intermediates for the synthesis of macromolecules; hence, a large percentage of the bacterial genome codes for proteins involved in metabolism and macromolecular synthesis [144,145,148–150]. Despite the large percentage of the genome dedicated to metabolism, bacteria require only 13 biosynthetic intermediates (Table 1.1) to synthesize all macromolecules in the cell. These 13 biosynthetic intermediates are derived from three metabolic pathways: the glycolytic pathway (Embden–Meyerhof–Parnas pathway), the pentose phosphate pathway (hexose monophosphate shunt), and the TCA cycle (Krebs cycle). While the glycolytic and pentose phosphate pathways are highly conserved throughout nature, the TCA cycle pathway is often found to be incomplete [151,152]. Both *S. aureus* and *S. epidermidis* possess complete glycolytic, pentose phosphate, and TCA cycle pathways; however, the TCA cycle lacks the glyoxylate shunt (discussed later in this chapter). The presence of these three pathways indicates that staphylococci can synthesize all the biosynthetic precursors necessary to make all macromolecules. In addition to being present in staphylococci, many of the genes encoding enzymes for the glycolytic and pentose phosphate pathways are essential for viability [153]; hence these data suggest that the amino acid auxotrophies are unlikely to be due to the absence of biosynthetic precursors generated by the glycolytic and pentose phosphate pathways. In contrast, the TCA cycle, which supplies the biosynthetic intermediates oxaloacetate, succinate, and α-ketoglutarate, can be genetically inactivated [136,148, 154,155] and "naturally occurring" TCA cycle mutants have been reported in *S. aureus* [152,156].

Biosynthetic intermediates and carbon catabolism

In staphylococci, the primary pathways for carbohydrate catabolism are the glycolytic pathway and pentose phosphate pathway [157,158]. The processing of glucose, in the form of glucose 6-phosphate, by the pentose phosphate pathway produces the biosynthetic intermediates ribose 5-phosphate, sedoheptulose 7-phosphate, and erythrose 4-phosphate and can also generate the glycolytic intermediates fructose 6-phosphate and glyceraldehyde 3-phosphate. Glycolysis produces two molecules of pyruvate for every molecule of glucose consumed and in the process reduces two molecules of NAD^+ to NADH. The catabolic fate of pyruvate is determined by the growth conditions; specifically, the availability of oxygen. During anaerobic growth, pyruvate is primarily reduced to lactic acid [159,160] with the concomitant reoxidation of NADH, thus allowing the continuation of glycolysis. During aerobic growth, pyruvate is enzymatically oxidized to acetyl-CoA and CO_2 by the pyruvate dehydrogenase complex [161]. Acetyl-CoA can be further oxidized by the TCA cycle when grown in the presence of certain citric acid cycle intermediates [162]; however, the amount of acetyl-CoA that enters the TCA cycle is low during the exponential growth phase [157,158,163]. In the exponential phase of growth, acetyl-CoA is usually converted into acetyl-phosphate by phosphotransacetylase, which is then used as a substrate for acetate kinase in substrate-level phosphorylation to generate ATP and acetate. The exponential phase of growth continues until the concentration of an essential nutrient (e.g., glucose, as shown in Figure 1.4) decreases to a level where it can no longer sustain rapid growth. Alternatively, entry into the postexponential growth phase can be caused by the accumulation of growth inhibitory molecules (e.g., lactic acid). If conditions are favorable, then entry into postexponential growth corresponds with the catabolism of nonpreferred carbon sources such as acetate [155].

On depletion of a preferred carbon source such as glucose, the postexponential growth of staphylococci will depend on the growth conditions, principally the availability of oxygen. Microaerobic or anaerobic growth will derepress the arginine deiminase pathway (*arcABDC*), generating energy via substrate-level phosphorylation using carbamoyl-phosphate as the phospho-donor [164]. Additionally, derepression of the histidine utilization pathway (*hutUI*, *hutG*, and *hutH*) will increase histidine catabolism, providing a source of glutamate [165]. If the culture is sufficiently anoxic and nitrate is present, then

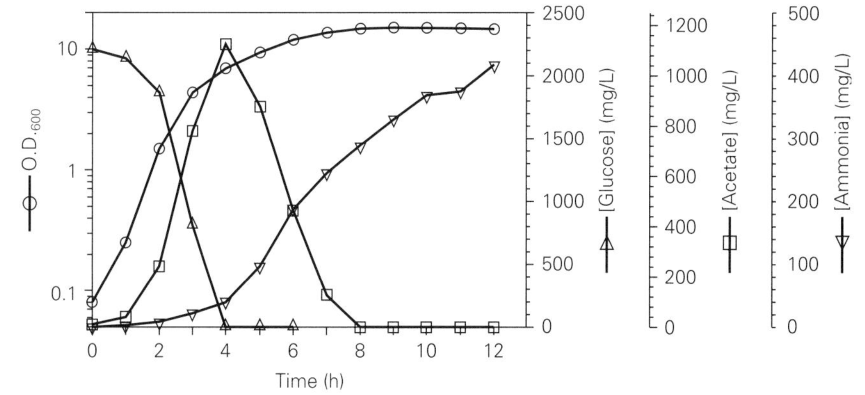

Figure 1.4 Temporal depletion and accumulation of ammonia, glucose, and acetate in *S. aureus* supernatants grown under aerobic conditions.

nitrate reductase-catalyzed nitrate reduction will maintain the proton motive force and generate ATP via anaerobic respiration [166,167]. Maintaining the proton motive force will also facilitate the oxidation of lactic acid into pyruvate by the NAD-independent lactate dehydrogenase, thus providing an important biosynthetic intermediate [168]. As stated, during aerobic growth, pyruvate undergoes oxidative decarboxylation to produce acetyl-CoA [161], which is converted into acetyl-phosphate and used for substrate-level phosphorylation, resulting in the accumulation of acetate in the culture medium (Figure 1.4). If oxygen is present, then the transition from exponential growth to postexponential growth is accompanied by a diauxic shift from glucose catabolism, or other rapidly catabolized carbohydrate, to acetate catabolism.

The first step in the catabolism of acetate is the ATP-dependent formation of a thioester bond between acetate and coenzyme A catalyzed by acetyl-CoA synthetase. The second step in acetate catabolism is the citrate synthase-catalyzed condensation of acetyl-CoA and oxaloacetate. Citrate synthase uses the energy of thioester hydrolysis to drive carbon–carbon bond formation to generate citric acid and nonesterified coenzyme A (CoASH). Citric acid is then catabolized by the TCA cycle; hence acetate catabolism is mediated by the TCA cycle [160,162,169]. In some bacteria, the glyoxylate shunt acts as a carbon salvage pathway that bypasses the two oxidative decarboxylation reactions catalyzed by isocitrate dehydrogenase and the α-ketoglutarate dehydrogenase complex. Because staphylococci lack a glyoxylate shunt, two carbons are lost as CO_2 for every two carbons (i.e., acetate) that enter the TCA cycle; for this reason, if carbons are withdrawn from the TCA cycle for biosynthesis, then anaplerotic reactions are required to maintain TCA cycle function. The substrates used in the anaplerotic reactions are most often amino acids (e.g., aspartate → oxaloacetate; glutamate → α-ketoglutarate; alanine → pyruvate → oxaloacetate), which require deamination prior to entry into the TCA cycle. The deamination of amino acids will result in the accumulation of ammonia in the culture medium; consequently, as TCA cycle activity increases during the postexponential growth phase, the rate of ammonia accumulation increases (Figure 1.4) [155]. In total, catabolism of acetate through the TCA cycle provides biosynthetic intermediates (α-ketoglutarate, succinyl-CoA, and oxaloacetate), ATP, and reducing potential, but consumes amino acids in the process.

The majority of ATP arising from TCA cycle activity is derived from the oxidation of NADH via the electron transport chain. During aerobic growth, electrons enter into the electron transport chain from NADH and are transferred to menaquinone by the NADH dehydrogenase complex [170]. Menaquinone transfers the electrons to oxidized cytochrome *c*, generating the reduced form of cytochrome *c*. The electrons are then transferred to oxygen by cytochrome *c* oxidase, generating water and driving protons across the membrane to produce a pH and electrochemical gradient. Protons return to the cytoplasm by way of the F_0 subunit of the F_0F_1-ATP synthase complex and drive the formation of ATP from inorganic phosphate, ADP, and free energy.

Amino acid auxotrophies and the TCA cycle

As previously stated, the biosynthesis of amino acids requires one or more precursors of pyruvate, acetyl-CoA, 3-phosphoglycerate, oxaloacetate, α-ketoglutarate, or succinyl-CoA. Pyruvate, acetyl-CoA, and 3-phosphoglycerate are derived from the glycolytic pathway, while the latter three molecules are intermediates of the TCA cycle (see Table 1.1). The glycolytic pathway is highly conserved and essential in staphylococci [153]; therefore, it is very unlikely that amino acid auxotrophies could be due to the absence of pyruvate, acetyl-CoA, or 3-phosphoglycerate. The TCA cycle is not essential in staphylococci and mutants can be readily identified based on their inability to catabolize acetate [152,156]. In addition to being unable to catabolize acetate, TCA cycle defective strains display multiple amino acid auxotrophies [163,171]; however, these auxotrophies can often be masked by growth in complex media. Although it is likely that TCA cycle mutants account for some of the stable amino acid auxotrophic staphylococci [152], TCA cycle mutants would be an unlikely cause of the transient amino acid auxotrophies [137,143] because TCA cycle mutants would require a suppressor mutation to restore prototrophy. An alternative to auxotrophy by mutation is prolonged repression of enzyme synthesis that limits biosynthetic intermediates. To understand this possibility, it is necessary to understand a little about the regulation of TCA cycle genes.

Synthesis of the first three enzymes of the TCA cycle is regulated by the availability of amino acids and carbohydrate(s) [161–163,172,173]. When amino acids and carbohydrates are exogenously available to staphylococci, TCA cycle activity is repressed [163]. Derepression of the TCA cycle occurs when the availability of exogenous amino acids and/or carbohydrates becomes growth limiting. In low-GC Gram-positive organisms like *S. aureus*, amino acid- and carbohydrate-dependent regulation of TCA cycle gene expression is largely mediated by the transcriptional regulators CodY and CcpA [174–180]. In addition to being regulated by the availability of amino acids and carbohydrates, TCA cycle genes are repressed by the two-component regulatory system SrhSR during anoxic growth [181,182]. In general, TCA cycle genes are repressed by a combination of amino acids, carbohydrates, and microaerobic/anaerobic conditions. Interestingly, carbohydrate-rich, amino acid replete, and microaerobic conditions were used to determine the length of time it took amino acid auxotrophic staphylococci to revert to a prototrophic state [137,138,143]. In other words, the staphylococci were grown under conditions that repress the major source of amino acid biosynthetic precursors at the same time researchers were trying to select for amino acid prototrophs. Although this explanation is unlikely to account for all the transient amino acid auxotrophies, it is a very plausible explanation for the prolonged repression of enzyme synthesis necessary to make biosynthetic intermediates.

Staphylococcal transport

In bacteria, there are four broad means by which molecules enter the cytoplasm: simple diffusion, secondary active transport (facilitated diffusion), ATP-dependent active transport, and group translocation.

Diffusion

Diffusion is the Brownian motion-driven movement of molecules from a higher concentration to a lower concentration. Bacteria gain oxygen and displace CO_2 by diffusion; however, a more important molecule that bacteria acquire or lose by diffusion is water. Sudden increases in the salt concentration of the culture medium or changes in the host environment can result in the rapid movement of water out through the cell membrane by osmosis, resulting in osmotic stress. Similarly, if the intracellular concentration of salt(s) dramatically increases relative to the external environment, then the diffusion of water into the bacterium can increase intracellular pressure causing the bacteria to burst. Diffusion-induced osmotic stress in *S. aureus* can alter the transport of other compounds, in particular the osmoprotectants glycine betaine, proline, and choline [13].

Secondary active transporters

Secondary active transporters allow transport of a molecule against a gradient by coupling it with the transport of another compound (e.g., Na, P_i, H^+, and ornithine) that flows with its gradient. One of the most commonly encountered members of the secondary active transporter family is the major facilitator superfamily transporters, which includes uniporters, antiporters, and symporters [183]. To continue the example of osmotic shock-induced transport of proline, proline enters the staphylococcal cytoplasm by one of two means: via a high-affinity major facilitator superfamily transporter known as the proline permease (PutP) [13,184,185] or via a low-affinity proline/betaine transporter like ProP [186]. In the case of the proline permease, PutP is a sodium/proline symporter, meaning that proline and sodium are transported together into the cytoplasm; thus for proline to be transported into the cytoplasm, a high extracellular sodium concentration is required [13,184]. From a clinical perspective, staphylococcal antiporters may have a greater impact on patient outcomes than do the symporters because of their involvement in antibiotic efflux from the cytoplasm [187]. Although the staphylococci contain several major facilitator superfamily antiporters, two well-studied examples are QacA, which is involved in multidrug resistance [188,189], and NorA, which mediates fluoroquinolone resistance [190]. As drug efflux-mediated antibiotic resistance mechanisms are covered more extensively in Chapter 9, they are not discussed further in this chapter. In addition to antibiotic efflux, staphylococcal antiporters have critical roles in nutrient acquisition.

Glycerophosphodiester phosphodiesterase (GlpQ) is a secreted protein [191] that can generate glycerol 3-phosphate by hydrolysis of deacylated phospholipids. This is important because glycerol 3-phosphate can be used to generate the biosynthetic intermediate dihydroxyacetone phosphate (see Table 1.1), via glycerol 3-phosphate dehydrogenase, which can be further metabolized to glyceraldehyde 3-phosphate by triosephosphate isomerase. Glycerol 3-phosphate dehydrogenase and triosephosphate isomerase are cytoplasmic proteins, meaning that glycerol 3-phosphate must be transported into the cytoplasm. To accomplish this, staphylococci utilize the GlpT antiporter [192]. GlpT uses the inorganic phosphate (P_i) gradient to drive the importation of glycerol 3-phosphate. In addition to glycerol 3-phosphate, antiporters import a wide array of solutes, including PEP, sugar-phosphates, and amino acids [183,193].

ATP-dependent active transport

ATP-dependent active transport utilizes the energy of ATP hydrolysis to overcome the electrochemical gradient and drive solute transport. ATP-dependent translocation is most often mediated by transporters belonging to the ATP-binding cassette (ABC) transporter superfamily. The basic structural unit of ABC transporters consists of two proteins containing transmembrane domains, which form the membrane channel, and a pair of cytoplasmic modules that bind and hydrolyze ATP to drive solute transport. In *S. aureus*, ABC transporters have been demonstrated to drive translocation of a wide array of solutes such as metal ions [194], heme [195], and oligopeptides [196] and are predicted to transport polyamines (e.g., spermine), maltose, and amino acids [197].

Group translocation

Group translocation, also known as the phosphotransferase system (PTS), is the process by which bacteria import different sugars into the cytoplasm using energy transferred from PEP [198]. PTS uses three enzymes to transfer the high-energy phosphate from PEP to the sugar being translocated: enzyme I (EI), enzyme II (EII), and a histidine-containing phosphocarrier protein (HPr) [198]. EI and HPr are soluble cytoplasmic proteins involved in the transport of all PTS transported sugars. In contrast to EI and HPr, EII components (domains EIIA, EIIB, and EIIC) are sugar-specific permeases; hence staphylococci contain multiple genes coding for EII components [147]. Transfer of the high-energy phosphate from PEP to a sugar starts with PEP transferring its phosphate to a histidine residue on EI, which is then transferred to a histidine residue on HPr. The phosphorylated HPr transfers the high-energy phosphate to EIIA, which then transfers it to the sugar. Transfer of phosphate from EIIA to the sugar has two primary consequences: first, the phosphorylated sugar is no longer recognized by the EII permease, preventing efflux of the sugar out of the cytoplasm; and second, the phosphorylated sugar is activated for catabolism. The exact number of sugars, sugar alcohols, and amino sugars transported by PTSs in staphylococci is not known; however, based on DNA sequence homology, the number is probably greater than 15 [147].

Acknowledgments

The authors are indebted to Hans-Georg Sahl for helpful suggestions about this chapter. We would also like to thank our colleagues, collaborators, and laboratory members for the many helpful and thought-provoking discussions. Lastly, we would like to thank the editors for their hard work in compiling this book. R.A.P. was supported by a grant from Kimberly Clark and by a subcontract on NIH grant R01 AI39108-05. G.A.S. was supported by grants from the National Institute of General Medical Sciences (GM076585) and the American Heart Association (0760005Z).

References

1 Melish ME, Glasgow LA. The staphylococcal scalded-skin syndrome. N Engl J Med 1970;282:1114–19.
2 Sakinç T, Kleine B, Gatermann SG. Biochemical characterization of the surface-associated lipase of *Staphylococcus saprophyticus*. FEMS Microbiol Lett 2007;274:335–41.
3 Tarazona RE, Padilla TP, Gomez JC, Sanchez JE, Hernandez MS. First report in Spain of linezolid non-susceptibility in a clinical isolate of *Staphylococcus haemolyticus*. Int J Antimicrob Agents 2007;30:277–8.
4 von Eiff C, Becker K, Machka K, Stammer H, Peters G. Nasal carriage as a source of *Staphylococcus aureus* bacteremia. N Engl J Med 2001;344:11–16.
5 von Eiff C, Peters G, Heilmann C. Pathogenesis of infections due to coagulase-negative staphylococci. Lancet Infect Dis 2002;2:677–85.
6 Tegmark K, Morfeldt E, Arvidson S. Regulation of *agr*-dependent virulence genes in *Staphylococcus aureus* by RNAIII from coagulase-negative staphylococci. J Bacteriol 1998;180:3181–6.
7 Jacobs SI, Willis AT. Some physiological characteristics of neomycin and kanamycin-resistant strains of *Staphylococcus aureus*. J Clin Pathol 1964;17:612–16.
8 Willis AT, Turner GC. Staphylococcal lipolysis and pigmentation. J Pathol Bacteriol 1962;84:337–47.
9 Pelz A, Wieland KP, Putzbach K, Hentschel P, Albert K, Götz F. Structure and biosynthesis of staphyloxanthin from *Staphylococcus aureus*. J Biol Chem 2005;280:32493–8.
10 Proctor RA, von Eiff C, Kahl BC *et al*. Small colony variants: a pathogenic form of bacteria that facilitates persistent and recurrent infections. Nat Rev Microbiol 2006;4:295–305.
11 Katzif S, Lee EH, Law AB, Tzeng YL, Shafer WM. CspA regulates pigment production in *Staphylococcus aureus* through a SigB-dependent mechanism. J Bacteriol 2005;187:8181–4.
12 O'Riordan K, Lee JC. *Staphylococcus aureus* capsular polysaccharides. Clin Microbiol Rev 2004;17:218–34.
13 Graham JE, Wilkinson BJ. *Staphylococcus aureus* osmoregulation: roles for choline, glycine betaine, proline, and taurine. J Bacteriol 1992;174:2711–16.
14 Vickers AA, Chopra I, O'Neill AJ. Intrinsic novobiocin resistance in *Staphylococcus saprophyticus*. Antimicrob Agents Chemother 2007;51:4484–5.
15 Owens JJ, John PC. The egg yolk and lipolytic reactions of coagulase positive staphylococci. J Appl Bacteriol 1975;39:23–30.
16 Karlsson A, Arvidson S. Variation in extracellular protease production among clinical isolates of *Staphylococcus aureus* due to different levels of expression of the protease repressor *sarA*. Infect Immun 2002;70:4239–46.
17 Geary C, Stevens M. Rapid lysostaphin test to differentiate *Staphylococcus* and *Micrococcus* species. J Clin Microbiol 1986; 23:1044–5.
18 Grundling A, Schneewind O. Cross-linked peptidoglycan mediates lysostaphin binding to the cell wall envelope of *Staphylococcus aureus*. J Bacteriol 2006;188:2463–72.

19 Klingenberg C, Ronnestad A, Anderson AS *et al*. Persistent strains of coagulase-negative staphylococci in a neonatal intensive care unit: virulence factors and invasiveness. Clin Microbiol Infect 2007;13:1100–11.

20 Becker K, von Eiff C, Keller B, Bruck M, Etienne J, Peters G. Thermonuclease gene as a target for specific identification of *Staphylococcus intermedius* isolates: use of a PCR-DNA enzyme immunoassay. Diagn Microbiol Infect Dis 2005;51:237–44.

21 Becker K, Haverkamper G, von Eiff C, Roth R, Peters G. Survey of staphylococcal enterotoxin genes, exfoliative toxin genes, and toxic shock syndrome toxin 1 gene in non-*Staphylococcus aureus* species. Eur J Clin Microbiol Infect Dis 2001;20:407–9.

22 Becker K, Roth R, Peters G. Rapid and specific detection of toxigenic *Staphylococcus aureus*: use of two multiplex PCR enzyme immunoassays for amplification and hybridization of staphylococcal enterotoxin genes, exfoliative toxin genes, and toxic shock syndrome toxin 1 gene. J Clin Microbiol 1998;36:2548–53.

23 Finck-Barbancon V, Duportail G, Meunier O, Colin DA. Pore formation by a two-component leukocidin from *Staphylococcus aureus* within the membrane of human polymorphonuclear leukocytes. Biochim Biophys Acta 1993;1182:275–82.

24 Kluytmans JA, Wertheim HF. Nasal carriage of *Staphylococcus aureus* and prevention of nosocomial infections. Infection 2005;33:3–8.

25 Hanselman BA, Kruth SA, Rousseau J *et al*. Methicillin-resistant *Staphylococcus aureus* colonization in veterinary personnel. Emerg Infect Dis 2006;12:1933–8.

26 Huijsdens XW, van Dijke BJ, Spalburg E *et al*. Community-acquired MRSA and pig-farming. Ann Clin Microbiol Antimicrob 2006;5:26.

27 Weese JS, Dick H, Willey BM *et al*. Suspected transmission of methicillin-resistant *Staphylococcus aureus* between domestic pets and humans in veterinary clinics and in the household. Vet Microbiol 2006;115:148–55.

28 Weese JS, Lefebvre SL. Risk factors for methicillin-resistant *Staphylococcus aureus* colonization in horses admitted to a veterinary teaching hospital. Can Vet J 2007;48:921–6.

29 Corrigan RM, Rigby D, Handley P, Foster TJ. The role of *Staphylococcus aureus* surface protein SasG in adherence and biofilm formation. Microbiology 2007;153:2435–46.

30 Mongodin E, Bajolet O, Cutrona J *et al*. Fibronectin-binding proteins of *Staphylococcus aureus* are involved in adherence to human airway epithelium. Infect Immun 2002;70:620–30.

31 Schaffer AC, Solinga RM, Cocchiaro J *et al*. Immunization with *Staphylococcus aureus* clumping factor B, a major determinant in nasal carriage, reduces nasal colonization in a murine model. Infect Immun 2006;74:2145–53.

32 Weidenmaier C, Kokai-Kun JF, Kristian SA *et al*. Role of teichoic acids in *Staphylococcus aureus* nasal colonization, a major risk factor in nosocomial infections. Nat Med 2004;10:243–5.

33 Harraghy N, Seiler S, Jacobs K, Hannig M, Menger MD, Herrmann M. Advances in *in vitro* and *in vivo* models for studying the staphylococcal factors involved in implant infections. Int J Artif Organs 2006;29:368–78.

34 Mertz D, Frei R, Zimmerli M *et al*. Risk factors for exclusive throat carriage of *Staphylococcus aureus*: A neglected site. K-449. Page 329. 47th ICAAC, Chicago, IL Sept 17–20, 2007.

35 Shurland SM, Johnson JK, Venezia RA, Stine OC, Roghmann M. Screening for USA300: Are the anterior nares adequate? K-448. Page 328. 47th ICAAC, Chicago, IL Sept 17–20, 2007.

36 Chen KT, Huard RC, Della-Latta P, Saiman L. Prevalence of methicillin-sensitive and methicillin-resistant *Staphylococcus aureus* in pregnant women. Obstet Gynecol 2006;108:482–7.

37 Chen KT, Campbell H, Borrell LN, Huard RC, Saiman L, Della-Latta P. Predictors and outcomes for pregnant women with vaginal-rectal carriage of community-associated methicillin-resistant *Staphylococcus aureus*. Am J Perinatol 2007;24:235–40.

38 Bogaert D, van Belkum A, Sluijter M *et al*. Colonisation by *Streptococcus pneumoniae* and *Staphylococcus aureus* in healthy children. Lancet 2004;363:1871–2.

39 Regev-Yochay G, Dagan R, Raz M *et al*. Association between carriage of *Streptococcus pneumoniae* and *Staphylococcus aureus* in Children. JAMA 2004;292:716–20.

40 Regev-Yochay G, Trzcinski K, Thompson CM, Malley R, Lipsitch M. Interference between *Streptococcus pneumoniae* and *Staphylococcus aureus*: in vitro hydrogen peroxide-mediated killing by *Streptococcus pneumoniae*. J Bacteriol 2006;188:4996–5001.

41 Herold BC, Immergluck LC, Maranan MC *et al*. Community-acquired methicillin-resistant *Staphylococcus aureus* in children with no identified predisposing risk. JAMA 1998;279:593–8.

42 Regev-Yochay G, Malley R, Rubinstein E, Raz M, Dagan R, Lipsitch M. In vitro bactericidal activity of *Streptococcus pneumoniae* and susceptibility of *Staphylococcus aureus* strains isolated from co-colonized vs. non-co-colonized children. J Clin Microbiol 2008;46:747–9.

43 Melles DC, Bogaert D, Gorkink RF *et al*. Nasopharyngeal co-colonization with *Staphylococcus aureus* and *Streptococcus pneumoniae* in children is bacterial genotype independent. Microbiology 2007;153:686–92.

44 Kushwaha SC, Kates M. Nonpolar lipids of a halotolerant species of *Staphylococcus epidermidis*. Can J Biochem 1976;54:79–85.

45 Nguyen DM, Bancroft E, Mascola L, Guevara R, Yasuda L. Risk factors for neonatal methicillin-resistant *Staphylococcus aureus* infection in a well-infant nursery. Infect Control Hosp Epidemiol 2007;28:406–11.

46 Raffi HS, Bates JM Jr, Laszik Z, Kumar S. Tamm–Horsfall protein acts as a general host-defense factor against bacterial cystitis. Am J Nephrol 2005;25:570–8.

47 Gatermann S, Meyer HG. *Staphylococcus saprophyticus* hemagglutinin binds fibronectin. Infect Immun 1994;62:4556–63.

48 Ohshima Y, Ko HL, Beuth J, Roszkowski K, Roszkowski W. Biological properties of staphylococcal lipoteichoic acid and related macromolecules. Zentralbl Bakteriol 1990;274:359–65.

49 Peake SL, Peter JV, Chan L, Wise RP, Butcher AR, Grove DI. First report of septicemia caused by an obligately anaerobic *Staphylococcus aureus* infection in a human. J Clin Microbiol 2006;44:2311–13.

50 Mukhopadhyay K, Whitmire W, Xiong YQ *et al*. In vitro susceptibility of *Staphylococcus aureus* to thrombin-induced platelet microbicidal protein-1 (tPMP-1) is influenced by cell membrane phospholipid composition and asymmetry. Microbiology 2007;153:1187–97.

51 Short SA, White DC. Metabolism of phosphatidylglycerol, lysylphosphatidylglycerol, and cardiolipin of *Staphylococcus aureus*. J Bacteriol 1971;108:219–26.

52 White DC, Tucker AN. Phospholipid metabolism during bacterial growth. J Lipid Res 1969;10:220–33.

53 Short SA, White DC. Metabolism of the glycosyl diglycerides and phosphatidylglucose of *Staphylococcus aureus*. J Bacteriol 1970;104:126–32.

54 Chintalapati S, Kiran MD, Shivaji S. Role of membrane lipid fatty acids in cold adaptation. Cell Mol Biol 2004;50:631–42.

55 Mykytczuk NC, Trevors JT, Leduc LG, Ferroni GD. Fluorescence polarization in studies of bacterial cytoplasmic membrane fluidity under environmental stress. Prog Biophys Mol Biol 2007;95:60–82.

56 Martin PK, Li T, Sun D, Biek DP, Schmid MB. Role in cell permeability of an essential two-component system in *Staphylococcus aureus*. J Bacteriol 1999;181:3666–73.

57 Kariyama R. Increase of cardiolipin content in *Staphylococcus aureus* by the use of antibiotics affecting the cell wall. J Antibiot (Tokyo) 1982;35:1700–4.

58 Eble KS, Coleman WB, Hantgan RR, Cunningham CC. Tightly associated cardiolipin in the bovine heart mitochondrial ATP synthase as analyzed by ^{31}P nuclear magnetic resonance spectroscopy. J Biol Chem 1990;265:19434–40.

59 Agarwal N, Kalra VK. Purification and functional properties of the DCCD-reactive proteolipid subunit of the H^+-translocating ATPase from *Mycobacterium phlei*. Biochim Biophys Acta 1983;723:150–9.

60 Joyce GH, Hammond RK, White DC. Changes in membrane lipid composition in exponentially growing *Staphylococcus aureus* during the shift from 37 to 25 C. J Bacteriol 1970;104:323–30.

61 Armstrong GA. Genetics of eubacterial carotenoid biosynthesis: a colorful tale. Annu Rev Microbiol 1997;51:629–59.

62 Marshall JH, Wilmoth GJ. Pigments of *Staphylococcus aureus*, a series of triterpenoid carotenoids. J Bacteriol 1981;147:900–13.

63 Giachino P, Engelmann S, Bischoff M. σ^B activity depends on RsbU in *Staphylococcus aureus*. J Bacteriol 2001;183:1843–52.

64 Chamberlain NR, Mehrtens BG, Xiong Z, Kapral FA, Boardman JL, Rearick JI. Correlation of carotenoid production, decreased membrane fluidity, and resistance to oleic acid killing in *Staphylococcus aureus* 18Z. Infect Immun 1991;59:4332–7.

65 Xiong Z, Ge S, Chamberlain NR, Kapral FA. Growth cycle-induced changes in sensitivity of *Staphylococcus aureus* to bactericidal lipids from abscesses. J Med Microbiol 1993;39:58–63.

66 Cebrian G, Sagarzazu N, Pagan R, Condon S, Manas P. Heat and pulsed electric field resistance of pigmented and non-pigmented enterotoxigenic strains of *Staphylococcus aureus* in exponential and stationary phase of growth. Int J Food Microbiol 2007;118:304–11.

67 Liu GY, Essex A, Buchanan JT *et al*. *Staphylococcus aureus* golden pigment impairs neutrophil killing and promotes virulence through its antioxidant activity. J Exp Med 2005;202:209–15.

68 Lee AC, Bergdoll MS. Spontaneous occurrence of *Staphylococcus aureus* mutants with different pigmentation and ability to produce toxic shock syndrome toxin 1. J Clin Microbiol 1985;22:308–9.

69 Peschel A, Sahl HG. The co-evolution of host cationic antimicrobial peptides and microbial resistance. Nat Rev Microbiol 2006;4:529–36.

70 Jones T, Yeaman MR, Sakoulas G *et al*. Failures in clinical treatment of *Staphylococcus aureus* infection with daptomycin are associated with alterations in surface charge, membrane phospholipid asymmetry, and drug binding. Antimicrob Agents Chemother 2008;52:269–78.

71 Mulkidjanian AY. Proton in the well and through the desolvation barrier. Biochim Biophys Acta 2006;1757:415–27.

72 Lohner K, Latal A, Degovics G, Garidel P. Packing characteristics of a model system mimicking cytoplasmic bacterial membranes. Chem Phys Lipids 2001;111:177–92.

73 Chang H, Saccomani G, Rabon E, Schackmann R, Sachs G. Proton transport by gastric membrane vesicles. Biochim Biophys Acta 1977;464:313–27.

74 Dufour S, Rousse N, Canioni P, Diolez P. Top-down control analysis of temperature effect on oxidative phosphorylation. Biochem J 1996;314:743–51.

75 Lewis K, Naroditskaya V, Ferrante A, Fokina I. Bacterial resistance to uncouplers. J Bioenerg Biomembr 1994;26:639–46.

76 Arechaga I, Miroux B, Karrasch S *et al*. Characterisation of new intracellular membranes in *Escherichia coli* accompanying large scale over-production of the b subunit of F_1F_0 ATP synthase. FEBS Lett 2000;482:215–19.

77 Haines TH, Dencher NA. Cardiolipin: a proton trap for oxidative phosphorylation. FEBS Lett 2002;528:35–9.

78 Ghuysen JM, Strominger JL. Structure of the cell wall of *Staphylococcus aureus*, strain Copenhagen. I. Preparation of fragments by enzymatic hydrolysis. Biochemistry 1963;2:1110–19.

79 Ghuysen JM, Strominger JL. Structure of the cell wall of *Staphylococcus aureus*, strain Copenhagen. II. Separation and structure of disaccharides. Biochemistry 1963;2:1119–25.

80 Ghuysen JM, Tipper DJ, Strominger JL. Structure of the cell wall of *Staphylococcus aureus*, strain Copenhagen. IV. The teichoic acid–glycopeptide complex. Biochemistry 1965;4:474–85.

81 Munoz E, Ghuysen JM, Heymann H. Cell walls of *Streptococcus pyogenes*, type 14. C polysaccharide-peptidoglycan and G polysaccharide–peptidoglycan complexes. Biochemistry 1967; 6:3659–70.

82 Tipper DJ, Strominger JL, Ensign JC. Structure of the cell wall of *Staphylococcus aureus*, strain Copenhagen. VII. Mode of action of the bacteriolytic peptidase from *Myxobacter* and the isolation of intact cell wall polysaccharides. Biochemistry 1967;6:906–20.

83 Tipper DJ. Structures of the cell wall peptidoglycans of *Staphylococcus epidermidis* Texas 26 and *Staphylococcus aureus* Copenhagen. II. Structure of neutral and basic peptides from hydrolysis with the *Myxobacter* al-1 peptidase. Biochemistry 1969;8:2192–202.

84 Berger-Bächi B, Tschierske M. Role of fem factors in methicillin resistance. Drug Resist Updat 1998;1:325–35.

85 Van Heijenoort Y, Derrien M, Van Heijenoort J. Polymerization by transglycosylation in the biosynthesis of the peptidoglycan of *Escherichia coli* K12 and its inhibition by antibiotics. FEBS Lett 1978;89:141–4.

86 Kuroda M, Nagasaki S, Ohta T. Sesquiterpene farnesol inhibits recycling of the C55 lipid carrier of the murein monomer precursor contributing to increased susceptibility to beta-lactams in methicillin-resistant *Staphylococcus aureus*. J Antimicrob Chemother 2007;59:425–32.

87 Stranden AM, Roos M, Berger-Bachi B. Glutamine synthetase and heteroresistance in methicillin-resistant *Staphylococcus aureus*. Microb Drug Resist 1996;2:201–7.

88 Schneider T, Senn MM, Berger-Bachi B, Tossi A, Sahl HG, Wiedemann I. In vitro assembly of a complete, pentaglycine interpeptide bridge containing cell wall precursor (lipid II-Gly5) of *Staphylococcus aureus*. Mol Microbiol 2004;53:675–85.

89 Frère J-M, Nguyen-Distèche M, Coyette J, Joris B. Mode of action: interaction with the penicillin binding proteins. In: Page M, ed. The Chemistry of Beta-lactams. Glasgow: Chapman & Hall, 1992:148–95.

90 Holtje JV. Growth of the stress-bearing and shape-maintaining murein sacculus of *Escherichia coli*. Microbiol Mol Biol Rev 1998;62:181–203.

91 Holtje JV. A hypothetical holoenzyme involved in the replication of the murein sacculus of *Escherichia coli*. Microbiology 1996;142:1911–18.

92 Pinho MG, Errington J. Dispersed mode of *Staphylococcus aureus* cell wall synthesis in the absence of the division machinery. Mol Microbiol 2003;50:871–81.

93 Hartman BJ, Tomasz A. Low-affinity penicillin-binding protein associated with beta-lactam resistance in *Staphylococcus aureus*. J Bacteriol 1984;158:513–16.

94 Reynolds PE, Brown DF. Penicillin-binding proteins of beta-lactam-resistant strains of *Staphylococcus aureus*. Effect of growth conditions. FEBS Lett 1985;192:28–32.

95 Pinho MG, Errington J. Recruitment of penicillin-binding protein PBP2 to the division site of *Staphylococcus aureus* is dependent on its transpeptidation substrates. Mol Microbiol 2005;55:799–807.

96 Pinho MG, Filipe SR, de Lencastre H, Tomasz A. Complementation of the essential peptidoglycan transpeptidase function of penicillin-binding protein 2 (PBP2) by the drug resistance protein PBP2A in *Staphylococcus aureus*. J Bacteriol 2001;183:6525–31.

97 Terrak M, Nguyen-Disteche M. Kinetic characterization of the monofunctional glycosyltransferase from *Staphylococcus aureus*. J Bacteriol 2006;188:2528–32.

98 Ghuysen JM. Serine β-lactamases and penicillin-binding proteins. Annu Rev Microbiol 1991;45:37–67.

99 Biswas R, Voggu L, Simon UK, Hentschel P, Thumm G, Götz F. Activity of the major staphylococcal autolysin Atl. FEMS Microbiol Lett 2006;259:260–8.

100 Neuhaus FC, Baddiley J. A continuum of anionic charge: structures and functions of D-alanyl-teichoic acids in gram-positive bacteria. Microbiol Mol Biol Rev 2003;67:686–723.

101 Navarre WW, Schneewind O. Surface proteins of gram-positive bacteria and mechanisms of their targeting to the cell wall envelope. Microbiol Mol Biol Rev 1999;63:174–229.

102 D'Elia MA, Pereira MP, Chung YS *et al*. Lesions in teichoic acid biosynthesis in *Staphylococcus aureus* lead to a lethal gain of function in the otherwise dispensable pathway. J Bacteriol 2006;188:4183–9.

103 Lazarevic V, Abellan FX, Moller SB, Karamata D, Mauel C. Comparison of ribitol and glycerol teichoic acid genes in *Bacillus subtilis* W23 and 168: identical function, similar divergent organization, but different regulation. Microbiology 2002;148:815–24.

104 Grundling A, Schneewind O. Genes required for glycolipid synthesis and lipoteichoic acid anchoring in *Staphylococcus aureus*. J Bacteriol 2007;189:2521–30.

105 Bierbaum G, Sahl HG. Autolytic system of *Staphylococcus simulans* 22: influence of cationic peptides on activity of *N*-acetylmuramoyl-L-alanine amidase. J Bacteriol 1987;169:5452–8.

106 Fischer W. Physiology of lipoteichoic acids in bacteria. Adv Microb Physiol 1998;29:233–302.

107 Jorasch P, Warnecke DC, Lindner B, Zahringer U, Heinz E. Novel processive and nonprocessive glycosyltransferases from *Staphylococcus aureus* and *Arabidopsis thaliana* synthesize glycoglycerolipids, glycophospholipids, glycosphingolipids and glycosylsterols. Eur J Biochem 2000;267:3770–83.

108 Grundling A, Schneewind O. Synthesis of glycerol phosphate lipoteichoic acid in *Staphylococcus aureus*. Proc Natl Acad Sci USA 2007;104:8478–83.

109 Fedtke I, Mader D, Kohler T *et al*. A *Staphylococcus aureus ypfP* mutant with strongly reduced lipoteichoic acid (LTA) content: LTA governs bacterial surface properties and autolysin activity. Mol Microbiol 2007;65:1078–91.

110 Stapleton PD, Shah S, Ehlert K, Hara Y, Taylor PW. The beta-lactam-resistance modifier (–)-epicatechin gallate alters the architecture of the cell wall of *Staphylococcus aureus*. Microbiology 2007;153:2093–103.

111 Rupp ME. Infections of intravascular catheters and vascular devices. In: Crossley KB, Archer GL, eds. The Staphylococci in Human Disease. New York: Churchill-Livingstone, 1997:379–99.

112 Rupp ME, Ulphani JS, Fey PD, Mack D. Characterization of *Staphylococcus epidermidis* polysaccharide intercellular adhesin/hemagglutinin in the pathogenesis of intravascular catheter-associated infection in a rat model. Infect Immun 1999;67:2656–9.

113 Heilmann C, Schweitzer O, Gerke C, Vanittanakom N, Mack D, Götz F. Molecular basis of intercellular adhesion in the biofilm-forming *Staphylococcus epidermidis*. Mol Microbiol 1996;20:1083–91.

114 Vuong C, Kocianova S, Voyich JM *et al*. A crucial role for exopolysaccharide modification in bacterial biofilm formation, immune evasion, and virulence. J Biol Chem 2004;279:54881–6.

115 Vuong C, Voyich JM, Fischer ER *et al*. Polysaccharide intercellular adhesin (PIA) protects *Staphylococcus epidermidis* against major components of the human innate immune system. Cell Microbiol 2004;6:269–75.

116 Maira-Litran T, Kropec A, Abeygunawardana C *et al*. Immunochemical properties of the staphylococcal poly-*N*-acetylglucosamine surface polysaccharide. Infect Immun 2002; 70:4433–40.

117 Mack D, Fischer W, Krokotsch A *et al*. The intercellular adhesin involved in biofilm accumulation of *Staphylococcus epidermidis* is a linear beta-1,6-linked glucosaminoglycan: purification and structural analysis. J Bacteriol 1996;178:175–83.

118 Gerke C, Kraft A, Sussmuth R, Schweitzer O, Götz F. Characterization of the *N*-acetylglucosaminyltransferase activity involved in the biosynthesis of the *Staphylococcus epidermidis* polysaccharide intercellular adhesin. J Biol Chem 1998; 273:18586–93.

119 Conlon KM, Humphreys H, O'Gara JP. *icaR* encodes a transcriptional repressor involved in environmental regulation of *ica* operon expression and biofilm formation in *Staphylococcus epidermidis*. J Bacteriol 2002;184:4400–8.

120 Jefferson KK, Cramton SE, Götz F, Pier GB. Identification of a 5-nucleotide sequence that controls expression of the *ica* locus in *Staphylococcus aureus* and characterization of the DNA-binding properties of IcaR. Mol Microbiol 2003;48:889–99.

121 Handke LD, Slater SR, Conlon KM *et al*. SigmaB and SarA independently regulate polysaccharide intercellular adhesin production in *Staphylococcus epidermidis*. Can J Microbiol 2007;53:82–91.

122 Tormo MA, Marti M, Valle J *et al*. SarA is an essential positive regulator of *Staphylococcus epidermidis* biofilm development. J Bacteriol 2005;187:2348–56.

123 Knobloch JK, Bartscht K, Sabottke A, Rohde H, Feucht HH, Mack D. Biofilm formation by *Staphylococcus epidermidis* depends on functional RsbU, an activator of the *sigB* operon: differential activation mechanisms due to ethanol and salt stress. J Bacteriol 2001;183:2624–33.

124 Knobloch JK, Jager S, Horstkotte MA, Rohde H, Mack D. RsbU-dependent regulation of *Staphylococcus epidermidis* biofilm formation is mediated via the alternative sigma factor sigmaB by repression of the negative regulator gene *icaR*. Infect Immun 2004;72:3838–48.

125 Rachid S, Ohlsen K, Wallner U, Hacker J, Hecker M, Ziebuhr W. Alternative transcription factor sigma(B) is involved in regulation of biofilm expression in a *Staphylococcus aureus* mucosal isolate. J Bacteriol 2000;182:6824–6.

126 Xu L, Li H, Vuong C *et al.* Role of the *luxS* quorum-sensing system in biofilm formation and virulence of *Staphylococcus epidermidis*. Infect Immun 2006;74:488–96.

127 Cramton SE, Ulrich M, Götz F, Doring G. Anaerobic conditions induce expression of polysaccharide intercellular adhesin in *Staphylococcus aureus* and *Staphylococcus epidermidis*. Infect Immun 2001;69:4079–85.

128 Deighton M, Borland R. Regulation of slime production in *Staphylococcus epidermidis* by iron limitation. Infect Immun 1993;61:4473–9.

129 Dobinsky S, Kiel K, Rohde H *et al.* Glucose-related dissociation between *icaADBC* transcription and biofilm expression by *Staphylococcus epidermidis*: evidence for an additional factor required for polysaccharide intercellular adhesin synthesis. J Bacteriol 2003;185:2879–86.

130 Götz F. *Staphylococcus* and biofilms. Mol Microbiol 2002; 43:1367–78.

131 Rachid S, Ohlsen K, Witte W, Hacker J, Ziebuhr W. Effect of subinhibitory antibiotic concentrations on polysaccharide intercellular adhesin expression in biofilm-forming *Staphylococcus epidermidis*. Antimicrob Agents Chemother 2000;44:3357–63.

132 Vuong C, Kidder JB, Jacobson ER, Otto M, Proctor RA, Somerville GA. *Staphylococcus epidermidis* polysaccharide intercellular adhesin production significantly increases during tricarboxylic acid cycle stress. J Bacteriol 2005;187:2967–73.

133 Chen Z, Luong TT, Lee CY. The *sbcDC* locus mediates repression of type 5 capsule production as part of the SOS response in *Staphylococcus aureus*. J Bacteriol 2007;189:7343–50.

134 Scovill WH, Schreier HJ, Bayles KW. Identification and characterization of the *pckA* gene from *Staphylococcus aureus*. J Bacteriol 1996;178:3362–4.

135 Dassy B, Fournier JM. Respiratory activity is essential for post-exponential-phase production of type 5 capsular polysaccharide by *Staphylococcus aureus*. Infect Immun 1996;64:2408–14.

136 Bae T, Banger AK, Wallace A *et al.* *Staphylococcus aureus* virulence genes identified by *bursa aurealis* mutagenesis and nematode killing. Proc Natl Acad Sci USA 2004;101:12312–17.

137 Emmett M, Kloos WE. Amino acid requirements of staphylococci isolated from human skin. Can J Microbiol 1975;21:729–33.

138 Fildes P, Richardson GM, Knight JG, Gladstone GP. A nutrient mixture suitable for the growth of *Staphylococcus aureus*. Br J Exp Pathol 1936;17:481–4.

139 Mah RA, Fung DY, Morse SA. Nutritional requirements of *Staphylococcus aureus* S-6. Appl Microbiol 1967;15:866–70.

140 Nychas GJ, Tranter HS, Brehm RD, Board RG. *Staphylococcus aureus* S-6: factors affecting its growth, enterotoxin B production and exoprotein formation. J Appl Bacteriol 1991;70:344–50.

141 Onoue Y, Mori M. Amino acid requirements for the growth and enterotoxin production by *Staphylococcus aureus* in chemically defined media. Int J Food Microbiol 1997;36:77–82.

142 Taylor D, Holland KT. Amino acid requirements for the growth and production of some exocellular products of *Staphylococcus aureus*. J Appl Bacteriol 1989;66:319–29.

143 Gladstone GP. The nutrition of *Staphylococcus aureus*: nitrogen requirements. Br J Exp Pathol 1937;18:322–33.

144 Baba T, Bae T, Schneewind O, Takeuchi F, Hiramatsu K. Genome sequence of *Staphylococcus aureus* strain Newman and comparative analysis of staphylococcal genomes: polymorphism and evolution of two major pathogenicity islands. J Bacteriol 2008;190:300–10.

145 Baba T, Takeuchi F, Kuroda M *et al.* Genome and virulence determinants of high virulence community-acquired MRSA. Lancet 2002;359:1819–27.

146 Diep BA, Gill SR, Chang RF *et al.* Complete genome sequence of USA300, an epidemic clone of community-acquired meticillin-resistant *Staphylococcus aureus*. Lancet 2006;367: 731–9.

147 Gill SR, Fouts DE, Archer GL *et al.* Insights on evolution of virulence and resistance from the complete genome analysis of an early methicillin-resistant *Staphylococcus aureus* strain and a biofilm-producing methicillin-resistant *Staphylococcus epidermidis* strain. J Bacteriol 2005;187:2426–38.

148 Holden MT, Feil EJ, Lindsay JA *et al.* Complete genomes of two clinical *Staphylococcus aureus* strains: evidence for the rapid evolution of virulence and drug resistance. Proc Natl Acad Sci USA 2004;101:9786–91.

149 Kuroda M, Ohta T, Uchiyama I *et al.* Whole genome sequencing of methicillin-resistant *Staphylococcus aureus*. Lancet 2001; 357:1225–40.

150 Lindsay JA, Holden MT. *Staphylococcus aureus*: superbug, super genome? Trends Microbiol 2004;12:378–85.

151 Huynen MA, Dandekar T, Bork P. Variation and evolution of the citric-acid cycle: a genomic perspective. Trends Microbiol 1999;7:281–91.

152 Somerville GA, Said-Salim B, Wickman JM, Raffel SJ, Kreiswirth BN, Musser JM. Correlation of acetate catabolism and growth yield in *Staphylococcus aureus*: implications for host–pathogen interactions. Infect Immun 2003;71:4724–32.

153 Forsyth RA, Haselbeck RJ, Ohlsen KL *et al.* A genome-wide strategy for the identification of essential genes in *Staphylococcus aureus*. Mol Microbiol 2002;43:1387–400.

154 Coulter SN, Schwan WR, Ng EY *et al.* *Staphylococcus aureus* genetic loci impacting growth and survival in multiple infection environments. Mol Microbiol 1998;30:393–404.

155 Somerville GA, Chaussee MS, Morgan CI *et al.* *Staphylococcus aureus* aconitase inactivation unexpectedly inhibits post-exponential-phase growth and enhances stationary-phase survival. Infect Immun 2002;70:6373–82.

156 Nelson JL, Rice KC, Slater SR *et al.* Vancomycin-intermediate *Staphylococcus aureus* strains have impaired acetate catabolism: implications for polysaccharide intercellular adhesin synthesis and autolysis. Antimicrob Agents Chemother 2007;51:616–22.

157 Collins FM, Lascelles J. The effect of growth conditions on oxidative and dehydrogenase activity in *Staphylococcus aureus*. J Gen Microbiol 1962;29:531–5.

158 Strasters KC, Winkler KC. Carbohydrate metabolism of *Staphylococcus aureus*. J Gen Microbiol 1963;33:213–29.

159 Kendall AI, Friedemann TE, Ishikawa M. Quantitative observations on the chemical activity of "resting" *Staphylococcus aureus*. J Infect Dis 1930;47:223–8.

160 Krebs HA. Dismutation of pyruvic acid in *Gonococcus* and *Staphylococcus*. Biochem J 1937;31:661–71.

161 Gardner JF, Lascelles J. The requirement for acetate of a streptomycin-resistant strain of *Staphylococcus aureus*. J Gen Microbiol 1962;29:157–64.

162 Goldschmidt MC, Powelson DM. Effect of the culture medium on the oxidation of acetate by *Micrococcus pyogenes* var. *aureus*. Arch Biochem Biophys 1953;46:154–63.

163 Somerville GA, Cockayne A, Durr M, Peschel A, Otto M, Musser JM. Synthesis and deformylation of *Staphylococcus aureus* delta-toxin are linked to tricarboxylic acid cycle activity. J Bacteriol 2003;185:6686–94.
164 Makhlin J, Kofman T, Borovok I *et al*. *Staphylococcus aureus* ArcR controls expression of the arginine deiminase operon. J Bacteriol 2007;189:5976–86.
165 Sinha AK, Chatterjee GC. Amino acid metabolism and protein synthesis in a pyrithiamine-requiring *Staphylococcus aureus* mutant. Biochem J 1967;104:888–92.
166 Burke KA, Lascelles J. Nitrate reductase system in *Staphylococcus aureus* wild type and mutants. J Bacteriol 1975;123:308–16.
167 Neubauer H, Götz F. Physiology and interaction of nitrate and nitrite reduction in *Staphylococcus carnosus*. J Bacteriol 1996;178:2005–9.
168 Stockland AE, San Clemente CL. Multiple forms of lactate dehydrogenase in *Staphylococcus aureus*. J Bacteriol 1969; 100:347–53.
169 Stedman RL, Kravitz E. Evidence for a common pathway for pyruvate and acetate oxidation by *Micrococcus pyogenes* var. *aureus*. Arch Biochem Biophys 1955;59:260–8.
170 Bayer AS, McNamara P, Yeaman MR *et al*. Transposon disruption of the complex I NADH oxidoreductase gene (*snoD*) in *Staphylococcus aureus* is associated with reduced susceptibility to the microbicidal activity of thrombin-induced platelet microbicidal protein 1. J Bacteriol 2006;188:211–22.
171 Heinemann M, Kummel A, Ruinatscha R, Panke S. In silico genome-scale reconstruction and validation of the *Staphylococcus aureus* metabolic network. Biotechnol Bioeng 2005;92:850–64.
172 Fortnagel P. The regulation of aconitase and isocitrate dehydrogenase in sporulation mutants of *Bacillus subtilis*. Biochim Biophys Acta 1970;222:290–8.
173 Hanson RS, Blicharska J, Arnaud M, Szulmajster J. Observation on the regulation of the synthesis of the tricarboxylic acid cycle enzymes in *Bacillus subtilis*, Marburg. Biochem Biophys Res Commun 1964;17:690–5.
174 Guedon E, Serror P, Ehrlich SD, Renault P, Delorme C. Pleiotropic transcriptional repressor CodY senses the intracellular pool of branched-chain amino acids in *Lactococcus lactis*. Mol Microbiol 2001;40:1227–39.
175 Jankovic I, Egeter O, Bruckner R. Analysis of catabolite control protein A-dependent repression in *Staphylococcus xylosus* by a genomic reporter gene system. J Bacteriol 2001;183:580–6.
176 Kim HJ, Kim SI, Ratnayake-Lecamwasam M, Tachikawa K, Sonenshein AL, Strauch M. Complex regulation of the *Bacillus subtilis* aconitase gene. J Bacteriol 2003;185:1672–80.
177 Kim HJ, Roux A, Sonenshein AL. Direct and indirect roles of CcpA in regulation of *Bacillus subtilis* Krebs cycle genes. Mol Microbiol 2002;45:179–90.
178 Slack FJ, Serror P, Joyce E, Sonenshein AL. A gene required for nutritional repression of the *Bacillus subtilis* dipeptide permease operon. Mol Microbiol 1995;15:689–702.
179 Sonenshein AL. CodY, a global regulator of stationary phase and virulence in Gram-positive bacteria. Curr Opin Microbiol 2005;8:203–7.
180 Tojo S, Satomura T, Morisaki K, Deutscher J, Hirooka K, Fujita Y. Elaborate transcription regulation of the *Bacillus subtilis ilv-leu* operon involved in the biosynthesis of branched-chain amino acids through global regulators of CcpA, CodY and TnrA. Mol Microbiol 2005;56:1560–73.
181 Nakano MM, Zuber P, Sonenshein AL. Anaerobic regulation of *Bacillus subtilis* Krebs cycle genes. J Bacteriol 1998;180:3304–11.
182 Throup JP, Zappacosta F, Lunsford RD *et al*. The *srhSR* gene pair from *Staphylococcus aureus*: genomic and proteomic approaches to the identification and characterization of gene function. Biochemistry 2001;40:10392–401.
183 Pao SS, Paulsen IT, Saier MH Jr. Major facilitator superfamily. Microbiol Mol Biol Rev 1998;62:1–34.
184 Townsend DE, Wilkinson BJ. Proline transport in *Staphylococcus aureus*: a high-affinity system and a low-affinity system involved in osmoregulation. J Bacteriol 1992;174:2702–10.
185 Wengender PA, Miller KJ. Identification of a PutP proline permease gene homolog from *Staphylococcus aureus* by expression cloning of the high-affinity proline transport system in *Escherichia coli*. Appl Environ Microbiol 1995;61:252–9.
186 Schwan WR, Lehmann L, McCormick J. Transcriptional activation of the *Staphylococcus aureus putP* gene by low-proline-high osmotic conditions and during infection of murine and human tissues. Infect Immun 2006;74:399–409.
187 Saidijam M, Benedetti G, Ren Q *et al*. Microbial drug efflux proteins of the major facilitator superfamily. Curr Drug Targets 2006;7:793–811.
188 Rouch DA, Cram DS, DiBerardino D, Littlejohn TG, Skurray RA. Efflux-mediated antiseptic resistance gene *qacA* from *Staphylococcus aureus*: common ancestry with tetracycline- and sugar-transport proteins. Mol Microbiol 1990;4:2051–62.
189 Tennent JM, Lyon BR, Midgley M, Jones IG, Purewal AS, Skurray RA. Physical and biochemical characterization of the *qacA* gene encoding antiseptic and disinfectant resistance in *Staphylococcus aureus*. J Gen Microbiol 1989;135:1–10.
190 Ubukata K, Itoh-Yamashita N, Konno M. Cloning and expression of the *norA* gene for fluoroquinolone resistance in *Staphylococcus aureus*. Antimicrob Agents Chemother 1989;33:1535–9.
191 Rogasch K, Ruhmling V, Pane-Farre J *et al*. Influence of the two-component system SaeRS on global gene expression in two different *Staphylococcus aureus* strains. J Bacteriol 2006; 188:7742–58.
192 Haga K, Liu H, Takahashi H, Yoshikawa H. Sequence analysis of a 45-kb segment in the 19 degrees-23 degrees region of the *Bacillus subtilis* chromosome containing *glpT* and *mpr* loci. DNA Res 1997;4:329–33.
193 Zhu Y, Weiss EC, Otto M, Fey PD, Smeltzer MS, Somerville GA. *Staphylococcus aureus* biofilm metabolism and the influence of arginine on polysaccharide intercellular adhesin synthesis, biofilm formation, and pathogenesis. Infect Immun 2007; 75:4219–26.
194 Lindsay JA, Foster SJ. *zur*: a Zn(2+)-responsive regulatory element of *Staphylococcus aureus*. Microbiology 2001;147:1259–66.
195 Skaar EP, Humayun M, Bae T, DeBord KL, Schneewind O. Iron-source preference of *Staphylococcus aureus* infections. Science 2004;305:1626–8.
196 Hiron A, Borezee-Durant E, Piard JC, Juillard V. Only one of four oligopeptide transport systems mediates nitrogen nutrition in *Staphylococcus aureus*. J Bacteriol 2007;189:5119–29.
197 Otto M, Götz F. ABC transporters of staphylococci. Res Microbiol 2001;152:351–6.
198 Kundig W, Ghosh S, Roseman S. Phosphate bound to histidine in a protein as an intermediate in a novel phospho-transferase system. Proc Natl Acad Sci USA 1964;52:1067–74.

Chapter 2
Genomics of the Staphylococci

Steven R. Gill

Infectious Disease and Genomics, Departments of Oral Biology/Microbiology and Immunology, Center of Excellence in Bioinformatics and Life Sciences, Buffalo, New York, USA

Introduction

Genome sequencing of the staphylococci has provided unprecedented insights into their success as significant bacterial pathogens. Genome sequences have enabled investigators to explore questions of virulence, resistance, physiology, and host interactions with rigor and efficiency previously not possible. Within the past decade, genomes of 13 *Staphylococcus aureus*, two *Staphylococcus epidermidis*, one *Staphylococcus haemolyticus*, and one *Staphylococcus saprophyticus* have been sequenced [1–9]. These staphylococcal genome sequences have been used for comparative analyses to identify both conserved metabolic and structural functions as well as species-specific functions enabling virulence and host-specific adaptation. The genome sequences have also been used as the basis for the development and application of postgenomic tools, including microarrays [10–17], protein arrays, and other high-throughput approaches [10] that have been used to explore genomic diversity and transcriptional responses, identify small RNAs, and examine the *S. aureus* proteome [11,16,18–22]. Emerging evidence of a dynamic staphylococcal genome in which horizontal gene transfer, nucleotide polymorphisms, and genetic mosaicism play pivotal roles in evolution of virulence and adaptation to host environments strongly supports the need for defining the genome sequence diversity within diverse collections of genetically and phenotypically distinct isolates. Characterization of the staphylococcal pan-genome or supergenome will be a significant step forward in our understanding of the dynamic relationship between the numerous staphylococcal virulence factors and their interactions with the host which determine the path toward either a commensal or pathogenic relationship.

Staphylococci in Human Disease, 2nd edition. Edited by Kent B. Crossley, Kimberly K. Jefferson, Gordon Archer, Vance G. Fowler, Jr.

Genomes of *Staphylococcus aureus*

The first *S. aureus* genome sequences were published in 2001 by Hiramatsu's group, comparing the genomes of two methicillin-resistant strains, N315 and Mu50 [7]. These genome sequences were followed in quick succession over the next 7 years by publication of the genome sequences of MW2 [2], MRSA252 and MSSA476 [6], COL [4], USA300-FPR3737 [3], USA300-HOU-MR [23], NCTC8325 [24], ET3-1 [5], JH1 and JH9 [25] and, most recently, Newman [1]. Phylogenetic analyses indicate that four of the sequenced genomes (COL, NCTC8325, USA300 and Newman) are in related clonal groups, with a greater evolutionary distance between strains N315, Mu50, MW2, MRSA252, MSSA476, JH1, JH9, and ET3-1 [1,26]. Despite the close evolutionary relationship between the sequenced strains, comparative genome analyses have identified not only core metabolic functions shared by all *S. aureus* strains, but also previously unidentified virulence factors with key roles in pathogenicity. A "typical" *S. aureus* genome contains a syntenous conserved core genome backbone and a collection of mobile genetic elements (MGEs), including bacteriophages and pathogenicity islands (*S. aureus* pathogenicity islands, or SaPI) that insert into site-specific locations across the genome and carry a majority of *S. aureus* virulence factors. Combinations of virulence factors carried by the MGEs and their exchange among strains results in evolution of clones able to infect selected hosts and cause specific diseases [5].

The core *Staphylococcus aureus* genome and population structure

The *S. aureus* genome core contains approximately 80% (~ 1930) of the genes conserved among strains, encoding essential metabolic and regulatory functions as well as surface proteins with roles in tissue adhesion and surface architecture. Within the core genome are core variable (CV) regions containing genes with a higher nucleotide substitution rate than core genes [14] and often showing variation associated with lineage. Included in the CV regions are surface proteins, *capHIJK* genes for *S. aureus* capsule production, and global virulence regulators (*agr*, *trap* and *sarT*) known to regulate expression of surface proteins. The surface proteins include staphylococcal protein A (Spa), fibronectin-binding proteins A and B (FnbA/B), collagen adhesion (CNA), *S. aureus* surface proteins A–G (SasA–G), serine-aspartate repeat domain proteins (SdrD-F), all which are LPXTG cell wall-anchored proteins, as well as coagulase (COA) and clumping factor A and B (ClfA/B) [27]. Selective variation generated by DNA recombination in the repeat regions of these surface proteins occurs as a result of interactions of *S. aureus* with the human host environment and as a means for evading the host immune system [28–31].

Two groups of genes contained within the core and core variable genome are used in DNA sequence-based methods to assess the highly clonal population structure of *S. aureus*. The first group includes seven housekeeping genes (*arcC*, *aroE*, *glpF*, *gmk*, *pta*, *tpi* and *yqiL*) in the core genome used for multilocus sequence typing (MLST) [32]. Sequence variation within these genes, which occurs primarily as a result of point mutations [33], provides an allelic profile that defines the sequence type (ST) and a determination of macro or long-term genetic variation and evolution. The second group includes families of surface proteins in the CV genome, including Spa [28] and ClfB [29], both based on sequence variation of variable repeat regions extending from the cell surface. Spa typing is capable of detecting both genetic microvariation and macrovariation and has discriminatory power similar to that of MLST [34]. In contrast, the highly evolving serine-aspartate (SD) repeat region in ClfB can be used to index genetic microvariation within closely related MSLT and Spa groups, enabling discrimination between newly emerging clinical clones.

The accessory genome

The remaining 20% of the *S. aureus* genome, often referred to as the accessory genome (dispensable genetic material), is assembled from MGEs that are integrated throughout the genome and carry about 50% of known *S. aureus* virulence factors. These elements, which include pathogenicity islands, bacteriophages, chromosomal cassettes, genomic islands, plasmids and transposons, transfer horizontally between strains and are thought to play significant roles in the evolution of *S. aureus* virulence and emergence of new strains with clinical implications. Particular lineages may dominate in carriage and disease as a result of MGE-mediated movement of toxin genes associated with these lineages [35,36]. Comparative analysis of the multiple *S. aureus* genome sequences has demonstrated evidence of substantial homologous recombination within MGEs, such that each MGE is composed of multiple short mosaic fragments that are randomly spread through other MGEs of the same type (phage or SaPI). As an example, comparative analysis of SaPI5 (from USA300) with other SaPIs suggest that evolution of SaPI5 likely involved recombination events between two pathogenicity islands from COL (SaPI1) and MW2 (SaPI3) [3]. Data from comparative genomic hybridization array (aCGH) analysis of multiple clinical isolates [14] further substantiates the mosaicism of MGEs and the mobility or loss and acquisition of MGEs among lineages. MGEs strongly associated with a particular lineage are likely stable and distributed by vertical transmission to daughter cells. In contrast, MGEs that are randomly distributed among multiple lineages are likely to be transferred horizontally.

Staphylococcus aureus pathogenicity islands

Ten SaPIs have been identified in the sequenced *S. aureus* genomes, all of which encode one or more superantigen toxins associated with symptoms ranging from food poisoning to a nonspecific T-cell response resulting in toxic shock [37]. The SaPIs include seven found in human *S. aureus* isolates – SaPI1 [4], SaPI2 type I [7] and SaPI2 type II [2,4], SaPI3 type I [7] and SaPI3 type II [2], SaPI4 [6], SaPI5 [3] – and three in bovine isolates, SaPIbov1 [23,38], SaPIbov2 [39], and SaPIbov3 [23]. The SaPIs are intimately dependent on coreplicating temperate bacteriophages for excision, replication, packaging into phage-like particles, and finally mobilization into recipient strains [40] where each SaPI is integrated at a specific attachment (*att*) site within the *S. aureus* genome. Essential functions shared by the SaPI and phage include an integrase, a replicon, an initiator protein, and a packaging module [40]. Systematic inactivation of the 17 open reading frames (ORFs) largely conserved between the distantly related SaPIs, SaPI1 and SaPIbov1, has been used to determine the functional groups and their role in the SaPI excision–replication–packaging cycle [41].

The *in vitro* movement of SaPIs is generally studied through mitomycin C induction of the SOS response in lysogenic SaPI-containing *S. aureus* [42–44]. However, the environmental and genetic factors that initiate high-frequency horizontal movement or transduction of SaPIs *in vivo* are largely unknown. The recent work demonstrating that SOS induction by fluoroquinolone antibiotics such as ciprofloxacin, as well as β-lactam antibiotics, leads to replication and high-frequency transfer of SaPI1 and SaPIbov1, respectively, suggests that *in vivo* movement may occur as a consequence of therapeutic treatment with these antibiotics [44,45].

Genomic islands

All sequenced *S. aureus* genomes contain sets of three genomic islands that, in contrast to the SaPIs, do not appear to be mobile and are stably integrated in the same position in all *S. aureus* genomes. These three islands, νSaα, νSaβ, and νSaγ [4], exhibit striking diversity between strains, each carrying variable families of lipoproteins, exotoxins, serine proteases, and an enterotoxin nursery encoding a cluster of cotranscribed enterotoxin genes [46]. As demonstrated in a study of the exotoxin genes in νSaα, gene diversification in the island occurs largely as a result of gene loss and recombination [47]. It is likely that diversification of enterotoxins and tandem lipoproteins in νSaα and νSaβ occurs through similar recombination mechanisms and the concept of gene nurseries in *S. aureus* should be extended to exotoxins and tandem lipoproteins. The third island, νSaγ, encodes the two β-type phenol soluble modulins (PSMβ1 and PSMβ2) in *S. aureus*. The *S. aureus* genome also contains a cluster of four α-type PSMs (PSMα1, PSMα2, PSMα3, PSMα4) which, together with the β-type PSMs, form a family of secreted peptides that function to diminish the neutrophil response, thereby removing the primary cellular defense against *S. aureus* [48]. Recent work by Wang *et al.* [48] has demonstrated that the PSMs contribute significantly to the enhanced virulence of community-acquired methicillin-resistant *S. aureus* (CA-MRSA) relative to hospital-acquired methicillin-resistant *S. aureus* (HA-MRSA).

Bacteriophages

Staphylococcus aureus harbor both temperate and lytic bacteriophages [49] that play key roles in mobilization of virulence factors between strains and genome evolution. These bacteriophages represent an untapped source of genetic diversity for *S. aureus*, with many of their ORFs having no similarity to other phage or bacterial sequences. The 13 sequenced *S. aureus* genomes contain 14 temperate bacteriophages, with at least one or up to three bacteriophages in each genome (Table 2.1). Aside from *S. aureus* whole-genome sequencing, a collection of 27 lytic bacteriophages has been sequenced with the goal of learning more about their molecular mechanisms of replication and their evolutionary relationships [49].

Two groups of *S. aureus* bacteriophage, generalized transducing phage [50] and temperate phage associated with SaPI [42,51,52], are likely responsible for the widespread horizontal gene transfer between strains. As an example, the generalized transducing phage identified in the *S. aureus* NCTC8325 genome, ϕ11 [24,50], packages and transfers up to 45 kb of plasmid or chromosomal genes. Two bacteriophages, ϕ11 and 80α [41], have been shown to induce replication of SaPI1 and SaPIbov1 and contribute packaging and structural proteins for encapsidation of these SaPI elements into phage particles [40]. Interestingly, in the dynamic relationship between these phages and SaPI, the SaPI element encodes proteins that remodel the phage capsid to accommodate the smaller SaPI genome [40].

A subgroup of temperate *S. aureus* bacteriophages insert into specific virulence genes, frequently leading to their inactivation in a phenomenon commonly referred to as lysogenic conversion. These include L54a (also identified as ϕCOL in *S. aureus* strain COL [4] and ϕNM4 in *S. aureus* strain Newman [53]) which inserts into the carboxy-terminal of the gene encoding lipase (*geh*) and a family of widely distributed serogroup F bacteriophages, which insert into and inactivate the β-hemolysin (Hlb) gene. The Hlb-converting phages are most frequently associated with clinical isolates of *S. aureus* and 10 of the 13 sequenced *S. aureus* strains carry these phages. The Hlb-converting phages include ϕSa3 (in N315, Mu50, MW2, MRSA252, MSSA476, JH1 and JH9), ϕSA3usa [3] (in USA300-FPR3737 and USA300-HOU-MR), and ϕNM3 [1,53] (in Newman) each of which carry staphylokinase [54] and a variable complement of enterotoxins [50], chemotaxis inhibitory protein (CHIP) [55], and the antiphagocytic protein (SCIN) [56] (see Table 2.1). Phage dynamics occurring *in vivo* in the human host (including recombination events, translocations, duplications, and transfer between hosts) leads to host adaptation by splitting of the phage population into two populations with differing virulence potentials: those that produce Hlb or alternatively the CHIP and SCIN immune evasion molecules [57]. A comparison of *S. aureus* strains from the sputum of patients with cystic fibrosis or bacteremia isolates with colonizing isolates from the anterior nares of healthy individuals demonstrated that phage movement is found primarily in the infecting or disease-related strains. In the disease-related isolates, the *sak*-containing phages are frequently not inserted in *hlb*, but rather in an atypical genome site [57].

Mobilization of bacteriophages encoding specific virulence factors, such as Panton–Valentine leukocidin (PVL), is another mechanism leading to the emergence of virulent *S. aureus* clinical isolates. PVL (*lukS-PV* and *lukF-PV*) is encoded by the bacteriophages ϕSa2 in MW2 [2] and ϕSa2usa in USA300 [3], CA-MRSA isolates associated with soft tissue infections and necrotizing pneumonia in children [58]. A comparison of MW2 with MSSA476, two closely related strains but differing in bacteriophage content and presence of ϕSa2, illustrates the central role of staphylococcal bacteriophages in evolution of virulent clinical isolates [2,6,59].

Staphylococcal cassette chromosome

The staphylococcal cassette chromosome (SCC) is a multifunctional MGE characterized by a set of site-specific recombinase genes (*ccrA* and *ccrB*), which promote site-specific integration into an *att* site within *orfX* near the *S. aureus* chromosome origin of replication [4]. Like other MGEs in *S. aureus*, the SCC element has evolved to carry multiple genes involved in virulence or antimicrobial resistance. The most common SCC element and the one first identified is the SCC*mec* element, which contains the *mecA* gene encoding methicillin resistance. Other forms of SCC include the SCC*cap1* element [60], SCC*far* (fusidic acid resistance) in the genome of MSSA476 [6], SCC12263 in *Staphylococcus hominis* [61], SCC*pbp4* in *S. epidermidis* ATCC12228 [62], SCC*cap*-enterotoxin in *S. aureus* ET3-1

Table 2.1 Major genomic islands, bacteriophages, and associated virulence factors in sequenced staphylococcal genomes.

Strain	*S. aureus*												*S. epidermidis*		*S. haemolyticus*	*S. saprophyticus*
	COL	NCTC8325	N315	Mu50	MW2	MSSA476	MRSA252	USA300-FPR3737	USA300-HOU-MR	Newman	JH1/JH9	ET3-1	RP62a	ATCC12228	JCSC1435	ATCC15305
Chromosome length (bp)	2 809 422	2 821 361	2 813 641	2 878 084	2 820 462	2 799 802	2 902 619	2 872 769	2 872 915	2 878 897	2 906 507/ 2 906 700	2 742 531	2 616 530	2 499 279	2 685 015	2 516 575
Number of ORFs	2673	2892	2593	2714	2632	2619	2744	2560	2657	2614	2747/2697	2589	2553	2381	2676	2446
Background	HA-MRSA	Laboratory strain	HA-MRSA	HA-MRSA	CA-MRSA	CA-MSSA	HA-MRSA	CA-MRSA	CA-MRSA	HA-MRSA		Bovine isolate	HA-MRSE	Typing strain		Typing strain
Reference	Gill *et al.* [4]	Iandolo *et al.* [50]	Kuroda *et al.* [7]	Kuroda *et al.* [7]	Baba *et al.* [1]	Holden *et al.* [6]	Holden *et al.* [6]	Diep *et al.* [3]	Highlander *et al.* [23]	Baba *et al.* [1]	Mwangi *et al.* [25]	Herron-Olson *et al.* [5]	Gill *et al.* [4]	Zhang *et al.* [84]	Takeuchi *et al.* [9]	Kuroda *et al.* [8]
GenBank accession	CP000046	CP000253	BA000018	BA000017	BA000033	BX571857	BX571856	CP000255	CP000730	AP009351	CP000736/ CP000703.1	AJ938182	CP000028	AE015929	AP006716	AP008934
Genomic islands																
vSaα	*set* (5)	*set* (10)	*set* (10)	*set* (9)	*set* (11)	*set* (11)	*set* (9)	*set* (10)	*set* (10)	*set* (10)	*set* (9)	*set* (9)	–	–	–	–
vSaβ	*spl* (5), *lukDE*, *bsa*	*spl* (5), *lukDE*, *bsa*	*spl* (5), *lukDE*, enterotoxin (6)	*spl* (5), *lukDE*, enterotoxin (6)	*spl* (4), *lukDE*, *bsa*	*spl* (4), *lukDE*, *bsa*	*spl* (5), *hysA*, enterotoxin (6)	*spl* (5), *lukDE*, *bsa*	*spl* (5), *lukDE*, *bsa*	*spl* (5), *lukDE*, *bsa*	*spl* (4), *lukDE*, enterotoxin (5)	*spl* (4), *lukDE*, enterotoxin, *bsa*	–	–	–	–
vSaγ	*set* (4), *eta*, *psm* β (2)	*set* (3), *eta*, *psm* β (2)	*set*, *eta*, *psm*β	*set*, *eta*, *psm*β	*set*, *eta*, *psm*β	*set*, *eta*, *psm*β	*set* (3), *eta*, *psm*β	*set*, *eta*, *psm*β	*set*, *eta*, *psm*β	*set*, *eta*, *psm*β	*set*, *eta*, *psm*β	*set*, *eta*	–	–	–	–
vSaBov	–	–	–	–	–	–	–	–	–	–	–	*sag* homologs	–	–	–	–
vSeγ	–	–	–	–	–	–	–	–	–	–	–	–	*psm*β	*psm*β	–	–
vSe1	–	–	–	–	–	–	–	–	–	–	–	–	*cadCD*	unknown ORF	–	–
vSe2	–	–	–	–	–	–	–	–	–	–	–	–	–	*srtA*, LPXTG	–	–
vSh1	–	–	–	–	–	–	–	–	–	–	–	–	–	–	A	–
vSh2	–	–	–	–	–	–	–	–	–	–	–	–	–	–	A	–
vSh3	–	–	–	–	–	–	–	–	–	–	–	–	–	–	A	–
vSs15305	–	–	–	–	–	–	–	–	–	–	–	–	–	–	–	*aadE*, *fofB*
Pathogenicity islands																
vSa1(SaPI1, SaPI3)	*seb*, *ear*, *sek*, *sei*	–	–	–	–	–	–	–	–	–	–	–	–	–	–	–
vSa3 (SaPI3)	–	–	–	*fhuD*	*ear*, *sel2*, *sec4*	–	–	–	–	–	–	–	–	–	–	–
vSa4 (SaPI2)	–	–	*sel*, *sec3*, *tsst*	*sel*, *sec3*, *tsst*	A	–	–	–	–	A	–	–	–	–	–	–
SaPI4	–	–	–	–	–	–	A	–	–	–	–	–	–	–	–	–
SaPI5	–	–	–	–	–	–	–	*seq*, *sek2*, *ear*	*seq*, *sek2*, *ear*	–	–	–	–	–	–	–
SaPIbov1	–	–	–	–	–	–	–	–	–	–	–	*sec-bovine*, *sel*, *tsst*	–	–	–	–
SaPIbov3	–	–	–	–	–	–	–	–	–	–	–	A	–	–	–	–

Other islands																
SCC*mec* type	type I	–	type II	type II	type IV	–	type II	type IV	type IV	–	type II	–	type II	–	–	–
SCC	–	–	–	–	–	SCC476 (*far1*)	–	–	–	–	–	–	–	SCC*pbp4*	–	–
ACME	–	–	–	–	–	–	–	type I	type I	–	–	–	–	type II	–	–
SCCcap-truncated	–	–	–	–	–	–	–	–	–	–	–	enterotoxin	–	–	–	–
SCC*mec haemolyticus*	–	–	–	–	–	–	–	–	–	–	–	–	–	–	B	–
SCC15305RM	–	–	–	–	–	–	–	–	–	–	–	–	–	–	–	C
SCC15305cap	–	–	–	–	–	–	–	–	–	–	–	–	–	–	–	D
Bacteriophages																
ϕSa1	–	–	–	A	–	–	–	–	–	–	–	–	–	–	–	–
ϕSa2	–	–	–	–	*lukSF-PV*	–	A	–	–	–	–	–	–	–	–	–
ϕSa3	–	–	*sak, sep, chp, scn*	*sak, sea, scn*	*sak, sea, seg2, sek2, scn*	*sak, sea, seg2, sek2, scn*	*sak, sea, chp, scn*	–	–	–	*chp, scn*	–	–	–	–	–
ϕSa4	–	–	–	–	–	A	–	–	–	–	–	–	–	–	–	–
ϕSa2usa	–	–	–	–	–	–	–	*lukSF-PV*	*lukSF-PV*	–	–	–	–	–	–	–
ϕSa3usa	–	–	–	–	–	–	–	*sak, chp*	*sak, chp*	–	–	–	–	–	–	–
ϕNM1	–	–	–	–	–	–	–	–	–	NV	–	–	–	–	–	–
ϕNM2	–	–	–	–	–	–	–	–	–	NV	–	–	–	–	–	–
ϕNM3	–	–	–	–	–	–	–	–	–	*sea, sak, chp, scn*	–	–	–	–	–	–
ϕNM4	–	–	–	–	–	–	–	–	–	NV	–	–	–	–	–	–
ϕ11	–	A	–	–	–	–	–	–	–	–	–	–	–	–	–	–
ϕ12	–	A	–	–	–	–	–	–	–	–	–	–	–	–	–	–
ϕ13	–	*sak, chp, scn*	–	–	–	–	–	–	–	–	–	–	–	–	–	–
ϕCOL	A	–	–	–	–	–	–	–	–	–	–	–	–	–	–	–
ϕ12Bov	–	–	–	–	–	–	–	–	–	–	–	A	–	–	–	–
ϕSaBov	–	–	–	–	–	–	–	–	–	–	–	A	–	–	–	–
SPβ	–	–	–	–	–	–	–	–	–	–	–	–	A	–	–	–
ϕSh1	–	–	–	–	–	–	–	–	–	–	–	–	–	–	β-lactamase	–
ϕSh2	–	–	–	–	–	–	–	–	–	–	–	–	–	–	A	–

HA-MRSA, hospital-acquired methicillin-resistant *S. aureus*; CA-MRSA, community-acquired methicillin-resistant *S. aureus*; CA-MSSA, community-acquired methicillin-sensitive *S. aureus*; HA-MRSE, hospital-acquired methicillin-resistant *S. epidermidis*.
A, genome elements are present, but do not encode virulence or drug resistance genes; B, assembled from integration of six independent SCC elements/remnants carrying *mecA* and multiple resistance genes; C, carries no resistance or virulence factors; D, carries orthologs of the *S. aureus* cap1 capsular polysaccharide synthesis locus; NV, contains virulence genes identified in the nemotode infection model.
Abbreviations: *aadE*, streptomycin resistance; *bsa*, bacteriocin biosynthesis genes; *cadCD*, cadmium resistance genes; *chp*, chemotaxis inhibitory protein; *ear*, putative β-lactamase protein; *eta*, exfoliative toxin A-like protein; *fhuD*, siderophore transporter; *fofB*, fosfomycin resistance; *hysA*, hyaluronate lyase; LPXTG, cell surface protein containing LPXTG motif; *lukDE*, two components of the leukocidin DE toxins; *lukSF-PV*, two components of the Panton–Valentine leukocidin toxin; *psmβ*, phenol soluble modulin; *sag* homologs, homologs of streptolysin; *sak*, staphylokinase; *sea*, enterotoxin A; *seb*, enterotoxin B; *sec3*, enterotoxin C3; *sec4*, enterotoxin C4; *seg2*, enterotoxin G2; *sei*, enterotoxin I; *sek*, enterotoxin K; *sek2*, enterotoxin K2; *sel*, enterotoxin L; *sel2*, enterotoxin L2; *sep*, enterotoxin P; *seq*, enterotoxin Q; *set*, staphylococcal exotoxins; *scn*, staphylococcal complement inhibitor; *spl*, staphylococcal serine proteases; *srtA*, sortase A; *yeeE*, putative transport system permease.

[23], and SCC15305RM and SCC15305cap in *S. saprophyticus* [8].

The SCC*mec* elements are classified into structurally distinct groups based on whether they are found in HA-MRSA or CA-MRSA isolates. Types I–III are HA-MRSA, with I and II present in COL (type I) and N315, Mu50 and MRSA252 (type II). Types IV–VII are CA-MRSA, with type IV found in MW2 and USA300-FPR3737/USA300-HOU-MR and types V–VII [63,64] in unsequenced *S. aureus* genomes. Evolutionary analysis suggests that SCC*mec* likely originated in coagulase-negative staphylococci (CoNS) [65]. However, unlike *S. aureus* bacteriophages and SaPIs, the transfer mechanism of *S. aureus* SCC*mec* forms with variable contents of insertion elements and plasmids, suggesting that ongoing recombination events are reshaping the element [66], perhaps towards a smaller element that is capable of being mobilized by transduction at a higher frequency.

ACME element

The ACME element has been identified in the *S. aureus* USA300-FPR3737/USA300-HOU-MR and *S. epidermidis* ATCC12228 genomes. The *S. aureus* USA300-FPR3737/USA300-HOU-MR ACME is 31 kb in length and referred to as the type I ACME allotype, while the *S. epidermidis* ACME is 34 kb in length and referred to as the type II ACME allotype. Both type I and type II ACME elements contain the six-gene *arc* cluster encoding a complete arginine deiminase pathway that converts L-arginine to carbon dioxide, ATP, and ammonia. This pathway likely plays several roles in virulence and survival of USA300-FPR3737/USA300-HOU-MR in an infection. For example, ATP production by the arginine deiminase pathway under anaerobic conditions may be important for energy production in wound environments low in oxygen. Arginine deiminase, the major enzyme in this pathway, is a major virulence factor in *Streptococcus pyogenes* where it plays an important role in survival at low pH and the capacity to invade and survive intracellularly. Depletion of L-arginine by arginine deiminase inhibits nitric oxide production, a molecule used in both the innate and adaptive immune responses against microbial infections.

The precise integration of both ACME elements into *orfX*, along with the presence of flanking repeats at the insertion site, led Diep *et al.* [3] to propose that the ACME element is a new member of the SCC family. The absence of SCC *ccrA/ccrB* recombinase genes in the ACME element suggests that it relies on *ccrA/ccrB* present in the SCC*mec* IV (USA300-FPR3737/USA300-HOU-MR) and SSC*pbp4* elements (ATCC12228) to catalyze the integration and excision of the element.

Plasmids

With the exception of Newman [1], ET3-1 [5], and NCTC8325 [24], all sequenced *S. aureus* genomes contain one or more extrachromosomal plasmids. A majority of these plasmids contain genes encoding resistance to antibiotics and heavy metals or antiseptics. The prevalence of similar antimicrobial plasmids in hospital-acquired *S. aureus* isolates underscores the central role they play in dispersion of resistant strains in the clinical setting. Unlike other Gram-positive pathogens such as *Streptococcus pneumoniae* and *Enterococcus faecalis*, *S. aureus* is not naturally competent and likely utilizes transduction for horizontal transfer of plasmids between isolates. Staphylococcal plasmids are classified into three groups based on size, gene complement, and presence of the *tra* genes required for conjugation between isolates [67]. Type I plasmids are small (1–5 kb) multicopy plasmids that either carry a single resistance determinant or are phenotypically cryptic. Type II plasmids are larger (15–40 kb), have a lower copy number than type I, and are multiresistant in that they frequently carry genes for multiple antimicrobial resistance factors. Type III plasmids are large (40–60 kb), often multiresistant and are conjugative. In some cases, extrachromosomal replicating plasmids have integrated into the *S. aureus* genome. For example, the pUB110 plasmid, which carries genes for resistance to bleomycin and kanamycin, has integrated into the *S. aureus* SCC*mec* type II.

Another group of plasmids carry virulence factors, including enterotoxins and exfoliative toxins. Initial analysis of staphylococcal enterotoxin D (SED)-producing strains led to the identification of a plasmid, pIB485, carrying the *sed* gene [68]. Subsequent analysis of pIB485 and pIB485-related plasmids has shown that they also encode enterotoxins SEJ and SER [69,70], with both genes immediately flanking each other. The close proximity of these enterotoxin genes on pIB485 is reminiscent of enterotoxin nursery in νSaβ, suggesting a similar recombination mechanism on these two distinct genomic elements. Staphylococcal exfoliative toxin B (ETB) is also carried by a plasmid, pRW001, which is specific to ETB-producing strains [71,72].

Emergence of the first vancomycin-resistant *S. aureus* (VRSA) occurred in 2002 in Michigan as a result of interspecies conjugative transfer of the *Tn1546* (*vanA*) MGE between vancomycin-resistant *E. faecalis* (VRE) and *S. aureus* co-isolates in a polymicrobial infection [73]. In *S. aureus*, the *Tn1546* (*vanA*) 10.8-kb element integrated into the resident tra+/conjugative multiresistant plasmid resulting in the formation of the 57.9-kb plasmid pLW1043. The pLW1043 plasmid shares significant homologous regions with the pSK41/pGO1 family of multiresistant conjugative staphylococcal plasmids [74]. Molecular analysis of a second 2002 VRSA isolate, this one from Pennsylvania [75], identified an approximately 120-kb mosaic plasmid containing *Tn1546* (*vanA*) and with nucleotide homologies to both VRE and *S. aureus* plasmids (S. Gill, unpublished data). The transfer of *Tn1546* (*vanA*) is an uncommon event with only seven total isolates identified since 2002, five of them from Michigan. Molecular analysis of the Michigan VRE donor isolates revealed that they all contain an Inc18-like *vanA* conjugative plasmid that is the likely factor in the geographically restricted emergence of VRSA [76].

Host-specific genomic determinants in *Staphylococcus aureus*: the bovine ET3-1 genome

Staphylococcus aureus is not solely a human bacterial pathogen, but colonizes and causes infections in multiple hosts, including rhesus macaque [77], cattle [78], and domesticated animals such as dogs and cats [79]. In cattle, *S. aureus* causes mastitis, an infection that results in significant economic loss to the dairy industries. Population genetic studies of mastitis-associated *S. aureus* isolates suggest that human-associated *S. aureus* clones were the evolutionary predecessors to the bovine clones. The clonal structure of bovine *S. aureus* isolates suggests that selected genotypes are more successful in causing mastitis [80,81]. To uncover the molecular basis of mastitis-associated *S. aureus* clones and identify genetic factors that select for bovine host specialization, Herron-Olson *et al.* [5] sequenced the genome of *S. aureus* ET3-1, a strain commonly isolated from bovine mastitis worldwide. The core genome of ET3-1 is remarkably similar in gene content and genome structure to that of sequenced human *S. aureus* isolates (see Table 2.1). The majority of ET3-1 unique genes, which includes 110 predicted proteins not found in existing *S. aureus* genome sequences, are restricted to a collection of MGEs that differ in gene content and genomic location compared with human *S. aureus* genomes. Included among these unique MGEs (see Table 2.1) is the genomic element vSaBov, which encodes homologs of two group A *Streptococcus* (GAS) streptolysins, SagB and SagD. A significant number of *S. aureus* virulence factors in ET3-1 (including surface adhesion proteins such as ClfA and Spa) have undergone substantial gene decay with premature truncations resulting in likely nonfunctional adhesins. This large-scale gene decay is suggestive of transition of *S. aureus* bovine mastitis isolates toward an intracellular lifestyle without the need for adhesion to host tissues.

Staphylococcus aureus genome nucleotide polymorphisms and their role in virulence

The molecular basis of host specificity and pathogenesis was previously thought to be related to variation in gene content and allelic variation between strains of *S. aureus*. Early genome sequencing and array comparative genomic hybridization experiments [11,19] demonstrated that individual *S. aureus* strains are often distinguished from one another by the presence or absence of hundreds of strain-specific nonessential genes, often encoding virulence factors, host- or niche-specific colonization factors, or proteins mediating antibiotic resistance. These nonessential genes, which are frequently carried on MGEs, represent up to 22% of *S. aureus* gene content and include significant virulence factors such as PVL [82,83] and the ACME element [3,59]. While these individual virulence factors play key roles in *S. aureus* pathogenesis, continuing comparative sequence analysis of *S. aureus* genomes suggests that DNA polymorphisms (single nucleotide polymorphisms including SNPs and indels) within the genome also have a direct and significant impact. A comparison of the *S. aureus* N315, Mu50, MW2, and COL genomes revealed thousands of SNPs and indels, with the majority clustered in MGEs and located in surface and envelope proteins [4]. Polymorphisms within these proteins, such as the LPXTG/NPQTN cell wall family proteins and ClfA, likely reflect pathoadaptive mutations that contribute to host interactions and evasion from the immune system [30]. The impact of nucleotide polymorphisms on virulence was more recently demonstrated by identification of indels and SNPs in comparative analyses of two *S. aureus* USA300 community isolates: USA300-FPR3737 [3] and USA300-HOU-MR [23]. For example, an indel in the *snoABCDEFG* operon in USA300-HOU-MR results in reduction in susceptibility to thrombin-induced platelet microbicidal protein 1 (tPMP-1), likely allowing USA300-HOU-MR to evade platelet-mediated killing and causing more severe disease [23]. A similar comparative whole-genome resequencing study of 10 USA300 isolates, two of which had reduced mortality in a mouse sepsis model, provided additional evidence that subtle nucleotide polymorphisms have profound effects on staphylococcal virulence [91]. In these 10 isolates, a total of 472 and 365 SNPs were present in the core *S. aureus* genome and MGEs, respectively. A total of 16 nonsynonymous SNPs were identified in core genome virulence determinants, including ClfA and ClfB and other genes encoding proteins with roles in pathogenesis. Collectively, the study revealed that the recent clonal expansion of a subset of USA300 isolates has been followed by diversification and emergence of increasingly virulent isolates as a result of SNPs and DNA polymorphisms. Overall, these recent studies effectively demonstrate that differences in pathogenesis are due not only to acquisition of virulence factor genes but also to SNPs and DNA polymorphisms occurring throughout the genome.

Other staphylococcal genomes

In addition to the 13 sequenced *S. aureus* genomes, the genomes of four additional staphylococcal strains have been

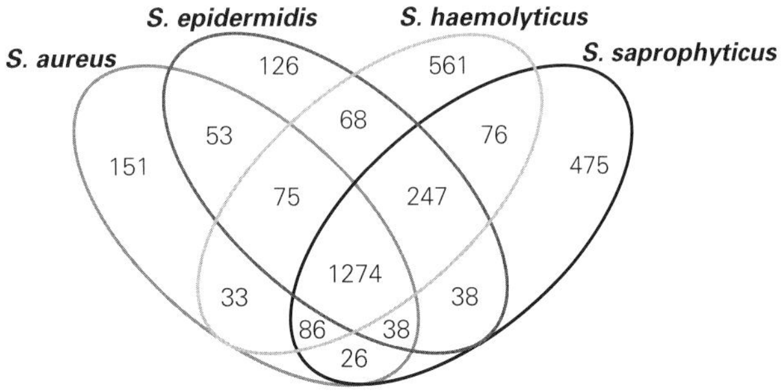

Figure 2.1 Identification of the staphylococcal core genome. Pairwise comparison among all 17 sequenced staphylococcal genomes was completed to identify a set of essential core open reading frames (ORFs). The *S. aureus* genomes were first compared by reciprocal blastp (e-value of 0.00001, 75% length match and 35% identity) to identify the core set of ORFs conserved between all 13 genomes. A similar analysis was completed for the two sequenced *S. epidermidis* genomes. The identified set of core ORFs from *S. aureus* and *S. epidermidis* were then compared by reciprocal blastp to the single *S. haemolyticus* and *S. saprophyticus* genomes to identify the core set of ORFs shared among all 17 staphylococcal genomes.

sequenced: *S. epidermidis* ATCC12228 [84], *S. epidermidis* RP62a [4], *S. haemolyticus* JCSC1435 [9], and *S. saprophyticus* [8]. Reciprocal blast comparison (Figure 2.1) identified a core of 1274 genes found in all 17 staphylococcal genomes. These core genes consist of essential metabolic and regulatory functions, including multiple two-component response regulatory systems, degradative functions (the Clp protease family), and ABC transporters (iron compound transporters SirB/C).

Staphylococcus epidermidis

Staphylococcus epidermidis is frequently considered a less-virulent member of the staphylococcal genus and is often associated with nosocomial and biomedical device infections. The genomes of two *S. epidermidis* isolates have been sequenced: (i) RP62a, a methicillin-resistant, biofilm-producing strain isolated during an outbreak of intravascular catheter-associated sepsis [4]; and (ii) ATCC12228, a laboratory strain that does not produce biofilm [84]. When compared with the *S. aureus* genomes, they are syntenous through their well-conserved core regions, with differences the result of genomic elements, including genome islands, integrated bacteriophages and plasmids (see Table 2.1), some of which are associated with virulence. The integrated plasmids in RP62a and ATCC12228, νSe1 and νSe2, contain integrase genes in a structure similar to that for *S. aureus* genome islands. While these *S. epidermidis* islands do not carry known virulence factors, they do carry factors that likely contribute to antimicrobial resistance and virulence. The RP62a νSe1 island carries genes encoding proteins for cadmium resistance. In ATCC12228, νSe1 carries a genus-unique sortase and two strain-specific LPXTG cell-surface attachment proteins with likely roles in adherence to host tissue. A type II SCC*mec* element is present in RP62a, while ATCC12228 harbors SCC*pbp4*, an SCC element that lacks *mec* but contains genes encoding penicillin-binding protein 4 (*pbp4*) and resistance to mercury and cadmium [62,84]. Increasing evidence of novel SCC elements, such as SCC*pbp4* and SCC*far* in *S. aureus* MSSA476, suggests that they play key roles in interspecies transfer of antimicrobial or virulence genes [61,85]. As previously discussed in this chapter, the ACME element present in *S. aureus* USA300 was first discovered in *S. epidermidis* ATCC12228, suggesting that *S. epidermidis* is a potential reservoir for both ACME and SCC.

Table 2.2 Virulence factors and surface proteins present in both *S. aureus* and *S. epidermidis*.

Virulence factors
Esterase
Serine V8 protease
Cysteine protease
Lipase
β-Hemolysin
δ-Hemolysin
Hemolysin III
Hemolysin
Nuclease
Clp protease
Phenol soluble modulins
Surface proteins
Serine-aspartate repeat domain proteins (Sdr)
SdrC,D,E in *S. aureus*
SdrF,G,H in *S. epidermidis*
LPXTG cell wall surface proteins
SasA–K in *S. aureus*
SesA–K in *S. epidermidis*
Fibrinogen-binding protein
Elastin-binding protein
Bifunctional autolysin

Although *S. epidermidis* is less virulent than *S. aureus*, there are several virulence factors and surface adhesin proteins that are shared between the two species (Table 2.2). These include the family of proinflammatory PSMs, which are more numerous in *S. epidermidis* where they appear to have expanded as a result of gene duplication within the νSeγ genomic island (three *psmβ1* and one *psmβ2*). Expression of PSMs is associated with persistence of *S. epidermidis* in the hospital environment [86].

Acquisition of virulence factors in *S. epidermidis* has occurred as a result of plasmid-mediated gene transfer between staphylococci and other Gram-positive pathogens. Both *S. epidermidis* RP62a and ATCC12228 have acquired the *cap* operon (*capABC*) and γ-glutamyltranspeptidase gene similar to that found on the *Bacillus anthracis* pX02 plasmid, where it encodes the polyglutamate capsule, a key virulence factor in anthrax. Similar to *B. anthracis*, the *S. epidermidis cap* operon produces a poly-γ-DL-glutamic acid, which protects the bacteria from components of innate host defense [87].

Comparative analysis of the *S. epidermidis* RP62a and ATCC12228 genomes revealed two key differences between the strains: (i) the intercellular adhesion locus (*icaABCD*), which is also present in *S. aureus*, and (ii) the cell wall-associated biofilm protein (Bap) or Bap homologous protein (Bhp), which is present in bovine *S. aureus* mastitis isolates [4]. The *ica* locus, which encodes the polysaccharide intercellular adhesin proteins that play a key role in biofilm formation, as well as Bap/Bhp, are present in the biofilm-associated isolate RP62a but absent in the commensal isolate ATCC12228.

Staphylococcus haemolyticus

Among the coagulase-negative staphylococci, *S. haemolyticus* is second to *S. epidermidis* in frequency of isolation from human blood cultures. Although recognized as less virulent than *S. aureus*, it is associated with urinary tract infections, peritonitis, septicemia, and peritonitis. Like *S. epidermidis*, *S. haemolyticus* is also a member of the normal human skin flora, primarily from the axillae, perineum, and inguinal areas [88]. Genome sequencing of the glycopeptide-resistant *S. haemolyticus* strain JCSC1435 has revealed the basis of its abundant multidrug resistance and the role of numerous IS elements in frequent genomic rearrangements [9]. The genome contains three genome islands (νSh1, νSh2, νSh3) that do not possess known virulence or resistance factors and two bacteriophages (ϕSh1 and ϕSh2), with ϕSh1 carrying a β-lactamase gene and ϕSh2 carrying a truncated mercuric reductase homolog. Two integrated plasmids, πSh1 and πSh2, that contribute to multidrug resistance were also found in the *S. haemolyticus* genome. The πSh1-integrated plasmid carries macrolide resistance genes (*msrSA* and *mphBM*) and cadmium resistance genes (*cadD* and *cadX*), while πSh2 carries a likely multidrug efflux pump. Another factor contributing to the multiresistance phenotype is the mosaic SCC element, which consists of up to six different SCCs, only one of which retains the cassette chromosome recombinase (*ccr*) genes needed for movement of the SCC. The six-part SCC element carries the *mecA* gene encoding methicillin resistance as well as the *ars* operon that encodes resistance to arsenic. A common feature shared by *S. haemolyticus* and *S. epidermidis* is the *cap* operon (described above). Similar to *S. epidermidis*, virulence genes in *S. haemolyticus* are not located on MGEs, but rather found throughout the genome.

Staphylococcus saprophyticus

Staphylococcus saprophyticus is frequently associated with uncomplicated urinary tract infections (UTIs) in young and middle-aged female outpatients [89]. Because *S. saprophyticus* UTIs do not require involvement of indwelling catheters, it is likely that it has the potential to adhere directly to the urinary tract where it can be a persistent colonizer [90]. The genome sequence of *S. saprophyticus* type strain ATCC 15305 was determined and compared with *S. aureus* and *S. epidermidis* to identify species-specific functions and genes potentially associated with its ability to cause UTIs [8]. The most striking feature of *S. saprophyticus* compared with *S. aureus* is its complete absence of virulence factors, such as coagulase, hemolysins, enterotoxins, extracellular matrix-binding proteins, and other exoenzymes. The genome contains a single 39.3-kb prophage remnant, one genomic island (νSs15305), and two SCC elements. The νSs15305 island carries resistance determinants for fosfomycin and streptomycin. The first SCC element, SCC15305cap, carries a capsular polysaccharide synthesis locus that includes orthologs to *S. aureus*-type I Cap enzymes. The second element, SCC15305RM, carries no antibiotic resistance determinant or virulence factor. The two elements share a single set of cassette chromosome recombinase (Ccr) genes (*ccrA*, *ccrB*, *ccrC*) and appear to have integrated into the genome in a two-step event similar to the SCC*mec* element in *S. haemolyticus* [9]. Contrary to the multiple sortase functions in *S. aureus* and *S. epidermidis*, *S. saprophyticus* contains a single sortase-A. This single sortase-A is likely responsible for mediating cell wall attachment of the single LPXTG cell wall anchored protein or adhesin in *S. saprophyticus*. This species-specific adhesin (UafA) is the single largest predicted ORF in the *S. saprophyticus* genome and is responsible for both hemagglutination and adherence to uroepithelial cells in the urinary tract.

Two additional features of the *S. saprophyticus* genome suggest that it has evolved to adapt to life in the urinary tract environment. In addition to the osomoprotectant orthologs shared among the sequenced staphylococcal species, including those for proline, choline and glycine betaine, *S. saprophyticus* carries an expanded family of osomoprotectant transport paralogs with potential roles in balancing intracellular osmotic pressure in the urinary environment. The second feature is high urease activity of the *ureABCEFGD* gene cluster. Although the same urease gene operon is present in other staphylococcal species, the urease activity is higher in *S. saprophyticus* suggesting an alternative regulatory mechanism adapted to the urinary tract environment.

Summary

The availability of multiple staphylococcal genome sequences has revolutionized studies in virulence and antimicrobial resistance. Comparative analysis of *S. aureus* genomes has demonstrated the role of MGEs in acquisition of virulence factors and evolution of increasingly virulent lineages. Comparison of the *S. aureus* genomes with those of the less virulent *S. epidermidis*, *S. haemolyticus*, and *S. saprophyticus* has revealed the genes that distinguish the lifestyle of the opportunistic pathogen from that of the commensal members of normal human flora. More recent studies have demonstrated the pivotal role that DNA polymorphisms (including SNPs and indels) play in emergence of new strains. Despite this vast wealth of genome sequence data, we have only begun to unravel the mechanisms that determine the ability for selected strains to succeed as pathogens and persist in their host. Emerging experimental approaches based on staphylococcal genome data will ultimately lead to discoveries that yield insights not only into this significant bacterial pathogen but also host responses that ultimately determine its pathogenic lifestyle.

Acknowledgments

I thank Rob Leach (Center for Computational Research) for his work on the bidirectional genome comparisons.

References

1 Baba T, Bae T, Schneewind O, Takeuchi F, Hiramatsu K. Genome sequence of *Staphylococcus aureus* strain Newman and comparative analysis of staphylococcal genomes: polymorphism and evolution of two major pathogenicity islands. J Bacteriol 2008;190:300–10.

2 Baba T, Takeuchi F, Kuroda M *et al.* Genome and virulence determinants of high virulence community-acquired MRSA. Lancet 2002;359:1819–27.

3 Diep BA, Gill SR, Chang RF *et al.* Complete genome sequence of USA300, an epidemic clone of community-acquired meticillin-resistant *Staphylococcus aureus*. Lancet 2006;367:731–9.

4 Gill SR, Fouts DE, Archer GL *et al.* Insights on evolution of virulence and resistance from the complete genome analysis of an early methicillin-resistant *Staphylococcus aureus* strain and a biofilm-producing methicillin-resistant *Staphylococcus epidermidis* strain. J Bacteriol 2005;187:2426–38.

5 Herron-Olson L, Fitzgerald JR, Musser JM, Kapur V. Molecular correlates of host specialization in *Staphylococcus aureus*. PLoS ONE 2007;2:e1120.

6 Holden MT, Feil EJ, Lindsay JA *et al.* Complete genomes of two clinical *Staphylococcus aureus* strains: evidence for the rapid evolution of virulence and drug resistance. Proc Natl Acad Sci USA 2004;101:9786–91.

7 Kuroda M, Ohta T, Uchiyama I *et al.* Whole genome sequencing of meticillin-resistant *Staphylococcus aureus*. Lancet 2001;357:1225–40.

8 Kuroda M, Yamashita A, Hirakawa H *et al.* Whole genome sequence of *Staphylococcus saprophyticus* reveals the pathogenesis of uncomplicated urinary tract infection. Proc Natl Acad Sci USA 2005;102:13272–7.

9 Takeuchi F, Watanabe S, Baba T *et al.* Whole-genome sequencing of *Staphylococcus haemolyticus* uncovers the extreme plasticity of its genome and the evolution of human-colonizing staphylococcal species. J Bacteriol 2005;187:7292–308.

10 Becker K, Bierbaum G, von Eiff C *et al.* Understanding the physiology and adaptation of staphylococci: a post-genomic approach. Int J Med Microbiol 2007;297:483–501.

11 Dunman PM, Mounts W, McAleese F *et al.* Uses of *Staphylococcus aureus* GeneChips in genotyping and genetic composition analysis. J Clin Microbiol 2004;42:4275–83.

12 Francois P, Hernandez D, Schrenzel J. Genome content determination in methicillin-resistant *Staphylococcus aureus*. Future Microbiol 2007;2:187–98.

13 Koessler T, Francois P, Charbonnier Y *et al.* Use of oligoarrays for characterization of community-onset methicillin-resistant *Staphylococcus aureus*. J Clin Microbiol 2006;44:1040–8.

14 Lindsay JA, Moore CE, Day NP *et al.* Microarrays reveal that each of the ten dominant lineages of *Staphylococcus aureus* has a unique combination of surface-associated and regulatory genes. J Bacteriol 2006;188:669–76.

15 Monecke S, Slickers P, Ellington MJ, Kearns AM, Ehricht R. High diversity of Panton–Valentine leukocidin-positive, methicillin-susceptible isolates of *Staphylococcus aureus* and implications for the evolution of community-associated methicillin-resistant *S. aureus*. Clin Microbiol Infect 2007;13:1157–64.

16 Pichon C, Felden B. Small RNA genes expressed from *Staphylococcus aureus* genomic and pathogenicity islands with specific expression among pathogenic strains. Proc Natl Acad Sci USA 2005;102:14249–54.

17 Torres VJ, Stauff DL, Pishchany G *et al.* A *Staphylococcus aureus* regulatory system that responds to host heme and modulates virulence. Cell Host Microbe 2007;1:109–19.

18 Cassat J, Dunman PM, Murphy E *et al.* Transcriptional profiling of a *Staphylococcus aureus* clinical isolate and its isogenic *agr* and *sarA* mutants reveals global differences in comparison to the laboratory strain RN6390. Microbiology 2006;152:3075–90.

19 Fitzgerald JR, Sturdevant DE, Mackie SM, Gill SR, Musser JM. Evolutionary genomics of *Staphylococcus aureus*: insights into the origin of methicillin-resistant strains and the toxic shock syndrome epidemic. Proc Natl Acad Sci USA 2001;98:8821–6.

20 Gatlin CL, Pieper R, Huang ST *et al.* Proteomic profiling of cell envelope-associated proteins from *Staphylococcus aureus*. Proteomics 2006;6:1530–49.

21 Mongodin E, Finan J, Climo MW, Rosato A, Gill S, Archer GL. Microarray transcription analysis of clinical *Staphylococcus aureus* isolates resistant to vancomycin. J Bacteriol 2003;185:4638–43.

22 Pieper R, Gatlin-Bunai CL, Mongodin EF *et al.* Comparative proteomic analysis of *Staphylococcus aureus* strains with differences in resistance to the cell wall-targeting antibiotic vancomycin. Proteomics 2006;6:4246–58.

23 Highlander SK, Hulten KG, Qin X *et al.* Subtle genetic changes enhance virulence of methicillin resistant and sensitive *Staphylococcus aureus*. BMC Microbiol 2007;7:99.

24 Gillaspy AF, Worrell V, Orvis J, Roe BA, Dyer DW, Iandolo JJ. The *Staphylococcus aureus* NCTC8325 genome. In: Fischetti VA, Novick RP, Ferretti JJ, Portnoy DA, J.I. Rood, eds. Gram-positive Pathogens. Washington, DC: ASM Press, 2006:381–412.

25 Mwangi MM, Wu SW, Zhou Y *et al.* Tracking the in vivo evolution of multidrug resistance in *Staphylococcus aureus* by whole-genome sequencing. Proc Natl Acad Sci USA 2007;104:9451–6.

26 Lindsay JA, Holden MT. Understanding the rise of the superbug: investigation of the evolution and genomic variation of *Staphylococcus aureus*. Funct Integr Genomics 2006;6:186–201.

27 Dedent AC, Marraffini LA, Schneewind O. Staphylococcal sortases and surface proteins. In: Fischetti VA, Novick RP, Ferretti JJ, Portnoy DA, Rood JI, eds. Gram-positive Pathogens. Washington, DC: ASM Press, 2006:486–95.

28 Koreen L, Ramaswamy SV, Graviss EA, Naidich S, Musser JM, Kreiswirth BN. *spa* typing method for discriminating among *Staphylococcus aureus* isolates: implications for use of a single

marker to detect genetic micro- and macrovariation. J Clin Microbiol 2004;42:792–9.

29 Koreen L, Ramaswamy SV, Naidich S *et al.* Comparative sequencing of the serine-aspartate repeat-encoding region of the clumping factor B gene (*clfB*) for resolution within clonal groups of *Staphylococcus aureus*. J Clin Microbiol 2005;43:3985–94.

30 Rivas JM, Speziale P, Patti JM, Hook M. MSCRAMM: targeted vaccines and immunotherapy for staphylococcal infection. Curr Opin Drug Discov Devel 2004;7:223–7.

31 Rivera J, Vannakambadi G, Hook M, Speziale P. Fibrinogen-binding proteins of Gram-positive bacteria. Thromb Haemost 2007;98:503–11.

32 Robinson DA, Enright MC. Multilocus sequence typing and the evolution of methicillin-resistant *Staphylococcus aureus*. Clin Microbiol Infect 2004;10:92–7.

33 Feil EJ, Cooper JE, Grundmann H *et al.* How clonal is *Staphylococcus aureus*? J Bacteriol 2003;185:3307–16.

34 Fowler VG Jr, Nelson CL, McIntyre LM *et al.* Potential associations between hematogenous complications and bacterial genotype in *Staphylococcus aureus* infection. J Infect Dis 2007;196: 738–47.

35 Moore PC, Lindsay JA. Genetic variation among hospital isolates of methicillin-sensitive *Staphylococcus aureus*: evidence for horizontal transfer of virulence genes. J Clin Microbiol 2001;39:2760–7.

36 Peacock SJ, Moore CE, Justice A *et al.* Virulent combinations of adhesin and toxin genes in natural populations of *Staphylococcus aureus*. Infect Immun 2002;70:4987–96.

37 Thomas D, Chou S, Dauwalder O, Lina G. Diversity in *Staphylococcus aureus* enterotoxins. Chem Immunol Allergy 2007;93:24–41.

38 Fitzgerald JR, Monday SR, Foster TJ *et al.* Characterization of a putative pathogenicity island from bovine *Staphylococcus aureus* encoding multiple superantigens. J Bacteriol 2001;183:63–70.

39 Ubeda C, Tormo MA, Cucarella C *et al.* Sip, an integrase protein with excision, circularization and integration activities, defines a new family of mobile *Staphylococcus aureus* pathogenicity islands. Mol Microbiol 2003;49:193–210.

40 Tormo MA, Ferrer MD, Maiques E *et al.* *Staphylococcus aureus* pathogenicity island DNA is packaged in particles composed of phage proteins. J Bacteriol 2008;190:2434–40.

41 Ubeda C, Maiques E, Barry P *et al.* SaPI mutations affecting replication and transfer and enabling autonomous replication in the absence of helper phage. Mol Microbiol 2008;67:493–503.

42 Lindsay JA, Ruzin A, Ross HF, Kurepina N, Novick RP. The gene for toxic shock toxin is carried by a family of mobile pathogenicity islands in *Staphylococcus aureus*. Mol Microbiol 1998;29:527–43.

43 Ruzin A, Lindsay J, Novick RP. Molecular genetics of SaPI1: a mobile pathogenicity island in *Staphylococcus aureus*. Mol Microbiol 2001;41:365–77.

44 Ubeda C, Maiques E, Knecht E, Lasa I, Novick RP, Penades JR. Antibiotic-induced SOS response promotes horizontal dissemination of pathogenicity island-encoded virulence factors in staphylococci. Mol Microbiol 2005;56:836–44.

45 Maiques E, Ubeda C, Campoy S *et al.* Beta-lactam antibiotics induce the SOS response and horizontal transfer of virulence factors in *Staphylococcus aureus*. J Bacteriol 2006;188:2726–9.

46 Jarraud S, Peyrat MA, Lim A *et al.* egc, a highly prevalent operon of enterotoxin gene, forms a putative nursery of superantigens in *Staphylococcus aureus*. J Immunol 2001;166:669–77.

47 Fitzgerald JR, Reid SD, Ruotsalainen E *et al.* Genome diversification in *Staphylococcus aureus*: molecular evolution of a highly variable chromosomal region encoding the staphylococcal exotoxin-like family of proteins. Infect Immun 2003;71:2827–38.

48 Wang R, Braughton KR, Kretschmer D *et al.* Identification of novel cytolytic peptides as key virulence determinants for community-associated MRSA. Nat Med 2007;13:1510–4.

49 Kwan T, Liu J, DuBow M, Gros P, Pelletier J. The complete genomes and proteomes of 27 *Staphylococcus aureus* bacteriophages. Proc Natl Acad Sci USA 2005;102:5174–9.

50 Iandolo JJ, Worrell V, Groicher KH *et al.* Comparative analysis of the genomes of the temperate bacteriophages phi 11, phi 12 and phi 13 of *Staphylococcus aureus* 8325. Gene 2002;289:109–18.

51 Novick RP, Subedi A. The SaPIs: mobile pathogenicity islands of *Staphylococcus*. Chem Immunol Allergy 2007;93:42–57.

52 Tallent SM, Langston TB, Moran RG, Christie GE. Transducing particles of *Staphylococcus aureus* pathogenicity island SaPI1 are comprised of helper phage-encoded proteins. J Bacteriol 2007;189:7520–4.

53 Bae T, Baba T, Hiramatsu K, Schneewind O. Prophages of *Staphylococcus aureus* Newman and their contribution to virulence. Mol Microbiol 2006;62:1035–47.

54 Coleman DC, Sullivan DJ, Russell RJ, Arbuthnott JP, Carey BF, Pomeroy HM. *Staphylococcus aureus* bacteriophages mediating the simultaneous lysogenic conversion of beta-lysin, staphylokinase and enterotoxin A: molecular mechanism of triple conversion. J Gen Microbiol 1989;135:1679–97.

55 de Haas CJ, Veldkamp KE, Peschel A *et al.* Chemotaxis inhibitory protein of *Staphylococcus aureus*, a bacterial antiinflammatory agent. J Exp Med 2004;199:687–95.

56 Rooijakkers SH, Ruyken M, Roos A *et al.* Immune evasion by a staphylococcal complement inhibitor that acts on C3 convertases. Nat Immunol 2005;6:920–7.

57 Goerke C, Wirtz C, Fluckiger U, Wolz C. Extensive phage dynamics in *Staphylococcus aureus* contributes to adaptation to the human host during infection. Mol Microbiol 2006;61:1673–85.

58 Gillet Y, Issartel B, Vanhems P *et al.* Association between *Staphylococcus aureus* strains carrying gene for Panton–Valentine leukocidin and highly lethal necrotising pneumonia in young immunocompetent patients. Lancet 2002;359:753–9.

59 Lindsay JA, Holden MT. *Staphylococcus aureus*: superbug, super genome? Trends Microbiol 2004;12:378–85.

60 Luong TT, Ouyang S, Bush K, Lee CY. Type 1 capsule genes of *Staphylococcus aureus* are carried in a staphylococcal cassette chromosome genetic element. J Bacteriol 2002;184:3623–9.

61 Katayama Y, Takeuchi F, Ito T *et al.* Identification in methicillin-susceptible *Staphylococcus hominis* of an active primordial mobile genetic element for the staphylococcal cassette chromosome mec of methicillin-resistant *Staphylococcus aureus*. J Bacteriol 2003;185:2711–22.

62 Mongkolrattanothai K, Boyle S, Murphy TV, Daum RS. Novel non-*mecA*-containing staphylococcal chromosomal cassette composite island containing *pbp4* and *tagF* genes in a commensal staphylococcal species: a possible reservoir for antibiotic resistance islands in *Staphylococcus aureus*. Antimicrob Agents Chemother 2004;48:1823–36.

63 Oliveira DC, Milheirico C, de Lencastre H. Redefining a structural variant of staphylococcal cassette chromosome mec, SCCmec type VI. Antimicrob Agents Chemother 2006;50:3457–9.

64 Takano T, Higuchi W, Otsuka T *et al.* Novel characteristics of community-acquired methicillin-resistant *Staphylococcus aureus*

strains belonging to multilocus sequence type 59 in Taiwan. Antimicrob Agents Chemother 2008;52:837–45.

65 Katayama Y, Ito T, Hiramatsu K. Genetic organization of the chromosome region surrounding *mecA* in clinical staphylococcal strains: role of IS431-mediated *mecI* deletion in expression of resistance in *mecA*-carrying, low-level methicillin-resistant *Staphylococcus haemolyticus*. Antimicrob Agents Chemother 2001; 45:1955–63.

66 Robinson DA, Enright MC. Evolutionary models of the emergence of methicillin-resistant *Staphylococcus aureus*. Antimicrob Agents Chemother 2003;47:3926–34.

67 Paulsen IT, Firth N, Skurray RA. Resistance to antimicrobial agents other than β-lactams. In: Crossley KB, Archer GL, eds. The Staphylococci in Human Disease. New York: Churchill Livingstone, 1997:175–212.

68 Bayles KW, Iandolo JJ. Genetic and molecular analyses of the gene encoding staphylococcal enterotoxin D. J Bacteriol 1989; 171:4799–806.

69 Omoe K, Hu DL, Takahashi-Omoe H, Nakane A, Shinagawa K. Identification and characterization of a new staphylococcal enterotoxin-related putative toxin encoded by two kinds of plasmids. Infect Immun 2003;71:6088–94.

70 Zhang S, Iandolo JJ, Stewart GC. The enterotoxin D plasmid of *Staphylococcus aureus* encodes a second enterotoxin determinant (*sej*). FEMS Microbiol Lett 1998;168:227–33.

71 Jackson MP, Iandolo JJ. Cloning and expression of the exfoliative toxin B gene from *Staphylococcus aureus*. J Bacteriol 1986;166:574–80.

72 Lee CY, Schmidt JJ, Johnson-Winegar AD, Spero L, Iandolo JJ. Sequence determination and comparison of the exfoliative toxin A and toxin B genes from *Staphylococcus aureus*. J Bacteriol 1987;169:3904–9.

73 Weigel LM, Clewell DB, Gill SR *et al*. Genetic analysis of a high-level vancomycin-resistant isolate of *Staphylococcus aureus*. Science 2003;302:1569–71.

74 Firth N, Skurray RA. Genetics: accessory elements and genetic exchange. In: Fischetti VA, Novick RP, Ferretti JJ, Portnoy DA, Rood JI, eds. Gram-positive Pathogens. Washington, DC: ASM Press, 2006:413–26.

75 Centers for Disease Control and and Prevention. Vancomycin-resistant *Staphylococcus aureus*: Pennsylvania, 2002. MMWR 2002;51:902.

76 Zhu W, Clark NC, McDougal LK, Hageman J, McDonald LC, Patel JB. Vancomycin-resistant *Staphylococcus aureus* isolates associated with Inc18-like vanA plasmids in Michigan. Antimicrob Agents Chemother 2008;52:452–7.

77 Kolappaswamy K, Shipley ST, Tatarov II, Detolla LJ. Methicillin-resistant *Staphylococcus* non-aureus infection in an irradiated rhesus macaque (*Macaca mulatta*). J Am Assoc Lab Anim Sci 2008;47:64–7.

78 Guinane CM, Sturdevant DE, Herron-Olson L *et al*. Pathogenomic analysis of the common bovine *Staphylococcus aureus* clone (ET3): emergence of a virulent subtype with potential risk to public health. J Infect Dis 2008;197:205–13.

79 Leonard FC, Markey BK. Meticillin-resistant *Staphylococcus aureus* in animals: a review. Vet J 2008;175:27–36.

80 Haveri M, Taponen S, Vuopio-Varkila J, Salmenlinna S, Pyorala S. Bacterial genotype affects the manifestation and persistence of bovine *Staphylococcus aureus* intramammary infection. J Clin Microbiol 2005;43:959–61.

81 Kapur V, Sischo WM, Greer RS, Whittam TS, Musser JM. Molecular population genetic analysis of *Staphylococcus aureus* recovered from cows. J Clin Microbiol 1995;33:376–80.

82 Labandeira-Rey M, Couzon F, Boisset S *et al*. *Staphylococcus aureus* Panton–Valentine leukocidin causes necrotizing pneumonia. Science 2007;315:1130–3.

83 Voyich JM, Otto M, Mathema B *et al*. Is Panton–Valentine leukocidin the major virulence determinant in community-associated methicillin-resistant *Staphylococcus aureus* disease? J Infect Dis 2006;194:1761–70.

84 Zhang YQ, Ren SX, Li HL *et al*. Genome-based analysis of virulence genes in a non-biofilm-forming *Staphylococcus epidermidis* strain (ATCC 12228). Mol Microbiol 2003;49:1577–93.

85 Katayama Y, Ito T, Hiramatsu K. A new class of genetic element, staphylococcus cassette chromosome mec, encodes methicillin resistance in *Staphylococcus aureus*. Antimicrob Agents Chemother 2000;44:1549–55.

86 Klingenberg C, Ronnestad A, Anderson AS *et al*. Persistent strains of coagulase-negative staphylococci in a neonatal intensive care unit: virulence factors and invasiveness. Clin Microbiol Infect 2007;13:1100–11.

87 Kocianova S, Vuong C, Yao Y *et al*. Key role of poly-gamma-DL-glutamic acid in immune evasion and virulence of *Staphylococcus epidermidis*. J Clin Invest 2005;115:688–94.

88 Tristan A, Lina G, Etienne J, Vandenesch F. Biology and pathogenicity of staphylococci other than *Staphylococcus aureus* and *Staphylococcus epidermidis*. In: Fischetti VA, Novick RP, Ferretti JJ, Portnoy DA, Rood JI, eds. Gram-positive Pathogens. Washington, DC: ASM Press, 2006:572–86.

89 Kahlmeter G. An international survey of the antimicrobial susceptibility of pathogens from uncomplicated urinary tract infections: the ECO.SENS Project. J Antimicrob Chemother 2003;51:69–76.

90 von Eiff C, Peters G, Heilmann C. Pathogenesis of infections due to coagulase-negative staphylococci. Lancet Infect Dis 2002;2:677–85.

91 Kennedy AD, Otto M, Braughton KR *et al*. Epidemic community-associated methicillin-resistant *Staphylococcus aureus*: recent clonal expansion and diversification. *Proc Natt Acad Sci* USA 2008; 105:1327–32.

Chapter 3
Evolution and Taxonomy of Staphylococci

Barun Mathema, José R. Mediavilla, Liang Chen and Barry N. Kreiswirth
Public Health Research Institute Tuberculosis Center, University of Medicine and Dentistry of New Jersey, Newark, New Jersey, USA

Introduction

Basics of bacterial evolution and genetics

Amidst the recent debate over the origins of life and human evolution stands the threat of (re)emerging pathogens, which include new species as well as strains with increasing levels of antibiotic resistance and epidemic potential. In fact, bacterial pathogens not only serve as a case in point for evolution, but also highlight the importance of understanding the biomedical implications of evolutionary processes. In the face of consistent environmental insults (e.g., antibiotics, immune response), the ability of bacteria to rapidly diversify their genetic content, thereby altering gene expression and proteomic profiles to enhance adaptability, underscores their innate survival strategies. Genetic variations in bacterial genomes are typically indexed by differences in gene content and nucleotide variation in or between structural and other coding regions. In general, differences in gene content are due to gene deletions or acquisition of mobile elements such as bacteriophages and plasmids [1]. Allelic variation arises from random nucleotide substitution, sometimes followed by selection, and from horizontal gene transfer and intergenic recombination events. Therefore, bacterial genomes generally evolve by substitution in existing genes, loss or rearrangement of genetic material, or interspecies and intraspecies lateral gene transfer.

Unlike eukaryotic systems, bacterial genomes are haploid, and therefore the link between genotype and phenotype is more apparent. Thus in the face of selective forces such as antibiotic therapy, cells that bear advantageous properties can persist, replicate and disseminate, subsequently predominating in the population. In contrast to adaptive evolution, which occurs by accumulation of mutations, lateral gene transfer is a quick process that enables acquisition of exogenous genetic material that may facilitate survival in specialized niches.

Our basic understanding of the underlying genetic characteristics of bacterial pathogens has been catapulted forward with the plethora of publicly available genomic information and molecular and bioinformatic tools. The list includes diverse bacterial species as well as multiple members of the same species. Interspecies and intraspecies comparison of complete bacterial genomes has deepened our understanding of the extent of genetic variation both within and between species. Moreover, comparative genomic analyses of closely related species, and of multiple strains within discrete phylogenetic lineages, enable a more thorough interrogation of bacterial genetics, trait-lineage relationships, and underlying evolutionary processes. In essence, evolutionary studies fall into two broad categories: short term (local) and long term (global) [2]. The former examines genetic variation of organisms that have been isolated within a restricted spatial and temporal framework, including studies of within-host evolution and genetic relatedness among isolates from outbreaks or transmission events. These studies are the basis of most molecular epidemiological investigations. Long-term or global studies aim to elucidate the overall genetic structure of pathogen populations that are spatiotemporally unrestricted. These studies not only propose a population genetic structure with detailed phylogenetic lineages and modes of evolution, but can also provide biomedically relevant information on pathogen response to selective forces, such as host immunity, both natural and vaccine-induced, and antibiotic therapy [2].

In this chapter we focus on *Staphylococcus aureus*, a bacterial pathogen that has a wide host range, diverse cellular and environmental lifestyles, and the ability to develop highly drug-resistant forms that can cause serious human disease with epidemic potential. There are > 14 published *S. aureus* genomes available, another thirty or so currently

Staphylococci in Human Disease, 2nd edition. Edited by Kent B. Crossley, Kimberly K. Jefferson, Gordon Archer, Vance G. Fowler, Jr.

in progress, and thousands of clinical isolates analyzed by various molecular methods, which have more clearly unraveled the population structure of the species. We describe the current taxonomic classification of staphylococcal species and particularly focus on the mechanisms of genetic variation and relatedness of *S. aureus* and its relation to virulence, pathogenesis, and epidemiology.

Staphylococcus aureus: a major human pathogen

Staphylococci are Gram-positive bacteria usually living as commensals on the skin of mammals and birds. To date, 41 species and several subspecies have been catalogued into the *Staphylococcus* genus. From a human health perspective, *S. aureus* and *S. epidermidis* are the most important. Indeed, *S. aureus* has long been recognized as a major human pathogen and remains a frequent cause of morbidity and mortality. According to the National Nosocomial Surveillance System report, *S. aureus* was the most common cause of nosocomial infections reported between 1996 and 2002 [3]. *Staphylococcus epidermidis*, particularly multidrug-resistant forms, is also a significant nosocomial pathogen often associated with indwelling devices, and can cause significant morbidity and mortality, especially among immunocompromised hosts. Infections caused by *S. aureus* are varied in their severity and tissue tropisms, ranging from relatively mild conditions such as skin and soft tissue infections, to more severe disease that includes necrotizing pneumonia, surgical-site and bloodstream infections, which can be complicated by endocarditis or septic shock [4]. In addition to hospital-acquired infections, *S. aureus* also causes community-acquired infections such as osteomyelitis, septic arthritis, and skin infections [5]. The versatile tissue tropism displayed by *S. aureus* is attributed to its remarkable array of cell-associated and secreted virulence factors involved in pathogenesis. As such, the aggregate healthcare-associated cost of *S. aureus* infections, especially multidrug-resistant forms, in hospital and community settings can range to well over US $1 billion per year [6].

Staphylococcus aureus has two distinct lifestyles: a commensal asymptomatic state where it is carried by 20–50% of the general population in the anterior nares; and an acute state where it invades specific tissues and pathogenicity ensues [4]. Individuals may be colonized persistently or transiently, or may never harbor *S. aureus* as a commensal. Clearly, there are host (susceptibility) and host–pathogen dynamics at play, although these phenomena are poorly understood. Infection, often preceded by colonization, occurs when the organisms enter soft tissues and establish an invasive infection on breaches in the skin or mucous membranes [4]. In general, *S. aureus* infections are acquired either by self-inoculation (when colonized organisms breach natural barriers) or by direct or indirect contact. Contact spread poses an enormous burden for infection control personnel in healthcare facilities, as universal precautions must be applied, and often contact isolation is recommended. In the community, contact spread, possibly due to environmental and personal hygiene or intimate contact, has been well documented among prison inmates, children, and athletes as well as within social networks [7–11]. Commonly cited risk factors for *S. aureus* infection include colonization, poor hygiene, substance abuse, and specific comorbidities (e.g., cystic fibrosis, dermatological conditions) [4]. In addition, risk factors for MRSA infection include prolonged hospital stay, extensive antibiotic usage, indwelling lines, and recent invasive procedures.

The control and prevention of *S. aureus* infections in recent years have been complicated by the pervasive spread of multidrug-resistant *S. aureus* strains known as methicillin-resistant *S. aureus* (MRSA) in nosocomial settings. Since the introduction of methicillin into clinical use in 1961, the occurrence of MRSA has steadily increased in healthcare institutions worldwide [4]. Typically, MRSA are increasingly resistant to all available classes of antibiotics. Treatment of infections caused by MRSA is often limited to vancomycin, linezolid, and daptomycin. However, resistance to these three drugs has been reported, making MRSA a formidable public health challenge. The epidemiology of MRSA infections has typically been restricted to nosocomial environments and individuals linked to healthcare institutions, although this ecological niche has expanded [12]. Since the late 1990s, there has been a bloom of *S. aureus*-associated skin and soft tissue infections, mostly caused by MRSA, in community settings among otherwise healthy individuals [8–11]. Some of these community-acquired MRSA (CA-MRSA) infections have resulted in serious medical complications with poor clinical outcomes [13–15]. The number of CA-MRSA infections isolated from the community has steadily risen and in some locales has become epidemic. Although CA-MRSA are methicillin resistant, a phenotypic characteristic distinguishing CA-MRSA from hospital-acquired MRSA (HA-MRSA) has been that CA-MRSA isolates are typically less resistant to other non-β-lactams; however this too is changing, with increasing resistance being reported. In fact, some epidemic clones of CA-MRSA are increasingly being isolated from healthcare settings, blurring the lines between community- and hospital-acquired infections, thereby further obscuring the epidemiology and control of this pathogen [12,16–19].

Staphylococcal taxonomy and systematics

Historical overview

Staphylococci have likely been associated with human beings since their evolution from hominid ancestors several million years ago, and with various orders of mammals and birds long before that. Indeed, Kloos [20] suggests that the evolution of different staphylococcal species appears to closely parallel that of the mammalian orders they colonize, with an apparent peak in adaptive radiation occurring among primates. It has been suggested that the sixth plague of Egypt described in Exodus (9: 8–12), that of "incurable boils" (Hebrew *shkhin*) afflicting both humans and livestock, may be attributed to the most pathogenic member of the genus, *S. aureus*.

In 1880, both Louis Pasteur and Sir Alexander Ogston provided the first description of "micrococci" isolated from furuncles and abscesses. While Pasteur believed them to be pathogenic, it was Ogston who observed that the introduction of pus into experimental subjects produced similar abscesses [20,21], and in 1883 he gave the offending microbes the name they still bear today, based on their appearance under the microscope. Since the clusters of cells he saw resembled bunches of grapes, he named them *Staphylococcus*, after the Greek *staphyle*, meaning grapes, and *kokkos*, meaning berry. The following year, the German physician Anton Rosenbach isolated two pigmented varieties in pure culture, and provided the first taxonomic description of the new genus, dividing it into a "golden" species (*Staphylococcus pyogenes* var. *aureus*) and a "white" species (*S. pyogenes* var. *albus*) [22]. The latter would eventually be renamed *S. epidermidis* [23], but the former designation, minus the "pyogenes," is still used to describe the type species of the genus.

Variation in colonial pigmentation dominated the field of staphylococcal taxonomy well into the twentieth century. The primary division between "aureus" and "albus" remained in effect for several decades, reflecting the importance of differentiating between the pathogenic *S. aureus* and other staphylococci regarded as commensals or saprophytes. The fundamental distinction between *S. aureus* and its less pathogenic relatives was thereby clearly enunciated, one which is still very much in evidence today, as demonstrated by the taxonomically imprecise use of the term "coagulase-negative staphylococci" to indicate all other staphylococci besides *S. aureus*. Nowadays it is recognized that many staphylococcal species contain pigment-bearing strains, and that even within *S. aureus* it is possible to observe the occasional "white" or "citrine" strain; indeed, the golden color only seems to manifest fully after prolonged growth on certain types of media. Nevertheless, in deference to these early attempts to relate pigmentation with pathogenicity, recent evidence suggests that colonial pigmentation in *S. aureus* may indeed correlate with enhanced virulence [24].

The discovery of additional biochemical and microbiological characteristics eventually led to formal descriptions of new *Staphylococcus* species. The use of the "coagulating principle" as a defining characteristic for *S. aureus* was introduced in 1925 by von Darány, and the potential for classification of staphylococci using serological characteristics was investigated by several authors [25–27]. In 1940, *S. saprophyticus* became the first new staphylococcal species to be described that is still formally recognized [28], followed by *S. saccharolyticus* in 1948 [29], and *S. hyicus* in 1953 [30]; however, no further species would be described until 1975. A review of staphylococcal taxonomy appeared around the same time [31], along with reports describing the use of bacteriophage- and penicillin-mediated lysis for purposes of classification [32,33]. These initiatives made use of technical developments stemming from two historical milestones associated with *S. aureus*: the discovery of the first bacteriophage in 1915 by Frederick Twort [34,35]; and the discovery of penicillin in 1928 by Alexander Fleming [36]. The development of bacteriophage typing for epidemiological purposes during the 1950s is described in an excellent review by Kathryn Hillier [37], and is discussed in further detail in a later section. Ironically, the varying susceptibilities of staphylococci to penicillin lysis were early harbingers of an unfortunate development in the evolutionary history of the genus that would ultimately supersede any potential utility as a taxonomic marker.

Despite progress in the delineation of staphylococcal species and strains, until the 1960s the taxonomic affiliation of the genus *Staphylococcus* was hampered by historical observations that grouped it together with other "micrococci." Zopf [38] originally assigned staphylococci to the genus *Micrococcus* and the family Coccaceae, insofar as both *Staphylococcus* and *Micrococcus* consisted of "group-forming cocci," although the following year Flügge [39] observed a fundamental distinction between the more pathogenic *Staphylococcus* and the saprophytic *Micrococcus*. From a biochemical standpoint, both genera are distinguished from other aerobic Gram-positive cocci by virtue of being catalase-positive, and members of the genus *Micrococcus* also exhibit pronounced colonial pigmentation that was believed to highlight their affiliation with the often pigmented staphylococci. It was not until the 1960s that differences in the guanine plus cytosine (GC) content of their respective DNA suggested a fundamental distinction, with staphylococci exhibiting a relatively low GC content (30–39%), whereas micrococci possess a GC content of 66–75% [20,40]. The distinction between low-GC and high-GC Gram-positive bacteria is now understood to represent a valid phylogenetic classification, and subsequent molecular analyses have confirmed the taxonomic separation of *Staphylococcus* and *Micrococcus*. Nevertheless, they are still grouped together in many manuals and textbooks of clinical microbiology, and it is still common to see staphylococci described erroneously as members of the family Micrococcaceae.

During the 1960s, Baird-Parker developed schemes that employed a variety of microbiological and biochemical assays, including cell wall structure, enzymatic activity, and growth requirements, in order to identify subgroups within the genus *Staphylococcus* and ascertain host ranges and clinical associations [20,41,42]. Using these schemes, he divided *S. epidermidis* into four "biotypes" named subgroups II, III, IV, and VI; *S. aureus* was assigned to a single subgroup (I), but was further subdivided into "ecotypes" on the basis of phage susceptibility, serology, and other biochemical properties [43]. Later versions of the scheme were modified to allow for the identification of *S. saprophyticus*. Baird-Parker's schemes were employed for many years in both the clinical and food microbiology fields, until new species began to be described and their limitations became apparent [20]. However, a selective medium containing potassium tellurite and lithium chloride, which he developed for the isolation of *S. aureus* from food, still bears his name and is used widely in that industry [44].

The 1970s and 1980s were characterized by further refinement of biochemical and morphological techniques, including carbohydrate fermentation patterns, cell wall composition, fatty acid analysis, intrinsic antibiotic resistance profiles, and other biochemical traits that could be combined in order to yield "phenetic" profiles [20]. This same period also witnessed the advent of DNA–DNA hybridization methods, in which whole-genome comparisons of different species could be performed by conducting reassociation experiments and measuring the extent of hybridization, thereby inferring relative measures of relatedness. The combination of these new approaches resulted in a veritable explosion in the number of newly described staphylococcal species from both humans and animals, beginning in 1975 with the formal description of no less than 10 novel species by Kloos and Schleifer. By the time volume 2 of the first edition of *Bergey's Manual of Systematic Bacteriology* was published in 1986 [45], 19 species and two subspecies had achieved formal recognition, and their putative phylogenetic relationships could be depicted in the form of a DNA hybridization dendrogram. The taxonomic proximity of the staphylococci to members of the genus *Bacillus*, as well as to the streptococci and lactobacilli, was likewise understood by the mid-1980s, although the genus *Staphylococcus* continued to be subsumed within the Micrococcaceae. Another noteworthy development during this period involved growing recognition of the clinical importance of coagulase-negative staphylococci, previously considered to be of a benign or commensal nature, but increasingly seen as responsible for infections associated with indwelling devices. *Staphylococcus epidermidis* is currently considered to account for an even larger percentage of hospital-acquired bloodstream infections than *S. aureus*, and other members of the genus are of increasing importance in veterinary microbiology.

The following decade bore witness to unabated discovery of new species and subspecies, with continuous reevaluation of taxonomic paradigms and dogma, driven largely by the 16S ribosomal RNA revolution [46]. In 1998, a novel species of *Staphylococcus* (*S. succinus*) was isolated from 25–35 million-year-old Dominican amber [47], while another species (*S. caseolyticus*) was reclassified into a novel genus, *Macrococcus*, which unlike its homonym Micrococcus appears to comprise the nearest relatives of the genus *Staphylococcus*. Although governing bodies of bacterial systematics still mandate a "polyphasic" approach [48] for formal descriptions of new species, the objectivity, reliability and ease of DNA sequencing has brought genetic identification of organisms within reach of many clinical laboratories [49], and curated quality-controlled databases devoted to ribosomal RNA identification exist for several species including staphylococci [50]. Therefore, aside from minor discrepancies highlighted by the use of different gene targets, the phylogenetic structure of most major prokaryotic groups has been convincingly resolved down to the genus and species levels.

Although new staphylococcal species (and subspecies) will continue to be described, the emphasis during the last decade has been on the population structure and microevolutionary dynamics of *S. aureus* at what is properly designated the "infra-subspecific" level. This refers to the in-depth analysis of specific strains, clones, and lineages of clinical and epidemiological importance, using molecular tools and approaches that can resolve genetic interrelationships below the level of resolution afforded by species-level methods such as 16S rRNA sequencing. Two such methods, pulsed-field gel electrophoresis (PFGE), and multilocus sequence typing (MLST), are discussed in later sections. The driving force for these types of investigations has been the global emergence and dissemination of multiple antibiotic-resistant epidemic clones within many pathogenic bacterial species, in both nosocomial and community settings, of which MRSA is quite possibly the principal example. These techniques have been applied to both infection control in localized outbreaks, as well as to global epidemiological studies of clonal spread. Additionally, the rapid growth and decreasing cost of high-throughput technologies is uncovering a wealth of information about the diversity that underlies particular species. Currently, 33 staphylococcal genomes have been completely sequenced, and at least thirty more are currently in progress, which averages out to eight new genomes per year since the first *S. aureus* genomes were published in 2001 [51]. Analysis of such sequences, coupled with microevolutionary studies based on population-level approaches, will doubtless enrich our understanding of the evolutionary structure of staphylococci on a level that our predecessors at the turn of the nineteenth century could not have imagined.

Description of the genus *Staphylococcus*

Staphylococci are Gram-positive cocci, approximately 0.5–1.5 μm in diameter, occurring singly, in pairs, tetrads, short chains, or grape-like clusters [40]. They are nonmotile, do not form spores or resting stages, and are typically unencapsulated, although some strains of *S. aureus* form an unusual capsule, and *S. epidermidis* is able to form biofilms on prosthetic devices. Most are also capable of growth on media containing 10% NaCl, and several species can grow at concentrations of up to 15% NaCl, which helps explain their predilection for the sebaceous surfaces of mammals. With respect to temperature, many species can grow at 15°C, others at temperatures as high as 45°C, and a few, including *S. aureus*, can grow at both extremes. Except for two members of the genus (*S. aureus* subsp. *anaerobius* and *S. saccharolyticus*), they tend to be catalase-positive, a feature that distinguishes them clinically from the streptococci and enterococci, although occasional reports of catalase-negative *S. aureus* strains have been described [52–57]. Unlike the obligately aerobic genus *Micrococcus* with which they have been historically confused, staphylococci are almost universally facultatively anaerobic, the exceptions again being the two catalase-negative species mentioned above. Also unlike *Micrococcus*, most clinically relevant staphylococci are oxidase-negative, although members of the *S. sciuri* group, which appears to be ancestral, do possess cytochome *c* oxidase.

On a macromolecular level, staphylococci have genomes in the range 2–3 Mb, with an overall GC content of 30–39%. They possess several prophages, but relatively few plasmids. Other characteristics include a particular cell wall structure that is resistant to lysozyme but susceptible to the action of lysostaphin, a glycylglycine metalloendopeptidase that specifically cleaves cross-linking pentaglycine bridges between peptidoglycan residues [58], and which is synthesized naturally by one member of the genus (*S. simulans*, formerly called *S. staphylolyticus*). This property has led to efforts to implement lysostaphin therapeutically, both in humans as a means of nasal decolonization, and in transgenic cows as a prophylactic defense against the development of mastitis [59].

In the clinical laboratory, staphylococci have traditionally been identified on the basis of cellular morphology, Gram-stain characteristics, ability to grow aerobically, and formation of catalase. Once a positive identification of *Staphylococcus* is made, the next priority is to determine if it is *S. aureus*, typically by observation of a positive coagulase reaction in rabbit plasma. Isolates exhibiting a negative reaction are therefore referred to as coagulase-negative staphylococci (CoNS), which has direct bearing on subsequent patient management, although as we shall see, this distinction is taxonomically inadequate; furthermore, the growing clinical significance of CoNS dictates that ruling out *S. aureus* is not necessarily indicative of a benign outcome. Another traditional means of differentiating *S. aureus* involves the use of mannitol-salt agar. Since most strains of *S. aureus* readily ferment mannitol, media containing a pH-based indicator will turn from red to yellow in the presence of *S. aureus*, while *S. epidermidis*, which does not ferment mannitol, forms white colonies instead. However, inspection of biochemical tables reveals that fermentation of mannitol is the norm rather than the exception for most members of the genus (Figure 3.1) and is therefore not diagnostic of *S. aureus*, although a negative reaction is strongly suggestive of *S. epidermidis*. Recently, various types of commercial media specific for *S. aureus* have been described [60,61]; these are largely based on proprietary chromogenic substrate formulations, some of which can also differentiate MRSA from methicillin-sensitive *S. aureus* (MSSA) [62]. While more expensive than traditional media, they are highly specific and can greatly reduce the time required for presumptive identification.

Algorithms for the differentiation of staphylococci from other genera, as well as the identification of particular *Staphylococcus* spp., are still published routinely [63]; however, most contemporary laboratories are likely to rely on commercial identification methods, rather than resort to manual biochemical profiling. More recently, the advent of molecular diagnostics in clinical laboratories has allowed many of these to invest in genotypic identification methods, such as those based on 16S rRNA sequencing. Additionally, as a result of the increasing need for rapid identification of MRSA (and methicillin-resistant CoNS) in bloodstream infections, several companies are developing real-time polymerase chain reaction (PCR)-based diagnostic platforms that can provide results in hours rather than days (e.g., Becton Dickinson's GeneOhm™ StaphSR assay).

Genus, species, subspecies, and infra-subspecies

The genus *Staphylococcus* is currently understood to lie within the same large order, Bacillales, that includes the familiar species *Bacillus* and *Listeria*, as shown in Figure 3.2b. Bacillales, in turn, forms part of the class Bacilli, along with the order Lactobacillales, wherein other important Gram-positive pathogens such as *Streptococcus* and *Enterococcus* are found. The nearest relatives of *Staphylococcus* appear to lie in the relatively novel genus *Macrococcus*, proposed in 1998 in order to resolve taxonomic ambiguities associated with the former species *Staphylococcus caseolyticus* [64], which was previously considered to occupy a position on the periphery of the genus [65]. As their name suggests, cells of the genus *Macrococcus* appear considerably larger (1.1–2.5 μm in diameter) than *Staphylococcus* when viewed under the microscope, but they are nevertheless closely related to staphylococci on

Staphylococcus spp.			colony pigment	oxidase	novobiocin resistance	coagulase	heat-stable nuclease	mannitol fermentation	pyrrolidonyl arylamidase	*mec A*
capitis-capitis	*	AY688037	–	–	–	–	–	+	–	+
capitis-urealyticus	*	AY688040	d	–	–	–	–	+	(d)	+
saccharolyticus	*	AY688087	–	–	–	–	ND	–	ND	
caprae	*	AY688036	–	–	–	–	–	d	d	+
epidermidis	*	AY688051	–	–	–	–	(–w)	–	–	+
simiae		AY727530	–	–	–	–	–	+	–	
aureus-anaerobius		AY688031	–	–	–	+	+	–	ND	
aureus-aureus	*	AY688032	(+w)	–	–	+	+	+	–	+
pasteuri		AY688082	w	–	–	–	–	w	–	
warneri	*	AY688105	d	–	–	–	–	d	–	+
muscae		AY688079	–	–	–	–	–	–	ND	
lugdunensis	*	AY688074	d	–	–	–	–	–	+	+
haemolyticus	*	AY688060	d	–	–	–	–	d	+	+
hominis-hominis	*	AY688063	d	–	–	–	–	d	–	+
hominis-novobiosepticus	*	AY688065	–	–	+	–	ND	–	–	+
cohnii-cohnii	*	AY688045	–	–	+	–	–	d	–	
cohnii-urealyticus		AY688047	d	–	+	–	–	d	d	
nepalensis		AY688080	–	–	+	–	–	+	+	
saprophyticus-bovis		AY688088	+	–	+	–	–	d	+	+
saprophyticus-saprophyticus	*	AY688089	d	–	+	–	–	d	–	+
xylosus	*	AY688107	d	–	+	–	–	d	d	
arlettae		AY688029	+	–	+	–	–	+	–	
gallinarum		AY688059	d	–	+	–	–	+	–	
equorum-equorum		AY688054	–	–	+	–	–	+	–	
equorum-linens		AY688056	–	–	–	–	–	+	–	
kloosii		AY688071	d	–	+	–	–	+	d	
succinus-casei		AY688102	–	–	+	ND	ND	ND	–	
succinus-succinus		AY688103	–	–	+	ND	ND	ND	–	
auricularis		AY688030	–	–	–	–	–	–	d	
felis		AY688057	–	–	–	–	(–w)	d	ND	
lutrae		AY688077	–	–	–	+	ND	+	ND	
chromogenes		AY688044	+	–	–	–	(–w)	d	–	
hyicus		AY688066	–	–	–	d	+	–	–	
schleiferi-coagulans	*	AY688091	ND	ND	–	+	+	ND	d	
schleiferi-schleiferi		AY688092	–	–	–	–	+	–	+	
pseudintermedius	*	**AJ780976**	–	–	–	+	ND	(w)	+	+
delphini		AY688050	–	ND	–	+	–	+	ND	
intermedius	*	AY688067	–	–	–	+	+	(d)	+	+
pettenkoferi	*	AY688083	d	–	–	–	ND	(d)	+	
pseudolugdunensis	*	EF053370	–	–	+	–	ND	d	+	+
simulans	*	AY688099	–	–	–	–	–	+	+	+
camosus-camosus		AY688041	–	–	–	–	d	+	+	
camosus-utilis		AY688042	+	ND	–	–	ND	+	ND	
condimenti		AY688048	+	ND	–	–	ND	d	ND	
piscifermentans		AY688085	+	–	–	–	ND	d	ND	
lentus		AY688073	d	+	+	–	ND	+	–	
sciuri-sciuri	*	AY688097	d	+	+	–	–	+	–	+
sciuri-camaticus		AY688095	d	+	+	–	–	+	–	+
sciuri-rodentium		AY688096	d	+	+	–	–	+	–	+
fleurettii		AY688058	–	+	+	–	–	ND	–	
pulvereri		AY688086	d	+	+	–	ND	+	–	
vitulinus		AY688104	+	+	+	–	ND	ND	–	+
Macrococcus caseolyticus		Y15711	–	+	+	–	ND	–	+	
Macrococcus equipercicus		Y15712	+	+	+	–	ND	+	–	

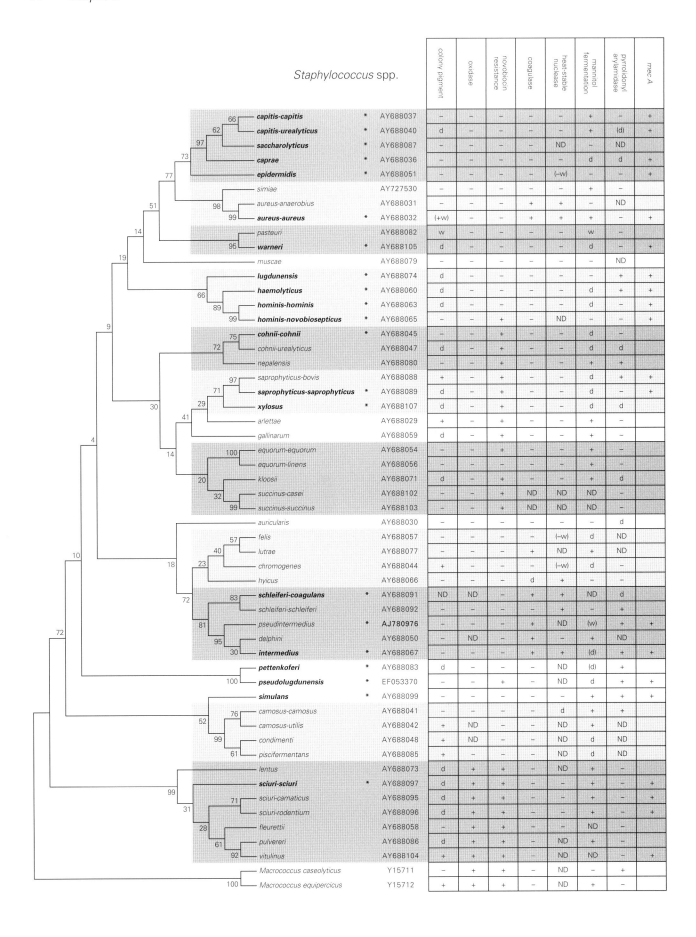

the basis of DNA–DNA hybridization and 16S rRNA sequence analysis. In particular, they appear to be closely related to members of the *S. sciuri* group, with which they share the biochemical characteristic of being oxidase-positive, and which in turn appears to represent an outgroup relative to the other staphylococcal species groups (Figure 3.1).

By comparison, the other members of the family Staphylococcaceae consist of less familiar-sounding organisms including *Gemella*, *Salinicoccus* and *Jeotgalicoccus*, the latter being named after a condiment made from seafood and used in kimchi and other elements of Korean cuisine. A quick glance at the names of various other neighbors within the order Bacillales is similarly suggestive of the halotolerant lifestyle characteristic of most staphylococci. Although the medically important genus *Gemella* is classified as a member of the Staphylococcaceae, it appears that on the basis of 16S rRNA sequence analysis it is more closely related to *Streptococcus*, as suggested by phenotypic characteristics and other phylogenetic studies [66–68]. As there do not seem to be any explicit systematic associations between *Gemella* and *Staphylococcus* in the literature, this classification should be further investigated.

Within the genus *Staphylococcus* itself, there are presently 41 species and 24 subspecies with standing in bacterial nomenclature, as mentioned earlier [69]; counting each species and/or subspecies individually, a total of 51 taxa can be enumerated. These are listed in Table 3.1 along with information about the source and/or host range, and references for their initial descriptions. Included also are the recently proposed *S. pseudolugdunensis* [70] and the somewhat ambiguous *S. pulvereri*, which has previously been suggested to be the same species as *S. vitulinus* [71]. Figure 3.2c shows a simplified 16S rRNA-based phylogenetic portrait of the various subgroupings in the genus, based on clusters with statistically significant bootstrap values. These groupings are in general agreement with those published in other studies [65], including those based on methods utilizing *rpoB* [72,73], *hsp60* [74–76], *tuf* [77], *sodA* [78], *GAPDH* [79], and DNA–DNA hybridization [20].

The relative phylogenetic distance exhibited by the *sciuri* group is readily apparent, although the location of the branch in Figure 3.2c is not reliable as the tree is unrooted; in Figure 3.1, rooting using *Macrococcus* as an outgroup places the *sciuri* group as a clear outgroup. Several of the subgroups appear to correlate to some extent with host range and/or environmental sources. For example, members of the *hyicus* and *intermedius* groups are composed largely of species associated with "lower" animals including carnivores, artiodactyls, and cetaceans, although these host ranges are also represented in other clusters; by contrast, the members of the *carnosus* group are of primary importance in the food industry. However, no exclusive host range associations can be inferred from phylogenetic analysis, and members of nearly every group have been reported to cause infections in humans. It is nevertheless clear that some species groups are more often found in humans and other primates, and all members of the *epidermidis* and *haemolyticus* groups are frequently implicated in clinical disease. Interestingly, *S. aureus* appears to occupy a somewhat solitary position, with the nearest relative being the recently described species *S. simiae*, isolated from South American squirrel monkeys [80]. Also of interest is the distribution of coagulase-positive species within the genus; as can be seen in Figure 3.2c and the table in Figure 3.1, several species within the *hyicus* and *intermedius* groups also exhibit coagulase activity, including several species of veterinary importance that are known to cause disease in humans. In particular, *S. intermedius* and *S. pseudintermedius* can be mistakenly identified as *S. aureus* when relying on phenotypic identification methods [81].

With respect to subspeciation, 10 species thus far have been subdivided into subspecies on the basis of both phenotypic and sequence-based differences. Both DNA–DNA hybridization and 16S rRNA approaches have traditionally employed threshold similarity cutoffs in order to differentiate between species and subspecies [20]. As an example, while 16S rRNA cannot differentiate between the *S. aureus* genome sequences currently available, it clearly suggests that *S. aureus* subsp. *anaerobius* is sufficiently

Figure 3.1 *(opposite)* (a) Neighbor-joining 16S rRNA phylogenetic tree depicting all currently recognized staphylococcal species and subspecies, including the recently proposed *S. pseudolugdunensis*; GenBank accession numbers are shown for all taxa. Of 52 staphylococcal sequences, 49 were downloaded according to the accession numbers provided by Becker *et al.* [50]; the remaining sequences were downloaded separately and trimmed to the same length. A 467-nucelotide alignment was used to construct a neighbor-joining tree with MEGA 4.0 [280], using the maximum composite likelihood method, and rooted using *Macrococcus* spp. as an outgroup. Bootstrap confidence intervals are indicated for 1000 replicates; taxa are right-justified to facilitate comparison with the table, and branch lengths do not reflect evolutionary distances. Species known to cause infections in humans are shown in bold and labeled with an asterisk. Selected phenotypic characteristics frequently used for differentiation of staphylococcal species and subspecies are organized according to the topology displayed by the tree; table rows and corresponding clusters in the tree are shaded alternately in order to highlight the same groups depicted in Figure 3.2c. Characters shown were obtained from a variety of sources, including Bannerman [40] and Freney *et al.* [48], and various monographs providing original descriptions of novel taxa; +, 90% or more strains are positive; –, 90% or more strains are negative; d, 11–89% of strains are positive; letters in parentheses indicate delayed reaction; w, weak reaction; (+w), positive to weak reaction; (–w), negative to weak reaction; ND, not determined. The last column shows taxa in which the presence of the *mecA* gene has been reported in the literature; a + sign indicates reported occurrence only, with no implication of frequency; taxa for which *mecA* has not been explicitly reported are left blank.

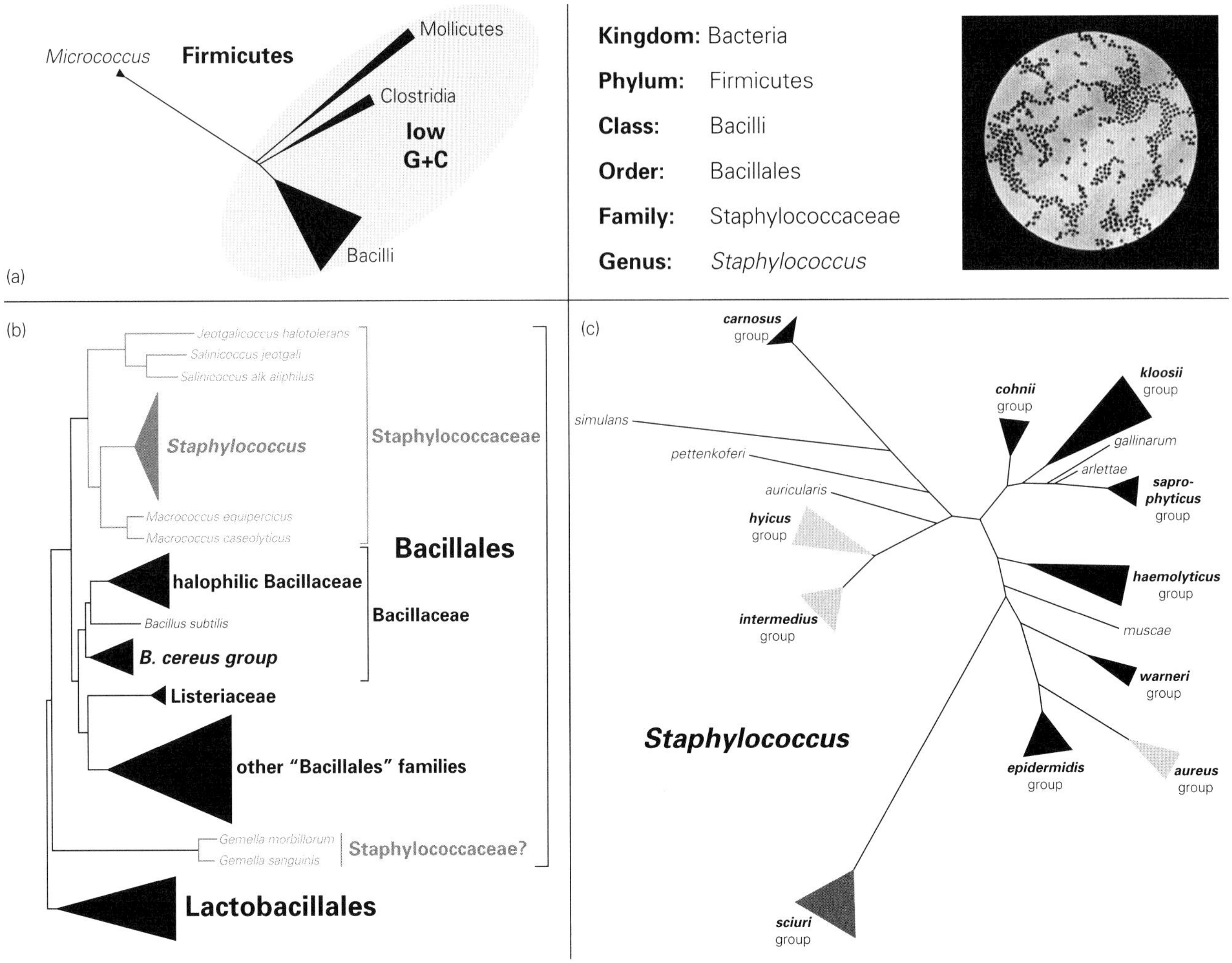

Figure 3.2 Phylogenetic context of the genus *Staphylococcus* based on 16S rRNA sequences. Sequences were downloaded from GenBank and aligned using MEGA 4.0 [280]; a 1386-nucelotide alignment was used to construct a neighbor-joining tree with MEGA 4.0, using the maximum composite likelihood method; 1000 bootstrap replicates were performed for all trees (values not shown here). (a) Simplified phylum-level view showing the three major classes of low-GC Gram-positive bacteria, and the relatively distant phylogenetic location of the genus *Micrococcus*. Class Bacilli consists of selected sequences from those described in (b); class Clostridia consists of *Clostridium botulinum* (L37585), *Clostridium difficile* (X73450), and *Eubacterium acidaminophilum* (AF071416); class Mollicutes consists of *Mycoplasma pneumoniae* (AF132740), *Acholeplasma laidlawii* (U14905), and *Spiroplasma lampyridicola* (AY189134); *Micrococcus* consists of *Micrococcus luteus* (DQ491453) and *Micrococcus flavus* (AJ536198). (b) Class Bacilli comprises two orders, Bacillales and Lactobacillales, with the family Staphylococcaceae shown in gray. Lactobacillales consists of *Aerococcus sanguinicola* (AJ276512), *Enterococcus faecalis* (AB012212), *Lactobacillus casei* (D86517), *Carnobacterium pleistocenium* (AF450136), *Leuconostoc fructosus* (AF360737), *Lactococcus lactis* (AB100804), and *Streptococcus pneumoniae* (AF003930). Bacillales comprises Listeriaceae, Bacillaceae, Staphylococcaceae, and other "Bacillales" families. Other "Bacillales" families consist of *Alicyclobacillus acidocaldarius* (AB271754), *Sulfobacillus thermosulfidooxidans* (AB089844), *Thermactinomyces vulgaris* (AF138739); *Planifilum yunannensis* (DQ119659), *Brevibacillus limnophilus* (AB112717); *Paenibacillus polymyxa* (D16276), *Anoxybacillus flavothermus* (AF004589), *Geobacillus stearothermophilus* (AB271757), *Exiguobacterium aurantiacum* (DQ019166), *Ureibacillus thermosphaericus* (AB101594), *Planococcus maritimus* (AF500007), and *Sporosarcina aquimarina* (AF202056). Listeriaceae consists of *Listeria monocytogenes* (X98530) and *Brochothrix* spp. TM5_5 (DQ279394). Bacillaceae comprises *B. cereus* group, consisting of *Bacillus megaterium* (D16273), *Bacillus anthracis* (AB190217), *Bacillus thuringiensis* (D16281), and *Bacillus cereus* (D16266); *Bacillus subtilis* (AB271744); and halophilic Bacillaceae, consisting of *Halobacillus salinus* (AF500003), *Gracilibacillus halotolerans* (AF036922), *Virgibacillus marismortui* (AJ009793), *Halalkalibacillus halophilus* (AB264529), *Alkalibacillus haloalkaliphilus* (AJ238041), and *Oceanobacillus iheyensis* (OB3546). Staphylococcaceae consists of *Gemella morbillorum* (L14327), *Gemella sanguinis* (Y13364), *Jeotgalicoccus halotolerans* (AY028925), *Salinicoccus jeotgali* (DQ471329), *Salinicoccus alkaliphilus* (AF275710), *Macrococcus caseolyticus* (Y15711), *Macrococcus equipercicus* (Y15712), and *Staphylococcus* (subset of sequences described in (c)). **(c)** Simplified phylogenetic representation of the genus *Staphylococcus*, with natural clusters exhibiting bootstrap values greater than 50% collapsed and named after the earliest member described; ungrouped species represent poorly resolved branches with low bootstrap values; branch lengths represent evolutionary distance; phylogenetic tree consists of all taxons displayed in Figure 3.1, with the exception of *Macrococcus* and the newly proposed species *S. pseudolugdunensis*; light gray indicates clusters containing coagulase-positive species; dark gray indicates clusters in which all members are oxidase-positive. Collapsed groups consist of the following species, in clockwise order (see Figure 3.1 for accession numbers): *sciuri* group comprises *S. sciuri* subsp. *sciuri*, *S. sciuri* subsp. *carnaticus*, *S. sciuri* subsp. *rodentium*, *S. lentus*, *S. fleuretti*, *S. pulvereri*, and *S. vitulinus*; *intermedius* group comprises *S. intermedius*, *S. pseudintermedius*, *S. delphini*, *S. schleiferi* subsp. *schleiferi*, and *S. schleiferi* subsp. *coagulans*; *hyicus* group comprises *S. hyicus*, *S. lutrae*, *S. felis*, and *S. chromogenes*; *carnosus* group comprises *S. carnosus* subsp. *carnosus*, *S. carnosus* subsp. *utilis*, *S. condimenti*, and *S. piscifermentans*; *cohnii* group comprises *S. cohnii* subsp. *cohnii*, *S. cohnii* subsp. *urealyticus*, and *S. nepalensis*; *kloosii* group comprises *S. kloosii*, *S. equorum* subsp. *equorum*, *S. equorum* subsp. *linens*, *S. succinus* subsp. *succinus*, and *S. succinus* subsp. casei; *saprophyticus* group comprises *S. saprophyticus* subsp. *saprophyticus*, *S. saprophyticus* subsp. *bovis*, and *S. xylosus*; *haemolyticus* group comprises *S. haemolyticus*, *S. lugdunensis*, *S. hominis* subsp. *hominis* and *S. hominis* subsp. *novobiosepticus*; *warneri* group = *S. warneri* and *S. pasteuri*; *aureus* group comprises *S. aureus* subsp. *aureus*, *S. aureus* subsp. *anaerobius*, and *S. simiae*; *epidermidis* group comprises *S. epidermidis*, *S. caprae*, *S. saccharolyticus*, *S. capitis* subsp. *capitis*, and *S. capitis* subsp. *urealyticus*. The panel in the upper-right corner displays the current Linnaean classification scheme for the genus *Staphylococcus*; the image is a methylene blue-stained micrograph of *S. aureus*, downloaded freely from the CDC Public Health Image Library (ID# 5144).

Table 3.1 Staphylococcal species and subspecies with standing in bacterial nomenclature [69] as of May 2009, along with the recently proposed *S. pseudolugdunensis* [70]; both *S. pulvereri* and *S. vitulinus* are included (indicated by *), although the synonymy between these two species is supported by the subcommittee on the taxonomy of staphylococci and streptococci of the international Committee on Systematics of Prokaryotes (ICSP).

Staphylococcus spp.	Isolated from	Initial description	
arlettae	Poultry	Schleifer *et al.* 1985	[281]
aureus subsp. *aureus*	Primates, domestic animals, poultry, rodents	Rosenbach 1884	[22]
aureus subsp. *anaerobius*	Domestic sheep	De La Fuente *et al.* 1985	[282]
auricularis	Primates, human external auditory meatus	Kloos & Schleifer 1983	[283]
capitis subsp. *capitis*	Human skin	Kloos & Schleifer 1975	[284]
capitis subsp. *urealyticus*	Primates	Bannerman & Kloos 1991	[285]
caprae	Goats, humans	Devriese *et al.* 1983	[286]
carnosus subsp. *carnosus*	Domestic artiodactyls	Schleifer & Fischer 1982	[287]
carnosus subsp. *utilis*	Domestic artiodactyls	Probst *et al.* 1998	[288]
chromogenes	Artiodactyls, horses	Devriese *et al.* 1978	[289]
cohnii subsp. *cohnii*	Humans	Schleifer & Kloos 1975	[290]
cohnii subsp. *urealyticus*	Primates, tree shrews	Kloos & Wolfshohl 1991	[291]
condimenti	Soy sauce mash	Probst *et al.* 1998	[288]
delphini	Dolphins	Varaldo *et al.* 1988	[292]
epidermidis	Human skin	Winslow & Winslow 1908	[23]
equorum subsp. *equorum*	Domestic horses, cattle	Schleifer *et al.* 1985	[281]
equorum subsp. *linens*	Surface-ripened cheese	Place *et al.* 2003	[293]
felis	Cats	Igimi *et al.* 1989	[294]
fleurettii	Goat milk cheese	Vernozy-Rozand *et al.* 2000	[295]
gallinarum	Poultry	Devriese *et al.* 1983	[286]
haemolyticus	Human skin, primates, horses, artiodactyls	Schleifer & Kloos 1975	[290]
hominis subsp. *hominis*	Human skin	Kloos & Schleifer 1975	[284]
hominis subsp. *novobiosepticus*	Human clinical specimens	Kloos *et al.* 1998	[64]
hyicus	Artiodactyls (swine, cattle), poultry	Sompolinsky 1953	[30]
intermedius	Carnivores, domestic horses, poultry	Hajek 1976	[296]
kloosii	Rodents, domestic artiodactyls	Schleifer *et al.* 1985	[281]
lentus	Artiodactyls, perissodactyls, cetaceans	Kloos *et al.* 1976	[297]
lugdunensis	Human clinical specimens	Freney *et al.* 1988	[298]
lutrae	Otters	Foster *et al.* 1997	[299]
muscae	Flies	Hajek *et al.* 1992	[300]
nepalensis	Goats	Spergser *et al.* 2003	[301]
pasteuri	Humans, animals, food, artiodactyls, horses	Chesneau *et al.* 1993	[302]
pettenkoferi	Human clinical specimens	Trülzsch *et al.* 2002	[303]
piscifermentans	Fermented fish	Tanasupawat *et al.* 1992	[304]
pseudintermedius	Domestic animals, humans	Devriese *et al.* 2005	[305]
pseudolugdunensis	Human blood cultures	Wei-Tang *et al.* 2008	[70]
*pulvereri**	Human and animal specimens	Zakrzewska-Czerwinska *et al.* 1995	[306]
saccharolyticus	Humans	Foubert & Douglas 1948	[29]
saprophyticus subsp. *saprophyticus*	Human skin, primates, tree shrews, rodents	Fairbrother 1940	[307]
saprophyticus subsp. *bovis*	Bovine nostrils	Hajek *et al.* 1996	[308]
schleiferi subsp. *schleiferii*	Human clinical specimens, carnivores	Freney *et al.* 1988	[298]
schleiferi subsp. *coagulans*	Dogs, external auditory meatus	Igimi *et al.* 1990	[309]
sciuri subsp. *sciuri*	Rodents, artiodactyls, cetaceans, marsupials	Kloos *et al.* 1976	[297]
sciuri subsp. *carnaticus*	Artiodactyls, cetaceans	Kloos *et al.* 1997	[310]
sciuri subsp. *rodentium*	Rodents, cetaceans	Kloos *et al.* 1997	[310]
simiae	S. American squirrel monkeys	Pantucek *et al.* 2005	[80]
simulans	Human skin, carnivores, artiodactyls	Kloos & Schleifer 1975	[284]
succinus subsp. *succinus*	Dominican amber (25–35 mya)	Lambert *et al.* 1998	[47]
succinus subsp. *casei*	Surface-ripened cheese	Place *et al.* 2003	[293]
*vitulinus**	Food, artiodactyls, perissodactyls, cetaceans	Webster *et al.* 1994	[311]
warneri	Human skin, artiodactyls, horses	Kloos & Schleifer 1975	[284]
xylosus	Human skin, rodents, mammals, birds	Schleifer & Kloos 1975	[290]

mya, million years ago.

distinct from all other *S. aureus* sequences to justify its classification as a bona-fide subspecies. Such considerations ultimately call into question concepts of prokaryotic "species," as they assume that evolutionary distance inferred from sequence comparisons correlates directly with taxonomic delimitation; from another perspective, *S. aureus* subsp. *anaerobius* can be seen as a catalase-negative mutant of *S. aureus* that is isolated only infrequently in nature.

Recently, a phylogenetic structure for the *S. aureus* species has been proposed, based on Bayesian phylogenetic analysis of 37 genes [82], a modified version of which is shown in Plate 3.1 and discussed in further detail later. The topology of this tree appears to support earlier descriptions suggesting a subdivision of the species into two major clusters [83], with one cluster subdivided further into two groups. However, whether these divisions can be considered equivalent to "subspecies" is unknown, especially since the tree is unrooted; conceivably, comparative sequencing of *S. aureus* subsp. *anaerobius* as a potential outgroup might shed further light on the actual relationships of different clusters within the species as a whole.

Clinical and epidemiological concerns have continued to focus attention on only a handful of species, most notably *S. aureus* and *S. epidermidis*, although other CoNS species such as *S. lugdunensis* [84] are becoming increasingly relevant in both clinical and veterinary settings. In particular, the global dissemination of MRSA has resulted in an acute need to comprehend the population structure and evolutionary dynamics of the uniquely pathogenic species *S. aureus*. The last two decades have witnessed the development of increasingly sophisticated approaches for characterizing genotypic diversity at the infra-subspecific level, thereby identifying particularly successful clonal lineages with widespread geographic distributions.

Genotyping of *Staphylococcus aureus*

According to Kathryn Hillier [37], the origins of both molecular epidemiology and infection control can be traced to the global pandemic of penicillin-resistant *S. aureus* that swept through hospital nurseries in Australia, North America, and the UK during the 1950s. The need to characterize the causative strain in order to identify and control outbreaks led to the categorization of strains according to their bacteriophage susceptibility profiles. Hence the pandemic strain is still referred to historically as 80/81, indicative of the two phage types to which it seemed consistently susceptible. Although there are several limitations associated with this approach, phage typing remained the method of choice for classification of nosocomial *S. aureus* strains until the development of PFGE during the mid to late 1980s, and is still used widely in some countries.

Another method for genotypic analysis and comparison of epidemic MRSA, introduced in the early 1990s, involved Southern blot analysis of *Cla*I-digested chromosomal fragments [85] with probes specific for the *mecA* gene and the insertion element Tn*554* [85–87]. The combination of *Cla*I-*mecA*::*Cla*I-Tn*554* patterns with PFGE (described below) resulted in the identification of globally disseminated epidemic MRSA clones, including the frequently described Iberian, Hungarian, Brazilian, Pediatric, and New York/Japan clones [88,89]. Additionally, it provided a foundation for deriving evolutionary inferences about the origin and spread of methicillin resistance in *S. aureus* [90,91]. As with DNA–DNA hybridization, PFGE allows for genome-level comparisons at the chromosomal level, but makes use of a comparatively limited amount of information. Restriction enzymes that recognize an informative number of sites are used to generate large fragments that are resolved by electrophoresis [92,93], thereby generating a strain-specific restriction fragment length polymorphism (RFLP) banding pattern or "fingerprint." Surprisingly, a high index of variation between closely related strains can be observed by this approach, as a result of point mutations, insertions, and deletions resulting in loss or gain of individual restriction sites and alteration of fragment sizes. In the case of *S. aureus* and other staphylococcal species, low GC content favors the use of restriction enzymes that recognize GC-rich sequences, and empirical analysis has led to the selection of *Sma*I as the enzyme of choice [94–97]. Plate 3.2a shows a *Sma*I restriction map of the USA300-FPR3757 genome, with the larger segments labeled according to the gel image in Plate 3.2b, by which it may be seen that many of the restriction sites coincide with regions of high GC content, including the locations of the five rRNA operons. Conversely, regions with low GC content are subject to undersampling by this method, although overall the technique has proven to be highly discriminating, and is still the method of choice for comparing closely related strains in localized outbreaks. Epidemic *S. aureus* strains have historically been catalogued on a national level as distinct "pulsed-field types" [98], in much the same way as is done for foodborne outbreaks, although the difficulties associated with interlaboratory comparisons, as well as the labor and time associated with performing PFGE on large numbers of samples, have led to investigation of alternative methods for large-scale genotyping.

Since its initial description in 1998 [99,100], MLST has become the gold standard for describing the large-scale population structure of prokaryotes. This method is based on comparative sequencing of at least seven conserved housekeeping genes, determined empirically for each species, with the assumption that variations accumulating in slowly evolving genes reflect the underlying evolutionary dynamics and "clock-speed" of the species as a whole. Each unique sequence recovered for a particular gene is denoted as a specific allele, and the concatenation of a given allelic profile is assigned a particular sequence type (designated ST followed by a number), with new sequence types assigned iteratively for each species. For *S. aureus*, for example, ST1 corresponds to the allelic profile 1-1-1-1-1-1-1, which is the sequence type of the community-acquired USA400 strain MW2 [13,101]. As of May 2009, more than 1300 unique sequence types have been reported for *S. aureus*, corresponding to > 2600 sequenced isolates, thereby making the *S. aureus* MLST database the fifth largest. This information is freely available via an online database located at http://saureus.mlst.net, along with primer sequences and protocols for performing MLST, and a variety of search engines and software, including the program eBURST, discussed in detail below.

The genes that have been selected for the *S. aureus* MLST scheme include *arcC* (carbamate kinase), *aroE* (shikimate 5-dehydrogenase), *glpF* (glycerol kinase), *gmk* (guanylate kinase), *pta* (phosphate acetyltransferase), *tpi* (triose phosphate isomerase), and *yqiL* (acetyl-CoA acetyltransferase). The locations of these genes on the chromosome of *S. aureus* USA300-FPR3757 are shown in Plate 3.2a; they are unevenly distributed throughout the chromosome, making this method sensitive to potential recombination events, as has been described previously [102].

An MLST scheme also exists for *S. epidermidis*, available at http://sepidermidis.mlst.net, although at present only 211 sequence types have been described. The *S. epidermidis* scheme, originally described by Wang *et al.* [103], presently uses four of the genes utilized in the *S. aureus* scheme (*arcC, aroE, tpiA, yqiL*), in addition to *gtr*, *mutS*, and *pyrR* [104]. Although there are not enough data at this time to adequately infer a population structure, several reports have suggested the existence of an epidemic clonal structure, and an apparent subdivision of the species into two major clusters [105,106].

The data generated by MLST are typically viewed using the freely available software eBURST [107] which, rather than relying on traditional clustering methods involving dendrograms or phylogenetic trees, links related sequence types on the basis of single nucleotide polymorphisms (SNPs) between one or more shared alleles, which are described as either single-locus variants (SLVs) or double-locus variants (DLVs). The sequence type with the greatest number of SLVs is assumed to represent the "founder" of a given cluster, with large clusters termed "clonal complexes" (designated CC followed by a number). Setting the minimum number of identical loci required for group definition to 0 allows the entire MLST database to be displayed in a single diagram, whereupon the relative distribution of clonal complexes, smaller clusters, and singletons may be appreciated; Plate 3.3 shows a modified example of such a representation. It is important to recognize that eBURST makes no attempt to link sequence types and clonal complexes beyond the SLV and DLV linkages portrayed, although it is obvious that these must all be related by an underlying phylogenetic structure. By avoiding the constraints imposed by clustering methods, eBURST facilitates the investigation of strain relatedness within individual clonal lineages without falling prey to assumptions implicit in phylogenetic analysis [108].

Taken together, PFGE and MLST represent two extremes of genotypic diversity: MLST is able to capture the large-scale population structure of an entire species but is unable to discriminate sufficiently between closely related isolates, whereas PFGE is the undisputed gold standard for indexing microvariation yet is unable to assess the overall population structure. Recently, a potential approach for addressing the middle ground between PFGE and MLST has emerged in the form of *spa*-typing [109,110], which is essentially a single-locus sequence typing method based on sequencing of a hypervariable repeat region within the coding sequence of protein A. Several reports describing the technique have been published, as well as various analyses comparing the relative levels of discrimination between *spa*-typing, MLST, and PFGE [111–116]. Empirical use seems to have validated the utility of this technique for indexing both microvariation and macrovariation, with comparable results to both PFGE and MLST respectively [117]. Indeed, the correlation with MLST is sufficiently close that the results of *spa*-typing can be considered predictive of major MLST lineages in almost all cases, as shown in Plate 3.1, in which *spa*-types corresponding to unique MLST sequence types can be seen to share similar repeat patterns.

As a result of its flexibility and ease of execution, *spa*-typing is proving to be useful for analysis of the global epidemiology of *S. aureus*, as well as for strain comparison in infection control and localized geographic studies [117]. It must be pointed out that there are two systems of nomenclature in use, which make direct comparisons between different datasets difficult. The original system described by Shopsin *et al.* [110] assigns alphabetic letters to individual repeats, as shown in Plate 3.1, and is freely available by contacting the developers at http://www.egenomics.com, whereas the system subsequently developed by Ridom in Europe uses numerical notation similar to MLST [109]. The Ridom *spa* website (http://spaserver.ridom.de) provides a direct interface with the *S. aureus* MLST database via the European SeqNet network (http://www.seqnet.org), and has accumulated > 5230 unique *spa*-types, corresponding to > 86 660 strains submitted from 64 countries. The developers have also created a graphic software tool called BURP (*B*ased *U*pon *R*epeat *P*attern), which utilizes an eBURST-style analysis in order to depict related *spa*-types and clonal complexes, and have demonstrated the utility of this method for infection control surveillance in hospital settings [118]. Lastly, software for the analysis of *spa* repeat patterns is also available as part of the BioNumerics software package (http://www.applied-maths.com/bionumerics/bionumerics.htm) as well as the Clondiag SPA TypeMapper application (http://www.clondiag.com/technologies/download.php?file=spa).

Various other genotyping methods have been proposed in the last few years for analysis of *S. aureus* and *S. epidermidis*, including amplified fragment length polymorphism (AFLP) [119,120], multiple-locus variable-number tandem repeat (VNTR) analysis [121–123], oligoarray analysis [124], single nucleotide polymorphisms (SNPs) [125], and a variety of other VNTR-based assays including coagulase-repeat (*coa*) sequencing [126], sequencing of *dru* repeats in the SCC*mec* (staphylococcal cassette chromosome *mec*) region [127], staphylococcal interspersed repeat units [128], and random PCR typing [129]. Recently, a double-locus sequence typing approach combining sequencing of repeats in both the *spa* and *clfB* (clumping factor B) genes has been described, in which the index of discrimination is reported to approach that exhibited by PFGE [130]. In addition to such approaches, there is an ongoing need for classification of the different SCC*mec* "types" described thus far for MRSA [131–133]. Since the initial description of SCC*mec* in 1999 [134], eight types labeled I–VIII have been described, along with several subtypes. Numerous multiplex PCR schemes have been proposed for rapid typing [135–138], but the extreme plasticity of the SCC element seems to dictate the continual permutation and identification of new "types" [131,139]. Most recently, Oliveira *et al.* [140] have created a web-based resource for SCC*mec* typing by comparative sequencing (available at http://www.ccrbtyping.net), and an International Working Group on the Classification of Staphylococcal Cassette Chromosome Elements (IWG-SCC) has been convened.

Molecular evolution of *Staphylococcus aureus*

Overview

Given the medical importance of *S. aureus* and the increasing affordability of sequencing, a number of genomes have been deciphered. Sequenced strains were isolated from diverse clinical settings, with varied antibiotic resistance and epidemic potential. In addition to clinical strains, common laboratory strains as well as isolates from bovine infections have been completely annotated. The availability of genomes allows direct comparison of the overall genetic structure within and between species. Such comparative analysis has revealed that the overall structure of the *S. aureus* genome is well conserved in order and genetic content. In comparison, there is a low level of gene order conservation between *S. aureus* and *S. epidermidis*, although genomic regions associated with central metabolism and housekeeping functions seem to be similar; most likely these regions were conserved within the genus before speciation.

Sequenced *S. aureus* genomes range from 2.8 to 2.9 Mb encoding 2565–2721 proteins [51,101,141–144]. Clearly, the availability of multiple genomes coupled with analysis of thousands of clinical isolates with other molecular classification techniques has provided a more succinct picture of the population structure of *S. aureus*. Within *S. aureus* species, the genome can be divided into two broad categories: core genome and accessory genome. The former, accounting for approximately 75% of the genome, is present in all, whereas the latter, the remaining 25% or so, is present uniquely or variably found in isolates [145]. The core consists of genes that encode essential housekeeping functions such as central metabolism as well as some virulence-associated factors that are expressed by nearly all strains, such as protein A (*spa*), clumping factor (*clfAB*), fibrinogen-binding protein A (*fnbA*), α-toxin (*hla*), coagulase (*coa*), lipase (*lip*), and superoxide dismutase (*sodM*). In addition, Fitzgerald *et al.* [145] reported that the most abundant *S. aureus* lineages, identified by multilocus enzyme electrophoresis (MLEE), all contain 2198 open reading frames (ORFs) that comprise the core genome; stated differently, all tested strains shared 78% of all *S. aureus* ORFs. The variably present genes were clustered in 18 regions of difference (RD) that in essence make up the accessory genome that contains insertion sequences, phages, plasmids, transposons, and genomic (pathogenicity) islands. Of the RDs identified, 10 encode antibiotic-resistance determinants (e.g., SCC*mec*) and virulence factors. In addition, some RDs varied significantly in their gene content and size suggesting that there exist in *S. aureus* hotspot regions where the genome is especially elastic and prone to deletions, integration, and recombination events. Overall, the phylogenetic structure of *S. aureus* has been elucidated by indexing the extent and nature of genomic elasticity of the core as well as presence/absence and variability within the accessory genome.

Core genome

The core region of *S. aureus* is made up of genes present in all strains and makes up approximately 75% of the genome. The core genome includes all genes that encode essential metabolic housekeeping and information processing functions. In addition, the core comprises all genes that are conserved at the species level with common species-associated function not linked with growth and survival, including virulence genes not present in other staphylococci, such as toxins, exoenzymes, and cell surface-binding proteins. Some of these genes, typically housekeeping genes, are maintained at the genus level (i.e., all staphylococci). When *S. aureus* is compared with CoNS strains (two *S. epiderimidis* strains, one *S. haemolyticus*, and one *S. saprophyticus* strain), a large proportion of genes are conserved in both sequence and order on the chromosome, comprising the backbone of the staphylococcal genome. A 0.4-Mb region downstream from the origin of replication, designated the "oriC environ," includes important *S. aureus* genes such as *spa* (encoding protein A) and *coa* (encoding coagulase), and has little homology among the species. Takeuchi *et al.* [146] suggested that this region is related to large-scale chromosomal inversion events that impacted the evolution and differentiation of the staphylococcal species.

While the core region implies genomic stability, some regions are more variable between strains and lineages. These variable regions may be more prone to diversifying events such as SNPs, partial or complete gene deletions likely by recombination events, and repeat variation. Such differences between closely related *S. aureus* strains can have meaningful biomedical implications. General mechanisms by which the core genome diversifies are highlighted below.

Single nucleotide polymorphisms

The core genome diversifies primarily by SNPs. The functional impact of a SNP depends on the position and nature. SNPs can occur in both coding and noncoding regions. In coding regions, two classes of substitution can occur in genes that encode proteins. Substitutions that result in amino acid replacements, or nonsynonymous SNPs (nsSNPs), provide the basis for evolutionary selection [147–149]. In contrast, substitutions that do not alter the structure of the proteins, or synonymous SNPs (sSNPs), are thought to be evolutionarily neutral or nearly so. Neutral alterations, when in structural or housekeeping genes, can provide the basis for studying genetic drift and evolutionary relationships among bacterial strains, especially among clonal species. In general, SNPs that occur in the first or second base pair of a codon are more likely to have a functional effect. As amino acid coding is redundant, most third position substitutions do not lead to changes in the structure of proteins. The functional effect and subsequent consequence of a particular substitution is heavily dependent on the selective forces at play.

At the species level, much of the DNA encoding the *S. aureus* core genome is very similar. In fact the stability of the core has been exploited to better understand the phylogenetic relationships between bacterial strains as well as for epidemiological investigations. Typically, MLEE, a classic method that measures allelic variation by examining the relative electrophoretic mobilities of a number of metabolic enzymes, has been used to index relatedness among bacterial species [150]. More recently, DNA sequence variation of a number of housekeeping genes dispersed around the bacterial genome (MLST) has been used to decipher the population structure of bacterial pathogens such as *Streptococcus pneumoniae* and *Neisseria meningitidis* [100]. Housekeeping genes are chosen because, being essential for survival, they are under moderate to intense purifying selection. Intraspecies phylogenetic reconstruction can be obscured by homologous recombination whereby replacement of a gene occurs with an ortholog from an unrelated lineage. Therefore, multiple loci are required for MLST to shield against confounding effects of a single locus. In *S. aureus*, MLST is based on detecting SNPs in sequence fragments of seven housekeeping genes (*arcC*, *aroE*, *glpF*, *gmk*, *pta*, *tpi*, and *yqiL*) [83,100,112]. The stability of the core region coupled with vertical inheritance allows allelic variation to index genetic relatedness. Comparative sequence analysis of alleles from a number of *S. aureus* strains enables generation of a numerical allelic profile or sequence type. In the case of *S. aureus*, strains sharing five or more identical alleles are grouped into a specific clonal complex, suggesting that isolates in the same clonal complex are related by descent (see section Population structure of *S. aureus*). Among monomorphic species such as *Mycobacterium tuberculosis* or *Bacillus anthracis*, where the molecular clock-speed or rate of change in housekeeping genes is relatively slow, the discriminatory power of MLST is limited. By contrast, *S. aureus* is an ideal species for MLST analysis as it is relatively diverse, with limited evidence of recombination [83]. Examination of sequence changes in several housekeeping genes indicates that point mutations (SNPs) give rise to new alleles at least 15-fold more frequently than recombination [83]. Consequently, MLST is able to address global epidemiological questions where the isolates have had substantial time to diversify, but is less discriminating in detecting changes in closely related strains. More importantly, large MLST databases allow comparison of sequenced strains to larger groups of genetically and geographically diverse strains thereby elucidating the population structure of *S. aureus*.

Point mutations that alter the encoding amino acid provide the basis of evolutionary selection. This is clearly illustrated with antimicrobial resistance. The widespread use of antibiotics to resolve *S. aureus* infections provides sufficient selection to maintain spontaneous mutants with reduced antibiotic susceptibility. For instance, fusidic acid is an antibiotic that blocks bacterial protein synthesis by inhibiting the function of elongation factor EF-G. NsSNPs within the gene encoding EF-G (*fusA*) confer fusidic acid resistance. Using clinical isolates and spontaneous mutants (grown under fusidic acid selection), Besier *et al.* [151] identified 13 amino acid residues within EF-G that could, if changed, confer resistance to fusidic acid. Similarly, quinolone resistance is primarily mediated through chromosomal nsSNPs in *gyrA* and *gyrB* (encoding subunits of DNA gyrase) and *grlA* (*parC*) and *grlB* (*parE*) (encoding subunits of DNA topoisomerase IV) [152].

Using comparative genomics, mutations that impact function, including frameshift and nonsense mutations as well as insertions/deletions that alter composition and number of amino acid residues, can be identified. Pseudogenes are typically recognized through a comparative approach by aligning homologs and searching for truncated or otherwise disrupted coding DNA sequences. In practice, pseudogenes are quite difficult to identify and characterize in genomes, since the two prerequisites, homology and nonfunctionality, are implied through DNA sequence calculations and alignments rather than experimentally. Thus, comparative analysis can greatly facilitate identification of putative pseudogenes that may be verified individually at the transcriptional and translational level. *Staphylococcus aureus* comprises a similar percentage of putative pseudogenes as most other annotated bacterial genomes [153]. Gene decay frequently results from random mutations, but may also be caused by insertion sequences or slip-strand mispairing resulting from short sequence repeats upstream of the gene [154]. Although the percentages of pseudogenes within *S. aureus* genomes are similar, they vary from approximately 0.7% in USA300 (FRP3757) and 0.8% in MSSA476 to over 2.5% in MRSA252 (other *S. aureus* genomes: MW2 1.0%, COL 1.3%, Mu50 1.5%, and N315 1.1%). Pseudogenes appear to be more common in the genomes of recent pathogens compared with their ancestral relatives. As such, some bacteria have accumulated a large number of pseudogenes likely as a consequence of recent evolutionary change. Gene decay has been described as a mechanism of adaptation among obligate intracellular and enteric Gram-negative pathogens, including *Helicobacter pylori*, *Yersinia pestis*, *Mycobacterium leprae* and others [155–158]. Evolutionarily divergent events leading to gene decay can facilitate host and/or niche specialization.

In general, the level and nature of pseudogenes within *S. aureus* genomes does not suggest such specialization has recently occurred. However, a recent report by Herron-Olson *et al.* [144] describes a number of well-characterized *S. aureus* virulence factors, including protein A and clumping factor A, that exist as pseudogenes in bovine mastitis strain ET3-1. Here these authors report that the majority of the annotated pseudogenes ($N = 70$) are a result of point mutations rather than insertion sequences and suggest that gene decay in the ET3-1 strain is associated with the transition to an intracellular lifestyle, whereby specific biosynthetic products are lost in favor of parasitizing nutrients, such as iron, from the host cell. These data support previous works that suggest the importance of intracellular life-style during *S. aureus* bovine mastitis [159,160]. Interestingly, strain MRSA252 (CC30) possesses the largest number of putative pseudogenes ($N = 88$) of all the human-associated *S. aureus* genomes published thus far [142]. MRSA252 and related strains from CC30 have caused extraordinary disease in the hospital setting, especially infections involving hematogenous complications [161]. It is possible that gene decay and subsequent loss of specific biosynthetic products allow these isolates to persist in the bloodstream, i.e., niche specialization. While most pseudogenes in *S. aureus* seem to be products of recent (random) mutational events likely under selection pressure, some events do allow for host or niche specialization, thereby optimizing virulence and pathogenic potential.

Diversity of gene content, repeat variation, and recombination

The genetic diversification of the *S. aureus* core genome can extend beyond SNPs to include larger regions of DNA diversity and polymorphic repetitive sequences. The differences in gene content or within operons between strains can range from a few nucleotides to several kilobase pairs that encompass complete or partial genes. Within these regions there are divergent DNA sequences suggestive of a mosaic genetic structure, most likely a result of homologous recombination. Such differences can have a significant impact on gene function.

Capsular genes in *S. aureus* provide an example of where the replacement within a conserved set of genes can alter the biological properties of the organism [162]. *Staphylococcus aureus* produces a capsular polysaccharide (CP) that enables resistance to the innate immune response. Clinically, CP5 and CP8 are most prevalent and are thought to contribute to the relative virulence *in vivo*; however, they differ in a number of biological properties including internal coding sequences (*cap5HIJK* and *cap8HIJK*) within a single operon located in the same chromosomal site [163].

Similarly, there are also examples of seemingly chimeric genes that contain internal regions of genetic variation. The staphylococcal accessory gene regulator (Agr) quorum-sensing system contains four genes involved in the regulation of virulence [164]: *agrA* and *agrC* make up a two-component signal transduction system [165], and *agrB* and *agrD* are required to produce an autoinducing peptide (AIP) that activates the quorum-sensing system [166]. Polymorphisms in the sequence of AIP and its corresponding receptor divide *S. aureus* into four *agr* groups that produce structurally distinct AIPs that have been identified on the basis of their ability to cross-inhibit *agr* quorum sensing [167]. Comparative sequence analysis of the four *agr* systems revealed an internal variable region that includes the entire *agrD*, the C-terminus of *agrB*, and the N-terminal half of *agrC* [168]. The functional integrity of the four *agr* systems are maintained by the covariation of the AIP structural gene and domains of the processing and sensing proteins, thereby providing a means by which strains could replace the specificity of their quorum signals and maintain the induction activity. Within each group, the specific AIP can activate the *agr* response in other related strains, whereas AIPs belonging to different groups are mutually inhibitory or interfering [167,169].

Strains from the same *agr* group are not necessarily related to each other, as evidenced by strains MRSA252 (CC30) and MW2 (CC1), both of which belong to *agr* group III [142,170]. However, Robinson *et al.* [171] proposed an evolutionary scenario using four stages and a two subspecies hypothesis by sequencing the complete *agr* locus of 27 diverse *S. aureus* strains. The first stage is the speciation event, which is followed by divergence of *S. aureus* into two subspecies groups, each having *agr* groups I, II and III. The third phase is the splintering of *agr* I to form *agr* IV, within subspecies I, and finally the recombination event between *agr* I and IV. The authors suggest that individual clonal complexes as well as broader subspecies groups are expected to have the same *agr* group due to simple clonal descent. However, recombination has been involved in distributing *agr* groups across the species. Furthermore, variation of *agr* at the amino acid level may provide for diversity in *agr* activity beyond that of the consensus activities of the four interference groups, and recombination of *agr* between lineages (i.e., clonal complexes) may offer some selectable traits under a larger evolutionary framework. As *agr* regulates an array of virulence genes, point mutations within the region may be deleterious or selected for in specialized environments. Kennedy *et al.* [172] recently reported on a variant of the epidemic USA300 isolate that has a missense mutation in *agrA* that lies within the putative DNA-binding domain of the encoded protein and likely alters the function of Agr.

The *S. aureus* core genome can also diversify by changes in repeated sequences, which are numerous and punctuated throughout the chromosome. Several studies have identified families of perfect repeats and tandem repeats that are mainly found within intergenic regions as well as within protein-coding sequences [128,173–176]. Genetic alterations in these repetitive sequences include point mutations as well as intragenic recombination events that presumably arise by slipped-strand mispairing during chromosomal replication [177], and in some cases result in a high degree of genetic polymorphism that can be used to differentiate isolates [110,126]. Well-studied VNTRs in *S. aureus* include genes encoding microbial surface components recognizing adhesive matrix molecules (MSCRAMMs). MSCRAMMs facilitate a key step in infection, namely attachment to host tissue by binding to fibrinogen, fibronectin, collagen, and other components of the host extracellular matrix [178], a role that is likely to be immunogenic [174,179]. A number of MSCRAMMs, such as the fibrinogen-binding protein ClfA and the collagen-binding protein Cna, contain repetitive protein motifs that are important for functional surface expression [180,181]. Similarly, many surface-associated proteins also contain repetitive regions that can vary between strains (e.g., SasA, SasC, SasI) [176] and are prone to slippage error in replication or induction of recombination events at these loci. Variation due to recombination in regions encoding repeats, especially in virulence genes, may allow *S. aureus* to evade the host immune response during systemic or long-term infections [182].

Recombination in *S. aureus* is thought to occur at a low frequency, although repetitive regions may have a higher rate. On occasion, a recombination event can alter the clonal structure. The relationships between sequence types are not always congruent. Over half of these inconsistent comparisons involve the *arcC* locus, which encodes carbamate kinase [83]. Interestingly, *arcC* is located near three putative virulence factors. Clumping factor B (*clfB*) is approximately 1 kb downstream, and aureolysin (*aur*) and *isaB* are roughly 6 kb upstream from the *arcC* locus. *isaB* encodes a 17-kDa immunodominant protein and *clfB* is associated with the cell wall [183,184]; both gene products are likely to be exposed to the host immune system and therefore will be under diversifying selection. Therefore, recombination events involving these genes that introduce genetic and antigenic variation will frequently involve the flanking genes and may influence the evolution of *arcC*, thereby obfuscating the population structure of *S. aureus* as informed by MLST analysis. Low recombination frequencies have been demonstrated by MLST analysis, where a recombinatorial event is detected between distinct lineages (i.e., clonal complex types) due to inconsistent sequence types or alleles at one or more of the MLST housekeeping genes. However, the ability to detect recombination events within the same lineage is unclear even when using seven housekeeping genes. Kuhn *et al.* [185], utilizing variable adhesion genes, suggest that recombination is more common within, rather than between, clonal complexes [185].

Interestingly, large chromosomal replacements have been identified in *S. aureus*, albeit occurring rarely. Robinson and Enright [102] reported on the mosaic chromosome of *S. aureus* strain ST239 that was founded by single chromosomal replacements of approximately 244 kb and 557 kb without the obvious involvement of mobile genetic elements (MGEs). Based on the annotated genome sequences of COL and MRSA252, the ST239 mosaic has approximately 557 kb straddling the origin of replication (*oriC*) from its ST30 parent and about 2220 kb spanning the *terC* (terminus of replication) from its ST8 parent. Much like both parental lineages, ST8 and ST30, ST239 has thrived to become a pandemic MRSA lineage that is represented by a number of clones, including epidemic EMRSA-1, -4, -7, -9 and -11, and the Hungarian, Brazilian, Portuguese and Vienna clones [102,186,187] (see Plate 3.3). To determine whether large chromosomal replacements are common in *S. aureus*, seven housekeeping genes (MLST targets), seven *sas* genes and *spa* were partially sequenced in 220 clinical isolates, representing lineages of MSSA and community-acquired MRSA. One strain, ST34, was identified that involved multiple replacements within the same lineage. ST34 differed from ST30 at one of the seven housekeeping genes (*arcC*), in three *sas* genes (*sasA*, *sasF* and *sasH*), and in the polymorphic *spa* repeat region. The five genes that distinguished ST30 from ST34 were shared by a pair of clones (ST10 and ST145), were contiguous, and spanned *oriC*. Interestingly, both replacements involved CC30 lineages, suggesting that these events may not occur randomly throughout the species. Indeed, the expression of lineage-specific genes or other molecular mechanisms may be required for replacements to occur. To date, the mechanisms underlying large chromosomal replacements are unknown, although such events can clearly have a dramatic impact on bacterial evolution and fitness as evidenced by the success of ST239.

Accessory genome

The accessory genome of *S. aureus*, which accounts for approximately 25% of the entire genome sequences, consists mostly of mobile (or once mobile) elements that are scattered throughout the genome. These elements include a wide range of putative mobile DNA elements, pathogenicity and genomic islands, up to 30 insertion sequences, staphylococcal cassette chromosome (SCC), five transposons, and several bacteriophages. Many of the regions found in the accessory genome are mobile genetic elements (MGEs) that can transfer horizontally between strains differentially, from high frequency to low frequency, while some do not transfer at all. In general, there are three mechanisms of lateral gene transfer in bacteria: conjugation, transformation, and transduction [188]. However, *S. aureus* is not naturally competent, and conjugative transfer of elements between strains does not appear to be common in nature.

Virulence and resistance genes are found in distinct genomic locales. The former tends to be found in *S. aureus* pathogenicity islands (SaPI) whereas the latter rely on SCC, plasmids and transposons for transfer. The distribution and lateral spread of these elements can be biomedically relevant. Studies further characterizing these elements provide insights into mechanisms of *S. aureus* pathogenesis as well as evolution. Some reports have noted that certain toxin genes are nonrandomly distributed along clonal lines (i.e., clonal complexes). These include toxic shock syndrome toxin-1 (*tst*), serine protease-like B (*splB*), and superantigens A, G and I (*sea*, *seg* and *sei*). The mechanism underlying the apparent association between such factors and clonal complexes is unclear; it is not due to vertical transmission alone as there is evidence for frequent acquisition or loss of specific elements within particular clonal complexes. It is possible that the ability of particular clonal lineages to acquire or lose specific elements may impact the success of certain strains in carriage and disease or enable niche specialization.

Bacteriophages

In nature, most *S. aureus* strains are polylysogenic. Following virus morphology, there are two groups of staphylococcal bacteriophages: Myoviridae (nonenveloped, contractile tail) and Siphoviridae (nonenveloped, long noncontractile tail). The bacteriophages of *S. aureus* belong to seven serological groups, A–D and F, G, and L. Staphylococcal prophages (the latent form of a bacteriophage in which the viral genes are incorporated into the bacterial chromosomes without causing disruption of the bacterial cell) can also be grouped into five families based on homology of the integrase gene that dictates insertion site, as well as into three classes by genomic size: class I (< 20 kb), class II (~ 40 kb), and class III (> 125 kb) [35]. Interestingly, no strain appears to have more than one phage of each family type, suggesting phage immunity or competition for insertion sites. Therefore, the presence of one phage may prevent the acquisition of another related phage, which has implications for evolution. Over 40 staphylococcal phage genomes have been deciphered, including those carrying important virulence determinants such as exfoliative toxin A, enterotoxin A, and Panton–Valentine leukocidin (PVL) [189–191]. Although the GC content of phages is similar to that of the host, most phages contain a large number of genes of unknown function and no homology to bacterial sequences [35]. The coding regions are tightly packed with over 90% capacity where the majority of genes are transcribed from one strand. In large phages, there may be a second DNA replication mode that is associated with lytic functions encoding amidase and holin genes, a factor that may be important for broad host range for these phages as they can infect both coagulase-positive and coagulase-negative staphylococci. Interestingly, bacteriophage genomes posses a mosaic structure, suggesting that recombination with other phages occurs frequently. Clearly, these attributes underscore the importance of phages for genomic elasticity of staphylococcal genomes.

Staphylococcus aureus bacteriophages often contain virulence genes, such as *chp* (chemotaxis inhibitory protein, an inhibitor of leukocyte migration) [192], *sea* (enterotoxin A, a common cause of food poisoning) [193], *eta* (exfoliative toxin A, a cause of scalded skin syndrome) [191], *sak* (staphylokinase, a thrombolytic enzyme) [194], and *lukSF-PV* (some evidence suggests that PVL is involved in hemolytic pneumonia and severe skin and soft tissue infections, although this is somewhat controversial) [190,195–198]. The lateral transfer of virulence factors by bacteriophages occurs by phage conversion (i.e., the transfer and integration of a phage that encodes the gene of interest on its genome) or generalized transduction.

Prophages are common in *S. aureus*, with most strains bearing between one and three [199]. These inactive lysogenic phages are replicated as part of bacterial replication and are vertically passed on to daughter cells. Here, prophages are induced by stress conditions, such as DNA-damaging agents and some antibiotics, presumably by the bacterial SOS response [200,201]. Induction involves excision of the phage from the chromosome and replication. As phage genomes replicate, the necessary components for the phage head and tail are produced and packaged. Replication is efficient and numerous phage particles are produced to cause bacterial cell lysis, thereby releasing infectious phage particles. These particles subsequently attach, by an unknown receptor, and enter *S. aureus* cells. Here the phage may enter the lytic cycle (replication) or enter the lysogenic cycle and integrate into the bacterial genome. Interestingly, the induction of phage and phage genome replication increases the copy number of phage-associated toxin genes and subsequently increases toxin production [202], thereby linking phage replication and life cycle directly with expression of virulence genes and pathogenicity.

All *S. aureus* phage genomes contain integrase promoter regions, much like the lambda phage model [203], that are thought to control the lytic/lysogenic switch and also presumably prevent reinfection with a similar phage. Integration sites are highly specific due to the specificity of the intergrase and the genome's conserved left and right junctions [204]. Two well-known virulence factors, β-hemolysin (*hlb*) and lipase (*geh*), contain phage integration sites, such that phage conversion renders the organism incapable of producing these gene products [204,205].

Lateral gene transfer of nonphage MGEs is thought to occur by generalized transduction. One of the best-studied staphylococcal phages is ϕ11, which has a 43.6-kb genome [199,206], is a member of serogroup B, and contains *int* and *xis* genes, similar to ϕL54a. Phage ϕ11 can package up to 45 kb of bacterial DNA instead of its own phage genome. The phage is able to package plasmids and chromosomal genes of the bacteria at low frequency, which in turn can be laterally injected into other *S. aureus* cells. Once delivered, the exogenous DNA needs to either replicate or integrate into a replicon such as a chromosome or a plasmid in order to survive. Since plasmids can replicate and integrate into the chromosome of the new host, transducing phages are important vehicles involved in lateral gene transfer. Although an inefficient process, survival of chromosomal DNA that lacks an encoded replication mechanism relies on recombination with the host (bacterial) chromosome via homologous recombination.

Currently, the phage carrying the PVL gene has received much attention as the underlying virulence factor associated with rise of CA-MRSA infections. PVL was first identified by Van deVelde in 1894 for its ability to lyse leukocytes and later, in 1932, by Panton and Valentine for its association with soft tissue infections. Until recently, PVL was rare and associated with less than 2% of the strains [207]. Recently, PVL-producing strains have been epidemiologically associated with an increase in severe boils and skin infections in diverse populations including prisoners, athletes, military recruits, children, native populations, and men who have sex with men [8–11]. Moreover, most of these cases were caused by MRSA in the community setting among otherwise healthy individuals. Phages carrying this toxin have likely transferred laterally to naive *S. aureus* MLST lineages, including ST1, ST8, ST30, ST59, and ST80, as well as by clonal expansion [208]. For example, strains MW2 and MSSA476 are closely related but bear different prophage profiles. Phage ϕSa2 (MW2), which carries the PVL subunits *lukS-lukF*, is absent from MSSA476, underscoring the role that bacteriophages can play in short-term *S. aureus* evolution and pathogenesis. However, the exact role PVL plays in the changing epidemiology of *S. aureus* and particularly MRSA infections in both the community and hospital settings is far from clear. Labandeira-Rey *et al.* [196] reported that PVL is sufficient to cause pneumonia in a murine infection model; however, a number of other reports have shown convincing data to suggest that PVL is not the major virulence determinant underlying CA-MRSA infections. Using the isogenic PVL-positive and -negative MRSA strains USA300 and MW2, Voyich *et al.* [197] showed no difference in both a murine bacteremia and an abscess model. In addition, no differences were noted between the isogenic PVL-positive and -negative strains' ability to cause lysis of human polymorphonuclear leukocytes (or neutrophils). These results have been supported using the same isogenic strains in a murine pneumonia model [198] as well as in a rabbit model of infection (H.F. Chambers, personal communication). Taken together, the studies suggest that PVL may have a role in the ongoing CA-MRSA epidemic, but that its role is a relatively minor one. At least in the USA, CA-MRSA infections are predominantly caused by a group of closely related strains called USA300 [172] that typically carry PVL. It is possible that PVL is erroneously associated with more severe disease and is actually just a proxy for other unidentified virulence determinants carried on the prophage itself or in the bacterial chromosome [16]. Other putative virulence factors include arginine catabolic mobile element (ACME) [141,209] and phenol-soluble modulins [210].

Pathogenicity islands and genomic islands

First described in *Escherichia coli*, pathogenicity islands are large chromosomal structures encoding virulence traits that have been acquired by lateral gene transfer [211,212]. Generally, pathogenicity islands are characterized by a GC content distinct from the organism's core genome, the presence of one or more virulence-associated genes, direct repeats at the flanking borders, the presence of mobility genes like transposases or recombinases, and putative mobility [213]. *Staphylococcus aureus* pathogenicity islands (SaPIs) have descended from bacteriophages as they bear some phage-related genes and demonstrate interaction with phages [214]. Importantly, SaPIs often carry superantigenic toxins and therefore clearly have biomedical implications. These islands carry approximately half of the *S. aureus* toxins or virulence factors, and allelic variations of these genes, which contribute to the pathogenic potential of *S. aureus* [215]. Eight SaPIs in human isolates (SaPIn1, SaPIm1, SaGIm, νSa3 (MW2), SaPI1, SaPI3, SaPI4, and SaPI5) and two in bovine isolates (SaPIbov and SaPIbov2) have been sequenced. Human SaPIs, much like bacteriophages, have a mosaic structure and can be classified into four groups based on integrase homology and insertion site. Interestingly, strains tend to carry no more than one copy of each SaPI type. SaPIs transfer horizontally in the presence of "helper" phage. SaPIs are approximately 15 kb in size and encode an integrase at one end [200]. The integrase promoter region is similar to bacteriophages and also has specific integration sites. SaPIs do not encode other genes for the transfer process and therefore rely on phage genes for induction. This process can be initiated by a helper phage infection or induction of helper prophages under stress [200]. Upon induction, the SaPI is excised and packaged into miniature phage-like particles concurrent with the production of typical-size infectious phage particles [216]. These particles deliver the SaPI DNA to the recipient *S. aureus* where efficient site-specific integration occurs.

The first pathogenicity island of *S. aureus*, as well as the first in Gram-positive pathogens, was described by Lindsay *et al.* [200]. The 15.2-kb SaPI1 encodes the toxic shock syndrome toxin TSST-1, a potent superantigen associated with most cases of menstrual toxic shock syndrome. SaPI1 is flanked by 17-bp long direct repeats and in addition to *tst* also contains other genes that encode for putative virulence determinants. SaPI1, much like other pathogenicity islands, carries a locus that is homologous to members of the bacteriophage integrase family. This type of SaPI has the ability to integrate in specific sites that are identical to the directly repeated sequences at the terminals of SaPIs in different *tst*-negative strains. SaPI1 uses excision, replication, and encapsulation functions of helper bacteriophages ϕ13 and 80α [200]; following excision, the islands are transduced efficiently to other strains. Other superantigen genes often carried by SaPIs include enterotoxins B and C, often a cause of food poisoning. Among sequenced genomes, N315 and Mu50 possess the superantigen genes *sel* (enterotoxin L), *sec3* (enterotoxin C3), and *tst* (TSST-1). A feature of the TSST island family is its close linkage to prophages ϕN315/ϕMu50A and ϕMu50B, respectively, which are integrated in close proximity to these islands and presumably utilized for lateral gene transfer. Mu50's pathogenicity island carries the *fhuD* gene that possibly encodes a ferrichrome-binding ABC transporter. This siderophore transporter may confer a selective advantage to Mu50 in human tissue [51,217]. The CA-MRSA strain MW2 carries two allelic forms of enterotoxin, *sel2* and *sel4*, that are unique and contribute to its increased virulence. MRSA252, a strain with epidemic potential, carries a SaPI-like element, SaPI4, which contains the same gene order and homologs of pathogenicity islands SaPI1 and SaPIbov. SaPI4 contains no protein homology to characterized virulence genes [142]. Interestingly, MSSA476, an invasive community-acquired methicillin-susceptible strain does not have a pathogenicity island in its genome. SaPI3, which is harbored by strain COL, is virtually identical to SaPI1 (from clinical isolate RN4282) as both islands share specific genes and have the same integration sites except that COL carries enterotoxin B gene (*seb*) instead of *tst* on the island [143,214].

Two types of genomic islands, νSaα and νSaβ, have been identified in all the sequenced genomes of *S. aureus* and are present in nearly all isolates from diverse clonal, geographic, and disease origins [51,101,143,145,218]. Although thought to have arisen by horizontal gene transfer, the origin and modes of transfer remain unclear. νSaα encodes a cluster of staphylococcal superantigen-like proteins, *set* clusters (now called *ssl* cluster), and a cluster of lipoproteins (*lpl* cluster) [182,219,220]. νSaβ encodes multiple exotoxin (*set*) and serine protease homolog (*spl*) gene clusters [221]. Despite the stability and the conserved integration site of these regions, the genomic content of these islands can differ between strains that often contain genes associated with pathogenicity. For instance, in MRSA252, νSaα contains nine *set* and seven putative *lpl* genes (one of which is a pseudogene), while in strain MSSA476 νSaα contains 11 *set* and five putative *lpl* genes. Similarly, in MRSA252, νSaβ contains three functional and two pseudo *spl* genes, and six *set* genes, whereas in MSSA476 νSaβ contains carries four *spl*, two leukotoxin homologs (*lukDE*) [222], and a lantibiotic biosynthesis cluster (*bsa*). The presence of this bacteriocin (also present in CA-MRSA strains MW2 and FPR3757) may confer advantage in the community as these strains compete with many other species on the skin and mucosal surfaces.

Given the number and variety of superantigens, it has been suggested that νSaα and νSaβ constitute an enterotoxin "nursery" that allows a diversity of toxin variants to be produced when needed [182]. Although the two genomic islands are likely ancient features of the *S. aureus* species, they are likely still evolving. The genomic elasticity is mainly driven by frequent recombination and deletion events leading to variation in copy number between isolates. Within the enterotoxin gene cluster, which usually has a common motif that carries two pseudoenterotoxins, φ*ent*1 and 2, recombination between the two pseudogenes can occur, giving rise to novel toxins [223]. It is possible that the accumulation of virulence genes may not always confer a selective advantage. Fitzgerald *et al.* [224] suggested an "independent loss" model for the *set* gene cluster, where the ancestral state of the *set* cluster may bear a full complement of *set* genes, which were lost independently multiple times leading to distinct gene sets in discrete lineages.

Plasmids and transposons

Most naturally occurring staphylococcal strains contain plasmids. These plasmids can be grouped into three major families based on size and ability to conjugate [225]. Class I are small (1–5 kb) multicopy plasmids that are either cryptic or carry a singe resistance determinant such as pT181, which encodes tetracycline resistance in COL [143, 226]. In some instances, class I plasmids may integrate into the chromosome; pT181, for example, is found in *S. aureus* strains with SCC*mec* type III elements, and pUB110 is associated with most SCC*mec* II strains [51,132,142]. Class II plasmids are 15–30 kb in size, have low copy number (four to six per cell), and generally carry several resistance determinants for β-lactams (*bla*), heavy metals (*ars*, *cad*, and *mer*), aminoglycosides (*aacA-aphD*), and/or antiseptics (*qac*). Resistance genes are often associated with transposons that have integrated into the plasmid genome, and plasmid variants are often due to rearrangement of such elements. Much like class I, class II plasmids are mainly transferred by generalized transduction [225,227]. Class III plasmids are conjugative (carrying transfer genes, *tra*) multiresistance plasmids that are comparatively large (30–60 kb) and carry a number of different resistance determinants for aminoglycosides (Tn*4001*), trimethoprim (Tn*4003*), quaternary ammonium compounds, and in some cases β-lactams (Tn*552*) [228–230]. The larger class III plasmids are often too big to be transferred by transduction. Two or more plasmids that share the same replication mechanism in a single cell can become unstable due to plasmid incompatibility [215]. Therefore, acquisition of novel plasmids depends on resident plasmids in a given strain, restriction modification barriers, and susceptibility to transduction and conjugation. Whereas plasmids generally carry many resistance determinants, they carry only a few virulence genes [231–233].

As described above, *S. aureus* transposons often encode resistance genes. All transposons encode a transposase gene that enables excision and/or replication and integration of the element. Lateral transfer from one *S. aureus* strain to another is believed to be facilitated by "piggybacking" onto another MGE that is subsequently transferred [234]. With respect to resistance determinants, Tn*554* encodes resistance to erythromycin and spectinomycin [86], often associated with SCC*mec* types II and III; Tn*552* encodes β-lactamase resistance and is typically associated with class II and III plasmids [235]; and Tn*5801* is a large integrated transposon in Mu50 that encodes tetracycline resistance (*tetM*) [51]. More recently, and of grave concern, clinical strains of vancomycin-resistant *S. aureus* (VRSA) have been reported [236–238]. Although rare, vancomycin resistance is a major medical and public health concern as it remains an important bactericidal antibiotic in the treatment of MRSA infections. The *vanA*, *vanH*, *vanX*, and *vanY* genes, which confer high-level vancomycin resistance, are encoded on a transposon that originated from *Enterococcus faecalis* [239]; the transposon likely jumped into a pheromone-responsive class III plasmid that was transferred into *S. aureus* via conjugation. Interestingly, *S. aureus*, much like *E. faecalis*, secretes a peptide that triggers lateral transfer of pheromone-responsive plasmids across species boundaries [239,240]. Once in *S. aureus*, the plasmid is unable to replicate, although it may still result in integration of the *vanA*-bearing transposon to the *S. aureus* chromosome or to another plasmid.

Staphylococcal cassette chromosome

A unique type of MGE in staphylococci is represented by the SCC, a heterogeneous element which integrates at a specific chromosomal site (*attBscc*) located approximately 35 kb downstream of *oriC* in *S. aureus* [132]. SCC elements are typically associated with methicillin resistance (SCC*mec*). Methicillin, a β-lactam antibiotic, acts by inhibiting penicillin-binding proteins (PBPs), which are involved in the synthesis of peptidoglycan, an essential cell-wall component. The *mecA* gene encodes an alternative low-affinity PBP, PBP2a (also referred to as PBP2′), that can perform the functions of the original PBP but is resistant to the action of methicillin and all other β-lactams. Large SCC*mec* elements can also carry additional MGEs such as plasmids and transposons that encode for various resistance markers. A family of site-specific recombinase genes (*ccrAB*, *ccrC*) are responsible for the mobility of SCC*mec*. Regions other than the *mec* and *ccr* gene complexes are designated J-regions (junkyard or joining), and do not appear to be essential, although some strains can bear resistance genes for non-β-lactam antibiotics or heavy metals, which are typically found in J-regions.

Although the origins of SCC*mec* are unknown, interspecies exchange of DNA between CoNS and *S. aureus* has been noted, and CoNS are thought to represent a reservoir for novel SCC elements [241–243]. MSSA can readily acquire SCC*mec* by lateral gene transfer to become MRSA, suggesting that MRSA may have evolved independently on multiple occasions [90,99,145,244]. However, MRSA is observed more often in certain lineages, suggesting that while these events may occur multiple times there is specificity for the recipient chromosomal background (see Plate 3.3), such that some MSSA lineages may have a greater affinity to accept *mecA* [245,246]. Katayama *et al.* [245] investigated the role of the host chromosome in the transformability and expression of *mecA* in 103 naturally occurring MSSA clinical isolates. Recipient MSSA strains from the major MRSA lineages were more transformable with pYK20 (low-copy-number plasmid with *mecA*), and better able to maintain the plasmid and express resistance in comparison with strains from other lineages, suggesting that the absence of *mecA* within certain lineages is partly due to genetic factors that are restrictive of *mecA* and its gene product [245]. This may be due to phage immunity or restriction modification, whereby foreign DNA is recognized and digested by restriction enzymes. Restriction modification can be mobilized, however, and therefore SCC*mec* may ultimately spread to all *S. aureus* clonal complexes [247]. Alternatively, it is possible, albeit unlikely, that lineages more likely to give rise to MRSA are more virulent and prevalent, and therefore have a higher chance of acquiring SCC*mec*, and that the hospital setting provides sufficient selection to maintain the element.

Currently, eight major types of SCC*mec* have been described, based on the combination of different variants of *mec* and *ccr* complex [138], with numerous subtypes assigned according to differences in J-regions. With the exception of strains USA300 and MW2 that bear SCC*mec* IV, all other sequenced MRSA strains contain SCC*mec* I or II. How the element replicates and transfers laterally is not clear. Type II SCC*mec* of N315, Mu50, and MRSA252 contain an integrated copy of plasmid pUB110 with kanamycin and bleomycin resistance genes, as well as transposon Tn*554* carrying erythromycin and spectinomycin resistance. The CA-MRSA strain MW2 has a type IVa element that is identical to that of USA300, and smaller in size than those of HA-MRSA strains (i.e., N315, Mu50, and MRSA252). Type IV SCC*mec* is made up of two allelic elements: class B *mec* gene complex (*mec*A and its regulatory genes), and type-2 *ccr* genes [101,141]. Type I SCC*mec*, by contrast, is composed of class B *mec* gene complex and type 1 *ccr* gene complex. It is interesting to note that movement of SCC*mec* elements may also be dependent on size and functional recombinases. For example, while type II and III SCC*mec* bear functional recombinases, they are too large to "package" into a generalized transducing phage head, which may explain why transfer seems to occur at low frequency. By contrast, SCC*mec* type IV and V elements are considerably smaller and contain functional recombinases, making them potentially transducible; consequently, these elements may spread between isolates more readily. Lastly, although type I SCC*mec* (COL) is relatively small and should be transducible, one of the recombinases is nonfunctional, thereby immobilizing this element [244,248].

SCC elements without *mecA* have also been described; a notable example is the methicillin-susceptible strain MSSA476 which carries a novel SCC-like element (SCC_{476}) that shows similarity to a previously described *S. hominis* non-*mec* SCC element (SCC_{12263}) [249]. Although SCC_{476} shares the same left and right boundaries (*attL* and *attR*) and similar inverted repeat sequences as SCC*mec* elements, it does not contain the *mecA* gene. It does carry a novel gene with homology to the fusidic acid resistance gene *far1* [250].

A unique feature of the FPR3757 genome is the 30.9 kb ACME element, which encodes an arginine deiminase pathway that converts L-arginine to carbon dioxide, ATP, and ammonia. The newly identified ACME is located immediately downstream of SCC*mec* in the FPR3757 genome, and has been proposed as a new member of the SCC family (see Plate 3.2) [141]. Studies have suggested that ACME is largely restricted to USA300 strains bearing SCC*mec* IVa, although a few examples have been found in other lineages, including ST5 (USA100), ST1, and ST97. In addition, ACME is thought to have been horizontally acquired from the ubiquitous skin commensal *S. epidermidis*, which may explain the enhanced growth and survival of USA300 in the host, particularly on human skin [141]. Interestingly, deletion of ACME resulted in attenuation of clinical USA300 infection in a rabbit infection model [209].

The insertion of mobile elements provides the potential for recombination hotspots, enabling rapid remodeling of the structure of SCC*mec* and giving rise to further diversity. Indeed, SCC*mec* seems to have high genomic plasticity given the mosaic structure of different SCC*mec* types, which are suggestive of recombination, deletion, and integration events, both within and across species boundaries. While types I–III are typically found in HA-MRSA strains, types IV and V seem to be associated primarily with CA-MRSA. Of late, this boundary seems to be more elusive as type IV SCC*mec* strains are increasingly associated with nosocomial infections [251]. Taken together, the evolution of the SCC*mec* element highlights the relevance of evolutionary dynamics to human health; novel forms can greatly reshape the epidemiology of *S. aureus* and in particular MRSA, as evidenced by the ongoing dominance of USA300 strains in the USA [172]. Detailed discussion of the SCC*mec* element is beyond the scope of this chapter, but several excellent reviews on the topic are available, as well as a dedicated website [139,252,253] (http://www.staphylococcus.net).

Population structure of *Staphylococcus aureus*

Pathogenic bacteria exist as populations wherein members exhibit varying levels of virulence, and at face value represent a deceptively simple prokaryotic population genetic model. That is, asexual reproduction by binary fission gives rise to identical daughter cells that can vary from each other by *de novo* mutations which can subsequently be passed on to descendants. Over time and after successful generations, new lineages emerge by the accumulation of such mutations. In the absence of sex or lateral movement of genetic material between cells that do not necessarily share a recent ancestor, the distribution of chromosomal polymorphisms within a population will be nonrandom (linkage disequilibrium). By contrast, in sexual organisms, where mutations are continually rearranged by recombination, linkage equilibrium occurs stochastically at distinct sites. Consequently, asexual bacterial populations exhibit stable independent lineages within which evolutionary changes occur by *de novo* mutations. Over time, differences in the frequencies of particular lineages in the population will occur due to selection or stochastic events. Mutations that increase bacterial fitness will promote these traits and the lineages that bear them, resulting in a loss or reduction of other competing lineages. This process, known as periodic selection, reduces the genetic diversity within the populations [254]. Bacterial populations are also prone to rapid expansions and severe bottlenecks that can reduce the diversity of clonal populations [255]. However, two facts regarding bacterial populations complicate this simple model: the presence of MGEs and a detectable level of recombination. Pathogens like *M. tuberculosis* represent one end of the clonal spectrum and are considered monomorphic, exhibiting very little recombination; by comparison, *H. pylori* is a freely recombining, naturally transformable organism that represents a nonclonal bacterial species [256,257].

Bacterial population structure can be deciphered using a number of different methods: analysis of linkage disequilibrium levels among alleles using MLEE data, phylogenetic inference from nucleotide sequence data (e.g., MLST), and studies of particular lineages as they diverge. Understanding of the phylogeny of bacterial populations can be used as a framework on which other characteristics, such as pathogenicity, host specificity, presence of virulence genes, and epidemic potential, can be mapped. Therein, critical insights into the origins of pathogenicity, enhanced fitness, and host/niche adaptation of lineages within a clonal or mostly clonal species can be elucidated [258–260].

The population structure of *S. aureus* has been studied by a variety of methods, including MLEE [91,258], PFGE [261], MLST [83,99], DNA microarrays [145], and *spa*-typing [117]. These studies have revealed a highly clonal population structure with limited evidence for recombination. Currently, the method most widely used to examine the population structure of *S. aureus* is MLST. Although true relationships between distantly related isolates can be obscured over time due to homologous recombination within housekeeping genes [262], recombination is unlikely to prevent recognition of clonal associations within shorter, biomedically relevant time-scales. However, while there is limited evidence for recombination, a few notable examples do exist (see Plates 3.1) [83,102].

Using seven loci, MLST analysis can provide a sound framework for examining the genetic relatedness of *S. aureus* strains. As described earlier, different sequences at each locus are assigned unique allele numbers, and each strain is defined by the alleles at the seven loci (the allelic profile). Each unique allelic profile (or genotype) is assigned a sequence type, which can be grouped into clonal complexes on the basis of threshold levels of allelic identity with at least one other sequence type (five or six identical loci). Clonal complexes are typically composed of a single predominant founding genotype, with a number of less common relatives (see Plate 3.3). As the founding genotype increases in frequency due to either fitness advantage or random genetic drift, it eventually diversifies to form a clonal complex. Putative descendants of a founder over time will continue to diversify into SLVs and DLVs, and may eventually become excluded from the founding clonal complex. Although MLST data were originally represented by a dendrogram on the basis of a matrix of pairwise differences in the allelic profile, this provides little or no information on the patterns of evolutionary descent within the clonal complex, or about the identity of the founder [107]. To that end, a modified version of BURST (*B*ased *U*pon *R*elated *S*equence *T*ypes), eBURST (http://eburst.mlst.net), is used to depict population snapshots and relatedness of sequence types.

Plate 3.3 shows a population snapshot of the entire *S. aureus* MLST database as of January 2008, with 13 sequenced human *S. aureus* strains mapping to four clonal complexes. The hospital-acquired strains N315, Mu50, Mu3, JH1, and JH9 [263] belong to CC5; community-acquired strains MW2 (USA400) and MSSA476 belong to CC1; and Newman [218], NCTC8325, FPR3757 (USA300), TCH1516 (USA300) [264], and COL belong to CC8. MRSA252, also hospital-associated, is the only representative of the CC30 lineage. Holden *et al.* [142] reported that 6% of the genome of MRSA252 was novel compared with the other sequenced strains. However, considering that most of the genomes map to only three clonal complexes, the diversity seen in MRSA252 is likely due to the relatedness of the other sequenced genomes rather than true divergence [142,234]. The one sequenced bovine *S. aureus* strain, RF122 (ET-3), appears as a singleton [144] in Plate 3.3, but is currently part of a minor clonal complex (CC151).

Assuming that clonal complexes represent biologically relevant groups rather than arbitrary divisions, it is unclear what the role of selection is in the origin and maintenance of these clusters. Descendants (e.g., SLVs) of a selectively adaptive founder will be more resistant to rapid changes from homologous recombination than to genetic drift. In sympatric populations, clonal complexes that emerge by acquiring adaptive mutation(s) likely represent distinct fitness peaks characteristic of a Sewall-Wright fitness landscape, i.e., existence of multiple (bacterial) populations exhibiting varying levels of fitness [265]. Some have suggested that clustering of bacterial populations reflects ecological specialization by individual clonal complexes (or "ecotypes"), which can be viewed as occupying different evolutionary trajectories, and may be considered separate species [266]. Although the definition of species, especially bacterial species, is highly debatable [267], Cohen's arguments underscore the importance of genotypic clusters that are biologically meaningful.

Cooper and Feil revisited the population structure of *S. aureus*, as depicted by MLST analysis, by comparing 37 additional loci representing an array of functional categories in 30 well-characterized strains [82]. Roughly 17.8 kb of DNA sequence data for each strain produced an unrooted Bayesian tree that confirms the population structure established by MLST, but with higher resolution and without unresolved branches (see Plate 3.1). The tree subdivides the *S. aureus* species into three genetic groups (1a, 1b, and 2), and within each group a subset of MLST sequence types are depicted as branches. The phylogenetic structure is largely consistent with groupings previously suggested by MLST housekeeping genes [83], adhesion genes [185], *sas* genes [171], PFGE [261], AFLP [119], and microarray analysis [268]. The authors suggest that for intraspecies phylogenetic markers, nucleotide diversity should first be considered, followed by gene function. That is, there is little evidence to justify the emphasis on housekeeping genes, at least for intraspecies phylogenetic comparisons. Moreover, in a highly clonal organism like *S. aureus* most genes will be informative for broad lineage assignments, as evidenced by corroborating data from PFGE and microarray analysis [261,268]. Indeed, this has proven to be the case when using *spa* to infer intraspecies relatedness [117].

A study by Koreen *et al.* reexamined a collection of 36 strains previously characterized by DNA microarray analysis using *spa*-typing [117,145]. The isolates were selected from over 2000 spatiotemporally diverse strains shown by MLEE to provide a likely population structure of *S. aureus*. The results revealed *spa*-typing to be highly discriminating in grouping strains based on sequence changes in the repeat region, which appears to have a molecular clock-speed in register with the overall evolutionary clock of the species. That is, point mutations accumulate at a lower rate than repeat number variation, and therefore the dual dynamics of slow point mutations in conjunction with faster changes in repeat number enable *spa*-typing to be used for studies of both microvariation and macrovariation [117,186]. For population studies, a direct comparison against the current gold standard, MLST, suggests that *spa*-typing is predictive of *S. aureus* sequence types and clonal complexes (see Plate 3.1), and its resolution approaches the discriminatory level of PFGE [113,114,117,269–271]. On occasion, recombination obscures the agreement of *spa* types with designated sequence types or clonal complexes [102].

Among nonsynonymous changes, the overall amino acid composition seems to be maintained, suggesting that SNPs are not under strong positive selection pressure. Analysis of 38 *spa* repeats showed a dS/dN value (ratio of the number of synonymous substitutions per potential synonymous site to the number of nonsynonymous substitutions per potential nonsynonymous site) of 6.4, where a ratio of less than 1 indicates positive selection, a value of 1 indicates neutral evolution, and a value greater than 1 indicates purifying selection. This result suggests that the variation seen in the polymorphic region is not the result of exogenous influences, but rather may reflect evolution of the species [117].

Concluding remarks

Understanding the evolutionary processes that give rise to the population genetic structure of *S. aureus* can greatly enhance our efforts towards control and prevention. *Staphylococcus aureus* has long been known to cause epidemics [16,272–275], some of which have involved single clones. Although bacteria are known to undergo periodic selection whereby adaptive mutants emerge and outcompete preexisting cells, thereby dramatically reducing the population diversity, the evolutionary events that follow the rise and fall of epidemics and particular clones are poorly understood. For instance, during the 1950s a penicillin-resistant clone of *S. aureus*, phage type 80/81, emerged and caused serious hospital-acquired and community infections worldwide [276,277]. This clone was largely eliminated in the 1960s following the introduction of methicillin, a semisynthetic penicillin, coupled with the inoculation of bacterial interference *S. aureus* strain 502A to control infections among infants (at least in the UK) [278]. Phage type 80/81 isolates carry PVL genes and belong to ST30 (CC30), a very common genotype [275]. Decades later, descendants of phage 80/81 reemerged in the community setting, and have become endemic in nosocomial environments (see Plate 3.3). Some of the descendants have gained methicillin resistance with the acquisition of type II SCC*mec* (e.g., MRSA252, also known as EMRSA-16) as well as type IV SCC*mec* (e.g., the South West Pacific clone [279]). Robinson *et al.* [275] present a parallel evolutionary hypothesis wherein both PVL-producing 80/81 and PVL-negative strains (that gave rise to MRSA252) are related to a common PVL-negative ancestor. The molecular underpinnings related to the decline of the pandemic 80/81 clone and the (re)emergence of community as well as hospital strains remains unclear. Notably, the MRSA252 genome contains the greatest number of pseudogenes, and may have undergone molecular remodeling, either by accumulating adaptive mutations, or even more dramatically by punctuated equilibrium, to become specialized for certain ecological niches. For example, strains from CC30 have been associated with bloodstream infections [161] as well as menstrual toxic shock syndrome [145].

The current epidemic of CA-MRSA, and in particular the rise of USA300 (FPR3757; see Plate 3.2), is likewise a major public health concern. While USA300 has novel genetic elements such as a smaller and more mobile type

Table 3.2 Staphylococcal genome sequences published as of May 2009, in order of sequence completion date.

Species	Strain	Other ID	Description	Isolated	Sequenced	Date	RefSeq	Ref.
S. aureus	N315	New York/ Japan	HA-MRSA: pharyngeal smear of a Japanese patient	Japan (1982)	National Institute of Technology and Evaluation (Japan)	Apr 2001	NC_002745	51
S. aureus	COL	Archaic	HA-MRSA: penicillinase (-) strain from hospital operating room	Colindale, UK (1961)	The Institute for Genomic Research (U.S.)	Sep 2001	NC_002951	143
S. aureus	Mu50	ATCC 700699	HA-MRSA: vancomycin-intermediate strain from pediatric surgical wound infection (first VISA isolated)	Japan (1996)	Juntendo University (Japan)	Oct 2001	NC_002758	51
S. aureus	MSSA476	Sanger 476	CA-MSSA: hypervirulent MSSA from 9-year-old boy with community-acquired osteomyelitis and bacteremia	UK (1998)	Sanger Institute (U.K.)	Nov 2001	NC_002953	142
S. aureus	MRSA252	EMRSA-16 Sanger 252	HA-MRSA: epidemic MRSA strain isolated from 64-year-old female with fatal post-operative septicemia	UK (1997)	Sanger Institute (U.K.)	Nov 2001	NC_002952	142
S. epidermidis	RP62A	ATCC 35984	MR-CoNS: biofilm isolate from intravascular catheter-associated sepsis	Tennessee, USA (1980)	The Institute for Genomic Research (U.S.)	Jan 2002	NC_002976	143
S. aureus	MW2	USA 400	CA-MRSA: fatal septicemia and septic arthritis in a 16-month-old Native American girl with no risk factors	North Dakota, USA (1998)	National Institute of Technology and Evaluation (Japan)	May 2002	NC_003923	101
S. epidermidis	ATCC 12228	FDA strain PCI 1200	non-biofilm forming, non-infection associated strain used to detect residual antibiotics in food		Chinese National HGSC, Shanghai (China)	Jan 2003	NC_004461	312
S. haemolyticus	JCSC1435		Japanese inpatient at Juntendo Hospital, Tokyo	Japan (2000)	National Institute of Technology and Evaluation (Japan)	Jul 2005	NC_007168	146
S. saprophyticus	ATCC 15305	NCTC 7292	type strain, isolated from human urine specimen (1951) J. Gen. Microbiol. 5, 1010-1023		Kitasato Institute for Life Sciences (Japan)	Aug 2005	NC_007350	313
S. aureus	RF122	ET3-1	bovine mastitis *(Bos taurus)*	Ireland (1993)	University of Minnesota (U.S.)	Nov 2005	NC_007622	144
S. aureus	USA300-FPR3757	USA 300	CA-MRSA: wrist abscess from 36-year-old white male HIV-positive intravenous drug user	San Francisco, USA (2000)	Univesity of California, San Francisco (U.S.)	Feb 2006	NC_007793	141

Table 3.2 (*cont'd*)

Species	Strain	Other ID	Description	Isolated	Sequence	Date	RefSeq	Ref.
S. aureus	NCTC 8325	RN1	MSSA: prototypical laboratory research strain: (1967) Virology 33:155-166.	UK (1960)	Microgen, Univ. of Oklahoma Health Sciences Center (U.S.)	Feb 2006	NC_007795	314
S. aureus	JH9		HA-MRSA: final isolate after therapy failure, showing decreased susceptibility to vancomycin *(see entry below)*	Baltimore, USA (2001)	U.S. Department of Energy Joint Genome Institute	May 2007	NC_009487	263
S. aureus	JH1		HA-MRSA: initial (vancomycin-susceptible) bloodstream isolate from patient with congenital heart disease	Baltimore, USA (2001)	U.S. Department of Energy Joint Genome Institute	Jul 2007	NC_009632	263
S. aureus	Newman		MSSA: isolated from human clinical specimen: (1952) J Gen Microbiol 6:95–107.		Juntendo University (Japan)	Jul 2007	NC_009641	218
S. aureus	Mu3	ATCC 700698	HA-MRSA: sputum of 64-year-old patient with post-operative pneumonia and vancomycin therapy failure	Japan (1996)	Juntendo University (Japan)	Sep 2007	NC_009782	315
S. aureus	USA300-TCH1516*	USA300 HOU-MR	CA-MRSA: adolescent patient with severe sepsis syndrome, Texas Children's Hospital, Houston	Houston, USA	Baylor College of Medicine Houston (U.S.)	Dec 2007	NC_010079	264
S. carnosus	subsp. *carnosus*	TM300	used as a meat starter culture in food industry (apathogenic), also used as a cloning vector in staphylococcal genetics		PathoGenoMik Univ. of Würzburg (Germany)	Feb 2009	NC_012121	316

As of May 2009, the following genome sequences are in progress: (strains highlighted with an asterisk (*) are designated as reference genomes for the Human Microbiome Project)

S. aureus	assembly: MN8 *, TCH60 *, TCH70 *, TCH130 *, TCH959 *, CF-Marseille, JKD6008, JKD6009, Mu50-omega draft: HMP0012 *, 930918-3, D30, 132, CGS00, CGS01, CGS03, Mu50 04-02981, 55/2053, 65-1322, 68-397, M876, E1410, A5937, A5948, A6224, A6300, A8115, A9299, A9635, A9719, A9763, A9781
S. epidermidis	assembly: W23144 *, M23864:W1 *, BCM-HMP0060 * draft: M23864:W2 *, M23590 *, CONS *, SK135 *, ATCC 14990
S. capitis	assembly: SK14 *
S. hominis	assembly: SK119 *
S. caprae	draft: JCVIHMP041 *
S. warneri	draft: L37603 *
S. xylosus	draft: DSM20267

IVa SCC*mec*, PVL, and ACME, the dominance of this clone remains obscure. Kennedy *et al.* [172] compared USA300 strains collected from geographically and demographically diverse sources by whole-genome sequencing, in order to understand the extent of genetic diversity underlying this epidemic clone. This study revealed that there has been recent clonal expansion (positive selection) of a subset of USA300 isolates followed by diversification. Although the study demonstrated that USA300 isolates all share a recent ancestor, there are subtle genetic changes between isolates that exhibit a measurable phenotype. Therefore, it is likely that the fitness landscape of epidemic USA300 isolates will include strains that differ in virulence potential and/or pathogenicity.

As highlighted in the USA300 and phage 80/81 examples, a comprehensive understanding of the extent and nature of genomic variation, as well as molecular evolutionary processes, is important for elucidating the events that define bacterial virulence, (re)emergence, epidemic potential, and drug resistance. While a number of *S. aureus* genomes are available, they are only partially representative of the overall population, and therefore the genetic make-up of the species may be distorted. For a more thorough picture, strains must be chosen carefully to represent the population structure. In addition, nearly all strains that have been sequenced thus far were isolated from diseased individuals (Table 3.2). This raises the question as to how representative the isolates are of the natural population structure of *S. aureus*, since this organism is mainly carried asymptomatically. Recently, genome sequence analysis of a Macrococcus caseolyticus strain from commercial poultry has confirmed the close relationship of this genus to the staphylococci, while suggesting a plausible mechanism for the origin of SCCmec [317]. Overall, comparative genomics has demonstrated that bacterial pathogens such as *S. aureus* contain extensive genome diversity, as well as multiple mechanisms of horizontal gene transfer and recombination that have contributed to variation within the species. The many strain-specific genes identified may facilitate colonization of specialized host and environmental niches, and could help explain the versatility of *S. aureus* in causing many different disease types in multiple host species.

References

1 Ochman H, Lawrence JG, Groisman EA. Lateral gene transfer and the nature of bacterial innovation. Nature 2000;405:299–304.

2 Levin BR, Lipsitch M, Bonhoeffer S. Population biology, evolution, and infectious disease: convergence and synthesis. Science 1999;283:806–9.

3 Fridkin SK, Hill HA, Volkova NV *et al.* Temporal changes in prevalence of antimicrobial resistance in 23 US hospitals. Emerg Infect Dis 2002;8:697–701.

4 Lowy FD. *Staphylococcus aureus* infections. N Engl J Med 1998;339:520–32.

5 Rubin RJ, Harrington CA, Poon A, Dietrich K, Greene JA, Moiduddin A. The economic impact of *Staphylococcus aureus* infection in New York City hospitals. Emerg Infect Dis 1999; 5:9–17.

6 Noskin GA, Rubin RJ, Schentag JJ *et al.* National trends in *Staphylococcus aureus* infection rates: impact on economic burden and mortality over a 6-year period (1998–2003). Clin Infect Dis 2007;45:1132–40.

7 Aiello AE, Lowy FD, Wright LN, Larson EL. Meticillin-resistant *Staphylococcus aureus* among US prisoners and military personnel: review and recommendations for future studies. Lancet Infect Dis 2006;6:335–41.

8 Fridkin SK, Hageman JC, Morrison M *et al.* Methicillin-resistant *Staphylococcus aureus* disease in three communities. N Engl J Med 2005;352:1436–44.

9 Naimi TS, LeDell KH, Como-Sabetti K *et al.* Comparison of community- and health care-associated methicillin-resistant *Staphylococcus aureus* infection. JAMA 2003;290:2976–84.

10 Zetola N, Francis JS, Nuermberger EL, Bishai WR. Community-acquired meticillin-resistant *Staphylococcus aureus*: an emerging threat. Lancet Infect Dis 2005;5:275–86.

11 Kazakova SV, Hageman JC, Matava M *et al.* A clone of methicillin-resistant *Staphylococcus aureus* among professional football players. N Engl J Med 2005;352:468–75.

12 Said-Salim B, Mathema B, Kreiswirth BN. Community-acquired methicillin-resistant *Staphylococcus aureus*: an emerging pathogen. Infect Control Hosp Epidemiol 2003;24:451–5.

13 Centers for Disease Control and Prevention. Four pediatric deaths from community-acquired methicillin-resistant *Staphylococcus aureus*: Minnesota and North Dakota, 1997–1999. JAMA 1999;282:1123–5.

14 Anon. Outbreaks of community-associated methicillin-resistant *Staphylococcus aureus* skin infections: Los Angeles County, California, 2002–2003. MMWR 2003;52:88.

15 Miller LG, Perdreau-Remington F, Rieg G *et al.* Necrotizing fasciitis caused by community-associated methicillin-resistant *Staphylococcus aureus* in Los Angeles. N Engl J Med 2005; 352:1445–53.

16 Chambers HF. Community-associated MRSA: resistance and virulence converge. N Engl J Med 2005;352:1485–7.

17 Klevens RM, Edwards JR, Tenover FC, McDonald LC, Horan T, Gaynes R. Changes in the epidemiology of methicillin-resistant *Staphylococcus aureus* in intensive care units in US hospitals, 1992–2003. Clin Infect Dis 2006;42:389–91.

18 Klevens RM, Morrison MA, Nadle J *et al.* Invasive methicillin-resistant *Staphylococcus aureus* infections in the United States. JAMA 2007;298:1763–71.

19 Moran GJ, Krishnadasan A, Gorwitz RJ *et al.* Methicillin-resistant *S. aureus* infections among patients in the emergency department. N Engl J Med 2006;355:666–74.

20 Kloos WE. Taxonomy and systematic of staphylococci indigenous to humans. In: Crossley KB, Archer GL, eds. The Staphylococci in Human Disease. New York: Churchill Livingstone, 1997:113–37.

21 Bureau of Tuberculosis Control. *Tuberculosis in New York City, 1997.* New York City: New York City Department of Health, 1998.

22 Rosenbach FJ. Mikro-Organismen bei den Wund-Infections-Krankheiten des Menschen. Bergman JF, ed. Wiesbaden, Germany, 1884:1–120.

23 Winslow CE, Winslow AR. The Systematic Relationships of the Coccaceae: With a Discussion of the Principles of Bacterial Classification. New York: John Wiley & Sons, 1908:1–300.

24 Liu GY, Essex A, Buchanan JT *et al*. *Staphylococcus aureus* golden pigment impairs neutrophil killing and promotes virulence through its antioxidant activity. J Exp Med 2005; 202:209–15.

25 R Christie, EV Keogh. Physiological and serological characteristics of staphylococci of human origin. J Pathol Bacteriol 1940; 51:189–97.

26 Cowan ST. The classification of staphylococci by precipitation and biological reactions. J Pathol Bacteriol 1938;46:31–45.

27 Blair JE, Hallman FA. Serologic grouping of Staphylococci. J Bacteriol 1936;31:81–82.

28 Fairbrother RW. Coagulase production as a criterion for the classification of the staphylococci. J Pathol Bacteriol 1940;50:83–8.

29 Foubert EL, Douglas HC. Studies on the anaerobic micrococci. I. Taxonomic considerations. J Bacteriol 1948;56:25–34.

30 Sompolinsky D. De l'impetigo contagiosa suis et du *Micrococcus hyicus* n. sp. Schweiz Arch Tierhilkd 1953;95:302–9.

31 Shaw C, Stitt JM, Cowan ST. Staphylococci and their classification. J Gen Microbiol 1951;5:1010–23.

32 Ingram GI. Classification of staphylococci by penicillin lysis. J Gen Microbiol 1951;5:30–8.

33 Wahl R, Lapeyre-Mensignac P. [Identification of staphylococci by bacteriophages: an attempt of staphylococci classification by the method of phages.] Ann Inst Pasteur (Paris) 1950; 78:765–777.

34 Twort FW. An investigation of the nature of ultra-microscopic viruses. Lancet 1915;186:1241–3.

35 Kwan T, Liu J, DuBow M, Gros P, Pelletier J. The complete genomes and proteomes of 27 *Staphylococcus aureus* bacteriophages. Proc Natl Acad Sci USA 2005;102:5174–9.

36 Fleming A. On the antibacterial action of cultures of a penicillium, with special reference to their use in the isolation of *B. influenzae*. Br J Exp Pathol 1929;10:226–36.

37 Hillier K. Babies and bacteria: phage typing, bacteriologists, and the birth of infection control. Bull Hist Med 2006;80:733–61.

38 Zopf W. Die Spaltpilze. Breslau: Edward Trewendt, 1885:1–127.

39 Flugge C. Die Mikroorganismen. Leipzig: F.C.W. Vogel, 1886.

40 Bannerman TL. *Staphylococcus*, *Micrococcus*, and other catalase-positive cocci that grow aerobically. In: Murray PR, Jorgensen EJ, Jolken MA, eds. Manual of Clinical Microbiology, 8th ed, Washington, DC: American Society for Microbiology, 2003.

41 Baird-Parker AC. A classification of micrococci and staphylococci based on physiological and biochemical tests. J Gen Microbiol 1963;30:409–27.

42 Baird-Parker AC. Staphylococci and their classification. Ann NY Acad Sci 1965;128:4–25.

43 Baird-Parker AC. The grouping of staphylococci and micrococci. J Clin Pathol 1971;24:769–70.

44 Baird-Parker AC. An improved diagnostic and selective medium for isolating coagulase positive Staphylococci. J Appl Bacteriol 1962;25:12–19.

45 Holt JG, ed. Bergey's Manual of Systematic Bacteriology Vol. 2. Gram-positive Bacteria other than Actinomycetes. Baltimore: Williams & Wilkins, 1986.

46 Woese CR, Fox GE. Phylogenetic structure of the prokaryotic domain: the primary kingdoms. Proc Natl Acad Sci USA 1977;74:5088–90.

47 Lambert LH, Cox T, Mitchell K *et al*. *Staphylococcus succinus* sp. nov., isolated from Dominican amber. Int J Syst Bacteriol 1998;48:511–18.

48 Freney J, Kloos WE, Hajek V *et al*. Recommended minimal standards for description of new staphylococcal species. Subcommittee on the taxonomy of staphylococci and streptococci of the International Committee on Systematic Bacteriology. Int J Syst Bacteriol 1999;49:489–502.

49 Janda JM, Abbott SL. 16S rRNA gene sequencing for bacterial identification in the diagnostic laboratory: pluses, perils, and pitfalls. J Clin Microbiol 2007;45:2761–4.

50 Becker K, Harmsen D, Mellmann A *et al*. Development and evaluation of a quality-controlled ribosomal sequence database for 16S ribosomal DNA-based identification of *Staphylococcus* species. J Clin Microbiol 2004;42:4988–95.

51 Kuroda M, Ohta T, Uchiyama I *et al*. Whole genome sequencing of meticillin-resistant *Staphylococcus aureus*. Lancet 2001; 357:1225–40.

52 Everall PH, Stacey PM. Catalase negative *Staphylococcus aureus*. J Med Lab Technol 1956;13:489–90.

53 Del'Alamo L, d'Azevedo PA, Strob AJ *et al*. An outbreak of catalase-negative methicillin-resistant *Staphylococcus aureus*. J Hosp Infect 2007;65:226–30.

54 Gruner BM, Han SR, Meyer HG, Wulf U, Bhakdi S, Siegel EK. Characterization of a catalase-negative methicillin-resistant *Staphylococcus aureus* strain. J Clin Microbiol 2007;45:2684–5.

55 Millar M, Wilcock A, Sanderson Y, Kite P, McDonnell MK. Catalase negative *Staphylococcus aureus*. J Clin Pathol 1986; 39:695.

56 Over U, Tuc Y, Soyletir G. Catalase-negative *Staphylococcus aureus*: a rare isolate of human infection. Clin Microbiol Infect 2000;6:681–2.

57 Tu KK, Palutke WA. Isolation and characterization of a catalase-negative strain of *Staphylococcus aureus*. J Clin Microbiol 1976;3:77–8.

58 Oluola O, Kong L, Fein M, Weisman LE. Lysostaphin in treatment of neonatal *Staphylococcus aureus* infection. Antimicrob Agents Chemother 2007;51:2198–200.

59 Wall RJ, Powell AM, Paape MJ *et al*. Genetically enhanced cows resist intramammary *Staphylococcus aureus* infection. Nat Biotechnol 2005;23:445–51.

60 Gaillot O, Wetsch M, Fortineau N, Berche P. Evaluation of CHROMagar Staph. aureus, a new chromogenic medium, for isolation and presumptive identification of *Staphylococcus aureus* from human clinical specimens. J Clin Microbiol 2000; 38:1587–91.

61 Perry JD, Rennison C, Butterworth LA, Hopley AL, Gould FK. Evaluation of *S. aureus* ID, a new chromogenic agar medium for detection of *Staphylococcus aureus*. J Clin Microbiol 2003; 41:5695–8.

62 Perry JD, Davies A, Butterworth LA, Hopley AL, Nicholson A, Gould FK. Development and evaluation of a chromogenic agar medium for methicillin-resistant *Staphylococcus aureus*. J Clin Microbiol 2004;42:4519–23.

63 Iorio NL, Ferreira RB, Schuenck RP *et al*. Simplified and reliable scheme for species-level identification of *Staphylococcus* clinical isolates. J Clin Microbiol 2007;45:2564–9.

64 Kloos WE, Ballard DN, George CG *et al*. Delimiting the genus *Staphylococcus* through description of *Macrococcus caseolyticus* gen. nov., comb. nov. and *Macrococcus equipercicus* sp. nov., and *Macrococcus bovicus* sp. no. and *Macrococcus carouselicus* sp. nov. Int J Syst Bacteriol 1998;48:859–77.
65 Takahashi T, Satoh I, Kikuchi N. Phylogenetic relationships of 38 taxa of the genus *Staphylococcus* based on 16S rRNA gene sequence analysis. Int J Syst Bacteriol 1999;49:725–8.
66 Collins MD, Hutson RA, Falsen E, Sjoden B, Facklam RR. *Gemella bergeriae* sp. nov., isolated from human clinical specimens. J Clin Microbiol 1998;36:1290–3.
67 Paster BJ, Falkler WA Jr, Enwonwu CO *et al*. Prevalent bacterial species and novel phylotypes in advanced noma lesions. J Clin Microbiol 2002;40:2187–91.
68 Woo PC, Lau SK, Fung AM, Chiu SK, Yung RW, Yuen KY. *Gemella* bacteraemia characterised by 16S ribosomal RNA gene sequencing. J Clin Pathol 2003;56:690–3.
69 Euzeby JP. List of bacterial names with standing in nomenclature: a folder available on the Internet. Int J Syst Bacteriol 1997;47:590–2.
70 Tang YW, Han J, McCormac MA, Li H, Stratton CW. *Staphylococcus pseudolugdunensis* sp. nov., a pyrrolidonyl arylamidase/ornithine decarboxylase-positive bacterium isolated from blood cultures. Diagn Microbiol Infect Dis 2008; 60:351–9.
71 Petras P. *Staphylococcus pulvereri = Staphylococcus vitulus*? Int J Syst Bacteriol 1998;48:617–18.
72 Drancourt M, Raoult D. *rpoB* gene sequence-based identification of *Staphylococcus* species. J Clin Microbiol 2002;40:1333–8.
73 Mellmann A, Becker K, von Eiff C, Keckevoet U, Schumann P, Harmsen D. Sequencing and staphylococci identification. Emerg Infect Dis 2006;12:333–6.
74 Goh SH, Potter S, Wood JO, Hemmingsen SM, Reynolds RP, Chow AW. HSP60 gene sequences as universal targets for microbial species identification: studies with coagulase-negative staphylococci. J Clin Microbiol 1996;34:818–23.
75 Kwok AY, Chow AW. Phylogenetic study of *Staphylococcus* and *Macrococcus* species based on partial *hsp60* gene sequences. Int J Syst Evol Microbiol 2003;53:87–92.
76 Kwok AY, Su SC, Reynolds RP *et al*. Species identification and phylogenetic relationships based on partial HSP60 gene sequences within the genus *Staphylococcus*. Int J Syst Bacteriol 1999;49:1181–92.
77 Martineau F, Picard FJ, Ke D *et al*. Development of a PCR assay for identification of staphylococci at genus and species levels. J Clin Microbiol 2001;39:2541–7.
78 Poyart C, Quesne G, Boumaila C, Trieu-Cuot P. Rapid and accurate species-level identification of coagulase-negative staphylococci by using the *sodA* gene as a target. J Clin Microbiol 2001;39:4296–301.
79 Ghebremedhin B, Layer F, König W, König B. Genetic classification and distinguishing of *Staphylococcus* species based on different partial gene sequences: gap, 16S rRNA, hsp60, rpoB, sodA, and tuf gene. J Clin Microbiol 2008;46:1019–25.
80 Pantucek R, Sedlacek I, Petras P *et al*. *Staphylococcus simiae* sp. nov., isolated from South American squirrel monkeys. Int J Syst Evol Microbiol 2005;55:1953–8.
81 Pottumarthy S, Schapiro JM, Prentice JL *et al*. Clinical isolates of *Staphylococcus intermedius* masquerading as methicillin-resistant *Staphylococcus aureus*. J Clin Microbiol 2004;42:5881–4.
82 Cooper JE, Feil EJ. The phylogeny of *Staphylococcus aureus*: which genes make the best intra-species markers? Microbiology 2006;152:1297–305.
83 Feil EJ, Cooper JE, Grundmann H *et al*. How clonal is *Staphylococcus aureus*? J Bacteriol 2003;185:3307–16.
84 Frank KL, Del Pozo JL, Patel R. From clinical microbiology to infection pathogenesis: how daring to be different works for *Staphylococcus lugdunensis*. Clin Microbiol Rev 2008;21:111–33.
85 Kreiswirth BN, Lutwick SM, Chapnick EK *et al*. Tracing the spread of methicillin-resistant *Staphylococcus aureus* by Southern blot hybridization using gene-specific probes of mec and Tn554. Microb Drug Resist 1995;1:307–13.
86 Phillips S, Novick RP. Tn554: a site-specific repressor-controlled transposon in *Staphylococcus aureus*. Nature 1979;278:476–8.
87 Chikramane SG, Matthews PR, Noble WC, Stewart PR, Dubin DT. Tn554 inserts in methicillin-resistant *Staphylococcus aureus* from Australia and England: comparison with an American methicillin-resistant group. J Gen Microbiol 1991;137:1303–11.
88 Mathema B, Kreiswirth BN. Genotyping bacteria by using variable-number tandem repeats. In: Persing DH, Tenover F, Versalovic J, Tang YW, Unger ER, Relman DA, White TJ, eds. Molecular Microbiology: Diagnostic Principles and Practice. Washington, DC: American Society for Microbiology Press, 2004:223–33.
89 Shopsin B, Kreiswirth BN. Molecular epidemiology of methicillin-resistant *Staphylococcus aureus*. Emerg Infect Dis 2001;7:323–6.
90 Kreiswirth B, Kornblum J, Arbeit RD *et al*. Evidence for a clonal origin of methicillin resistance in *Staphylococcus aureus*. Science 1993;259:227–30.
91 Musser JM, Kapur V. Clonal analysis of methicillin-resistant *Staphylococcus aureus* strains from intercontinental sources: association of the *mec* gene with divergent phylogenetic lineages implies dissemination by horizontal transfer and recombination. J Clin Microbiol 1992;30:2058–63.
92 Goering RV. Molecular epidemiology of nosocomial infection: analysis of chromosomal restriction fragment patterns by pulsed-field gel electrophoresis. Infect Control Hosp Epidemiol 1993;14:595–600.
93 Schwartz DC, Cantor CR. Separation of yeast chromosome-sized DNAs by pulsed field gradient gel electrophoresis. Cell 1984;37:67–75.
94 Linhardt F, Ziebuhr W, Meyer P, Witte W, Hacker J. Pulsed-field gel electrophoresis of genomic restriction fragments as a tool for the epidemiological analysis of *Staphylococcus aureus* and coagulase-negative staphylococci. FEMS Microbiol Lett 1992;74:181–5.
95 Pantucek R, Götz F, Doskar J, Rosypal S. Genomic variability of *Staphylococcus aureus* and the other coagulase-positive *Staphylococcus* species estimated by macrorestriction analysis using pulsed-field gel electrophoresis. Int J Syst Bacteriol 1996;46:216–22.
96 Poddar SK, McClelland M. Restriction fragment fingerprint and genome sizes of *Staphylococcus* species using pulsed-field gel electrophoresis and infrequent cleaving enzymes. DNA Cell Biol 1991;10:663–9.
97 Prevost G, Pottecher B, Dahlet M, Bientz M, Mantz JM, Piemont Y. Pulsed field gel electrophoresis as a new epidemiological tool for monitoring methicillin-resistant *Staphylococcus aureus* in an intensive care unit. J Hosp Infect 1991;17:255–69.

98 McDougal LK, Steward CD, Killgore GE, Chaitram JM, McAllister SK, Tenover FC. Pulsed-field gel electrophoresis typing of oxacillin-resistant *Staphylococcus aureus* isolates from the United States: establishing a national database. J Clin Microbiol 2003;41:5113–20.
99 Enright MC, Day NP, Davies CE, Peacock SJ, Spratt BG. Multilocus sequence typing for characterization of methicillin-resistant and methicillin-susceptible clones of *Staphylococcus aureus*. J Clin Microbiol 2000;38:1008–15.
100 Maiden MC, Bygraves JA, Feil E *et al*. Multilocus sequence typing: a portable approach to the identification of clones within populations of pathogenic microorganisms. Proc Natl Acad Sci USA 1998;95:3140–5.
101 Baba T, Takeuchi F, Kuroda M *et al*. Genome and virulence determinants of high virulence community-acquired MRSA. Lancet 2002;359:1819–27.
102 Robinson DA, Enright MC. Evolution of *Staphylococcus aureus* by large chromosomal replacements. J Bacteriol 2004; 186:1060–4.
103 Wang XM, Noble L, Kreiswirth BN *et al*. Evaluation of a multilocus sequence typing system for *Staphylococcus epidermidis*. J Med Microbiol 2003;52:989–98.
104 Thomas JC, Vargas MR, Miragaia M, Peacock SJ, Archer GL, Enright MC. Improved multilocus sequence typing scheme for *Staphylococcus epidermidis*. J Clin Microbiol 2007;45:616–19.
105 Miragaia M, Carrico JA, Thomas JC, Couto I, Enright MC, de Lencastre H. Comparison of molecular typing methods for characterization of *Staphylococcus epidermidis*: proposal for clone definition. J Clin Microbiol 2008;46:118–29.
106 Miragaia M, Thomas JC, Couto I, Enright MC, de Lencastre H. Inferring a population structure for *Staphylococcus epidermidis* from multilocus sequence typing data. J Bacteriol 2007; 189:2540–52.
107 Feil EJ, Li BC, Aanensen DM, Hanage WP, Spratt BG. eBURST: inferring patterns of evolutionary descent among clusters of related bacterial genotypes from multilocus sequence typing data. J Bacteriol 2004;186:1518–30.
108 Hall BG, Barlow M. Phylogenetic analysis as a tool in molecular epidemiology of infectious diseases. Ann Epidemiol 2006;16:157–69.
109 Harmsen D, Claus H, Witte W *et al*. Typing of methicillin-resistant *Staphylococcus aureus* in a university hospital setting by using novel software for *spa* repeat determination and database management. J Clin Microbiol 2003;41:5442–8.
110 Shopsin B, Gomez M, Montgomery SO *et al*. Evaluation of protein A gene polymorphic region DNA sequencing for typing of *Staphylococcus aureus* strains. J Clin Microbiol 1999;37:3556–63.
111 Mathema B, Mediavilla J, Kreiswirth BN. Sequence Analysis of the Variable Number Tandem Repeat in *Staphylococcus aureus* Protein Gene. Totowa, NJ: Humana Press, 2008.
112 Feil EJ, Enright MC. Analyses of clonality and the evolution of bacterial pathogens. Curr Opin Microbiol 2004;7:308–13.
113 Strommenger B, Kettlitz C, Weniger T, Harmsen D, Friedrich AW, Witte W. Assignment of *Staphylococcus* isolates to groups by *spa* typing, *Sma*I macrorestriction analysis, and multilocus sequence typing. J Clin Microbiol 2006;44:2533–40.
114 Oliveira DC, Crisostomo I, Santos-Sanches I *et al*. Comparison of DNA sequencing of the protein A gene polymorphic region with other molecular typing techniques for typing two epidemiologically diverse collections of methicillin-resistant *Staphylococcus aureus*. J Clin Microbiol 2001;39:574–80.
115 Strommenger B, Braulke C, Heuck D *et al*. *spa* typing of *Staphylococcus aureus* as a frontline tool in epidemiological typing. J Clin Microbiol 2008;46:574–81.
116 Tang YW, Waddington MG, Smith DH *et al*. Comparison of protein A gene sequencing with pulsed-field gel electrophoresis and epidemiologic data for molecular typing of methicillin-resistant *Staphylococcus aureus*. J Clin Microbiol 2000;38:1347–51.
117 Koreen L, Ramaswamy SV, Graviss EA, Naidich S, Musser JM, Kreiswirth BN. *spa* typing method for discriminating among *Staphylococcus aureus* isolates: implications for use of a single marker to detect genetic micro- and macrovariation. J Clin Microbiol 2004;42:792–9.
118 Mellmann A, Friedrich AW, Rosenkotter N *et al*. Automated DNA sequence-based early warning system for the detection of methicillin-resistant *Staphylococcus aureus* outbreaks. *PLoS Med* 2006;3:e33.
119 Melles DC, Gorkink RF, Boelens HA *et al*. Natural population dynamics and expansion of pathogenic clones of *Staphylococcus aureus*. J Clin Invest 2004;114:1732–40.
120 Melles DC, van Leeuwen WB, Snijders SV *et al*. Comparison of multilocus sequence typing (MLST), pulsed-field gel electrophoresis (PFGE), and amplified fragment length polymorphism (AFLP) for genetic typing of *Staphylococcus aureus*. J Microbiol Methods 2007;69:371–5.
121 Francois P, Hochmann A, Huyghe A *et al*. Rapid and high-throughput genotyping of *Staphylococcus epidermidis* isolates by automated multilocus variable-number of tandem repeats: a tool for real-time epidemiology. J Microbiol Methods 2008; 72:296–305.
122 Francois P, Huyghe A, Charbonnier Y *et al*. Use of an automated multiple-locus, variable-number tandem repeat-based method for rapid and high-throughput genotyping of *Staphylococcus aureus* isolates. J Clin Microbiol 2005;43:3346–55.
123 Tenover FC, Vaughn RR, McDougal LK, Fosheim GE, McGowan JE Jr. Multiple-locus variable-number tandem-repeat assay analysis of methicillin-resistant *Staphylococcus aureus* strains. J Clin Microbiol 2007;45:2215–19.
124 Koessler T, Francois P, Charbonnier Y *et al*. Use of oligoarrays for characterization of community-onset methicillin-resistant *Staphylococcus aureus*. J Clin Microbiol 2006;44:1040–8.
125 Stephens AJ, Huygens F, Inman-Bamber J *et al*. Methicillin-resistant *Staphylococcus aureus* genotyping using a small set of polymorphisms. J Med Microbiol 2006;55:43–51.
126 Shopsin B, Gomez M, Waddington M, Riehman M, Kreiswirth BN. The use of coagulase gene (*coa*) repeat region nucleotide sequences for the typing of methicillin-resistant *Staphylococcus aureus*. J Clin Microbiol 2000;38:3453–6.
127 Nahvi MD, Fitzgibbon JE, John JF, Dubin DT. Sequence analysis of dru regions from methicillin-resistant *Staphylococcus aureus* and coagulase-negative staphylococcal isolates. Microb Drug Resist 2001;7:1–12.
128 Hardy KJ, Ussery DW, Oppenheim BA, Hawkey PM. Distribution and characterization of staphylococcal interspersed repeat units (SIRUs) and potential use for strain differentiation. Microbiology 2004;150:4045–52.
129 Mishaan AM, Mason EO Jr, Martinez-Aguilar G *et al*. Emergence of a predominant clone of community-acquired

Staphylococcus aureus among children in Houston, Texas. Pediatr Infect Dis J 2005;24:201–6.

130 Kuhn G, Francioli P, Blanc DS. Double-locus sequence typing using *clfB* and *spa*, a fast and simple method for epidemiological typing of methicillin-resistant *Staphylococcus aureus*. J Clin Microbiol 2007;45:54–62.

131 Deurenberg RH, Vink C, Kalenic S, Friedrich AW, Bruggeman CA, Stobberingh EE. The molecular evolution of methicillin-resistant *Staphylococcus aureus*. Clin Microbiol Infect 2007; 13:222–35.

132 Ito T, Katayama Y, Asada K *et al*. Structural comparison of three types of staphylococcal cassette chromosome mec integrated in the chromosome in methicillin-resistant *Staphylococcus aureus*. Antimicrob Agents Chemother 2001;45:1323–36.

133 Ito T, Ma XX, Takeuchi F, Okuma K, Yuzawa H, Hiramatsu K. Novel type V staphylococcal cassette chromosome mec driven by a novel cassette chromosome recombinase, ccrC. Antimicrob Agents Chemother 2004;48:2637–51.

134 Katayama Y, Ito T, Hiramatsu K. A new class of genetic element, staphylococcus cassette chromosome mec, encodes methicillin resistance in *Staphylococcus aureus*. Antimicrob Agents Chemother 2000;44:1549–55.

135 Stephens AJ, Huygens F, Giffard PM. Systematic derivation of marker sets for staphylococcal cassette chromosome mec typing. Antimicrob Agents Chemother 2007;51:2954–64.

136 Oliveira DC, de Lencastre H. Multiplex PCR strategy for rapid identification of structural types and variants of the mec element in methicillin-resistant *Staphylococcus aureus*. Antimicrob Agents Chemother 2002;46:2155–61.

137 Milheiriço C, Oliveira DC, de Lencastre H. Multiplex PCR strategy for subtyping the staphylococcal cassette chromosome mec type IV in methicillin-resistant *Staphylococcus aureus*: 'SCCmec IV multiplex'. J Antimicrob Chemother 2007;60:42–8.

138 Kondo Y, Ito T, Ma XX *et al*. Combination of multiplex PCRs for staphylococcal cassette chromosome mec type assignment: rapid identification system for mec, ccr, and major differences in junkyard regions. Antimicrob Agents Chemother 2007;51:264–74.

139 Hanssen AM, Ericson Sollid JU. SCCmec in staphylococci: genes on the move. FEMS Immunol Med Microbiol 2006;46: 8–20.

140 Oliveira DC, Milheirico C, Vinga S, de Lencastre H. Assessment of allelic variation in the ccrAB locus in methicillin-resistant *Staphylococcus aureus* clones. J Antimicrob Chemother 2006;58:23–30.

141 Diep BA, Gill SR, Chang RF *et al*. Complete genome sequence of USA300, an epidemic clone of community-acquired meticillin-resistant *Staphylococcus aureus*. Lancet 2006;367:731–9.

142 Holden MT, Feil EJ, Lindsay JA *et al*. Complete genomes of two clinical *Staphylococcus aureus* strains: evidence for the rapid evolution of virulence and drug resistance. Proc Natl Acad Sci USA 2004;101:9786–91.

143 Gill SR, Fouts DE, Archer GL *et al*. Insights on evolution of virulence and resistance from the complete genome analysis of an early methicillin-resistant *Staphylococcus aureus* strain and a biofilm-producing methicillin-resistant *Staphylococcus epidermidis* strain. J Bacteriol 2005;187:2426–38.

144 Herron-Olson L, Fitzgerald JR, Musser JM, Kapur V. Molecular correlates of host specialization in *Staphylococcus aureus*. PLoS ONE 2007;2:e1120.

145 Fitzgerald JR, Sturdevant DE, Mackie SM, Gill SR, Musser JM. Evolutionary genomics of *Staphylococcus aureus*: insights into the origin of methicillin-resistant strains and the toxic shock syndrome epidemic. Proc Natl Acad Sci USA 2001; 98:8821–6.

146 Takeuchi F, Watanabe S, Baba T *et al*. Whole-genome sequencing of *Staphylococcus haemolyticus* uncovers the extreme plasticity of its genome and the evolution of human-colonizing staphylococcal species. J Bacteriol 2005;187:7292–308.

147 Gut IG. Automation in genotyping of single nucleotide polymorphisms. Hum Mutat 2001;17:475–92.

148 Kimura M. The Neutral Theory of Molecular Evolution. Cambridge, UK: Cambridge University Press, 1983.

149 Schork NJ, Fallin D, Lanchbury JS. Single nucleotide polymorphisms and the future of genetic epidemiology. Clin Genet 2000;58:250–64.

150 Selander RK, Caugant DA, Ochman H, Musser JM, Gilmour MN, Whittam TS. Methods of multilocus enzyme electrophoresis for bacterial population genetics and systematics. Appl Environ Microbiol 1986;51:873–84.

151 Besier S, Ludwig A, Brade V, Wichelhaus TA. Molecular analysis of fusidic acid resistance in *Staphylococcus aureus*. Mol Microbiol 2003;47:463–9.

152 Drlica K, Malik M. Fluoroquinolones: action and resistance. Curr Top Med Chem 2003;3:249–82.

153 Liu Y, Harrison PM, Kunin V, Gerstein M. Comprehensive analysis of pseudogenes in prokaryotes: widespread gene decay and failure of putative horizontally transferred genes. *Genome Biol* 2004;5:R64.

154 Moxon R, Bayliss C, Hood D. Bacterial contingency loci: the role of simple sequence DNA repeats in bacterial adaptation. Annu Rev Genet 2006;40:307–33.

155 Bayliss CD, Field D, Moxon ER. The simple sequence contingency loci of *Haemophilus influenzae* and *Neisseria meningitidis*. J Clin Invest 2001;107:657–62.

156 O'Brien DP, Israel DA, Krishna U *et al*. The role of decay-accelerating factor as a receptor for *Helicobacter pylori* and a mediator of gastric inflammation. J Biol Chem 2006;281: 13317–23.

157 Parkhill J, Wren BW, Thomson NR *et al*. Genome sequence of *Yersinia pestis*, the causative agent of plague. Nature 2001;413:523–7.

158 Cole ST, Eiglmeier K, Parkhill J *et al*. Massive gene decay in the leprosy bacillus. Nature 2001;409:1007–11.

159 Bayles KW, Wesson CA, Liou LE, Fox LK, Bohach GA, Trumble WR. Intracellular *Staphylococcus aureus* escapes the endosome and induces apoptosis in epithelial cells. Infect Immun 1998; 66:336–42.

160 Lowy FD. Is *Staphylococcus aureus* an intracellular pathogen? Trends Microbiol 2000;8:341–3.

161 Fowler VG Jr, Nelson CL, McIntyre LM *et al*. Potential associations between hematogenous complications and bacterial genotype in *Staphylococcus aureus* infection. J Infect Dis 2007; 196:738–47.

162 Sau S, Bhasin N, Wann ER, Lee JC, Foster TJ, Lee CY. The *Staphylococcus aureus* allelic genetic loci for serotype 5 and 8 capsule expression contain the type-specific genes flanked by common genes. Microbiology 1997;143:2395–405.

163 O'Riordan K, Lee JC. *Staphylococcus aureus* capsular polysaccharides. Clin Microbiol Rev 2004;17:218–34.

164 Novick RP, Projan SJ, Kornblum J *et al*. The *agr* P2 operon: an autocatalytic sensory transduction system in *Staphylococcus aureus*. Mol Gen Genet 1995;248:446–58.
165 Lina G, Jarraud S, Ji G *et al*. Transmembrane topology and histidine protein kinase activity of AgrC, the *agr* signal receptor in *Staphylococcus aureus*. Mol Microbiol 1998;28:655–62.
166 Ji G, Beavis RC, Novick RP. Cell density control of staphylococcal virulence mediated by an octapeptide pheromone. Proc Natl Acad Sci USA 1995;92:12055–9.
167 Ji G, Beavis R, Novick RP. Bacterial interference caused by autoinducing peptide variants. Science 1997;276:2027–30.
168 Dufour P, Jarraud S, Vandenesch F *et al*. High genetic variability of the *agr* locus in *Staphylococcus* species. J Bacteriol 2002;184:1180–6.
169 Jarraud S, Lyon GJ, Figueiredo AM *et al*. Exfoliatin-producing strains define a fourth agr specificity group in *Staphylococcus aureus*. J Bacteriol 2000;182:6517–22.
170 Hughes AL, Friedman R. Nucleotide substitution and recombination at orthologous loci in *Staphylococcus aureus*. J Bacteriol 2005;187:2698–704.
171 Robinson DA, Monk AB, Cooper JE, Feil EJ, Enright MC. Evolutionary genetics of the accessory gene regulator (*agr*) locus in *Staphylococcus aureus*. J Bacteriol 2005;187:8312–21.
172 Kennedy AD, Otto M, Braughton KR *et al*. Epidemic community-associated methicillin-resistant *Staphylococcus aureus*: recent clonal expansion and diversification. Proc Natl Acad Sci USA 2008;105:1327–32.
173 Cramton SE, Schnell NF, Gotz F, Bruckner R. Identification of a new repetitive element in *Staphylococcus aureus*. Infect Immun 2000;68:2344–8.
174 Schneewind O, Model P, Fischetti VA. Sorting of protein A to the staphylococcal cell wall. Cell 1992;70:267–81.
175 Uhlen M, Guss B, Nilsson B, Gatenbeck S, Philipson L, Lindberg M. Complete sequence of the staphylococcal gene encoding protein A. A gene evolved through multiple duplications. J Biol Chem 1984;259:1695–702.
176 Roche FM, Meehan M, Foster TJ. The *Staphylococcus aureus* surface protein SasG and its homologues promote bacterial adherence to human desquamated nasal epithelial cells. Microbiology 2003;149:2759–67.
177 Brigido M de M, Barardi CR, Bonjardin CA, Santos CL, Junqueira ML, Brentani RR. Nucleotide sequence of a variant protein A of *Staphylococcus aureus* suggests molecular heterogeneity among strains. J Basic Microbiol 1991;31:337–45.
178 Foster TJ, Hook M. Surface protein adhesins of *Staphylococcus aureus*. Trends Microbiol 1998;6:484–8.
179 Mazmanian SK, Ton-That H, Schneewind O. Sortase-catalysed anchoring of surface proteins to the cell wall of *Staphylococcus aureus*. Mol Microbiol 2001;40:1049–57.
180 Hartford O, Francois P, Vaudaux P, Foster TJ. The dipeptide repeat region of the fibrinogen-binding protein (clumping factor) is required for functional expression of the fibrinogen-binding domain on the *Staphylococcus aureus* cell surface. Mol Microbiol 1997;25:1065–76.
181 Hartford O, McDevitt D, Foster TJ. Matrix-binding proteins of *Staphylococcus aureus*: functional analysis of mutant and hybrid molecules. Microbiology 1999;145:2497–505.
182 Jarraud S, Peyrat MA, Lim A *et al*. egc, a highly prevalent operon of enterotoxin gene, forms a putative nursery of superantigens in *Staphylococcus aureus*. J Immunol 2001;166:669–77.
183 Ni Eidhin D, Perkins S, Francois P, Vaudaux P, Hook M, Foster TJ. Clumping factor B (ClfB), a new surface-located fibrinogen-binding adhesin of *Staphylococcus aureus*. Mol Microbiol 1998;30:245–57.
184 Lorenz U, Ohlsen K, Karch H, Hecker M, Thiede A, Hacker J. Human antibody response during sepsis against targets expressed by methicillin resistant *Staphylococcus aureus*. FEMS Immunol Med Microbiol 2000;29:145–53.
185 Kuhn G, Francioli P, Blanc DS. Evidence for clonal evolution among highly polymorphic genes in methicillin-resistant *Staphylococcus aureus*. J Bacteriol 2006;188:169–78.
186 Aires de Sousa M, Conceicao T, Simas C, de Lencastre H. Comparison of genetic backgrounds of methicillin-resistant and -susceptible *Staphylococcus aureus* isolates from Portuguese hospitals and the community. J Clin Microbiol 2005;43:5150–7.
187 Witte W. Antibiotic resistance in gram-positive bacteria: epidemiological aspects. J Antimicrob Chemother 1999;44(suppl A): 1–9.
188 Thomas CM, Nielsen KM. Mechanisms of, and barriers to, horizontal gene transfer between bacteria. Nat Rev Microbiol 2005;3:711–21.
189 Betley MJ, Mekalanos JJ. Nucleotide sequence of the type A staphylococcal enterotoxin gene. J Bacteriol 1988;170:34–41.
190 Kaneko J, Kimura T, Narita S, Tomita T, Kamio Y. Complete nucleotide sequence and molecular characterization of the temperate staphylococcal bacteriophage phiPVL carrying Panton–Valentine leukocidin genes. Gene 1998;215:57–67.
191 Yamaguchi T, Hayashi T, Takami H *et al*. Phage conversion of exfoliative toxin A production in *Staphylococcus aureus*. Mol Microbiol 2000;38:694–705.
192 de Haas CJ, Veldkamp KE, Peschel A *et al*. Chemotaxis inhibitory protein of *Staphylococcus aureus*, a bacterial antiinflammatory agent. J Exp Med 2004;199:687–95.
193 Betley MJ, Mekalanos JJ. Staphylococcal enterotoxin A is encoded by phage. Science 1985;229:185–7.
194 Collen D. Staphylokinase: a potent, uniquely fibrin-selective thrombolytic agent. Nat Med 1998;4:279–84.
195 Narita S, Kaneko J, Chiba J *et al*. Phage conversion of Panton–Valentine leukocidin in *Staphylococcus aureus*: molecular analysis of a PVL-converting phage, phiSLT. Gene 2001;268:195–206.
196 Labandeira-Rey M, Couzon F, Boisset S *et al*. *Staphylococcus aureus* Panton Valentine leukocidin causes necrotizing pneumonia. Science 2007;315:1130–3.
197 Voyich JM, Otto M, Mathema B *et al*. Is Panton–Valentine leukocidin the major virulence determinant in community-associated methicillin-resistant *Staphylococcus aureus* disease? J Infect Dis 2006;194:1761–70.
198 Wardenburg JB, Bae T, Otto M, Deleo FR, Schneewind O. Poring over pores: alpha-hemolysin and Panton–Valentine leukocidin in *Staphylococcus aureus* pneumonia. Nat Med 2007;13:1405–6.
199 Iandolo JJ, Worrell V, Groicher KH *et al*. Comparative analysis of the genomes of the temperate bacteriophages phi 11, phi 12 and phi 13 of *Staphylococcus aureus* 8325. Gene 2002;289:109–18.
200 Lindsay JA, Ruzin A, Ross HF, Kurepina N, Novick RP. The gene for toxic shock toxin is carried by a family of mobile pathogenicity islands in *Staphylococcus aureus*. Mol Microbiol 1998;29:527–43.
201 Ubeda C, Maiques E, Knecht E, Lasa I, Novick RP, Penades JR. Antibiotic-induced SOS response promotes horizontal

dissemination of pathogenicity island-encoded virulence factors in staphylococci. Mol Microbiol 2005;56:836–44.

202 Sumby P, Waldor MK. Transcription of the toxin genes present within the staphylococcal phage phiSa3ms is intimately linked with the phage's life cycle. J Bacteriol 2003;185:6841–51.

203 Carroll D, Kehoe MA, Cavanagh D, Coleman DC. Novel organization of the site-specific integration and excision recombination functions of the *Staphylococcus aureus* serotype F virulence-converting phages phi 13 and phi 42. Mol Microbiol 1995;16:877–93.

204 Lee CY, Iandolo JJ. Integration of staphylococcal phage L54a occurs by site-specific recombination: structural analysis of the attachment sites. Proc Natl Acad Sci USA 1986;83:5474–8.

205 Coleman DC, Sullivan DJ, Russell RJ, Arbuthnott JP, Carey BF, Pomeroy HM. *Staphylococcus aureus* bacteriophages mediating the simultaneous lysogenic conversion of beta-lysin, staphylokinase and enterotoxin A: molecular mechanism of triple conversion. J Gen Microbiol 1989;135:1679–97.

206 Novick RP. Analysis by transduction of mutations affecting penicillinase formation in *Staphylococcus aureus*. J Gen Microbiol 1963;33:121–36.

207 Prevost G, Couppie P, Prevost P *et al*. Epidemiological data on *Staphylococcus aureus* strains producing synergohymenotropic toxins. J Med Microbiol 1995;42:237–45.

208 O'Hara FP, Guex N, Word JM *et al*. A geographic variant of the *Staphylococcus aureus* Panton–Valentine leukocidin toxin and the origin of community-associated methicillin-resistant *S. aureus* USA300. J Infect Dis 2008;197:187–94.

209 Diep BA, Stone GG, Basuino L *et al*. The ACME and SCC*mec* linkage: convergence of virulence and resistance in the USA300 clone of methicillin-resistant *Staphylococcus aureus*. J Infect Dis 2008;197:1523–30.

210 Wang R, Braughton KR, Kretschmer D *et al*. Identification of novel cytolytic peptides as key virulence determinants for community-associated MRSA. Nat Med 2007;13:1510–14.

211 Dobrindt U, Hochhut B, Hentschel U, Hacker J. Genomic islands in pathogenic and environmental microorganisms. Nat Rev Microbiol 2004;2:414–24.

212 Blum G, Ott M, Lischewski A *et al*. Excision of large DNA regions termed pathogenicity islands from tRNA-specific loci in the chromosome of an *Escherichia coli* wild-type pathogen. Infect Immun 1994;62:606–14.

213 Hacker J, Blum-Oehler G, Muhldorfer I, Tschape H. Pathogenicity islands of virulent bacteria: structure, function and impact on microbial evolution. Mol Microbiol 1997;23:1089–97.

214 Yarwood JM, McCormick JK, Paustian ML, Kapur V, Schlievert PM. Repression of the *Staphylococcus aureus* accessory gene regulator in serum and in vivo. J Bacteriol 2002;184:1095–101.

215 Novick RP. Plasmid incompatibility. Microbiol Rev 1987; 51:381–95.

216 Ruzin A, Lindsay J, Novick RP. Molecular genetics of SaPI1: a mobile pathogenicity island in *Staphylococcus aureus*. Mol Microbiol 2001;41:365–77.

217 Sebulsky MT, Speziali CD, Shilton BH, Edgell DR, Heinrichs DE. FhuD1, a ferric hydroxamate-binding lipoprotein in *Staphylococcus aureus*: a case of gene duplication and lateral transfer. J Biol Chem 2004;279:53152–9.

218 Baba T, Bae T, Schneewind O, Takeuchi F, Hiramatsu K. Genome sequence of *Staphylococcus aureus* strain Newman and comparative analysis of staphylococcal genomes: polymorphism and evolution of two major pathogenicity islands. J Bacteriol 2008;190:300–10.

219 Williams RJ, Ward JM, Henderson B *et al*. Identification of a novel gene cluster encoding staphylococcal exotoxin-like proteins: characterization of the prototypic gene and its protein product, SET1. Infect Immun 2000;68:4407–15.

220 Lina G, Bohach GA, Nair SP, Hiramatsu K, Jouvin-Marche E, Mariuzza R. Standard nomenclature for the superantigens expressed by *Staphylococcus*. J Infect Dis 2004;189:2334–6.

221 Reed SB, Wesson CA, Liou LE *et al*. Molecular characterization of a novel *Staphylococcus aureus* serine protease operon. Infect Immun 2001;69:1521–7.

222 Gravet A, Colin DA, Keller D, Girardot R, Monteil H, Prevost G. Characterization of a novel structural member, LukE-LukD, of the bi-component staphylococcal leucotoxins family. FEBS Lett 1998;436:202–8.

223 Thomas DY, Jarraud S, Lemercier B *et al*. Staphylococcal enterotoxin-like toxins U2 and V, two new staphylococcal superantigens arising from recombination within the enterotoxin gene cluster. Infect Immun 2006;74:4724–34.

224 Fitzgerald JR, Reid SD, Ruotsalainen E *et al*. Genome diversification in *Staphylococcus aureus*: molecular evolution of a highly variable chromosomal region encoding the staphylococcal exotoxin-like family of proteins. Infect Immun 2003; 71:2827–38.

225 Novick RP. Staphylococcal plasmids and their replication. Annu Rev Microbiol 1989;43:537–65.

226 Khan SA, Novick RP. Complete nucleotide sequence of pT181, a tetracycline-resistance plasmid from *Staphylococcus aureus*. Plasmid 1983;10:251–9.

227 Shalita Z, Murphy E, Novick RP. Penicillinase plasmids of *Staphylococcus aureus*: structural and evolutionary relationships. Plasmid 1980;3:291–311.

228 Thomas WD Jr, Archer GL. Identification and cloning of the conjugative transfer region of *Staphylococcus aureus* plasmid pGO1. J Bacteriol 1989;171:684–91.

229 Townsend DE, Bolton S, Ashdown N, Grubb WB. Transfer of plasmid-borne aminoglycoside-resistance determinants in staphylococci. J Med Microbiol 1985;20:169–85.

230 Archer GL, Coughter JP, Johnston JL. Plasmid-encoded trimethoprim resistance in staphylococci. Antimicrob Agents Chemother 1986;29:733–40.

231 Bayles KW, Iandolo JJ. Genetic and molecular analyses of the gene encoding staphylococcal enterotoxin D. J Bacteriol 1989; 171:4799–806.

232 Zhang S, Iandolo JJ, Stewart GC. The enterotoxin D plasmid of *Staphylococcus aureus* encodes a second enterotoxin determinant (sej). FEMS Microbiol Lett 1998;168:227–33.

233 Yamaguchi T, Hayashi T, Takami H *et al*. Complete nucleotide sequence of a *Staphylococcus aureus* exfoliative toxin B plasmid and identification of a novel ADP-ribosyltransferase, EDIN-C. Infect Immun 2001;69:7760–71.

234 Lindsay JA, Holden MT. Understanding the rise of the superbug: investigation of the evolution and genomic variation of *Staphylococcus aureus*. Funct Integr Genomics 2006;6:186–201.

235 Rowland SJ, Dyke KG. Characterization of the staphylococcal beta-lactamase transposon Tn552. EMBO J 1989;8:2761–73.

236 Anon. *Staphylococcus aureus* resistant to vancomycin: United States, 2002. MMWR 2002;51:565–7.

237 Anon. Vancomycin-resistant *Staphylococcus aureus*: Pennsylvania, 2002. MMWR 2002;51:902.
238 Chang S, Sievert DM, Hageman JC *et al.* Infection with vancomycin-resistant *Staphylococcus aureus* containing the vanA resistance gene. N Engl J Med 2003;348:1342–7.
239 Weigel LM, Clewell DB, Gill SR *et al.* Genetic analysis of a high-level vancomycin-resistant isolate of *Staphylococcus aureus*. Science 2003;302:1569–71.
240 Clewell DB, An FY, White BA, Gawron-Burke C. *Streptococcus faecalis* sex pheromone (cAM373) also produced by *Staphylococcus aureus* and identification of a conjugative transposon (Tn918). J Bacteriol 1985;162:1212–20.
241 Hanssen AM, Kjeldsen G, Sollid JU. Local variants of staphylococcal cassette chromosome mec in sporadic methicillin-resistant *Staphylococcus aureus* and methicillin-resistant coagulase-negative staphylococci: evidence of horizontal gene transfer? Antimicrob Agents Chemother 2004;48:285–96.
242 Wielders CL, Vriens MR, Brisse S *et al.* In-vivo transfer of mecA DNA to *Staphylococcus aureus*. Lancet 2001;357:1674–5.
243 Wisplinghoff H, Rosato AE, Enright MC, Noto M, Craig W, Archer GL. Related clones containing SCCmec type IV predominate among clinically significant *Staphylococcus epidermidis* isolates. Antimicrob Agents Chemother 2003;47:3574–9.
244 Robinson DA, Enright MC. Evolutionary models of the emergence of methicillin-resistant *Staphylococcus aureus*. Antimicrob Agents Chemother 2003;47:3926–34.
245 Katayama Y, Robinson DA, Enright MC, Chambers HF. Genetic background affects stability of *mecA* in *Staphylococcus aureus*. J Clin Microbiol 2005;43:2380–3.
246 Katayama Y, Zhang HZ, Hong D, Chambers HF. Jumping the barrier to beta-lactam resistance in *Staphylococcus aureus*. J Bacteriol 2003;185:5465–72.
247 Lindsay JA, Holden MTG. *Staphylococcus aureus*: superbug, super genome? Trends Microbiol 2004;12:378.
248 Ma XX, Ito T, Tiensasitorn C *et al.* Novel type of staphylococcal cassette chromosome *mec* identified in community-acquired methicillin-resistant *Staphylococcus aureus* strains. Antimicrob Agents Chemother 2002;46:1147–52.
249 Katayama Y, Takeuchi F, Ito T *et al.* Identification in methicillin-susceptible *Staphylococcus hominis* of an active primordial mobile genetic element for the staphylococcal cassette chromosome mec of methicillin-resistant *Staphylococcus aureus*. J Bacteriol 2003;185:2711–22.
250 O'Brien FG, Price C, Grubb WB, Gustafson JE. Genetic characterization of the fusidic acid and cadmium resistance determinants of *Staphylococcus aureus* plasmid pUB101. J Antimicrob Chemother 2002;50:313–21.
251 Seybold U, Kourbatova EV, Johnson JG *et al.* Emergence of community-associated methicillin-resistant *Staphylococcus aureus* USA300 genotype as a major cause of health care-associated blood stream infections. Clin Infect Dis 2006;42:647–56.
252 de Lencastre H, Oliveira D, Tomasz A. Antibiotic resistant *Staphylococcus aureus*: a paradigm of adaptive power. Curr Opin Microbiol 2007;10:428–35.
253 Ito T, Okuma K, Ma XX, Yuzawa H, Hiramatsu K. Insights on antibiotic resistance of *Staphylococcus aureus* from its whole genome: genomic island SCC. Drug Resist Updat 2003;6:41–52.
254 Levin BR. Periodic selection, infectious gene exchange and the genetic structure of *E. coli* populations. Genetics 1981;99:1–23.
255 Achtman M. Microevolution and epidemic spread of serogroup A *Neisseria meningitidis*: a review. Gene 1997;192:135–40.
256 Gutacker MM, Mathema B, Soini H *et al.* Single-nucleotide polymorphism-based population genetic analysis of *Mycobacterium tuberculosis* strains from 4 geographic sites. J Infect Dis 2006;193:121–8.
257 Suerbaum S, Smith JM, Bapumia K *et al.* Free recombination within *Helicobacter pylori*. Proc Natl Acad Sci USA 1998; 95:12619–24.
258 Musser JM. Molecular population genetic analysis of emerged bacterial pathogens: selected insights. Emerg Infect Dis 1996; 2:1–17.
259 Selander RK, Beltran P, Smith NH *et al.* Genetic population structure, clonal phylogeny, and pathogenicity of *Salmonella paratyphi B*. Infect Immun 1990;58:1891–901.
260 Selander RK, Beltran P, Smith NH *et al.* Evolutionary genetic relationships of clones of *Salmonella* serovars that cause human typhoid and other enteric fevers. Infect Immun 1990;58:2262–75.
261 Grundmann H, Hori S, Enright MC *et al.* Determining the genetic structure of the natural population of *Staphylococcus aureus*: a comparison of multilocus sequence typing with pulsed-field gel electrophoresis, randomly amplified polymorphic DNA analysis, and phage typing. J Clin Microbiol 2002;40:4544–6.
262 Feil EJ, Spratt BG. Recombination and the population structures of bacterial pathogens. Annu Rev Microbiol 2001;55:561–90.
263 Mwangi MM, Wu SW, Zhou Y *et al.* Tracking the in vivo evolution of multidrug resistance in *Staphylococcus aureus* by whole-genome sequencing. Proc Natl Acad Sci USA 2007;104:9451–6.
264 Highlander SK, Hulten KG, Qin X *et al.* Subtle genetic changes enhance virulence of methicillin resistant and sensitive *Staphylococcus aureus*. BMC Microbiol 2007;7:99.
265 Feil EJ. Small change: keeping pace with microevolution. Nat Rev Microbiol 2004;2:483–95.
266 Cohan FM. What are bacterial species? Annu Rev Microbiol 2002;56:457–87.
267 Gevers D, Cohan FM, Lawrence JG *et al.* Opinion: Re-evaluating prokaryotic species. Nat Rev Microbiol 2005;3:733–9.
268 Lindsay JA, Moore CE, Day NP *et al.* Microarrays reveal that each of the ten dominant lineages of *Staphylococcus aureus* has a unique combination of surface-associated and regulatory genes. J Bacteriol 2006;188:669–76.
269 Crisostomo MI, Westh H, Tomasz A, Chung M, Oliveira DC, de Lencastre H. The evolution of methicillin resistance in *Staphylococcus aureus*: similarity of genetic backgrounds in historically early methicillin-susceptible and -resistant isolates and contemporary epidemic clones. Proc Natl Acad Sci USA 2001;98:9865–70.
270 Oliveira DC, Tomasz A, de Lencastre H. The evolution of pandemic clones of methicillin-resistant *Staphylococcus aureus*: identification of two ancestral genetic backgrounds and the associated *mec* elements. Microb Drug Resist 2001;7:349–61.
271 Robinson DA, Enright MC. Multilocus sequence typing and the evolution of methicillin-resistant *Staphylococcus aureus*. Clin Microbiol Infect 2004;10:92–7.
272 Stewart GT, Holt RJ. Evolution of natural resistance to the newer penicillins. BMJ 1963;5326:308–11.
273 Chambers HF. The changing epidemiology of *Staphylococcus aureus*? Emerg Infect Dis 2001;7:178–82.

274 Enright MC, Robinson DA, Randle G, Feil EJ, Grundmann H, Spratt BG. The evolutionary history of methicillin-resistant *Staphylococcus aureus* (MRSA). Proc Natl Acad Sci USA 2002; 99:7687–92.

275 Robinson DA, Kearns AM, Holmes A *et al*. Re-emergence of early pandemic *Staphylococcus aureus* as a community-acquired meticillin-resistant clone. Lancet 2005;365:1256–8.

276 Donahue JA, Baldwin JN. Hemolysin and leukocidin production by 80/81 strains of *Staphylococcus aureus*. J Infect Dis 1966;116:324–8.

277 Rountree PM, Beard MA. Further observations on infection with phage type 80 staphylococci in Australia. Med J Aust 1958;45:789–95.

278 Light IJ, Walton RL, Sutherland JM, Shinefield HR, Brackvogel V. Use of bacterial interference to control a staphylococcal nursery outbreak. Deliberate colonization of all infants with the 502A strain of *Staphylococcus aureus*. Am J Dis Child 1967;113: 291–300.

279 Coombs GW, Nimmo GR, Bell JM *et al*. Genetic diversity among community methicillin-resistant *Staphylococcus aureus* strains causing outpatient infections in Australia. J Clin Microbiol 2004;42:4735–43.

280 Tamura K, Dudley J, Nei M, Kumar S. MEGA4: Molecular Evolutionary Genetics Analysis (MEGA) software version 4.0. Mol Biol Evol 2007;24:1596–9.

281 Schleifer KH, Kilpper-Bälz R, Devriese LA. *Staphylococcus arlettae* sp. nov., *S. equorum* sp. nov. and *S. kloosii* sp. nov.: three new coagulase-negative, novobiocin-resistant species from animals. Syst Appl Microbiol 1985;5:501–9.

282 De la Fuente R, Suarez G, Schleifer KH. *Staphylococcus aureus* subsp. *anaerobius* subsp. nov., the causal agent of abscess disease of sheep. Int J Syst Bacteriol 1985;35:99–102.

283 Kloos WE, Schleifer KH. *Staphylococcus auricularis* sp. nov.: an inhabitant of the human external ear. Int J Syst Bacteriol 1983;33:9–14.

284 Kloos WE, Schleifer KH. Isolation and characterization of staphylococci from human skin. II. Description of four new species: *Staphylococcus warneri*, *Staphylococcus capitis*, *Staphylococcus hominis*, and *Staphylococcus simulans*. Int J Syst Bacteriol 1975;25:62–79.

285 Bannerman TL, Kloos WE. *Staphylococcus capitis* subsp. *ureolyticus* subsp. nov. from human skin. Int J Syst Bacteriol 1991;41:144–7.

286 Devriese LA, Poutrel B, Kilpper-Bälz R, Schleifer KH. *Staphylococcus gallinarum* and *Staphylococcus caprae*, two new species from animals. Int J Syst Bacteriol 1983;33:480–6.

287 Schleifer KH, Fischer U. Description of a new species of the genus *Staphylococcus*: *Staphylococcus carnosus*. Int J Syst Bacteriol 1982;32:153–6.

288 Probst AJ, Hertel C, Richter L, Wassill L, Ludwig W, Hammes WP. *Staphylococcus condimenti* sp. nov., from soy sauce mash, and *Staphylococcus carnosus* (Schleifer and Fischer 1982) subsp. utilis subsp. nov. Int J Syst Bacteriol 1998;48:651–8.

289 Devriese LA, Hajec V, Oeding P, Meyer SA, Schleifer KH. *Staphylococcus hyicus* (Sompolinsky 1953) comb. nov. and *Staphylococcus hyicus* subsp. chromogenes subsp. nov. Int J Syst Bacteriol 1978;28:482–90.

290 Schleifer KH, Kloos WE. Isolation and characterization of staphylococci from human skin. I. Amended descriptions of *Staphylococcus epidermidis* and *Staphylococcus saprophyticus* and descriptions of three new species: *Staphylococcus cohnii*, *Staphylococcus haemolyticus*, and *Staphylococcus xylosus*. Int J Syst Bacteriol 1975;26:50–61.

291 Kloos WE, Wolfshohl JF. *Staphylococcus cohnii* subspecies: *Staphylococcus cohnii* subsp. cohnii subsp. nov. and *Staphylococcus cohnii* subsp. *urealyticum* subsp. nov. Int J Syst Bacteriol 1991;41:284–9.

292 Varaldo PE, Kilpper-Bälz R, Biavasco F, Satta G, Schleifer KH. *Staphylococcus delphini* sp. nov., a coagulase-positive species isolated from dolphins. Int J Syst Bacteriol 1988;38:436–9.

293 Place RB, Hiestand D, Gallmann HR, Teuber M. *Staphylococcus equorum* subsp. *linens*, subsp. nov., a starter culture component for surface ripened semi-hard cheeses. Syst Appl Microbiol 2003;26:30–7.

294 Igimi S, Kawamura S, Takahashi E, Mitsuoka T. *Staphylococcus felis*, a new species from clinical specimens from cats. Int J Syst Bacteriol 1989;39:373–7.

295 Vernozy-Rozand C, Mazuy C, Meugnier H *et al*. *Staphylococcus fleurettii* sp. nov., isolated from goat's milk cheeses. Int J Syst Evol Microbiol 2000;50:1521–7.

296 Hájek V. *Staphylococcus intermedius*, a new species isolated from animals. Int J Syst Bacteriol 1976;26:401–8.

297 Kloos WE, Schleifer KH, Smith RF. Characterization of *Staphylococcus sciuri* sp. nov. and its subspecies. Int J Syst Bacteriol 1976;26:22–37.

298 Freney J, Brun Y, Bes M *et al*. *Staphylococcus lugdunensis* sp. nov. and *Staphylococcus schleiferi* sp. nov., two species from human clinical specimens. Int J Syst Bacteriol 1988;38:168–72.

299 Foster G, Ross HM, Hutson RA, Collins MD. *Staphylococcus lutrae* sp. nov., a new coagulase-positive species isolated from otters. Int J Syst Bacteriol 1997;47:724–6.

300 Hajek V, Ludwig W, Schleifer KH *et al*. *Staphylococcus muscae*, a new species isolated from flies. Int J Syst Bacteriol 1992;42:97–101.

301 Spergser J, Wieser M, Taubel M, Rossello-Mora RA, Rosengarten R, Busse HJ. *Staphylococcus nepalensis* sp. nov., isolated from goats of the Himalayan region. Int J Syst Evol Microbiol 2003;53:2007–11.

302 Chesneau O, Morvan A, Grimont F, Labischinski H, el Solh N. *Staphylococcus pasteuri* sp. nov., isolated from human, animal, and food specimens. Int J Syst Bacteriol 1993;43:237–44.

303 Trulzsch K, Grabein B, Schumann P *et al*. *Staphylococcus pettenkoferi* sp. nov., a novel coagulase-negative staphylococcal species isolated from human clinical specimens. Int J Syst Evol Microbiol 2007;57:1543–8.

304 Tanasupawat S, Hashimoto Y, Ezaki T, Kozaki M, Komagata K. *Staphylococcus piscifermentans* sp. nov., from fermented fish in Thailand. Int J Syst Bacteriol 1992;42:577–81.

305 Devriese LA, Vancanneyt M, Baele M *et al*. *Staphylococcus pseudintermedius* sp. nov., a coagulase-positive species from animals. Int J Syst Evol Microbiol 2005;55:1569–73.

306 Zakrzewska-Czerwinska J, Gaszewska-Mastalarz A, Lis B, Gamian A, Mordarski M. *Staphylococcus pulvereri* sp. nov., isolated from human and animal specimens. Int J Syst Bacteriol 1995;45:169–72.

307 Fairbrother RW. Coagulase production as a criterion for the classification of the staphylococci. J Pathol Bacteriol 1940; 50:83–8.

308 Hajek V, Meugnier H, Bes M *et al*. *Staphylococcus saprophyticus* subsp. *bovis* subsp. nov., isolated from bovine nostrils. Int J Syst Bacteriol 1996;46:792–6.

309 Igimi S, Takahashi E, Mitsuoka T. *Staphylococcus schleiferi* subsp. *coagulans* subsp. nov., isolated from the external auditory meatus of dogs with external ear otitis. Int J Syst Bacteriol 1990;40:409–11.

310 Kloos WE, Ballard DN, Webster JA *et al*. Ribotype delineation and description of *Staphylococcus sciuri* subspecies and their potential as reservoirs of methicillin resistance and staphylolytic enzyme genes. Int J Syst Bacteriol 1997;47:313–23.

311 Webster JA, Bannerman TL, Hubner RJ *et al*. Identification of the *Staphylococcus sciuri* species group with *Eco*RI fragments containing rRNA sequences and description of *Staphylococcus vitulus* sp. nov. Int J Syst Bacteriol 1994;44:454–60.

312 Zhang YQ, Ren SX, Li HL *et al*. Genome-based analysis of virulence genes in a non-biofilm-forming *Staphylococcus epidermidis* strain (ATCC 12228). Mol Microbiol 2003;49:1577–93.

313 Kuroda M, Yamashita A, Hirakawa H *et al*. Whole genome sequence of *Staphylococcus saprophyticus* reveals the pathogenesis of uncomplicated urinary tract infection. Proc Natl Acad Sci USA 2005;102:13272–7.

314 Fischetti VA, Novick RP, Ferretti JJ, Portnoy DA, Rood JI. Grampositive Pathogens, 2nd edn. Washington DC: ASM Press, 2006.

315 Hiramatsu K, Aritaka N, Hanaki H *et al*. Dissemination in Japanese hospitals of strains of *Staphylococcus aureus* heterogeneously resistant to vancomycin. Lancet 1997;350:1670–3.

316 Rosenstein R, Nerz C, Biswas L, Resch A, Raddatz G, Schuster SC, Götz F. Genome analysis of the meat starter culture bacterium Staphylococcus carnosus TM300. Appl Environ Microbiol. 2009 Feb; 75(3):811–22.

317 Baba T, Kuwahara-Arai K, Uchiyama I, Takeuchi F, Ito T, Hiramatsu K. Complete genome sequence of Macrococcus caseolyticus strain JCSCS5402, reflecting the ancestral genome of the human-pathogenic staphylococci. J Bacteriol. 2009 Feb; 191(4):1180–90.

Chapter 4
Molecular Basis of Pathogenicity

Mark S. Smeltzer[1], *Chia Y. Lee*[1], *Nada Harik*[2] *and Mark E. Hart*[3]

[1] Department of Microbiology and Immunology, University of Arkansas for Medical Sciences, Little Rock, Arkansas, USA
[2] Department of Pediatrics, Arkansas Children's Hospital, Little Rock, Arkansas, USA
[3] National Center for Toxicological Research, Division of Microbiology, Jefferson, Arkansas, USA

Introduction

Although all staphylococcal species are capable of causing disease, *Staphylococcus aureus* is clearly the predominant pathogen. The classic distinction between *S. aureus* and most other species is the production of coagulase, but there is little evidence to suggest that this accounts for its pathogenic predominance. Indeed, studies that directly examined this issue concluded that mutation of the coagulase gene (*coa*) itself has little impact on virulence [1–4]. The enhanced virulence of *S. aureus* relative to other staphylococcal species must therefore be a function of other factors. Comparison of the genomes of *S. aureus* and the coagulase-negative species *S. epidermidis* demonstrated that they share a syntenic core genome that includes 1681 open-reading frames (ORFs) but that *S. aureus* has strain-dependent combinations of 18 "genome islands," each of which encodes various virulence factors and most of which are absent in *S. epidermidis* [5]. One general observation in this regard is that many of these virulence factors contribute to the subversion of host defenses [6]. This may explain, at least in part, why disease caused by *S. epidermidis* is primarily limited to biofilm-associated infections, with the biofilm itself providing a certain level of intrinsic resistance to host defenses [6,7]. At the same time, it is important to recognize the dynamic nature of the staphylococcal genome and the fact that most types of virulence factor are represented to some degree in both *S. aureus* and at least some strains of coagulase-negative species [5].

Our overall goal in this chapter is to summarize current knowledge of the involvement of specific *S. aureus* virulence factors in ability to cause disease (Table 4.1). It is important to recognize from the outset that different studies have often reached contradictory conclusions. For instance, while α-toxin is an important virulence factor of *S. aureus* [8–16], strains that do not produce α-toxin are capable of causing disease [17,18], and one report concluded that "hyperproduction" of α-toxin results in decreased virulence in a rabbit endocarditis model [19]. One reason for such contradictory results is strain-dependent variability, which is discussed in some detail below. The other is the simple observation that all staphylococcal species, including *S. aureus*, are opportunistic pathogens, and by definition disease caused by such pathogens is an algebraic equation. There are, after all, multiple ways to add two things to get the same result, and the only way to define one of these things (e.g., the bacterial part of the equation) is to know the other (e.g., the host part of the equation). Indeed, medical advances of the twentieth and twenty-first centuries have had the paradoxical effect of keeping people alive under circumstances that, from an infectious disease point of view, make the bacterial pathogen the lesser part of the equation.

Is there a *Staphylococcus aureus* virulence paradigm?

Much of the work to identify the *S. aureus* virulence factors that define its pathogenicity has been done with a limited number of strains, the most prominent of which are derived directly from NCTC-8325 [20]. Examples include RN4220, which is a chemically mutagenized strain used almost universally by staphylococcal geneticists as a primary transformation host, and 8325-4, which was generated by curing the ϕ11, ϕ12, and ϕ13 prophages from the 8325 chromosome. The relatedness of these strains, together with the fact that RN4220 is a restriction-deficient strain that more readily accepts foreign DNA [20,21], make it relatively easy to carry out primary manipulations in RN4220 and to then move the relevant constructs into 8325-4 strains by electroporation or phage-mediated transduction. However, important differences exist between 8325-derived strains and clinical isolates of *S. aureus* [17,22]. One example is the absence of ϕ13, which is one of a group of temperate phages that integrate into the *S. aureus* chromosome via an *att* site within the gene (*hlb*) encoding β-toxin [23–25]. The curing of ϕ13 to generate 8325-4 therefore restored the capacity to produce β-toxin. This is

Staphylococci in Human Disease, 2nd edition. Edited by Kent B. Crossley, Kimberly K. Jefferson, Gordon Archer, Vance G. Fowler, Jr.
 ISBN 978-14051-6332-3.

Table 4.1 Virulence factors of *S. aureus*.[1]

Gene	Product	Study	Role in virulence
Cell wall components	Teichoic acid	Animal model [79]	Nasal colonization
	Lipoteichoic acid	Animal model [92]	Septic shock
		Cell culture [86–91]	
	Peptidoglycan	Animal model [92]	Septic shock
		Cell culture [89]	
Surface adhesins			
cna	Collagen adhesin	Epidemiological [42, 46, 166]	Adhesin: collagen
		Animal model [167–172]	
bbp	Bone sialoprotein-binding protein	Epidemiological [48]	Adhesin: bone sialoprotein
sdrE	Serine–aspartate-rich protein E	Epidemiological [46]	Adhesin: unknown
spa	Protein A	Cell culture [114]	Inhibits opsonophagocytosis
		Animal model [115]	Binds TNFR1
fnbA, fnB	Fibronectin-binding proteins A and B	Epidemiological [46, 117]	Adhesin: fibronectin
		Animal model [123, 127–130]	
clfA, clfB	Clumping factors A and B	Animal model [2, 129, 145, 147]	Adhesin: fibrinogen
			Nasal colonization
		Cell culture [148, 149]	Evasion of phagocytosis
sdrC, sdrD, sdrE	Serine–aspartate repeat proteins	Epidemiological [157]	Adhesin: unknown
sas genes	*S. aureus* surface proteins	Epidemiological [47]	Adhesin: unknown
		Animal model [178]	SasG: biofilm
			SasA: platelet binding
Secreted adhesins			
efb	Extracellular fibrinogen-binding protein		
emp	Extracellular matrix-binding protein		
eap (*map, p70*)	Extracellular adhesive protein (EAP)	*In vitro* [190]	
		Cell culture [192, 193]	
		Animal model [192, 194]	
Exopolysaccharides			
cap genes	Capsular polysaccharide	Animal model [202, 205–210]	Inhibits opsonophagocytosis
icaADBC	Polysaccharide intercellular adhesin	*In vitro* [228, 231]	Biofilm formation
		Epidemiological [46]	Resistance to phagocytosis and antimicrobial peptides
Exotoxins			
hla	α-Toxin	Animal model [8–16, 248]	Cell lysis
hlb	β-Toxin	Animal model [248]	Cell lysis
hld	δ-Toxin	Animal model [70]	Cell lysis
lukF-PV, lukS-PV	Panton–Valentine leukotoxin	Animal model [15, 68–70]	
etA, etB, etC, etD	Exfoliative toxins	[255–258]	Sloughing of superficial dermal layer
			Immune evasion through superantigenicity
tstH	Toxic shock syndrome toxin (TSST)-1	Animal model [248]	Superantigenicity
seA, seB, seC, seD, seE, seG, sel selH, and *sel-J-sel-V*	Staphylococcal enterotoxins	Animal model [248, 249]	Superantigenicity
			Emesis
Enzymes			
sspA	Serine protease	Animal model [34]	Unknown
sspB	Cysteine protease	Animal model [34]	Unknown
clpX, clpP	ClpX, ClpP	[295, 296]	Virulence factor regulation
Iron acquisition			
isd genes	Iron-responsive surface determinants	Animal model [109, 334]	Hemoglobin binding
sbnABCDEFGHI	Staphylobactin	Animal model [315]	Siderophore
stbA	Staphylococcal transferrin-binding protein A	*In vitro* [326]	Transferrin binding
Regulators			
agr	Accessory gene regulator	Animal model [398–403]	Quorum sensing
sar genes	Staphylococcal accessory regulator	*In vitro* [73, 359, 361, 389, 422–425]	Regulation of Agr
		Animal model [42, 400, 438, 439]	Regulation of extracellular and surface-associated virulence factors
saeRS	*S. aureus* exoprotein expression	Animal model [464]	Regulation of exotoxins
srrAB	Staphylococcal respiratory response	Animal model [471–473]	Response to oxygen levels
vraSR	Two-component response regulator	*In vitro* [348]	Regulation of Agr
		In vitro [484–486]	Response to cell wall-active antibiotics; increases resistance to vancomycin and β-lactams
graRS	Two-component response regulator	*In vitro* [490, 491]	Resistance to vancomycin and antimicrobial peptides
apsRS	Two-component response regulator	Animal model [491]	Resistance to antimicrobial peptides
alsSD	Two-component response regulator	*In vitro* [17, 496]	Cell wall integrity and biofilm formation
Spx	Regulation of metabolic pathways	*In vitro*	Stress response, biofilm formation
Msa	Modulator of *sarA*	*In vitro* [503]	Increases expression of *sarA* and virulence factors under *sarA* control
murF	Peptidoglycan synthesis	*In vitro* [506]	Affects expression of cell-associated and extracellular virulence factors

[1] The table lists factors of *S. aureus* that have been implicated in virulence and the models that suggest their role in virulence. Note that studies exist which challenge the role of some of these factors in virulence and that only supportive studies are shown here. The reader is referred to the text for references to contradictory studies. TNFR, tumor necrosis factor α receptor.

relevant in that the vast majority of human clinical isolates are lysogenized and consequently β-toxin negative [25–27]. Conversely, the group of phages that utilize the *hlb att* site also positively convert for various combinations of genes (e.g., *sea, sak, scn, chp*) that contribute to virulence and the subversion of host defenses [25,28].

All strains derived from 8325 also carry mutations in at least two genes (*rsbU* and *tcaR*) that modulate the production of specific *S. aureus* virulence factors [29–34]. Once again, contradictions exist in that some studies have concluded that the *rsbU* mutation, or more precisely the impact of the *rsbU* mutation on production of the alternative sigma factor SigB, has no impact on virulence [30,35,36], while others found that mutation of *rsbU* or *sigB* results in reduced capacity to cause disease [37]. In comparison with the global impact of *sigB*, the role of *tcaR* appears to be more limited [33,38–40]. We used genome-scale transcriptional profiling to compare the most commonly studied 8325-4 strain (RN6390) with a clinical isolate (UAMS-1) that does not have the *rsbU* or *tcaR* mutations and identified almost 300 genes that were present in both strains but which were differentially expressed in a strain-dependent manner [17,22]. Less than half of these were identified as part of the *sigB* regulon in independent genome-scale transcriptional profiling experiments [39]. To date, there are no published transcriptional profiling studies comparing clinical isolates, but comparisons based on gene content demonstrate that about 20% of the *S. aureus* genome differs in a strain-dependent manner [22,41]. This translates to over 500 variable genes among clinical isolates, some of which also serve regulatory roles [41].

A number of studies have attempted to determine whether a correlation exists between the occurrence of these variable genes and virulence. For instance, Booth *et al.* [42] examined 405 clinical isolates using pulsed-field gel electrophoresis (PFGE) and identified 90 "lineages," five of which accounted for more than 65% of all infections. Three of these five were characterized by the presence of the collagen-binding adhesin gene *cna*, which is absent in most strains including those derived from 8325 [43–45]. A subsequent study examined the distribution of 33 genes encoding recognized virulence factors among a total of 334 strains and found that *cna* was one of seven genes that was more common among invasive isolates [46]. Booth *et al.* [42] also found that none of the strains in *cna*-positive lineages encoded the fibronectin-binding protein gene *fnbB*. Given the conservation of *fnbA* (see below), and the fact that the presence of one or both *fnb* genes has little impact on the ability to bind fibronectin [46], this would not be expected to have a phenotypic effect in terms of binding fibronectin. However, the absence of *fnbB* remains potentially significant in that it is part of a "region of difference" (RD5) that also includes the surface-associated protein SasG and the regulatory elements *sarT* and *sarU* [41,47].

More recently, Otsuka *et al.* [48] examined strains from 15 clonal lineages of community-acquired methicillin-resistant *Staphylococcus aureus* (CA-MRSA), all of which were defined as prominent clinical isolates on a continent-specific if not global scale, and nine of these 15, including all five of the pandemic lineages, were found to encode *cna*. All five pandemic lineages were also found to lack *fnbB*. While this study focused specifically on genes encoding adhesins, the latter implies the absence of RD5 and therefore the absence of the RD5-linked genes *sasG*, *sarT* and *sarU*. Otsuka *et al.* [48] also found that all pandemic lineages encode *bbp*, which encodes an adhesin that binds bone sialoprotein [49]. It was suggested that the presence of *bbp*, perhaps in combination with *cna*, might promote colonization and spread to the point that such strains become pandemic.

While such studies suggest that certain clonal lineages of *S. aureus* are prominent if not predominant causes of infection, there are contradictory reports. For example, using genome-scale microarrays, Lindsay *et al.* [50] identified 10 dominant lineages of *S. aureus*, each of which was distinguished by "a unique combination of 'core variable' (CV) genes scattered throughout the chromosome," but in no case was any specific lineage or gene found to be associated with invasive disease. Similarly, Feil *et al.* [51] concluded on the basis of multilocus sequence typing (MLST), which focuses on sequence divergence in seven unrelated housekeeping genes contained within the core genome [52,53], that there were no significant correlations between different clonal lineages and commensal versus invasive isolates. Most recently, Feng *et al.* [54] also failed to find any genotypic distinction that defines pathogenic strains, and based on this it was concluded that virulence differences were likely to be defined by different patterns of gene expression and that "commensal and pathogenic strains are the same organism of two different states rather than two different types of organisms."

One possible explanation for such disparate results is the simple observation that *S. aureus* is, in fact, an opportunistic pathogen. The practical implication is that isolation of a strain from a diseased host could reflect compromise of the host rather than virulence of the strain. Conversely, isolation of a strain from a healthy donor does not mean that the strain lacks the capacity to cause invasive disease. Perhaps with this in mind, Fowler *et al.* [55] used MLST to characterize 379 *S. aureus* isolates using an additional level of discrimination that distinguished between isolates from "uncomplicated infection" and isolates from "bacteremia with hematogenous complications." These 379 isolates were placed into 18 clonal complexes (CC), two of which (CC5 and CC30) "exhibited a significant trend toward increasing levels of hematogenous complications." Most prominent among the CC30 isolates were strains of MLST 36 (ST36). A prototype example of an ST36 isolate is the sequenced strain EMRSA-16 (Sanger-252), which lacks RD5 but encodes both *cna* and *bbp* [17]. EMRSA-16 is representative of one of two groups of strains that collectively account for the overwhelming majority of all MRSA bacteremias in the UK [56–58]. Much of our own work has focused on the *S. aureus* clinical isolates UAMS-1 (ATCC 49230) and UAMS-601, and we found that these strains, which have no epidemiological connection to each other or to EMRSA-16, are nevertheless closely related both to each other and to EMRSA-16 [22]. Interestingly, all these strains encode *cna* but not RD5, and none produce α-toxin due to a nonsense mutation in *hla* [17,18].

We also found that EMRSA-16 (Sanger-252) and our UAMS isolates are the most distantly related of the admittedly limited number of strains we examined in comparison with the 8325 lineage [22]. At the same time, a recent report describing the genome sequence of the clinical isolate Newman concluded that this strain is more similar to 8325 than EMRSA-16 and, based on MLST typing and variation in two genomic islands (νSAα and νSAβ), that EMRSA-16 is relatively distinct in comparison with essentially all other sequenced strains [59]. Recent years have also seen the almost explosive emergence of CA-MRSA, one prominent example of which are strains of the USA300 lineage [60,61], and the genome sequence of one such isolate (FPR3757) confirmed that this lineage is also more similar to 8325 than to EMRSA-16 [62]. However, both Newman and USA300 have specific characteristics that distinguish them from strains derived directly from NCTC-8325. This includes the absence of the *rsbU* and *tcaR* mutations and the presence of an *hlb*-converting prophage which, in the specific case of FPR3757, includes the positively converted genes *sak* and *scn* [62]. In the case of Newman, it also includes point mutations in both genes (*fnbA* and *fnbB*) encoding the primary fibronectin-binding proteins of *S. aureus* [63]. As a result, neither adhesin is anchored to the cell surface, which as discussed below has far-reaching implications for the pathogenesis of Newman in comparison with other clinical isolates.

Many CA-MRSA strains also encode the arginine catabolite mobile element (ACME), which is thought to have been recently acquired from *S. epidermidis* and is not present in most lineages of *S. aureus* [64]. The precise role of the ACME element in virulence is not known. The element contains the arginine deiminase (*arc*) operon, which is also present in *S. aureus* strains that do not encode ACME [22]. Mutation of the arginine/ornithine antiporter gene (*arcD*) in a strain that does not encode ACME completely inhibited arginine transport but had little impact on pathogenesis at least in the context of biofilm-associated infection [65]. However, the "native" *arc* operon differs from that in the ACME element, and it is certainly possible that the latter contributes to virulence due to a gene dosage effect and/or differential regulation of the two operons [62]. Additionally, the 30.9-kb ACME element contains additional genes, at least one of which (*opp3*) encodes a putative oligopeptide permease that is functionally similar to genes previously shown to contribute to virulence in animal models of *S. aureus* infection [66].

A number of studies have also demonstrated that many CA-MRSA isolates contain the *lukS-PV* and *lukF-PV* genes, which encode the two components of the Panton–Valentine leukocidin (PVL) [48,67]. It has been widely speculated that PVL makes a major contribution to the severity of infections caused by such strains, but this remains yet another controversial topic. For instance, Labandeira-Rey *et al.* [68] concluded that PVL plays a primary role in the pathogenesis of the necrotizing pneumonia associated with CA-MRSA strains. In fact, these authors found that purified PVL alone was sufficient to cause lethal pneumonia in a mouse model. At the same time, Voyich *et al.* [69] concluded that PVL-producing strains are no more virulent than their PVL-negative counterparts, while Wang *et al.* [70] concluded that the increased virulence of CA-MRSA strains is due, at least in part, to the increased production of small peptides classified as "phenol-soluble modulins" (see below) rather than to PVL. Bubeck Wardenburg *et al.* [15] also found that the PVL-negative strain Newman causes lethal pneumonia in a mouse model and that its lethality is a collective function of both surface-associated proteins (e.g., protein A) and extracellular toxins other than PVL (e.g., α-toxin). In fact, these authors subsequently compared isogenic derivatives of Newman expressing either PVL or α-toxin and found that it is α-toxin rather than PVL that accounts for their virulence in a murine pneumonia model [15]. The same conclusion was reached based on comparison of isogenic derivatives of the community-acquired isolates USA300 and MW2 carrying mutations in either *hla* or *pvl*.

Labandeira-Rey *et al.* [68] also found that production of PVL was associated with global phenotypic changes including decreased production of several proteases and increased production of the surface-associated proteins SdrD and protein A (Spa). The fact that these changes also contribute to virulence was evident in the observation that *pvl*-positive, *spa*-negative mutants have reduced virulence compared with their isogenic, *pvl*-positive, *spa*-positive counterparts. Similar global effects on the production of *S. aureus* virulence factors have been observed with strains that produce other strain-dependent staphylococcal toxins including SEB and toxic shock syndrome toxin (TSST)-1 [71]. Altered expression of certain proteases (e.g., ClpP) also has a global impact that is reflected in clinically relevant phenotypes including biofilm formation and intercellular survival (see below). Thus, even studies comparing isogenic strains carrying single mutations must be interpreted in context, and this adds yet another complicating factor to efforts to define the most relevant *S. aureus* virulence factors and their contribution to disease.

The studies discussed above support the hypothesis that *S. aureus* has indeed taken more than one path to the same end. Direct support for this hypothesis comes from Diep *et al.* [67], who assessed the distribution of 34 virulence genes among six clonal lineages that collectively accounted for 88.2% of all MRSA infections over an 8.5-year period in San Francisco. The results led the authors to propose a series of genetic events that resulted in the emergence of two predominant lineages, one of which arose from an ancestral ST30 clone and is similar to ST36 MRSA, and one of which arose from the 8325 ST8 lineage and includes USA300. Whether these lineages can be definitively associated with relevant clinical correlates remains to be determined, but extending experiments to include such strains, which are undeniably important if not clinically predominant, and making direct comparisons using relevant animal models will help resolve many of the conflicting reports regarding the contribution of specific virulence factors to the molecular pathogenesis of *S. aureus* infection.

Irrespective of the issues discussed above, studies done with 8325-derived strains like RN6390 have led to the development of a virulence paradigm that provides a convenient framework from which to formulate the most relevant questions for future studies. The general, rather obvious tenet of this paradigm is that the ability of *S. aureus* to cause its diverse array of infections is dependent on its ability to modulate the production of its diverse array of virulence factors in response to changing conditions in the host. These virulence factors have been categorized based on several considerations including (i) cellular localization (surface-exposed vs. extracellular), (ii) temporal pattern of production (produced during exponential vs. postexponential growth *in vitro*), and (iii) primary contribution to the disease process (toxins vs. colonization and evasion of host defenses). While none of these categories are mutually exclusive, all of them have some relevance, and there is in fact a common theme that ties them all together. Specifically, the surface-exposed virulence factors are generally produced *in vitro* during the exponential growth phase while production of most toxins and extracellular enzymes is delayed until postexponential growth. In the previous edition of this book, it was proposed that this temporal pattern has an *in vivo* corollary that reflects the need to produce surface-exposed factors early in the course of infection to avoid innate host defenses and promote colonization, while production of extracellular toxins and degradative enzymes becomes more important later in the disease process to facilitate tissue invasion and acquisition of nutrients in the face of an ongoing immune response [72]. Although this has been called into question by recent reports demonstrating that regulatory events defined *in vitro* may not accurately reflect *in vivo* events [73–76], this paradigm remains a convenient starting point, and we have chosen to organize this updated chapter accordingly. Where appropriate, we have noted recognized contradictions not in an attempt to resolve them but rather in the hope that acknowledging their existence will prompt research that ultimately leads to their resolution in a therapeutically relevant fashion.

Surface-associated virulence factors of *Staphylococcus aureus*

Surface-associated virulence factors of *S. aureus* include structural components of the cell wall; surface-exposed proteins, most of which are covalently linked to cell wall peptidoglycan; and extracellular polysaccharides. Collectively, these virulence factors play important roles in helping *S. aureus* avoid host defenses and promote colonization.

Structural components of the cell wall

The host innate defenses produce various cytokines and chemokines in response to *S. aureus* infection, and several components of the cell wall potentially contribute to this process. This includes wall teichoic acid (WTA), lipoteichoic acid (LTA), lipoprotein, and peptidoglycan (PG) [77].

Wall teichoic acid

WTA is a major component of the *S. aureus* cell wall, but it does not appear to play a significant role in immune modulation [78]. However, there are reports suggesting that it makes an important contribution to nasal colonization, which is antecedent to many if not most *S. aureus* infections [79,80]. Mutants that lack WTA also exhibit reduced adherence to endothelial cells, and this has been associated with reduced virulence in a rabbit endocarditis model [81].

Lipoteichoic acid and peptidoglycan

Several studies have concluded that both LTA and PG induce an inflammatory response and contribute markedly to the onset of septic shock [77,82,83]. It was recently suggested that lipoprotein, rather than LTA, plays the immunologically dominant role in that regard and that contaminating lipoprotein present in LTA preparations may account, at least partly, for the activity previously ascribed to LTA [84,85]. However, highly purified LTA induces cytokine release from neutrophils [86–89], and even synthetic LTA has the same effect [90,91]. At the same time, there is evidence to suggest that the independent effects of LTA and PG observed *in vitro* may not reflect *in vivo* events. More directly, there are reports suggesting that LTA and PG have relatively little individual impact *in vivo* but have synergistic effects *in vivo* that ultimately lead to the recruitment of neutrophils and the onset of septic shock [83,92,93].

Whether acting alone or in combination with each other, the nature of the inflammatory response induced by LTA and PG is similar to that observed with the lipopolysaccharide (LPS) of Gram-negative bacteria. Considerably less LPS is required to achieve the same effect, but in comparison with LPS, LTA and PG are much more concentrated in the *S. aureus* cell wall such that the level of induction on the basis of cell equivalents is similar [77]. As a result, *S. aureus* has the capacity to cause septic shock as severe as that more commonly associated with Gram-negative bacteria. Some reports have concluded that Toll-like receptor (TLR)2 plays a primary role in the host response to LTA and PG [77,87], but recent *in vivo* studies suggest that this pathway may not be as important as previously thought [86,94,95].

Fedtke *et al.* [96] recently demonstrated that strains with reduced LTA content also have altered physicochemical properties including reduced autolysin activity and altered cell-surface hydrophobicity. The latter was correlated with a reduced capacity to form a biofilm. However, marked strain-dependent differences were observed in this study, which was limited to strains SA113 (ATCC 35556) and RN4220, both of which are chemically mutagenized derivatives of 8325 [21,97], and it is unclear whether similar changes occur in clinical isolates. Nevertheless, a recent study demonstrated that mutation of *ltaS*, a gene required for LTA biosynthesis, results in complete growth arrest [98]. This suggests that targeted inhibition of LTA synthesis could have therapeutic utility. In fact, it was initially suggested that the cyclic lipopeptide antibiotic daptomycin may function by inhibiting LTA synthesis [99], but this was subsequently called into question by a study that identified point mutations contributing to daptomycin resistance, none of which were in LTA biosynthesis genes [100].

Cell surface adhesins

The surface of *S. aureus* is coated with a variety of adhesins capable of binding different host proteins present in plasma and/or the extracellular matrix. Indeed, a recent review listed 28 different *S. aureus* surface proteins that promote the binding of at least 18 different host proteins [101]. Most of these have specific properties that define them as MSCRAMM adhesins, denoting their role as *m*icrobial *s*urface *c*omponents *r*ecognizing *a*dhesive *m*atrix *m*olecules [102–104]. This includes a C-terminal sorting signal containing an LPXTG motif followed by a hydrophobic membrane-spanning region and a positively charged cytoplasmic tail. The LPXTG motif is used to covalently anchor the MSCRAMM to cell wall PG via a reaction catalyzed by sortase A [105]. The predominance of this anchoring system makes it convenient to assess the collective contribution of MSCRAMMs to virulence by examining strains carrying mutations in the relevant gene (*srtA*), and such comparisons have confirmed that *srtA* mutants are significantly less virulent than their isogenic parent strains in animal models of *S. aureus* infection [15,106–108]. There is a second sortase encoded by *srtB*, but a very limited number of *S. aureus* surface proteins are anchored by this alternative mechanism (see below). The relative contribution of sortase A and B is reflected in their impact on virulence. Specifically, *srtB* contributes to virulence in at least some models, but its contribution is minor in comparison with *srtA* [106,108,109].

Protein A

In comparison with sortase A, it has been more difficult to define the role of individual MSCRAMMs in pathogenesis. One example is Spa, a well-characterized surface protein that has been used as a prototype for sortase A-mediated anchoring studies [105,110]. The classic functional description is that Spa binds the Fc region of IgG and thereby limits antibody-mediated opsonization. Based on this, it has been proposed that the primary contribution of Spa to virulence is to limit phagocytosis [6]. However, Spa also binds both von Willebrand factor, a large serum glycoprotein that mediates adherence of platelets upon endothelial damage [111], and TNFR1, a receptor for tumor necrosis factor α that plays an important role in the signaling pathways of innate immunity [112,113]. Although early studies failed to demonstrate a major role for Spa in virulence [72], more recent studies have concluded that Spa plays an important role in murine models of both septic arthritis and pneumonia [15,114–116]. As noted above, Labandeira-Rey *et al.* [68] also concluded that the increased production of Spa observed in PVL-positive CA-MRSA isolates contributes to their virulence in a murine pneumonia model. At present, the relative contribution of the different binding properties of Spa to virulence is not clear, but there is evidence to suggest that Spa binding to TNFR1 plays a major role in the pathogenesis of staphylococcal pneumonia [114].

Fibronectin-binding proteins

Fibronectin is a major, high-molecular-weight glycoprotein of the host extracellular matrix that is also found in soluble form in plasma and other body fluids. *Staphylococcus aureus* produces several surface-associated and secreted proteins that bind fibronectin [101], but the two primary adhesins in this respect are FnbA and FnbB. These MSCRAMM adhesins are encoded by genes designated *fnbA* and *fnbB* respectively, and in strains that produce both adhesins, the two genes are contiguous in the *S. aureus* chromosome. The presence of one or both genes has little phenotypic consequence with respect to the overall capacity to bind fibronectin [117]; however, the two adhesins are not entirely redundant. For instance, FnbA, but not FnbB, mediates platelet aggregation [118]. These adhesins are also multifunctional, with FnbA also binding fibrinogen and elastin and FnbB also binding elastin

[119–121]. The binding of different host proteins is mediated by different Fnb domains such that binding one host protein is not competitive with respect to binding another [120,121].

Peacock *et al.* [117] concluded that strains encoding both *fnbA* and *fnbB* are more commonly associated with invasive disease, and to the extent that the presence of one or both *fnb* genes has little impact on fibronectin binding, this would suggest that the alternative functions of FnbA versus FnbB might be important. A subsequent study from the same group found that *fnbA* was also one of the seven virulence factor genes (the others noted thus far being *cna* and *sdrE*) correlated with the ability to cause invasive infection [46]. However, the significance of this correlation is difficult to assess for two reasons. First, while there are reports to the contrary [43,122], *fnbA* appears to be highly conserved among *S. aureus* strains [48]. This makes it difficult to envision how its presence could be used to discriminate between any two groups of *S. aureus* strains. Secondly, the prevalence of *fnbB* was not assessed, so it is not possible to determine whether the test strains had one or both *fnb* genes. While this would not be expected to have an impact on fibronectin binding [117], the absence of *fnbB* could still be relevant based either on the ability of each adhesin to bind other host proteins (e.g., fibrinogen and/or elastin) or because it reflects the absence of other RD5-associated genes (e.g., *sasG*, *sarT*/*sarU*).

Early studies attempting to more directly define the role of FnbA and FnbB in virulence reached contradictory conclusions, with some concluding that fibronectin binding makes an important contribution to virulence [123] and others disputing that claim [124]. In fact, one report concluded that mutation of *fnbA* and *fnbB* results in enhanced rather than reduced virulence [125]. Palmqvist *et al.* [126] concluded that *S. aureus* fibronectin-binding proteins make little direct contribution to the pathogenesis of septic arthritis but nevertheless contribute significantly to the induction of systemic inflammation. Although it could be argued that the only way to accurately assess the contribution of a specific virulence factor to pathogenesis is to directly examine the species in question, particularly when that species produces such a diverse and sometimes redundant array of virulence factors, one approach to resolving these contradictions is to introduce the genes encoding *S. aureus* virulence factors into less pathogenic bacterial species. For instance, Que *et al.* [127] demonstrated that expression of *fnbA* in *Lactococcus lactis* resulted in enhanced capacity to infect rats and cause catheter-associated cardiac vegetations. Similarly, Kerdudou *et al.* [128] demonstrated that expression of *fnbA* or *fnbB* in *S. carnosus* significantly enhanced adherence to intact endothelium *in vivo*.

Que *et al.* [129] subsequently demonstrated that FnbA-expressing *L. lactis* caused persistent infection and promoted tissue invasion and dissemination to distant sites. The multifunctional nature of FnbA was apparent in these studies in that deletion of the fibrinogen-binding domain of FnbA did not affect fibronectin binding or internalization by host cells *in vitro* but abolished valve infectivity *in vivo*. This defect could be restored by inserting the fibrinogen-binding domain of ClfA (see below) into the truncated FnbA adhesin or by coexpressing full-length ClfA with the truncated FnbA. It was proposed on this basis that fibronectin and fibrinogen binding cooperate to promote valve colonization and invasion of adjacent endothelial cells. However, Heying *et al.* [130] concluded that expression of FnbA or FnbB alone in *L. lactis* was sufficient to promote internalization and activation of endothelial cells while expression of ClfA had little effect. To the extent that FnbB has not been shown to bind fibrinogen, this would suggest that fibronectin plays the primary role with respect to internalization. Other reports directly examining *S. aureus fnb* mutants have reached the same conclusion [131–133]. Classically *S. aureus* is considered an extracellular pathogen, and the contribution of internalization to pathogenesis remains unclear, but it could promote bacterial persistence by sequestering *S. aureus* into the intracellular environment and thereby allowing it to avoid host immune surveillance. *Staphylococcus aureus* can replicate intracellularly [134–136], and recent studies have demonstrated that internalized *S. aureus* adopts the phenotype of a small-colony variant (SCV) including reduced susceptibility to antibiotics [134,137,138].

Fibrinogen-binding proteins

Staphylococcus aureus also produces two primary fibrinogen-binding proteins designated ClfA and ClfB. As noted above, there is some degree of functional redundancy between these adhesins and the fibronectin-binding proteins, particularly FnbA. Unlike *fnbA* and *fnbB*, the *clfA* and *clfB* genes are not contiguous in the *S. aureus* chromosome, and both appear to be highly conserved among different strains [48,122]. ClfA and ClfB also differ with respect to the nature of their binding interaction with fibrinogen [139,140], and while the binding of either to fibrinogen has similar biological effects, ClfA appears to play a predominant role in comparison with ClfB. For instance, both ClfA and ClfB promote platelet aggregation by fibrinogen-dependent and fibrinogen-independent mechanisms, the latter depending on the presence of complement and/or adhesin-specific antibodies [139,141,142], but ClfA has the greater overall impact with respect to both pathways [143]. Platelet aggregation contributes to the development of infective endocarditis [144], and ClfA and to a lesser extent ClfB were shown to promote virulence in an experimental endocarditis model [2,129,145,146]. ClfA also plays a role in the pathogenesis of sepsis and septic arthritis [147], and it was suggested that this is a function of its ability to bind soluble fibrinogen and thereby limit deposition of opsonins [6,148,149]. It has also been suggested that ClfA contributes to virulencein experimental septic arthritis through a fibrinogen-independent mechanism [150].

Although ClfB appears to make a relatively limited contribution to virulence in comparison with ClfA, *clfB* is expressed *in vitro* during exponential growth while *clfA* is expressed uncharacteristically (compared with most other surface-associated proteins) during postexponential growth [151], and based on this it has been proposed that these adhesins may serve similar roles during different stages of infection [6]. However, as with FnbA and FnbB, ClfA and ClfB also have distinct functional properties. For instance, O'Brien *et al.* [152] demonstrated that ClfB also binds cytokeratin 10 and that this promotes adherence to desquamated nasal epithelial cells. Schaffer *et al.* [153] subsequently demonstrated using a mouse model that *clfB* mutants do in fact have a reduced capacity for nasal colonization. The same was true of an *srtA* mutant, but it was not true of isogenic strains carrying mutations in *clfA*, *fnbA*, *fnbB* or the collagen-binding adhesin gene *cna*. Active immunization with purified ClfB or passive immunization with a ClfB-specific monoclonal antibody was also correlated with reduced nasal colonization. Once again, this emphasizes the fact that while many *S. aureus* virulence factors have functionally redundant properties (e.g., fibrinogen binding), they are not necessarily functionally redundant in the overall context of their contribution to pathogenesis.

Other adhesins

ClfA and ClfB are structurally characterized by the presence of extensive serine-aspartate (SD) repeats, and *S. aureus* also produces an additional group of MSCRAMMs (SdrC, SdrD, and SdrE) with the same structural properties [101]. The genes encoding these adhesins (*sdrCDE*) are contiguous in the *S. aureus* chromosome, and they should not be confused with *sdrM* (staphylococcus *d*rug *r*esistance), which encodes an *S. aureus* multidrug efflux pump that is structurally unrelated to the *sdr* adhesins [154]. At present, the ligand-binding specificity of the Sdr adhesins remains unknown, but a recent report demonstrated that they collectively contribute to the ability to bind fibrinogen, albeit to a limited extent compared with ClfA [155]. SdrE has also been shown to induce platelet aggregation but, in comparison with ClfA and ClfB, SdrE-mediated platelet aggregation is less efficient and appears to be dependent on one or more plasma proteins (perhaps fibrinogen) serving as a "bridge" between the adhesin and its as yet unknown platelet target [143].

Early reports suggested that all three *sdr* genes are highly conserved [156]. However, Sabat *et al.* [157] recently concluded that *sdrC* is the only gene present in all strains. At the same time, strains encoding only *sdrC* were exclusively methicillin-sensitive *S. aureus* isolates, and even then they were relatively rare (< 10%). In contrast, all MRSA isolates encoded at least two if not all three genes. The presence of *sdrD* was specifically correlated with both methicillin resistance and bone infection, while the presence of *sdrE* was not definitively correlated with resistance status or the ability to cause different types of infection. However, Sabat *et al.* [157] did not distinguish between the *sdrE* and *bbp* allelic variants, and the latter has also been correlated with bone and joint infection [122]. As noted above, the *bbp* variant encodes an adhesin that binds bone sialoprotein [49,158], but at present it is unclear whether the allelic variation between *sdrE* and *bbp* alters binding specificity or has an impact on the specificity of the immune response.

Variants of the Sdr adhesins are also present in coagulase-negative species including *S. epidermidis*, *S. capitis*, and *S. saprophyticus*, and in at least some cases they contribute to collagen binding in these species [159–163]. However, there is no evidence to suggest that any of the *S. aureus* Sdr adhesins exhibit the same binding specificity. Rather, the collagen-binding capacity of *S. aureus* is closely associated with the presence of *cna* [44]. There are reports suggesting that *cna*-negative strains also bind collagen [164], but the relative level of collagen binding in such strains is very low in comparison with *cna*-positive strains, and in the strains we have examined it cannot be competitively inhibited [44]. This suggests that *cna* is the predominant if not the only collagen-binding adhesin produced by *S. aureus*. Although *cna* is not present in all *S. aureus* strains [165], there are reports suggesting that it is common among isolates from bone and joint infection [166], and mutation of *cna* resulted in reduced virulence not only in murine models of septic arthritis and osteomyelitis [167–170] but also in a rat model of catheter-associated endocarditis [171] and a rabbit model of bacterial keratitis [172].

Studies examining the genome sequence of six *S. aureus* strains identified a number of other genes encoding proteins with an LPXTG-like anchoring motif [47,173]. Most of these have not yet been functionally characterized and are referred to in the current literature as Sas (*S. aureus* surface) proteins. Eight of 10 *sas* genes were present in all six strains, while one (*sasG*) was present in all strains other than EMRSA-16 and another (*sasK*) was present only in the vancomycin-intermediate *S. aureus* (VISA) isolates Mu50 and N315 [47]. This is consistent with the observation that *sasG* is part of the RD5 genetic element that includes *fnbB*, *sarT* and *sarU*, which as noted above is also absent in EMRSA-16. SasG has the apparently opposing properties of promoting biofilm formation but masking the ability of Spa, ClfB, and the Fnb adhesins to bind IgG, cytokeratin 10, and fibronectin respectively [174]. At the same time, SasG promotes adherence to nasal epithelial cells, and it was proposed that this might compensate for masking the ability of ClfB to bind cytokeratin 10 (once again, *S. aureus* appears to have found multiple paths to the same end). The mechanism responsible for both the masking and adherence properties of SasG appears to involve formation of peritrichous surface fibrils, the length and density of which are correlated with both its masking and adherence properties [174].

SasG binding is dependent on processing by proteases, which is consistent with the observation that it exhibits significant similarities to the accumulation-associated protein (Aap) of *S. epidermidis* [47]. SasG is also similar to the *S. aureus* surface-associated protein Pls, which is closely associated with the SCC*mec* element type I and has also been shown to limit bacterial adherence to certain host proteins [175,176]. To our knowledge, the role of *sasG* in virulence has not been directly assessed, but mutation of *pls* has been correlated with reduced capacity to cause septic arthritis [175] and reduced invasion of host cells [177]. Interestingly, a recent study found that only 18 of 66 (27%) clinical MRSA isolates encoded *pls* [177]. This included all SCC*mec* type I strains, which are typically hospital-acquired MRSA (HA-MRSA), but only one SCC*mec* type IV isolate. SCC*mec* type IV variants are common among CA-MRSA, which would suggest that such strains generally lack *pls* and may therefore have an enhanced capacity for cellular invasion at least in comparison with SCC*mec* type I strains.

SasA is yet another protein that promotes the interaction between *S. aureus* and platelets, and this presumably accounts for the reduced virulence of a *sasA* mutant in a rabbit endocarditis model [178]. Screening of convalescent human serum demonstrated that patients who have recovered from *S. aureus* infection have higher titers of antibody to a number of Sas proteins including SasA, SasG, SasH, SasI, and SasJ, which suggests that these adhesins are expressed *in vivo* during the course of infection [47]. Subsequent expansion of the original studies, which were limited to *in silico* analysis of the genome sequence data available at the time, to direct analysis of invasive versus carriage isolates also revealed an apparent correlation between the presence of *sasG* and *sasH* and invasive disease. These correlations appeared to be independent of each other [47], suggesting that SasG and SasH contribute independently to the overall capacity to cause invasive disease. SasE, SasJ, and SasI were subsequently redesignated IsdA, IsdB, and IsdH respectively to denote the fact that they are *i*ron-responsive *s*urface *d*eterminants [179,180]. Not surprisingly, all these surface proteins are involved in some aspect of iron acquisition as discussed below.

Cucarella *et al.* [181] described an MSCRAMM designated Bap (*b*iofilm-*a*ssociated *p*rotein) that, like SasG, interferes with the function of other adhesins as evidenced by a reduced capacity of *bap*-expressing strains to bind fibrinogen and fibronectin. Nevertheless, *bap* promotes biofilm formation [182,183], and Tormo *et al.* [184] recently demonstrated that Bap production is subject to phase variation and suggested that this may serve as a specific means of detachment from biofilms *in vivo*. This is discussed below in the context of the polysaccharide intercellular adhesin (PIA), but it is important to note that *bap* is associated with bovine mastitis isolates and to date has not been reported in any human clinical isolate [185,186].

Staphylococcus aureus also produces a number of surface proteins that are distinguished from MSCRAMMs in that they are not covalently anchored to the cell wall. This includes the elastin-binding protein EbpS, which remains associated with the cell surface as an integral transmembrane protein [187], and Ebh (*e*xtracellular matrix-*b*inding *h*omolog), which holds the distinction of being encoded by the largest gene in the *S. aureus* genome [188]. Ebh contributes to fibronectin binding, and while its contribution to virulence has not been directly assessed, it has been demonstrated that patients with *S. aureus* infection have elevated antibody levels to Ebh [188].

Secreted adhesins

There are also a number of adhesive proteins collectively referred to as SERAM (secretable expanded repertoire adhesive molecules) [189]. Included in this group are adhesins designated Efb (*e*xtracellular *f*ibrinogen-*b*inding protein), Emp (*e*xtracellular *m*atrix-binding *p*rotein), and Eap (*e*xtracellular *a*dhesive *p*rotein, also known as MAP and p70). At present, the contribution of SERAM proteins to virulence remains undefined, but there is evidence to suggest that they promote the interaction of *S. aureus* with host cells and that this contributes to both internalization and immune modulation [190,191]. There are also reports indicating that Eap has an impact on host physiological processes including wound healing and angiogenic responses of endothelial cells [192–194].

Adhesins as vaccine candidates

Stranger-Jones *et al.* [180] recently carried out a comprehensive experiment in which mice were immunized with each of 19 purified MSCRAMM adhesins and then challenged by intraperitoneal infection. Some degree of protection was observed in mice immunized with ClfA, ClfB, FnbA, IsdA, IsdB, IsdC, IsdH, SasD, SasF, SasG, SdrD, SdrC, SdrE, or Spa. In contrast, immunization with FnbB, SasA, SasB, SasC, or SasK did not provide a significant degree of protection. The level of protection was closely correlated with the level of MSCRAMM-specific antibody and its impact on opsonophagocytic killing. A multivalent vaccine consisting of IsdA, IsdB, SdrD, and SdrE, which were four of the individual adhesins that elicited the greatest antibody response, also conferred protection against an otherwise lethal infection. This was evaluated by challenging with multiple strains of *S. aureus*, including the *pvl*-positive CA-MRSA isolate USA400, and the level of protection did vary to some extent in a strain-dependent manner [180]. Whether this variation is a function of strain-dependent differences with respect to specific adhesins (e.g., *sdrE* vs. *bbp*) was not addressed.

Autolysin/adhesins

There are at least two *S. aureus* proteins (Atl and Aaa) that serve the dual roles of functioning as autolysins important in cell wall turnover and in modulating adherence to host proteins [195,196]. Aaa, which has also been referred to as Sle1, binds several host proteins including fibrinogen, fibronectin, and vitronectin, and mutation of *aaa* has been associated with reduced virulence in a mouse model [195,197]. Although mutation of *atl* has a major impact on cell wall turnover, the limited pathogenesis studies performed to date indicate that that it does not contribute to the virulence of *S. aureus* at least as judged using a murine peritonitis model [196].

Surface-associated polysaccharides

The staphylococcal literature makes reference to 11 capsular serotypes of *S. aureus*, but only four of these (serotypes 1, 2, 5, and 8) are clinically relevant [198]. In addition to the structural differences that define these serotypes, strains of serotype 1 and 2 express their capsule genes constitutively and at high levels [199,200]. In contrast, expression of the capsule genes in strains of serotype 5 and 8 is tightly regulated in a complex manner involving a number of regulatory loci [201]. The increased production of capsular polysaccharides in serotype 1 and 2 strains clearly contributes to virulence as evidenced by studies demonstrating that expression of type 8 *cap* genes under the regulatory control of a type 1 promoter results in both increased capsule production and increased virulence [202]. Nevertheless, the overwhelming majority of human clinical isolates are serotype 5 or 8 [198]. This suggests that the constitutive production of large amounts of capsular polysaccharide is not necessary and may even be detrimental in human infection.

The operons encoding the enzymes required for the biosynthesis of type 5 and type 8 capsules are allelic and contain 16 genes, 12 of which are common among both serotypes [203,204]. These 12 genes are almost identical, which reflects the overall structural similarity between serotypes 5 and 8 capsular polysaccharides. Early studies attempting to define the role of capsular polysacchrides in pathogenesis were controversial [198], but more recent studies have confirmed that capsule production makes an important contribution to virulence in several animal models including bacteremia, renal abscess, subcutaneous abscess, intraabdominal abscess, and septic arthritis [202,205–209]. A more recent study demonstrated that isogenic strains expressing serotype 5 or 8 capsular polysaccharides were more persistent in the bloodstream and more resistant to phagocytosis that an isogenic capsule mutant [210]. However, serotype 5 and 8 strains were not equivalent in that regard. Specifically, a strain producing serotype 5 capsule exhibited an enhanced capacity to persist in the bloodstream even in comparison with an isogenic strain producing serotype 8 capsular polysaccharides [210]. Strains expressing serotype 8 capsule were also more susceptible to phagocytic killing *in vitro*.

The primary contribution of capsular polysaccharides to virulence is to limit opsonization and phagocytosis [202,208,210,211]. In studies done with type 1 strains, this appears to be a function of masking C3b deposited on the bacterial surface and thereby limiting recognition by C3b receptors on phagocytic cells [212]. Serotype 5 and 8 strains produce reduced amounts of capsule in comparison with type 1 strains, but recent data indicate that this has a similar masking effect even in these strains [210]. Production of capsular polysaccharides also limits complement deposition even in serotype 5 and 8 strains [210,213]. In addition to limiting opsonization and activation of the alternative complement pathway, capsules may contribute to virulence in more direct ways. For example, Tzianabos *et al.* [209] demonstrated that purified type 8 capsular polysaccharides caused abscess formation when administered intraabdominally to rats. This was associated with a zwitterionic structural motif that was a potent activator of both rat and human $CD4^+$ T cells. Moreover, passive transfer of activated T cells could be used to moderate abscess formation.

Paradoxically, production of capsular polysaccharides was associated with reduced virulence in a rat endocarditis model [214,215]. One possible explanation is that capsular polysaccharides mask adhesins as well as opsonins on the surface of *S. aureus*. Indeed, Pohlmann-Dietze *et al.* [216] demonstrated that capsular polysaccharides mask adhesins to an extent that limits attachment to endothelial cells. We have also demonstrated that the *cna*-positive, heavily encapsulated serotype 1 strain Smith diffuse does not bind collagen while its corresponding *cap* mutant does [217]. While Smith diffuse was more virulent than the serotype 8 strain UAMS-1 in a murine peritonitis model, the opposite was true when they were compared in an osteomyelitis model [218]. Such results emphasize the need not only to consider different strains but also different clinical contexts when defining the pathogenesis of *S. aureus*.

A second *S. aureus* exopolysaccharide that has also been associated with virulence, particularly in the context of biofilm-associated infection, is PIA. Although there is evidence to suggest that PIA contributes to the initial attachment to biomaterials [219], the PIA nomenclature reflects what appears to be its primary function of promoting cell-to-cell adherence and the accumulation stage of biofilm formation [220]. PIA has also been referred to as PNAG to reflect its structural identity as a β-1,6-poly-*N*-acetylglucosamine. It is synthesized by enzymes encoded in the *icaADBC* operon, which is present in most but not all strains of *S. aureus* [221–224].

The original focus on *ica* and PIA production was based on its role in biofilm formation in *S. epidermidis* [225]. This is not surprising since *S. epidermidis* infections are almost exclusively associated with biofilms and implanted medical devices. Although most studies have concluded that PIA does in fact play an important role in *S. epidermidis* foreign-body infections [226–228], there are contradictory reports [229,230]. While PIA also contributes to biofilm formation in at least some strains of *S. aureus*, it was found to have little impact on *S. aureus* foreign-body infections [230–233]. It is also clear that some strains of both *S. epidermidis* and *S. aureus* form biofilms in a PIA-independent manner [234–237], and it has been suggested that several other cellular components, including teichoic acids, cell wall autolysins, extracellular DNA, and various surface-associated proteins, may compensate for the absence of PIA [238–240]. Included among the surface-associated proteins proposed to play a role in that regard are Atl, Aap, and various MSCRAMMs including Bap [220,239,241]. As a specific example, analysis of *S. aureus* strains that encode *bap* and/or *ica* suggest that Bap and PIA represent independent means of accomplishing the same goal in that the impact of mutating *ica* on biofilm formation was dependent on the presence or absence of *bap* [186]. The existence of such alternative means to promote accumulation is consistent with reports indicating that a functional *ica* operon is not required for biofilm formation or the maintenance of biofilm-associated infection in at least some strains of *S. aureus* [229,237,238,242].

PIA may also serve other functions that contribute to the ability of *S. aureus* to cause disease. For instance, there are reports indicating that it contributes to the resistance of both *S. aureus* and *S. epidermidis* to antimicrobial peptides and phagocytosis [228,243,244]. This suggests that PIA may have a role in immune evasion similar to capsular polysaccharides. Moreover, both active and passive immunization with PIA protected mice against metastatic kidney infection after intravenous inoculation [245]. A subsequent study confirmed that PIA-producing strains of *S. aureus* are more virulent in a murine bacteremia model and that this is correlated with reduced susceptibility to opsonic killing [246]. Begun *et al.* [247] also concluded that PIA is an essential virulence factor in a *Caenorhabditis elegans* infection model. What is perhaps most important about this study is that these authors also demonstrated that the impact of PIA was not evident in *C. elegans* mutants with defects in the p38 MAP kinase signaling pathway. This not only emphasizes that PIA may contribute to staphylococcal pathogenesis beyond its contribution to biofilm formation but also the utility of using alternative models to define the host response and its contribution to the pathogenesis of *S. aureus* infection.

Extracellular virulence factors of *Staphylococcus aureus*

Although from a global perspective the pathogenesis of *S. aureus* is far from defined, it is clear that an important distinguishing characteristic among the staphylococci is that *S. aureus* has the capacity to produce a remarkable array of extracellular proteins, many of which can be definitively considered toxins based on their ability to cause disease when administered as sterile purified preparations [248]. These include the exfoliative toxins, enterotoxins, and TSST-1. The genes encoding these toxins are strain-dependent, but several of the most prevalent *S. aureus* diseases are clearly associated with the production of specific toxins. Examples include the exfoliative toxins in staphylococcal scalded skin syndrome (SSSS) and bullous impetigo, enterotoxins in staphylococcal food poisoning, and TSST-1 in toxic shock syndrome. Many of these exotoxins also share the property of superantigenicity [249], the pathological impact of which is described elsewhere (see Chapter 6). This includes many of the enterotoxins, some subset of which is produced by virtually all *S. aureus* strains [22]. As a result, most *S. aureus* strains, including those that do not produce TSST-1, have some capacity to cause superantigen-mediated disease [250].

Exfoliative/epidermolytic toxins

Although exfoliation is a characteristic sign of several forms of *S. aureus* disease, including toxic shock syndrome (see below), classic staphylococcal exfoliative disease is caused by strains producing one of four antigenically distinct exfoliative toxins designated ETA, ETB, ETC, and ETD [251–253]. However, ETA and ETB are the only variants commonly associated with human disease, with about 5% of clinical isolates producing one or both toxins [254]. All exfoliative toxins share properties with staphylococcal serine proteases [255], but their pathological effects are much more specific in that the proteolytic domain is exposed only after binding to the desmosome cadherin protein desmoglein 1, which results in a conformational change that exposes the proteolytic active site resulting in the characteristic separation of the epidermis at the stratum granulosum [255–257]. There are reports suggesting that the exfoliative toxins are superantigens with a broader impact on pathogenesis [258], but more recent reports have concluded that this is not the case [259].

Although early descriptions of staphylococcal exfoliative disease referred to these infections by various names including Ritter disease [260], the current nomenclature is much simpler and refers either to SSSS or bullous impetigo, both of which are most common in infants and are characterized by sloughing of the outer epidermal layers resulting in the characteristic skin lesions of staphylococcal exfoliative disease [255,261]. The important distinguishing characteristic is that SSSS is due to widespread dissemination of the toxin from an infected or even commensal site (e.g., anterior nares), which means the skin lesions themselves are typically sterile. In contrast, bullous impetigo is a localized infection in which staphylococci spread within the epidermal layer [254]. As a result,

S. aureus can generally be isolated from the lesions of bullous impetigo patients. However, *S. aureus* is a commensal species, so its isolation does not necessarily confirm a diagnosis of SSSS or bullous impetigo. For this reason, the most definitive diagnostic method remains skin biopsy showing epidermal cleavage with limited inflammation [262]. This allows differentiation of exfoliative toxin-mediated disease from other forms of exfoliative disease including the physical damage of scalding itself and staphylococcal toxic shock syndrome [260].

Staphylococcal superantigens

Staphylococcus aureus exotoxins that clearly have superantigenic properties include TSST-1 and many of the enterotoxins. Along with similar exotoxins produced by *Streptococcus pyogenes*, these have been collectively referred to as pyrogenic toxin superantigens (PTSAgs). PTSAgs share the characteristics of superantigenicity, pyrogenicity, and the capacity to dramatically enhance the lethality of endotoxin in rabbits [248]. At the same time, the enterotoxins are distinguished from other PTSAgs, including TSST-1, by their emetic effects, which accounts for their predominance as agents of staphylococcal food poisoning [249]. The enterotoxins include antigenic variants designated SEA through SEE and SEG through SEJ, with SEF having subsequently been designated TSST-1 to distinguish it from the emetic enterotoxins [248,249]. There is also a growing number of staphylococcal enterotoxin-like (SEl) proteins that share structural properties with other enterotoxins but either lack emetic properties or have not yet been examined in that respect [263,264].

Staphylococcal food poisoning results from ingesting contaminated food containing a preformed heat-stable enterotoxin. It is characterized by rapid onset (6–8 hours) of diarrhea and vomiting without fever and because it is a toxemia rather than an infection, the symptoms are typically resolved spontaneously within 1–2 days. Cellular receptors in the abdominal viscera, and the mechanism by which enterotoxins induce emesis, have not been defined [249]. Unlike TSST-1, the enterotoxins cannot cross mucosal surfaces [265], but there is evidence to suggest they can penetrate the intestinal lining and initiate a local immune response that includes activation of mast cells leading to histamine release [266]. In fact, histamine H_2 and calcium channel blockers, which block histamine release, attenuate the emetic response [267].

Staphylococcal toxic shock syndrome was first recognized by Todd *et al.* [268] and is characterized by high fever, diffuse erythematous rash, hypotension, desquamation of the skin, and multiorgan failure often leading to death [249]. While TSST-1 is the best-known toxin associatied with toxic shock syndrome, the superantigenic enterotoxins, most notably SEA, SEB and SEC, have the capacity to cause the same clinical syndrome when introduced via some route other than food [269]. One important difference is that TSST-1 is the only staphylococcal superantigen capable of crossing the vaginal mucosa, and as a result is the only toxin associated with menstruation-associated toxic shock syndrome [249]. However, owing to the removal of high absorbancy tampons from the market, nonmenstrual toxic shock syndrome, which is typically associated with infected surgical wounds, is currently the most prominent form of superantigen-mediated staphylococcal disease. Whether caused by strains producing TSST-1 or one of the enterotoxins, the pathology of toxic shock syndrome is clearly a function of the superantigenicity of these toxins and their impact on the host cytokine response (see Chapter 6).

Hemolytic/cytolytic toxins

Although less definitively associated with specific diseases, *S.aureus* also produces several membrane-damaging toxins that lyse various types of host cell. These can generally be divided into the single-component and bicomponent toxins, with the most prominent examples of the former being α-, β- and δ-toxins and the most prominent examples of the latter being γ-toxin and PVL.

With respect to hemolytic activity, the two primary toxins are α-toxin and β-toxin. α-Toxin is both dermonecrotic and neurotoxic, but it has been functionally defined based primarily on its hemolytic properties. From a mechanistic point of view, it is a pore-forming toxin and as such causes ion imbalances and ultimately lysis of various types of host cell. As a hemolysin, it is most active against rabbit erythrocytes, with approximately 1000-fold greater activity compared with human erythrocytes [248]. In contrast, β-toxin is a sphingomyelinase, its activity being higher against sheep than rabbit or human erythrocytes due to the relative sphingomyelin content [248,270]. Based on these differential activities, production of α-toxin versus β-toxin is often assessed by hemolysis of rabbit and sheep blood without further confirmation (e.g., direct transcriptional analysis and/or western blotting with toxin-specific antibody). This is potentially problematic in that the erythrocyte specificity of neither toxin is absolute. Additionally, α- and β-toxin are antagonistic, with β-toxin disrupting membrane integrity to an extent that precludes α-toxin pore formation [271]. Thus, strains that produce high levels of α-toxin can be hemolytic on sheep blood agar, particularly if they also fail to produce β-toxin. One distinguishing characteristic in this respect is the "hot–cold" phenotype of β-toxin. Specifically, β-toxin causes incomplete lysis at 37°C that fully clears after incubation at 4°C [270].

All *S. aureus* strains contain the genes encoding both α- and β-toxin (*hla* and *hlb* respectively), and production of both toxins has been associated with enhanced virulence in animal models of staphylococcal disease [248]. There is also one report concluding that α-toxin is required for biofilm formation [272]. At the same time, there are biofilm-positive virulent clinical isolates (e.g., UAMS-1, Sanger-252) that do not produce either toxin owing to a nonsense mutation in *hla* and the presence of a lysogenic prophage that disrupts *hlb* [17,26,270]. This clearly demonstrates that neither toxin is required to cause staphylococcal disease. Nevertheless, when they are produced, both toxins clearly contribute to the pathogenesis of *S. aureus* infection. The reasons for this are poorly defined, but one possible explanation is that either or both provide a source of heme-iron proteins (see below).

δ-Toxin is a small, helical, amphipathic peptide that has the capacity to lyse a wide variety of mammalian cells including erythrocytes [248]. Its hemolytic activity is often overlooked on blood agar plates owing to the greater activity of α- and β-toxin, but it can be specifically detected based on its synergism with β-toxin [271]. The δ-toxin gene (*hld*) is encoded within the RNAIII effector molecule of the accessory gene regulator (*agr*) regulatory system (see below), but it does not play a functional role with respect to *agr*-mediated regulation [70,273]. For this reason, most of the focus with respect to pathogenesis has been on *agr* rather than δ-toxin itself. However, Wang *et al.* [70] recently demonstrated that CA-MRSA mutants unable to produce δ-toxin but fully capable of *agr*-mediated regulation are attenuated in a murine bacteremia model. This clearly indicates that δ-toxin contributes to pathogenesis in a manner that is independent of the impact of the regulatory impact of RNAIII.

δ-Toxin is also one of a group of phenol-soluble modulins (PSMs) produced by both *S. aureus* and *S. epidermidis* [274]. *Staphylococcus aureus* produces six additional PSMs [70], two of which (β-type) are relatively long (about 40 amino acids) while the other four (α-type) are shorter (about 20 amino acids). The genetic loci encoding these two types of PSM are distinct with respect to each other but contiguous within each group [70]. PSMs function as chemoattractants and have proinflammatory properties similar to LPS, and all seven *S. aureus* PSMs (including δ-toxin) have some capacity to activate neutrophils and initiate an inflammatory response [70,275,276]. However, they are not equivalent in this regard, with the greatest activity observed with α-type PSMs, most notably PSMα3 [70]. A PSMα mutant also had reduced capacity to lyse neutrophils that was almost completely restored by complementation with a plasmid expressing PSMα3 alone. PSMα, and to a lesser extent δ-toxin, mutants also exhibited reduced virulence in a murine bactermia model but only the PSMα mutant was significantly attenuated in a murine model of skin infection. Importantly, production of PSMs is elevated in CA-MRSA in comparison with HA-MRSA, and it has been suggested that increased production of PSMs in general, and PSMα3 in particular, may explain, at least in part, the increased virulence of CA-MRSA strains [70].

γ-Toxin and PVL are bicomponent toxins produced via the association of two separate protein subunits. These subunits, which are referred to as S and F to reflect the fact that they are "slow" and "fast" eluting proteins in an ion-exchange column, assemble into heptameric or hexameric oligomers in the host cell membrane [248]. The γ-toxin S components are encoded by *hlgA* and *hlgC* while the F component is encoded by *hlgB*. All three genes are highly conserved while those encoding the components of PVL (*lukS-PV*, *lukF-PV*) are relatively rare [277]. Having said this, it should be reemphasized that *lukS-PV* and *lukF-PV* are common among CA-MRSA [278,279], and there is some evidence to suggest that PVL contributes to the virulence of these strains [68].

Two additional pairs of genes (*lukE/lukD* and *lukM/lukF′-PV*) encode S and F components of bicomponent leukotoxins [280,281]. The *lukE/lukD* genes are present in most but not all strains while the *lukM/lukF′-PV* genes are confined primarily if not exclusively to bovine mastitis isolates [282,283]. In addition to their own virulence properties, there is evidence to suggest that *lukE/lukD* is associated with other potentially significant genetic differences including *agr* subtype and genes encoding additional *S. aureus* exotoxins [283,284].

Perhaps the most intriguing property of the bicomponent leukotoxins is their ability to form functional heterologous pairs of S and F components that exhibit unique biological properties. For instance, Prevost *et al.* [285] demonstrated that the Hlg and Luk-PV S and F components can form six different combinations of functional toxin, all of which are leukocytic, three of which (HlgA/HlgB, HlgC/HlgB, and HlgA/LukF-PV) are hemolytic on rabbit blood, and two of which (LukS-PV/LukF-PV and HlgA/LukF-PV) are dermonecrotic. Similarly, Konig *et al.* [286] found that all six combinations induced production of inflammatory mediators from human granulocytes but that LukS-PV/LukF-PV and LukS-PV/HlgB complexes are the most active in this regard. Another report confirmed the functionality of heterologous S and F components but found that relative activity defined by the severity of infection in a rabbit eye model differed, with the combination of HlgA/LukF-PV being the most active of the six possible combinations [287]. Most recently, Barrio *et al.* [280] demonstrated that the LukE/LukD and LukM/LukF′-PV components could also form heterologous complexes both with each other and with other S and F components. Thus, a total of five S components (HlgA, HlgC, LukS-PVL, LukE, and LukM) and four F components (HlgB, LukF-PVL, LukD, and LukF′-PVL) allow for up to 20 different functional toxins, any or all of which could contribute to virulence by virtue of their cytolytic properties and its impact on the host inflammatory response. However, studies demonstrating formation of functional heterologous combinations have been limited to *in vitro* assays with purified S and F components, and to date there is no evidence to indicate that these combinations are formed *in vivo* during the course of *S. aureus* infection.

Enzymes

Exoenzymes

Staphylococcus aureus also produces a number of exoproteins that are not toxigenic or cytolytic but are widely presumed to contribute to pathogenesis by promoting nutrient acquisition and tissue invasion. These include proteases, lipases, hyaluronidases, and nucleases. In most cases, there is relatively little evidence to support a direct role for these enzymes in virulence. One exception are the proteases, which when broadly defined include the exfoliative toxins and staphylokinase, both of which have been associated with virulence [257,288]. Also included is a diverse array of extracellular serine and cysteine proteases and metalloproteases, production of which is tightly coordinated by both specific staphylococcal regulatory elements (see below) and the interplay of the proteases themselves [34,289,290]. Studies examining the contribution of these proteases to virulence have reached differing conclusions. For instance, Calander *et al.* [291] found that SspA, SspB, and aureolysin did not play a significant role in the pathogenesis of septic arthritis. Similarly, Reed *et al.* [292] found that deletion of the *spl* operon, which encodes six serine protease-like genes, had no effect on virulence in a murine model of intraperitoneal infection. However, Shaw *et al.* [34] found that while aureolysin and the cysteine protease ScpA did not play a significant role, production of both the serine protease SspA and the cysteine protease SspB contributed to virulence in a murine model of abscess formation. One possible explanation for these contrasting results is that some forms of *S. aureus* infection (e.g., septic arthritis) are more dependent than others (e.g., abscess formation) on the production of adhesins that are particularly sensitive to protease degradation. More directly, the increased presence of certain adhesins (e.g., the fibronectin-binding proteins) in protease-deficient strains may offset the lack of the proteases themselves in at least some models including septic arthritis.

Proteases as virulence factor regulators

Proteases also play an important role in modulating intracellular events. This is particularly true of the Clp proteolytic complexes, which are functionally defined by the complex of a Clp ATPase and its Clp proteolytic partner. These systems are highly conserved in low-GC Gram-positive bacteria and serve a primary role in maintaining protein integrity, particularly during periods of stress [293]. As a result, *clp* mutants exhibit diverse phenotypic changes. Given the stress of *in vivo* growth, this includes a reduced capacity to cause disease. Their importance is further illustrated by the fact that acyldepsipeptide antibiotics function by binding one of these proteases (ClpP) resulting in dysregulation of proteolysis [294].

Frees *et al.* [295] demonstrated that mutation of the ClpP proteolytic subunit or its ClpX ATPase resulted in reduced virulence in a murine skin abscess model. Both *clpX* and *clpP* mutants also exhibited reduced expression of *agr* and consequently *hla*. Michel *et al.* [296] subsequently confirmed that mutation of *clpP* results in global changes in gene expression that include reduced expression of *agr*. Given the regulatory roles of *agr* (see below), this would presumably contribute to their reduced virulence and account in large part for why *clpP* mutants generally produce elevated amounts of surface protein and decreased amounts of exoprotein. The serine protease SspA is included among the exoproteins produced in reduced amounts in a *clpP* mutant, and Frees *et al.* [297] subsequently demonstrated that mutation of *rot* restores SspA production even in a *clpXP* mutant. Based on this, a model was proposed in which accumulation of the *agr*-encoded regulatory molecule RNAIII targets Rot for degradation by ClpXP resulting in increased transcription of *sspA*. At the same time, mutation of *clpP* also results in altered expression of other regulatory genes including increased expression of *sarA*, and since SarA represses protease production (see below), this could also contribute to the reduced production of proteases in *clpP* mutants [296].

ClpP and ClpX also have independent regulatory functions. This is perhaps best evidenced by the fact that mutation of *clpX* resulted in reduced capacity to form a biofilm while mutation of *clpP* had the opposite effect [298]. This is in contrast to studies done in *S. epidermidis*, where mutation of *clpP* resulted in reduced capacity to form a biofilm and reduced virulence in a rat model of biofilm-associated infection [299]. Mutation of *agr* also results in increased biofilm formation, at least in strains like RN6390 that produce RNAIII at high levels [242], and it was suggested on this basis that the increased biofilm formation observed in a *clpP* mutant may reflect the reduced expression of *agr* [298]. Mutation of *clpP* also resulted in reduced expression of the *ica* operon but increased expression of *clfA*, *clfB*, *ebpS*, *fnbA*, and *fnbB* [296]. The latter encode adhesins sensitive to SspA-mediated degradation, and one possible scenario is that the combined effect of the increased production of these adhesins and decreased production of RNAIII and consequently SspA accounts for the enhanced ability of a *clpP* mutant to form a biofilm in an *ica*-independent manner. Mutation of *clpP* also resulted in reduced production of nuclease, which may be relevant in light of recent reports demonstrating that extracellular DNA also contributes to biofilm formation in *S. aureus* [238,240].

Because both *clpX* and *clpP* enhance expression of *agr* [297], it is not obvious why mutation of *clpP* and *clpX* would have opposite effects on biofilm formation. However, Frees *et al.* [295] also demonstrated that ClpX is required independently of *agr* for the production of Spa. Indeed, the increased expression of *spa* characteristic of an *agr* mutant was completely reversed by concomitant mutation of *clpX* [297]. It was suggested that the inability of *clpX* mutants to produce Spa and perhaps other MSCRAMMs may account for their reduced biofilm formation. The *clpC* gene is highly expressed in biofilms [300], and mutation of *clpC* also reduced biofilm formation [298]. It also had profound effects on central metabolic pathways that included the loss of aconitase activity and an inability to catabolize acetate during the stationary growth phase [301]. Reduced aconitase activity has been associated with reduced *agr* function [302], and it was subsequently suggested that ClpC may contribute to regulation of the tricarboxylic acid cycle in a manner that results in reduced expression of *agr* [303]. While this is consistent with the reduced capacity of a *clpC* mutant to form a biofilm, it is inconsistent with the observation that mutation of *clpC* has little effect on the production of *S. aureus* toxins [298].

While mutation of the *clpQ* protease or its *clpY* ATPase partner has little phenotypic effect, mutation of *clpP*, *clpX*, *clpB* and, to a lesser extent, *clpC* and *clpL* results in reduced intracellular replication [297,298]. Since uptake by host cells is unaffected, it was suggested that these mutants are unable to respond to the stress of the intracellular environment. Intracellular replication of *S. aureus* requires escape from the endosome, and *agr* is required for escape, presumably because it activates production of cytolytic exoproteins that lyse the endosomal membrane [304]. Because they are required for *agr*-mediated induction of extracellular toxins, it has been proposed that the reduced intracellular replication of *clpP* and *clpX* mutants may be a function of their reduced expression of *agr* and consequent inability to escape from the endosome [293].

Iron acquisition and its contribution to disease

We have chosen to give iron acquisition specific consideration based on the amount of information generated since the previous edition of this book. Indeed, it has become clear that *S. aureus* has at its disposal multiple iron acquisition systems that include both siderophore-based systems and systems for direct uptake via surface-associated proteins [305–307]. The four siderophores identified to date are staphyloferrin A [308,309], staphyloferrin B [310,311], aureochelin [312], and staphylobactin [313,314]. The enzymes required for production of staphylobactin are encoded within the nine-gene *sbnABCDEFGHI* operon, and mutation of one of these genes (*sbnE*) was shown to result in reduced growth in iron-limited media and reduced virulence in a murine kidney abscess model [315].

Once siderophores bind extracellular iron, they are moved back into the cell by a number of iron-regulated ABC transporter systems that include iron-binding lipoproteins, an ATPase, and integral membrane proteins [316–318]. One of the best-known transporters is the ferric hydroxamate uptake (Fhu) system, which is composed of five genes, three of which (*fhuCBG*) are part of an operon and two of which (*fhuD1* and *fhuD2*) are genetically unlinked [318,319]. These genes encode proteins that transport iron(III)-hydroxamate siderophores including ferrichrome, coprogen, aerobactin, desferal, and rhodotorulic acid [318,320]. None of the siderophores produced by *S. aureus* are of the hydroxamate type, which suggests that *S. aureus* can scavenge iron(III)-hydroxamate siderophores produced by other bacteria. This was confirmed by Speziali *et al.* [314], who demonstrated uptake of iron(III)-hydroxamate complexes by the wild-type strains RN6390 and Newman but not their corresponding *fhuCBG* mutants. It was also demonstrated that iron(III)-staphylobactin, a nonhydroxamate-type siderophore, was not transported into the *fhuCBG* mutant unless the *fhuC* gene was provided in *trans* [314].

Transport of iron(III)-staphylobactin also requires products of the *sirABC* operon, which is upstream of the *sbn* operon encoding the enzymes required for staphylobactin synthesis [313,315]. The *sirA* gene encodes a lipoprotein while *sirBC* encodes two membrane-spanning proteins [313,315,316]. What is missing from the SirABC iron transport system is a cognate ATPase to produce the necessary energy to move iron(III)-staphylobactin into the cell, and FhuC appears to serve this function. Specifically, Speziali *et al.* [314] demonstrated that FhuC possesses all the characteristics of an ATP-binding protein and that it not only promotes uptake of hydroxamate siderophores by way of the Fhu system but also uptake of iron(III)-staphylobactin via SirABC. Sir-mediated uptake appears to be specific in that uptake of other siderophores, including hydroxamates, is not altered in *sirA* or *sirB* mutants [313,315]. This suggests that FhuC plays an important multifunctional role in *S. aureus* iron uptake. However, while mice infected with *fhuCBG* mutants exhibit reduced clinical signs (alertness, activity, and coat condition) during the early stages of infection, there are no significant differences in comparison with the isogenic parent strains with respect to abscess formation or the number of bacteria recovered from the kidney [314]. Once again, this suggests that *S. aureus* does in fact have multiple paths to the same end.

Morrissey *et al.* [317] described a third operon (*sstABCD*) that is preceded by a consensus Fur (*f*erric *u*ptake *r*epressor) box and encodes products with significant homology to other siderophore transport systems. These include two cytoplasmic membrane proteins (SstA and SstB), an ATPase (SstC), and a membrane-bound lipoprotein (SstD). Subsequent experiments confirmed that SstD is produced *in vivo* in a rat intraperitoneal chamber model and that its production is partially repressed by addition of ferric iron to the growth medium. However, little is known about the siderophore specificity of Sst-mediated uptake, largely because attempts to generate an *sstD* mutant were not successful. Morrissey *et al.* [317] did examine strains in which production of SstD was repressed using antisense technology, but no significant differences were observed with respect to uptake of any of the siderophores examined, perhaps owing to the fact that this approach did not result in complete repression of SstD production. Other possibilities include uptake of an as yet unrecognized siderophore or compensation via an alternative uptake system in a manner similar to FhuC.

Although Park *et al.* [321] concluded that siderophore-mediated uptake plays a "dominant and essential role" in acquiring iron from transferrin, *S. aureus* also produces a number of cell wall-associated proteins that promote the direct uptake of iron from host proteins. For instance, Modun *et al.* [322] identified a 42-kDa cell wall-associated protein (Tpn) that binds human transferrin and is produced by both *S. aureus* and *S. epidermidis*. Further characterization confirmed that this protein is actually the glycolytic enzyme glyceraldehyde 3-phosphate dehydrogenase (GAPDH) and that it can bind transferrin without compromising its enzymatic activity [323]. This is similar to the GAPDH of group A streptococci (subsequently renamed the streptococcal surface dehydrogenase), which is also capable of binding the extracellular matrix protein fibronectin while maintaining its enzymatic activity [324,325].

Taylor and Heinrichs [326] generated a GAPDH (*gap*) mutant in *S. aureus* RN6390 and demonstrated that cell wall fractions from the mutant were indeed devoid of GAPDH enzymatic activity. However, the same cell wall fractions retained the capacity to bind transferrin. This led to identification of a 38.5-kDa transferrin-binding protein (StbA) that is produced only when *S. aureus* is grown under iron-limited conditions. Mutation of the corresponding gene (*StbA*, *s*taphylococcal *t*ransferrin-*b*inding protein A) suggested that StbA rather than Tpn (GAPDH) is responsible for transferrin binding in *S. aureus*. Even if this is true, it does not preclude a role for GAPDH in iron acquisition in that its enzymatic activity (conversion of glyceraldehyde 3-phosphate to 1,3-diphosphoglycerate) may result in an acidic environment that promotes the removal of iron from transferrin [325]. It is also interesting to note that all sequenced staphylococci (including *S. epidermidis* and *S. haemolyticus*) contain two genes (*gapA1* and *gapA2*) encoding GAPDH. In *Bacillus subtilis*, GAPDH isoenzymes have the same enzymatic function, but one isozyme functions preferentially during glycolysis and the other during gluconeogenesis [327]. The *gapA1* and *gapA2* products in *S. aureus* may function in a similar manner, perhaps with one isozyme also being preferentially localized to the cell wall where it promotes transferrin binding either directly or indirectly by virtue of its enzymatic activity.

Staphylococcus aureus also has at least two systems capable of acquiring iron from heme proteins [307]. These are potentially the most important of all *S. aureus* iron acquisition systems considering that the majority (> 95%) of iron in the human host is bound by heme proteins located inside host cells [328]. In fact, this may be a primary function of the hemolytic toxins discussed above. The first of these systems was designated Isd and includes five transcriptional units (*isdA*, *isdB*, *isdCDEFsrtBisdG*, *isdH*, and *isdI*) [109,326,329]. The second (HtsABC, for *h*eme *t*ransport *s*ystem) was identified in a genome search for proteins similar to ABC-type iron transporters (see below).

The genes of the Isd system were first identified in an attempt to find sortase A (*srtA*) homologs in the *S. aureus* genome. This led to identification of *srtB*, which is part of a six-gene operon designated *isdCDEFsrtBisdG* [109]. One of these genes (*isdC*) encodes a protein with a unique NPQTN anchoring motif that is the only recognized substrate of sortase B [179]. Unlike sortase A substrates, which are displayed on the staphylococcal surface, IsdC is attached within the peptidoglycan layer such that the protein is not accessible to extracellular proteolysis [179,330]. Utilizing a murine renal abscess model, Mazmanian *et al.* [109] demonstrated that mutation of *srtB* had little effect on virulence during the early stages of infection but resulted in a significant defect compared with the parent strain as the infection progressed. This led to the suggestion that IsdC may not be important for initiating infection but rather makes its primary contribution with respect to maintaining infection in the face of ongoing changes in the host.

Two additional genes (*isdA* and *isdB*) are located upstream of the *isdCDEFsrtBisdG* operon and are divergently transcribed as monocistronic messages. Each of these genes, as well as the *isdCDEFsrtBisdG* operon itself, was subsequently shown to contain a Fur box and to be tightly regulated by the availability of iron [109,179]. Morrissey *et al.* [329] independently identified the same proteins, which they designated FrpA and FrpB (*f*ur-*r*egulated *p*roteins), and demonstrated that they are expressed *in vivo* as evidenced by the presence of specific antibodies in human sera from patients with *S. aureus* septicemia. IsdA/FrpA was subsequently shown to be identical to StbA (see above), and analysis of the region flanking *StbA* revealed a well-conserved region that includes a four-gene operon that Taylor and Heinrichs [326] designated *sirDEFG* for *s*taphylococcal *i*ron-*r*egulated (in keeping with the previously reported *sirABC* loci; see above). Thus, *sirDEFG* and *isdCDEF* would appear to be two different designations for the same genes.

The functions of the Isd proteins were recently reviewed by Maresso and Schneewind [305]. The system includes three heme or heme protein receptors covalently linked to the cell wall by sortase A (IsdA, IsdB, and IsdH) and a fourth (IsdC) covalently linked to the cell wall but by sortase B. IsdA binds hemoglobin, transferrin, and the extracellular matrix proteins fibronectin and fibrinogen [179,326,331,332]. This suggests that IsdA may function both in iron acquisition and as an adhesin. With respect to acquiring iron from transferrin, Park *et al.* [321] concluded that it plays an ancillary role in comparison with siderophore-mediated uptake. IsdA also binds heme in an atypical fashion [333], and Torres *et al.* [334] found that mutation of *isdA* has little impact on the ability to acquire iron from heme-containing proteins, at least in comparison with IsdB (see below). Mutation of *isdA* also had no effect on virulence in a murine model of abscess formation [334]. However, Clarke *et al.* [335] demonstrated that humans who are nasal carriers of *S. aureus* have reduced antibody titers to IsdA in comparison with noncarriers, and immunization with purified IsdA reduced nasal colonization in a rat model. A recent report also demonstrated that IsdA on the cell surface decreases cellular hydrophobicity and increases resistance to human skin fatty acids and antimicrobial peptides [336].

Kuklin *et al.* [337] demonstrated that immunization with IsdB also protects against staphylococcal sepsis in both a murine model and in rhesus macaques. IsdB and IsdH are immunologically similar in that antibodies raised against IsdB are cross-reactive with IsdH, and immunization with purified IsdH also resulted in reduced nasal colonization in the cotton rat model [335]. Elevated antibody levels to IsdH have been observed in humans who are not nasal carriers and in human convalescent sera [338]. An alternative nomenclature also exists for IsdH, which was independently identified when DNA fragments of *S. aureus* COL were cloned into an *Escherichia coli* surface display system and screened with human sera from patients suffering from staphylococcal disease [338]. In this case, the protein was designated HarA (*ha*ptoglobin *r*eceptor *A*) based on its ability to bind haptoglobin, hemoglobin, and the haptoglobin–hemoglobin complex [339]. Growth studies demonstrated that *S. aureus* can use hemoglobin as a sole iron source, and *in vitro* studies using purified IsdB also confirmed its ability to bind both hemoglobin [179] and the haptoglobin–hemoglobin complex [340].

The significance of binding hemoglobin–haptoglobin can be appreciated by the fact that during erythrocyte turnover in the host, a large amount of hemoglobin is released into the plasma. Hemoglobin is efficiently bound by haptoglobin ($K_a > 10^{15}$ mol/L) and transported to the liver by way of the reticuloendothelial system in order to prevent kidney damage, conserve iron pools, and recycle heme [341]. Thus, IsdB and/or IsdH may help *S. aureus* compete for this iron independently of the production of the α or β hemolytic toxins. This is consistent with the results of Torres *et al.* [334], who demonstrated that purified hemoglobin as well as intracellular erythrocyte hemoglobin is bound by IsdB on the surface of *S. aureus* and that the heme moiety is subsequently removed and transported into the cell. These authors also demonstrated that *isdB* and *isdH* mutants generated in strain Newman are attenuated in a mouse model. However, the defects were not equivalent in that a significant reduction (10-fold) was observed in spleen and kidneys harvested from mice inoculated with *isdB/isdBH* mutants whereas only a marginal reduction was observed for the *isdH* mutant and even then only in the kidney and not the spleen [334]. This clearly suggests that IsdB plays the predominant role in comparison with IsdH.

The remaining members of the Isd system are responsible for transporting heme iron across the cytoplasmic membrane or for removing iron from heme once inside the cell [305]. Specifically, IsdD is a membrane protein, IsdE is a hemin-binding lipoprotein, and IsdF is a heme-permease, with these proteins collectively functioning as an ABC-type iron transport system [307]. IsdG and IsdI are heme monooxygenases found in the cytoplasm, and both have been shown to degrade hemin releasing free iron [342]. Although *isdG* is part of the larger *isd* operon while *isdI* is part of a different transcriptional unit, expression of both is controlled by Fur in response to iron limitation. These enzymes resemble the ABM family of monooxygenases, which catalyze the oxidation of aromatic polyketides in *Streptomyces* [16]. However, IsdG and IsdI have a different substrate specificity making them the first members of a novel group of heme monooxygenases found exclusively in Gram-positive bacteria (e.g., *Bacillus anthracis*, *Listeria monocytogenes*, and *S. epidermidis*) [306,307].

Because *S. aureus* can acquire iron from different host proteins, Skaar *et al.* [343] examined whether one source was preferred over another. Results from this analysis indicated that the preferred iron source was heme, although the ratio of heme to transferrin uptake decreased with samples taken later in growth. This was attributed to a growth phase-dependent upregulation of other iron acquisition systems (e.g., siderophores and/or direct binding of transferrin). In addition, Skaar *et al.* [343] analyzed the available *S. aureus* genomes for other ABC-type iron transporters and found seven such systems. This included the *isdDEF*-, *sirABC*-, *fhuCBG*- and *sstABCD*-encoded systems discussed above, two systems that have not yet been functionally investigated and which are designated only as ORFs *sav0609-0610* and *sav1554-1557*, and a system designated *hts* (heme transport system). The last encodes two permeases (HtsB and HtsC) and a membrane lipoprotein (HtsA). Subsequent studies focusing on strain Newman indicated that the iron preference of *isdDEF*, *sirABC*, *fhuCBG*, *sav0609-0610*, and *sav1554-1557* mutants was no different from that of the parent strain in that heme was preferred over transferrin. This clearly suggests that *isdDEF* does not encode the primary heme transport system. In the case of the *sstABCD* mutant, the heme to transferrin ratio was the same as that of the parent strain early, but at later time points there was an apparent increase in the preference for heme [343]. It was suggested that this reflects a shift toward siderophore-mediated iron uptake during the later stages of infection, with the increased heme preference reflecting the inability of an *sstABCD* mutant to moderate this shift. In contrast, a decrease in the ratio of heme to transferrin uptake was observed in the *htsABC* mutant at all time points. This suggests that HtsABC plays the primary role in heme transport. The importance of this system was further evidenced by the fact that *htsB* and *htsC* mutants were significantly attenuated in a murine model [343]. This included abscess formation in the liver, which is the primary site of iron storage and heme recycling in mammals. Taken together, these observations led Skaar *et al.* [343] to suggest that *S. aureus* preferentially utilizes heme uptake via the HtsABC transport system during the early stages of infection and at sites rich in heme proteins but then shifts to siderophore-mediated iron uptake once the availability of heme proteins becomes limited.

Reniere *et al.* [306] proposed three possible fates of heme iron once it is inside the cell. First, intracellular heme is degraded by the IsdG and IsdI monooxygenases releasing free iron that would more than likely be bound by staphylococcal ferritin (FtnA), a protein that stores iron in a nontoxic form for use when iron becomes restricted [344]. Second, intact heme is complexed with a membrane-associated heme-binding factor and used as a cofactor for specific *S. aureus* enzymes involved in energy production and/or protection against reactive oxygen species (e.g., cytochromes and catalase). This "molecular hijacking" hypothesis [306] is consistent with the observation that heme is segregated into the *S. aureus* cytoplasmic membrane whereas transferrin is preferentially sorted to the cytoplasm [343]. Third, given the toxicity of heme at high concentration, excess intracellular heme needs to be removed. Indeed, Mazmanian *et al.* [179] demonstrated that when *S. aureus* is given exogenous heme, cells are saturated in as little as 15 min. Therefore, any heme that is not degraded by IsdG and IsdI or incorporated into heme-requiring proteins must be efficiently removed.

In *S. aureus*, heme is transported out of the cell by the ABC-type efflux pump HrtAB (*h*eme-*r*egulated *t*ransporter). Mutants defective in either HrtA (ATP-binding protein) or HrtB (permease) have a reduced capacity to grow in media with heme as the sole iron source [100]. However, an *hrtA* mutant exhibited increased virulence in a murine model [345]. This hypervirulence was correlated with a reduction in the number of phagocytes recruited to the site of infection. Additionally, the *hrtA* mutant produced elevated amounts of a number of extracellular proteins with immunomodulatory functions that include inhibition of phagocyte recruitment/activation and opsonophagocytosis. Based on this, it was hypothesized that once *S. aureus* encounters a heme-rich environment, it avoids heme toxicity by activating the HrtAB system to promote efflux of heme iron while simultaneously reducing the production of specific virulence factors that would otherwise promote host tissue damage and further release of heme.

Torres *et al.* [345] examined the region upstream of *hrtAB* and found two genes (*hssRS*) whose products are related to the response regulator (HssR) and sensor components (HssS) of bacterial two-component signal transduction systems. Expression of *hrtAB* was dependent on *hssRS*, and HssR was subsequently shown to bind a direct repeat within the *hrtAB* promoter resulting in increased expression of *hrtAB* [345,346]. Mutation of *hssR* also resulted in a phenotype identical to that of an *hrtA* mutant including increased virulence in a murine model of hematogenous infection [345]. This appears to be a highly specific regulatory system in that previous studies found that expression of *hrtAB* was not affected by other environmental cues including low pH [347], nitric oxide concentration [348], the cold shock, heat shock, stringent or SOS response [349], or the global regulators *agr*, *mgrA*, *sigB* or *sarA* [39,350,351].

Regulation of *Staphylococcus aureus* virulence factors

Equally important as the ability to produce a virulence factor is the ability to produce it in a controlled manner appropriate for the task at hand. In their analysis of the N315 and Mu50 genomes, Kuroda *et al.* [352] identified 124 genes encoding what they considered "transcription regulators." This included 17 two-component signal-transduction systems and 63 regulators presumed to be DNA-binding proteins based on the presence of helix-turn-helix motifs. Based on our search of the literature, mutations have been generated in just over 30 of these genes. Reports describing three of these (*svrA*, *traP*, *xpr*) have subsequently been called into question based on previously undetected mutations in *agr* [271,353–357]. Other than *traP*, which we address based on its persistence in the staphylococcal literature, we have limited our comments to those remaining regulatory elements that have been examined in the specific context of pathogenesis. It should be noted that some of these (e.g., *hssRS*) have already been discussed elsewhere in this chapter. For detailed mechanistic studies, we defer to the primary papers cited below and several recent and relatively comprehensive reviews [73,74,358–361].

Accessory gene regulator

The original *agr* mutant (ISP546) was isolated by Peter Pattee and colleagues as a chromosomal Tn*551* insertion in an 8325-4 strain. It was initially concluded that the insertion occurred in the *hla* gene based on the failure of this mutant to produce α-toxin [362], but it was later determined that *hla* was intact in ISP546 and that the Tn*551* insertion had a pleiotropic effect that included decreased production of several exoproteins and increased production of SpA [363]. The insertion site was characterized by two groups, with one designating it *exp* [364] and the other *agr* [365]. The insertion was subsequently localized to what became designated *agrA*, which encodes the response regulator of the *agr* system as described below.

The *agr* regulatory system includes two divergent promoters (P2 and P3) that drive production of transcripts designated RNAII and RNAIII respectively [361]. The RNAII transcript spans the operon (*agrACDB*) that encodes the individual elements of the two-component regulatory system itself. Specifically, AgrA and AgrC are the response regulator and membrane sensor respectively. These proteins are responsive to accumulation of an *agrD*-encoded autoinducing peptide (AIP), production of which requires processing and export by the membrane-embedded AgrB along with the SpsB signal peptidase [366]. AIP consists of a thiolactone "macrocycle" and an "exocyclic tail," both of which are functionally important [367]. AIP binding to the AgrC membrane sensor initiates a phosphorylation cascade that results in activation of the AgrA response regulator and increased transcription from both the P2 and P3 promoters. The AgrA binding sites within the intergenic region between P2 and P3 have been mapped, and biochemical studies have confirmed that phosphorylation promotes homodimerization of AgrA and binding to both the P2 and P3 promoters [368]. To date, this is the only recognized function of AgrA.

Strain-dependent subtypes of *agr* have been identified based on genetic polymorphisms that match the *agrD*-encoded AIP, the *agrB*-encoded enzyme required for AIP processing, and the *agrC*-encoded membrane histidine kinase sensor [369]. While binding of AIP to its cognate AgrC sensor results in activation of *agr*, binding of "mismatched" variants generally results in inhibition rather than activation [370,371]. A recent report examining mixed populations in an insect (*Manduca sexta*) model found that this interference occurs *in vivo* [372]. It could be argued that an *agr* subtype associated with a constellation of genes that confers an *in vivo* advantage could exert its dominance not only by controlling production of its own *agr*-regulated virulence factors but also by inhibiting the ability of other staphylococci in the same microenvironment to do the same thing, but to date there is little evidence to suggest that *agr*-mediated interference plays a direct role in human infection. Indeed, Robinson *et al.* [373] proposed on the basis of population studies that host–pathogen interactions selecting among different patterns of gene expression drive the divergence of *agr* subtypes and that this is the more important evolutionary force in comparison with bacterial interference. This is consistent with the observation that certain *agr* subtypes can be associated, albeit loosely, with the ability to cause certain types of infection [374]. This is particularly true in the context of toxin-mediated diseases including exfoliative disease and toxic shock syndrome, but certain *agr* subtypes have also been associated with infections that are less obviously toxin-mediated including endocarditis [370,371,374,375].

Attempts have also been made to determine whether *agr*-mediated interference plays a role in other aspects of pathogenesis. For instance, Lina *et al.* [376] found that nasal carriers of *S. aureus* were always colonized with only one *agr* variant and that colonization with *S. epidermidis*, which is capable of cross-species *agr*-mediated interference [377], generally precluded concomitant colonization with *S. aureus*. However, based on comparison with inhibitory profiles defined *in vitro*, these authors also concluded that this was a function of something other than *agr*-mediated bacterial interference. As with the production of specific exotoxins, this suggests that *agr* subtype may not be the defining characteristic but rather a marker of clonal lineages that possess specific properties that impact colonization and/or virulence. Similarly, there is evidence to suggest a correlation between certain *agr* subtypes and antibiotic resistance, although once again this correlation is far from absolute [378–381].

The functional result of *agr* activation is increased expression from the P3 promoter, resulting in increased production of RNAIII. The RNAIII transcript spans the *hld* gene, which encodes δ-toxin [382], but it has been conclusively demonstrated that the regulatory effects of *agr* are mediated by RNAIII irrespective of the production of δ-toxin [70,273,383]. The mechanism by which RNAIII functions is not fully understood but appears to involve both transcriptional and posttranscriptional effects [360,361,383–386]. With respect to the latter, the best-studied examples are α-toxin (Hla) and Spa, production of which is inversely regulated by RNAIII. In the case of α-toxin, RNAIII interacts with the *hla* transcript in a fashion that exposes the ribosome-binding site and thereby facilitates translation [386]. In contrast, RNAIII down-regulates Spa production by binding the *spa* transcript and inhibiting translation and by forming an RNAIII–*spa* mRNA complex that is degraded by RNase III [387]. A recent study confirmed that RNAIII binds a variety of mRNAs and that this both limits translation and triggers RNase III cleavage [384].

RNAIII also modulates the production of virulence factors indirectly through its impact on other regulatory elements. For instance, *rot* (*r*epressor *o*f *t*oxins, see below) encodes a protein (Rot) with a global but generally opposite regulatory effect in comparison with *agr* [388], and it was recently demonstrated that RNAIII binds *rot* mRNA in a manner that blocks translation [384,385]. Additionally, Arvidson and Tegmark [358] suggested that RNAIII may function, at least in part, by binding and inactivating the

DNA-binding protein SarA (see below). Such results suggest that it may not be the absolute amount of RNAIII but rather the amount of RNAIII relative to other regulatory factors that defines the overall gene expression profile in *S. aureus*.

The overall regulatory effect of RNAIII is characterized by the increased production of exoproteins and decreased production of surface-associated virulence factors [72,361]. Although there are exceptions, particularly with respect to certain surface proteins [389,390], this is by and large a global effect that reflects the need to delay the metabolic expense of producing exoproteins in favor of colonization until the infection achieves a quorum of bacteria capable of maintaining the infection in light of an ongoing immune response [361]. However, this paradigm is based primarily on studies done *in vitro*, and there are numerous reports suggesting that regulatory events observed *in vitro* may not be representative of those observed *in vivo*. For instance, Yarwood *et al.* [76] found that expression of *agr* is repressed both in serum and *in vivo*. In fact, these authors failed to reveal a statistical correlation between the expression of *agr* and expression of any *S. aureus* virulence factor *in vivo*. Similarly, Xiong *et al.* [75] found that expression of *hla* in cardiac vegetations is essentially unchanged by mutation of *agr*. There is also evidence to suggest that RNAIII can be activated *in vivo* through an RNAII-independent mechanism [391]. Such studies emphasize the importance of examining regulatory events *in vivo* rather than solely by extension of *in vitro* observations [73,74,392].

Expression of *agr* has also been associated with a reduced capacity to form a biofilm in both *S. aureus* and *S. epidermidis* [393,394]. In strains that produce RNAIII at high levels, including RN6390, mutation of *agr* results in an increased capacity to form a biofilm [242], and there is evidence to suggest that activation of *agr* may constitute a specific means of dispersal from a biofilm [395]. In fact, Yarwood *et al.* [396] recently demonstrated that *agr*-negative variants arise spontaneously in *S. aureus* biofilms and that, over time, these variants become the dominant subpopulation. To the extent that surface-associated adhesins contribute to biofilm formation, these results are consistent with the observation that *agr* mutants exhibit increased production of most surface proteins. However, unlike *agr*-mediated regulation, there is evidence to suggest that the negative impact of *agr* on biofilm formation is a function of the surfactant properties of δ-toxin rather than RNAIII itself [397]. At the same time, there is also evidence to suggest that addition of exogenous AIP to *S. aureus* biofilms results in dissociation due to the induction of *agr* transcription and the consequent increase in the production of specific proteases (Dr Alex Horswill, University of Iowa, personal communication). Presumably, the combined effect of repression of surface protein synthesis and induction of proteases that degrade adhesins on the cell surface would promote release of bacterial cells from the biofilm.

Despite evidence that *agr* has a negative impact on biofilm formation and may not function as predicted under *in vivo* conditions, the fact remains that mutation of *agr* has resulted in reduced virulence in every animal model examined [398–403]. This clearly demonstrates that *agr* plays a central role in the production of *S. aureus* virulence factors both *in vitro* and *in vivo*. However, that does not preclude the possibility that it plays different roles in different strains. Indeed, recent data suggest that the increased virulence of CA-MRSA isolates may be a function of their increased expression of *agr*. Specifically, one possible explanation for the increased virulence of CA-MRSA isolates is their increased production of PSMs (see above), and Wang *et al.* [70] demonstrated that PSM production is positively regulated by *agr* and that expression of *agr* is also elevated in CA-MRSA in comparison with HA-MRSA. This was not an absolute correlation, which suggests the existence of an *agr*-independent regulatory pathway that also modulates PSM production, but it nevertheless emphasizes that the relative level of gene expression may be as important in pathogenesis as the presence or absence of different virulence factors.

The inverse effect of *agr* on PSM production and biofilm formation is interesting because it suggests two relatively distinct pathways to disease. These clearly are not mutually exclusive pathways as evidenced by the fact that at least some CA-MRSA strains, including USA300, retain some capacity to form a biofilm [357]. Expression of *agr* is also tightly regulated, so a single strain can presumably modulate its phenotype to promote biofilm formation or PSM production depending on its immediate needs. Nevertheless, the distinction between HA-MRSA and CA-MRSA with respect to production of RNAIII was apparent even during the postexponential growth phase when *agr* expression would presumably be highest for any given strain [70]. This suggests that the level of *agr* expression may in fact define two relatively distinct phenotypic groups, one of which is geared toward biofilm formation while the other is geared toward toxin production. The existence of such groups may help explain the distinction between the opportunistic nature of HA-MRSA infection and the fact that CA-MRSA cause disease even in uncompromised hosts [278,404].

Target of RNAIII-activating protein

There are reports indicating that other regulatory loci also modulate transcription from the *agr* P2 and P3 promoters. One of these is *traP*, which is described in numerous reports as an activator of *agr* expression [405–410]. Specifically, accumulation of a protein designated RAP (RNAIII-activating peptide) reportedly results in phosphorylation of an intracellular protein designated TraP (*t*arget of *R*NAIII-*a*ctivating *p*rotein), which in turn leads to activation of RNAII production, accumulation of the *agr*-encoded AIP, and ultimately increased production of RNAIII [411]. These reports are in direct contrast to studies demonstrating that mutation of *traP* has no impact on expression of *agr* [356,357]. There is also evidence to suggest that the original *traP* mutation was in fact a spontaneous *agr* mutant [271].

There are also numerous studies suggesting that a peptide designated RIP (RNAIII-inhibitory peptide) can be used to inhibit *traP* phosphorylation and both limit expression of *agr* [412] and inhibit biofilm formation [406,413,414]. Despite the preponderance of data indicating that *agr* has a negative impact on biofilm formation (see above), one issue that has never been addressed in the *traP* literature is why RIP/*traP*-mediated inhibition of *agr* expression would inhibit rather than enhance biofilm formation. Moreover, mutation of *traP* in clinical isolates also had no significant impact on biofilm formation [357]. This suggests that any inhibitory effect observed with RIP is a function of something other than inhibition of an *S. aureus* regulatory pathway involving *traP* and/or *agr*. However, this does not preclude the possibility that synthetic RIP could be used therapeutically to limit *S. aureus* biofilm formation *in vivo* [415].

Staphylococcal accessory regulator

A second regulatory locus that impacts expression of *agr* is the staphylococcal accessory regulator (*sarA*). The *sarA* locus was identified by screening a transposon-insertion library generated in strain DB [416]. Analysis of genome sequence data has revealed the existence of many genes encoding structurally similar proteins (e.g., *sarR*, *sarT*, *sarU*, *sarV*, *sarX*, *sarZ*, *rot* and *mgrA*), and these factors act through the *agr* system and independently of *agr* in a complex signaling web to regulate the expression of virulence determinants (Figure 4.1).

The *sarA* locus encodes three overlapping transcripts, all of which share a common terminus and include the *sarA* gene [417]. These transcripts have been designated *sarA* (0.56 kb), *sarC* (0.8 kb), and *sarB* (1.2 kb), with the corresponding promoters designated P1, P3 and P2

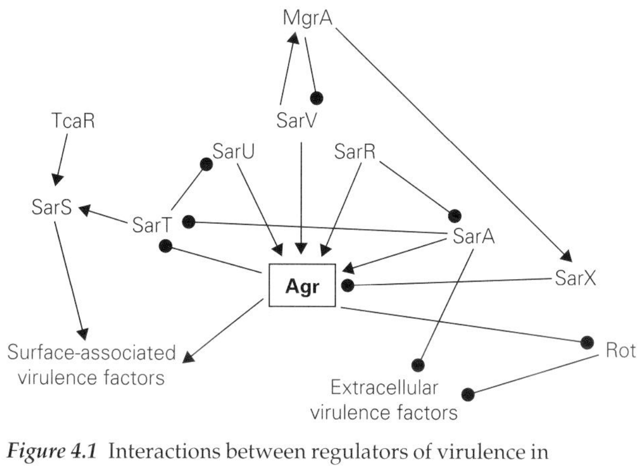

Figure 4.1 Interactions between regulators of virulence in *S. aureus*. Schematic of the complex pathways involved in the expression of both surface-associated and extracellular virulence factors.

respectively [418]. The *sarA* and *sarB* transcripts are produced preferentially during the exponential growth phase while the *sarC* transcript is produced preferentially during post-exponential growth [418]. This is consistent with the observation that transcription from the P3 promoter is at least partially *sigB*-dependent [38]. Other regulatory elements that contribute to the temporal pattern of *sarA* transcription include SarR, which reportedly inhibits transcription from the P1 promoter [419], and SarA itself, which represses its own production by limiting transcription from both P1 and P3 [420]. Different studies have reached different conclusions with respect to the overall impact of the temporal regulation of *sarA* transcription on the production of SarA, with some concluding that SarA is produced in a growth phase-dependent manner [421,422] and others concluding that it is produced in roughly equivalent amounts irrespective of growth phase [389]. There are two small ORFs (designated ORF3 and ORF4) upstream of the *sarA* ORF, and Chien *et al.* [422] concluded that mutation of ORF3, which is located immediately upstream of the P1 promoter, results in reduced production of SarA. However, Blevins *et al.* [389] did not find a significant difference in the amount of SarA produced based on the presence of either upstream ORF.

SarA and its homologs are winged helix DNA-binding proteins [423]. Attempts to define the SarA binding site have met with limited success beyond demonstrating a strong preference for AT-rich DNA [424,425], and it is clear that SarA has the ability to bind DNA in a relatively indiscriminate manner. Based on this, it has been suggested that SarA may function through its ability to alter DNA topology in a manner similar to HN-S rather than as a classic transcription factor [426,427]. It has also been shown that mutation of *sarA* affects mRNA stability in a global manner [428]. Of 145 mRNA transcripts affected, 138 had a longer half-life in wild-type cells (UAMS-1) than in the corresponding *sarA* mutant, suggesting that in general SarA stabilizes mRNA. More detailed analysis of the *cna* and *spa* transcripts confirmed that both are significantly destabilized in a *sarA* mutant. SarA also represses transcription of both *cna* and *spa* [17,389,429], which means that it has the apparently opposing effects of repressing transcription but stabilizing those transcripts that are produced. At the same time, stabilization may occur in a manner that limits translation, in which case SarA would limit production of the corresponding proteins at both the transcriptional and posttranscriptional levels.

Mutation of *sarA* in the 8325-4 strains RN450 and RN6390 was found to limit expression of *agr* and a number of *agr*-regulated genes, particularly under microaerophilic growth conditions [421,422,430–432]. SarA has been shown to bind the intergenic region between the *agr* P2 and P3 promoters [433–436], and based on this the current regulatory paradigm is that SarA binding activates transcription of *agr* and that this accounts in large part for the impact of *sarA* on expression of *S. aureus* virulence factors

[73,359,361,422–424,433]. SarA also reportedly has an indirect effect on expression of *agr* via its impact on expression of other *sarA* homologs. Specifically, Schmidt *et al.* [437] proposed a model in which SarU induces production of RNAIII while SarT represses expression of *sarU*. Mutation of *sarT* would therefore enhance expression of RNAIII by virtue of the depression of *sarU*. Since SarA represses production of SarT, it would indirectly activate production of RNAIII by repressing production of SarT and thereby increasing production of SarU. This secondary amplification loop is potentially important in that *sarT* and *sarU* are part of RD5, which, as noted above, is absent in prominent lineages of *S. aureus* clinical isolates. The presence or absence of RD5 could therefore be one factor defining strain-dependent differences in the overall level of *agr* transcription.

The relative contributions of the direct and indirect pathways of SarA-mediated *agr* activation have not been defined, and it is possible that strain-dependent variation in the level of *agr* transcription is a function of factors unrelated to *sarA* or its homologs. Bischoff *et al.* [38] concluded that SigB increases expression of *sarA* while simultaneously reducing expression of *agr*. This would not be expected if the major regulatory impact of SarA on *agr* expression was mediated by direct activation of *agr* transcription. It also would not be expected based on the *sarT*/*sarU* secondary amplification loop since the increased production of SarA would result in reduced expression of *sarT*, which would lead in turn to increased expression of *sarU* and presumably RNAIII. This suggests that the *rsbU* mutation in 8325-4 strains may play a primary role in *agr* expression in comparison with *sarA* irrespective of whether the effect of the latter is direct or indirect. This is consistent with the results of Horsburgh *et al.* [40], who found that *agr* expression was reduced in an *rsbU*-repaired derivative of 8325-4 (SH1000) despite the fact that SarA levels were unchanged by repair of *rsbU* in 8325-4 or mutation of *sigB* in SH1000.

The more important point with respect to the impact of *sarA* on expression of *agr* is that the current paradigm, like the *S. aureus* regulatory paradigm in general, is defined almost exclusively by studies done with 8325-4 strains. This is true despite the fact that the phenotype of the original *sarA* mutant, which was generated in the clinical isolate DB, was completely at odds with this paradigm. Specifically, the phenotype of the original DB *sarA* mutant (11D2) was characterized by increased production of extracellular virulence factors and decreased production of surface-associated virulence factors, and it was proposed on this basis that *sarA* acts as a "counter-regulatory system" with respect to *agr* [416].

While its impact with respect to *agr* remains unclear, it is clear that *sarA* has *agr*-independent regulatory effects. The impact of SarA on expression of *sarT* has been mentioned, and this also has regulatory effects independent of *agr*. Specifically, SarT also induces transcription of *sarS* [437]. Since SarS is an activator of Spa production, this suggests that strains lacking *sarT* would express *sarS* and therefore *spa* at reduced levels, but we have not found this to be the case [429]. Rather, we found that RN6390 expresses *sarS* at greatly reduced levels in comparison with clinical isolates irrespective of whether the clinical isolates encode RD5 (unpublished results). One possible explanation for this is the *tcaR* mutation in all 8325-4 strains including RN6390 (see below).

SarA also binds *cis* elements associated with the promoters of other *S. aureus* virulence factors [389,424,425]. The importance of the *agr*-independent regulatory functions of SarA are best evidenced by the fact that *sarA*/*agr* mutants have reduced virulence even in comparison with *agr* mutants [42,400,438,439]. In some cases (e.g., *agr*, *hla*, *fnbA*), mutation of *sarA* results in reduced transcription, while in others (e.g., *cna*, *spa*, *sspA*) transcription is increased. However, Arvidson and Tegmark [358] concluded that SarA and its homologs are essentially repressors, with the difference between activation and repression being dependent on whether the activity of SarA is mediated by a direct interaction with the relevant promoter or indirectly via the impact of SarA on some downstream gene (e.g., direct repression of *sarT* resulting indirectly in activation of *sarU*). We believe the cumulative evidence to date suggests that SarA is primarily if not exclusively a repressor and that the *agr*-independent regulatory functions of *sarA* play the more important role in comparison with the impact of *sarA* on transcription of *agr*. For example, mutation of *sarA* in RN6390 results in decreased expression of *hla* but has the opposite effect in clinical isolates [17,429]. Since *agr* activates *hla* transcription and the production of α-toxin (see above), this clearly suggests that the impact of *sarA* on *hla* transcription, at least in clinical isolates, is independent of its impact on expression of *agr*. Additionally, mutation of *sarA* results in reduced capacity to bind fibronectin, and while there are reports concluding this is a direct effect [390,424], other reports have concluded that the impact of *sarA* on fibronectin binding is indirect in that it is mediated primarily through increased production of proteases in *sarA* mutants resulting in degradation of the Fnb adhesins [429,440,441].

The inverse effect of *sarA* on *hla* transcription in RN6390 versus clinical isolates is important in that several studies focusing on 8325-4 strains have concluded that mutation of *sarA* or *hla* attenuates the virulence of *S. aureus*. Based on the paradigm defined by such strains, it is reasonable to suggest that the reduced production of α-toxin in *sarA* mutants would contribute to their reduced virulence. However, this would not be expected in clinical isolates, where *sarA* mutants express *hla* and produce α-toxin at increased rather than decreased levels [429]. Although we demonstrated that mutation of *sarA* attenuated the virulence of the clinical isolate UAMS-1 in a murine model of septic arthritis despite the fact that it resulted in increased capacity to bind collagen and increased hemolytic activity [438], it remains important to explain the mechanistic basis for this disparity.

One possible explanation for this disparity, at least according to the current regulatory paradigm, is the presence of RD5 and consequently *sarT* and *sarU*. More directly, SarA represses transcription of *sarT* which in turn represses transcription of *hla* [437]. At the same time, SarA binds the *hla* promoter directly, and mutation of putative SarA-binding sites upstream of *hla* was correlated with reduced expression of *hla* and reduced production of α-toxin [424]. This suggests that the impact of SarA on production of α-toxin may be dependent on whether SarA interacts directly with the *hla* promoter or indirectly through *sarT*. Specifically, mutation of *sarA* in a *sarT*-positive strain would result in increased production of SarT and decreased expression of *hla*, while mutation of *sarA* in a *sarT*-negative strain would result directly in decreased repression, and therefore increased expression, of *hla* transcription.

Despite the logic of this hypothesis, it is unlikely to be relevant since mutation of *sarA* results in increased *hla* transcription even in strains that encode RD5 [429]. In fact, Oscarsson *et al.* [442] have demonstrated that mutation of *sarA* in the *rsbU*-repaired 8325-4 strain SH1000 results in increased rather than decreased hemolytic activity. While this suggests that the *rsbU* mutation in 8325-4 contributes to the disparate effect of *sarA* on *hla* transcription, expression of *hla* was also increased when *sarA* was mutated in the strain V8, which also carries an *rsbU* mutation [442]. This implies some additional difference that defines the impact of *sarA* on transcription of *hla*. One possibility is the *tcaR* mutation in 8325-4 strains, which is not present in V8 [33]. As noted above, TcaR plays an important role in expression of *sarS* [33], which is consistent with the observation that RN6390 produces less SarS than clinical isolates (unpublished results). Based on this, Oscarsson *et al.* [442] proposed a model in which SarS and SarA both repress transcription of *hla*, with SarA serving the dual role of also acting indirectly as a repressor of SarS production [437]. In 8325-4 strains like RN6390, where the level of SarS is limited, mutation of *sarA* would result in a net increase in the amount of repressor by virtue of increasing production of SarS. Thus, transcription of *hla* would decrease. However, in clinical isolates, where the amount of SarS is already high, mutation of *sarA* would result in a net decrease in the amount of repressor (owing to the absence of SarA) and consequently increased expression of *hla*.

TcaR also regulates expression of *sasF* (SACOL2668), which encodes a surface protein of unknown function [33], and we have also confirmed that clinical isolates express *sasF* at levels that far exceed those observed in RN6390 [17]. At present, the possible impact of this on pathogenesis has not been investigated, but taken together these results clearly suggest that the *tcaR* mutation in 8325-derived strains is potentially important with respect to the overall pathogenesis of *S. aureus*. Subsequent studies have demonstrated that mutation of *tcaR* in at least some *S. aureus* strains (e.g., NCTC-10833) also results in enhanced transcription of the intercellular adhesin (*ica*) operon [31]. To the extent that PIA contributes to *S. aureus* biofilm formation [231], this would suggest that strains with reduced *tcaR* function would have enhanced capacity to form a biofilm, but this is clearly not the case with RN6390 [242]. Once again, this may be a function of multiple, overlapping regulatory pathways, with the impact of one being dependent on the relative level of another. More directly, the elevated production of RNAIII in RN6390 may limit biofilm formation irrespective of any impact the *tcaR* mutation has on the production of PIA. The fact that mutation of *agr* enhances biofilm formation in RN6390 provides support for this hypothesis [242].

Unlike RN6390, mutation of *sarA* results in reduced capacity to form a biofilm in clinical isolates while mutation of *agr* has relatively little effect [242]. This is important for several reasons. First, it may well explain why *sarA*-negative clinical isolates exhibit reduced virulence despite the fact that they produce toxins (including α-toxin) and extracellular proteins at elevated levels [429,438]. Second, it is difficult to envision how these disparate phenotypes would arise if the primary impact of *sarA* on *S. aureus* regulatory circuits were mediated through its ability to enhance transcription of *agr*, and this is true irrespective of whether the impact of *sarA* on *agr* transcription is mediated through a direct or indirect pathway. Finally, irrespective of the mechanism involved (e.g., δ-toxin acting as a surfactant or the induction of *agr* and consequent production of proteases), mutation of *agr* enhances biofilm formation in RN6390 but has little effect in clinical isolates, which suggests that *agr* expression in RN6390 can be functionally defined as excessive at least in the context of biofilm formation. Genome-scale transcriptional profiling studies clearly demonstrate that mutation of *agr* has a greater impact in the 8325-derived strain RN27 [350] than in the clinical isolate UAMS-1 [17], but to date the relative impact in other isolates, including CA-MRSA, has not been examined. The 8325-4 strains like RN6390 are obviously virulent, and this is to be expected given the fact that such strains produce essentially all toxins (including β-toxin) and extracellular proteins (e.g., proteases) at high levels. However, this does not mean that other strains have not chosen a different path to the same end or that the path they have chosen is not more representative of a prominent if not predominant type of *S. aureus* clinical isolate.

Other SarA homologs

Staphylococcus aureus also produces a number of other SarA homologs including SarR, SarV, SarX, SarZ, Rot, and MgrA. These systems interact in complex and as yet incompletely understood ways. The primary function of SarR appears to be repression of *sarA* transcription [419], but another report suggests it also activates transcription of *agr* by binding to sites in the intergenic region between the P2 and P3 promoters [443]. In fact, SarR bound this region with higher affinity than SarA, and it was suggested based on analysis of an RN6390 *sarA*/*sarR* double mutant that the two proteins have an additive effect on transcription of *agr*. A recent report concluded that SarA and SarR also cooperate to modulate transcription of *sarA*, although in this case they appear to function as repressors rather than activators [420]. It has been proposed on the basis of such studies that SarA and SarR may modulate transcription of target genes as heterodimers with the ultimate effect (activation vs. repression) depending on the relative position of binding sites with respect to each other [443].

In contrast to SarR, most other *sarA* homologs appear to function downstream of SarA. This includes SarT, production of which is repressed by SarA, as well as SarU and SarS, production of which is modulated by SarA indirectly by virtue of its effect on SarT [437]. SarA, along with MgrA (see below), also represses production of SarV. Mutation of *sarV* was associated with reduced expression of both *mgrA* and *agr*, with the former contributing to altered autolytic activity and the latter being associated with decreased expression of *hla* and the genes encoding several proteases [444]. With respect to autolytic activity, it was proposed that *sarV* and *mgrA* (also known as *rat* and *norR*) constitute an important feedback loop, which is consistent with other studies demonstrating that mutation of *mgrA* results in increased autolysis [445]. With respect to the production of other virulence factors, it was proposed on the basis of transcriptional profiling studies that *mgrA* acts in concert with *agr* to increase production of exoproteins and decrease production of surface proteins [351]. At the same time, there is evidence to suggest that *mgrA*, like *sarA*, has *agr*-independent regulatory functions that include modulating transcription of both *hla* and *sarS* [446]. In fact, the transcriptional profiling results of Luong *et al.* [351], which were done with Newman rather than RN6390, confirmed that mutation of *mgrA* has a global effect on the production of virulence factors but relatively little impact on expression of *agr*. To the extent that mutation of *agr* enhances biofilm formation, this is consistent with the observation that mutation of *mgrA* was recently shown to limit biofilm formation [447]. Another report has also demonstrated that MgrA is responsive to oxidative changes that induce, among other things, resistance to certain antibiotics [448].

In contrast to *sarV*, MgrA activates transcription of *sarX* [443]. SarX in turn negatively regulates expression of *agr*. This would be the third *sarA* homolog (the other two being SarA and SarR) that bind the *agr* intergenic region, the difference being that the binding of SarX represses rather than activates *agr* expression [443]. Yet another is *sarZ*, mutation of which results in decreased production of RNAIII and decreased expression of the *agr*-regulated genes *hla* and *hlb* [449]. Although the reduced hemolytic activity of a *sarZ* mutant could be explained by the impact of SarZ on production of RNAIII, binding studies also indicated that SarZ is capable of binding the *hla* promoter directly, once again suggesting the existence of both *agr*-dependent and *agr*-independent regulatory pathways for most if not all *sarA* homologs.

SarZ was identified in a screen for genes that suppress the nonhemolytic phenotype of a mutant designated *cvfA* (*c*onserved *v*irulence *f*actor A). Specifically, Kaito *et al.* [450] identified three genes (*cvfA*, *cvfB*, and *cvfC*) that are required for full virulence in a silkworm pathogenesis model. Hemolysin production was reduced in all three mutants, and mutations in *cvfA* and *cvfC* were also shown to result in reduced virulence in a murine model. Subsequent studies confirmed that the *cvfA* and *cvfB* mutations result in a phenotype consistent with *agr*-dependent regulation but that both also have *agr*-independent functions [449,451]. In the case of *cvfA*, this is apparently mediated through *sarZ* in that mutation of *cvfA* resulted in reduced transcription of *sarZ* and consequently reduced expression of *agr*. Nagata *et al.* [452] demonstrated that CvfA has phosphodiesterase activity and that the reduced virulence of a *cvfA* mutant cannot be complemented with CvfA variants lacking this activity. To date, these studies have been limited to 8325-4 strains, most commonly the chemically mutagenized derivative RN4220, and the relevance of these observations in clinical isolates remains to be determined.

In contrast to many *sarA* homologs, rot functions in an opposing fashion to *agr*. Specifically, McNamara *et al.* [453] identified a transposon-insertion mutant in which exoprotein production was restored even in an *agr*-null background. The corresponding gene was designated *rot* (*r*epressor *o*f *t*oxins). McNamara and Bayer [403] subsequently demonstrated that mutation of *rot* restored virulence to an *agr* mutant in a rabbit endocarditis model. Said-Salim *et al.* [388] used genome-scale microarrays to confirm that *rot* has global effects on gene expression that are essentially opposite to those observed in *agr* mutants. Geisinger *et al.* [385] demonstrated that RNAIII directly inhibits production of Rot by binding the *rot* transcript and inhibiting translation. This would suggest that *rot* and *agr* function in direct opposition to each other to fine tune the transition between production of the surface proteins and production of exoproteins. This is consistent with the hypothesis that the overall gene expression profile in *S. aureus* is defined by the relative level of multiple regulatory elements rather than the absolute amount of any single gene product. Indeed, Geisinger *et al.* [385] also suggested that the increased production of RNAIII relative to Rot may account for the increased production of exoproteins in RN6390 and, conversely, that clinical isolates exhibit a phenotype dominated by production of surface proteins rather owing to the increased production and/or activity of Rot.

A recent report concluded that *rot* is expressed from a single promoter throughout the growth cycle of *S. aureus* [454]. However, experiments employing promoter fusions concluded that *rot* expression is influenced by multiple regulatory elements including *sigB*, *agr*, sarA, *sarR*, and *sarS*. These effects were growth-phase dependent, with mutation of *sigB* resulting in a modest increase in promoter activity during exponential growth and mutation of *agr* having the same effect in the postexponential growth phase [454]. As was the case for the *agr* and *sarA* promoter regions, both SarA and SarR were also shown to bind the *rot* promoter. However, the primary regulatory impact appeared to be mediated by by *sarS*, mutation of which resulted in a significant increase in *rot* expression. Interestingly, this effect was dependent on *agr* and *sarA* as evidenced by the fact that concomitant mutation of either largely eliminated the increased *rot* expression observed in a *sarS* mutant [454]. Based on the 8325-defined regulatory paradigm, *sarA* is upstream of *sarS* [437], so the impact of *sarA* on *rot* expression would presumably be independent of its impact on *sarS*, but at present the mechanism by which this occurs remains unclear. It is also unclear whether the impact of *sarS* on *rot* expression is mediated by direct binding of SarS, but irrespective of whether the regulatory effect is direct or indirect, it remains important to emphasize once again that expression of *sarS* is greatly reduced in 8325-4 strains in comparison with clinical isolates, presumably owing to the *tcaR* mutation (see above).

It is difficult, at best, to combine all the observations regarding *agr* and the *sarA* homologs into a cohesive regulatory model. Gao and Stewart [455] focused on detailed studies of the *spa* promoter and presented a model in which expression of *spa* is maximal when the *agr*-encoded AIP has not yet reached its threshold concentration. Production of SarT and Rot is repressed by *agr*, so during the period prior to AIP-mediated induction of *agr* transcription, these regulatory proteins would be present at functional levels, thus promoting expression of *sarS*. SarS in turn binds to defined sites upstream of the *spa* promoter in a fashion that precludes binding of SarA. As cell density increases resulting in activation of *agr*, functional levels of both SarT and Rot decline resulting in reduced production of SarS. SarA now becomes the predominant protein bound to the *spa* promoter, resulting in reduced transcription. Production of SpA would be further limited by the increased production of RNAIII, which as noted above downregulates production of Spa by binding the *spa* transcript resulting in reduced translation and formation of an RNAIII–*spa* mRNA complex that is specifically degraded by RNase III [387]. According to this model, the increased production of RNAIII, together with the reduced production of Rot, would promote translation of *hla* and production of α-toxin. Presumably, some variation on this theme would also account for the increased production of other *S. aureus* exoproteins.

Oscarsson *et al.* [456] went even further to suggest that *agr*, *sarA*, *sarR*, *sarT*, *sarU*, *mgrA*, and *rot* all contribute to the expression of *sarS* and the production of Spa either directly (*sarA*, *sarT*, *mgrA*, and *rot*) or indirectly (*agr*, *sarR*, and *sarU*). These authors proposed an interactive regulatory network in which SarA, SarT, Rot, and possibly MgrA all bind the *sarS* promoter, with the influence of *sarU* being mediated by its impact on production of RNAIII, the influence of RNAIII being mediated by its interaction with Rot, and the influence of SarR being mediated by its repression of *sarA* transcription. The same group subsequently concluded that these regulatory elements, with the addition of *arlRS* (see below) and *sarV*, also contribute either directly or indirectly to production of the *S. aureus* proteases aureolysin and the *sspA*-encoded serine protease [457]. However, with the exception of the *sigB*-deficient strain V8, these studies focused on 8325-4 strains including the *rsbU*-repaired strain SH1000, and while we agree with the suggestion that "the much-studied and genetically well characterized strain 8325-4 and its derivatives seem unrepresentative of most clinical *S. aureus* isolates because of the mutations in *rsbU* and *tcaR*, they are still very useful in the exploration of the regulatory networks governing virulence gene expression if compared to other strains," we do not believe these issues can be addressed without the direct analysis of other strains, with a specific emphasis on clinical isolates like those discussed in the introductory sections of this chapter.

The *saeRS* two-component regulatory system

Giraudo *et al.* [458] isolated yet another mutant defined by a Tn*551* insertion in a gene they designated *sae* (*S. aureus* exoprotein expression). Subsequent analysis confirmed the presence of two genes designated *saeR* and *saeS*, which encode the response regulator and histidine kinase respectively of a two-component signal transduction system [459,460]. Later studies demonstrated that transcription of *saeRS* is highly complex and under certain circumstances includes transcripts that span two upstream ORFs designated *saeP* and *saeQ* [461]. It was also suggested that *saeRS* is directly downstream of *agr* but that its expression is not dependent on production of RNAIII. Based on this, it was proposed that *saeRS* functions in an epistatic fashion to *agr* to activate exoprotein synthesis in response to certain environmental signals [461].

Rogasch *et al.* [462] also concluded that mutation of *saeRS* has no effect on expression of *agr* or *sarA* but that it nevertheless has a global impact on expression of *S. aureus* virulence factors. In most cases, the impact of *saeRS* and *agr* were similar although there were exceptions. For example, production of the serine protease SspA was increased in an *saeRS* mutant but is characteristically decreased in an *agr* mutant. However, transcription of *sspA* was unaffected by mutation of *saeRS*, which suggests its regulatory effect occurs at a posttranscriptional level. Thus, like *agr* and *sarA*, the *saeRS* regulatory system also appears to have both transcriptional and posttranscriptional regulatory effects. How *saeRS* exerts these effects remains unknown. Transcriptional regulation would presumably involve binding of SaeR to *cis* sites upstream of target genes, but alignment of upstream sequences from genes found to be regulated at the transcriptional level failed to identify a consensus binding site [462].

Unlike earlier studies, Liang *et al.* [463] concluded from studies on the human clinical isolate WCUH29 that mutation of *saeRS* results in increased expression of *agr*. However, expression of genes known to be positively regulated by *agr* (e.g., *hla*) was decreased in the corresponding *saeRS* mutant. These authors also found that expression of the genes encoding several adhesins, including the fibronectin-binding proteins, was reduced in an *saeRS* mutant, and it was proposed that this accounts for their reduced capacity to invade epithelial cells and that this in turn contributes to their reduced virulence in a murine model of hematogenous pyelonephritis. Perhaps most importantly, Goerke *et al.* [392] found that mutation of *agr* or *sarA* in both Newman and RN6390 had little effect on expression of *hla in vivo* while mutation of *saeRS* resulted in reduced *hla* expression both *in vitro* and *in vivo*. It was concluded on this basis that "*S. aureus* seems to be provided with regulatory circuits different from those characterized *in vitro* to ensure α-toxin synthesis during infections." Goerke *et al.* [464] also concluded that *saeRS* plays a "dominant" role, at least in comparison with *sigB*, in modulating gene expression during device-related infection.

The *arlRS* two-component regulatory system

Fournier and Hooper [465] isolated a mutant that exhibited reduced protease production, increased autolysin activity and, in comparison with its 8325 parent, an increased capacity to form a biofilm. The mutation occurred in a gene designated *arlS* (*a*utolysis-*r*elated *l*ocus) which appeared to be part of an operon that also includes *arlR*. Fournier *et al.* [466] subsequently generated an *arlR* mutant and demonstrated that this abolished transcription of both *arlR* and the downstream gene *arlS*, thus confirming that these two genes are part of an operon. However, these experiments were done with 8325-4 rather than 8325, and the results demonstrated that in this background mutation of mutation of *arlR* or *arlS* resulted in increased production of several secreted proteins including α-toxin, β-toxin, lipase, and serine protease. Further analysis demonstrated that this was a function of increased transcription of the corresponding genes [466].

Mutation of *arlRS* in 8325-4 also resulted in increased production of Spa, and it was proposed that this effect, as well as the increased production of serine protease, could be explained by the impact of *arlRS* on expression of *sarA* [466]. Specifically, mutation of *arlRS* resulted in decreased expression of *sarA*, which as discussed above is associated with increased production of both Spa and SspA. Conversely, mutation of *arlRS* resulted in increased expression of *agr*, which is classically associated with increased production of SspA but reduced production of Spa. To the extent that *sarA* enhances *agr* expression in 8325-4 strains (see above), the inverse effect of *arlRS* on *sarA* and *agr* suggests that *arlRS* modulates expression of these loci independently. The fact that mutation of *arlRS* resulted in increased rather than decreased production of Spa would also suggest that its impact on *sarA* is dominant in comparison with its impact on *agr*. However, mutation of *arlRS* did not alter expression of *spa* in either an *agrA* or *sarA* mutant, which demonstrates that both loci are required for the regulatory impact of *arlRS* on *spa* [466].

In a more recent study, Toledo-Arana *et al.* [467] examined biofilm formation using multiple strains and two different media formulations, one of which was a chemically defined medium designated HHWm (Hussain–Hastings–White modified medium). Biofilm formation was limited in HHWm in comparison with glucose-supplemented tryptic soy broth in essentially all strains. In an attempt to identify the genes involved in this repression, these authors generated mutations in 15 of 17 two-component systems, the two exceptions being the essential two-component systems *yycGF* (see below) and SA0067-SA0066 (based on the N315 sequence), which is absent in the clinical isolate (designated 15981) targeted in their mutagenesis experiments. Only the *arlRS* mutation restored the ability of 15981 to form a biofilm in HHWm [467]. This phenotype was enhanced by mutation of *agr*, which suggests that the level of *agr* expression even in the *rsbU*-positive clinical isolate 15981 limits biofilm formation. In contrast, the phenotype was reversed by concomitant mutation of *sarA*. Based on this, it was concluded that *sarA* was epistatic to *arlRS* at least in the context of biofilm formation. It was also suggested that the "accumulation of one or more proteins" in an *arlRS* mutant might enhance biofilm formation, an effect that would presumably be reversed by mutation of *sarA*. This is consistent with the observation that biofilm formation in the *arlRS* mutant was "sensitive to detachment by proteases" [467]. However, this hypothesis is based on results observed in 8325 [465], and it does not account for studies demonstrating that mutation of *arlRS* resulted in increased rather than decreased production of proteases in 8325-4 strains [466]. Mutation of *arlRS* also enhanced biofilm formation in ISP479r, a derivative of 8325-4 in which the *rsbU* mutation has been repaired, and this effect was further augmented by concomitant mutation of *agr* [467]. Protease production was not directly assessed in this study, so it is unclear whether the ISP479r *arlRS* mutant, unlike the 8325-4 mutant, produced decreased amounts of protease, but the results taken together suggest that the impact of *arlRS* on protease production may be at least somewhat dependent on a fully functional *sigB* operon.

Further evidence to support the involvement of *sigB* in *arlRS*-mediated regulation comes from studies examining regulation of capsule production. Regulation of *cap* transcription is highly complex, which reflects the need for *S. aureus* to fine tune capsule production under different conditions and thereby balance the need to limit phagocytosis with the need to avoid masking adhesins and limiting colonization of host tissues (see above). The *arlRS* operon was recently shown to positively regulate the production of *S. aureus* capsular polysaccharides, and it was suggested that this is mediated at the transcriptional level but indirectly through *mgrA* [201], a transcriptional regulator previously identified as an activator of capsule production [468]. In an independent study investigating regulation of capsule production, Ingavale *et al.* [445] identified a protein that binds the *arlRS* promoter. The original designation for this protein was Rat (regulator of autolytic activity), but this was later changed to MgrA [446] in the interests of consistency. Based on binding data, it was proposed that MgrA regulates *arlRS* transcription directly, but a subsequent reported concluded that this is mediated through SarV [444]. Whether mediated by a direct or indirect mechanism, these results are in contrast to studies concluding that mutation of *mgrA* has no effect on expression of *arlRS* [201]. To the extent that the earlier studies were done with an 8325-4 strain while the latter were done with the *rsbU*-positive strain Newman, this suggests that the impact of *mgrA* on expression of *arlRS* is also *sigB*-dependent.

This was subsequently confirmed by Meier *et al.* [469], who demonstrated the existence of five *arlRS* transcripts, two of which were absent in all *rsbU*-negative strains. These same authors also confirmed that *arlRS* modulates capsule production in *S. aureus* and that this effect is, in fact, influenced by *sigB* as well as products of the *yabJ-spoVG* locus. More specifically, it was suggested that *arlRS*, together with *yabJ-spoVG*, "may serve as effectors that modulate sigma(B) control over sigma(B)-dependent genes lacking an apparent sigma(B) promoter." Interestingly, mutation of *arlRS* or *spoVG* in the *rsbU*-positive strain Newman also resulted in decreased protease production and, in VISA isolates, reduced resistance against β-lactam antibiotics and glycopeptides. Unfortunately, these authors did not assess the impact of either mutation on biofilm formation, so the hypothesis that the primary impact of *arlRS* on biofilm formation is mediated by its impact on protease production [467] remains unresolved. However, a recent paper described yet another locus (*sbcDC*), mutation of which also resulted in increased expression of the *cap* genes and increased production of capsular polysaccharides [470]. This effect was attributed to increased expression of *arlRS* and *mgrA*. This suggests that the increased capacity of an *arlRS* mutant to form a biofilm could be a function of decreased production of capsular polysaccharides resulting in an enhanced capacity to bind host proteins rather than any effect mediated by altered production of proteases. Interestingly, expression of *sbcDC* was induced by subinhibitory concentrations of ciprofloxacin and mitomycin C. Mutation of *sbcDC* also resulted in increased sensitivity to ultraviolet irradiation. Taken together, this suggests that *sbcDC* may be involved in some fashion with DNA repair [470].

The *srrAB* (*srhSR*) two-component regulatory system

Two reports published almost simultaneously described an *S. aureus* regulatory locus similar to the *B. subtilis resDE* system. One of these reports designated this locus *srhSR* [471] while the other designated it *srrAB* [472]. The latter reflects its role in the staphylococcal respiratory response and has become the accepted nomenclature. These reports demonstrated that *srrAB* plays an important role in both central metabolic pathways and expression of specific virulence factors. Specifically, Throup *et al.* [471] demonstrated that mutation of *srrAB* resulted in reduced growth under anaerobic conditions and altered production of several proteins involved in energy metabolism, while Yarwood *et al.* [472] demonstrated that it also resulted in increased levels of RNAIII but decreased production of TSST-1, particularly under microaerophilic conditions. In contrast, SpA production was increased in an *srrAB* mutant under microaerophilic conditions but decreased under aerobic conditions. Because increased levels of RNAIII would not be expected to result in decreased production of TSST-1 or increased production of Spa under any condition, it was suggested that these effects might be mediated by a general metabolic defect rather than a specific regulatory event involving *agr*.

Subsequent studies confirmed that SrrAB does in fact function as a two-component system, with SrrB serving as the membrane-associated histidine kinase and SrrA serving as the response regulator that binds *cis* DNA elements associated with its target genes. Specifically, Pragman and Schlievert [74] demonstrated that, under anaerobic conditions, SrrA binds the promoter regions of *agr*, *tst*, and *spa* resulting in reduced transcription as well as reduced virulence in a rabbit endocarditis model [472,473]. SrrA also binds the *agr*, *tst*, and *spa* promoters under aerobic conditions, but in this case binding results in increased rather than decreased transcription [474]. The same is true of the *ica* operon even under anaerobic conditions [244]. Mutation of *sarA* also results in decreased transcription of *ica* [475], and a model was proposed in which SrrA and SarA cooperatively enhance production of PIA by both activating transcription of the *icaADBC* operon and repressing transcription of *icaR* [244,476]. It was also suggested that SrrA-mediated PIA production protects *S. aureus* from nonoxidative killing inside neutrophils [244]. Moreover, Richardson *et al.* [348] demonstrated that *srrAB* protects *S. aureus* from the toxic effects of reactive nitric oxide due in part to the regulatory effects of SrrAB on expression of *hmp*, which encodes a nitric oxide-scavenging flavohemoprotein. Mutation of *srrAB* or *hmp* attenuated virulence in a murine sepsis model, and mutation of *ssrAB* has also been associated with reduced virulence in a murine pyelonephritis model [471].

The *yycGF* two-component regulatory system

Of all the *S. aureus* two-component systems studied to date, the only one found to be essential is *yycGF*. Martin *et al.* [477] identified this system as a conditional lethal mutation in genes involved in maintenance of the cell envelope. YycG and YycF were subsequently confirmed to function as a histidine kinase and response regulator respectively [478]. A consensus binding site for YycF has been defined, and analysis of *S. aureus* genome data based on this sequence identified 12 potential YycF targets, five of which (*isaA*, *ssaA*, *sdrD*, *ebpS*, and *sak*) have been previously associated in some fashion with virulence [479]. Two of these (*isaA* and *ssaA*) were subsequently shown to encode proteins involved in peptidoglycan hydrolysis, and the remaining genes in the *yycGF* regulon (e.g., *lytM*, *atlA*) are also generally involved in cell wall metabolism. Specific binding of YycF has been confirmed for at least three of these targets [479].

YycGF is required for expression of both *lytM* and *atlA*, which encode the two primary *S. aureus* autolysins. This is consistent with the observation that inactivation of *yycGF* is lethal but does not result in cell lysis [480]. In general, reduced levels of *yycGF* expression result in increased peptidoglycan cross-linking and lowered rates of peptidoglycan synthesis and cell wall turnover. Based on this, the alternative nomenclature *walKR* has been proposed [480]. Expression of *yycGF* is also associated with enhanced ability to form a biofilm; to the extent that *yycGF* enhances expression of *atlA*, this is consistent with the observation that mutation of *atlA* in *S. aureus* also impairs biofilm formation [480,481]. Importantly, derivatives of thiazolidinone that inhibit function of the YycG histidine kinase were recently shown to be bactericidal against *S. epidermidis* even in the context of a biofilm [482].

The *vraSR* and *graRS* two-component systems

Kuroda *et al.* [483] identified the *vraSR* two-component system based on its increased expression in VISA strains. It was subsequently shown that of 139 genes expressed at higher levels in the presence of vancomycin, 46 were expressed in a *vraSR*-dependent manner [484]. This included a number of genes involved in cell wall biosynthesis including penicillin-binding proteins, which is consistent with the fact that *vraSR* also modulates the response of *S. aureus* to β-lactam antibiotics [485,486].

Similar studies led to identification of *graRS*, expression of which was also induced in VISA isolates [487]. Overexpression of *graR* was also associated with increased resistance to other antibiotics including oxacillin and daptomycin [487,488]. Meehl *et al.* [489] recently demonstrated that *graRS* functions, at least in part, by regulating transcription of *vraFG*, which is located adjacent to *graRS* and encodes an ABC transporter. Mutation of *graRS* or *vraFG* resulted in increased susceptibility not only to vancomycin but also to cationic antimicrobial peptides [489,490]. With respect to the latter, Li *et al.* [491] described a three-component regulatory system (the two-component *apsRS* system together with a third gene of unknown function designated *apsX*) that is located adjacent to *vraFG* and is also involved in resistance to antimicrobial peptides. Moreover, mutation of *apsS* was shown to result in reduced virulence in a murine model of kidney infection [491]. Thus, this regulatory circuit not only contributes to the ability of *S. aureus* to cause disease but also the ability to treat the resulting infection.

Other regulatory loci affecting cell wall biosynthesis

Brunskill and Bayles [492] identified a regulatory locus designated *lytSR* that also regulates expression of genes involved in cell wall metabolism. The primary genes regulated by *lytSR* are *lrgAB* and *scdA*, all of which are immediately adjacent to *lytSR* [492,493]. Mutation of *lrgAB* results in increased murein hydrolase activity and increased sensitivity to penicillin-mediated killing [494]. Mutation of a second locus designated *cidABC* has the opposite effect, and it was proposed based both on this and sequence similarities that the *cidABC* and *lrgAB* operons encode proteins analogous to phage-encoded holins and antiholins respectively [495]. A second locus designated *cidR* also positively regulates expression of *cidABC* and *lrgAB* as well as *alsSD*, an unlinked operon encoding enzymes involved in acetoin production [496]. Mutation of *alsSD* also results in reduced murein hydrolase activity and stationary phase survival, and there is some evidence to suggest that it also limits the ability to form a biofilm [17]. Thus, it seems clear that maintenance of the *S. aureus* cell wall is important enough to justify multiple overlapping regulatory pathways (e.g., *graRS*, *lytSR*, *vraFG*, and *yycGF*) and that disruption of any of these pathways has the potential to alter biofilm formation.

Other regulatory loci affecting biofilm formation

Pamp *et al.* [497] demonstrated that mutation of *spx* limits the stress response of *S. aureus* and results in altered production of multiple proteins, most of which are involved in central metabolic pathways. This included reduced production of thioredoxin reductase, which is encoded by the essential gene *trxB*, and in this case the regulatory effect was shown to be transcriptional. Mutation of *spx* also enhanced biofilm formation, and it was proposed that this was a function of enhanced transcription of the *ica* operon resulting from reduced transcription of *icaR*. In contrast to *spx*, Lim *et al.* [498] found that mutation of *rbf* in the 8325-4 strain RN450 results in increased rather than decreased biofilm formation. Rbf has a "consensus region signature" of the AraC/XylS family of transcriptional regulators, but at present the mechanism by which *rbf* modulates biofilm formation remains unknown. In our hands, 8325-4 strains do not form a robust biofilm, a phenotype we attribute to their increased expression of *agr*. In this regard it is perhaps worth noting that RN450 is "partially *agr* defective" (based on the website of the Network on Antimicrobial Resistance in *S. aureus*, or NARSA).

A recent report demonstrated that mutation of *codY* in clinical isolates has a global effect on gene expression that includes increased biofilm formation [499]. This was attributed, at least in part, to increased production of PIA. Mutation of *codY* also resulted in increased expression of *agr* and increased hemolytic activity. One possible explanation for the enhanced ability of a *codY* mutant to form a biofilm even in the context of increased expression to of *agr* is that the increased production of PIA is sufficient to overcome any inhibition associated with *agr*. However, this also appears to be a strain-dependent effect in that Tu Quoc *et al.* [447] found that mutation of *codY* in the clinical isolate S30 resulted in reduced rather than enhanced biofilm formation. These same authors identified a number of additional mutants that had the same effect, several of which (e.g., *bfd1* and *bfd4*) appear to be involved in cyclic di-GMP signaling. It is interesting to note in this regard that cyclic di-GMP has been reported to inhibit *S. aureus* biofilm formation both *in vitro* and *in vivo* [500,501]. This is in contrast to the effect observed in Gram-negative bacteria, where cyclic di-GMP typically promotes rather than inhibits biofilm formation [502].

Other regulatory loci affecting production of *Staphylococcus aureus* virulence factors

Mutations in at least four other genes have been shown to result in altered expression of *S. aureus* virulence factors. These include *msa* (*m*odulator of sar*A*), mutation of which resulted in reduced expression of *sarA* in both RN6390 and the clinical isolate UAMS-1 [503]. The fact that the regulatory impact of *msa* is mediated primarily through its impact on *sarA* is reflected by the fact that mutation of *msa* had the same disparate effect on transcription of *hla* in RN6390 versus UAMS-1. Mutation of *msa* also resulted in increased production of RNAIII in UAMS-1 but not RN6390, particularly in the late-exponential growth phase. This could explain why the UAMS-1 *msa* mutant expressed *hla* at increased levels, but as noted above there is also evidence to suggest that this is a function of the relative levels of SarS produced by the two strains [442]. Either way, the reduced expression of *sarA* in an *msa* mutant together with the increased expression of *agr* provides further support for the hypothesis that *sarA* plays a limited role in activating transcription of *agr* in clinical isolates.

Rossi *et al.* [504] described a locus designated *msrR*, mutation of which resulted in increased transcription of *sarA*, RNAIII, and *hla* and decreased transcription of *spa*. This phenotype is perfectly consistent with the current, RN6390-defined regulatory paradigm in that increased transcription of *sarA* would be expected to result in increased production of RNAIII, which in turn would be expected to result in increased expression of *hla* and decreased expression of *spa*. Based on this, it was proposed that this was a cause-and-effect relationship in that attenuation of *sarA* transcription defined the phenotype of an *msrR* mutant [504]. Importantly, transcription of *msrR* was induced by cell wall inhibitors including β-lactam and glycopeptide antibiotics. This provides yet another link between cell wall metabolism and expression of *S. aureus* virulence factors.

Mutations in *ccpA* and *murF* also resulted in altered expression of multiple *S. aureus* virulence factors. In the case of *ccpA*, this included reduced expression of *agr*, particularly in the absence of glucose [505]. Based on these results, it was suggested that glucose depletion may serve as a signal for induction of *agr* expression and that this may account for the altered expression of genes encoding multiple virulence factors including *hla* and *spa*. Reduced expression of *murF* had an even more global impact in that it resulted in altered expression of 79 virulence-related genes [506]. This included genes encoding both surface-associated and extracellular virulence factors, all of which were expressed at elevated levels. In contrast, all genes in the *isd* operon were expressed at reduced levels. Mutation of *murF* also resulted in increased susceptibility to β-lactam antibiotics [507], and in this case there is a more obvious link. Specifically, MurF catalyzes the last step (addition of the D-alanyl-D-alanyl dipeptide) in synthesis of the peptidoglycan precursor UDP-linked MurNAc pentapeptide [508], and it was recently suggested that *murF* transcription may be linked to the accumulation of premature cell wall precursors, thus providing a single-step link between cell wall biosynthesis and production of *S. aureus* virulence factors [506]. However, to date, the contribution of *ccpA* or *murF* to virulence has not been directly examined in a relevant animal model of *S. aureus* infection.

Acknowledgments

As of December 25, 2007, a PubMed search using the general search terms *staphylococcus* and *virulence* yielded 4281 papers dating to 1951. This number can be reduced to 2082 if the search is done more specifically ("staphylococcus" AND "virulence"). Either way, it is a daunting task to summarize the volume of studies that could be considered relevant to this chapter. We have attempted to be reasonably comprehensive while maintaining a specific emphasis on papers published in the twenty-first century, and we apologize to investigators who think we failed in that regard.

We thank the National Institute of Allergy and Infectious Disease, the American Heart Association, and the Orthopaedic Research and Education Foundation for funding. We would also like to thank our colleagues who have been generous in sharing the fruits of their labor. We reserve special thanks for our students and post-docs and, most importantly, for Dr John J. Iandolo, who trained three of us directly (M.S.S., C.Y.L., and M.E.H.) and the fourth (N.H.) by extension. There could be no better friend or mentor. The views presented in this chapter do not necessarily reflect those of the US Food and Drug Administration.

References

1 Baddour LM, Tayidi MM, Walker E, McDevitt D, Foster TJ. Virulence of coagulase-deficient mutants of *Staphylococcus aureus* in experimental endocarditis. J Med Microbiol 1994;41:259–63.

2 Moreillon P, Entenza JM, Francioli P *et al*. Role of *Staphylococcus aureus* coagulase and clumping factor in pathogenesis of experimental endocarditis. Infect Immun 1995;63:4738–43.

3 Phonimdaeng P, O'Reilly M, Nowlan P, Bramley AJ, Foster TJ. The coagulase of *Staphylococcus aureus* 8325-4. Sequence analysis and virulence of site-specific coagulase-deficient mutants. Mol Microbiol 1990;4:393–404.

4 Stutzmann MP, Entenza JM, Vaudaux P, Francioli P, Glauser MP, Moreillon P. Study of *Staphylococcus aureus* pathogenic genes by transfer and expression in the less virulent organism *Streptococcus gordonii*. Infect Immun 2001;69:657–64.

5 Gill SR, Fouts DE, Archer GL *et al*. Insights on evolution of virulence and resistance from the complete genome analysis of an early methicillin-resistant *Staphylococcus aureus* strain and a biofilm-producing methicillin-resistant *Staphylococcus epidermidis* strain. J Bacteriol 2005;187:2426–38.

6 Foster TJ. Immune evasion by staphylococci. Nat Rev Microbiol 2005;3:948–58.

7 Lewis K. Persister cells, dormancy and infectious disease. Nat Rev Microbiol 2007;5:48–56.

8 Bramley AJ, Patel AH, O'Reilly M, Foster R, Foster TJ. Roles of alpha-toxin and beta-toxin in virulence of *Staphylococcus aureus* for the mouse mammary gland. Infect Immun 1989;57:2489–94.

9 Dajcs JJ, Austin MS, Sloop GD *et al*. Corneal pathogenesis of *Staphylococcus aureus* strain Newman. Invest Ophthalmol Vis Sci 2002;43:1109–15.

10 Dajcs JJ, Thibodeaux BA, Girgis DO, O'Callaghan RJ. Corneal virulence of *Staphylococcus aureus* in an experimental model of keratitis. DNA Cell Biol 2002;21:375–82.

11 Girgis DO, Sloop GD, Reed JM, O'Callaghan RJ. Effects of toxin production in a murine model of *Staphylococcus aureus* keratitis. Invest Ophthalmol Vis Sci 2005;46:2064–70.

12 Kielian T, Cheung A, Hickey WF. Diminished virulence of an alpha-toxin mutant of *Staphylococcus aureus* in experimental brain abscesses. Infect Immun 2001;69:6902–11.

13 Nilsson IM, Hartford O, Foster T, Tarkowski A. Alpha-toxin and gamma-toxin jointly promote *Staphylococcus aureus* virulence in murine septic arthritis. Infect Immun 1999;67:1045–9.

14 O'Callaghan RJ, Callegan MC, Moreau JM *et al*. Specific roles of alpha-toxin and beta-toxin during *Staphylococcus aureus* corneal infection. Infect Immun 1997;65:1571–8.

15 Bubeck Wardenburg JB, Patel RJ, Schneewind O. Surface proteins and exotoxins are required for the pathogenesis of *Staphylococcus aureus* pneumonia. Infect Immun 2007;75:1040–4.

16 Wu PZ, Zhu H, Stapleton F *et al*. Effects of alpha-toxin-deficient *Staphylococcus aureus* on the production of peripheral corneal ulceration in an animal model. Curr Eye Res 2005;30:63–70.

17 Cassat J, Dunman PM, Murphy E *et al*. Transcriptional profiling of a *Staphylococcus aureus* clinical isolate and its isogenic *agr* and *sarA* mutants reveals global differences in comparison to the laboratory strain RN6390. Microbiology 2006;152:3075–90.

18 Holden MT, Feil EJ, Lindsay JA *et al*. Complete genomes of two clinical *Staphylococcus aureus* strains: evidence for the rapid evolution of virulence and drug resistance. Proc Natl Acad Sci USA 2004;101:9786–91.

19 Bayer AS, Ramos MD, Menzies BE, Yeaman MR, Shen AJ, Cheung AL. Hyperproduction of alpha-toxin by *Staphylococcus aureus* results in paradoxically reduced virulence in experimental endocarditis: a host defense role for platelet microbicidal proteins. Infect Immun 1997;65:4652–60.

20 Traber K, Novick R. A slipped-mispairing mutation in AgrA of laboratory strains and clinical isolates results in delayed activation of *agr* and failure to translate delta- and alpha-haemolysins. Mol Microbiol 2006;59:1519–30.

21 Novick R. Properties of a cryptic high-frequency transducing phage in *Staphylococcus aureus*. Virology 1967;33:155–66.

22 Cassat JE, Dunman PM, McAleese F, Murphy E, Projan SJ, Smeltzer MS. Comparative genomics of *Staphylococcus aureus* musculoskeletal isolates. J Bacteriol 2005;187:576–92.

23 Coleman DC, Sullivan DJ, Russell RJ, Arbuthnott JP, Carey BF, Pomeroy HM. *Staphylococcus aureus* bacteriophages mediating the simultaneous lysogenic conversion of beta-lysin, staphylokinase and enterotoxin A: molecular mechanism of triple conversion. J Gen Microbiol 1989;135:1679–97.

24 Smeltzer MS, Pratt FL, Gillaspy AF, Young LA. Genomic fingerprinting for epidemiological differentiation of *Staphylococcus aureus* clinical isolates. J Clin Microbiol 1996;34:1364–72.

25 van Wamel WJ, Rooijakkers SH, Ruyken M, van Kessel KP, van Strijp JA. The innate immune modulators staphylococcal complement inhibitor and chemotaxis inhibitory protein of *Staphylococcus aureus* are located on beta-hemolysin-converting bacteriophages. J Bacteriol 2006;188:1310–15.

26 Aarestrup FM, Larsen HD, Eriksen NH, Elsberg CS, Jensen NE. Frequency of alpha- and beta-haemolysin in *Staphylococcus aureus* of bovine and human origin. A comparison between pheno- and genotype and variation in phenotypic expression. APMIS 1999;107:425–30.

27 Novick RP. Staphylococcal pathogenesis and pathogenicity factors: genetics and regulation. In: Fischetti VA, Novick RP, Ferretti JJ, Portnoy DA, Rood JI, eds. Gram-positive Pathogens. Washington, DC: ASM Press, 2006:496–516.

28 Rooijakkers SH, Ruyken M, van Roon J, van Kessel KP, van Strijp JA, van Wamel WJ. Early expression of SCIN and CHIPS drives instant immune evasion by *Staphylococcus aureus*. Cell Microbiol 2006;8:1282–93.

29 Gertz S, Engelmann S, Schmid R, Ohlsen K, Hacker J, Hecker M. Regulation of sigmaB-dependent transcription of *sigB* and *asp23* in two different *Staphylococcus aureus* strains. Mol Gen Genet 1999;261:558–66.

30 Giachino P, Engelmann S, Bischoff M. Sigma(B) activity depends on RsbU in *Staphylococcus aureus*. J Bacteriol 2001;183:1843–52.

31 Jefferson KK, Pier DB, Goldmann DA, Pier GB. The teicoplanin-associated locus regulator (TcaR) and the intercellular adhesin locus regulator (IcaR) are transcriptional inhibitors of the *ica* locus in *Staphylococcus aureus*. J Bacteriol 2004;186:2449–56.
32 Kullik I, Giachino P, Fuchs T. Deletion of the alternative sigma factor sigmaB in *Staphylococcus aureus* reveals its function as a global regulator of virulence genes. J Bacteriol 1998;180:4814–20.
33 McCallum N, Bischoff M, Maki H, Wada A, Berger-Bachi B. TcaR, a putative MarR-like regulator of *sarS* expression. J Bacteriol 2004;186:2966–72.
34 Shaw L, Golonka E, Potempa J, Foster SJ. The role and regulation of the extracellular proteases of *Staphylococcus aureus*. Microbiology 2004;150:217–28.
35 Chan PF, Foster SJ, Ingham E, Clements MO. The *Staphylococcus aureus* alternative sigma factor sigmaB controls the environmental stress response but not starvation survival or pathogenicity in a mouse abscess model. J Bacteriol 1998;180:6082–9.
36 Nicholas RO, Li T, McDevitt D *et al*. Isolation and characterization of a *sigB* deletion mutant of *Staphylococcus aureus*. Infect Immun 1999;67:3667–9.
37 Jonsson IM, Arvidson S, Foster S, Tarkowski A. Sigma factor B and RsbU are required for virulence in *Staphylococcus aureus*-induced arthritis and sepsis. Infect Immun 2004;72:6106–11.
38 Bischoff M, Entenza JM, Giachino P. Influence of a functional *sigB* operon on the global regulators *sar* and *agr* in *Staphylococcus aureus* . J Bacteriol 2001;183:5171–9.
39 Bischoff M, Dunman P, Kormanec J *et al*. Microarray-based analysis of the *Staphylococcus aureus* sigmaB regulon. J Bacteriol 2004;186:4085–99.
40 Horsburgh MJ, Aish JL, White IJ, Shaw L, Lithgow JK, Foster SJ. sigmaB modulates virulence determinant expression and stress resistance: characterization of a functional *rsbU* strain derived from *Staphylococcus aureus* 8325-4. J Bacteriol 2002;184:5457–67.
41 Fitzgerald JR, Sturdevant DE, Mackie SM, Gill SR, Musser JM. Evolutionary genomics of *Staphylococcus aureus*: insights into the origin of methicillin-resistant strains and the toxic shock syndrome epidemic. Proc Natl Acad Sci USA 2001;98:8821–6.
42 Booth MC, Pence LM, Mahasreshti P, Callegan MC, Gilmore MS. Clonal associations among *Staphylococcus aureus* isolates from various sites of infection. Infect Immun 2001;69:345–52.
43 Arciola CR, Campoccia D, Gamberini S, Baldassarri L, Montanaro L. Prevalence of *cna*, *fnbA* and *fnbB* adhesin genes among *Staphylococcus aureus* isolates from orthopedic infections associated to different types of implant. FEMS Microbiol Lett 2005;246:81–6.
44 Gillaspy AF, Lee CY, Sau S, Cheung AL, Smeltzer MS. Factors affecting the collagen binding capacity of *Staphylococcus aureus*. Infect Immun 1998;66:3170–8.
45 Patti JM, Jonsson H, Guss B *et al*. Molecular characterization and expression of a gene encoding a *Staphylococcus aureus* collagen adhesin. J Biol Chem 1992;267:4766–72.
46 Peacock SJ, Moore CE, Justice A *et al*. Virulent combinations of adhesin and toxin genes in natural populations of *Staphylococcus aureus*. Infect Immun 2002;70:4987–96.
47 Roche FM, Massey R, Peacock SJ *et al*. Characterization of novel LPXTG-containing proteins of *Staphylococcus aureus* identified from genome sequences. Microbiology 2003;149:643–54.
48 Otsuka T, Saito K, Dohmae S *et al*. Key adhesin gene in community-acquired methicillin-resistant *Staphylococcus aureus*. Biochem Biophys Res Commun 2006;346:1234–44.
49 Tung H, Guss B, Hellman U, Persson L, Rubin K, Ryden C. A bone sialoprotein-binding protein from *Staphylococcus aureus*: a member of the staphylococcal Sdr family. Biochem J 2000; 345:611–19.
50 Lindsay JA, Moore CE, Day NP *et al*. Microarrays reveal that each of the ten dominant lineages of *Staphylococcus aureus* has a unique combination of surface-associated and regulatory genes. J Bacteriol 2006;188:669–76.
51 Feil EJ, Cooper JE, Grundmann H *et al*. How clonal is *Staphylococcus aureus*? J Bacteriol 2003;185:3307–16.
52 Feil EJ, Enright MC. Analyses of clonality and the evolution of bacterial pathogens. Curr Opin Microbiol 2004;7:308–13.
53 Turner KM, Feil EJ. The secret life of the multilocus sequence type. Int J Antimicrob Agents 2007;29:129–35.
54 Feng Y, Chen CJ, Su LH, Hu S, Yu J, Chiu CH. Evolution and pathogenesis of *Staphylococcus aureus*: lessons learned from genotyping and comparative genomics. FEMS Microbiol Rev 2008;32:23–37.
55 Fowler VG, Nelson CL, McIntyre LM *et al*. Potential associations between hematogenous complications and bacterial genotype in *Staphylococcus aureus* infection. J Infect Dis 2007;196:738–47.
56 Johnson AP, Aucken HM, Cavendish S *et al*. Dominance of EMRSA-15 and -16 among MRSA causing nosocomial bacteraemia in the UK: analysis of isolates from the European Antimicrobial Resistance Surveillance System (EARSS). J Antimicrob Chemother 2001;48:143–4.
57 Johnson AP, Pearson A, Duckworth G. Surveillance and epidemiology of MRSA bacteraemia in the UK. J Antimicrob Chemother 2005;56:455–62.
58 Moore PC, Lindsay JA. Molecular characterisation of the dominant UK methicillin-resistant *Staphylococcus aureus* strains, EMRSA-15 and EMRSA-16. J Med Microbiol 2002;51:516–21.
59 Baba T, Bae T, Schneewind O, Takeuchi F, Hiramatsu K. Genome sequence of *Staphylococcus aureus* strain Newman and comparative analysis of staphylococcal genomes: polymorphism and evolution of two major pathogenicity islands. J Bacteriol 2008;190:300–10.
60 Davis SL, Perri MB, Donabedian SM *et al*. Epidemiology and outcomes of community-associated methicillin-resistant *Staphylococcus aureus* infection. J Clin Microbiol 2007;45:1705–11.
61 Moran GJ, Krishnadasan A, Gorwitz RJ *et al*. Methicillin-resistant *S. aureus* infections among patients in the emergency department. N Engl J Med 2006;355:666–74.
62 Diep BA, Gill SR, Chang RF *et al*. Complete genome sequence of USA300, an epidemic clone of community-acquired meticillin-resistant *Staphylococcus aureus*. Lancet 2006;367:731–9.
63 Grundmeier M, Hussain M, Becker P, Heilmann C, Peters G, Sinha B. Truncation of fibronectin-binding proteins in *Staphylococcus aureus* strain Newman leads to deficient adherence and host cell invasion due to loss of the cell wall anchor function. Infect Immun 2004;72:7155–63.
64 Goering RV, McDougal LK, Fosheim GE, Bonnstetter KK, Wolter DJ, Tenover FC. Epidemiologic distribution of the arginine catabolic mobile element among selected methicillin-resistant and methicillin-susceptible *Staphylococcus aureus* isolates. J Clin Microbiol 2007;45:1981–4.
65 Zhu Y, Weiss EC, Otto M, Fey PD, Smeltzer MS, Somerville GA. *Staphylococcus aureus* biofilm metabolism and the influence of arginine on polysaccharide intercellular adhesin synthesis, biofilm formation, and pathogenesis. Infect Immun 2007;75:4219–26.

66 Coulter SN, Schwan WR, Ng EY *et al*. *Staphylococcus aureus* genetic loci impacting growth and survival in multiple infection environments. Mol Microbiol 1998;30:393–404.
67 Diep BA, Carleton HA, Chang RF, Sensabaugh GF, Perdreau-Remington F. Roles of 34 virulence genes in the evolution of hospital- and community-associated strains of methicillin-resistant *Staphylococcus aureus*. J Infect Dis 2006;193:1495–503.
68 Labandeira-Rey M, Couzon F, Boisset S *et al*. *Staphylococcus aureus* Panton–Valentine leukocidin causes necrotizing pneumonia. Science 2007;315:1130–3.
69 Voyich JM, Otto M, Mathema B *et al*. Is Panton–Valentine leukocidin the major virulence determinant in community-associated methicillin-resistant *Staphylococcus aureus* disease? J Infect Dis 2006;194:1761–70.
70 Wang R, Braughton KR, Kretschmer D *et al*. Identification of novel cytolytic peptides as key virulence determinants for community-associated MRSA. Nat Med 2007;13:1510–14.
71 Vojtov N, Ross HF, Novick RP. Global repression of exotoxin synthesis by staphylococcal superantigens. Proc Natl Acad Sci USA 2002;99:10102–7.
72 Projan SJ, Novick RP. The molecular basis of pathogenicity. In: Crossley KB, Archer GL, eds. The Staphylococci in Human Disease. New York: Churchill Livingstone, 1997:55–81.
73 Cheung AL, Bayer AS, Zhang G, Gresham H, Xiong YQ. Regulation of virulence determinants *in vitro* and *in vivo* in *Staphylococcus aureus*. FEMS Immunol Med Microbiol 2004;40:1–9.
74 Pragman AA, Schlievert PM. Virulence regulation in *Staphylococcus aureus*: the need for *in vivo* analysis of virulence factor regulation. FEMS Immunol Med Microbiol 2004;42:147–54.
75 Xiong YQ, Willard J, Yeaman MR, Cheung AL, Bayer AS. Regulation of *Staphylococcus aureus* alpha-toxin gene (*hla*) expression by *agr*, *sarA*, and *sae in vitro* and in experimental infective endocarditis. J Infect Dis 2006;194:1267–75.
76 Yarwood JM, McCormick JK, Paustian ML, Kapur V, Schlievert PM. Repression of the *Staphylococcus aureus* accessory gene regulator in serum and *in vivo*. J Bacteriol 2002; 184:1095–101.
77 Fournier B, Philpott DJ. Recognition of *Staphylococcus aureus* by the innate immune system. Clin Microbiol Rev 2005;18:521–40.
78 Majcherczyk PA, Rubli E, Heumann D, Glauser MP, Moreillon P. Teichoic acids are not required for *Streptococcus pneumoniae* and *Staphylococcus aureus* cell walls to trigger the release of tumor necrosis factor by peripheral blood monocytes. Infect Immun 2003;71:3707–13.
79 Weidenmaier C, Kokai-Kun JF, Kristian SA *et al*. Role of teichoic acids in *Staphylococcus aureus* nasal colonization, a major risk factor in nosocomial infections. Nat Med 2004;10:243–5.
80 Wertheim HF, Melles DC, Vos MC *et al*. The role of nasal carriage in *Staphylococcus aureus* infections. Lancet Infect Dis 2005;5:751–62.
81 Weidenmaier C, Peschel A, Xiong YQ *et al*. Lack of wall teichoic acids in *Staphylococcus aureus* leads to reduced interactions with endothelial cells and to attenuated virulence in a rabbit model of endocarditis. J Infect Dis 2005;191:1771–7.
82 Ginsburg I. Role of lipoteichoic acid in infection and inflammation. Lancet Infect Dis 2002;2:171–9.
83 Kengatharan KM, De Kimpe S, Robson C, Foster SJ, Thiemermann C. Mechanism of Gram-positive shock: identification of peptidoglycan and lipoteichoic acid moieties essential in the induction of nitric oxide synthase, shock, and multiple organ failure. J Exp Med 1998;188:305–15.
84 Hashimoto M, Tawaratsumida K, Kariya H *et al*. Not lipoteichoic acid but lipoproteins appear to be the dominant immunobiologically active compounds in *Staphylococcus aureus*. J Immunol 2006;177:3162–9.
85 Hashimoto M, Furuyashiki M, Kaseya R *et al*. Evidence of immunostimulating lipoprotein existing in the natural lipoteichoic acid fraction. Infect Immun 2007;75:1926–32.
86 Hattar K, Grandel U, Moeller A *et al*. Lipoteichoic acid (LTA) from *Staphylococcus aureus* stimulates human neutrophil cytokine release by a CD14-dependent, Toll-like-receptor-independent mechanism: autocrine role of tumor necrosis factor-α in mediating LTA-induced interleukin-8 generation. Crit Care Med 2006;34:835–41.
87 Kinsner A, Boveri M, Hareng L *et al*. Highly purified lipoteichoic acid induced pro-inflammatory signalling in primary culture of rat microglia through Toll-like receptor 2: selective potentiation of nitric oxide production by muramyl dipeptide. J Neurochem 2006;99:596–607.
88 Lotz S, Aga E, Wilde I *et al*. Highly purified lipoteichoic acid activates neutrophil granulocytes and delays their spontaneous apoptosis via CD14 and TLR2. J Leukoc Biol 2004;75:467–77.
89 Paik YH, Lee KS, Lee HJ *et al*. Hepatic stellate cells primed with cytokines upregulate inflammation in response to peptidoglycan or lipoteichoic acid. Lab Invest 2006;86:676–86.
90 Deininger S, Stadelmaier A, von Aulock S, Morath S, Schmidt RR, Hartung T. Definition of structural prerequisites for lipoteichoic acid-inducible cytokine induction by synthetic derivatives. J Immunol 2003;170:4134–8.
91 Morath S, Stadelmaier A, Geyer A, Schmidt RR, Hartung T. Synthetic lipoteichoic acid from *Staphylococcus aureus* is a potent stimulus of cytokine release. J Exp Med 2002;195:1635–40.
92 Leemans JC, Heikens M, van Kessel KP, Florquin S, van der Poll T. Lipoteichoic acid and peptidoglycan from *Staphylococcus aureus* synergistically induce neutrophil influx into the lungs of mice. Clin Diagn Lab Immunol 2003;10:950–3.
93 Thiemermann C. Interactions between lipoteichoic acid and peptidoglycan from *Staphylococcus aureus*: a structural and functional analysis. Microbes Infect 2002;4:927–35.
94 Mullaly SC, Kubes P. The role of TLR2 *in vivo* following challenge with *Staphylococcus aureus* and prototypic ligands. J Immunol 2006;177:8154–63.
95 Travassos LH, Girardin SE, Philpott DJ *et al*. Toll-like receptor 2-dependent bacterial sensing does not occur via peptidoglycan recognition. EMBO Rep 2004;5:1000–6.
96 Fedtke I, Mader D, Kohler T *et al*. A *Staphylococcus aureus ypfP* mutant with strongly reduced lipoteichoic acid (LTA) content: LTA governs bacterial surface properties and autolysin activity. Mol Microbiol 2007;65:1078–91.
97 Iordanescu S, Surdeanu M. Two restriction and modification systems in *Staphylococcus aureus* NCTC8325. J Gen Microbiol 1976;96:277–81.
98 Grundling A, Schneewind O. Synthesis of glycerol phosphate lipoteichoic acid in *Staphylococcus aureus*. Proc Natl Acad Sci USA 2007;104:8478–83.
99 Canepari P, Boaretti M, Lleo MM, Satta G. Lipoteichoic acid as a new target for activity of antibiotics: mode of action of daptomycin (LY146032). Antimicrob Agents Chemother 1990;34:1220–6.
100 Friedman DB, Stauff DL, Pishchany G, Whitwell CW, Torres VJ, Skaar EP. *Staphylococcus aureus* redirects central metabolism to increase iron availability. PLoS Pathog 2006;2:e87.

101 Clarke SR, Foster SJ. Surface adhesins of *Staphylococcus aureus*. Adv Microb Physiol 2006;51:187–224.
102 Foster TJ, Hook M. Surface protein adhesins of *Staphylococcus aureus*. Trends Microbiol 1998;6:484–8.
103 Patti JM, Allen BL, McGavin MJ, Hook M. MSCRAMM-mediated adherence of microorganisms to host tissues. Annu Rev Microbiol 1994;48:585–617.
104 Rivas JM, Speziale P, Patti JM, Hook M. MSCRAMM-targeted vaccines and immunotherapy for staphylococcal infection. Curr Opin Drug Discov Devel 2004;7:223–7.
105 Schneewind O, Mihaylova-Petkov D, Model P. Cell wall sorting signals in surface proteins of Gram-positive bacteria. EMBO J 1993;12:4803–11.
106 Jonsson IM, Mazmanian SK, Schneewind O, Bremell T, Tarkowski A. The role of *Staphylococcus aureus* sortase A and sortase B in murine arthritis. Microbes Infect 2003;5:775–80.
107 Mazmanian SK, Liu G, Jensen ER, Lenoy E, Schneewind O. *Staphylococcus aureus* sortase mutants defective in the display of surface proteins and in the pathogenesis of animal infections. Proc Natl Acad Sci USA 2000;97:5510–15.
108 Weiss WJ, Lenoy E, Murphy T *et al*. Effect of *srtA* and *srtB* gene expression on the virulence of *Staphylococcus aureus* in animal models of infection. J Antimicrob Chemother 2004;53:480–6.
109 Mazmanian SK, Ton-That H, Su K, Schneewind O. An iron-regulated sortase anchors a class of surface protein during *Staphylococcus aureus* pathogenesis. Proc Natl Acad Sci USA 2002;99:2293–8.
110 Dent AC, McAdow M, Schneewind O. Distribution of protein A on the surface of *Staphylococcus aureus*. J Bacteriol 2007;189:4473–84.
111 Hartleib J, Kohler N, Dickinson RB *et al*. Protein A is the von Willebrand factor binding protein on *Staphylococcus aureus*. Blood 2000;96:2149–56.
112 Gomez MI, O'Seaghdha M, Magargee M, Foster TJ, Prince AS. *Staphylococcus aureus* protein A activates TNFR1 signaling through conserved IgG binding domains. J Biol Chem 2006; 281:20190–6.
113 Gomez MI, O'Seaghdha M, Prince AS. *Staphylococcus aureus* protein A activates TACE through EGFR-dependent signaling. EMBO J 2007;26:701–9.
114 Gomez MI, Lee A, Reddy B *et al*. *Staphylococcus aureus* protein A induces airway epithelial inflammatory responses by activating TNFR1. Nat Med 2004;10:842–8.
115 Palmqvist N, Foster T, Tarkowski A, Josefsson E. Protein A is a virulence factor in *Staphylococcus aureus* arthritis and septic death. Microb Pathog 2002;33:239–49.
116 Wardenburg JB, Bae T, Otto M, DeLeo FR, Schneewind O. Poring over pores: alpha-hemolysin and Panton–Valentine leukocidin in *Staphylococcus aureus* pneumonia. Nat Med 2007;13:1405–6.
117 Peacock SJ, Day NP, Thomas MG, Berendt AR, Foster TJ. Clinical isolates of *Staphylococcus aureus* exhibit diversity in fnb genes and adhesion to human fibronectin. J Infect 2000; 41:23–31.
118 Heilmann C, Niemann S, Sinha B, Herrmann M, Kehrel BE, Peters G. *Staphylococcus aureus* fibronectin-binding protein (FnBP)-mediated adherence to platelets, and aggregation of platelets induced by FnBPA but not by FnBPB. J Infect Dis 2004;190:321–9.
119 Keane FM, Loughman A, Valtulina V, Brennan M, Speziale P, Foster TJ. Fibrinogen and elastin bind to the same region within the A domain of fibronectin binding protein A, an MSCRAMM of *Staphylococcus aureus*. Mol Microbiol 2007; 63:711–23.
120 Roche FM, Downer R, Keane F, Speziale P, Park PW, Foster TJ. The N-terminal A domain of fibronectin-binding proteins A and B promotes adhesion of *Staphylococcus aureus* to elastin. J Biol Chem 2004;279:38433–40.
121 Wann ER, Gurusiddappa S, Hook M. The fibronectin-binding MSCRAMM FnbpA of *Staphylococcus aureus* is a bifunctional protein that also binds to fibrinogen. J Biol Chem 2000; 275:13863–71.
122 Tristan A, Ying L, Bes M, Etienne J, Vandenesch F, Lina G. Use of multiplex PCR to identify *Staphylococcus aureus* adhesins involved in human hematogenous infections. J Clin Microbiol 2003;41:4465–7.
123 Kuypers JM, Proctor RA. Reduced adherence to traumatized rat heart valves by a low-fibronectin-binding mutant of *Staphylococcus aureus*. Infect Immun 1989;57:2306–12.
124 Flock JI, Hienz SA, Heimdahl A, Schennings T. Reconsideration of the role of fibronectin binding in endocarditis caused by *Staphylococcus aureus*. Infect Immun 1996;64:1876–8.
125 McElroy MC, Cain DJ, Tyrrell C, Foster TJ, Haslett C. Increased virulence of a fibronectin-binding protein mutant of *Staphylococcus aureus* in a rat model of pneumonia. Infect Immun 2002;70:3865–73.
126 Palmqvist N, Foster T, Fitzgerald JR, Josefsson E, Tarkowski A. Fibronectin-binding proteins and fibrinogen-binding clumping factors play distinct roles in staphylococcal arthritis and systemic inflammation. J Infect Dis 2005;191:791–8.
127 Que YA, Francois P, Haefliger JA, Entenza JM, Vaudaux P, Moreillon P. Reassessing the role of *Staphylococcus aureus* clumping factor and fibronectin-binding protein by expression in *Lactococcus lactis*. Infect Immun 2001;69:6296–302.
128 Kerdudou S, Laschke MW, Sinha B, Preissner KT, Menger MD, Herrmann M. Fibronectin binding proteins contribute to the adherence of *Staphylococcus aureus* to intact endothelium in vivo. Thromb Haemost 2006;96:183–9.
129 Que YA, Haefliger JA, Piroth L *et al*. Fibrinogen and fibronectin binding cooperate for valve infection and invasion in *Staphylococcus aureus* experimental endocarditis. J Exp Med 2005; 201:1627–35.
130 Heying R, van de Gevel J, Que YA, Moreillon P, Beekhuizen H. Fibronectin-binding proteins and clumping factor A in *Staphylococcus aureus* experimental endocarditis: FnBPA is sufficient to activate human endothelial cells. Thromb Haemost 2007; 97:617–26.
131 Dziewanowska K, Patti JM, Deobald CF, Bayles KW, Trumble WR, Bohach GA. Fibronectin binding protein and host cell tyrosine kinase are required for internalization of *Staphylococcus aureus* by epithelial cells. Infect Immun 1999;67:4673–8.
132 Jett BD, Gilmore MS. Internalization of *Staphylococcus aureus* by human corneal epithelial cells: role of bacterial fibronectin-binding protein and host cell factors. Infect Immun 2002; 70:4697–700.
133 Khalil H, Williams RJ, Stenbeck G, Henderson B, Meghji S, Nair SP. Invasion of bone cells by *Staphylococcus epidermidis*. Microbes Infect 2007;9:460–5.
134 Ellington JK, Harris M, Hudson MC, Vishin S, Webb LX, Sherertz R. Intracellular *Staphylococcus aureus* and antibiotic resistance: implications for treatment of staphylococcal osteomyelitis. J Orthop Res 2006;24:87–93.

135 Hauck CR, Ohlsen K. Sticky connections: extracellular matrix protein recognition and integrin-mediated cellular invasion by *Staphylococcus aureus*. Curr Opin Microbiol 2006;9:5–11.
136 Schwarz-Linek U, Hook M, Potts JR. Fibronectin-binding proteins of Gram-positive cocci. Microbes Infect 2006;8:2291–8.
137 Alexander EH, Hudson MC. Factors influencing the internalization of *Staphylococcus aureus* and impacts on the course of infections in humans. Appl Microbiol Biotechnol 2001;56:361–6.
138 Krut O, Sommer H, Kronke M. Antibiotic-induced persistence of cytotoxic *Staphylococcus aureus* in non-phagocytic cells. J Antimicrob Chemother 2004;53:167–73.
139 Miajlovic H, Loughman A, Brennan M, Cox D, Foster TJ. Both complement- and fibrinogen-dependent mechanisms contribute to platelet aggregation mediated by *Staphylococcus aureus* clumping factor B. Infect Immun 2007;75:3335–43.
140 Ni ED, Perkins S, Francois P, Vaudaux P, Hook M, Foster TJ. Clumping factor B (ClfB), a new surface-located fibrinogen-binding adhesin of *Staphylococcus aureus*. Mol Microbiol 1998;30:245–57.
141 Fitzgerald JR, Foster TJ, Cox D. The interaction of bacterial pathogens with platelets. Nat Rev Microbiol 2006;4:445–57.
142 Loughman A, Fitzgerald JR, Brennan MP *et al*. Roles for fibrinogen, immunoglobulin and complement in platelet activation promoted by *Staphylococcus aureus* clumping factor A. Mol Microbiol 2005;57:804–18.
143 O'Brien L, Kerrigan SW, Kaw G *et al*. Multiple mechanisms for the activation of human platelet aggregation by *Staphylococcus aureus*: roles for the clumping factors ClfA and ClfB, the serine-aspartate repeat protein SdrE and protein A. Mol Microbiol 2002;44:1033–44.
144 Moreillon P, Que YA. Infective endocarditis. Lancet 2004; 363:139–49.
145 Entenza JM, Foster TJ, Ni ED, Vaudaux P, Francioli P, Moreillon P. Contribution of clumping factor B to pathogenesis of experimental endocarditis due to *Staphylococcus aureus*. Infect Immun 2000;68:5443–6.
146 Vernachio J, Bayer AS, Le T *et al*. Anti-clumping factor A immunoglobulin reduces the duration of methicillin-resistant *Staphylococcus aureus* bacteremia in an experimental model of infective endocarditis. Antimicrob Agents Chemother 2003; 47:3400–6.
147 Josefsson E, Hartford O, O'Brien L, Patti JM, Foster T. Protection against experimental *Staphylococcus aureus* arthritis by vaccination with clumping factor A, a novel virulence determinant. J Infect Dis 2001;184:1572–80.
148 Higgins J, Loughman A, van Kessel KP, van Strijp JA, Foster TJ. Clumping factor A of *Staphylococcus aureus* inhibits phagocytosis by human polymorphonuclear leucocytes. FEMS Microbiol Lett 2006;258:290–6.
149 Palmqvist N, Patti JM, Tarkowski A, Josefsson E. Expression of staphylococcal clumping factor A impedes macrophage phagocytosis. Microbes Infect 2004;6:188–95.
150 Palmqvist N, Josefsson E, Tarkowski A. Clumping factor A-mediated virulence during *Staphylococcus aureus* infection is retained despite fibrinogen depletion. Microbes Infect 2004;6: 196–201.
151 McAleese FM, Walsh EJ, Sieprawska M, Potempa J, Foster TJ. Loss of clumping factor B fibrinogen binding activity by *Staphylococcus aureus* involves cessation of transcription, shedding and cleavage by metalloprotease. J Biol Chem 2001;276:29969–78.
152 O'Brien LM, Walsh EJ, Massey RC, Peacock SJ, Foster TJ. *Staphylococcus aureus* clumping factor B (ClfB) promotes adherence to human type I cytokeratin 10: implications for nasal colonization. Cell Microbiol 2002;4:759–70.
153 Schaffer AC, Solinga RM, Cocchiaro J *et al*. Immunization with *Staphylococcus aureus* clumping factor B, a major determinant in nasal carriage, reduces nasal colonization in a murine model. Infect Immun 2006;74:2145–53.
154 Yamada Y, Hideka K, Shiota S, Kuroda T, Tsuchiya T. Gene cloning and characterization of SdrM, a chromosomally-encoded multidrug efflux pump, from *Staphylococcus aureus*. Biol Pharm Bull 2006;29:554–6.
155 George NP, Wei Q, Shin PK, Konstantopoulos K, Ross JM. *Staphylococcus aureus* adhesion via Spa, ClfA, and SdrCDE to immobilized platelets demonstrates shear-dependent behavior. Arterioscler Thromb Vasc Biol 2006;26:2394–400.
156 Josefsson E, McCrea KW, Ni ED *et al*. Three new members of the serine-aspartate repeat protein multigene family of *Staphylococcus aureus*. Microbiology 1998;144:3387–95.
157 Sabat A, Melles DC, Martirosian G, Grundmann H, van Belkum A, Hryniewicz W. Distribution of the serine-aspartate repeat protein-encoding *sdr* genes among nasal-carriage and invasive *Staphylococcus aureus* strains. J Clin Microbiol 2006;44: 1135–8.
158 Ryden C, Yacoub AI, Maxe I *et al*. Specific binding of bone sialoprotein to *Staphylococcus aureus* isolated from patients with osteomyelitis. Eur J Biochem 1989;184:331–6.
159 Arrecubieta C, Lee MH, Macey A, Foster TJ, Lowy FD. SdrF, a *Staphylococcus epidermidis* surface protein, binds type I collagen. J Biol Chem 2007;282:18767–76.
160 Bowden MG, Heuck AP, Ponnuraj K *et al*. Evidence for the "dock, lock and latch" ligand binding mechanism of the staphylococcal MSCRAMM SdrG. J Biol Chem 2008;283:638–47.
161 Liu Y, Ames B, Gorovits E *et al*. SdrX, a serine-aspartate repeat protein expressed by *Staphylococcus capitis* with collagen VI binding activity. Infect Immun 2004;72:6237–44.
162 McCrea KW, Hartford O, Davis S *et al*. The serine-aspartate repeat (Sdr) protein family in *Staphylococcus epidermidis*. Microbiology 2000;146:1535–46.
163 Sakinc T, Kleine B, Gatermann SG. SdrI, a serine-aspartate repeat protein identified in *Staphylococcus saprophyticus* strain 7108, is a collagen-binding protein. Infect Immun 2006;74:4615–23.
164 Nilsson IM, Bremell T, Ryden C, Cheung AL, Tarkowski A. Role of the staphylococcal accessory gene regulator (*sar*) in septic arthritis. Infect Immun 1996;64:4438–43.
165 Gillaspy AF, Patti JM, Pratt FL Jr, Iandolo JJ, Smeltzer MS. The *Staphylococcus aureus* collagen adhesin-encoding gene (*cna*) is within a discrete genetic element. Gene 1997;196:239–48.
166 Buxton TB, Rissing JP, Horner JA *et al*. Binding of a *Staphylococcus aureus* bone pathogen to type I collagen. Microb Pathog 1990;8:441–8.
167 Elasri MO, Thomas JR, Skinner RA *et al*. *Staphylococcus aureus* collagen adhesin contributes to the pathogenesis of osteomyelitis. Bone 2002;30:275–80.
168 Patti JM, Bremell T, Krajewska-Pietrasik D *et al*. The *Staphylococcus aureus* collagen adhesin is a virulence determinant in experimental septic arthritis. Infect Immun 1994;62:152–61.
169 Switalski LM, Patti JM, Butcher W, Gristina AG, Speziale P, Hook M. A collagen receptor on *Staphylococcus aureus* strains

isolated from patients with septic arthritis mediates adhesion to cartilage. Mol Microbiol 1993;7:99–107.
170 Xu Y, Rivas JM, Brown EL, Liang X, Hook M. Virulence potential of the staphylococcal adhesin CNA in experimental arthritis is determined by its affinity for collagen. J Infect Dis 2004; 189:2323–33.
171 Hienz SA, Schennings T, Heimdahl A, Flock JI. Collagen binding of *Staphylococcus aureus* is a virulence factor in experimental endocarditis. J Infect Dis 1996;174:83–8.
172 Rhem MN, Lech EM, Patti JM *et al*. The collagen-binding adhesin is a virulence factor in *Staphylococcus aureus* keratitis. Infect Immun 2000;68:3776–9.
173 Mazmanian SK, Ton-That H, Schneewind O. Sortase-catalysed anchoring of surface proteins to the cell wall of *Staphylococcus aureus*. Mol Microbiol 2001;40:1049–57.
174 Corrigan RM, Rigby D, Handley P, Foster TJ. The role of *Staphylococcus aureus* surface protein SasG in adherence and biofilm formation. Microbiology 2007;153:2435–46.
175 Josefsson E, Juuti K, Bokarewa M, Kuusela P. The surface protein Pls of methicillin-resistant *Staphylococcus aureus* is a virulence factor in septic arthritis. Infect Immun 2005;73:2812–17.
176 Savolainen K, Paulin L, Westerlund-Wikstrom B, Foster TJ, Korhonen TK, Kuusela P. Expression of *pls*, a gene closely associated with the *mecA* gene of methicillin-resistant *Staphylococcus aureus*, prevents bacterial adhesion *in vitro*. Infect Immun 2001;69:3013–20.
177 Werbick C, Becker K, Mellmann A *et al*. Staphylococcal chromosomal cassette *mec* type I, *spa* type, and expression of Pls are determinants of reduced cellular invasiveness of methicillin-resistant *Staphylococcus aureus* isolates. J Infect Dis 2007;195:1678–85.
178 Siboo IR, Chambers HF, Sullam PM. Role of SraP, a serine-rich surface protein of *Staphylococcus aureus*, in binding to human platelets. Infect Immun 2005;73:2273–80.
179 Mazmanian SK, Skaar EP, Gaspar AH *et al*. Passage of heme-iron across the envelope of *Staphylococcus aureus*. Science 2003;299:906–9.
180 Stranger-Jones YK, Bae T, Schneewind O. Vaccine assembly from surface proteins of *Staphylococcus aureus*. Proc Natl Acad Sci USA 2006;103:16942–7.
181 Cucarella C, Tormo MA, Knecht E *et al*. Expression of the biofilm-associated protein interferes with host protein receptors of *Staphylococcus aureus* and alters the infective process. Infect Immun 2002;70:3180–6.
182 Lasa I, Penades JR. Bap: a family of surface proteins involved in biofilm formation. Res Microbiol 2006;157:99–107.
183 Tormo MA, Knecht E, Gotz F, Lasa I, Penades JR. Bap-dependent biofilm formation by pathogenic species of *Staphylococcus*: evidence of horizontal gene transfer? Microbiology 2005;151:2465–75.
184 Tormo MA, Ubeda C, Marti M *et al*. Phase-variable expression of the biofilm-associated protein (Bap) in *Staphylococcus aureus*. Microbiology 2007;153:1702–10.
185 Cucarella C, Solano C, Valle J, Amorena B, Lasa I, Penades JR. Bap, a *Staphylococcus aureus* surface protein involved in biofilm formation. J Bacteriol 2001;183:2888–96.
186 Cucarella C, Tormo MA, Ubeda C *et al*. Role of biofilm-associated protein *bap* in the pathogenesis of bovine *Staphylococcus aureus*. Infect Immun 2004;72:2177–85.
187 Downer R, Roche F, Park PW, Mecham RP, Foster TJ. The elastin-binding protein of *Staphylococcus aureus* (EbpS) is expressed at the cell surface as an integral membrane protein and not as a cell wall-associated protein. J Biol Chem 2002;277: 243–50.
188 Clarke SR, Harris LG, Richards RG, Foster SJ. Analysis of Ebh, a 1.1-megadalton cell wall-associated fibronectin-binding protein of *Staphylococcus aureus*. Infect Immun 2002;70:6680–7.
189 Chavakis T, Wiechmann K, Preissner KT, Herrmann M. *Staphylococcus aureus* interactions with the endothelium: the role of bacterial "secretable expanded repertoire adhesive molecules" (SERAM) in disturbing host defense systems. Thromb Haemost 2005;94:278–85.
190 Hansen U, Hussain M, Villone D *et al*. The anchorless adhesin Eap (extracellular adherence protein) from *Staphylococcus aureus* selectively recognizes extracellular matrix aggregates but binds promiscuously to monomeric matrix macromolecules. Matrix Biol 2006;25:252–60.
191 Harraghy N, Hussain M, Haggar A *et al*. The adhesive and immunomodulating properties of the multifunctional *Staphylococcus aureus* protein Eap. Microbiology 2003;149:2701–7.
192 Athanasopoulos AN, Economopoulou M, Orlova VV *et al*. The extracellular adherence protein (Eap) of *Staphylococcus aureus* inhibits wound healing by interfering with host defense and repair mechanisms. Blood 2006;107:2720–7.
193 Sobke AC, Selimovic D, Orlova V *et al*. The extracellular adherence protein from *Staphylococcus aureus* abrogates angiogenic responses of endothelial cells by blocking Ras activation. FASEB J 2006;20:2621–3.
194 Xie C, Alcaide P, Geisbrecht BV *et al*. Suppression of experimental autoimmune encephalomyelitis by extracellular adherence protein of *Staphylococcus aureus*. J Exp Med 2006;203:985–94.
195 Kajimura J, Fujiwara T, Yamada S *et al*. Identification and molecular characterization of an *N*-acetylmuramyl-L-alanine amidase Sle1 involved in cell separation of *Staphylococcus aureus*. Mol Microbiol 2005;58:1087–101.
196 Takahashi J, Komatsuzawa H, Yamada S *et al*. Molecular characterization of an *atl* null mutant of *Staphylococcus aureus*. Microbiol Immunol 2002;46:601–12.
197 Heilmann C, Hartleib J, Hussain MS, Peters G. The multifunctional *Staphylococcus aureus* autolysin *aaa* mediates adherence to immobilized fibrinogen and fibronectin. Infect Immun 2005;73:4793–802.
198 O'Riordan K, Lee JC. *Staphylococcus aureus* capsular polysaccharides. Clin Microbiol Rev 2004;17:218–34.
199 Lin WS, Cunneen T, Lee CY. Sequence analysis and molecular characterization of genes required for the biosynthesis of type 1 capsular polysaccharide in *Staphylococcus aureus*. J Bacteriol 1994;176:7005–16.
200 Ouyang S, Lee CY. Transcriptional analysis of type 1 capsule genes in *Staphylococcus aureus*. Mol Microbiol 1997;23:473–82.
201 Luong TT, Lee CY. The *arl* locus positively regulates *Staphylococcus aureus* type 5 capsule via an *mgrA*-dependent pathway. Microbiology 2006;152:3123–31.
202 Luong TT, Lee CY. Overproduction of type 8 capsular polysaccharide augments *Staphylococcus aureus* virulence. Infect Immun 2002;70:3389–95.
203 Jones C. Revised structures for the capsular polysaccharides from *Staphylococcus aureus* Types 5 and 8, components of novel glycoconjugate vaccines. Carbohydr Res 2005;340:1097–106.
204 Sau S, Bhasin N, Wann ER, Lee JC, Foster TJ, Lee CY. The *Staphylococcus aureus* allelic genetic loci for serotype 5 and 8

capsule expression contain the type-specific genes flanked by common genes. Microbiology 1997;143:2395–2405.
205 Kiser KB, Cantey-Kiser JM, Lee JC. Development and characterization of a *Staphylococcus aureus* nasal colonization model in mice. Infect Immun 1999;67:5001–6.
206 Nilsson IM, Lee JC, Bremell T, Ryden C, Tarkowski A. The role of staphylococcal polysaccharide microcapsule expression in septicemia and septic arthritis. Infect Immun 1997;65:4216–21.
207 Portoles M, Kiser KB, Bhasin N, Chan KH, Lee JC. *Staphylococcus aureus* Cap5O has UDP-ManNAc dehydrogenase activity and is essential for capsule expression. Infect Immun 2001;69:917–23.
208 Thakker M, Park JS, Carey V, Lee JC. *Staphylococcus aureus* serotype 5 capsular polysaccharide is antiphagocytic and enhances bacterial virulence in a murine bacteremia model. Infect Immun 1998;66:5183–9.
209 Tzianabos AO, Wang JY, Lee JC. Structural rationale for the modulation of abscess formation by *Staphylococcus aureus* capsular polysaccharides. Proc Natl Acad Sci USA 2001;98:9365–70.
210 Watts A, Ke D, Wang Q, Pillay A, Nicholson-Weller A, Lee JC. *Staphylococcus aureus* strains that express serotype 5 or serotype 8 capsular polysaccharides differ in virulence. Infect Immun 2005;73:3502–11.
211 Karakawa WW, Sutton A, Schneerson R, Karpas A, Vann WF. Capsular antibodies induce type-specific phagocytosis of capsulated *Staphylococcus aureus* by human polymorphonuclear leukocytes. Infect Immun 1988;56:1090–5.
212 Verbrugh HA, Peterson PK, Nguyen BY, Sisson SP, Kim Y. Opsonization of encapsulated *Staphylococcus aureus*: the role of specific antibody and complement. J Immunol 1982;129:1681–7.
213 Cunnion KM, Lee JC, Frank MM. Capsule production and growth phase influence binding of complement to *Staphylococcus aureus*. Infect Immun 2001;69:6796–803.
214 Baddour LM, Lowrance C, Albus A, Lowrance JH, Anderson SK, Lee JC. *Staphylococcus aureus* microcapsule expression attenuates bacterial virulence in a rat model of experimental endocarditis. J Infect Dis 1992;165:749–53.
215 Nemeth J, Lee JC. Antibodies to capsular polysaccharides are not protective against experimental *Staphylococcus aureus* endocarditis. Infect Immun 1995;63:375–80.
216 Pohlmann-Dietze P, Ulrich M, Kiser KB *et al.* Adherence of *Staphylococcus aureus* to endothelial cells: influence of capsular polysaccharide, global regulator *agr*, and bacterial growth phase. Infect Immun 2000;68:4865–71.
217 Snodgrass JL, Mohamed N, Ross JM, Sau S, Lee CY, Smeltzer MS. Functional analysis of the *Staphylococcus aureus* collagen adhesin B domain. Infect Immun 1999;67:3952–9.
218 Smeltzer MS, Thomas JR, Hickmon SG *et al.* Characterization of a rabbit model of staphylococcal osteomyelitis. J Orthop Res 1997;15:414–21.
219 Olson ME, Garvin KL, Fey PD, Rupp ME. Adherence of *Staphylococcus epidermidis* to biomaterials is augmented by PIA. Clin Orthop Relat Res 2006;451:21–4.
220 Gotz F. Staphylococcus and biofilms. Mol Microbiol 2002; 43:1367–78.
221 Arciola CR, Baldassarri L, Montanaro L. Presence of *icaA* and *icaD* genes and slime production in a collection of staphylococcal strains from catheter-associated infections. J Clin Microbiol 2001;39:2151–6.
222 Fowler VG Jr, Fey PD, Reller LB, Chamis AL, Corey GR, Rupp ME. The intercellular adhesin locus *ica* is present in clinical isolates of *Staphylococcus aureus* from bacteremic patients with infected and uninfected prosthetic joints. Med Microbiol Immunol 2001;189:127–31.
223 Martin-Lopez JV, Perez-Roth E, Claverie-Martin F *et al.* Detection of *Staphylococcus aureus* clinical isolates harboring the *ica* gene cluster needed for biofilm establishment. J Clin Microbiol 2002;40:1569–70.
224 Satorres SE, Alcaraz LE. Prevalence of *icaA* and *icaD* genes in *Staphylococcus aureus* and *Staphylococcus epidermidis* strains isolated from patients and hospital staff. Cent Eur J Public Health 2007;15:87–90.
225 Mack D, Fischer W, Krokotsch A *et al.* The intercellular adhesin involved in biofilm accumulation of *Staphylococcus epidermidis* is a linear beta-1,6-linked glucosaminoglycan: purification and structural analysis. J Bacteriol 1996;178:175–83.
226 Li H, Xu L, Wang J *et al.* Conversion of *Staphylococcus epidermidis* strains from commensal to invasive by expression of the *ica* locus encoding production of biofilm exopolysaccharide. Infect Immun 2005;73:3188–91.
227 Rupp ME, Fey PD, Heilmann C, Gotz F. Characterization of the importance of *Staphylococcus epidermidis* autolysin and polysaccharide intercellular adhesin in the pathogenesis of intravascular catheter-associated infection in a rat model. J Infect Dis 2001;183:1038–42.
228 Vuong C, Voyich JM, Fischer ER *et al.* Polysaccharide intercellular adhesin (PIA) protects *Staphylococcus epidermidis* against major components of the human innate immune system. Cell Microbiol 2004;6:269–75.
229 Chokr A, Leterme D, Watier D, Jabbouri S. Neither the presence of *ica* locus, nor *in vitro*-biofilm formation ability is a crucial parameter for some *Staphylococcus epidermidis* strains to maintain an infection in a guinea pig tissue cage model. Microb Pathog 2007;42:94–7.
230 Francois P, Tu Quoc PH, Bisognano C *et al.* Lack of biofilm contribution to bacterial colonisation in an experimental model of foreign body infection by *Staphylococcus aureus* and *Staphylococcus epidermidis*. FEMS Immunol Med Microbiol 2003;35: 135–40.
231 Cramton SE, Gerke C, Schnell NF, Nichols WW, Gotz F. The intercellular adhesion (*ica*) locus is present in *Staphylococcus aureus* and is required for biofilm formation. Infect Immun 1999;67:5427–33.
232 Heilmann C, Schweitzer O, Gerke C, Vanittanakom N, Mack D, Gotz F. Molecular basis of intercellular adhesion in the biofilm-forming *Staphylococcus epidermidis*. Mol Microbiol 1996; 20:1083–91.
233 Kristian SA, Golda T, Ferracin F *et al.* The ability of biofilm formation does not influence virulence of *Staphylococcus aureus* and host response in a mouse tissue cage infection model. Microb Pathog 2004;36:237–45.
234 Beenken KE, Dunman PM, McAleese F *et al.* Global gene expression in *Staphylococcus aureus* biofilms. J Bacteriol 2004; 186:4665–84.
235 Hennig S, Nyunt WS, Ziebuhr W. Spontaneous switch to PIA-independent biofilm formation in an *ica*-positive *Staphylococcus epidermidis* isolate. Int J Med Microbiol 2007;297:117–22.
236 Qin Z, Yang X, Yang L *et al.* Formation and properties of *in vitro* biofilms of *ica*-negative *Staphylococcus epidermidis* clinical isolates. J Med Microbiol 2007;56:83–93.
237 Rohde H, Burandt EC, Siemssen N *et al.* Polysaccharide intercellular adhesin or protein factors in biofilm accumulation of

Staphylococcus epidermidis and *Staphylococcus aureus* isolated from prosthetic hip and knee joint infections. Biomaterials 2007;28:1711–20.

238 Izano EA, Amarante MA, Kher WB, Kaplan JB. Differential roles of poly-*N*-acetylglucosamine surface polysaccharide and extracellular DNA in *Staphylococcus aureus* and *Staphylococcus epidermidis* biofilms. Appl Environ Microbiol 2008;74:470–6.

239 O'Gara JP. *ica* and beyond: biofilm mechanisms and regulation in *Staphylococcus epidermidis* and *Staphylococcus aureus*. FEMS Microbiol Lett 2007;270:179–88.

240 Rice KC, Mann EE, Endres JL *et al*. The *cidA* murein hydrolase regulator contributes to DNA release and biofilm development in *Staphylococcus aureus*. Proc Natl Acad Sci USA 2007; 104:8113–18.

241 Fitzpatrick F, Humphreys H, O'Gara JP. The genetics of staphylococcal biofilm formation: will a greater understanding of pathogenesis lead to better management of device-related infection? Clin Microbiol Infect 2005;11:967–73.

242 Beenken KE, Blevins JS, Smeltzer MS. Mutation of *sarA* in *Staphylococcus aureus* limits biofilm formation. Infect Immun 2003;71:4206–11.

243 Kropec A, Maira-Litran T, Jefferson KK *et al*. Poly-*N*-acetylglucosamine production in *Staphylococcus aureus* is essential for virulence in murine models of systemic infection. Infect Immun 2005;73:6868–76.

244 Ulrich M, Bastian M, Cramton SE *et al*. The staphylococcal respiratory response regulator SrrAB induces *ica* gene transcription and polysaccharide intercellular adhesin expression, protecting *Staphylococcus aureus* from neutrophil killing under anaerobic growth conditions. Mol Microbiol 2007;65:1276–87.

245 McKenney D, Pouliot K, Wang Y *et al*. Vaccine potential of poly-1–6 beta-D-*N*-succinylglucosamine, an immunoprotective surface polysaccharide of *Staphylococcus aureus* and *Staphylococcus epidermidis*. J Biotechnol 2000;83:37–44.

246 Cerca N, Jefferson KK, Maira-Litran T *et al*. Molecular basis for preferential protective efficacy of antibodies directed to the poorly acetylated form of staphylococcal poly-*N*-acetyl-beta-(1-6)-glucosamine. Infect Immun 2007;75:3406–13.

247 Begun J, Gaiani JM, Rohde H *et al*. Staphylococcal biofilm exopolysaccharide protects against *Caenorhabditis elegans* immune defenses. PLoS Pathog 2007;3:e57.

248 Dinges MM, Orwin PM, Schlievert PM. Exotoxins of *Staphylococcus aureus*. Clin Microbiol Rev 2000;13:16–34.

249 Thomas D, Chou S, Dauwalder O, Lina G. Diversity in *Staphylococcus aureus* enterotoxins. Chem Immunol Allergy 2007;93:24–41.

250 Jarraud S, Peyrat MA, Lim A *et al*. *egc*, a highly prevalent operon of enterotoxin gene, forms a putative nursery of superantigens in *Staphylococcus aureus*. J Immunol 2001;166:669–77.

251 Lee CY, Schmidt JJ, Johnson-Winegar AD, Spero L, Iandolo JJ. Sequence determination and comparison of the exfoliative toxin A and toxin B genes from *Staphylococcus aureus*. J Bacteriol 1987;169:3904–9.

252 Sato H, Matsumori Y, Tanabe T, Saito H, Shimizu A, Kawano J. A new type of staphylococcal exfoliative toxin from a *Staphylococcus aureus* strain isolated from a horse with phlegmon. Infect Immun 1994;62:3780–5.

253 Yamaguchi T, Nishifuji K, Sasaki M *et al*. Identification of the *Staphylococcus aureus* etd pathogenicity island which encodes a novel exfoliative toxin, ETD, and EDIN-B. Infect Immun 2002;70:5835–45.

254 Plano LR. *Staphylococcus aureus* exfoliative toxins: how they cause disease. J Invest Dermatol 2004;122:1070–7.

255 Hanakawa Y, Stanley JR. Mechanisms of blister formation by staphylococcal toxins. J Biochem (Tokyo) 2004;136:747–50.

256 Hanakawa Y, Schechter NM, Lin C, Nishifuji K, Amagai M, Stanley JR. Enzymatic and molecular characteristics of the efficiency and specificity of exfoliative toxin cleavage of desmoglein 1. J Biol Chem 2004;279:5268–77.

257 Nishifuji K, Sugai M, Amagai M. Staphylococcal exfoliative toxins: "molecular scissors" of bacteria that attack the cutaneous defense barrier in mammals. J Dermatol Sci 2008; 49:21–31.

258 Monday SR, Vath GM, Ferens WA *et al*. Unique superantigen activity of staphylococcal exfoliative toxins. J Immunol 1999; 162:4550–9.

259 Plano LR, Gutman DM, Woischnik M, Collins CM. Recombinant *Staphylococcus aureus* exfoliative toxins are not bacterial superantigens. Infect Immun 2000;68:3048–52.

260 Ladhani S. Understanding the mechanism of action of the exfoliative toxins of *Staphylococcus aureus*. FEMS Immunol Med Microbiol 2003;39:181–9.

261 Prevost G, Couppie P, Monteil H. Staphylococcal epidermolysins. Curr Opin Infect Dis 2003;16:71–6.

262 Ladhani S, Joannou CL. Difficulties in diagnosis and management of the staphylococcal scalded skin syndrome. Pediatr Infect Dis J 2000;19:819–21.

263 Al-Shangiti AM, Naylor CE, Nair SP, Briggs DC, Henderson B, Chain BM. Structural relationships and cellular tropism of staphylococcal superantigen-like proteins. Infect Immun 2004; 72:4261–70.

264 Lina G, Bohach GA, Nair SP, Hiramatsu K, Jouvin-Marche E, Mariuzza R. Standard nomenclature for the superantigens expressed by *Staphylococcus*. J Infect Dis 2004;189:2334–6.

265 Hamad AR, Marrack P, Kappler JW. Transcytosis of staphylococcal superantigen toxins. J Exp Med 1997;185:1447–54.

266 Shupp JW, Jett M, Pontzer CH. Identification of a transcytosis epitope on staphylococcal enterotoxins. Infect Immun 2002; 70:2178–86.

267 Scheuber PH, Golecki JR, Kickhofen B, Scheel D, Beck G, Hammer DK. Skin reactivity of unsensitized monkeys upon challenge with staphylococcal enterotoxin B: a new approach for investigating the site of toxin action. Infect Immun 1985; 50:869–76.

268 Todd J, Fishaut M, Kapral F, Welch T. Toxic-shock syndrome associated with phage group I staphylococci. Lancet 1978; ii:1116–18.

269 McCormick JK, Yarwood JM, Schlievert PM. Toxic shock syndrome and bacterial superantigens: an update. Annu Rev Microbiol 2001;55:77–104.

270 Huseby M, Shi K, Brown CK *et al*. Structure and biological activities of beta toxin from *Staphylococcus aureus*. J Bacteriol 2007;189:8719–26.

271 Adhikari RP, Arvidson S, Novick RP. A nonsense mutation in *agrA* accounts for the defect in *agr* expression and the avirulence of *Staphylococcus aureus* 8325–4 *traP::kan*. Infect Immun 2007;75:4534–40.

272 Caiazza NC, O'Toole GA. Alpha-toxin is required for biofilm formation by *Staphylococcus aureus*. J Bacteriol 2003;185:3214–17.

273 Janzon L, Arvidson S. The role of the delta-lysin gene (*hld*) in the regulation of virulence genes by the accessory gene regulator (*agr*) in *Staphylococcus aureus*. EMBO J 1990;9:1391–9.

274 Mehlin C, Headley CM, Klebanoff SJ. An inflammatory polypeptide complex from *Staphylococcus epidermidis*: isolation and characterization. J Exp Med 1999;189:907–18.
275 Liles WC, Thomsen AR, O'Mahony DS, Klebanoff SJ. Stimulation of human neutrophils and monocytes by staphylococcal phenol-soluble modulin. J Leukoc Biol 2001;70:96–102.
276 Otto M, O'Mahoney DS, Guina T, Klebanoff SJ. Activity of *Staphylococcus epidermidis* phenol-soluble modulin peptides expressed in *Staphylococcus carnosus*. J Infect Dis 2004;190: 748–55.
277 Prevost G, Couppie P, Prevost P *et al*. Epidemiological data on *Staphylococcus aureus* strains producing synergohymenotropic toxins. J Med Microbiol 1995;42:237–45.
278 Gillet Y, Issartel B, Vanhems P *et al*. Association between *Staphylococcus aureus* strains carrying gene for Panton–Valentine leukocidin and highly lethal necrotising pneumonia in young immunocompetent patients. Lancet 2002;359:753–9.
279 Tristan A, Bes M, Meugnier H *et al*. Global distribution of Panton–Valentine leukocidin-positive methicillin-resistant *Staphylococcus aureus*, 2006. Emerg Infect Dis 2007;13:594–600.
280 Barrio MB, Rainard P, Prevost G. LukM/LukF'-PV is the most active *Staphylococcus aureus* leukotoxin on bovine neutrophils. Microbes Infect 2006;8:2068–74.
281 Gravet A, Colin DA, Keller D, Girardot R, Monteil H, Prevost G. Characterization of a novel structural member, LukE-LukD, of the bi-component staphylococcal leucotoxins family. FEBS Lett 1998;436:202–8.
282 Arciola CR, Baldassarri L, Von Eiff C *et al*. Prevalence of genes encoding for staphylococcal leukocidal toxins among clinical isolates of *Staphylococcus aureus* from implant orthopedic infections. Int J Artif Organs 2007;30:792–7.
283 Von Eiff C, Friedrich AW, Peters G, Becker K. Prevalence of genes encoding for members of the staphylococcal leukotoxin family among clinical isolates of *Staphylococcus aureus*. Diagn Microbiol Infect Dis 2004;49:157–62.
284 Gravet A, Couppie P, Meunier O *et al*. *Staphylococcus aureus* isolated in cases of impetigo produces both epidermolysin A or B and LukE-LukD in 78% of 131 retrospective and prospective cases. J Clin Microbiol 2001;39:4349–56.
285 Prevost G, Cribier B, Couppie P *et al*. Panton–Valentine leucocidin and gamma-hemolysin from *Staphylococcus aureus* ATCC 49775 are encoded by distinct genetic loci and have different biological activities. Infect Immun 1995;63:4121–9.
286 Konig B, Prevost G, Konig W. Composition of staphylococcal bi-component toxins determines pathophysiological reactions. J Med Microbiol 1997;46:479–85.
287 Siqueira JA, Speeg-Schatz C, Freitas FI, Sahel J, Monteil H, Prevost G. Channel-forming leucotoxins from *Staphylococcus aureus* cause severe inflammatory reactions in a rabbit eye model. J Med Microbiol 1997;46:486–94.
288 Bokarewa MI, Jin T, Tarkowski A. *Staphylococcus aureus*: staphylokinase. Int J Biochem Cell Biol 2006;38:504–9.
289 Dubin G. Extracellular proteases of *Staphylococcus* spp. Biol Chem 2002;383:1075–86.
290 Nickerson NN, Prasad L, Jacob L, Delbaere LT, McGavin MJ. Activation of the SspA serine protease zymogen of *Staphylococcus aureus* proceeds through unique variations of a trypsinogen-like mechanism and is dependent on both autocatalytic and metalloprotease-specific processing. J Biol Chem 2007;282:34129–38.
291 Calander AM, Jonsson IM, Kanth A *et al*. Impact of staphylococcal protease expression on the outcome of infectious arthritis. Microbes Infect 2004;6:202–6.
292 Reed SB, Wesson CA, Liou LE *et al*. Molecular characterization of a novel *Staphylococcus aureus* serine protease operon. Infect Immun 2001;69:1521–7.
293 Frees D, Savijoki K, Varmanen P, Ingmer H. Clp ATPases and ClpP proteolytic complexes regulate vital biological processes in low GC, Gram-positive bacteria. Mol Microbiol 2007;63:1285–95.
294 Brotz-Oesterhelt H, Beyer D, Kroll HP *et al*. Dysregulation of bacterial proteolytic machinery by a new class of antibiotics. Nat Med 2005;11:1082–7.
295 Frees D, Qazi SN, Hill PJ, Ingmer H. Alternative roles of ClpX and ClpP in *Staphylococcus aureus* stress tolerance and virulence. Mol Microbiol 2003;48:1565–78.
296 Michel A, Agerer F, Hauck CR *et al*. Global regulatory impact of ClpP protease of *Staphylococcus aureus* on regulons involved in virulence, oxidative stress response, autolysis, and DNA repair. J Bacteriol 2006;188:5783–96.
297 Frees D, Sorensen K, Ingmer H. Global virulence regulation in *Staphylococcus aureus*: pinpointing the roles of ClpP and ClpX in the sar/agr regulatory network. Infect Immun 2005;73:8100–8.
298 Frees D, Chastanet A, Qazi S *et al*. Clp ATPases are required for stress tolerance, intracellular replication and biofilm formation in *Staphylococcus aureus*. Mol Microbiol 2004;54:1445–62.
299 Wang C, Li M, Dong D *et al*. Role of ClpP in biofilm formation and virulence of *Staphylococcus epidermidis*. Microbes Infect 2007;9:1376–83.
300 Becker P, Hufnagle W, Peters G, Herrmann M. Detection of differential gene expression in biofilm-forming versus planktonic populations of *Staphylococcus aureus* using micro-representational-difference analysis. Appl Environ Microbiol 2001;67:2958–65.
301 Chatterjee I, Becker P, Grundmeier M *et al*. *Staphylococcus aureus* ClpC is required for stress resistance, aconitase activity, growth recovery, and death. J Bacteriol 2005;187:4488–96.
302 Somerville GA, Cockayne A, Durr M, Peschel A, Otto M, Musser JM. Synthesis and deformylation of *Staphylococcus aureus* delta-toxin are linked to tricarboxylic acid cycle activity. J Bacteriol 2003;185:6686–94.
303 Chatterjee I, Herrmann M, Proctor RA, Peters G, Kahl BC. Enhanced post-stationary-phase survival of a clinical thymidine-dependent small-colony variant of *Staphylococcus aureus* results from lack of a functional tricarboxylic acid cycle. J Bacteriol 2007;189:2936–40.
304 Shompole S, Henon KT, Liou LE, Dziewanowska K, Bohach GA, Bayles KW. Biphasic intracellular expression of *Staphylococcus aureus* virulence factors and evidence for Agr-mediated diffusion sensing. Mol Microbiol 2003;49:919–27.
305 Maresso AW, Schneewind O. Iron acquisition and transport in *Staphylococcus aureus*. Biometals 2006;19:193–203.
306 Reniere ML, Torres VJ, Skaar EP. Intracellular metalloporphyrin metabolism in *Staphylococcus aureus*. Biometals 2007;20:333–45.
307 Skaar EP, Schneewind O. Iron-regulated surface determinants (Isd) of *Staphylococcus aureus*: stealing iron from heme. Microbes Infect 2004;6:390–7.
308 Konetschny-Rapp S, Jung G, Meiwes J, Zahner H. Staphyloferrin A: a structurally new siderophore from staphylococci. Eur J Biochem 1990;191:65–74.

309 Meiwes J, Fiedler HP, Haag H, Zahner H, Konetschny-Rapp S, Jung G. Isolation and characterization of staphyloferrin A, a compound with siderophore activity from *Staphylococcus hyicus* DSM 20459. FEMS Microbiol Lett 1990;55:201–5.

310 Drechsel H, Freund S, Nicholson G *et al*. Purification and chemical characterization of staphyloferrin B, a hydrophilic siderophore from staphylococci. Biometals 1993;6:185–92.

311 Haag H, Fiedler HP, Meiwes J, Drechsel H, Jung G, Zahner H. Isolation and biological characterization of staphyloferrin B, a compound with siderophore activity from staphylococci. FEMS Microbiol Lett 1994;115:125–30.

312 Courcol RJ, Trivier D, Bissinger MC, Martin GR, Brown MR. Siderophore production by *Staphylococcus aureus* and identification of iron-regulated proteins. Infect Immun 1997;65:1944–8.

313 Dale SE, Sebulsky MT, Heinrichs DE. Involvement of SirABC in iron-siderophore import in *Staphylococcus aureus*. J Bacteriol 2004;186:8356–62.

314 Speziali CD, Dale SE, Henderson JA, Vines ED, Heinrichs DE. Requirement of *Staphylococcus aureus* ATP-binding cassette-ATPase FhuC for iron-restricted growth and evidence that it functions with more than one iron transporter. J Bacteriol 2006;188:2048–55.

315 Dale SE, Doherty-Kirby A, Lajoie G, Heinrichs DE. Role of siderophore biosynthesis in virulence of *Staphylococcus aureus*: identification and characterization of genes involved in production of a siderophore. Infect Immun 2004;72:29–37.

316 Henrichs JH, Gatlin LE, Kunsch C, Choi GH, Hanson MS. Identification and characterization of SirA, an iron-regulated protein from *Staphylococcus aureus*. J Bacteriol 1999;181:1436–43.

317 Morrissey JA, Cockayne A, Hill PJ, Williams P. Molecular cloning and analysis of a putative siderophore ABC transporter from *Staphylococcus aureus*. Infect Immun 2000;68:6281–8.

318 Sebulsky MT, Hohnstein D, Hunter MD, Heinrichs DE. Identification and characterization of a membrane permease involved in iron-hydroxamate transport in *Staphylococcus aureus*. J Bacteriol 2000;182:4394–400.

319 Sebulsky MT, Heinrichs DE. Identification and characterization of *fhuD1* and *fhuD2*, two genes involved in iron-hydroxamate uptake in *Staphylococcus aureus*. J Bacteriol 2001;183:4994–5000.

320 Xiong A, Singh VK, Cabrera G, Jayaswal RK. Molecular characterization of the ferric-uptake regulator, *fur*, from *Staphylococcus aureus*. Microbiology 2000;146:659–68.

321 Park RY, Sun HY, Choi MH, Bai YH, Shin SH. *Staphylococcus aureus* siderophore-mediated iron-acquisition system plays a dominant and essential role in the utilization of transferrin-bound iron. J Microbiol 2005;43:183–90.

322 Modun B, Kendall D, Williams P. Staphylococci express a receptor for human transferrin: identification of a 42-kilodalton cell wall transferrin-binding protein. Infect Immun 1994;62:3850–8.

323 Modun B, Williams P. The staphylococcal transferrin-binding protein is a cell wall glyceraldehyde-3-phosphate dehydrogenase. Infect Immun 1999;67:1086–92.

324 Pancholi V, Fischetti VA. A major surface protein on group A streptococci is a glyceraldehyde-3-phosphate-dehydrogenase with multiple binding activity. J Exp Med 1992;176:415–26.

325 Pancholi V, Chhatwal GS. Housekeeping enzymes as virulence factors for pathogens. Int J Med Microbiol 2003;293:391–401.

326 Taylor JM, Heinrichs DE. Transferrin binding in *Staphylococcus aureus*: involvement of a cell wall-anchored protein. Mol Microbiol 2002;43:1603–14.

327 Fillinger S, Boschi-Muller S, Azza S, Dervyn E, Branlant G, Aymerich S. Two glyceraldehyde-3-phosphate dehydrogenases with opposite physiological roles in a nonphotosynthetic bacterium. J Biol Chem 2000;275:14031–7.

328 Otto BR, Verweij-van Vught AM, MacLaren DM. Transferrins and heme-compounds as iron sources for pathogenic bacteria. Crit Rev Microbiol 1992;18:217–33.

329 Morrissey JA, Cockayne A, Hammacott J *et al*. Conservation, surface exposure, and *in vivo* expression of the Frp family of iron-regulated cell wall proteins in *Staphylococcus aureus*. Infect Immun 2002;70:2399–407.

330 Marraffini LA, Schneewind O. Anchor structure of staphylococcal surface proteins. V. Anchor structure of the sortase B substrate IsdC. J Biol Chem 2005;280:16263–71.

331 Clarke SR, Wiltshire MD, Foster SJ. IsdA of *Staphylococcus aureus* is a broad spectrum, iron-regulated adhesin. Mol Microbiol 2004;51:1509–19.

332 Grigg JC, Vermeiren CL, Heinrichs DE, Murphy ME. Haem recognition by a *Staphylococcus aureus* NEAT domain. Mol Microbiol 2007;63:139–49.

333 Vermeiren CL, Pluym M, Mack J, Heinrichs DE, Stillman MJ. Characterization of the heme binding properties of *Staphylococcus aureus* IsdA. Biochemistry 2006;45:12867–75.

334 Torres VJ, Pishchany G, Humayun M, Schneewind O, Skaar EP. *Staphylococcus aureus* IsdB is a hemoglobin receptor required for heme iron utilization. J Bacteriol 2006;188:8421–9.

335 Clarke SR, Brummell KJ, Horsburgh MJ *et al*. Identification of *in vivo*-expressed antigens of *Staphylococcus aureus* and their use in vaccinations for protection against nasal carriage. J Infect Dis 2006;193:1098–108.

336 Clarke SR, Mohamed R, Bian L *et al*. The *Staphylococcus aureus* surface protein IsdA mediates resistance to innate defenses of human skin. Cell Host Microbe 2007;1:199–212.

337 Kuklin NA, Clark DJ, Secore S *et al*. A novel *Staphylococcus aureus* vaccine: iron surface determinant B induces rapid antibody responses in rhesus macaques and specific increased survival in a murine *S. aureus* sepsis model. Infect Immun 2006;74:2215–23.

338 Etz H, Minh DB, Henics T *et al*. Identification of *in vivo* expressed vaccine candidate antigens from *Staphylococcus aureus*. Proc Natl Acad Sci USA 2002;99:6573–8.

339 Dryla A, Gelbmann D, von Gabain A, Nagy E. Identification of a novel iron regulated staphylococcal surface protein with haptoglobin-haemoglobin binding activity. 2003;49:37–53.

340 Dryla A, Hoffmann B, Gelbmann D *et al*. High-affinity binding of the staphylococcal HarA protein to haptoglobin and hemoglobin involves a domain with an antiparallel eight-stranded beta-barrel fold. J Bacteriol 2007;189:254–64.

341 Kristiansen M, Graversen JH, Jacobsen C *et al*. Identification of the haemoglobin scavenger receptor. Nature 2001;409:198–201.

342 Skaar EP, Gaspar AH, Schneewind O. IsdG and IsdI, heme-degrading enzymes in the cytoplasm of *Staphylococcus aureus*. J Biol Chem 2004;279:436–43.

343 Skaar EP, Humayun M, Bae T, DeBord KL, Schneewind O. Iron-source preference of *Staphylococcus aureus* infections. Science 2004;305:1626–8.

344 Morrissey JA, Cockayne A, Brummell K, Williams P. The staphylococcal ferritins are differentially regulated in response to iron and manganese and via PerR and Fur. Infect Immun 2004;72:972–9.
345 Torres VJ, Stauff DL, Pishchany G *et al*. A *Staphylococcus aureus* regulatory system that responds to host heme and modulates virulence. Cell Host Microbe 2007;1:109–19.
346 Stauff DL, Torres VJ, Skaar EP. Signaling and DNA-binding activities of the *Staphylococcus aureus* HssR-HssS two-component system required for heme sensing. J Biol Chem 2007;282:26111–21.
347 Weinrick B, Dunman PM, McAleese F *et al*. Effect of mild acid on gene expression in *Staphylococcus aureus*. J Bacteriol 2004; 186:8407–23.
348 Richardson AR, Dunman PM, Fang FC. The nitrosative stress response of *Staphylococcus aureus* is required for resistance to innate immunity. Mol Microbiol 2006;61:927–39.
349 Anderson KL, Roberts C, Disz T *et al*. Characterization of the *Staphylococcus aureus* heat shock, cold shock, stringent, and SOS responses and their effects on log-phase mRNA turnover. J Bacteriol 2006;188:6739–56.
350 Dunman PM, Murphy E, Haney S *et al*. Transcription profiling-based identification of *Staphylococcus aureus* genes regulated by the agr and/or *sarA* loci. J Bacteriol 2001;183:7341–53.
351 Luong TT, Dunman PM, Murphy E, Projan SJ, Lee CY. Transcription profiling of the *mgrA* regulon in *Staphylococcus aureus*. J Bacteriol 2006;188:1899–910.
352 Kuroda M, Ohta T, Uchiyama I *et al*. Whole genome sequencing of meticillin-resistant *Staphylococcus aureus*. Lancet 2001; 357:1225–40.
353 Chen J, Novick RP. *svrA*, a multi-drug exporter, does not control *agr*. Microbiology 2007;153:1604–8.
354 Garvis S, Mei JM, Ruiz-Albert J, Holden DW. *Staphylococcus aureus svrA*: a gene required for virulence and expression of the *agr* locus. Microbiology 2002;148:3235–43.
355 McNamara PJ, Iandolo JJ. Genetic instability of the global regulator *agr* explains the phenotype of the *xpr* mutation in *Staphylococcus aureus* KSI9051. J Bacteriol 1998;180:2609–15.
356 Shaw LN, Jonsson IM, Singh VK, Tarkowski A, Stewart GC. Inactivation of *traP* has no effect on the *agr* quorum-sensing system or virulence of *Staphylococcus aureus*. Infect Immun 2007;75:4519–27.
357 Tsang LH, Daily ST, Weiss EC, Smeltzer MS. Mutation of traP in *Staphylococcus aureus* has no impact on expression of *agr* or biofilm formation. Infect Immun 2007;75:4528–33.
358 Arvidson S, Tegmark K. Regulation of virulence determinants in *Staphylococcus aureus*. Int J Med Microbiol 2001;291:159–70.
359 Bronner S, Monteil H, Prevost G. Regulation of virulence determinants in *Staphylococcus aureus*: complexity and applications. FEMS Microbiol Rev 2004;28:183–200.
360 George EA, Muir TW. Molecular mechanisms of *agr* quorum sensing in virulent staphylococci. Chembiochem 2007;8:847–55.
361 Novick RP. Autoinduction and signal transduction in the regulation of staphylococcal virulence. Mol Microbiol 2003; 48:1429–49.
362 Mallonee DH, Glatz BA, Pattee PA. Chromosomal mapping of a gene affecting enterotoxin A production in *Staphylococcus aureus*. Appl Environ Microbiol 1982;43:397–402.
363 Recsei P, Kreiswirth B, O'Reilly M, Schlievert P, Gruss A, Novick RP. Regulation of exoprotein gene expression in *Staphylococcus aureus* by agar. Mol Gen Genet 1986;202:58–61.
364 Morfeldt E, Janzon L, Arvidson S, Lofdahl S. Cloning of a chromosomal locus (*exp*) which regulates the expression of several exoprotein genes in *Staphylococcus aureus*. Mol Gen Genet 1988;211:435–40.
365 Peng HL, Novick RP, Kreiswirth B, Kornblum J, Schlievert P. Cloning, characterization, and sequencing of an accessory gene regulator (*agr*) in *Staphylococcus aureus*. J Bacteriol 1988; 170:4365–72.
366 Kavanaugh JS, Thoendel M, Horswill AR. A role for type I signal peptidase in *Staphylococcus aureus* quorum sensing. Mol Microbiol 2007;65:780–98.
367 Lyon GJ, Wright JS, Muir TW, Novick RP. Key determinants of receptor activation in the *agr* autoinducing peptides of *Staphylococcus aureus*. Biochemistry 2002;41:10095–104.
368 Koenig RL, Ray JL, Maleki SJ, Smeltzer MS, Hurlburt BK. *Staphylococcus aureus* AgrA binding to the RNAIII-*agr* regulatory region. J Bacteriol 2004;186:7549–55.
369 Jarraud S, Lyon GJ, Figueiredo AM *et al*. Exfoliatin-producing strains define a fourth *agr* specificity group in *Staphylococcus aureus*. J Bacteriol 2000;182:6517–22.
370 Ji G, Beavis R, Novick RP. Bacterial interference caused by autoinducing peptide variants. Science 1997;276:2027–30.
371 Wright JS III, Traber KE, Corrigan R, Benson SA, Musser JM, Novick RP. The *agr* radiation: an early event in the evolution of staphylococci. J Bacteriol 2005;187:5585–94.
372 Fleming V, Feil E, Sewell AK, Day N, Buckling A, Massey RC. Agr interference between clinical *Staphylococcus aureus* strains in an insect model of virulence. J Bacteriol 2006;188:7686–8.
373 Robinson DA, Monk AB, Cooper JE, Feil EJ, Enright MC. Evolutionary genetics of the accessory gene regulator (*agr*) locus in *Staphylococcus aureus*. J Bacteriol 2005;187:8312–21.
374 Jarraud S, Mougel C, Thioulouse J *et al*. Relationships between *Staphylococcus aureus* genetic background, virulence factors, *agr* groups (alleles), and human disease. Infect Immun 2002; 70:631–41.
375 Chini V, Dimitracopoulos G, Spiliopoulou I. Occurrence of the enterotoxin gene cluster and the toxic shock syndrome toxin 1 gene among clinical isolates of methicillin-resistant *Staphylococcus aureus* is related to clonal type and *agr* group. J Clin Microbiol 2006;44:1881–3.
376 Lina G, Boutite F, Tristan A, Bes M, Etienne J, Vandenesch F. Bacterial competition for human nasal cavity colonization: role of staphylococcal *agr* alleles. Appl Environ Microbiol 2003;69:18–23.
377 Otto M. *Staphylococcus aureus* and *Staphylococcus epidermidis* peptide pheromones produced by the accessory gene regulator *agr* system. Peptides 2001;22:1603–8.
378 Moise-Broder PA, Sakoulas G, Eliopoulos GM, Schentag JJ, Forrest A, Moellering RC Jr. Accessory gene regulator group II polymorphism in methicillin-resistant *Staphylococcus aureus* is predictive of failure of vancomycin therapy. Clin Infect Dis 2004;38:1700–5.
379 Rose WE, Rybak MJ, Tsuji BT, Kaatz GW, Sakoulas G. Correlation of vancomycin and daptomycin susceptibility in *Staphylococcus aureus* in reference to accessory gene regulator (*agr*) polymorphism and function. J Antimicrob Chemother 2007;59:1190–3.
380 Sakoulas G, Eliopoulos GM, Moellering RC Jr *et al*. *Staphylococcus aureus* accessory gene regulator (*agr*) group II: is there a

relationship to the development of intermediate-level glycopeptide resistance? J Infect Dis 2003;187:929–38.
381 Tsuji BT, Rybak MJ, Lau KL, Sakoulas G. Evaluation of accessory gene regulator (*agr*) group and function in the proclivity towards vancomycin intermediate resistance in *Staphylococcus aureus*. Antimicrob Agents Chemother 2007;51:1089–91.
382 Janzon L, Lofdahl S, Arvidson S. Identification and nucleotide sequence of the delta-lysin gene, *hld*, adjacent to the accessory gene regulator (*agr*) of *Staphylococcus aureus*. Mol Gen Genet 1989;219:480–5.
383 Novick RP, Ross HF, Projan SJ, Kornblum J, Kreiswirth B, Moghazeh S. Synthesis of staphylococcal virulence factors is controlled by a regulatory RNA molecule. EMBO J 1993; 12:3967–75.
384 Boisset S, Geissmann T, Huntzinger E *et al*. *Staphylococcus aureus* RNAIII coordinately represses the synthesis of virulence factors and the transcription regulator Rot by an antisense mechanism. Genes Dev 2007;21:1353–66.
385 Geisinger E, Adhikari RP, Jin R, Ross HF, Novick RP. Inhibition of *rot* translation by RNAIII, a key feature of *agr* function. Mol Microbiol 2006;61:1038–48.
386 Morfeldt E, Taylor D, von Gabain A, Arvidson S. Activation of alpha-toxin translation in *Staphylococcus aureus* by the trans-encoded antisense RNA, RNAIII. EMBO J 1995;14:4569–77.
387 Huntzinger E, Boisset S, Saveanu C *et al*. *Staphylococcus aureus* RNAIII and the endoribonuclease III coordinately regulate *spa* gene expression. EMBO J 2005;24:824–35.
388 Said-Salim B, Dunman PM, McAleese FM *et al*. Global regulation of *Staphylococcus aureus* genes by Rot. J Bacteriol 2003; 185:610–19.
389 Blevins JS, Gillaspy AF, Rechtin TM, Hurlburt BK, Smeltzer MS. The staphylococcal accessory regulator (*sar*) represses transcription of the *Staphylococcus aureus* collagen adhesin gene (*cna*) in an *agr*-independent manner. Mol Microbiol 1999;33:317–26.
390 Wolz C, Pohlmann-Dietze P, Steinhuber A *et al*. Agr-independent regulation of fibronectin-binding protein(s) by the regulatory locus *sar* in *Staphylococcus aureus*. Mol Microbiol 2000;36:230–43.
391 Xiong YQ, Van Wamel W, Nast CC, Yeaman MR, Cheung AL, Bayer AS. Activation and transcriptional interaction between *agr* RNAII and RNAIII in *Staphylococcus aureus in vitro* and in an experimental endocarditis model. J Infect Dis 2002;186:668–77.
392 Goerke C, Fluckiger U, Steinhuber A, Zimmerli W, Wolz C. Impact of the regulatory loci *agr*, *sarA* and *sae* of *Staphylococcus aureus* on the induction of alpha-toxin during device-related infection resolved by direct quantitative transcript analysis. Mol Microbiol 2001;40:1439–47.
393 Kong KF, Vuong C, Otto M. *Staphylococcus* quorum sensing in biofilm formation and infection. Int J Med Microbiol 2006;296:133–9.
394 Vuong C, Kocianova S, Yao Y, Carmody AB, Otto M. Increased colonization of indwelling medical devices by quorum-sensing mutants of *Staphylococcus epidermidis in vivo*. J Infect Dis 2004;190:1498–505.
395 Yarwood JM, Bartels DJ, Volper EM, Greenberg EP. Quorum sensing in *Staphylococcus aureus* biofilms. J Bacteriol 2004; 186:1838–50.
396 Yarwood JM, Paquette KM, Tikh IB, Volper EM, Greenberg EP. Generation of virulence factor variants in *Staphylococcus aureus* biofilms. J Bacteriol 2007;189:7961–7.
397 Vuong C, Saenz HL, Gotz F, Otto M. Impact of the *agr* quorum-sensing system on adherence to polystyrene in *Staphylococcus aureus*. J Infect Dis 2000;182:1688–93.
398 Abdelnour A, Arvidson S, Bremell T, Ryden C, Tarkowski A. The accessory gene regulator (*agr*) controls *Staphylococcus aureus* virulence in a murine arthritis model. Infect Immun 1993;61:3879–85.
399 Booth MC, Atkuri RV, Nanda SK, Iandolo JJ, Gilmore MS. Accessory gene regulator controls *Staphylococcus aureus* virulence in endophthalmitis. Invest Ophthalmol Vis Sci 1995; 36:1828–36.
400 Cheung AL, Eberhardt KJ, Chung E *et al*. Diminished virulence of a *sar–/agr–* mutant of *Staphylococcus aureus* in the rabbit model of endocarditis. J Clin Invest 1994;94:1815–22.
401 Gillaspy AF, Hickmon SG, Skinner RA, Thomas JR, Nelson CL, Smeltzer MS. Role of the accessory gene regulator (*agr*) in pathogenesis of staphylococcal osteomyelitis. Infect Immun 1995;63:3373–80.
402 Mayville P, Ji G, Beavis R *et al*. Structure–activity analysis of synthetic autoinducing thiolactone peptides from *Staphylococcus aureus* responsible for virulence. Proc Natl Acad Sci USA 1999;96:1218–23.
403 McNamara PJ, Bayer AS. A rot mutation restores parental virulence to an *agr*-null *Staphylococcus aureus* strain in a rabbit model of endocarditis. Infect Immun 2005;73:3806–9.
404 Gillet Y, Vanhems P, Lina G *et al*. Factors predicting mortality in necrotizing community-acquired pneumonia caused by *Staphylococcus aureus* containing Panton–Valentine leukocidin. Clin Infect Dis 2007;45:315–21.
405 Balaban N, Goldkorn T, Gov Y *et al*. Regulation of *Staphylococcus aureus* pathogenesis via target of RNAIII-activating Protein (TRAP). J Biol Chem 2001;276:2658–67.
406 Balaban N, Cirioni O, Giacometti A *et al*. Treatment of *Staphylococcus aureus* biofilm infection by the quorum-sensing inhibitor RIP. Antimicrob Agents Chemother 2007;51:2226–9.
407 Gilot P, Lina G, Cochard T, Poutrel B. Analysis of the genetic variability of genes encoding the RNA III-activating components Agr and TRAP in a population of *Staphylococcus aureus* strains isolated from cows with mastitis. J Clin Microbiol 2002;40:4060–7.
408 Gov Y, Borovok I, Korem M *et al*. Quorum sensing in staphylococci is regulated via phosphorylation of three conserved histidine residues. J Biol Chem 2004;279:14665–72.
409 Han YH, Kim YG, Kim DY, Ha SC, Lokanath NK, Kim KK. The target of RNAIII-activating protein (TRAP) from *Staphylococcus aureus*: purification, crystallization and preliminary X-ray analysis. Biochim Biophys Acta 2005;1748:134–6.
410 Korem M, Gov Y, Kiran MD, Balaban N. Transcriptional profiling of target of RNAIII-activating protein, a master regulator of staphylococcal virulence. Infect Immun 2005;73:6220–8.
411 Korem M, Sheoran AS, Gov Y, Tzipori S, Borovok I, Balaban N. Characterization of RAP, a quorum sensing activator of *Staphylococcus aureus*. FEMS Microbiol Lett 2003;223:167–75.
412 Vieira-da-Motta O, Ribeiro PD, Dias da Silva W, Medina-Acosta E. RNAIII inhibiting peptide (RIP) inhibits *agr*-regulated toxin production. Peptides 2001;22:1621–7.
413 Balaban N, Stoodley P, Fux CA, Wilson S, Costerton JW, Dell'Acqua G. Prevention of staphylococcal biofilm-associated infections by the quorum sensing inhibitor RIP. Clin Orthop Relat Res 2005;(437):48–54.

414 Giacometti A, Cirioni O, Gov Y *et al.* RNA III inhibiting peptide inhibits *in vivo* biofilm formation by drug-resistant *Staphylococcus aureus*. Antimicrob Agents Chemother 2003;47:1979–83.
415 Cirioni O, Ghiselli R, Minardi D *et al.* RNAIII-inhibiting peptide affects biofilm formation in a rat model of staphylococcal ureteral stent infection. Antimicrob Agents Chemother 2007;51:4518–20.
416 Cheung AL, Koomey JM, Butler CA, Projan SJ, Fischetti VA. Regulation of exoprotein expression in *Staphylococcus aureus* by a locus (*sar*) distinct from *agr*. Proc Natl Acad Sci USA 1992;89:6462–6.
417 Bayer MG, Heinrichs JH, Cheung AL. The molecular architecture of the *sar* locus in *Staphylococcus aureus*. J Bacteriol 1996;178:4563–70.
418 Manna AC, Bayer MG, Cheung AL. Transcriptional analysis of different promoters in the *sar* locus in *Staphylococcus aureus*. J Bacteriol 1998;180:3828–36.
419 Manna A, Cheung AL. Characterization of *sarR*, a modulator of *sar* expression in *Staphylococcus aureus*. Infect Immun 2001;69:885–96.
420 Cheung AL, Nishina K, Manna AC. SarA of *S. aureus* binds to its own promoter to regulate gene expression. J Bacteriol 2008;190:2239–43.
421 Chan PF, Foster SJ. Role of SarA in virulence determinant production and environmental signal transduction in *Staphylococcus aureus*. J Bacteriol 1998;180:6232–41.
422 Chien Y, Manna AC, Cheung AL. SarA level is a determinant of *agr* activation in *Staphylococcus aureus*. Mol Microbiol 1998; 30:991–1001.
423 Cheung AL, Zhang G. Global regulation of virulence determinants in *Staphylococcus aureus* by the SarA protein family. Front Biosci 2002;7:d1825–d1842.
424 Chien Y, Manna AC, Projan SJ, Cheung AL. SarA, a global regulator of virulence determinants in *Staphylococcus aureus*, binds to a conserved motif essential for *sar*-dependent gene regulation. J Biol Chem 1999;274:37169–76.
425 Sterba KM, Mackintosh SG, Blevins JS, Hurlburt BK, Smeltzer MS. Characterization of *Staphylococcus aureus* SarA binding sites. J Bacteriol 2003;185:4410–17.
426 Fujimoto DF, Brunskill EW, Bayles KW. Analysis of genetic elements controlling *Staphylococcus aureus lrgAB* expression: potential role of DNA topology in SarA regulation. J Bacteriol 2000;182:4822–8.
427 Schumacher MA, Hurlburt BK, Brennan RG. Crystal structures of SarA, a pleiotropic regulator of virulence genes in S. aureus. Nature 2001;409:215–19.
428 Roberts C, Anderson KL, Murphy E *et al.* Characterizing the effect of the *Staphylococcus aureus* virulence factor regulator, SarA, on log-phase mRNA half-lives. J Bacteriol 2006;188:2593–603.
429 Blevins JS, Beenken KE, Elasri MO, Hurlburt BK, Smeltzer MS. Strain-dependent differences in the regulatory roles of *sarA* and *agr* in *Staphylococcus aureus*. Infect Immun 2002;70:470–80.
430 Cheung AL, Ying P. Regulation of alpha- and beta-hemolysins by the *sar* locus of *Staphylococcus aureus*. J Bacteriol 1994; 176:580–5.
431 Cheung AL, Projan SJ. Cloning and sequencing of *sarA* of *Staphylococcus aureus*, a gene required for the expression of *agr*. J Bacteriol 1994;176:4168–72.
432 Lindsay JA, Foster SJ. Interactive regulatory pathways control virulence determinant production and stability in response to environmental conditions in *Staphylococcus aureus*. Mol Gen Genet 1999;262:323–31.
433 Chien Y, Cheung AL. Molecular interactions between two global regulators, *sar* and *agr*, in *Staphylococcus aureus*. J Biol Chem 1998;273:2645–52.
434 Heinrichs JH, Bayer MG, Cheung AL. Characterization of the *sar* locus and its interaction with *agr* in *Staphylococcus aureus*. J Bacteriol 1996;178:418–23.
435 Morfeldt E, Tegmark K, Arvidson S. Transcriptional control of the *agr*-dependent virulence gene regulator, RNAIII, in *Staphylococcus aureus*. Mol Microbiol 1996;21:1227–37.
436 Rechtin TM, Gillaspy AF, Schumacher MA, Brennan RG, Smeltzer MS, Hurlburt BK. Characterization of the SarA virulence gene regulator of *Staphylococcus aureus*. Mol Microbiol 1999;33:307–16.
437 Schmidt KA, Manna AC, Cheung AL. SarT influences *sarS* expression in *Staphylococcus aureus*. Infect Immun 2003; 71:5139–48.
438 Blevins JS, Elasri MO, Allmendinger SD *et al.* Role of *sarA* in the pathogenesis of *Staphylococcus aureus* musculoskeletal infection. Infect Immun 2003;71:516–23.
439 Van Wamel W, Xiong YQ, Bayer AS, Yeaman MR, Nast CC, Cheung AL. Regulation of *Staphylococcus aureus* type 5 capsular polysaccharides by *agr* and *sarA in vitro* and in an experimental endocarditis model. Microb Pathog 2002;33:73–9.
440 Karlsson A, Saravia-Otten P, Tegmark K, Morfeldt E, Arvidson S. Decreased amounts of cell wall-associated protein A and fibronectin-binding proteins in *Staphylococcus aureus sarA* mutants due to up-regulation of extracellular proteases. Infect Immun 2001;69:4742–8.
441 McGavin MJ, Zahradka C, Rice K, Scott JE. Modification of the *Staphylococcus aureus* fibronectin binding phenotype by V8 protease. Infect Immun 1997;65:2621–8.
442 Oscarsson J, Kanth A, Tegmark-Wisell K, Arvidson S. SarA is a repressor of *hla* (alpha-hemolysin) transcription in *Staphylococcus aureus*: its apparent role as an activator of *hla* in the prototype strain NCTC 8325 depends on reduced expression of *sarS*. J Bacteriol 2006;188:8526–33.
443 Manna AC, Cheung AL. Transcriptional regulation of the *agr* locus and the identification of DNA binding residues of the global regulatory protein SarR in *Staphylococcus aureus*. Mol Microbiol 2006;60:1289–301.
444 Manna AC, Ingavale SS, Maloney M, Van Wamel W, Cheung AL. Identification of sarV (SA2062), a new transcriptional regulator, is repressed by SarA and MgrA (SA0641) and involved in the regulation of autolysis in *Staphylococcus aureus*. J Bacteriol 2004;186:5267–80.
445 Ingavale SS, Van Wamel W, Cheung AL. Characterization of RAT, an autolysis regulator in *Staphylococcus aureus*. Mol Microbiol 2003;48:1451–66.
446 Ingavale S, Van Wamel W, Luong TT, Lee CY, Cheung AL. Rat/MgrA, a regulator of autolysis, is a regulator of virulence genes in *Staphylococcus aureus*. Infect Immun 2005;73:1423–31.
447 Tu Quoc PH, Genevaux P, Pajunen M *et al.* Isolation and characterization of biofilm formation-defective mutants of *Staphylococcus aureus*. Infect Immun 2007;75:1079–88.
448 Chen PR, Bae T, Williams WA *et al.* An oxidation-sensing mechanism is used by the global regulator MgrA in *Staphylococcus aureus*. Nat Chem Biol 2006;2:591–5.

449 Kaito C, Morishita D, Matsumoto Y, Kurokawa K, Sekimizu K. Novel DNA binding protein SarZ contributes to virulence in *Staphylococcus aureus*. Mol Microbiol 2006;62:1601–17.
450 Kaito C, Kurokawa K, Matsumoto Y *et al*. Silkworm pathogenic bacteria infection model for identification of novel virulence genes. Mol Microbiol 2005;56:934–44.
451 Matsumoto Y, Kaito C, Morishita D, Kurokawa K, Sekimizu K. Regulation of exoprotein gene expression by the *Staphylococcus aureus cvfB* gene. Infect Immun 2007;75:1964–72.
452 Nagata M, Kaito C, Sekimizu K. Phosphodiesterase activity of CvfA is required for virulence in *Staphylococcus aureus*. J Biol Chem 2008;283:2176–84.
453 McNamara PJ, Milligan-Monroe KC, Khalili S, Proctor RA. Identification, cloning, and initial characterization of *rot*, a locus encoding a regulator of virulence factor expression in *Staphylococcus aureus*. J Bacteriol 2000;182:3197–203.
454 Hsieh HY, Tseng CW, Stewart GC. Regulation of Rot expression in *Staphylococcus aureus*. J Bacteriol 2008;190:546–54.
455 Gao J, Stewart GC. Regulatory elements of the *Staphylococcus aureus* protein A (Spa) promoter. J Bacteriol 2004;186:3738–48.
456 Oscarsson J, Harlos C, Arvidson S. Regulatory role of proteins binding to the *spa* (protein A) and *sarS* (staphylococcal accessory regulator) promoter regions in *Staphylococcus aureus* NTCC 8325-4. Int J Med Microbiol 2005;295:253–66.
457 Oscarsson J, Tegmark-Wisell K, Arvidson S. Coordinated and differential control of aureolysin (*aur*) and serine protease (*sspA*) transcription in *Staphylococcus aureus* by *sarA*, *rot* and *agr* (RNAIII). Int J Med Microbiol 2006;296:365–80.
458 Giraudo AT, Raspanti CG, Calzolari A, Nagel R. Characterization of a Tn551-mutant of *Staphylococcus aureus* defective in the production of several exoproteins. Can J Microbiol 1994;40:677–81.
459 Giraudo AT, Calzolari A, Cataldi AA, Bogni C, Nagel R. The *sae* locus of *Staphylococcus aureus* encodes a two-component regulatory system. FEMS Microbiol Lett 1999;177:15–22.
460 Steinhuber A, Goerke C, Bayer MG, Doring G, Wolz C. Molecular architecture of the regulatory locus *sae* of *Staphylococcus aureus* and its impact on expression of virulence factors. J Bacteriol 2003;185:6278–86.
461 Novick RP, Jiang D. The staphylococcal *saeRS* system coordinates environmental signals with *agr* quorum sensing. Microbiology 2003;149:2709–17.
462 Rogasch K, Ruhmling V, Pane-Farre J *et al*. Influence of the two-component system SaeRS on global gene expression in two different *Staphylococcus aureus* strains. J Bacteriol 2006; 188:7742–58.
463 Liang X, Yu C, Sun J *et al*. Inactivation of a two-component signal transduction system, SaeRS, eliminates adherence and attenuates virulence of *Staphylococcus aureus*. Infect Immun 2006;74:4655–65.
464 Goerke C, Fluckiger U, Steinhuber A *et al*. Role of *Staphylococcus aureus* global regulators *sae* and sigmaB in virulence gene expression during device-related infection. Infect Immun 2005;73:3415–21.
465 Fournier B, Hooper DC. A new two-component regulatory system involved in adhesion, autolysis, and extracellular proteolytic activity of *Staphylococcus aureus*. J Bacteriol 2000;182:3955–64.
466 Fournier B, Klier A, Rapoport G. The two-component system ArlS-ArlR is a regulator of virulence gene expression in *Staphylococcus aureus*. Mol Microbiol 2001;41:247–61.
467 Toledo-Arana A, Merino N, Vergara-Irigaray M, Debarbouille M, Penades JR, Lasa I. *Staphylococcus aureus* develops an alternative, *ica*-independent biofilm in the absence of the *arlRS* two-component system. J Bacteriol 2005;187:5318–29.
468 Luong TT, Newell SW, Lee CY. Mgr, a novel global regulator in *Staphylococcus aureus*. J Bacteriol 2003;185:3703–10.
469 Meier S, Goerke C, Wolz C *et al*. sigmaB and the sigmaB-dependent *arlRS* and *yabJ-spoVG* loci affect capsule formation in *Staphylococcus aureus*. Infect Immun 2007;75:4562–71.
470 Chen Z, Luong TT, Lee CY. The *sbcDC* locus mediates repression of type 5 capsule production as part of the SOS response in *Staphylococcus aureus*. J Bacteriol 2007;189:7343–50.
471 Throup JP, Zappacosta F, Lunsford RD *et al*. The *srhSR* gene pair from *Staphylococcus aureus*: genomic and proteomic approaches to the identification and characterization of gene function. Biochemistry 2001;40:10392–401.
472 Yarwood JM, McCormick JK, Schlievert PM. Identification of a novel two-component regulatory system that acts in global regulation of virulence factors of *Staphylococcus aureus*. J Bacteriol 2001;183:1113–23.
473 Pragman AA, Yarwood JM, Tripp TJ, Schlievert PM. Characterization of virulence factor regulation by SrrAB, a two-component system in *Staphylococcus aureus*. J Bacteriol 2004; 186:2430–8.
474 Pragman AA, Herron-Olson L, Case LC *et al*. Sequence analysis of the *Staphylococcus aureus srrAB* loci reveals that truncation of *srrA* affects growth and virulence factor expression. J Bacteriol 2007;189:7515–19.
475 Valle J, Toledo-Arana A, Berasain C *et al*. SarA and not sigmaB is essential for biofilm development by *Staphylococcus aureus*. Mol Microbiol 2003;48:1075–87.
476 Pragman AA, Ji Y, Schlievert PM. Repression of *Staphylococcus aureus* SrrAB using inducible antisense *srrA* alters growth and virulence factor transcript levels. Biochemistry 2007;46:314–21.
477 Martin PK, Li T, Sun D, Biek DP, Schmid MB. Role in cell permeability of an essential two-component system in *Staphylococcus aureus*. J Bacteriol 1999;181:3666–73.
478 Clausen VA, Bae W, Throup J, Burnham MK, Rosenberg M, Wallis NG. Biochemical characterization of the first essential two-component signal transduction system from *Staphylococcus aureus* and *Streptococcus pneumoniae*. J Mol Microbiol Biotechnol 2003;5:252–60.
479 Dubrac S, Msadek T. Identification of genes controlled by the essential YycG/YycF two-component system of *Staphylococcus aureus*. J Bacteriol 2004;186:1175–81.
480 Dubrac S, Boneca IG, Poupel O, Msadek T. New insights into the WalK/WalR (YycG/YycF) essential signal transduction pathway reveal a major role in controlling cell wall metabolism and biofilm formation in *Staphylococcus aureus*. J Bacteriol 2007;189:8257–69.
481 Biswas R, Voggu L, Simon UK, Hentschel P, Thumm G, Gotz F. Activity of the major staphylococcal autolysin Atl. FEMS Microbiol Lett 2006;259:260–8.
482 Qin Z, Lee B, Yang L *et al*. Antimicrobial activities of YycG histidine kinase inhibitors against *Staphylococcus epidermidis* biofilms. FEMS Microbiol Lett 2007;273:149–56.
483 Kuroda M, Kuwahara-Arai K, Hiramatsu K. Identification of the up- and down-regulated genes in vancomycin-resistant *Staphylococcus aureus* strains Mu3 and Mu50 by cDNA differential

hybridization method. Biochem Biophys Res Commun 2000; 269:485–90.
484 Kuroda M, Kuroda H, Oshima T, Takeuchi F, Mori H, Hiramatsu K. Two-component system VraSR positively modulates the regulation of cell-wall biosynthesis pathway in *Staphylococcus aureus*. Mol Microbiol 2003;49:807–21.
485 Gardete S, Wu SW, Gill S, Tomasz A. Role of VraSR in antibiotic resistance and antibiotic-induced stress response in *Staphylococcus aureus*. Antimicrob Agents Chemother 2006;50:3424–34.
486 Yin S, Daum RS, Boyle-Vavra S. VraSR two-component regulatory system and its role in induction of *pbp2* and *vraSR* expression by cell wall antimicrobials in *Staphylococcus aureus*. Antimicrob Agents Chemother 2006;50:336–43.
487 Cui L, Lian JQ, Neoh HM, Reyes E, Hiramatsu K. DNA microarray-based identification of genes associated with glycopeptide resistance in *Staphylococcus aureus*. Antimicrob Agents Chemother 2005;49:3404–13.
488 Neoh HM, Cui L, Yuzawa H, Takeuchi F, Matsuo M, Hiramatsu K. Mutated response regulator *graR* is responsible for phenotypic conversion of *Staphylococcus aureus* from heterogeneous vancomycin-intermediate resistance to vancomycin-intermediate resistance. Antimicrob Agents Chemother 2008; 52:45–53.
489 Meehl M, Herbert S, Gotz F, Cheung A. Interaction of the GraRS two-component system with the VraFG ABC transporter to support vancomycin-intermediate resistance in *Staphylococcus aureus*. Antimicrob Agents Chemother 2007;51:2679–89.
490 Herbert S, Bera A, Nerz C *et al*. Molecular basis of resistance to muramidase and cationic antimicrobial peptide activity of lysozyme in staphylococci. PLoS Pathog 2007;3:e102.
491 Li M, Cha DJ, Lai Y, Villaruz AE, Sturdevant DE, Otto M. The antimicrobial peptide-sensing system *aps* of *Staphylococcus aureus*. Mol Microbiol 2007;66:1136–47.
492 Brunskill EW, Bayles KW. Identification and molecular characterization of a putative regulatory locus that affects autolysis in *Staphylococcus aureus*. J Bacteriol 1996;178:611–18.
493 Brunskill EW, de Jonge BL, Bayles KW. The *Staphylococcus aureus scdA* gene: a novel locus that affects cell division and morphogenesis. Microbiology 1997;143:2877–82.
494 Groicher KH, Firek BA, Fujimoto DF, Bayles KW. The *Staphylococcus aureus lrgAB* operon modulates murein hydrolase activity and penicillin tolerance. J Bacteriol 2000;182:1794–801.
495 Rice KC, Firek BA, Nelson JB, Yang SJ, Patton TG, Bayles KW. The *Staphylococcus aureus cidAB* operon: evaluation of its role in regulation of murein hydrolase activity and penicillin tolerance. J Bacteriol 2003;185:2635–43.
496 Yang SJ, Dunman PM, Projan SJ, Bayles KW. Characterization of the *Staphylococcus aureus* CidR regulon: elucidation of a novel role for acetoin metabolism in cell death and lysis. Mol Microbiol 2006;60:458–68.
497 Pamp SJ, Frees D, Engelmann S, Hecker M, Ingmer H. Spx is a global effector impacting stress tolerance and biofilm formation in *Staphylococcus aureus*. J Bacteriol 2006;188:4861–70.
498 Lim Y, Jana M, Luong TT, Lee CY. Control of glucose- and NaCl-induced biofilm formation by *rbf* in *Staphylococcus aureus*. J Bacteriol 2004;186:722–9.
499 Majerczyk CD, Sadykov MR, Luong TT, Lee C, Somerville GA, Sonenshein AL. *Staphylococcus aureus* CodY negatively regulates virulence gene expression. J Bacteriol 2008;190:2257–65.
500 Brouillette E, Hyodo M, Hayakawa Y, Karaolis DK, Malouin F. 3′,5′-Cyclic diguanylic acid reduces the virulence of biofilm-forming *Staphylococcus aureus* strains in a mouse model of mastitis infection. Antimicrob Agents Chemother 2005;49:3109–13.
501 Karaolis DK, Rashid MH, Chythanya R, Luo W, Hyodo M, Hayakawa Y. c-di-GMP (3′-5′-cyclic diguanylic acid) inhibits *Staphylococcus aureus* cell–cell interactions and biofilm formation. Antimicrob Agents Chemother 2005;49:1029–38.
502 Tamayo R, Pratt JT, Camilli A. Roles of cyclic diguanylate in the regulation of bacterial pathogenesis. Annu Rev Microbiol 2007;61:131–48.
503 Sambanthamoorthy K, Smeltzer MS, Elasri MO. Identification and characterization of *msa* (SA1233), a gene involved in expression of SarA and several virulence factors in *Staphylococcus aureus*. Microbiology 2006;152:2559–72.
504 Rossi J, Bischoff M, Wada A, Berger-Bachi B. MsrR, a putative cell envelope-associated element involved in *Staphylococcus aureus sarA* attenuation. Antimicrob Agents Chemother 2003; 47:2558–64.
505 Seidl K, Stucki M, Ruegg M *et al*. *Staphylococcus aureus* CcpA affects virulence determinant production and antibiotic resistance. Antimicrob Agents Chemother 2006;50:1183–94.
506 Sobral RG, Jones AE, Des Etages SG *et al*. Extensive and genome-wide changes in the transcription profile of *Staphylococcus aureus* induced by modulating the transcription of the cell wall synthesis gene *murF*. J Bacteriol 2007;189:2376–91.
507 Sobral RG, Ludovice AM, Gardete S, Tabei K, De Lencastre H, Tomasz A. Normally functioning *murF* is essential for the optimal expression of methicillin resistance in *Staphylococcus aureus*. Microb Drug Resist 2003;9:231–41.
508 Sobral RG, Ludovice AM, De Lencastre H, Tomasz A. Role of *murF* in cell wall biosynthesis: isolation and characterization of a *murF* conditional mutant of *Staphylococcus aureus*. J Bacteriol 2006;188:2543–53.

Chapter 5
Adaptation to Stress: Biofilms and Small-colony Variants

Karl M. Thompson and Kimberly K. Jefferson
Department of Microbiology and Immunology, Virginia Commonwealth University School of Medicine, Richmond, Virginia, USA

Introduction

No earthly niche represents a completely static environment and consequently the ability to adapt to changes in the surrounding milieu is a fundamental component of life. Many pathogenic bacterial species must be particularly adaptable, as they may be faced with tremendous fluctuations in nutrient and oxygen availability and temperature as they transition between their environmental niche and the human host, and as metabolic changes and immune defenses are encountered within the host. Bacterial adaptation occurs primarily through the highly developed orchestration of gene expression, and chemical or physical cues can rapidly set into motion an elaborate cascade of alterations in the cell's physiology.

Staphylococcus aureus has an astonishingly plastic genome and is able to adapt to almost any imaginable hazard. Whereas the development of resistance to antibiotics such as penicillin, methicillin, and vancomycin depends on the acquisition of mutations and new DNA, alterations in the expression of existing genetic material function more subtly in adaptation, but play an even more critical role in the success of the pathogen. *Staphylococcus aureus* has an overwhelming arsenal of virulence factors and expression of these factors at the appropriate times leads to physiological changes involved in pathogenesis. A better understanding of these phenomena is needed to develop novel and more effective therapeutic agents to combat infection.

Coagulase-negative staphylococcal species are also able to alter their physiology to adapt to offensive environmental conditions. Unlike *S. aureus*, *Staphylococcus epidermidis* possesses few virulence factors; however, iatrogenic infections pose a serious emerging threat due to the pervasive presence of this species on human skin and to its propensity to assume the biofilm mode of growth, especially in the presence of an indwelling medical device.

Staphylococci in Human Disease, 2nd edition. Edited by Kent B. Crossley, Kimberly K. Jefferson, Gordon Archer, Vance G. Fowler, Jr.

Staphylococcal physiology is multifaceted and complex and efforts are underway to unravel these complexities. A thorough understanding of the physiology of this pathogen will arm researchers with a larger toolkit with which to garner potential targets for antibiotics, vaccines, or other therapeutic targets. This toolkit needs to be built upon current knowledge and rapidly expanded in order to combat eminent threats such as methicillin and vancomycin resistance. The goal of this chapter is therefore to review and expound the current data about two important alternative physiological states that play a role in staphylococcal pathogenesis: the biofilm mode of growth and the small-colony variant phenotype.

The stress response

Stressors present in the environment of a bacterial cell strongly influence its homeostatic and adaptive physiology. Volatility in the environment can lead to a sudden shift in physiology known as a stress response. Stress responses are often facilitated by global changes in transcriptional or posttranscriptional gene expression. *Staphylococcus aureus*, and other potentially pathogenic staphylococcal species, have developed mechanisms to adapt to environmental volatility including shifts in temperature and osmolarity, mechanical stimulation, carbon availability, and metal (e.g., iron and magnesium) availability. Sudden shifts in any of these, or other noteworthy important environmental conditions, can act as stressors for bacteria. When a bacterium is exposed to a stressor, a dramatic and specific change in their internal physiology, the stress response, is initiated to ensure survival in the harsh conditions created by the presence of the stressor.

Biofilm formation

Certain stressors including increased temperature, osmotic shock, low oxygen tension, changes in the availability of glucose, glucosamine, *N*-acetylglucosamine or nitrite, changes in bis-(3′,5′)-cyclic-dimeric-guanosine monophosphate (cyclic-di-GMP) levels, and exposure to toxic chemicals such as ethanol and antibiotics can induce global changes in gene expression that initiate the switch to what is referred to as the biofilm mode of growth [1–6].

Recently, biofilms have garnered increased attention because of their significant role in bacterial physiology, gene regulation, and ecology. A biofilm is an adherent community of bacteria with an organized structure and chemistry, surrounded by an extracellular biochemical polymer. The close proximity of bacteria within a biofilm maximizes the potential of extracellular proteases. In addition, the physiological heterogeneity throughout the biofilm results in a form of "division of labor." Together, these properties endow the community with a higher metabolic potential than an equivalent planktonic population. Biofilms also afford a bacterial community increased resistance to mechanical manipulation and antiinfective agents. This undoubtedly plays a role in the suboptimal efficacy of antibiotics against biofilm-associated infections and impacts the prevalence of persistent and recurrent bacterial infections. Both *S. aureus* and coagulase-negative staphylococci (CoNS) can form biofilms, and this mode of growth plays an important role in certain pathogenic processes. In fact, for CoNS, which do not possess the outstanding array of virulence factors characteristic of *S. aureus*, biofilm formation is considered the major virulence factor. Biofilms appear to be the preferred physiological state for staphylococci during many types of infections, including not only device-related infections but also native valve endocarditis, otitis media, and pneumonia [7].

The transition of a bacterial population from a planktonic (free-floating) to a biofilm state can be somewhat arbitrarily divided into five stages: (i) initial reversible surface association, (ii) irreversible surface attachment mediated by bacterial surface adhesins, (iii) expression of intercellular adhesins, (iv) development of biofilm architecture, and (v) dispersion of cells from the biofilm [8].

In the initial stage of biofilm formation, bacteria reversibly adhere to a solid surface via nonspecific charge-related interactions. The second stage, irreversible adherence, is a necessary step in the pathogenesis of all bacterial infections as bacteria must first adhere to host tissues to avoid clearance by host defenses that physically remove non-self entities, such as the mucociliary escalator. *Staphylococcus aureus* produces a wide variety of surface adhesins called microbial surface components recognizing adhesive matrix molecules (MSCRAMMs) that mediate irreversible adhesion [9]. MSCRAMMs, by definition, are surface-associated proteins that specifically bind to some component of the extracellular matrix of host tissues. The MSCRAMM family includes two fibronectin-binding proteins, FnbA and FnbB, the collagen-binding protein Cna, and the fibrinogen-binding proteins clumping factor (Clf)A and ClfB. For a more detailed discussion of surface adhesins refer to Chapter 4.

The third stage of biofilm formation distinguishes this phenotype from bacteria that are simply adherent. In the third stage, the staphylococci initiate expression of intercellular adhesins that allow the bacterial cells to adhere to one another and to aggregate and begin to form microcolonies. Staphylococcal intercellular adhesins that promote biofilm formation include surface proteins such as biofilm-associated protein (Bap), *S. aureus* surface protein G (SasG), and accumulation/adhesion-associated protein (Aap) as well as a carbohydrate adhesin known as polysaccharide intercellular adhesin (PIA) in *S. epidermidis* and poly-*N*-acetylglucosamine (PNAG) in *S. aureus* [10–13].

During the fourth stage, maturation of the biofilm architecture, the structure becomes larger and more porous. Bacterial microcolonies separated by water channels become encased within a protective exopolymeric matrix. The exopolymeric matrix is most commonly composed of polysaccharides, predominantly PIA/PNAG, but recent studies have shown that in the absence of polysaccharide production, staphylococcal biofilm matrices can be proteinaceous [14–16]. Even more recently, extracellular bacterial DNA, presumably released by lysed bacteria, has been observed as a component of the matrix of staphylococcal biofilms [17].

The fifth and final stage of biofilm development, dispersal of individual cells or clusters from the biofilm, allows the bacteria to either resume the planktonic lifestyle or to establish a new biofilm within an alternate location [18]. Some bacterial species produce an enzyme that actively degrades the biofilm matrix so that bacteria can disperse, but dispersal has not been shown to be an active process in the staphylococci.

Each stage of biofilm formation requires synchronized changes in gene expression and environmental factors set these changes in motion. Bacteria may switch to the biofilm mode of growth for a number of reasons but it is frequently a stressful environmental stimulus that triggers the phenotypic change. Biofilms are uniquely resistant to a large variety of mechanical, physical, nutritional, and chemical insults, as well as to host immune defenses, and bacteria likely evolved this growth state, at least in part, as a defense mechanism.

Biofilm determinants

Intercellular adhesin locus

The *ica* (*i*ntra*c*ellular *a*dhesin) locus is necessary for the synthesis of PIA/PNAG in *S. epidermidis* and *S. aureus* and is a major genetic determinant involved in staphylococcal biofilm formation [19]. The environmental factors that modulate biofilm formation also modulate the expression

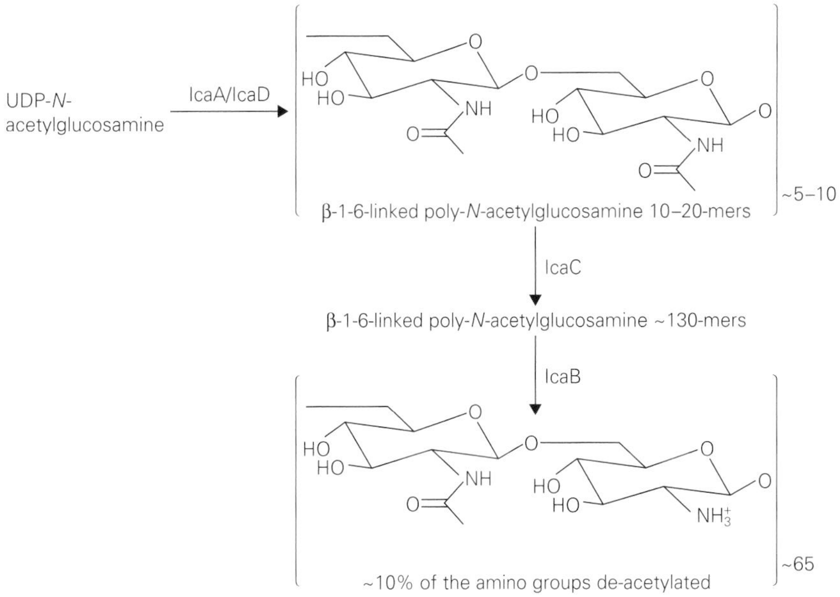

Figure 5.1 Synthesis of PIA/PNAG. The proteins encoded by the intercellular adhesin locus are responsible for the synthesis of poly-*N*-acetylglucosamine. IcaA and IcaD together synthesize short oligomers, IcaC polymerizes the short oligomers into longer oligomers, and IcaB deacetylates approximately 10% of the residues, giving the molecule an overall net positive charge.

of the *ica* locus, and there appears to be a direct correlation between the modulation of the *ica* locus and the modulation of biofilm formation by many of these factors.

There are four proteins encoded within the *ica* locus that mediate PNAG/PIA synthesis (Figure 5.1). IcaA, IcaC, and IcaD are all membrane proteins, while IcaB is a secreted protein. IcaA functions as an *N*-acetylglucosaminyltransferase, with UDP-*N*-acetylglucosamine as its substrate. However, IcaA alone does not exhibit maximum enzymatic activity. IcaD, in combination with IcaA, creates a significant increase in *N*-acetylglucosaminyltransferase activity and facilitates the synthesis of 10–20-mers of *N*-acetylglucosamine [20]. Although the function of IcaC is not fully characterized, *N*-acetylglucosamine oligomers longer than 20 residues can be synthesized *in vitro* when IcaC is coexpressed with IcaAD [20,21]. IcaC is therefore thought to be necessary for the synthesis of *N*-acetylglucosamine oligomers longer than 20 residues, and is hypothesized to play a role in the export of these polymers from the cell. Finally, IcaB is a deacetylase. In the absence of IcaB, PNAG/PIA is fully acetylated and fails to adhere to the bacterial cell surface or to contribute to biofilm formation or immune evasion [22]. When IcaB is produced, however, approximately 3–8% of the amino groups are deacetylated and the polysaccharide adheres to the cell surface and contributes to bacterial aggregation and biofilm formation [11]. Interestingly, antibodies against PNAG that has been chemically deacetylated (85% of amino groups deacetylated) are more effective at opsonizing *S. aureus* for phagocytosis [23]. This suggests that there is an optimal level of deacetylation for immune evasion, and that IcaB activity must be regulated somehow.

The regulation of expression of the staphylococcal *ica* locus is multifaceted. There are both positive and negative regulators of *ica* expression. Seven genetic factors have been shown to play a role in the regulation of expression of the *ica* locus. Six of these factors, the intercellular adhesin regulator (IcaR), the teicoplanin-associated locus regulator (TcaR), the staphylococcal accessory regulator A (SarA), the general stress alternative sigma factor Sigma B (SigB or σ^B), the staphylococcal respiratory response regulator (SrrB) and the phase-variable regulation of *ica* expression, are all *trans* acting. The remaining factor, a 5-nucleotide (TATTT) motif in the *ica* promoter, is distinctly *cis* acting in that it has not been shown to be necessary for the action of any of the other *trans*-acting *ica* regulators.

Two of the *trans*-acting regulators of the *ica* operon are negative regulators that have been shown to act at the level of transcription. IcaR acts as a transcriptional repressor of the *ica* operon in both *S. epidermidis* and *S. aureus* [24,25]. The *icaR* gene is located immediately upstream of the *icaADBC* operon, but is transcribed divergently from it. The expression of *icaR* is repressed by ethanol [24,26]. As one would logically predict from the repression of a repressor, the *ica* operon is induced in the presence of ethanol. NaCl induces expression of the *ica* operon in an IcaR-independent manner [24,26]. It is not clear which *icaA* regulator the NaCl-dependent induction signals through. TcaR was picked up in a biochemical screen for additional regulators of the *ica* operon [27]. Northern blot analysis of the *ica* transcript in the absence of *tcaR*, and electrophoretic mobility shift analysis with purified TcaR and the *ica* promoter, confirmed that TcaR acts as a transcriptional repressor of the *ica* operon [27]. Phase variation also affects the expression of the *ica* locus and is discussed in a separate section below [28,29].

The positive transcriptional regulators of the *ica* operon are SarA and SigB. SarA is a virulence gene regulator necessary for the expression of the *agr* locus [30,31]. SarA is necessary for the transcription of the *ica* operon, but it is not known whether it directly or indirectly activates *ica* transcription [31,32]. A typical binding sequence for SarA is not found upstream of the *ica* operon, although there remains some controversy regarding the binding specificity of SarA [33]. SigB is one of only two staphylococcal alternative sigma factors, along with SigH, reported thus far [34,35]. The role of SigB in the positive regulation of the *ica* operon in *S. epidermidis* is due to its negative regulation of *icaR* [31]. SigB influences biofilm formation in an *ica*-independent manner as well. However, there are conflicting reports of the role of SigB in biofilm formation. In the absence of *sigB*, biofilm formation and salt-dependent induction of biofilms were defective in mucosal isolates of *S. aureus* [36]. *Staphylococcus epidermidis* biofilm-negative phenotypes were isolated from Tn*917* insertions into the positive regulator of *sigB*, *rsbU*, further supporting an argument for SigB in biofilm formation [37]. Bateman *et al.* [38] demonstrated that expression of *sigB* in *trans*, from a tetracycline-inducible promoter, resulted in dose-dependent attachment to polystyrene microtiter wells. The SigB effect on biofilm formation occurs, at least in part, through the *ica* locus in *S. epidermidis*, and Knobloch *et al.* [39] demonstrated that *rsbU*-dependent biofilm formation is related to a negative regulatory effect of SigB on *icaR* expression. In contrast, Valle *et al.* [32] reported that an *S. aureus sigB* mutant showed no difference in its ability to form biofilms compared with the wild-type parental strain, and Kies *et al.* [40] reported no effect on the overexpression of SigB in *S. epidermidis* Tu3298, in *trans*, on bacterial aggregation as observed by light microscopy, suggesting that SigB did not influence biofilm formation in this strain background. This lack of an effect of SigB on aggregation was likely due to the fact that the strain background, Tu3298, was *ica* negative, but the basis for a lack of SigB influence on biofilm formation as reported by Valle *et al.* is unclear.

In addition to IcaR, SigB, and SarA, an additional as yet uncharacterized regulator of *icaA* transcript levels exerts tricarboxylic acid cycle-dependent control over PIA/PNAG production [41]. Although the mechanism has not yet been thoroughly characterized, the relationship between *icaADBC* expression and metabolism has been well established. Glucose affects *icaADBC* expression and PIA/PNAG production, and the catabolite control protein A (CcpA) is required for aggregation and biofilm formation [42,43].

Global regulators of protein stability also play a role. The Clp ATPases function in the staphylococci as chaperones and in the regulation of protein stability through a mechanism similar to eukaryotic proteasome function. The Clp ATPases ClpX and ClpC are required for intercellular adhesion and biofilm formation in *S. aureus* [44]. Whether this role is through PIA/PNAG expression has not yet been determined.

Staphylococcal biofilms are generally sensitive to dispersal by sodium metaperiodate, a chemical that non-specifically hydrolyzes polysaccharides, whereas they are generally resistant to proteolytic dispersal. This is due to the fact that the staphylococcal biofilm matrix is generally composed predominantly of the polysaccharide PIA/PNAG. However, *ica*-negative strains of *S. epidermidis* have been shown recently to produce sodium periodate-resistant, protease-sensitive biofilms [15]. This stems from the fact that in addition to the *ica* locus and PIA/PNAG, proteinaceous intercellular adhesins play a role in staphylococcal biofilm formation. Surface protein-dependent biofilm formation is negatively regulated by the pleiotropic regulator of autolytic activity, toxin production and efflux pump expression MgrA [45]. Proteins implicated in biofilm formation include Bap, SasG, Aap, and autolysin E (AtlE).

Proteinaceous biofilm adhesins

Biofilm-associated protein

Bap family proteins play an important role in biofilm formation in a various Gram-positive and Gram-negative bacteria [46]. The staphylococcal Bap protein, with 2276 amino acid residues, 13 successive 86-amino-acid repeats and a Gram-positive signal sequence (LPXTG motif), attains a remarkable size and boasts interesting characteristics [47]. The staphyloccocal Bap protein was identified in a genetic screen for factors involved in biofilm formation; two Tn*917* insertion mutants that resulted in a biofilm-negative phenotype in a strain of *S. aureus* known for its strong ability to produce a biofilm were mapped to the *bap* gene [47]. Bap is necessary for intercellular adhesion, primary surface attachment to inanimate surfaces, as well as biofilm formation in bovine mastitis isolates; however, the gene is not generally associated with human isolates of *S. aureus* and consequently no data currently support a role for Bap in biofilm formation by strains that cause human infections [47]. Although Bap facilitates adhesion to inanimate objects, the presence of Bap interferes with the binding of *S. aureus* to certain host cell receptors [48]. However, it has also been shown that the presence of Bap increases colonization in bovine intramammary glands [49].

The Bap protein is regulated at the level of expression and activity. The regulation of *bap* gene expression has been explored and partially characterized. SarA binds to the *bap* promoter and acts as a direct transcriptional activator of *bap* gene expression [50]. Consequently, SarA is particularly critical for Bap expression during late log phase. The activity of Bap is also affected by calcium. Calcium and manganese inhibit biofilm formation in *bap*-positive *S. aureus* strains but do not affect *bap*-negative strains [51]. This is due to the EF calcium-binding domains in the Bap proteins. The EF domain was originally characterized and named alphabetically as the third loop in carp muscle calcium-binding protein [52]. EF domains have been found in a number of staphylococcal adhesins, and millimolar concentrations of calcium appear to interfere with adhesion. Therefore, calcium-bound Bap is defective for intercellular adhesion and biofilm formation [51].

Accumulation-associated protein

The Aap protein of *S. epidermidis* appears to stimulate biofilm formation under conditions that are unfavorable for PIA/PNAG-dependent biofilm formation. The role of Aap in biofilm formation was originally defined when an isogenic mutant of *S. epidermidis* RP62A (ATCC 35984), strain M7, was shown to be defective in accumulation on plastic or glass [53]. One of the two extracellular proteins absent from this strain, according to SDS-PAGE analysis, was a 140-kDa protein that was subsequently named accumulation-associated protein due to the phenotype [53,54]. Polyclonal antisera raised against Aap abrogated biofilm formation in the wild-type parental strain, strongly suggestive of a role for Aap in biofilm formation [54]. This effect was later confirmed and augmented with the observation that monoclonal antibodies against Aap also block biofilm formation in the wild-type parental strain [55]. Aap transcription is increased in *ica*-independent proteinaceous biofilms, suggesting that Aap plays a role in proteinaceous biofilm formation in *S. epidermidis* [16].

Staphylococcus aureus surface protein G

SasG is another large surface protein with a series of repeats, and it exhibits significant homology to *S. epidermidis* Aap [13,56]. Deletion of *sasG* reduces aggregation and biofilm formation, implicating the gene product in intercellular adhesion [57]. Furthermore, *Lactococcus lactis* expressing SasG exhibits a significant increase in adherence to desquamated nasal epithelial cells [56] and overexpression of SasG stimulates biofilm formation even in the absence of an *ica* locus [13].

Autolysin E

AtlE has a predicted size of 148 kDa [58]. AtlE derived its name mainly from its high degree (61%) of similarity to the major autolysin gene of *S. aureus* (*atl*) [58]. AtlE, like Bap and Aap, was found in a genetic screen for biofilm-defective mutants of *S. epidermidis* [58]. Two classes of biofilm-defective Tn*917* mutants were found: one class was defective for intercellular adhesion while the other was defective for initial attachment [58]. The *altE*::Tn*917* mutant was the only mutant of its class and was specifically defective for initial attachment to a polystyrene surface [58]. A homologous and functionally similar protein was also discovered in *S. saprohyticus* [59]. Another interesting observation with regard to AtlE is its potential role in the accumulation of extracellular DNA in *S. epidermidis* biofilms. Qin *et al.* [17] reported that addition of DNaseI to growth media before the establishment of a biofilm prevented biofilm formation in most strains of *S. epidermidis* but that the enzyme was not able to disperse mature biofilms. In the same study these authors detected extracellular DNA in wild-type *S. epidermidis* biofilms by fluorescence microscopy but noted a significant decrease in the amount of extracellular DNA in an *atlE* deletion mutant strain. Extracellular DNA release may be mediated through AtlE-mediated autolysis but this has not yet been confirmed. The role of extracellular DNA in biofilm formation is in the infant stages of investigation in staphylococcal species and the precise link and mechanism is unclear.

Phase variation and biofilm formation

Staphylococcal biofilm formation can exhibit phase variability that can be either *ica*-dependent or *ica*-independent. Phase variation is a dramatic and rapid change in any general or specific phenotypic expression of a bacterial cell or population [60]. It is characterized as a reversible switch between full expression of the respective phenotype and absence of expression of the respective phenotype (on–off switch) [60]. Consequently, phase variation can act as a regulatory factor for gene expression. The mechanisms resulting in phase variation are nearly as broad as the number of phase-variable phenotypes. Genomic DNA rearrangements such as insertion events, inversions, and nucleotide additions or subtractions in regulatory elements or the open reading frame of a gene are causative agents of phase-variable "switches" [60].

The synthesis of PNAG/PIA-dependent biofilms are subject to phase variation of *ica* expression in both *S. epidermidis* and *S. aureus* [28,29]. The mechanism responsible for this phase variation is reversible insertion and excision of IS256 into the *icaC* gene [28,29]. There are IS256 insertions within other regions of the chromosome that result in decreased *ica* expression in *S. epidermidis* [61]. IS256 insertions in *rsbU*, the positive activator of *sigB*, and *sarA* result in decreased expression of the *ica* operon [61]. This is consistent with the positive regulatory roles that SigB and SarA play in *ica* expression [31]. Biofilm-negative variants caused by *sarA*::IS256 insertions revert back to a biofilm-positive phenotype after excision of IS256 from *sarA*, which is consistent with the role of IS256 in causing a phase-variable biofilm phenotype through reversible insertion and excision in *icaC* [61]. In contrast to the mechanism of the *sarA* and *icaC* insertions, biofilm-negative variants caused by *rsbU*::IS256 insertion reverted back to a biofilm-positive phenotype after one passage, without the excision of IS256 from *rsbU* [61].

Cell surface proteins that influence *ica*-independent biofilm formation in staphylococcal species are also influenced by phase variation. Bap, Aap, and AltE are involved in *ica*-independent biofilm formation. The regulation of Bap expression is subject to phase variation [62]. Hence, Bap-associated biofilm formation is a phase-variable phenotype. A genetic screen for phenotypic variants of *S. aureus* V329, on Congo Red agar plates, was successful in identifying biofilm-negative variants [62]. Since the *bap* gene is encoded within the staphylococcal pathogenicity island bovine 2 (SaPIbov2) mobile genetic element, these biofilm variants were tested for the presence of the *bap* gene to rule out the possibility that excision of SaPIbov2 was responsible for the biofilm-negative phenotypic variant [62,63]. The *bap* gene was present in the biofilm-negative variants but Northern blot analysis revealed that Bap transcript levels were significantly decreased in these variants suggesting that the variation was influenced by switching a transcriptional regulator on or off [62]. The mechanism of this has not yet been described and it is not clear whether transcript modulation in this circumstance is SarA-dependent or SarA-independent.

Quorum sensing and biofilm formation

Quorum sensing is the perception of a critical density of a secreted signaling molecule (autoinducers) by a bacterial cell that results in a change in gene expression. This will occur when the bacterial population reaches a certain density, or "quorum," within a confined space. However, the signal concentration can also increase locally if the bacteria is localized to a viscous environment, which led to the suggestion of the alternate term "diffusion sensing" [64]. The receptor for the autoinducer either acts directly as a sensor/regulator or stimulates a signal transduction system. This leads to autophosphorylation of a histidine residue on the sensor kinase and the subsequent transfer of the phosphate group to a response regulator [65]. The phosphorylated response regulator then binds to DNA and acts as a transcriptional activator or repressor. This is the canonical mechanism of all bacterial two-component signal transduction systems. Although quorum sensing is not generally classified as a stress response, it does occur in "overpopulated" conditions, which is a stress-inducing condition itself. Increased population density, along with limited oxygen or nutrients, are often associated with general stress and starvation for a bacterial population. In addition, an increase in byproducts of metabolism can be associated with free radical formation and macromolecular damage.

Quorum sensing is associated with biofilm formation and virulence in both Gram-negative and Gram-positive bacteria but the systems differ [65]. In Gram-negative bacteria, an organic chemical autoinducer is secreted through the membrane by diffusion and its sensor acts to modulate gene expression in response to binding the autoinducer. In Gram-positive bacteria like the staphylococci, short autoinducing peptides (AIPs) are transported outside the cell by an ATP-binding cassette associated transporter. The extracellular signal binds to a sensor histidine kinase, stimulating signal transduction to its cognate response regulator that modulates expression of its target gene [65].

Staphylococci possess two quorum-sensing systems, the *agr* system and the *luxS* system [66]. While the *agr* system is specific to the genus *Staphylococcus*, the *luxS* system is found in both Gram-negative and Gram-positive bacteria [66]. The *agr* locus is necessary for synthesis of the octapeptide, AIP, involved in *agr*-dependent quorum sensing [67,68]. The two divergent promoters of the *agr* locus, P2 and P3, drive transcription of *agrACDB* (RNAII) and RNAIII (also encoding the *hld* open reading frame), respectively [7]. The *hld* gene also encodes δ-hemolysin [7]. Each of the *agr* genes encodes specific proteins necessary for AIP synthesis, secretion, and activity. The AIP coding sequence is encoded in *agrD* [7,68,69]. The *agrB* gene product is involved in posttranslational modification and/or export of AIP [68,69]. The *agrC* and *agrA* gene products encode typical sensor histidine kinase and response regulator components of a bacterial two-component signal transduction system, respectively [68,70,71]. AgrC is a receptor for AIP. On recognition of AIP binding, AgrC becomes autophosphorylated. Phosphorylated AgrC transfers its phosphate group to AgrA, which then regulates the transcription of RNAIII and *hld*. RNAIII directly regulates a couple of important virulence factors in a posttranscriptional manner. RNAIII inhibits posttranscriptional expression of Spa and Rot in conjunction with endoribonuclease III [72–74].

There are reports of a small peptide called RNAIII-inhibiting peptide (RIP) that allegedly regulates the *agr* system through a second quorum-sensing protein TraP [75]. Balaban and colleagues reported that RIP inhibits *agr* and subsequently suppresses biofilm formation. However, these studies have recently come under scrutiny as it has been shown that the *traP* mutant that originally led to the hypothesis that TraP regulates *agr* also contains a mutation in *agrA* [76]. It appears that the *agrA* mutation accounts for the loss of *agr* function rather than the mutation in *traP*. Therefore the basis for biofilm inhibition by RIP is currently unclear and may be a nonspecific effect [77,78]. In fact, there is evidence that inhibition of *agr* actually increases biofilm formation rather than inhibiting it [79–81]. In comparing *agr*-positive and *agr*-negative *S. aureus* for biofilm formation, 78% of *agr*-negative and 6% of *agr*-positive strains formed biofilms on polystyrene, although the negative effect of the *agr* locus seemed to be due to expression of δ-hemolysin rather than to quorum sensing [79]. In the clinical isolate MN8, the absence of *agrD* caused a threefold to fourfold increase in biofilm formation [82]. However, a negative role for *agr* has not yet been definitively demonstrated and it seems that while *agr* may limit the thickness of biofilms under certain conditions, the *agr* system is active within biofilms. Yarwood *et al.* [82] demonstrated, using *agr* P3::*gfp* fusions, that all five stages of biofilm formation are coincident with *agr* expression. In sum, it is likely that the role and effect of the quorum-sensing system is complex and depends on strain differences, *agr* type, and environmental conditions [83].

In Gram-negative bacteria, a quorum-sensing system based on an organic chemical autoinducer is most frequently used. One of these systems uses *N*-acyl-homoserine lactone (AHL) as its autoinducer molecule. LuxI and LuxR act as the AHL synthase and sensor, respectively. The other system uses a different organic chemical autoinducer, a furanosyl borate diester, called AI-2. AI-2, which has been characterized mostly in *Vibrio harveyi*, is synthesized by LuxS. LuxS homologs are found in both Gram-negative and Gram-positive bacteria, including *S. aureus* and *S. epidermidis*. Biochemical evidence suggests that the purified LuxS proteins from *S. aureus* and *Escherichia coli* catalyze identical reactions in *vitro* [69,84]. The role of LuxS in quorum sensing in staphylococci is in the initial stages of exploration. Genetic evidence suggests that, like the effect of the *agr* locus on biofilm formation, the LuxS system has a negative effect on biofilm formation and virulence [85,86].

In considering biofilm formation and adaptive physiology of *Staphylococcus*, quorum sensing is an important phenomenon. The two staphylococcal quorum-sensing systems, *agr* and LuxS, appear to negatively influence biofilm formation. Population critical mass, limited physical space, limited nutrients, and increased toxic byproducts, which are all associated with high population density and lead to activation of quorum-sensing systems, could serve as a feedback mechanism for preventing the biofilm from becoming too large or as a mechanism for dispersal.

Cyclic-di-GMP and *Staphylococcus aureus* biofilm formation

In addition to the extracellular signaling that influences biofilm formation during quorum sensing, there are also intracellular signaling events that widely influence the physiology of the bacterial cell. The cyclic dinucleotide cyclic-di-GMP is a widely utilized intracellular second messenger influencing many pathways and phenotypes in bacteria, including motility, virulence gene expression, and biofilm formation [87–89]. Prior to investigations into the role of cyclic-di-GMP in *S. aureus* biofilm formation, investigations into *Vibrio cholerae* virulence yielded data that demonstrated a role for this important intracellular second messenger in *V. cholerae* biofilm formation [90]. Tischler and Camilli [90] demonstrated that Vie, the transcriptional repressor of *Vibrio* exopolysaccharide synthesis (*vps*) genes necessary for *Vibrio* biofilm formation, modulates intracellular levels of cyclic-di-GMP. Karaolis and colleagues demonstrated that chemically synthesized cyclic-di-GMP inhibited aggregation of *S. aureus*, biofilm formation, and adherence to HeLa epithelial cells [91,92]. This suggests that externally added cyclic-di-GMP has an inhibitory effect on biofilm formation on both abiotic and biotic surfaces. The therapeutic efficacy of cyclic-di-GMP treatment against infection with biofilm-producing *S. aureus* strains was subsequently tested in an intramamary gland mouse model of infection [92]. The addition of cyclic-di-GMP to mammary glands inoculated with *S. aureus* Newbould resulted in a significant decrease in the number of infected mammary glands, suggesting that cyclic-di-GMP addition can decrease virulence of *S. aureus* infection.

The mechanism of action of cyclic-di-GMP-dependent inhibition of biofilm formation is not completely clear. However, investigations into the role of cyclic-di-GMP in *Pseudomonas aeruginosa* and immune cell function yield some potentially insightful clues. In a previous section of this chapter, the role of exopolysaccharides in staphylococcal biofilms was discussed. *Pseudomonas aeruginosa* biofilm formation is influenced by the production of extracellular PEL polysaccharide. *Pseudomonas aeruginosa* PelD is a cyclic-di-GMP receptor protein and the cyclic-di-GMP-binding activity of PelD is necessary for PEL polysaccharide production [93]. It is possible that the negative effect of cyclic-di-GMP on biofilm formation in *S. aureus* is facilitated through modulation of PNAG production. However, none of the *ica*-encoded proteins has been shown to bind cyclic-di-GMP. Furthermore, there have been no reports characterizing putative cyclic-di-GMP-binding proteins in *S. aureus* or *S. epidermidis*. Until such investigations are consummated, the full potential of cyclic-di-GMP and putative cyclic-di-GMP-binding proteins in staphylcoccal biofilm formation will remain unknown. Karaolis *et al.* [94] reported that cyclic-di-GMP is an immunomodulatory molecule. This accounts for the reduction in *S. aureus* virulence in the presence of cyclic-di-GMP reported by Brouillette *et al.* [92].

Mobile genetic elements and biofilm formation

Mobile genetic elements such as insertion elements, transposons, plasmids, and bacteriophages can significantly influence bacterial cellular physiology. Transformation, transduction, and conjugation are the three processes that facilitate horizontal gene transfer in bacterial biology. Horizontal gene transfer, via mobile genetic elements, does not appear to be influential in biofilm formation or dispersion in *Staphylococcus*. However, there are some examples of the presence of mobile genetic elements influencing staphylococcal biofilms.

Insertion sequences and bacteriophages are the only mobile genetic elements thus far reported to be associated with *Staphylococcus* biofilms. Insertion sequences cannot independently transfer themselves between cells in the absence of a genetic vector such as a bacteriophage or plasmid. Hence, they are usually transferred via conjugation or transduction. Once present within a chromosome, insertion sequences can move from one genetic locus to another. As stated in a previous section of this chapter, insertion sequence IS256 plays a significant role in the phase variation of the biofilm phenotype. It executes this by intracellular transfer from one genetic locus to another.

IS256-dependent phase variation is caused by reversible insertion/excision into the *icaC*, *rsbU*, or *sarA* genes.

While transduction within biofilms has not been reported or shown to play a significant role within the phenotype, bacteriophages appear to influence biofilms in ways that are yet to be fully characterized. In the section that discussed Bap, it was noted that the *bap* gene is located on a mobile genetic element, the cryptic prophage SaPIbov2. SaPIs can be mobilized by phage 80α. With this in mind, it is not unreasonable to assume that transduction of SaPIbov2 between different strains of *S. aureus*, within their respective environments, may contribute to the dissemination of the *bap* gene to strain variants that are SaPI-negative or biofilm-negative. The dissemination of *bap* to beneficiaries that would otherwise have been Bap-negative may lead to the propagation of biofilm-positive strains.

The biofilm synthesis and dispersal process appears to be affected by bacteriophages in ways distinctly separate from gene transfer. Various investigations suggest that phages may play a role in biofilm dispersal. It is clear that bacteriophages have developed ways to escape a biofilm of *Staphylococcus* as well as other bacteria. Resch *et al.* [95] detected about 10^5 plaque-forming units from both planktonic and biofilm cultures of *S. aureus* SA113 and Newman strains grown for 4 hours. By 8 hours, the planktonic cultures had decreased to about 10^1 plaque-forming units. In contrast, 48–72 hours passed before the same decrease in plaque-forming units was seen in the biofilm cultures. This suggests that although the *S. aureus* biofilm state decreases the rate of staphylococcal bacteriophage progeny production in reference to the planktonic state, the exopolysaccharide structure of a biofilm matrix is not sufficient to totally abrogate bacteriophage progeny formation or dispersal from biofilms. *Staphylococcus* phages also exhibit lytic activity against biofilm-associated structures. Cerca *et al.* [96] demonstrated that *Staphylococcus* bacteriophage K has the ability to reduce *S. epidermidis* biofilm formation after 24 hours of treatment. Phage therapy was used to treat bacterial infections prior to the development of chemical antibiotics [97]. The use of whole phages or, more recently, phage components has been proposed as a novel alternative treatment for multidrug-resistant bacterial infections [98]. In a potential segue into this therapeutic application as it pertains to biofilm associated infection, Curtin and Donlan [99] used bacteriophage 456 to prevent *S. epidermidis* biofilm formation on catheters in *vitro*.

Clinical implications of biofilms

Biofilms are more resistant than their free-floating counterparts to nearly every imaginable chemical and physical hazard. The viscoelasticity imparted by the exopolymeric matrix allows them to withstand shear forces such as those caused by the flow of blood past a catheter. Biofilms are more resistant to desiccation and pH extremes, and they can tolerate much higher concentrations of most antibiotics and disinfectants. They are also resistant to phagocytosis, and while neutrophils can migrate into the biofilm, they are ineffective and fail to ingest the bacteria [100]. This makes infections involving biofilms very difficult to treat; antibiotic therapy often fails, or the infection relapses following cessation of antibiotics, and removal and invasive treatment such as replacement of the infected tissue or medical device are frequently required.

Antibiotic resistance

Biofilms tolerate antibiotics and disinfectants at concentrations 10-fold to 1000-fold higher than the concentrations needed to kill or inhibit the growth of genetically equivalent phenotypic bacteria. Unfortunately, standard methods for analyzing antibiotic susceptibility are performed on planktonic bacterial populations and do not take biofilm-mediated resistance into account. For this reason, a biofilm-related infection with a strain that appears to be sensitive to an antibiotic may not be completely resolved by antimicrobial therapy. To further complicate matters, subinhibitory doses of disinfectants and antibiotics can actually induce the biofilm phenotype [101]. The disinfectants chlorhexidine and benzalkonium chloride and ethanol have been shown to increase biofilm formation in *S. epidermidis* [24,37,102].

The basis for the increased tolerance of biofilms to disinfectants and antibiotics has not been well defined but, as illustrated in Plate 5.1, it is almost certainly multifactorial [103]. Studies using microarray analysis of global gene expression in *S. aureus* biofilm versus planktonic cultures reveal alterations in the expression of 580 genes, which represents more than 20% of the genome [6]. Clearly there is a sizeable phenotypic disparity between biofilm and planktonic bacteria, and homing in on the differences that are responsible for tolerance to various chemical insults has proven to be a difficult task.

Bacteria within biofilms grow more slowly than exponential-phase bacteria, partly due to limitations on mass transfer within the biofilm but also due to alterations in gene expression that are characteristic of the phenotype. Slow growth may contribute to increased resistance to cell wall-active antibiotics that depend on rapid growth for activity [104]. Indeed, biofilm bacteria exhibit a striking increase in resistance to many cell wall-active antibiotics such as vancomycin whereas some protein synthesis inhibitors such as minocycline and tigecycline, which do not depend on cell division to exert their activity, retain fairly good efficacy against biofilms [105,106]. However, the target of an antibiotic does not reliably predict whether it will be effective in killing biofilm bacteria, and other protein synthesis inhibitors, such as linezolid, exhibit very poor activity against biofilms. Overall, tolerance to every class of antibiotics is at least somewhat higher in biofilms than in planktonic cultures so other factors must be at play.

The exopolymeric matrix of biofilms may sequester, exclude, or inactivate certain antibiotics; however, biofilms are designed to be fairly porous to allow nutrients in and metabolites out, so the diffusion of most small molecules, including antibiotics, is not significantly inhibited within biofilms [107,108]. However, we found that while the rate of diffusion of the antibiotic vancomycin through biofilms was similar to the rate through water, the force of convection was significantly limited [109]. This resulted in slow accumulation of vancomycin within the deeper layers of the biofilm and we hypothesized that the bacteria that were gradually exposed to increasing concentrations of the antibiotic would be afforded an opportunity to alter the expression of certain genes that would augment their tolerance.

The existence of a small subpopulation of bacteria that exhibits high tolerance to antibiotics was recognized more than 60 years ago [110]. A culture that has been treated with penicillin may fail to grow but if plated on media that does not contain antibiotics, colonies will be recovered, even if the penicillin concentration was much higher than the minimum bactericidal concentration. The bacteria in this small subpopulation are referred to as persister cells [111]. They are not antibiotic-resistant mutants but rather a dormant subpopulation that exhibits tolerance to different classes of antibiotics and other chemical hazards. These bacteria are not merely nondividing but also exhibit reduced cell activity; therefore, antibiotics that affect transcription and translation are also ineffective against them. Persister bacteria are present not only in biofilms but also in stationary phase planktonic polulations [112]. Lewis [113] hypothesized that antibiotic therapy fails to kill persister cells in any bacterial population, be it planktonic or biofilm, but that remaining planktonic cells that tolerate the antibiotic *in vivo* are destroyed by the immune system. However, biofilm persisters would be protected from immune defenses and once antibiotic therapy is withdrawn, these bacteria would exit the persister state and repopulate the biofilm. The physiological basis behind the persister phenotype is only just beginning to be unraveled as is its role in biofilm resistance.

Finally, changes in the expression of permeases and efflux pumps may play a role in the resistance of biofilm bacteria to certain antbtiotics. Reduced permease expression could potentially inhibit the ability of certain antibiotics to enter cells and interact with their targets. It has also been postulated that increased expression of efflux pumps could augment antibiotic resistance, although studies in *P. aeruginosa* indicate that efflux pumps are not induced in biofilms [114].

Resistance to immune defenses

Resistance of biofilms to host defenses is not well understood either, but it is evident that the biofilm exopolysaccharide matrix, comprising PIA/PNAG, plays a role in increased resistance to phagocytosis and to antimicrobial peptides [115]. PIA/PNAG within the biofilm matrix that is not intimately associated with bacterial cells may act as a false target for opsonophagocytosis [116]. Certain immune factors may also be inactivated within the biofilm, and studies using *Caenorhabditis elegans* as a model for virulence suggest that neutrophil-independent components of innate immunity are also inhibited by the polysaccharide [117]. There may also be PIA/PNAG-independent biofilm characteristics that aid in immune evasion but this has yet to be investigated.

Potential solutions to the biofilm problem

A number of strategies to deal with the problem of refractory or relapsing biofilm infections have been investigated. One such strategy is to interfere with the cellular processes that induce the biofilm phenotype in bacteria. As discussed above, quorum sensing plays a positive role in the formation of biofilms by a number of bacterial species, but the role of quorum sensing in staphylococcal biofilm formation is still somewhat unclear. Despite the fact that most studies indicate a negative effect of quorum sensing on biofilm formation, there have been reports of quorum-sensing inhibitors effectively preventing the establishment of a biofilm on solid surfaces. Balaban *et al.* [118,119] reported that coating dialysis catheters with the alleged *agr* inhibitor RIP prevented biofilm formation, whereas uncoated catheters became rapidly colonized. The same group even found that RIP acted synergistically with antibiotics to clear recalcitrant biofilm infections, suggesting that the peptide can exert its effect on established biofims in addition to preventing biofilm formation [120]. However, as mentioned above, the effects of RIP have not yet been sufficiently characterized and there is evidence that the anti-biofilm effect is not related to quorum-sensing inhibition.

In addition, Baveja *et al.* [121] reported that a furanone antimicrobial compound was able to inhibit *S. epidermidis* biofilm formation on biomaterials. Furanones inhibit organic chemical autoinducers, suggesting that the observed effect occurred through the LuxS system. However, as mentioned above, LuxS appears to play a negative role in biofilm formation in the staphylococci, so it would seem that a LuxS inhibitor would actually augment biofilm formation. The use of furanones to inhibit biofilm formation on biomaterials therefore needs to be tested further.

Quorum-sensing inhibitors may or may not prove an effective means of preventing biofilm formation but either way this approach is not very useful in cases where the formation of a biofilm would not necessarily be predicted. In other words, inhibitors of biofilm formation may be useful for coating catheters and other medical devices, but for spontaneous infections in host tissues there would be no call for prophylactic therapy. A more practical approach in such cases would be to disrupt established biofilms in an effort to increase their sensitivity to antimicrobial agents. The divalent cation chelator EDTA causes PIA/PNAG to dissociate from the bacterial cell surface. If the polysaccharide does not adhere to the cell surface, then it cannot act as an intercellular adhesin and the biofilm will dissolve. A combination of EDTA, minocycline, and ethanol effectively eradicated biofilms from catheter segments, whereas minocycline and ethanol were not effective when used alone [122]. The enzyme dispersin B is produced by the oral bacterial species *Actinobacillus actinomycetemcomitans* as a means of releasing bacteria from its own PNAG-based biofilms. Dispersin B can degrade staphylococcal PIA/PNAG and has been shown to increase the efficacy of the antibiotic cefamandole nafate against staphylococcal biofilms [123]. Finally, lysostaphin, an enzyme that degrades staphylococcal peptidoglycan, has been shown to disrupt *S. aureus* and *S. epidermidis* biofilms and subsequently restores their sensitivity to antibiotics [124].

Small-colony variants

Similar to bacteria that express the biofilm phenotype, staphylococci with the small-colony variant (SCV) phenotype are more resistant to antibiotics, phagocytosis (as a result of intracellular survival), and antimicrobial peptides, and they are associated with recalcitrant or relapsing infections [125]. In addition, there is evidence to suggest that subinhibitory doses of antimicrobial agents can induce both the SCV and biofilm phenotypes. For example, aminoglycoside antibiotics stimulate generation of *S. aureus* SCVs (discussed in more detail below), and *P. aeruginosa* biofilm formation is also induced by treatment with subinhibitory concentrations of aminoglycoside antibiotics [126]. The aminoglycoside response regulator (Arr), which has a predicted cyclic-di-GMP phosphodiesterase domain, is necessary for aminoglycoside-dependent biofilm formation in *P. aeruginosa* [126]. In addition, bacteria expressing the SCV phenotype tend to form strong biofilms [127,128]. Together, these characteristics suggest underlying similarities between these two altered physiological states. An important distinction is that the SCV phenotype is generally induced by a mutation within a gene, whereas the biofilm phenotype is generally regulated at the level of gene expression in the absence of a genotypic alteration.

Staphylococcal SCVs exhibit physiological changes that result in a decline in growth rate and colonies with a significant decrease in diameter relative to normal colonies [129]. Bacterial cells that develop into SCVs typically represent a physiologically distinctive subset of an otherwise normal bacterial population [130,131]. Although most frequently associated with *Staphylococcus*, SCVs are observed in many other bacterial genera [130,131]. SCVs were first observed in *Salmonella enterica* serovar *typhi* in 1910 [132]. SCVs of *S. aureus* have a diameter of approximately 0.2 mm compared with a diameter of 2 mm for normal colonies [129]; fail to produce coagulase, the pigment staphyloxanthin, and hemolysin; and are also characterized by various auxotrophies, decreased sensitivity to antibiotics, and intracellular survival [129]. Studies on SCVs of *S. aureus* were reported as early as 1935 [133]. Since then much research has been executed to characterize the SCV phenotype in *Staphylococcus*.

Genetic and physiological analysis of SCV clinical isolates has led to the identification of the etiological defects in *S. aureus* physiology that lead to this phenotype [134]. SCV clinical isolates were shown to be auxotrophs for hemin, thymidine, and/or menadione [134]. These auxotrophies reflect a defect in one of two physiological pathways: the electron transport chain (ETC) and thymidine biosynthesis [130]. ETC-defective SCVs are unable to synthesize menaquinone, hemin, heme A, or thiamine. Some of these biosynthetic defects have been confirmed by supplementation of ETC-defective SCVs with hemin or menadione.

Thymidine auxotrophic, or thymidine-dependent, SCVs can emerge in *S. aureus*-infected cystic fibrosis patients undergoing long-term treatment with trimethoprim–sulfamethoxazole [134,135]. Trimethoprim acts by inhibiting the tetrahydrofolic acid pathway leading to the synthesis of deoxythymidine monophosphate (dTMP). Expression of *thyA*, encoding thymidylate synthase, in *trans* results in complementation of the thymidine biosynthesis-defective SCV phenotype [130,136,137]. There is a correlation between the amount of thymidine in growth media and the growth rate of these thymidine-dependent SCVs [134]. When excess thymidine is available, the growth rate of SCVs more closely resembles the growth rate of wild-type cells [134]. It is suspected that the thymidine biosynthesis-defective SCVs may be defective in thymidine uptake [130]. More specifically, they may have mutations in the *Bacillus subtilis nupC* homolog, which is necessary for full pyrimidine uptake in *B. subtilis* [130,138]. Recently, a couple of research groups have demonstrated that thymidine-dependent SCVs have an increased frequency of mutations in *thyA* [136,137].

The ETC-defective SCV phenotype can be caused by a number of different genetic lesions in the chromosome. Mutations in *hemB*, *menD*, and *ctaA* are necessary for synthesis of hemin, menadione, and heme A [130]. Menadione is used in the synthesis of menaquinone (vitamin K) [130]. Heme and hemin A are necessary for cytochrome biosynthesis [130]. Other mutations in the hemin biosynthesis locus, such as partial deletions in *hemH*, can result in ETC-defective SCVs [139]. Both cytochromes and menaquinone are major components of the ETC, explaining the link between these particular auxotrophies and ETC-defective SCVs.

Small-colony variants and pathogenesis

Intracellular persistence

There are some significant pathogenesis-related phenotypes associated with SCVs. Proctor *et al.* [140] proposed that the phenotypic characteristics associated with SCVs correlated with persistent infection. Two major virulence-associated phenotypes connected with SCVs that could account for their persistence include intracellular survival and antibiotic resistance. Balwit *et al.* [141] demonstrated that menadione and hemin auxotrophs, now known to indicate an ETC-defective SCV phenotype, had increased intracellular survival in bovine aortic endothelial cells compared with wild-type strains. In addition, this phenotype could be reversed by the addition of menadione or hemin exogenously. Another early clue into the relationship between SCVs and intracellular survival was obtained by Vesga *et al.* [142]. Wild-type *S. aureus* cells were incubated with bovine endothelial cells in the presence of lysostaphin for 72 hours; intracellular *S. aureus* developed SCVs at a much higher frequency than *S. aureus* cells not exposed to the endothelial cells. ETC-defective *S. aureus* 8325-4 SCVs, generated manually via the construction of a *hemB::ermB* insertion mutation, can persist in bovine aortic endothelial cells [143]. *Staphylococcus aureus* is known to lyse these cells and it was hypothesized that the persistence in this cell line was due to lack of hemolytic activity in the *hemB::ermB* mutants. SCVs exhibited a 100-fold increase in intracellular persistence in a transformed human keratinocyte cell line (HaCaT) compared with the wild-type parental strain (isolated from a patient with Darier disease, i.e., keratosis follicularis) [144].

The role of MSCRAMMs in biofilm formation was discussed briefly above. These proteins contribute to adherence, which is a prerequisite step, not only to biofilm formation but for invasion and intracellular persistence as well. Vaudaux *et al.* [145] demonstrated that *S. aureus hemB* mutants, exhibiting the SCV phenotype, demonstrated increased expression of the mRNAs for ClfA and FnbA by quantitative reverse-transcriptase polymerase chain reaction (RT-PCR) [145]. This correlated with increased ClfA and FnbA protein expression, demonstrated by a 7.6-fold increase in binding of anti-ClfA antibodies and 2.1-fold increase in FITC-labeled fibronectin to *hemB* mutants, respectively. Increased adhesion of *hemB* mutants to fibrinogen- and fibronectin-coated coverslips compared with the 8325-4 wild type was observed [145]. Finally, a 10-fold increase in *S. aureus* cells internalized into human embryonic kidney cells was seen in the *hemB* mutant compared with the wild-type parental strain [145]. Together these results suggest that increased adherence plays a role in intracellular persistence of *S. aureus* SCVs. However, this may be tissue-dependent as Brouillette *et al.* [146] demonstrated that *hemB* mutants are defective for colonization of mouse mammary glands. Furthermore, the *hemB* effect on *clfA* expression may be indirect and SigB-dependent, as Senn *et al.* [147] demonstrated that a *hemB/sigB* double mutant abolishes the ClfA mRNA expression seen in a *hemB* mutant [147]. SigB appears to be largely influential in the intracellular persistence phenotype of *S. aureus* SCVs [148].

Intracellular persistence is an advantage that is dangerously effective for the pathogenic bacteria and detrimental to the host. It allows for evasion of the host response system and decreased exposure to antibiotics. Some compounds appear to be effective against intracellular *S. aureus*. Malouin *et al.* [149] performed a screen for compounds with bactericidal activity against *S. aureus hemB* mutants residing intracellularly in cultured NMuMG cells. Of 921 potential candidates, nine had bactericidal activity against intracellular *S. aureus hemB* mutants, suggesting that potential therapeutics for intracellular *S. aureus* infections (wild type or SCVs) may become available in the future [149].

Antibiotic resistance

Similar to biofilms, SCVs exhibit increased resistance to different classes of antibiotics. Increased antibiotic resistance is partly due to intracellular persistence where antibiotics cannot reach the bacteria. However, even extracellular SCVs are less susceptible to certain antibiotics. Aminoglycoside (gentamicin) treatment can select for SCVs [146,150,151]. Aminoglycoside-resistant *S. aureus* SCVs share characteristics of ETC-defective SCVs. Schaaf *et al.* [139] observed that approximately 80% of gentamicin-induced SCVs were hemin auxotrophic compared with approximately 20% of spontaneous SCVs. PCR amplification and DNA sequence analysis of the hemin biosynthetic operon of gentamicin-induced SCVs revealed a 113-bp deletion within *hemH*. This deletion led to a frameshift mutation and a premature stop codon, resulting in the protein being shortened from 357 amino acids to 22 amino acids [139].

Other antibiotics, including methicillin, teicoplanin, triclosan, lactoferricin B, fluoroquinolones and rifampicin, have been reported to be less effective against SCV isolates and may select for the SCV phenotype. Methicillin-resistant *S. aureus* (MRSA) SCVs have been studied from as early as 1969, when Bulger and Bulger determined thar SCVs had an intact cell wall and were distinct from protoplasts (L forms) [152,153]. Glycopeptide-resistant SCVs of *S. epidermidis* were isolated from a leukemia patient undergoing vancomycin therapy for a catheter-induced bacteremia [154]. Triclosan-resistant SCVs of MRSA clinical isolates and methicillin-susceptible *S. aureus* strains were selected for on Mueller–Hinton media supplemented with 1 mg/L triclosan [155]. Triclosan-resistant SCVs have also been isolated from triclosan-treated polymers inoculated with MRSA clinical isolates [156]. Mitsuyama *et al.* [157] isolated SCVs of *S. aureus* after exposure to a minimal inhibitory concentration of the broad-spectrum fluoroquinolone pazufloxacin.

Global regulation in small-colony variants: the role of SigB

SigB influences the expression of many factors that affect diverse physiological pathways. For the SCV phenotype,

SigB activity is also extremely influential in the modulation of pathways and the expression of other global regulators [158]. Kahl *et al.* demonstrated that expression of the SigB-dependent *asp23* promoter was significantly abrogated in thymidine-dependent SCVs isolated from cystic fibrosis patients versus wild-type strains, suggesting that SigB activity is suppressed in these strains [158]. However, Moisan *et al.* [148] reported results from microarray analysis of *S. aureus* clinical SCVs isolated from cystic fibrosis patients, which revealed an increase in the expression of genes that were previously shown to be upregulated by SigB and/or biofilm formation. Because the study by Kahl *et al.* used *asp23* expression as a marker for SigB activity whereas the study by Moisan *et al.* detected an increase in transcript levels of multiple SigB targets, it is possible that repression of *asp23* transcript levels was a SigB-independent event. Alternatively, the contradictory results could be related to differences in growth conditions. As stated above, the increase in *clfA* expression seen in *hemB* SCVs is SigB dependent [147]. This is consistent with the reports of Moisan *et al.* [148], suggesting a larger role for SigB in global gene expression with SCVs. The intracellular persistence of SCVs appears to be influenced by SigB as well [148]. A *sigB* mutant of *S. aureus* Newbould was severely defective for invasion of, and persistence in, mammalian cells (bovine epithelial MAC-T cells) compared with the wild-type parental strain, while the *hemB* mutant strain had increased persistence compared with the wild-type parental strain [148]. This result suggests that upregulation or increased activity of SigB would cause an increase in intracellular persistence. Furthermore, upregulation of SigB and its regulon is most likely a major contributor to the overall SCV phenotype.

Conclusion

Both biofilm formation and the SCV phenotype provide mechanisms for *S. aureus* and *S. epidermidis* to evade the host response and thrive in the presence of antibiotics. They are a reflection of the remarkable capacity of this organism to adapt to change and stress. Novel therapeutic agents that target these specific phenotypes or act synergistically with conventional antimicrobial agents are being pursued and will likely come to fruition as our knowledge about the regulation of these alternative phenotypic states continues to increase.

References

1 Shanks RM, Donegan NP, Graber ML *et al.* Heparin stimulates *Staphylococcus aureus* biofilm formation. Infect Immun 2005; 73:4596–606.

2 Shanks RM, Sargent JL, Martinez RM, Graber ML, O'Toole GA. Catheter lock solutions influence staphylococcal biofilm formation on abiotic surfaces. Nephrol Dial Transplant 2006; 21:2247–55.

3 Cramton SE, Ulrich M, Götz F, Doring G. Anaerobic conditions induce expression of polysaccharide intercellular adhesin in *Staphylococcus aureus* and *Staphylococcus epidermidis*. Infect Immun 2001;69:4079–85.

4 Lim Y, Jana M, Luong TT, Lee CY. Control of glucose and NaCl-induced biofilm formation by rbf in *Staphylococcus aureus*. J Bacteriol 2004;186:722–9.

5 Resch A, Rosenstein R, Nerz C, Gotz F. Differential gene expression profiling of *Staphylococcus aureus* cultivated under biofilm and planktonic condition. Appl Environ Microbiol 2005;71:2663–76.

6 Beenken KE, Dunman PM, McAleese F *et al.* Global gene expression in *Staphylococcus aureus* biofilms. J Bacteriol 2004; 186:4665–84.

7 George EA, Muir TW. Molecular mechanisms of *agr* quorum sensing in virulent staphylococci. Chembiochem 2007;8:847–55.

8 Stoodley P, Sauer K, Davies DG, Costerton JW. Biofilms as complex differentiated communities. Annu Rev Microbiol 2002; 56:187–209.

9 Foster SJ, Hook M. Surface protein adhesins of *Staphylococcus aureus*. Trends Microbiol 1998;6:484–8.

10 Mack D, Fischer W, Krokotsch A *et al.* The intercellular adhesin involved in biofilm accumulation of *Staphylococcus epidermidis* is a linear beta-1,6-linked glucosaminoglycan: purification and structural analysis. J Bacteriol 1996;178:175–83.

11 Maira-Litràn T, Kropec A, Abeygunawardana C *et al.* Immunochemical properties of the staphylococcal poly-*N*-acetylglucosamine surface polysaccharide. Infect Immun 2002; 70:4433–40.

12 Roche FM, Massey R, Peacock SJ *et al.* Characterization of novel LPXTG-containing proteins of *Staphylococcus aureus* identified from genome sequences. Microbiology 2003;149:643–54.

13 Corrigan RM, Rigby D, Handley P, Foster TJ. The role of *Staphylococcus aureus* surface protein SasG in adherence and biofilm formation. Microbiology 2007;153:2435–46.

14 Frank KL, Patel R. Poly-*N*-acetylglucosamine is not a major component of the extracellular matrix in biofilms formed by *icaADBC*-positive *Staphylococcus lugdunensis* isolates. Infect Immun 2007;75:4728–42.

15 Rohde H, Burandt EC, Siemssen N *et al.* Polysaccharide intercellular adhesin or protein factors in biofilm accumulation of *Staphylococcus epidermidis* and *Staphylococcus aureus* isolated from prosthetic hip and knee joint infections. Biomaterials 2007;28:1711–20.

16 Hennig S, Nyunt Wai S, Ziebuhr W. Spontaneous switch to PIA-independent biofilm formation in an *ica*-positive *Staphylococcus epidermidis* isolate. Int J Med Microbiol 2007;297:117–22.

17 Qin Z, Ou Y, Yang L *et al.* Role of autolysin-mediated DNA release in biofilm formation of *Staphylococcus epidermidis*. Microbiology 2007;153:2083–92.

18 Stoodley P, Wilson S, Hall-Stoodley L, Boyle JD, Lappin-Scott HM, Costerton JW. Growth and detachment of cell clusters from mature mixed species biofilms. Appl Environ Microbiol 2001;67:5608–13.

19 Cramton SE, Gerke C, Schnell NF, Nichols WW, Götz F. The intercellular adhesion (*ica*) locus is present in *Staphylococcus aureus* and is required for biofilm formation. Infect Immun 1999;67:5427–33.

20 Gerke C, Kraft A, Sussmuth R, Schweitzer O, Götz F. Characterization of the *N*-acetylglucosaminyltransferase activity involved in the biosynthesis of the *Staphylococcus epidermidis* polysaccharide intercellular adhesin. J Biol Chem 1998;273: 18586–93.

21 Götz F. *Staphylococcus* and biofilms. Mol Microbiol 2002;43: 1367–78.

22 Vuong C, Kocianova S, Voyich JM *et al*. A crucial role for exopolysaccharide modification in bacterial biofilm formation, immune evasion, and virulence. J Biol Chem 2004;279:54881–6.

23 Maira-Litran T, Kropec A, Goldmann DA, Pier GB. Comparative opsonic and protective activities of *Staphylococcus aureus* conjugate vaccines containing native or deacetylated staphylococcal poly-*N*-acetyl-beta-(1–6)-glucosamine. Infect Immun 2005;73:6752–62.

24 Conlon KM, Humphreys H, O'Gara JP. *icaR* encodes a transcriptional repressor involved in environmental regulation of *ica* operon expression and biofilm formation in *Staphylococcus epidermidis*. J Bacteriol 2002;184:4400–8.

25 Jefferson KK, Cramton SE, Gotz F, Pier GB. Identification of a 5-nucleotide sequence that controls expression of the ica locus in *Staphylococcus aureus* and characterization of the DNA-binding properties of IcaR. Mol Microbiol 2003;48:889–99.

26 Conlon KM, Humphreys H, O'Gara JP. Regulation of icaR gene expression in *Staphylococcus epidermidis*. FEMS Microbiol Lett 2002;216:171–7.

27 Jefferson KK, Pier DB, Goldmann DA, Pier GB. The teicoplanin-associated locus regulator (TcaR) and the intercellular adhesin locus regulator (IcaR) are transcriptional inhibitors of the ica locus in *Staphylococcus aureus*. J Bacteriol 2004;186:2449–56.

28 Ziebuhr W, Krimmer V, Rachid S, Lossner I, Götz F, Hacker J. A novel mechanism of phase variation of virulence in *Staphylococcus epidermidis*: evidence for control of the polysaccharide intercellular adhesin synthesis by alternating insertion and excision of the insertion sequence element IS256. Mol Microbiol 1999;32:345–56.

29 Kiem S, Oh WS, Peck KR *et al*. Phase variation of biofilm formation in *Staphylococcus aureus* by IS 256 insertion and its impact on the capacity adhering to polyurethane surface. J Korean Med Sci 2004;19:779–82.

30 Rechtin TM, Gillaspy AF, Schumacher MA, Brennan RG, Smeltzer MS, Hurlburt BK. Characterization of the SarA virulence gene regulator of *Staphylococcus aureus*. Mol Microbiol 1999;33:307–16.

31 Handke LD, Slater SR, Conlon KM *et al*. SigmaB and SarA independently regulate polysaccharide intercellular adhesin production in *Staphylococcus epidermidis*. Can J Microbiol 2007; 53:82–91.

32 Valle J, Toledo-Arana A, Berasain C *et al*. SarA and not sigmaB is essential for biofilm development by *Staphylococcus aureus*. Mol Microbiol 2003;48:1075–87.

33 Sterba KM, Mackintosh SG, Blevins JS, Hurlburt BK, Smeltzer MS. Characterization of *Staphylococcus aureus* SarA binding sites. J Bacteriol 2003;185:4410–17.

34 Wu S, de Lencastre H, Tomaz A. Sigma-B, a putative operon encoding alternative sigma factor of *Staphylococcus aureus* RNA polymerase: molecular cloning and DNA sequencing. J Bacteriol 1996;178:6036–42.

35 Morikawa K, Inose Y, Okamura H *et al*. A new staphylococcal sigma factor in the conserved gene cassette: functional significance and implication for the evolutionary processes. *Genes Cells* 2003;8:699–712.

36 Rachid S, Ohlsen K, Wallner U, Hacker J, Hecker M, Ziebuhr W. Alternative transcription factor sigma(B) is involved in regulation of biofilm expression in a *Staphylococcus aureus* mucosal isolate. J Bacteriol 2000;182:6824–6.

37 Knobloch JK, Bartscht K, Sabottke A, Rohde H, Feucht HH, Mack D. Biofilm formation by *Staphylococcus epidermidis* depends on functional RsbU, an activator of the sigB operon: differential activation mechanisms due to ethanol and salt stress. J Bacteriol 2001;183:2624–33.

38 Bateman BT, Donegan NP, Jarry TM, Palma M, Cheung AL. Evaluation of a tetracycline-inducible promoter in *Staphylococcus aureus* in vitro and in vivo and its application in demonstrating the role of *sigB* in microcolony formation. Infect Immun 2001;69:7851–7.

39 Knobloch JK, Jager S, Horstkotte MA, Rohde H, Mack D. RsbU-dependent regulation of *Staphylococcus epidermidis* biofilm formation is mediated via the alternative sigma factor sigmaB by repression of the negative regulator gene *icaR*. Infect Immun 2004;72:3838–48.

40 Kies S, Otto M, Vuong C, Gotz F. Identification of the sigB operon in *Staphylococcus epidermidis*: construction and characterization of a sigB deletion mutant. Infect Immun 2001;69:7933–6.

41 Sadykov MR, Olson ME, Halouska S *et al*. Tricarboxylic acid cycle-dependent regulation of *Staphylococcus epidermidis* polysaccharide intercellular adhesin synthesis. J Bacteriol 2008;190: 7621–32.

42 Dobinsky S, Kiel K, Rohde H *et al*. Glucose-related dissociation between *ica*ADBC transcription and biofilm expression by *Staphylococcus epidermidis*: evidence for an additional factor required for polysaccharide intercellular adhesin synthesis. J Bacteriol 2003;185:2879–86.

43 Seidl K, Goerke C, Wolz C, Mack D, Berger-Bachi B, Bischoff M. *Staphylococcus aureus* CcpA affects biofilm formation. Infect Immun 2008;76:2044–50.

44 Frees D, Chastanet A, Qazi SN *et al*. Clp ATPases are required for stress tolerance, intracellular replication and biofilm formation in *Staphylococcus aureus*. Mol Microbiol 2004;54:1445–62.

45 Trotonda MP, Tamber S, Memmi G, Cheung AL. MgrA represses biofilm formation in *Staphylococcus aureus*. Infect Immun 2008;76:5645–54.

46 Latasa C, Solano C, Penadés JR, Lasa I. Biofilm-associated proteins. C R Biol 2006;329:849–57.

47 Cucarella C, Solano C, Valle J, Amorena B, Lasa I, Penades JR. Bap, a *Staphylococcus aureus* surface protein involved in biofilm formation. J Bacteriol 2001;183:2888–96.

48 Cucarella C, Tormo MA, Knecht E *et al*. Expression of the biofilm-associated protein interferes with host protein receptors of *Staphylococcus aureus* and alters the infective process. Infect Immun 2002;70:3180–6.

49 Cucarella C, Tormo MA, Ubeda C *et al*. Role of biofilm-associated protein *bap* in the pathogenesis of bovine *Staphylococcus aureus*. Infect Immun 2004;72:2177–85.

50 Trotonda MP, Manna AC, Cheung AL, Lasa I, Penades JR. SarA positively controls bap-dependent biofilm formation in *Staphylococcus aureus*. J Bacteriol 2005;187:5790–8.

51 Arrizubieta MJ, Toledo-Arana A, Amorena B, Penades JR, Lasa I. Calcium inhibits bap-dependent multicellular behavior in *Staphylococcus aureus*. J Bacteriol 2004;186:7490–8.

52 Kretsinger RH, Nockolds CE. Carp muscle calcium-binding protein. II. Structure determination and general description. J Biol Chem 1973;248:3313–26.

53 Schumacher-Perdreau F, Heilmann C, Peters G, Gotz F, Pulverer G. Comparaive analysis of a biofilm forming *Staphylococcus epidermidis* strain and its adhesion-positive, accumulation-negative isogenic mutant. FEMS Microbiol Lett 1994;117:71–8.

54 Hussain M, Herrmann M, von Eiff C, Perdreau-Remington F, Peters G. A 140-kilodalton extracellular protein is essential for the accumulation of *Staphylococcus epidermidis* strains on surfaces. Infect Immun 1997;65:519–24.

55 Sun D, Accavitti MA, Bryers JD. Inhibition of biofilm formation by monoclonal antibodies against *Staphylococcus epidermidis* RP62A accumulation-associated protein. Clin Diagn Lab Immunol 2005;12:93–100.

56 Roche FM, Meehan M, Foster TJ. The *Staphylococcus aureus* surfaces protein SasG and its homologues promote bacterial adherence to human desquamated nasal epithelial cells. Microbiology 2003;149:2759–67.

57 Kuroda M, Ito R, Tanaka Y *et al*. *Staphylococcus aureus* surface protein SasG contributes to intercellular autoaggregation of *Staphylococcus aureus*. Biochem Biophys Res Commun 2008; 377:1102–6.

58 Heilmann C, Hussain M, Peters G, Gotz F. Evidence for autolysin-mediated primary attachment of *Staphylococcus epidermidis* to polystyrene surface. Mol Microbiol 1997;24:1013–24.

59 Hell W, Meyer HG, Gaterman SG. Cloning of *aas*, a gene encoding a *Staphylococcus saprophyticus* surface protein with adhesive and autolytic properties. Mol Microbiol 1998;29:871–81.

60 van der Woude MW, Baumler AJ. Phase and antigenic variation in bacteria. Clin Microbiol Rev 2004;17:581–611.

61 Conlon KM, Humphreys H, O'Gara JP. Inactivations of *rsbU* and *sarA* by IS256 represent novel mechanisms of biofilm phenotypic variation in *Staphylococcus epidermidis*. J Bacteriol 2004;186:6208–19.

62 Tormo MA, Ubeda C, Marti M *et al*. Phase-variable expression of the biofilm-associated protein (Bap) in *Staphylococcus aureus*. Microbiology 2007;153:1702–10.

63 Ubeda C, Tormo MA, Cucarella C *et al*. Sip, an integrase protein with excision, circularization and integration activities, defines a new family of mobile *Staphylococcus aureus* pathogenicity islands. Mol Microbiol 2003;49:193–210.

64 Redfield RJ. Is quorum sensing a side effect of diffusion sensing? Trends Microbiol 2002;10:365–70.

65 Miller MB, Bassler BL. Quorum sensing in bacteria. Annu Rev Microbiol 2001;55:165–99.

66 Kong KF, Vuong C, Otto M. *Staphylococcus* quorum sensing in biofilm formation and infection. Int J Med Microbiol 2006;296:133–9.

67 Otto M, Sussmuth R, Jung G, Gotz F. Structure of the pheromone peptide of the *Staphylococcus epidermidis* agr system. FEBS Lett 1998;424:89–94.

68 Otto M. *Staphylococcus aureus* and *Staphylococcus epidermidis* peptide pheromones produced by the accessory gene regulator agr system. Peptides 2001;22:1603–8.

69 Novick RP, Muir TW. Virulence gene regulation by peptides in staphylococci and other gram-positive bacteria. Curr Opin Microbiol 1999;2:40–5.

70 Lina G, Jarraud S, Ji G *et al*. Transmembrane topology and histidine protein kinase activity of AgrC, the agr signal receptor in *Staphylococcus aureus*. Mol Microbiol 1998;28:655–62.

71 Janson L, Arvidson S. The role of the d-lysin (hld) in the regulation of virulence genes by the accessory gene regulator (agr) in *Staphylococcus aureus*. EMBO J 1990;9:1391–9.

72 Boisset S, Geissmann T, Huntzinger E *et al*. *Staphylococcus aureus* RNAIII coordinately represses the synthesis of virulence factors and the transcription regulator Rot by an antisense mechanism. Genes Dev 2007;21:1351–66.

73 Geisinger E, Adhikari RP, Jin R, Ross HF, Novick RP. Inhibition of *rot* translation by RNAIII, a key feature of *agr* function. Mol Microbiol 2006;61:1038–48.

74 Huntzinger E, Boisset S, Saveanu C *et al*. *Staphylococcus aureus* RNAIII and the endoribonuclease III coordinately regulate *spa* gene expression. EMBO J 2005;24:824–35.

75 Balaban N. Regulation of *Staphylococcus aureus* pathogenesis via target of RNAIII-activating peptide protein (TraP). J Biol Chem 2001;276:2658–67.

76 Adhikari RP, Arvidson S, Novick RP. A nonsense mutation in agrA accounts for the defect in agr expression and the avirulence of *Staphylococcus aureus* 8325-4 traP:kan. Infect Immun 2007;75:4534–50.

77 Tsang LH, Daily ST, Weiss EC, Smeltzer MS. Mutation of *traP* in *Staphylococcus aureus* has no impact on expression of *agr* or biofilm formation. Infect Immun 2007;75:4528–33.

78 Otto M. Quorum-sensing control in staphylococci: a target for antimicrobial drug therapy? FEMS Microbiol Lett 2004; 241:135–41.

79 Vuong C, Saenz HL, Gotz F, Otto M. Impact of the agr quorum-sensing system on adherence to polystyrene in *Staphylococcus aureus*. J Infect Dis 2000;182:1688–93.

80 Vuong C, Gerke C, Somerville GA, Fischer ER, Otto M. Quorum-sensing control of biofilm factors in *Staphylococcus epidermidis*. J Infect Dis 2003;188:706–18.

81 Vuong C, Kocianova S, Yao Y, Carmody AB, Otto M. Increased colonization of indwelling medical devices by quorum-sensing mutants of *Staphylococcus epidermidis* in vivo. J Infect Dis 2004;190:1498–505.

82 Yarwood JM, Bartels DJ, Volper EM, Greenberg EP. Quorum sensing in *Staphylococcus aureus* biofilms. J Bacteriol 2004;186:1838–50.

83 Coelho LR, Souza RR, Ferreira FA, Guimaraes MA, Ferreira-Carvalho BT, Figueiredo AM. agr RNAIII divergently regulates glucose-induced biofilm formation in clinical isolates of *Staphylococcus aureus*. Microbiology 2008;154:3480–90.

84 Winzer K, Hardie KR, Burgess N *et al*. LuxS: its role in central metabolism and the in vitro synthesis of 4-hydroxy-5-methyl-3(2H)-furanone. Microbiology 2002;148:909–22.

85 Xu L, Li H, Vuong C *et al*. Role of the luxS quorum-sensing system in biofilm formation and virulence of *Staphylococcus epidermidis*. Infect Immun 2006;74:488–96.

86 Doherty N, Holden MTG, Qazi SN, Williams P, Winzer K. Functional analysis of *luxS* in *Staphylococcus aureus* reveals a role in metabolism but not quorum sensing. Infect Immun 2006;188:2885–97.

87 Camilli A, Bassler BL. Bacterial small-molecule signaling pathways. Science 2006;311:1113–16.

88 Cotter PA, Stibitz S. c-di-GMP-mediated regulation of virulence and biofilm formation. Curr Opin Microbiol 2007;10: 17–23.

89 Tamayo R, Pratt JT, Camilli A. Roles of cyclic diguanylate in the regulation of bacterial pathogenesis. Annu Rev Microbiol 2007;61:131–48.

90 Tischler AD, Camilli A. Cyclic diguanylate (c-di-GMP) regulates *Vibrio cholerae* biofilm formation. Mol Microbiol 2004; 53:857–69.

91 Karaolis DK, Rashid MH, Chythanya R, Luo W, Hyodo M, Hayakawa Y. c-di-GMP (3′-5′-cyclic diguanylic acid) inhibits *Staphylococcus aureus* cell–cell interacterions and biofilm. Antimicrob Agents Chemother 2005;49:1029–38.

92 Brouillette E, Hyodo M, Hayakawa Y, Karaolis DK, Malouin F. 3′,5′-Cyclic diguanylic acid reduces the virulence of biofilm-forming *Staphylococcus aureus* strains in a mouse model of mastitis infection. Antimicrob Agents Chemother 2005;49:3109–13.

93 Lee VT, Matewish JM, Kessler JL, Hyodo M, Hayakawa Y. A cyclic-di-GMP receptor required for bacterial exopolysaccharide production. Mol Microbiol 2007;65:1474–84.

94 Karaolis DK, Means TK, Yand D *et al*. Bacterial c-di-GMP is an immunostimulatory molecule. J Immunol 2007;178:2171–81.

95 Resch A, Fehrenbacher B, Eisele K, Schaller M, Gotz F. Phage release from biofilm and planktonic *Staphylococcus aureus* cells. FEMS Microbiol Lett 2005;252:89–96.

96 Cerca N, Oliveira R, Azeredo J. Susceptibility of *Staphylococcus epidermidis* planktonic cells and biofilms to the lytic action of *Staphylococcus* bacteriophage K. Lett Appl Microbiol 2007; 45:313–17.

97 Summers WC. Bacteriophage therapy. Annu Rev Microbiol 2001;55:437–51.

98 Fishetti VA, Nelson D, Schuch R. Reinventing phage therapy: are the parts greater than the sum? Nat Biotechnol 2006; 24:1508–11.

99 Curtin JJ, Donlan RM. Using bacteriophages to reduce formation of catheter-associated biofilms by *Staphylococcus epidermidis*. Antimicrob Agents Chemother 2006;50:1268–75.

100 Leid JG, Shirtliff ME, Costerton JW, Stoodley AP. Human leukocytes adhere to, penetrate, and respond to *Staphylococcus aureus* biofilms. Infect Immun 2002;70:6339–45.

101 O'Toole GA, Stewart PS. Biofilms strike back. Nat Biotechnol 2005;23:1378–9.

102 Houari A, Di Martino P. Effect of chlorhexidine and benzalkonium chloride on bacterial biofilm formation. Lett Appl Microbiol 2007;45:652–6.

103 Fux CA, Costerton JW, Stewart PS, Stoodley P. Survival strategies of infectious biofilms. Trends Microbiol 2005;13:34–40.

104 Anderl JN, Franklin MJ, Stewart PS. Role of antibiotic penetration limitation in *Klebsiella pneumoniae* biofilm resistance to ampicillin and ciprofloxacin. Antimicrob Agents Chemother 2000;44:1818–24.

105 Raad I, Hanna H, Jiang Y *et al*. Comparative activities of daptomycin, linezolid, and tigecycline against catheter-related methicillin-resistant *Staphylococcus* bacteremic isolates embedded in biofilm. Antimicrob Agents Chemother 2007;51:1656–60.

106 Monzon M, Oteiza C, Leiva J, Lamata M, Amorena B. Biofilm testing of *Staphylococcus epidermidis* clinical isolates: low performance of vancomycin in relation to other antibiotics. Diagn Microbiol Infect Dis 2002;44:319–24.

107 Zheng Z, Stewart PS. Penetration of rifampin through *Staphylococcus epidermidis* biofilms. Antimicrob Agents Chemother 2002;46:900–3.

108 Stewart PS. Theoretical aspects of antibiotic diffusion into microbial biofilms. Antimicrob Agents Chemother 1996;40:2517–22.

109 Jefferson KK, Goldmann DA, Pier GB. Use of confocal microscopy to analyze the rate of vancomycin penetration through *Staphylococcus aureus* biofilms. Antimicrob Agents Chemother 2005;49:2467–73.

110 Bigger JW. Treatment of staphylococcal infections with penicillin. Lancet 1944;244:497–500.

111 Lewis K. Persister cells and the riddle of biofilm survival. Biochemistry (Mosc) 2005;70:267–74.

112 Keren I, Kaldalu N, Spoering A, Wang Y, Lewis K. Persister cells and tolerance to antimicrobials. FEMS Microbiol Lett 2004;230:13–18.

113 Lewis K. Persister cells, dormancy and infectious disease. Nat Rev Microbiol 2007;5:48–56.

114 De Kievit TR, Parkins MD, Gillis RJ *et al*. Multidrug efflux pumps: expression patterns and contribution to antibiotic resistance in *Pseudomonas aeruginosa* biofilms. Antimicrob Agents Chemother 2001;45:1761–70.

115 Vuong C, Voyich JM, Fischer ER *et al*. Polysaccharide intercellular adhesin (PIA) protects *Staphylococcus epidermidis* against major components of the human innate immune system. Cell Microbiol 2004;6:269–75.

116 Cerca N, Jefferson KK, Oliveira R, Pier GB, Azeredo J. Comparative antibody-mediated phagocytosis of *Staphylococcus epidermidis* cells grown in a biofilm or in the planktonic state. Infect Immun 2006;74:4849–55.

117 Begun J, Gaiani JM, Rohde H *et al*. Staphylococcal biofilm exopolysaccharide protects against *Caenorhabditis elegans* immune defenses. PLoS Pathog 2007;3:e57.

118 Balaban N, Gov Y, Bitler A, Boelaert JR. Prevention of *Staphylococcus aureus* biofilm on dialysis catheters and adherence to human cells. Kidney Int 2003;63:340–5.

119 Balaban N, Giacometti A, Cirioni O *et al*. Use of the quorum-sensing inhibitor RNAIII-inhibiting peptide to prevent biofilm formation in vivo by drug-resistant *Staphylococcus epidermidis*. J Infect Dis 2003;187:625–30.

120 Balaban N, Stoodley P, Fux CA, Wilson S, Costerton JW, Dell'Acqua G. Prevention of staphylococcal biofilm-associated infections by the quorum sensing inhibitor RIP. Clin Orthop Relat Res 2005;(437):48–54.

121 Baveja JK, Willcox MD, Hume EB, Kumar N, Odell R, Poole-Warren LA. Furanones as potential anti-bacterial coatings on biomaterials. Biomaterials 2004;25:5003–12.

122 Raad I, Hanna H, Dvorak T, Chaiban G, Hachem R. Optimal antimicrobial catheter lock solution, using different combinations of minocycline, EDTA, and 25-percent ethanol, rapidly eradicates organisms embedded in biofilm. Antimicrob Agents Chemother 2007;51:78–83.

123 Donelli G, Francolini I, Romoli D *et al*. Synergistic activity of dispersin B and cefamandole nafate in inhibition of staphylococcal biofilm growth on polyurethanes. Antimicrob Agents Chemother 2007;51:2733–40.

124 Wu JA, Kusuma C, Mond JJ, Kokai-Kun JF. Lysostaphin disrupts *Staphylococcus aureus* and *Staphylococcus epidermidis* biofilms on artificial surfaces. Antimicrob Agents Chemother 2003;47:3407–14.

125 Samuelsen O, Haukland HH, Kahl B *et al*. *Staphylococcus aureus* small colony variants are resistant to the antimicrobial peptide lactoferricin B. J Antimicrob Chemother 2005;56:1126–9.

126 Hoffman LR, D'Argenio DA, MacCoss MJ, Zhang A, Jones RA, Miller SI. Aminoglycoside antibiotics induce bacterial biofilm formation. Nature 2005;436:1171–5.

127 Deziel E, Comeau Y, Villemur R. Initiation of biofilm formation by *Pseudomonas aeruginosa* 57RP correlates with emergence of hyperpiliated and highly adherent phenotypic variants deficient in swimming, swarming, and twitching motilities. J Bacteriol 2001;183:1195–204.
128 Haussler S. Biofilm formation by the small colony variant phenotype of *Pseudomonas aeruginosa*. Environ Microbiol 2004;6:546–51.
129 Neut D, Van Der Mei HC, Bulstra SK, Busscher HJ. The role of small colony variants in failure to diagnose and treat biofilm infections in orthopedics. Acta Orthop 2007;78:299.
130 Proctor RA, von Eiff C, Kahl BC *et al*. Small colony variants: a pathogenic form of bacteria that facilitates persistent and recurrent infections. Nat Rev Microbiol 2006;4:295–305.
131 von Eiff C, Peters G, Becker K. The small colony variant (SCV) concept: the role of staphylococcal SCVs in persistent infections. Injury 2006;37:S26–S33.
132 Eisenberg P. Untersuchungen uber die variablen Typhusstamm (Bacterium typhi mutabile), sowie uber eine eigentumliche hemmende Wirkung des gewohnlichen Agar, verursacht durch Autoklavierung, abstr. 56. Zentbl Bakteriol Abt 1910;1:208.
133 Swingle EL. Studies on small colony variants of *Staphylococcus aureus*. J Bacteriol 1935;29:467–89.
134 Kahl B, Herrmann M, Everding AS *et al*. Persistent infection with small colony variant strains of *Staphylococcus aureus* in patients with cystic fibrosis. J Infect Dis 1998;177:1023–9.
135 Besier S, Smaczny C, von Mallinckrodt C *et al*. Prevalence and clinical significance of *Staphylococcus aureus* small-colony variants in cystic fibrosis lung disease. J Clin Microbiol 2007;45:168–72.
136 Chatterjee I, Kriegeskorte A, Fischer A *et al*. *In vivo* mutations of thymidylate synthase (*thyA*) are responsible for thymidine dependency in clinical small colony variants (TD-SCVs) of *Staphylococcus aureus*. J Bacteriol 2008;190:834–42.
137 Besier S, Ludwig A, Ohlsen K, Brade V, Wichelhaus TA. Molecular analysis of the thymidine-auxotrophic small colony variant phenotype of *Staphylococcus aureus*. Int J Med Microbiol 2007;297:217–25.
138 Saxild HH, Anderon LN, Hammer K. *dra-nupC-pdp* operon of *Bacillus subtilis*: nucleotide sequence, induction by deoxyribonucleosides, and transcriptional regulation by the *deoR*-encoded DeoR repressor protein. J Bacteriol 1996;178:424–34.
139 Schaaff F, Bierbaum G, Baumert N, Bartmann P, Sahl H-G. Mutations are involved in emergence of aminoglycoside-induced small colony variants of *Staphylococcus aureus*. Int J Med Microbiol 2003;293:427–35.
140 Proctor RA, van Langevelde P, Kristjansson M, Maslow JN, Arbeit RD. Persistant and relapsing infections associated with small-colony variants of *Staphylococcus aureus*. Clin Infect Dis 1995;20:95–102.
141 Balwit JM, van Langevelde P, Vann JM, Proctor RA. Gentamicin-resistant menadione and hemin auxotrophic *Staphylococcus aureus* persist within cultured endothelial cells. J Infect Dis 1994;170:1033–7.
142 Vesga O, Groeschel MC, Otten MF, Brar DW, Vann JM, Proctor RA. *Staphylococcus aureus* small colony variants are induced by the endothelial cell intracellular milieu. J Infect Dis 1996; 173:739–42.
143 von Eiff C, Heilmann C, Proctor RA, Woltz C, Peters G, Gotz F. A site-directed *Staphylococcus aureus hemB* mutant is a small-colony variant which persists intracellularly. J Bacteriol 1997; 179:4706–12.
144 von Eiff C, Becker K, Metze D *et al*. Intracellular persistence of *Staphylococcus aureus* small-colony variants within keratinocytes: a cause for antibiotic treatment failure in a patient with Darier's disease. Clin Infect Dis 2001;32:1643–7.
145 Vaudaux P, Francois P, Bisognano C *et al*. Increased expression of clumping factor and fibronectin-binding proteins by hemB mutants of *Staphylococcus aureus* expressing small colony variant phenotypes. Infect Immun 2002;70:5428–37.
146 Brouillette E, Martinez A, Boyll BJ, Allen NE, Malouin F. Persistence of a *Staphylococcus aureus* small-colony variant under antibiotic pressure in vivo. FEMS Immunol Med Microbiol 2004;41:35–41.
147 Senn MM, Bischoff M, von Eiff C, Berger-Bachi B. s^B activity in a *Staphylococcus aureus hemB* mutant. J Bacteriol 2005; 187:7397–406.
148 Moisan H, Brouillette E, Jacob CL, Langlois-Begin P, Michaud S, Malouin F. Transcription of virulence factors in *Staphylococcus aureus* small-colony variants isolated from cystic fibrosis patients is influenced by SigB. J Bacteriol 2006;188:64–76.
149 Malouin F, Brouillette E, Martinez RM *et al*. Identification of antimicrobial compounds active against intracellular *Staphylococcus aureus*. FEMS Immunol Med Microbiol 2005;45:245–52.
150 Miller MM, Wexler MA, Steigbigel NH. Single and combination antibiotic therapy of *Staphylococcus aureus* experimental endocarditis: emergence of gentamicin-resistant mutants. Antimicrob Agents Chemother 1978;14:336–43.
151 Pelleter LL Jr, Richardson M, Feist M. Virulent gentamicin-induced small colony variants of *Staphylococcus aureus*. J Lab Clin Med 1979;94:324–34.
152 Bulger RJ, Bulger RE. Ultrastructure of small colony variants of a methicillin-resistant *Staphylococcus aureus*. J Bacteriol 1969; 94:1244–6.
153 Bulger RJ. In vitro studies on highly resistant small colony variants of *Staphylococcus aureus* resistant to methicillin. J Infect Dis 1969;120:491–4.
154 Adler H, Widmer A, Frei R. Emergence of a teicoplanin-resistant small colony variant of *Staphylococcus epidermidis* during vancomycin therapy. Eur J Clin Microbiol Infect Dis 2003;22:746–8.
155 Seaman PF, Ochs D, Day MJ. Small-colony variants: a novel mechanism for triclosan resistance in methicillin-resistant *Staphylococcus aureus*. J Antimicrob Chemother 2007;59:43–50.
156 Bayston R, Ashraf W, Smith S. Triclosan resistance in methicillin-resistant *Staphylococcus aureus* expressed as small colony variants: a novel mode of evasion of susceptibility to antiseptics. J Antimicrob Chemother 2007;59:848–53.
157 Mitsuyama J, Yamada H, Maehana J *et al*. Characteristics of quinolone-induced small colony variants in *Staphylococcus aureus*. J Antimicrob Chemother 1997;39:697–705.
158 Kahl B, Belling G, Becker P *et al*. Thymidine-dependent *Staphylococcus aureus* small-colony variants are associated with extensive alterations in regulator and virulence gene expression profiles. Infect Immun 2005;73:4119–26.

Chapter 6
Exotoxins

Patrick M. Schlievert[1], *John K. McCormick*[2], *Gregory A. Bohach*[3] *and Douglas H. Ohlendorf*[4]

[1] Department of Microbiology, University of Minnesota, Minneapolis, Minnesota, USA
[2] Department of Microbiology, University of Western Ontario, London, Ontario, Canada
[3] Department of Microbiology, Molecular Biology, and Biochemistry, University of Idaho, Moscow, Idaho, USA
[4] Department of Biochemistry, Molecular Biology, and Biophysics, University of Minnesota, Minneapolis, Minnesota, USA

Introduction

Staphylococcus aureus is a highly versatile organism in its ability to cause human diseases that range from mild skin furuncles to life-threatening toxic shock syndromes. This pathogenic capacity results from production of a myriad of cell-surface and secreted virulence factors. These virulence determinants can be categorized into (i) superantigen exotoxins that act systemically to alter normal immune function dramatically, (ii) cytotoxic exotoxins that act locally to provide nutrients and disrupt immune function of host cells that have withstood superantigen immune alteration, and (iii) antiphagocytic microbial surface-associated virulence factors that provide the last line of microbial defense against the host immune response. While the second group of exotoxins, the cytotoxins and enzymes (comprising α-hemolysin, β-hemolysin, γ-hemolysin, δ-hemolysin, nucleases, proteases, lipases, hyaluronidase, and collagenase), are made by all or nearly all strains of *S. aureus*, the first group of exotoxins typically lack enzymatic function and are variable traits, made by some strains but not others. These proteins include the superantigens toxic shock syndrome toxin (TSST)-1, staphylococcal enterotoxins, and staphylococcal enterotoxin-like proteins; exfoliative toxins; and Panton–Valentine leukocidin (PVL). This chapter reviews the structure and function of several of the staphylococcal exoproteins, specifically the superantigens, exfoliative toxins, hemolysins, and PVL.

Superantigens

Introduction and biological activities

The superantigen family of proteins comprises true exotoxins that include staphylococcal TSST-1; staphylococcal enterotoxin serotypes SEA, SEB, SEC*n*, SED, SEE, SEG, and SEI; staphylococcal enterotoxin-like serotypes SEl-H and SEl-J to SEl-V; and the streptococcal pyrogenic exotoxins (SPEs) synthesized by group A *Streptococcus* strains and certain other β-hemolytic streptococci [1]. The superantigen SEF was renamed TSST-1 and therefore the SEF serotype has been retired [2]. These toxins are all characterized by their shared capacities to induce high fever, enhance host susceptibility to the lethal effects of endotoxin, and induce T-lymphocyte proliferation as superantigens [1,3]. All share the ability to cause serious life-threatening toxic shock syndromes and related illnesses. The staphylococcal enterotoxins possess the additional property, not shared with other members of the family, of causing emesis when given orally to monkeys [4]. Thus, staphylococcal enterotoxins are major causes of food poisoning, characterized by vomiting and diarrhea with onset 2–8 hours after ingestion of preformed toxin in contaminated food. The staphylococcal enterotoxin-like proteins are related to staphylococcal enterotoxins in both primary amino acid sequence and three-dimensional structure, but the staphylococcal enterotoxin-like proteins either lack emetic activity or have not been tested [5]. Table 6.1 summarizes the biological activities of these toxins.

Figure 6.1 summarizes three probable mechanisms by which superantigens contribute to hypotension, the most serious symptom of toxic shock syndrome and related illnesses. First, the toxins are potent T-lymphocyte superantigens, based on their shared but unusual mechanism of action [3]. The mechanism of T-lymphocyte stimulation differs from typical antigen activation in three important ways. Superantigens do not require proteolytic processing by antigen-presenting cells (APCs), in contrast to processing that is required for typical antigenic peptide presentation. Superantigens bind directly to invariant regions on major histocompatibility complex (MHC) class II molecules displayed on the surface of APCs. The toxins have the ability to bind to a wide variety of these molecules, although there is some preference depending on the superantigen involved. Finally, the superantigens stimulate

Staphylococci in Human Disease, 2nd edition. Edited by Kent B. Crossley, Kimberly K. Jefferson, Gordon Archer, Vance G. Fowler, Jr.
 ISBN 978-14051-6332-3.

Table 6.1 Shared biological activities of superantigens.[1]

Pyrogenicity through interleukin (IL)-1β
Enhancement of host susceptibility to lethal endotoxin shock via tumor necrosis factor (TNF)-α resulting in capillary leak and hypotension
T-lymphocyte superantigenicity resulting in cytokine production with:
Capillary leak and hypotension
B-lymphocyte immunosuppression (failure to develop neutralizing antibodies on recovery from disease)
Rash formation (possibly due to IL-2 and interferon γ)
Direct effects on endothelial cells resulting in capillary leak and hypotension
Direct effects on epithelial cells resulting in cytokine production resulting in mucosal permeability

[1] Staphylococcal enterotoxins have the unique property of being emetic.

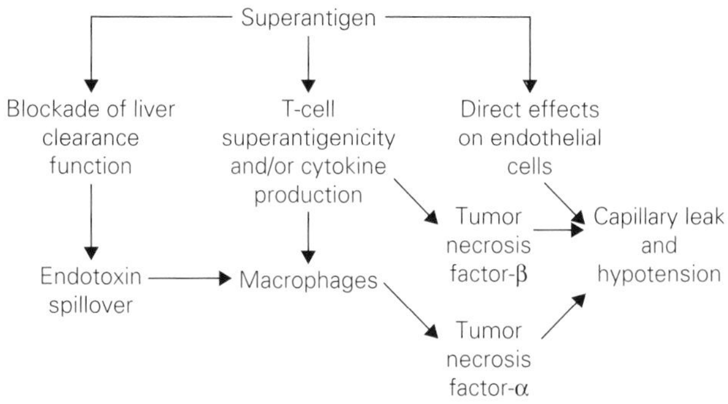

Figure 6.1 Model for the production of superantigen-induced hypotension and shock in toxic shock syndrome.

T-lymphocyte proliferation without regard to the antigenic specificity of the T-lymphocyte, but rather only as a function of the composition of the variable part of the β-chain (Vβ) of the T-cell receptor (TCR) complex (Vβ-TCR) [1,3,6]. Typically, an antigenic peptide stimulates approximately 1 in 10 000 T lymphocytes after specific interaction of the antigenic peptide–class II MHC complex with both the α- and β-chains of the TCR. In contrast, superantigens such as TSST-1, which stimulates all human T lymphocytes bearing Vβ2, may activate up to 20% or more of all T cells [7]. The consequence of an interaction between an APC and a T lymphocyte, whether it involves a typical antigen or a superantigen, is activation of the same signal transduction pathways that ultimately lead to interleukin (IL)-2 production and cell division. In addition, superantigens are also capable of utilizing an alternative T-lymphocyte activation pathway, different from the canonical T-cell activation pathway, such that in the absence of the Src family kinase Lck, superantigens activate T lymphocytes through a $G_{\alpha 11}$, phospholipase Cβ-dependent pathway [8]. This alternative pathway converges with the conventional pathway at the level of ERK-1/2 activation. Differences between antigenic peptide stimulation and superantigenic activation of T lymphocytes is also one of magnitude, with antigenic peptides causing controlled cytokine release while superantigens lead to massive release of cytokines. The mechanism of T-lymphocyte stimulation by superantigens is summarized in Figure 6.2.

The massive T-lymphocyte proliferation induced by superantigens results in the release of high levels of a variety of cytokines from both macrophages and Th1 lymphocytes, with major systemic effects [1,3,6]. These include IL-1β and tumor necrosis factor (TNF)-α from macrophages and TNF-β, IL-2 and interferon (IFN)-γ from Th1 cells. Importantly, although interaction of Th1 lymphocytes with macrophages is critical for maximal cytokine production by both cell types, Th1 lymphocyte proliferation is not required. This explains why some studies have observed that T-cell proliferation is not required for development of toxic shock syndrome in animal model systems [9]. All these important cytokines have deleterious effects on the host when present in high concentrations, including the production of the most serious consequence of toxic shock syndromes and related illnesses, as well as hypotension through capillary leakage. It is noteworthy

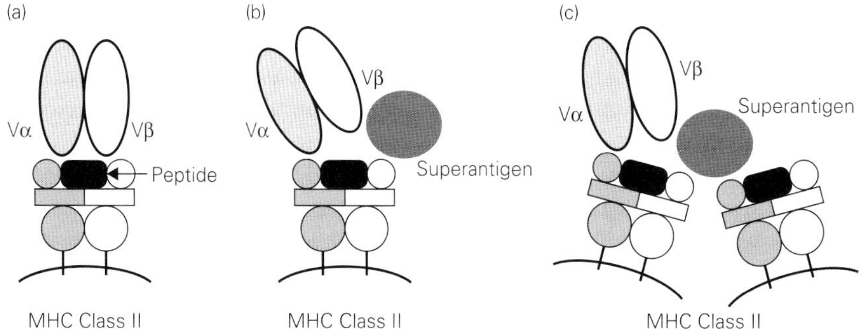

Figure 6.2 (a) Interaction of a typical antigenic peptide with major histocompatibility complex (MHC) class II molecules on antigen-presenting cells and the T-cell receptor α- and β-chains compared with the interaction of superantigens with MHC class II and T-cell receptor. (b) Some superantigens, such as TSST-1, SEB and SEC, interact with the α-chain of MHC II and the β-chain of the T-cell receptor. (c) Other superantigens, such as SEA, may interact with either the α-chain or β-chain of MHC II and the β-chain of the T-cell receptor. In those instances where the superantigen interacts with the β-chain of MHC II and the β-chain of the T-cell receptor, the superantigen lies across the antigenic peptide contact area, and as much as one-third of the MHC II contact may be with the antigenic peptide.

that host skin exposure to superantigens in many individuals leads to local atopic dermatitis reactions [10,11]; in others systemic exposure leads to extremely severe anaphylaxis-related toxic shock syndromes. These type I hypersensitivity effects likely result from overactivation (via exacerbated Blymphocyte help) from Th2 lymphocyte activation.

The second major property of superantigens that appears to be an important contributory factor to hypotension in toxic shock syndromes is their ability to enhance susceptibility to lethal endotoxin shock by up to 1 million-fold [12]. For example, pretreatment of rabbits with a bolus injection of 50 μg/kg of TSST-1 renders the animals susceptible to the lethal effects of 0.01 μg/kg endotoxin. It is our experience that rabbits can be administered more than 1 mg/kg of TSST-1 in a single intravenous injection without lethality. The LD_{50} of endotoxin in rabbits is approximately 500 μg/kg. Thus, the above combination treatment with TSST-1 and endotoxin represents a 50 000-fold enhancement of susceptibility to endotoxin.

The mechanism underlying the endotoxin enhancement phenomenon remains to be elucidated but appears to involve superantigen interference with both liver clearance function and interaction in the liver between T lymphocytes and macrophages (Kupffer cells) [12]. It is well known that many agents that interfere with liver function, such as cycloheximide, actinomycin D, lead, $CC1_4$, α-amanitin, hepatitis virus, and ethanol, greatly amplify susceptibility to the lethal effects of endotoxin. In this regard, superantigens have been shown to inhibit RNA synthesis in isolated liver cells and their nuclei [13]. All species of RNA were inhibited by the toxins, and the nuclei from superantigen-treated rabbits were significantly less dense than nuclei from untreated controls. The capacity of superantigens to amplify the lethal effects of endotoxin parallels that of α-amanitin, which also interferes with RNA synthesis [14] in that pretreatment with superantigen or α-amanitin for approximately 2 hours is required before administration of endotoxin [13]. Whether superantigen blockade of RNA synthesis is the primary effect amplifying susceptibility to endotoxin is unclear. It has been proposed that blockade of liver function permits endotoxin "spillover" into the circulation, which also contributes to TNF-α release, with consequent production of capillary leak and hypotension. The source of endotoxin may be either gut or vagina, or other body sites [15]. It is noteworthy that mammalian species which are susceptible to the toxic shock syndrome-inducing effects of superantigens, such as humans, chimpanzees and rabbits, have gut flora with large numbers of facultative Gram-negative rods, whereas mammalian species that are highly resistant, such as rodents and monkeys, have gut flora with very few facultative Gram-negative rods. Lastly, rabbits less than 8 months of age are highly resistant to single-bolus injections of superantigens (milligram quantities), but animals older than about 8 months become highly susceptible (microgram quantities). This change in susceptibility is independent of sexual maturity, but rather coincides with the time that rabbits become a thousand times more susceptible to endotoxin shock.

The role of the endotoxin enhancement phenomenon in human toxic shock syndromes remains debatable. However, the effect is by far the most dramatic activity of superantigens in experimental animals, with individuals succumbing within only a few hours after treatment. A study has shown that the endotoxin enhancement phenomenon results from the synergistic action of superantigen and endotoxin on TNF-α production by macrophages [16]. It is also noteworthy that laboratory accidents suggest that the lethal dose of endotoxin in humans may be 1–2 μg [17]. The amplification effect of superantigens could reduce the lethal amount of endotoxin in humans into the picogram range.

The third effect of superantigens that may contribute to lethality is direct effects on endothelial cells. TSST-1 has been shown to bind to human and porcine endothelial cells [18,19]. Furthermore, the toxin is cytotoxic for porcine endothelial cells, and at lower toxin concentrations causes leakage across endothelial cell monolayers without causing significant toxicity.

A final shared biological property of all superantigens is their ability to cause toxic shock syndromes in animals [20,21]. This has also been observed in studies of disease in humans, clearly demonstrating the ability of superantigens to cause toxic shock syndrome and related illnesses [1,22]. These effects can be neutralized by antitoxin antibodies [23,24]. Although superantigens are not particularly toxic to young adult rabbits when given in single-bolus injections, the toxins are highly lethal to these rabbits when administered continuously over a period of 1 week [21]. Thus, the LD_{50} of TSST-1 in young 1–2 kg adult rabbits is approximately 75 μg when that total 75 μg is given over a period of 1 week (in contrast to greater than 1 mg/kg in a single injection). Furthermore, in our experience multiple superantigens administered together are more toxic than any one superantigen alone, even when matched for dose. Animals exposed to superantigens develop the clinical signs of toxic shock syndrome, with the exception of rash. Experience indicates that animals treated with toxins in this way die in two major groups: one group on days 1–2 and another group on days 4–5. The early group is hypothesized to succumb as a result of direct effects of the toxins on the endothelium or as a result of endotoxin enhancement. The latter group probably succumbs as a result of superantigenicity combined with the other two effects.

Some superantigens have unique biological effects. For example, staphylococcal enterotoxins induce emesis when given orally to monkeys [4]. TSST-1, staphylococcal enterotoxin-like proteins, and SPEs do not. SPEs induce highly significant myocardial necrosis [25], although the majority of superantigens likely induce lethality dependent on direct or indirect effects on the heart. TSST-1 has also been shown to amplify the lethal effects of endotoxin for renal tubular cells [26]. In addition, SPE-A is toxic to immune cells in the presence of endotoxin and binds tightly to endotoxin [27]. These latter two effects have not been assessed for other superantigens. The remainder of the discussion of superantigens focuses on recent structure–function studies.

Structure–function studies

Staphylococcal and streptococcal superantigens fall into five major subfamilies of proteins, based on amino acid sequence similarities and unique structural features. These subfamilies are categorized in Table 6.2 and form the basis for this discussion. Much of the discussion will focus on TSST-1, but comparisons of other superantigens with TSST-1 are also highlighted.

Biology and biochemistry of TSST-1

TSST-1 is proposed to form a separate group (group I) due to the weak homology within the overall superantigen family, the unique peptide dependence of the low-affinity MHC II binding domain, and an altered Vβ-TCR binding domain [1,28]. TSST-1 does not contain a high-affinity MHC II binding domain unlike that found in groups III, IV and V (discussed below). TSST-1, along with SEB and SEC (both members of the group II subfamily), are considered to be the principal causes of human toxic shock syndrome and related illnesses [1].

Toxic shock syndrome is a staphylococcal illness characterized by acute onset of high fever, diffuse erythematous rash, desquamation of the skin 1–2 weeks after onset (if not fatal), hypotension, and involvement of three or more organ systems [1]. The syndrome was first reported by Todd *et al.* [29] in 1978 as a major systemic illness associated with noninvasive *S. aureus* colonization of mucosal surfaces and was designated "toxic shock syndrome" by these investigators. During the 1980s an epidemic of toxic shock syndrome was described among young women who were using tampons, particularly those of higher absorbency [30–32].

The illness was initially associated with the presence of toxigenic *S. aureus* strains, primarily of phage group I, localized to cervical or vaginal colonization [29]. TSST-1 was the first toxin shown to be involved in toxic shock syndrome and today is accepted as the cause of approximately 75% of all cases [33,34]. The toxin was identified and characterized as a new *S. aureus* exotoxin in 1981 by the independent investigations of Bergdoll *et al.* [33] and Schlievert *et al.* [34]. TSST-1 is produced by nearly all the *S. aureus* strains isolated from vaginal or cervical cultures in cases of menstruation-associated toxic shock syndrome, and by approximately 50% of *S. aureus* isolates obtained from other body sites in nonmenstrual cases of toxic shock syndrome [35–37]. Coagulase-negative staphylococci do not produce TSST-1 [38]. The toxin is encoded by the gene *tstH* (where H refers to human isolate) and is encoded on a pathogenicity island [39]. TSST-1 is translated as a protein that consists of 234 residues of which the first 40 amino acids comprise a signal peptide [40–42]. Like many other *S. aureus* exotoxins, TSST-1 is made primarily during the postexponential phase of growth [43,44]. The mature secreted protein is a single polypeptide chain with a molecular mass of 22 kDa and an isoelectric point (pI) of 7.2. The protein occurs as two forms, differing slightly in pI (attributed to microheterogeneity), but having the same biochemical properties and encoded by a single gene [40,41]. Despite its functional relatedness to other superantigens, TSST-1 shares relatively weak primary sequence similarity and does not share antibody-binding epitopes with other superantigens. The toxin contains no cysteines, has a high percentage of hydrophobic amino acids, and is generally resistant to heat and proteolysis. For example, the protein can be heated to 100°C for more than 1 hour without demonstrable loss of biological activity [40,41]. Similarly, the toxin is not susceptible to trypsin, despite the presence of many lysine and arginine residues [45].

Table 6.2 Subfamily groups of staphylococcal and streptococcal superantigens with structural characteristics that define the groups.

Superantigen group	Prototype	Low-affinity MHC II	Zn^{2+}-dependent high-affinity MHC II	Emesis cystine loop	15-Amino-acid insert
I	TSST-1	Present	Absent	Absent	Absent
II	SEB	Present	Absent	Present; cysteines separated by 10–19 amino acids	Absent
III	SEA	Present	Present	Present; cysteines separated by 9 amino acids	Absent
IV	SPE-C	Present	Present	Absent	Absent
V	SEI-Q	Present	Present	Absent	Present

MHC, major histocompatibility complex; SE, staphylococcal enterotoxin; SEI, staphylococcal enterotoxin-like; SPE, streptococcal pyrogenic exotoxin; TSST-1, toxic shock syndrome toxin 1.

Production of TSST-1 and other postexponential-phase virulence factors of *S. aureus* is positively and negatively regulated by multiple global regulatory systems.

- Accessory gene regulator (*agr*): pleiotropic effects; exotoxin production generally upregulated and cell surface factors downregulated [43,46,47].
- Staphylococcal accessory element R/S (*saeR-saeS*): virulence factors generally upregulated; downstream of *agr* [48–51].
- Staphylococcal accessory regulator (*sar*): pleiotropic effects; required for full expression of *agr*, but independently represses production of some exotoxins [52–69].
- Staphylococcal respiratory response A/B (*srrA-srrB*): master switch repressor of exotoxins under low pH, low oxygen, and high glucose [70–72]; upstream of *agr*.
- Repressor of toxin (*rot*): primarily a repressor of exotoxins [73].
- Arl R/S (*arlR-arlS*): exhibits pleiotropic effects on virulence factors [74].
- Multiple gene regulator (*mgrA*): pleiotropic effects on virulence factors [75].
- *svrA*: primarily upregulates *agr* and exotoxin production [76].

There are other global regulators, including sigma factors, that participate in regulation of exotoxin production, but the above groups form many of the major regulatory systems. The *srrA-srrB*, *agr*, and *sar* systems are discussed below in more detail. Readers are referred to other excellent reviews for more complete discussions of these global regulatory systems.

We refer to Srr as the "master switch" regulator of exotoxin production. SrrA-SrrB is a typical two-component system comprising a plasma membrane-spanning histidine kinase (SrrB) and a phosphorylated response regulator (SrrA) that binds DNA promoter regions to affect gene function. SrrA-SrrB appears to function as an O_2/CO_2 and pH sensing system that represses production of TSST-1, other superantigens, and all other exotoxins under low oxygen and low pH conditions [70–72]. It appears that the role of tampons in association with menstrual toxic shock syndrome is to introduce oxygen to a typically anaerobic vaginal environment, with derepression of TSST-1 production through inactivation of Srr. Interestingly, a recent study suggested that TSST-1 is not produced by *S. aureus* in the presence of blood [77]. This finding is counterintuitive, given the association of toxic shock syndrome with menstruation and tampon use. The study showed that TSST-1 is produced by *S. aureus* growing in parts of tampons that do not contain menses. The lack of TSST-1 production in blood appeared dependent on the interaction of SrrA-SrrB with the α- and β-globin chains of hemoglobin (acting as corepressors), and suggested that *S. aureus* may be sequestered from blood (e.g., by residence on mucosal surfaces or within walled-off abscesses) during superantigen production leading to toxic shock syndrome [77].

The *agr* system, which is described in greater detail in Chapter 4, positively regulates secreted postexponential phase-produced exotoxins but negatively regulates cell surface-associated virulence factors [43,44]. The genes for *agr* include *agrA*, *agrB*, *agrC*, *agrD*, and the gene for δ-hemolysin (*hld*) [43,44,78]. Like Srr, *agr* contains a two-component regulatory system, with *agrC* encoding a sensor histidine kinase and *agr*A encoding the transcription activator (response regulator). Two major transcripts are produced, one designated RNAII (*agrBDCA*) and the second RNAIII (*hld*). The products of *agrB* and *agrD* together constitute a quorum-sensing system, with *agrD* encoding the autoinducing peptide (AIP) that is processed and secreted by AgrB. The AIP interacts with the AgrC histidine kinase leading to expression of the transcript RNAIII, which consists of 514 nucleotides and acts primarily to initiate transcription of virulence factors in postexponential phase.

Exotoxins regulated by *agr* are either not produced or are significantly reduced in *agr*-defective mutants. RNAIII encodes the exotoxin δ-hemolysin and therefore expression of δ-hemolysin is dependent on an intact *agr* system; however, it is the RNAIII transcript itself and not the δ-hemolysin protein that exerts a regulatory function. Production of α-hemolysin and TSST-1 are also strictly dependent on the *agr* system [78]. These toxins are produced in high amounts in *agr*-positive strains and but in only minimal amounts in *agr*-negative mutants (referred to as class I toxins). β-Toxin (hemolysin), enterotoxins B and C, exfoliative toxin A, and group A SPE-A (when cloned into *S. aureus*) appear to be less dependent on *agr* in that these proteins are made in high amounts in *agr*-positive strains and in moderate amounts in *agr*-negative mutants (referred to as class II toxins). Enterotoxin A appears to be made independent of *agr* in some strains; in other strains it appears to be a class II toxin. Class III proteins include protein A, coagulase, and fibronectin-binding proteins, which are produced in high amounts in *agr*-negative mutants but in low amounts in *agr*-positive strains.

The global regulator *sarA* also appears to regulate exotoxin production positively in that mutations in this locus result in reduced mRNA for exotoxins. The locus appears to regulate levels of RNAII and RNAIII but it also has *agr*-independent effects [79]. SarA has a molecular mass of approximately 15 kDa and is clearly a DNA-binding protein that interacts directly with the promoters of *agr* and certain virulence factors. SarT, another member of a family of transcription factors with homology to SarA, represses transcription of the secreted virulence factor α-hemolysin.

Highly purified TSST-1 has been obtained from cultures of *S. aureus* by the use of several published protocols [33,42]. Since toxin production is subject to catabolite repression in high concentrations of glucose, producing strains, such as MN8, FRI1169 or RN4220 (pCE107), are grown to stationary phase in complex media containing animal protein and only low levels of glucose, such as dialyzable beef heart medium [1,42]. Toxin is produced across a pH range of 6.5–8.0, at temperatures of 37–40°C, with increased production reported at 40°C, and under aerobic (but not anaerobic) conditions [42,80]. We find the simplest method to prepare highly purified toxin includes precipitation of cultures (including cells) with four volumes of ethanol, resolubilization in pyrogen-free water, and separation by preparative isoelectric focusing in a pH gradient of 3–10 and then 6–8. Thus purified, TSST-1 is homogeneous when tested by sodium dodecyl sulfate-polyacrylamide gel electrophoresis (SDS-PAGE) and protein sequencing. Furthermore, the toxin yields diffraction-quality crystals that have led to the solution of the three-dimensional structure [81,82]. Yields of 10–20 mg/L from strain RN4220 (pCE107) are achievable by this method. Other methods of TSST-1 purification have employed ion-exchange and gel-filtration chromatography techniques, as well as recombinant expression from *Escherichia coli.*

TSST-1 is a member of the large family of superantigens that also includes staphylococcal enterotoxins, staphylococcal enterotoxin-like proteins, and SPEs [1,3]. The lack of sequence and serological similarity between TSST-1 and other superantigens has not been predictive of structural similarity. The crystal structure of TSST-1 is representative of the prototypical structure observed in each superantigen, for most of which structural data are available [1,81,82]. It is noteworthy that all superantigens share 13 amino acids that are positioned identically in three-dimensional space, allowing the molecules to be folded with relatively great accuracy by first positioning those residues [28]. TSST-1 is folded into two closely associated domains, as illustrated in the ribbon diagram shown in Plate 6.1.

Domain A (residues 1–17 and 90–194) contains a five-strand β-sheet surrounding a long central α-helix (residues 125–140), which approaches a short N-terminal α-helix near the top of domain A. Domain B (residues 18–89) is folded into a barrel motif composed of five β-strands (referred to as O/B fold for oligosaccharide-oligonucleotide-binding fold). As viewed from the front in the TSST-1 ribbon diagram, the central α-helix forms the base of two major grooves, referred to as the frontside and backside grooves. The N-terminal α-helix and loops located on opposite sides of the central α-helix define the walls of these grooves. The backside groove of TSST-1 is larger and more exposed to the external environment than the frontside groove. TSST-1 and other superantigens appear to have arisen from the merging of two major protein folds: domain A, a β-grasp domain that is present in Fc immunoglobulin-binding proteins; and O/B fold, present in many other exotoxins [28]. No enzymatic activity has been associated with superantigens.

Highly detailed pictures of the interaction between TSST-1 and MHC molecules and Vβ2-TCR have come from the published crystal structure of TSST-1 complexed with HLA-DRI and Vβ2-TCR (see Plate 6.2) [83]. In agreement with other lines of evidence, including mutational analysis, residues within the β-barrel structure of domain B bind primarily to the α-chain of HLA-DR1 [84]. Unexpectedly, however, interactions between TSST-1 and the antigenic peptide present within the groove of HLA-DR1 were also detected. The regions of potential intermolecular contact were observed in the binding interface. Contact points in region I center around residue Leu30 of TSST-1 and appear to involve hydrogen bonding between residues in two loops of the HLA-DR1 α-chain (α_{13}–α_{18} and α_{36}–α_{39}) and TSST-1 residues Asp27, Lys58, Ser53, and Pro50. Region II consists of four TSST-1 β-strands (β2, β3, β5, β4) and external face of the α-helix in the HLA-DR1 α-domain. Region III contains two sets of interactions. Residues in the loop between strands β4 and β5 of TSST-1 (i.e., Thr75 and Ser76) may interact with the C-terminal end of the HLA-DR1-bound peptide, while Gln73 of TSST-1 may interact with residues at the top of one turn of the α-helix in the β-chain of HLA-DR1.

TSST-1 was recently co-crystallized with an affinity-matured variant of the human Vβ-TCR 2.1 chain that bound TSST-1 with an affinity three orders of magnitude higher than wild-type Vβ-TCR 2.1 [85,86]. From this structure, a complex between TSST-1 and the wild-type Vβ-TCR 2.1 chain was modeled (see Plate 6.2), and importantly the model was completely consistent with prior mutational analyses [84,87–90]. The majority of intermolecular contacts occur between the β-chain complementarity-determining region (CDR)2 loop, which is a common target among all characterized superantigens, and the β-chain third framework region (FR3), which makes the interaction of TSST-1 with Vβ2-TCR unique. Thus, the β-chain contact surfaces are shifted laterally away from the elements necessary for binding peptide–MHC. TSST-1 is the most specific known superantigen, activating only Vβ2-positive T cells [7]. The Vβ2.1–TSST-1 structure revealed a number of intermolecular contacts with residues unique to the Vβ2 chain, primarily in FR3, providing the molecular basis by which TSST-1 displays such stringent β-chain specificity [86].

Collectively, structural and mutational analyses of TSST-1 indicate the following findings: (i) the O/B fold barrel structure present in domain B interacts with class II MHC molecules, which are required for superantigenicity; and (ii) the Vβ2-TCR interaction with TSST-1 depends on amino acids from the TSST-1 central α-helix within the deep groove on the backside of the toxin that contact the apical loop of Vβ-TCR 2.1 FR3, and residues from the TSST-1 α1-β1 and β5-β6 loops that contact CDR2.

Recent studies suggest that TSST-1 interacts with human vaginal epithelial cells in order to penetrate mucosal surfaces [91–93]. This penetration also appears to be enhanced by other exotoxins such as α--hemolysin. The ability of

TSST-1 to bind epithelial cells has been documented for many years, and the sites on the superantigen that appear to be required for this interaction have now been elucidated [26,94]. These residues include amino acids within a stretch of 12 residues, beginning with Phe119 and extending to Asp130. This group of amino acids is exposed on the underside (residues 121 and 122) and backside groove (residues 127–130) [93]. The receptor on epithelial cells for TSST-1 remains to be determined.

Staphylococcal enterotoxin and staphylococcal enterotoxin-like superantigens

Staphylococcal enterotoxin and staphylococcal enterotoxin-like superantigens are produced by several coagulase-expressing *Staphylococcus* species but are not routinely reported to be produced by coagulase-negative strains. Despite their long association with a form of gastroenteritis known as staphylococcal food poisoning (SFP), in recent years staphylococcal enterotoxins have received more attention for causing toxic shock syndromes [1,4,35,37]. Like other superantigens, the staphylococcal enterotoxins have immunomodulatory and lethal properties necessary for toxic shock syndromes. Although some investigators have suggested that the superantigen activity of staphylococcal enterotoxins is also responsible for SFP, it is fairly well established that SFP gastroenteritis and superantigenicity are determined by separate parts of the staphylococcal enterotoxin molecule [95,96]. This section focuses on (i) the biological and physicochemical properties of staphylococcal enterotoxins and staphylococcal enterotoxin-like proteins; (ii) the structural features involved in superantigen activity and gastroenteritis; and (iii) the mechanisms of pathogenesis in SFP. Other information pertinent to staphylococcal enterotoxins and staphylococcal enterotoxin-like proteins may be obtained from several thorough reviews [1,6,97] and from Chapter 25 of this book.

Important properties shared by all staphylococcal enterotoxins include their ability to induce emesis and gastroenteritis on oral administration to primates, superantigenicity, moderate stability to heat and pepsin, and conformational similarities including an intramolecular disulfide bond. Despite their similarities, staphylococcal enterotoxins and staphylococcal enterotoxin-like proteins display antigenic heterogeneity that provides the criteria for differentiating them into their major currently recognized types (staphylococcal enterotoxins SEA, SEB, SEC, SED, SEE, SEG, and SEI; staphylococcal enterotoxin-like proteins SEl-H and SEl-J to SEl-V). Based on minor differences in antigenicity, SEC can be further differentiated into multiple subtypes (SEC1, SEC2, and SEC*n*) [98–102]. The primary sequences of the major antigenic forms of staphylococcal enterotoxins and staphylococcal enterotoxin-like proteins are known. In some cases, antigenic epitopes have been mapped to the responsible residues. It is evident from the sequence alignment of the currently known staphylococcal enterotoxins and staphylococcal enterotoxin-like proteins that a great deal of similarity exists among these toxins, most of the conserved amino acid residues being located in central and C-terminal portions of the sequences. Based on sequence comparison, staphylococcal enterotoxins can be divided into at least three subfamilies (groups II, III, and V; see Table 6.2), with an additional subfamily comprising exclusively streptococcal superantigens (group IV) [1]. Group II contains SEB and the SEC subtypes and molecular variants (see Table 6.2). Toxins in this group are highly related to each other and to several streptococcal superantigens (e.g., SPE-A and streptococcal superantigen). Group II superantigens contain the low-affinity MHC II-binding site in the same approximate region as that for TSST-1 (see Plate 6.2c). They contain a Vβ-TCR-binding domain that is on the top frontside of the superantigens (see Plate 6.2c) [103–108]. These superantigens contain a cystine loop structure of variable size that is required for emetic activity [109]. Finally, as with all superantigens, group II superantigens contain the relatively highly conserved dodecapeptide domain proposed for epithelial cell binding [93].

Group III contains SEA and SEE, which are 84% identical, and the more distantly related SED [1]. These superantigens contain the same basic structural features as group II superantigens, except that group III superantigens contain a second high-affinity MHC II-binding site [110,111]. This second MHC II site requires the cation Zn^{2+} and is located on the opposite side of the superantigen, compared with the low-affinity site (see Plate 6.2d). The high-affinity MHC II site interacts with MHC II residues in the β-chain as opposed to the α-chain for group I and II superantigens. The consequence of the high-affinity MHC II site is a 10-fold increase in superantigenic activity and the requirement for the superantigen to lie across the antigenic peptide within the groove areas of the MHC II molecule [112,113]. Currently, the structural basis by which group III superantigens engage the TCR is unknown. Of note, however, is SEl-H, which has been shown to be Vα [114,115] rather than Vβ specific and although classified as a group III superantigen, it is more distantly related to the other group III members [116].

The superantigens in group IV are produced exclusively by β-hemolytic streptococci and do not include any staphylococcal enterotoxins [1]. These superantigens lack the cystine loop structure, are not emetic, and contain both low- and high-affinity MHC II-binding sites.

Finally, a subfamily of staphylococcal enterotoxin-like proteins (group V, including SEl-K to SEl-Q) has been recently described that lack the cystine loop structure, are not emetic, have both low- and high-affinity MHC II-binding sites, and contain an approximately 15-amino-acid extension which results in an additional loop at the top left front of the superantigen [1,116–120]. Recent structural studies have shown that this loop binds to residues in both the third and fourth framework regions (FR4). FR4 is a region of the TCR β-chain not engaged by the other superantigen groups and this interaction further extends the possible recognition site for superantigens on the TCR β-chain [120]. Functionally, the length and conformation of this additional superantigen loop is important for optimal activation of T cells [116], and that engagement of FR3/FR4 is required for T-cell activation [120].

The differences between SFP and toxic shock syndrome are best demonstrated in humans and monkeys and are a reflection of alternate routes of exposure to the staphylococcal enterotoxins. When ingested, staphylococcal enterotoxins do not typically produce life-threatening toxemia unless massive doses are consumed [95]. The major features of SFP gastroenteritis are vomiting, diarrhea, and characteristic histopathological abnormalities [121]. On ingestion, the effects of staphylococcal enterotoxins are noted in several parts of the gastrointestinal tract, although the major pathological lesions are in the stomach and upper part of the small intestine [122]. In these areas, one observes hyperemic lesions with a neutrophil influx into the lamina propria and epithelium. A mucopurulent exudate appears in the lumen. The jejunum shows signs of crypt extension, disruption or loss of the brush border, and an extensive infiltrate of neutrophils and macrophages into the lamina propria.

In primates, the staphylococcal enterotoxin target responsible for producing the emetic reflex is located in the abdominal viscera [123]. Although the cellular and molecular events leading to emesis are not completely known, multiple factors are involved. For example, staphylococcal enterotoxin-induced vomiting is known to be mediated by the medullary emetic center, which is stimulated by impulses transmitted through the vagus and sympathetic nerves. However, inflammatory mediators also correlate with SFP symptoms. Jett *et al.* [124] showed that orally administered SEB induces elevated levels of prostaglandin E_2, leukotriene B_4, and 5-hydroxyeicosatetraenoic acid, whereas Scheuber *et al.* [125] proposed that cysteinyl leukotrienes such as leukotriene E_4 are more important in SFP. The question still remains as to whether synthesis of these mediators is induced directly or indirectly by staphylococcal enterotoxins. Much of our uncertainty regarding the mechanism of SFP induction stems from the fact that the cellular target for staphylococcal enterotoxins in the gastrointestinal tract has not been identified. Several groups of investigators have proposed a role for mast cells, and evidence for the existence of a staphylococcal enterotoxin receptor on these cells has been provided [126,127]. If the role of the mast cell in SFP is eventually confirmed, several lines of evidence suggest that mast cell stimulation by staphylococcal enterotoxins occurs through a novel mechanism. One current proposal is that staphylococcal enterotoxins act directly on their receptor and circumvent the typical two-stage mast cell IgE antibody–antigen interaction [124]. Alber *et al.* [128] were unable to directly stimulate monkey mast cells to release inflammatory mediators. It was suggested that stimulation of mast cells *in vivo* occurs through a nonimmunological mechanism requiring the generation of neuropeptides released from primary sensory nerves. At least one putative mast cell-stimulating peptide, substance P, has been implicated in SEB-induced toxicity [129]. Although this model of mast cell activation is consistent with earlier investigations implicating nerve stimulation in SFP pathogenesis, a firm mechanistic link between staphylococcal enterotoxins and neuropeptide induction has not been established. Beery *et al.* [130] were unable to demonstrate neural binding of SEA in the rat gastrointestinal tract after oral administration of the toxin.

Despite being laborious and expensive, the monkey feeding assay as described by Bergdoll [131] is the gold standard assay for mimicking human SFP. Over the years, several nonprimate animal models (kitten, piglet, ferret, and mouse shrew) have been used to demonstrate staphylococcal enterotoxin-induced emesis [132–134]. Because of overlap in symptoms between SFP and toxic shock syndrome, further confirmation of these models for SFP is warranted, in particular those requiring systemic administration. Furthermore, their relevance for human illness needs to be evaluated by direct comparison with results in primates. For example, the oral doses of staphylococcal enterotoxins required to induce emesis (5 mg in ferrets) are much higher than those required in monkeys.

The lack of a confirmed inexpensive animal model has hindered progress toward understanding the structure and function of staphylococcal enterotoxins in relation to SFP. However, in recent years sequence data and crystallographic results have facilitated the planning of logical mutagenesis, so that these studies are now more feasible. One structural feature of staphylococcal enterotoxins that has received the most attention is their intermolecular disulfide linkage [109]. While several investigations have focused on the mutagenesis of cystine residues in staphylococcal enterotoxins, the disulfide bond in SEC has received the most thorough analysis with regard to emesis. Interestingly, SEC1 mutants with serine substituted for one or both cysteines (positions 93 and 110) are emetic. In contrast, the substitution of alanine at the same location(s) produces nonemetic mutants. The differences in toxicity between alanine and serine mutants are suspected to result from the ability of serine hydrogen bonds to substitute for the disulfide linkage. Thus, in the absence of a disulfide bond, residual native structure stabilized by serine substitutions holds critical residues in proper orientation. The question that remains to be answered is which crucial residues, affected by the disulfide bond, must be properly oriented for emesis to occur? Since the cystine loops are not highly conserved, residues within them are unlikely candidates. Iandolo [135] recognized a stretch of residues immediately downstream from the disulfide bond that are highly conserved among the staphylococcal enterotoxins. These residues are located within the β5 strand of SEC1 and analogous region of other staphylococcal enterotoxins and could be influenced by stability of the disulfide bond.

Two final areas of research have been initiated with respect to superantigens. First, now that most interactions of superantigens with MHC II and Vβ-TCRs are known, studies have been undertaken to produce small-molecule inhibitors of the interaction [136,137]. Recent studies with SEB as the representative superantigen have shown that super-high-affinity Vβ-TCRs can be produced that have the ability to neutralize both superantigenicity and development of toxic shock syndrome in rabbits. The super-high-affinity Vβ-TCRs can even be administered up to 2 hours after superantigen and neutralize activity. Finally, the Vβ-TCR is 2200 times more effective than commercially available intravenous immunoglobulin in neutralization of SEB, requiring a one-to-one molar ratio of Vβ-TCR and SEB in rabbits.

The second new area of intense research includes studies to more clearly define the full spectrum of staphylococcal superantigen-associated illnesses. These are thoroughly discussed in a recent review [138], but one aspect of these studies merits additional consideration: the potential role of superantigens in infections caused by community-associated methicillin-resistant *S. aureus* (CA-MRSA) strains. Until recently, MRSA was considered a problem associated with hospitals (i.e., HA-MRSA). Recently, however, CA-MRSA strains have emerged as a significant health concern. These CA-MRSA strains differ significantly from HA-MRSA strains in that CA-MRSA strains produce high levels of superantigens, notably TSST-1, SEB, SEC, or SEl-Q [139]. These four superantigens may be made *in vitro* in concentrations up to 1000 μg/mL, or approximately 1 million-fold higher than other superantigens. HA-MRSA strains do not typically produce these four superantigens [139]. The significance of these findings is that CA-MRSA strains should have a much greater ability to induce toxic shock syndrome than HA-MRSA strains. Our experience is that in causing toxic shock syndromes and related illnesses, CA-MRSA strain USA200 produces TSST-1, USA300 strain produces SEl-Q, and USA400 strain produces either SEB or SEC [140]. Unfortunately, these strains are also now present in hospitals.

Exfoliative toxins A and B

Three major serologically distinct exfoliative toxins have been described in association with human strains of *S. aureus*, designated exfoliative toxin (ET)A, ETB, and ETD. ETA, ETB, ETC, and ETD have been reported in *S. hyicus* strains [141]. ETA and ETB cause staphylococcal scalded skin syndrome (SSSS), usually seen in newborns and characterized by intraepidermal separation of layers of the skin at the desmosomes [142]. The illness begins abruptly with generalized erythema, often near the mouth and spreading over the entire body in the course of a few days. When the skin is lightly rubbed, the epidermal layer wrinkles irreversibly, giving rise to the characteristic positive Nikolsky sign. Later, large flaccid sterile bullae appear that lead to separation through the stratum granulosum layer. The entire sequence from disease onset to recovery is 7–10 days. There is no permanent scarring on areas of the skin, and the causative toxins are not themselves lethal to the host; as many as 5% of affected neonates may succumb due to production of superantigens and other factors by causative *S. aureus*. ETD, a recently recognized exfoliative toxin, has not been highly associated with production of SSSS. Instead, the toxin was associated with *S. aureus* strains from skin abscesses and furuncles [143]. ETC and ETD are not discussed further in this chapter.

In 1972, Melish and Glasgow [144] provided an animal model for the study of SSSS, the newborn mouse, and were thus able to fulfill Koch's postulates for the role of both *S. aureus* and toxin in the illness. ETA was purified by several investigators during the early 1970s, with Kondo *et al.* in 1974 identifying and purifying ETB [145–149]. Both genes, designated *etA* and *etB*, have been cloned and the nucleotide sequences determined [150]. ETA is encoded on a lysogenic bacteriophage element integrated into the chromosome and is the more commonly seen of the two toxins [151]. ETB is encoded by a gene present on a large plasmid [152]. Both genes encode exfoliative toxins with signal peptides that are removed on secretion. ETA and ETB are both synthesized as proteins of 280 residues, with the first 38 comprising signal peptides. The mature proteins have molecular masses of 27 kDa, in good agreement with previously determined values by SDS-PAGE. These two toxins are serologically distinct and share only 45% sequence similarity, located almost entirely in three regions of the molecules: N-terminal 46–70 (80% similar), middle 106–134 (58% similar), and C-terminus 201–221 (81% similar). Antibody against the toxins is neutralizing. ETA has a pI of approximately 7.0 and ETB a pI of approximately 4.0.

Both exfoliative toxins are produced in large amounts in standard media such as trypticase yeast extract broth in the presence of 10% CO_2 or in beef heart medium without added CO_2 [153]. Clones such as *S. aureus* RN4220 containing exfoliative toxin genes produce 10–20 times more toxin than clinical isolates in which yields of 10–20 mg/L are easily achievable [154,155]. As with other staphylococcal exotoxins, diverse methods have been used to purify exfoliative toxins. These include combinations of precipitation, gel filtration, ion-exchange chromatography, and isoelectric focusing. These methods have been reviewed extensively [142,153]. We find that the simplest method to produce large quantities of ETA and ETB is to precipitate toxins made in RN4220 with four volumes of ethanol and subject the resolubilized toxins to successive isoelectric focusing in pH gradients of 3–10 and then a narrower range. Toxins thus obtained are homogeneous in SDS-PAGE.

Although it has been definitively established for many years that exfoliative toxins cause SSSS, the molecular mechanism of action of the toxins has only recently been elucidated. Lillibridge *et al.* [156] reported that injection of exfoliative toxins into the skin of newborn mice resulted in positive Nikolsky signs by 25 min after injection. At 20 min after injection, light-density oval bubbles in the region of the stratum granulosum widened and lost their oval appearance. By 25 min, the desmosomes, which are specialized thickenings of cell membranes that hold cells together, began to split and separate. At 150 min after injection, all desmosomes along the region of cleavage were split; the cleavage plane was in the stratum granulosum layer. These researchers proposed that exfoliative toxins may affect the ovoid bubbles and activate proteolytic enzymes contained therein to cleave at the desmosomes.

Electron microscopic studies conducted by Elias *et al.* [157] suggest that the desmosome region is not the primary site of exfoliative toxin action. During early separation in the stratum granulosum, desmosomes often clung together, whereas interdesmosomal regions ballooned. In other sites, separation occurred simultaneously along entire cell surfaces. Cleaved surfaces showed intact plasma membranes. These researchers also demonstrated that perfused tracers did not penetrate cells, and cells cultured with exfoliative toxins showed no signs of injury. Exfoliative toxins failed to alter concanavalin A binding, ruthenium red staining, pemphigus antibody binding, and HLA surface antigens in cultures containing keratinocytes, fibroblasts, sperm cells or lymphocytes and in human or mouse skin *in vivo*. Thus, exfoliative toxins appeared to act extracellularly rather than by altering the cells themselves.

McLay *et al.* [158] also suggested that the desmosomal region was not the major target of exfoliative toxin action. Ultrastructural studies were performed on mice challenged with exfoliative toxins. For up to 130 min after injection, wide gaps developed between cells in the horizontal planes of the stratum granulosum and, as noted by Lillibridge *et al.* [156], the oval bubbles normally present in the intercellular spaces were no longer present. Splitting of the desmosomes occurred after development of distended intercellular spaces. After 20 hours, the appearance suggested alterations in the maturation of keratinocytes. The proteinase inhibitor aprotinin did not inhibit the effect of exfoliative toxins, suggesting that proteolytic enzyme action on the desmosomes did not occur. Wuepper *et al.* [159] noted that complement activation and competent thymocytes were not necessary for the action of exfoliative toxins. These researchers also reported that protease inhibitors failed to block the exfoliation caused by exfoliative toxins. Baker *et al.* [160] showed that radioiodinated exfoliative toxins failed to bind erythrocytes, leukocytes, keratinocytes, heat-separated epidermis, or whole newborn mouse skin.

In 1980, the lymphocyte mitogenic activity of exfoliative toxins was described. It was shown that the toxin primarily stimulated T cells to proliferate, but B cells from nude (T-cell-deficient) mice were also significantly stimulated. Several other laboratories have confirmed the finding that exfoliative toxins are mitogenic, culminating in the report by Marrack and Kappler [3] that exfoliative toxins are superantigens. We have also noted the very strong mitogenic activity associated with ETA [155,161,162]. However, the study by Fleischer *et al.* [163] suggests that ETA is not mitogenic; rather, its apparent superantigenic activity results from contamination with enterotoxins. This is based on the following observations: a commercial ETA preparation failed to bind to class II MHC molecules and, when more extensively purified, failed to stimulate T cells from humans. The mitogenic activity was localized into a different fraction. Further studies are needed to clarify this issue. If the toxin is shown to be superantigenic, it is possible that the separation of layers of the skin results in part from capillary leakage and pressure as a result of fluid accumulation.

A final note on the potential superantigenicity of exfoliative toxins: the definition of superantigens does not require that the toxins be structurally related to the pyrogenic toxin family (TSST-1, staphylococcal enterotoxins, staphylococcal enterotoxin-like proteins or SPEs). Indeed, many more recently identified superantigens lack similarities with pyrogenic toxins. Similarly, there is no requirement that all superantigens cause T-cell proliferation at the same minimum concentration; indeed, differences in activity are seen between superantigens with high-affinity MHC II-binding sites and those with low-affinity MHC II-binding sites. Thus, it is formally possible and worth testing to assess whether a population of Vβ-TCRs is cleavable by exfoliative toxins and if this accounts for their apparent superantigenicity.

A series of studies has shown that ETA and ETB bind to the intracellular proteins profilaggrin, filaggrin (components of keratohyalin granules) and a histone-like protein [164–167]. The link between this binding and skin separation was not demonstrated. Other reports have noted amino acid sequence similarities between ETA and ETB and serine proteases such as staphylococcal V8 protease, suggesting that these toxins may be proteolytic [167]. Experiments using diisopropylfluorophosphate (DFP) to inhibit serine protease activity did not result in complete loss of biological activity, although binding of DFP to a peptide containing Ser195 was demonstrated. Subsequently, Prevost *et al.* [168] substituted a cysteine in place of serine at position 195 of ETA. This led to the complete inactivation of the toxin, in that it did not induce a positive

Nikolsky sign in mice. These investigators also evaluated 10 chromogens as protease substrates for ETA; however, no activity was demonstrated. They also failed to detect lipase activity in ETA.

Finally, we have solved the three-dimensional structures of both ETA and ETB [154,155]. Both structures are consistent with chymotrypsin-like serine proteases that cleave substrates after acidic residues, often glutamic acid. In both exfoliative toxins, the studies confirmed the importance of the catalytic triad of amino acids (His72, Asp120, Ser195 in ETA; His65, Asp114, Ser186 in ETB) as important in the active sites. The structural studies suggested that the active site of the molecules may be very small and partially blocked by a loop, permitting only very small peptides or unique proteins to be susceptible to proteolysis. With this in mind, our group tested a variety of small peptides containing glutamic acid residues for ability to be cleaved by exfoliative toxins. Both α- and β-melanocyte-stimulating hormone peptides were cleaved by ETA, after the Glu residue; it was thus shown for the first time that exfoliative toxins are serine proteases [169]. Subsequently, it has been shown that desmoglein 1, but not desmoglein 3, is cleaved by exfoliative toxins, suggesting that this activity accounts for the clinical illness SSSS [170–172]. Desmoglein 1 functions as a desmosomal cadherin that mediates cell–cell adhesion, just below the stratum corneum, whereas desmoglein 3 is expressed in the lower epidermis, thus explaining the superficial skin peeling seen in SSSS.

Cytotoxins

Strains of *S. aureus* may produce up to four classes of cytotoxin, comprising α-hemolysin, β-hemolysin, γ-hemolysin, and δ-hemolysin, as well as PVL. Each of the four classes of cytotoxins is discussed separately.

α-Toxin (α-hemolysin)

α-Toxin is the most studied of the cytotoxins produced by *S. aureus*. It is produced by a large percentage of strains, is toxic to a wide range of mammalian cells and animals, is highly hemolytic for rabbit erythrocytes, and is dermonecrotic and neurotoxic. Major reviews of α-toxin, notably by Freer and Arbuthnott [173] and Bhakdi and Tranum-Jensen [174], have discussed much of the early work on this toxin. This chapter focuses on more recent developments.

The gene for α-hemolysin, *hla*, was cloned from the chromosome and sequenced by Gray and Kehoe in 1984 [175]. The amino-terminal 26 residues of the α-toxin protein comprise a signal peptide. The mature secreted protein has a molecular mass of 33 kDa with a pI of approximately 8.5. The protein contains no cytsteine residues, has an abundance of β-sheets (68%), and a paucity of α-helices (10%). α-Toxin is under *agr*, *sar*, and *srr* control and is produced in the postexponential phase of growth. O'Reilly *et al.* [176] suggested that some strains, particularly toxic shock syndrome isolates, have the α-toxin gene but do not produce protein; this partly results from mutations arising in the structural gene such that protein cannot be translated. However, it is our experience that the majority of menstrual toxic shock syndrome isolates produce α-toxin, and this protein may facilitate TSST-1 penetration of mucosal barriers (discussed earlier in this chapter).

Numerous methods have been described for producing and purifying α-toxin. The yeast extract dialysate medium of Bernheimer and Schwartz is the most frequently used, and the Wood 46 strain is the organism of choice for toxin production [177]. Harshman *et al.* [178] described the most straightforward methods for obtaining highly purified toxin: the first included preparative gel electrophoresis, the second selective adsorption and elution from glasspore beads followed by gel filtration. The second procedure is simple and rapid and gives high yields (10–20 mg/L) of homogeneous protein.

α-Toxin is made as a monomer but forms cylindrical oligomeric heptamers that are important for functional activity (see Plate 6.3) [179]. The toxin is defined by its ability to lyse erythrocytes, notably those from rabbits, in which the red blood cells are least 100 times more susceptible than those from other species and 1000 times more susceptible than human red blood cells [174,177,180,181]. The formation of cylindrical oligomers in the cell membrane accompanies formation of a pore with an internal diameter of 1–2 nm. Pore formation is described as a stepwise process, beginning with a monomer and ending with a heptameric complex [179]. Initially, the toxin binds to the cell membrane [178,182,183]. Two types of binding have been observed: at low concentrations, nonspecific adsorption to lipid membranes occurs. The monomers appear to open to form amphipathic rods with the ability to penetrate the bilayer. Finally, the monomers diffuse in the membrane until they collide with other monomers or form oligomeric structures, wherein they become part of the oligomer. In this process the monomers become even more hydrophobic, causing membrane pertubations and hexamer or heptamer formation with a central pore. No major structural changes are believed to occur in the toxin monomers upon oligomer formation. The small pores formed permit rapid efflux of K^+, Na^+, Ca^{2+} and other small molecules of less than 1 kDa. Finally, rupture of the cell with release of hemoglobin occurs as a result of osmotic swelling.

Not all cell types form the pores described above. Keratinocytes and lymphocytes appear to develop smaller pores, permeable only to monovalent ions [184–186]. Fibroblasts have the ability to repair lesions formed by low-dose exposure to α-toxin. The mechanism of repair appears to be exclusion of much, but not all, of the oligomeric toxin complexes and closing of the pores. Studies have shown that deletion of five C-terminal amino acids leads to loss of oligomerization, but binding to red blood cell membranes occurs normally [187].

As α-toxin is both dermonecrotic and neurotoxic and is responsible for lethality in a variety of animals, it is likely that this protein is important in the causation of a variety of disease conditions, but this has not been established with complete certainty. The toxin has a myriad of effects on the host, primarily due to the effects of ion imbalances created as a result of pore formation in a variety of cell types [174,188–190]. For example, α-toxin activates arachidonic acid metabolism in endothelial cells due to Ca^{2+} influx. This leads to thromboxane and prostacyclin formation, which are vasoconstrictive. Cell integrity breaks down due to osmotic swelling, ultimately resulting in increased vascular permeability and pulmonary edema or adult respiratory distress syndrome. In addition, α-toxin, which causes Ca^{2+} influx in platelets, leads to the release of procoagulatory factors. Calcium is important in the contraction of actin–myosin filaments, and ATP is required for relaxation. α-Toxin-induced calcium influx and leakage of ATP induces endothelial cell contraction, with leaky gaps forming between cells, and ultimately edema. Finally, the calcium influx may trigger cellular endonucleases, leading to programmed cell death.

Other effects of α-toxin include macrophage secretion of IL-1β and disruption of myelin sheaths in rabbit nerve and mouse brain [174]. Because the toxin interacts both specifically and nonspecifically to form pores in cell membranes in general, it is likely that α-toxin has additional important effects on the host that are mediated by altered ion balance.

β-Toxin (β-hemolysin, sphingomyelinase C)

The β-toxin of *S. aureus* was the first hemolysin identified in 1935 by Glenny and Stevens [191] who also showed the toxin to be highly hemolytic for sheep but not rabbit red blood cells, and not dermonecrotic in guinea-pig skin or lethal for mice. These researchers noted that the hemolytic effect was greatly enhanced by refrigerating the red blood cells below 10°C after treating them with toxin at 37°C, giving rise to the designation "hot–cold hemolysin."

β-Toxin is an exotoxin with a molecular mass of 35 kDa when secreted into the culture medium [192,193]. The gene for the toxin was cloned and nucleotide sequence determined by Projan *et al.* [193] and cloned by Coleman *et al.* [192]. The *hlb* gene is located on a 4-kb *Cla*I chromosomal DNA fragment; it contains 330 amino acids with a predicted molecular mass of 39 kDa. The toxin shares 55.7% similarity over 200 residues with *Bacillus cereus* sphingomyelinase. In unpublished studies in our laboratory, we determined the N-terminal sequence of secreted β-hemolysin to be Glu-Ser-Lys-Lys-Asp-Asp-Thr-Asp-Leu-Lys, which unambiguously corresponds to residues 35–44 of the protein predicted by Projan *et al.* Thus, the first 33 residues of their sequence comprise a signal peptide yielding a mature protein of approximately 35 kDa, in agreement with data achieved by SDS-PAGE. The toxin has an estimated pI above pH 9.0.

β-Toxin is made in high concentration by both animal and human strains of *S. aureus*. The conditions required for production have been extensively reviewed [173]. Media appropriate for production of α-toxin, such as yeast extract dialysate, or beef heart dialysate medium as we use, yield large amounts of toxin. As with most other secreted exoproteins, β-toxin is produced during postexponential phase.

The methods used to purify β-toxin have also been extensively reviewed and involve combinations of precipitation, gel filtration, ion-exchange chromatrography, electrophoresis, and isoelectric focusing [173]. Yields of purified toxin of 1–2 mg/L of culture fluid have been reported, but in our hands yields of 15–20 mg/L may be obtained simply by ethanol precipitation (75% final concentration), followed by isolectric focusing in pH gradients of 3–10 and then 7–9. Toxin thus purified is homogeneous when tested in SDS-PAGE and protein sequencing.

In 1963, β-toxin was shown to exhibit phosphorylase C activity requiring Mg^{2+} [194]. The enzyme has a limited range of activity, with specificity for sphingomyelin and lysophosphatidylcholine. Thus, the activity of β-toxin can be described as follows:

$$\text{Sphingomyelin} + H_2O \xrightarrow[\beta\text{-toxin} + Mg^{2+}]{} N\text{-acyl-sphingosine} + \text{phosphorylcholine}$$

Recently, we solved the structure of β-toxin to a resolution of 0.24 nm [195]. The data indicate the protein belongs to the larger DNase I superfamily and acts as a neutral sphingomyelinase. The report also indicated that the ability to lyse red blood cells and kill human lymphocytes depends on the sphingomyelinase activity, involving an active site that includes residues His150 and His189.

The differences in susceptibility of red blood cells to β-toxin may be explained by the sphingomyelin content of red blood cells. Low *et al.* [196] suggested a mechanism to explain the hot–cold phenomenon associated with the toxin. At 20°C, cohesive forces associated with intact red blood cell membranes are capable of holding the hydrolysis products in position in the membranes, whereas cooling to 10°C induces phase separation and pooling of hydrolysis products resulting in bilayer collapse.

The role of β-toxin in disease is poorly understood. The fact that the toxin is made in such high concentrations by strains suggests that the protein must provide some form of selective advantage to the microbe. It has been reported to be nondermonecrotic in guinea pigs and nonlethal for mice. The toxin has been shown to be cytotoxic for human cells [195,197].

β-Toxin is also used in diagnostic microbiology in a presumptive test for group B streptococci. This test, referred to as CAMP (Christie, Atlkins, Munch-Petersen), involves one of two processes. One approach is to drop purified β-toxin or culture extract containing β-toxin on a lawn of presumptive group B streptococci and then examine it for enhanced β-hemolysis on blood agar after 30 min to a few hours at 35°C. Alternatively, the presumptive group B streptococci and β-toxin-producing *S. aureus* are streaked perpendicular to, but not touching, each other; the blood agar plate is then examined after growth for an arrow of enhanced β-toxin near the intersection of the two organisms.

γ-Hemolysin and PVL: bicomponent toxins

Strains of *S. aureus* produce two classes of bicomponent toxins composed of two independently secreted, nonassociated proteins (referred to as class S and class F components, i.e., slow eluting and fast eluting from an ion-exchange column) [198,199]. These toxins, γ-hemolysin and PVL, are synergistically toxic (with respect to S and F components) to polymorphonuclear leukocytes and monocytes and macrophages; γ-hemolysin is additionally lytic for red cells from a variety of mammalian species. Studies indicate that nearly all *S. aureus* strains manufacture γ-hemolysin, which is inactivated by agar and therefore not demonstrable on blood agar plates, while 2–3% of strains also make PVL [200]. The literature concerning the physicochemical and biological properties and relatedness to each other of γ-hemolysin and PVL has been confusing at best. However, studies by Prevost and colleagues have clarified the literature considerably and provide the basic reference point for this part of the chapter [201–210].

The results of the studies conducted by Prevost *et al.* and earlier investigators indicate that strains contain separate loci, giving rise to γ-hemolysins and PVLs. Within strains capable of making both toxins, seven S components (HlgA, HlgC, LukS-PV, LukS-R, LukE, LukM, and LukS-I) and six F components (HlgB, LukF-PV, LukF-R, LukD, LukF′-PV, and LukF-I) may be produced. These products display a high degree of sequence similarity, and various members are associated with certain disease types.

Genes for γ-hemolysin

Three open reading frames comprise the gene for γ-hemolysin, *hlg*, encompassing a locus located on a 4.5-kb *Sca*I chromosomal DNA fragment. Crude extracts from a clone containing this DNA fragment were both hemolytic and leukotoxic. The three open reading frames are designated in order *hlgA*, *hlgC*, and *hlgB* and correspond to genes identified previously, most notably by Cooney *et al.* [211,212]. Two of the open reading frames, *hlgC* and *hlgB*, are cotranscribed, whereas *hlgA* is transcribed separately.

The proteins encoded by the three genes contain signal peptides, the molecular masses of the mature proteins being 32 kDa for HlgA, 34 kDa for HlgB, and 32.5 kDa for HlgC. Their estimated pI values are 9.4, 9.1, and 9.0, respectively. The mature HlgA protein corresponds to the γ_1 component of γ-hemolysin identified previously. HlgC appears to encode the γ_2 component. HlgB together with HlgC have typically been referred to as γ-hemolysin. The locus encompassing *hlgA*, *hlgC*, and *hlgB* is nearly identical with that of the *lukR* locus encoding leukocidin R. Although there are a few nucleotide differences between the *hlg* and *lukR* loci, only the HlgA protein shows any amino acid differences (R258K and H284P).

γ-Hemolysin was first described in 1938. A variety of review articles have since been published concerning its production [213]. *Staphylococcus aureus* strain 5R appears to be an excellent source of γ-hemolysin, as the strain does not produce α-, β-, or δ-hemolysins. Plommet [213] suggests that production is dependent on three factors: (i) the *S. aureus* clone selected for use; (ii) the growth medium and, in particular, a yeast extract dialysate; and (iii) aeration consisting of O_2/CO_2 in a ratio of 80 : 20.

Purification of γ-hemolysin may be achieved by batch adsorption onto hydroxyapatite and subsequent elution with potassium phosphate. Separation of the two components may be accomplished by adsorption onto hydroxyapatite and then eluting with two different potassium phosphate buffers.

Panton–Valentine leukocidin

Prevost *et al.* [214] also cloned and sequenced the genes encoding PVL, termed *lukS-PV* and *lukF-PV*. The locus, *luk-PV*, consisted of two open reading frames. Extracts from the clone exhibited leukotoxic but not hemolytic activity. The *lukS-PV* and *lukF-PV* genes are cotranscribed in order and are similar to *hlgC* and *hlgB*. No *hlgA* analog was present in the *luk-PV* locus. The *lukS-PV* gene encodes a protein of 312 amino acids, of which the first 28 comprise a signal peptide. The mature LukS-PV protein has a molecular mass of 32 kDa and a pI of 9.0. The *lukF-PV* gene encodes a 325-amino-acid protein, of which the first 24 comprise a signal peptide. The mature protein has a molecular mass of 34 kDa and a pI of 9.

Noda and Kato [215] summarized the techniques used to produce PVL. The V8 strain of *S. aureus* is useful for production. The organisms are cultured in a yeast extract casamino acid medium. Purification of PVL is complex but involves precipitation with $ZnCl_2$ and ammonium sulfate, followed by various chromatographic and electrophoretic procedures. With the multiple S and F components, it is possible for a particular *S. aureus* strain to make many combinations of toxins, each with S and F components. Prevost *et al.* [214] noted that when assayed alone, these proteins lacked both hemolytic and leukotoxic activities. The three-dimensional structures of multiple S and F components of the family have been determined. Like α-toxin, this family of proteins, both hemolysins and leukocidins, form multimeric pores in membranes; the pores are smaller in diameter than those produced by α-toxin [216–218].

Although it is clear that γ-hemolysin and PVL are cytotoxic, their role in disease is unclear. However, the high association of PVL with necrotizing pneumonia and MRSA has been noted [219–221]. Here we provide some key references that have noted this association, although a complete list of publications is impossible. Recent studies have attempted to resolve whether the association of PVL with necrotizing pneumonia is causative or simply a strain and trait association. The first of these studies [222], performed in mice, suggested that PVL is not critical for the development of necrotizing pneumonia. A second study [223], though less well controlled, indicated that PVL is the critical toxin in necrotizing pneumonia. Finally, very recently, it has been suggested that α-toxin is a critical player in the illness [224]. A comment on these studies is merited. Both PVL and α-toxin are multimeric pore-forming toxins, produced by many but not all necrotizing pneumonia isolates. They are redundant members of the large pore-forming family of cytotoxins made by these organisms. Thus, it is not surprising that, if present, both toxins would contribute to disease. However, since the above studies have used mice as animal models, none has evaluated the role of superantigens in necrotizing pneumonia with clinical features also consistent with toxic shock syndrome; mice are resistant to the lethal effects of superantigens. An association has been reported between SEB and SEC and deaths in four Upper Midwest children with lung infections and necrotizing pneumonia [225], and we have noted an association of staphylococcal purpura fulminans (with necrotizing pneumonia and toxic shock syndrome) with superantigens [226]. Thus, as stated earlier in this chapter, four superantigens produced in high concentrations are nearly always present in CA-MRSA, namely TSST-1, SEB, SEC, and SEl-Q. Studies to assess the role of superantigens in necrotizing pneumonia will require alternative animal models, such as the rabbit, and should be performed.

δ-Hemolysin (δ-lysin, δ-toxin)

δ-Hemolysin is a 26-amino-acid peptide that causes membrane damage in a wide range of mammalian cell types. The toxin obtained from human strains of *S. aureus* differs from that made by canine strains by nine amino acids despite the fact that both toxins have 26 residues (Figure 6.3) and are approximately 3 kDa. These hemolysins conserve their interesting charge properties, and both are biologically active, although they are serologically only partially identical. In addition to being made by approximately 97% of *S. aureus* strains, *S. haemolyticus* strains also produce an immunologically related protein [227].

δ-Hemolysin is encoded by the *hld* gene, which gives rise to a transcript of 514 nucleotides [78]. The structural gene for δ-hemolysin is the 3′ part of a 45-codon open reading frame that occupies the first 160 nucleotides of the large transcript. The regulatory role of the larger transcript has been discussed previously as an important part of the *agr* system that regulates expression of both cell-associated and secreted virulence factors. δ-Hemolysin itself is under *agr* control and is therefore maximally produced in the late logarithmic phase (postexponential phase), along with many other staphylococcal exoproteins.

δ human N formyl met	ala	gln	asp	ile	ile	ser	thr	ile	gly	asp	leu	val	
δ canine N formyl met	ala	ala	asp	ile	ile	ser	thr	ile	val	glu	phe	val	
	lys	trp	ile	ile	asp	thr	val	asn	lys	phe	thr	lys	lys
	lys	leu	ile	ala	glu	thr	val	glu	lys	phe	ile	lys	lys

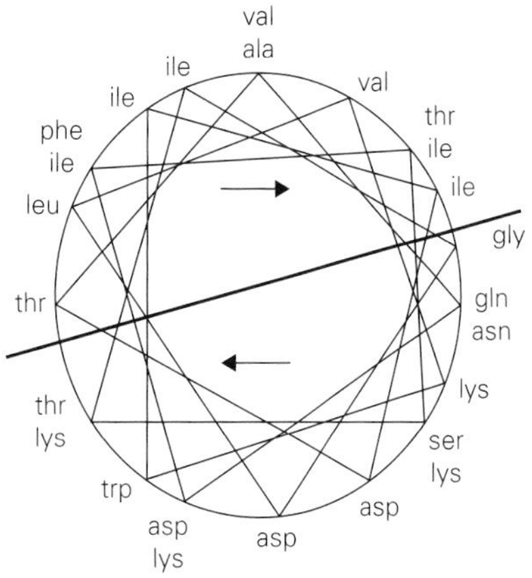

Figure 6.3 Primary amino acids sequence and proposed structure for delta (symbol) toxin.

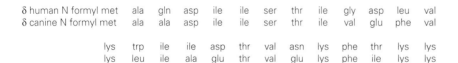

Interestingly, δ-hemolysin is secreted without a signal peptide; indeed, it has been suggested that the toxin itself may function as an excellent signal peptide.

δ-Hemolysin is produced today in two major ways: (i) from cultures of *S. aureus* deficient in α-hemolysin (e.g., strains NCTC 10345 and 186X), and (ii) by peptide synthesis, as we and others have done. For production by bacteria, the yeast extract dialysate culture medium of Bernheimer and Schwartz [177] provides excellent yields, approximately 300 μg/L of purified protein. Toxin made in this medium can be purifed most easily by one of two techniques: purification on a hydroxyapatite column with sequential elution of contaminants and then δ-hemolysin with phosphate buffers or by partitioning the toxin in either the aqueous or chloroform–methanol phases of extraction. The location of the toxin in this latter method is pH dependent, in the lower phase under acidic conditions and in the upper phase under basic conditions. Detailed descriptions of both methods have been reported by Birkbeck and Freer [228,229]. Toxin purified by either method appears to be highly pure as analyzed by SDS-PAGE and migrates as a diffuse band with molecular mass of approximately 6 kDa, or about twice that expected on the basis of sequence analysis. This difference likely results either from the tendency of δ-hemolysin to aggregate, with the band in the gel representing a dimer, or from altered mobility due to charge or shape properties. Gram quantities of δ-hemolysin can be synthesized in the laboratory by the use of either automated or manual peptide synthesis techniques. Dhople and Nagaraj [230] synthesized δ-hemolysin without amino-formyl methionine, showing no demonstrable loss of characteristics of the protein.

δ-Hemolysin is made by 97% of *S. aureus*. It may also be produced by 50–70% of coagulase-negative staphylococci. The precise role of δ-hemolysin in the causation of human disease remains unclear, but it has a wide range of cytolytic effects. The toxin has broad-spectrum lytic activity for erythrocytes, other eukaryotic cells, organelles, and spheroplasts and protoplasts. It has also been reported to be dermonecrotic and lethal in experimental animals when used in high concentrations [173]. It is possible, however, that these latter effects result from contamination with minute amounts of α-hemolysin. The activity of δ-hemolysin is inhibited by phospholipids [231].

There has been considerable interest in the mechanism of cell lysis by δ-hemolysin. As indicated in Figure 6.3, the toxin forms an amphipathic α-helix such that hydrophilic and hydrophobic domains form on opposing sides [229,231]. This has led to the presumption that δ-hemolysin acts as a surfactant. Consistent with this is the rapidity with which cells are lysed. Low-molecular-weight substances (< 1 kDa) are released first, followed by large molecules after prolonged exposure.

Thelestam and Mollby [232] showed that δ-hemolysin is similar both structurally and in its mechanism of action to the bee venom mellitin. Other members with similar properties have been identified, some displaying antimicrobial activity. However, δ-hemolysin is not antimicrobial. The similarities of these molecules and their ability to aggregate suggest that they may aggregate to form channels in planar lipid bilayers. Mellor *et al.* [233] showed that 0.3 μmol/L δ-hemolysin causes cation-selective channels to form in membranes. Mellor's group proposed that the toxin may aggregate, forming a hexagonal cluster of six α-helices. In this way, δ-hemolysin may also serve as a model system for the study of ion channels of excitable membranes, such as the nicotinic acetylcholine receptor.

Acknowledgments

This work was supported by USPHS research grants AI64611 and AI074283 from the National Institute of Allergy and Infectious Diseases and RR15587 and RR016454 from the National Center for Research Resources.

References

1 McCormick JK, Yarwood JM, Schlievert PM. Toxic shock syndrome and bacterial superantigens: an update. Annu Rev Microbiol 2001;55:77–104.
2 Bergdoll MS, Schlievert PM. Toxic-shock syndrome toxin. Lancet 1984;ii:691.
3 Marrack P, Kappler J. The staphylococcal enterotoxins and their relatives. Science 1990;248:705–11.
4 McCormick JK, Bohach GA, Schlievert PM. Pyrogenic, lethal, and emetic properties of superantigens in rabbits and primates. Methods Mol Biol 2003;214:245–53.
5 Lina G, Bohach GA, Nair SP *et al.* Standard nomenclature for the superantigens expressed by *Staphylococcus*. J Infect Dis 2004;189:2334–6.
6 Kotzin BL, Leung DY, Kappler J, Marrack P. Superantigens and their potential role in human disease. Adv Immunol 1993;54:99–166.
7 Choi Y, Lafferty JA, Clements JR *et al.* Selective expansion of T cells expressing V beta 2 in toxic shock syndrome. J Exp Med 1990;172:981–4.
8 Bueno C, Lemke CD, Criado G *et al.* Bacterial superantigens bypass Lck-dependent T cell receptor signaling by activating a Galpha11-dependent, PLC-beta-mediated pathway. Immunity 2006;25:67–78.
9 Dinges MM, Gregerson DS, Tripp TJ, McCormick JK, Schlievert PM. Effects of total body irradiation and cyclosporin A on the lethality of toxic shock syndrome toxin-1 in a rabbit model of toxic shock syndrome. J Infect Dis 2003;188:1142–5.
10 Hofer MF, Harbeck RJ, Schlievert PM, Leung DY. Staphylococcal toxins augment specific IgE responses by atopic patients exposed to allergen. J Invest Dermatol 1999;112:171–6.
11 Hofer MF, Lester MR, Schlievert PM, Leung DY. Upregulation of IgE synthesis by staphylococcal toxic shock syndrome toxin-1 in peripheral blood mononuclear cells from patients with atopic dermatitis. Clin Exp Allergy 1995;25:1218–27.

12 Schlievert PM. Enhancement of host susceptibility to lethal endotoxin shock by staphylococcal pyrogenic exotoxin type C. Infect Immun 1982;36:123–8.
13 Schlievert PM, Bettin KM, Watson DW. Inhibition of ribonucleic acid synthesis by group A streptococcal pyrogenic exotoxin. Infect Immun 1980;27:542–8.
14 Fiume L, Stirpe F. Decreased RNA content in mouse liver nuclei after intoxication with alpha-amanitin. Biochim Biophys Acta 1966;123:643–5.
15 Chow AW, Bartlett KH, Percival-Smith R, Morrison BJ. Vaginal colonization with *Staphylococcus aureus*, positive for toxic-shock marker protein, and *Escherichia coli* in healthy women. J Infect Dis 1984;150:80–4.
16 Dinges MM, Schlievert PM. Comparative analysis of lipopolysaccharide-induced tumor necrosis factor alpha activity in serum and lethality in mice and rabbits pretreated with the staphylococcal superantigen toxic shock syndrome toxin 1. Infect Immun 2001;69:7169–72.
17 Sauter C, Wolfensberger C. Interferon in human serum after injection of endotoxin. Lancet 1980;ii:852–3.
18 Kushnaryov VM, MacDonald HS, Reiser RF, Bergdoll MS. Reaction of toxic shock syndrome toxin 1 with endothelium of human umbilical cord vein. Rev Infect Dis 1989;11(suppl 1): S282–S287; discussion S287–S288.
19 Lee PK, Vercellotti GM, Deringer JR, Schlievert PM. Effects of staphylococcal toxic shock syndrome toxin 1 on aortic endothelial cells. J Infect Dis 1991;164:711–19.
20 Lee PK, Deringer JR, Kreiswirth BN, Novick RP, Schlievert PM. Fluid replacement protection of rabbits challenged subcutaneously with toxic shock syndrome toxins. Infect Immun 1991;59:879–84.
21 Parsonnet J, Gillis ZA, Richter AG, Pier GB. A rabbit model of toxic shock syndrome that uses a constant, subcutaneous infusion of toxic shock syndrome toxin 1. Infect Immun 1987;55:1070–6.
22 Giantonio BJ, Alpaugh RK, Schultz J *et al.* Superantigen-based immunotherapy: a phase I trial of PNU-214565, a monoclonal antibody–staphylococcal enterotoxin A recombinant fusion protein, in advanced pancreatic and colorectal cancer. J Clin Oncol 1997;15:1994–2007.
23 Kaul R, McGeer A, Norrby-Teglund A *et al.* Intravenous immunoglobulin therapy for streptococcal toxic shock syndrome: a comparative observational study. Clin Infect Dis 1999;28:800–7.
24 Schlievert PM. Use of intravenous immunoglobulin in the treatment of staphylococcal and streptococcal toxic shock syndromes and related illnesses. J Allergy Clin Immunol 2001; 108:107S–110S.
25 Schwab JH, Watson DW, Cromartie WJ. Further studies of group A streptococcal factors with lethal and cardiotoxic properties. J Infect Dis 1955;96:14–18.
26 Keane WF, Gekker G, Schlievert PM, Peterson PK. Enhancement of endotoxin-induced isolated renal tubular cell injury by toxic shock syndrome toxin 1. Am J Pathol 1986;122:169–76.
27 Leonard BA, Schlievert PM. Immune cell lethality induced by streptococcal pyrogenic exotoxin A and endotoxin. Infect Immun 1992;60:3747–55.
28 Mitchell DT, Levitt DG, Schlievert PM, Ohlendorf DH. Structural evidence for the evolution of pyrogenic toxin superantigens. J Mol Evol 2000;51:520–31.
29 Todd JK, Kapral FA, Fishaut M, Welch TR. Toxic shock syndrome associated with phage group 1 staphylococci. Lancet 1978;ii:1116–18.
30 Davis JP, Chesney PJ, Wand PJ, LaVenture M. Toxic-shock syndrome: epidemiologic features, recurrence, risk factors, and prevention. N Engl J Med 1980;303:1429–35.
31 Osterholm MT, Davis JP, Gibson RW *et al.* Tri-state toxic-state syndrome study. I. Epidemiologic findings. J Infect Dis 1982;145:431–40.
32 Shands KN, Schmid GP, Dan BB *et al.* Toxic-shock syndrome in menstruating women: association with tampon use and *Staphylococcus aureus* and clinical features in 52 cases. N Engl J Med 1980;303:1436–42.
33 Bergdoll MS, Crass BA, Reiser RF, Robbins RN, Davis JP. A new staphylococcal enterotoxin, enterotoxin F, associated with toxic-shock-syndrome *Staphylococcus aureus* isolates. Lancet 1981;i:1017–21.
34 Schlievert PM, Shands KN, Dan BB, Schmid GP, Nishimura RD. Identification and characterization of an exotoxin from *Staphylococcus aureus* associated with toxic-shock syndrome. J Infect Dis 1981;143:509–16.
35 Schlievert PM, Tripp TJ, Peterson ML. Reemergence of staphylococcal toxic shock syndrome in Minneapolis-St. Paul, Minnesota, during the 2000–2003 surveillance period. J Clin Microbiol 2004;42:2875–6.
36 Schlievert PM, Kim MH. Reporting of toxic shock syndrome *Staphylococcus aureus* in 1982 to 1990. J Infect Dis 1991; 164:1245–6.
37 Schlievert PM. Staphylococcal enterotoxin B and toxic-shock syndrome toxin-1 are significantly associated with non-menstrual TSS. Lancet 1986;i:1149–50.
38 Kreiswirth BN, Schlievert PM, Novick RP. Evaluation of coagulase-negative staphylococci for ability to produce toxic shock syndrome toxin 1. J Clin Microbiol 1987;25:2028–9.
39 Lindsay JA, Ruzin A, Ross HF, Kurepina N, Novick RP. The gene for toxic shock toxin is carried by a family of mobile pathogenicity islands in *Staphylococcus aureus*. Mol Microbiol 1998;29:527–43.
40 Blomster-Hautamaa DA, Kreiswirth BN, Kornblum JS, Novick RP, Schlievert PM. The nucleotide and partial amino acid sequence of toxic shock syndrome toxin-1. J Biol Chem 1986;261:15783–6.
41 Blomster-Hautamaa DA, Kreiswirth BN, Novick RP, Schlievert PM. Resolution of highly purified toxic-shock syndrome toxin 1 into two distinct proteins by isoelectric focusing. Biochemistry 1986;25:54–9.
42 Blomster-Hautamaa DA, Schlievert PM. Preparation of toxic shock syndrome toxin-1. Methods Enzymol 1988;165:37–43.
43 Novick RP. Autoinduction and signal transduction in the regulation of staphylococcal virulence. Mol Microbiol 2003; 48:1429–49.
44 Recsei P, Kreiswirth B, O'Reilly M, Schlievert P, Gruss A, Novick RP. Regulation of exoprotein gene expression in *Staphylococcus aureus* by agr. Mol Gen Genet 1986;202:58–61.
45 Blomster-Hautamaa DA, Novick RP, Schlievert PM. Localization of biologic functions of toxic shock syndrome toxin-1 by use of monoclonal antibodies and cyanogen bromide-generated toxin fragments. J Immunol 1986;137:3572–6.
46 Pragman AA, Schlievert PM. Virulence regulation in *Staphylococcus aureus*: the need for in vivo analysis of virulence

factor regulation. FEMS Immunol Med Microbiol 2004;42:147–54.

47 Yarwood JM, Schlievert PM. Quorum sensing in *Staphylococcus* infections. J Clin Invest 2003;112:1620–5.

48 Steinhuber A, Goerke C, Bayer MG, Doring G, Wolz C. Molecular architecture of the regulatory locus *sae* of *Staphylococcus aureus* and its impact on expression of virulence factors. J Bacteriol 2003;185:6278–86.

49 Giraudo AT, Cheung AL, Nagel R. The *sae* locus of *Staphylococcus aureus* controls exoprotein synthesis at the transcriptional level. Arch Microbiol 1997;168:53–8.

50 Giraudo AT, Mansilla C, Chan A, Raspanti C, Nagel R. Studies on the expression of regulatory locus *sae* in *Staphylococcus aureus*. Curr Microbiol 2003;46:246–50.

51 Giraudo AT, Raspanti CG, Calzolari A, Nagel R. Characterization of a Tn551-mutant of *Staphylococcus aureus* defective in the production of several exoproteins. Can J Microbiol 1994;40:677–81.

52 Dunman PM, Murphy E, Haney S *et al*. Transcription profiling-based identification of *Staphylococcus aureus* genes regulated by the *agr* and/or *sarA* loci. J Bacteriol 2001;183:7341–53.

53 Bayer AS, Ramos MD, Menzies BE, Yeaman MR, Shen AJ, Cheung AL. Hyperproduction of alpha-toxin by *Staphylococcus aureus* results in paradoxically reduced virulence in experimental endocarditis: a host defense role for platelet microbicidal proteins. Infect Immun 1997;65:4652–60.

54 Cheung AL, Bayer MG, Heinrichs JH. *sar* genetic determinants necessary for transcription of RNAII and RNAIII in the *agr* locus of *Staphylococcus aureus*. J Bacteriol 1997;179:3963–71.

55 Cheung AL, Koomey JM, Butler CA, Projan SJ, Fischetti VA. Regulation of exoprotein expression in *Staphylococcus aureus* by a locus (*sar*) distinct from *agr*. Proc Natl Acad Sci USA 1992;89:6462–6.

56 Cheung AL, Schmidt K, Bateman B, Manna AC. SarS, a SarA homolog repressible by *agr*, is an activator of protein A synthesis in *Staphylococcus aureus*. Infect Immun 2001;69:2448–55.

57 Cheung AL, Ying P. Regulation of alpha- and beta-hemolysins by the *sar* locus of *Staphylococcus aureus*. J Bacteriol 1994; 176:580–5.

58 Cheung AL, Zhang G. Global regulation of virulence determinants in *Staphylococcus aureus* by the SarA protein family. Front Biosci 2002;7:d1825–d1842.

59 Chien Y, Cheung AL. Molecular interactions between two global regulators, *sar* and *agr*, in *Staphylococcus aureus*. J Biol Chem 1998;273:2645–52.

60 Chien Y, Manna AC, Projan SJ, Cheung AL. SarA, a global regulator of virulence determinants in *Staphylococcus aureus*, binds to a conserved motif essential for *sar*-dependent gene regulation. J Biol Chem 1999;274:37169–76.

61 Chan PF, Foster SJ. Role of SarA in virulence determinant production and environmental signal transduction in *Staphylococcus aureus*. J Bacteriol 1998;180:6232–41.

62 Chan PF, Foster SJ, Ingham E, Clements MO. The *Staphylococcus aureus* alternative sigma factor σB controls the environmental stress response but not starvation survival or pathogenicity in a mouse abscess model. J Bacteriol 1998; 180:6082–9.

63 Deora R, Tseng T, Misra TK. Alternative transcription factor σB of *Staphylococcus aureus*: characterization and role in transcription of the global regulatory locus *sar*. J Bacteriol 1997;179:6355–9.

64 Heinrichs JH, Bayer MG, Cheung AL. Characterization of the *sar* locus and its interaction with *agr* in *Staphylococcus aureus*. J Bacteriol 1996;178:418–23.

65 Manna AC, Cheung AL. *sarU*, a *sarA* homolog, is repressed by SarT and regulates virulence genes in *Staphylococcus aureus*. Infect Immun 2003;71:343–53.

66 Manna AC, Cheung AL. Expression of SarX, a negative regulator of *agr* and exoprotein synthesis, is activated by MgrA in *Staphylococcus aureus*. J Bacteriol 2006;188:4288–99.

67 Rechtin TM, Gillaspy AF, Schumacher MA, Brennan RG, Smeltzer MS, Hurlburt BK. Characterization of the SarA virulence gene regulator of *Staphylococcus aureus*. Mol Microbiol 1999;33:307–16.

68 Schmidt KA, Manna AC, Gill S, Cheung AL. SarT, a repressor of α-hemolysin in *Staphylococcus aureus*. Infect Immun 2001; 69:4749–58.

69 Tormo MA, Martí M, Valle J *et al*. SarA is an essential positive regulator of *Staphylococcus epidermidis* biofilm development. J Bacteriol 2005;187:2348–56.

70 Pragman AA, Herron-Olson L, Case LC *et al*. Sequence analysis of the *Staphylococcus aureus srrAB* loci reveals that truncation of *srrA* affects growth and virulence factor expression. J Bacteriol 2007;189:7515–19.

71 Pragman AA, Yarwood JM, Tripp TJ, Schlievert PM. Characterization of virulence factor regulation by SrrAB, a two-component system in *Staphylococcus aureus*. J Bacteriol 2004;186:2430–8.

72 Yarwood JM, McCormick JK, Schlievert PM. Identification of a novel two-component regulatory system that acts in global regulation of virulence factors of *Staphylococcus aureus*. J Bacteriol 2001;183:1113–23.

73 Said-Salim B, Dunman PM, McAleese FM *et al*. Global regulation of *Staphylococcus aureus* genes by Rot. J Bacteriol 2003;185:610–19.

74 Fournier B, Klier A, Rapoport G. The two-component system ArlS-ArlR is a regulator of virulence gene expression in *Staphylococcus aureus*. Mol Microbiol 2001;41:247–61.

75 Luong TT, Newell SW, Lee CY. Mgr, a novel global regulator in *Staphylococcus aureus*. J Bacteriol 2003;185:3703–10.

76 Garvis S, Mei JM, Ruiz-Albert J, Holden DW. *Staphylococcus aureus svrA*: a gene required for virulence and expression of the *agr* locus. Microbiology 2002;148:3235–43.

77 Schlievert PM, Case LC, Nemeth KA *et al*. Alpha and beta chains of hemoglobin inhibit production of *Staphylococcus aureus* exotoxins. Biochemistry 2007;46:14349–58.

78 Peng HL, Novick RP, Kreiswirth B, Kornblum J, Schlievert P. Cloning, characterization, and sequencing of an accessory gene regulator (*agr*) in *Staphylococcus aureus*. J Bacteriol 1988; 170:4365–72.

79 Cheung AL, Projan SJ. Cloning and sequencing of *sarA* of *Staphylococcus aureus*, a gene required for the expression of *agr*. J Bacteriol 1994;176:4168–72.

80 Schlievert PM, Blomster DA. Production of staphylococcal pyrogenic exotoxin type C: influence of physical and chemical factors. J Infect Dis 1983;147:236–42.

81 Acharya KR, Passalacqua EF, Jones EY *et al*. Structural basis of superantigen action inferred from crystal structure of toxic-shock syndrome toxin-1. Nature 1994;367:94–7.

82 Prasad GS, Earnhart CA, Murray DL, Novick RP, Schlievert PM, Ohlendorf DH. Structure of toxic shock syndrome toxin 1. Biochemistry 1993;32:13761–6.

83 Kim J, Urban RG, Strominger JL, Wiley DC. Toxic shock syndrome toxin-1 complexed with a class II major histocompatibility molecule HLA-DR1. Science 1994;266:1870–4.
84 Hurley JM, Shimonkevitz R, Hanagan A *et al.* Identification of class II major histocompatibility complex and T cell receptor binding sites in the superantigen toxic shock syndrome toxin 1. J Exp Med 1995;181:2229–35.
85 Moza B, Buonpane RA, Zhu P *et al.* Long-range cooperative binding effects in a T cell receptor variable domain. Proc Natl Acad Sci USA 2006;103:9867–72.
86 Moza, B. Varma AK, Buonpane RA *et al.* Structural basis of T-cell specificity and activation by the bacterial superantigen TSST-1. EMBO J 2007;26:1187–97.
87 Murray DL, Earhart CA, Mitchell DT, Ohlendorf DH, Novick RP, Schlievert PM. Localization of biologically important regions on toxic shock syndrome toxin 1. Infect Immun 1996;64:371–4.
88 Murray DL, Prasad GS, Earhart CA *et al.* Immunobiologic and biochemical properties of mutants of toxic shock syndrome toxin-1. J Immunol 1994;152:87–95.
89 McCormick JK, Tripp TJ, Llera AS *et al.* Functional analysis of the TCR binding domain of toxic shock syndrome toxin-1 predicts further diversity in MHC class II/superantigen/TCR ternary complexes. J Immunol 2003;171:1385–92.
90 Bonventre PF, Heeg H, Edwards CK III, Cullen CM. A mutation at histidine residue 135 of toxic shock syndrome toxin yields an immunogenic protein with minimal toxicity. Infect Immun 1995;63:509–15.
91 Davis CC, Kremer MJ, Schlievert PM, Squier CA. Penetration of toxic shock syndrome toxin-1 across porcine vaginal mucosa ex vivo: permeability characteristics, toxin distribution, and tissue damage. Am J Obstet Gynecol 2003;189:1785–91.
92 Squier CA, Mantz MJ, Schlievert PM, Davis CC. Porcine vagina ex vivo as a model for studying permeability and pathogenesis in mucosa. J Pharm Sci 2008;97:9–21.
93 Peterson M, Ault K, Kremer MJ *et al.* Innate immune system is activated by stimulation of vaginal epithelial cells with *Staphylococcus aureus* and toxic shock syndrome toxin-1. Infect Immun 2005;73:2164–74.
94 Kushnaryov VM, MacDonald HS, Reiser R, Bergdoll MS. Staphylococcal toxic shock toxin specifically binds to cultured human epithelial cells and is rapidly internalized. Infect Immun 1984;45:566–71.
95 Schlievert PM, Jablonski LM, Roggiani M *et al.* Pyrogenic toxin superantigen site specificity in toxic shock syndrome and food poisoning in animals. Infect Immun 2000;68:3630–34.
96 Harris TO, Grossman D, Kappler JW, Marrack P, Rich RR, Betley MJ. Lack of complete correlation between emetic and T-cell-stimulatory activities of staphylococcal enterotoxins. Infect Immun 1993;61:3175–83.
97 Dinges MM, Orwin PM, Schlievert PM. Exotoxins of *Staphylococcus aureus*. Clin Microbiol Rev 2000;13:16–34.
98 Hovde CJ, Hackett SP, Bohach GA. Nucleotide sequence of the staphylococcal enterotoxin C3 gene: sequence comparison of all three type C staphylococcal enterotoxins. Mol Gen Genet 1990;220:329–33.
99 Turner TN, Smith CL, Bohach GA. Residues 20, 22, and 26 determine the subtype specificities of staphylococcal enterotoxins C1 and C2. Infect Immun 1992;60:694–7.
100 Marr JC, Lyon JD, Roberson JR, Lupher M, Davis WC, Bohach GA. Characterization of novel type C staphylococcal enterotoxins: biological and evolutionary implications. Infect Immun 1993;61:4254–62.
101 Deringer JR, Ely RJ, Stauffacher CV, Bohach GA. Subtype-specific interactions of type C staphylococcal enterotoxins with the T-cell receptor. Mol Microbiol 1996;22:523–34.
102 Edwards VM, Deringer JR, Callantine SD *et al.* Characterization of the canine type C enterotoxin produced by *Staphylococcus intermedius* pyoderma isolates. Infect Immun 1997;65: 2346–52.
103 Fields BA, Malchiodi EL, Li H *et al.* Crystal structure of a T-cell receptor beta-chain complexed with a superantigen. Nature 1996;384:188–92.
104 Andersen PS, Lavoie PM, Séklay RP *et al.* Role of the T cell receptor alpha chain in stabilizing TCR–superantigen–MHC class II complexes. Immunity 1999;10:473–83.
105 Leder L, Llera A, Lavoie PM *et al.* A mutational analysis of the binding of staphylococcal enterotoxins B and C3 to the T cell receptor beta chain and major histocompatibility complex class II. J Exp Med 1998;187:823–33.
106 Malchiodi EL, Eisenstein E, Fields BA *et al.* Superantigen binding to a T cell receptor beta chain of known three-dimensional structure. J Exp Med 1995;182:1833–45.
107 Li H, Llera A, Tsuchiya D *et al.* Three-dimensional structure of the complex between a T cell receptor beta chain and the superantigen staphylococcal enterotoxin B. Immunity 1998; 9:807–16.
108 Li H, Llera A, Malchiodi EL, Mariuzza RA. The structural basis of T cell activation by superantigens. Annu Rev Immunol 1999;17:435–66.
109 Hovde CJ, Marr JC, Hoffmann ML *et al.* Investigation of the role of the disulphide bond in the activity and structure of staphylococcal enterotoxin C1. Mol Microbiol 1994;13:897–909.
110 Sundström M, Hallén D, Svensson A *et al.* The co-crystal structure of staphylococcal enterotoxin type A with Zn^{2+} at 2.7 Å resolution. Implications for major histocompatibility complex class II binding. J Biol Chem 1996;271:32212–16.
111 Schad EM, Papageorgiou AC, Svensson LA, Acharya KR. A structural and functional comparison of staphylococcal enterotoxins A and C2 reveals remarkable similarity and dissimilarity. J Mol Biol 1997;269:270–80.
112 Li Y, Li H, Dimasi N *et al.* Crystal structure of a superantigen bound to the high-affinity, zinc-dependent site on MHC class II. Immunity 2001;14:93–104.
113 Sundberg EJ, Li H, Llera AS *et al.* Structures of two streptococcal superantigens bound to TCR beta chains reveal diversity in the architecture of T cell signaling complexes. Structure 2002;10:687–99.
114 Petersson K, Pettersson H, Skartved NJ, Walse B, Forsberg G. Staphylococcal enterotoxin H induces V alpha-specific expansion of T cells. J Immunol 2003;170:4148–54.
115 Pumphrey N, Vuidepot A, Jakobsen B, Forsberg G, Walse B, Lindkvist-Petersson K. Cutting edge: Evidence of direct TCR alpha-chain interaction with superantigen. J Immunol 2007; 179:2700–4.
116 Brouillard JN, Günther S, Varma AK *et al.* Crystal structure of the streptococcal superantigen SpeI and functional role of a novel loop domain in T cell activation by group V superantigens. J Mol Biol 2007;367:925–34.

117 Orwin PM, Fitzgerald JR, Leung DY, Gutierrez JA, Bohacj GA, Schlievert PM. Characterization of *Staphylococcus aureus* enterotoxin L. Infect Immun 2003;71:2916–19.
118 Orwin PM, Leung DY, Donahue HL, Novick RP, Schlievert PM. Biochemical and biological properties of staphylococcal enterotoxin K. Infect Immun 2001;69:360–6.
119 Orwin PM, Leung DY, Tripp TJ *et al*. Characterization of a novel staphylococcal enterotoxin-like superantigen, a member of the group V subfamily of pyrogenic toxins. Biochemistry 2002;41:14033–40.
120 Günther S, Varma AK, Moza B *et al*. A novel loop domain in superantigens extends their T cell receptor recognition site. J Mol Biol 2007;371:210–21.
121 Holmberg SD, Blake PA. Staphylococcal food poisoning in the United States. New facts and old misconceptions. JAMA 1984;251:487–9.
122 Kent TH. Staphylococcal enterotoxin gastroenteritis in rhesus monkeys. Am J Pathol 1966;48:387–407.
123 Sugiyama H, Hayama T. Abdominal viscera as site of emetic action for staphylococcal enterotoxin in the monkey. J Infect Dis 1965;115:330–6.
124 Jett M, Brinkley W, Neill R, Gemski P, Hunt R. *Staphylococcus aureus* enterotoxin B challenge of monkeys: correlation of plasma levels of arachidonic acid cascade products with occurrence of illness. Infect Immun 1990;58:3494–9.
125 Scheuber PH, Golecki JR, Kickhöfen B, Scheel D, Beck G, Hammer DK. Skin reactivity of unsensitized monkeys upon challenge with staphylococcal enterotoxin B: a new approach for investigating the site of toxin action. Infect Immun 1985;50:869–76.
126 Reck B, Scheuber PH, Longdong W, Sailer-Kramer B, Bartsch K, Hammer DK. Protection against the staphylococcal enterotoxin-induced intestinal disorder in the monkey by anti-idiotypic antibodies. Proc Natl Acad Sci USA 1988;85:3170–4.
127 Komisar J, Rivera J, Vega A, Tseng J. Effects of staphylococcal enterotoxin B on rodent mast cells. Infect Immun 1992;60: 2969–75.
128 Alber G, Hammer DK, Fleischer B. Relationship between enterotoxic- and T lymphocyte-stimulating activity of staphylococcal enterotoxin B. J Immunol 1990;144:4501–6.
129 Alber G, Scheuber PH, Reck B, Sailer-Kramer B, Hartmann A, Hammer DK. Role of substance P in immediate-type skin reactions induced by staphylococcal enterotoxin B in unsensitized monkeys. J Allergy Clin Immunol 1989;84:880–5.
130 Beery JT, Taylor SL, Schlunz LR, Freed RC, Bergdoll MS. Effects of staphylococcal enterotoxin A on the rat gastrointestinal tract. Infect Immun 1984;44:234–40.
131 Bergdoll MS. Monkey feeding test for staphylococcal enterotoxin. Methods Enzymol 1988;165:324–33.
132 Wright A, Andrews PL, Titball RW. Induction of emetic, pyrexic, and behavioral effects of *Staphylococcus aureus* enterotoxin B in the ferret. Infect Immun 2000;68:2386–9.
133 van Gessel YA, Mani S, Bi S *et al*. Functional piglet model for the clinical syndrome and postmortem findings induced by staphylococcal enterotoxin B. Exp Biol Med (Maywood) 2004; 229:1061–71.
134 Hu DL, Omoe K, Shimura H, Ono K, Sugii S, Shinagawa K. Emesis in the shrew mouse (*Suncus murinus*) induced by peroral and intraperitoneal administration of staphylococcal enterotoxin A. J Food Prot 1999;62:1350–3.
135 Iandolo JJ. Genetic analysis of extracellular toxins of *Staphylococcus aureus*. Annu Rev Microbiol 1989;43:375–402.
136 Buonpane RA, Churchhill HR, Moza B *et al*. Neutralization of staphylococcal enterotoxin B by soluble, high-affinity receptor antagonists. Nat Med 2007;13:725–9.
137 Buonpane RA, Moza B, Sundberg EJ, Kranz DM. Characterization of T cell receptors engineered for high affinity against toxic shock syndrome toxin-1. J Mol Biol 2005;353:308–21.
138 Schlievert PM, Bohach GA. Staphylococcal and streptococcal superantigens: an update. In: Kotb M, Fraser JD, eds. Superantigens. Molecular Basis for Their Role in Human Diseases. Washington, DC: American Society for Microbiology Press, 2007:21–36.
139 Fey PD, Said-Salim B, Rupp ME *et al*. Comparative molecular analysis of community- or hospital-acquired methicillin-resistant *Staphylococcus aureus*. Antimicrob Agents Chemother 2003;47:196–203.
140 Tenover FC, Gaynes RP. The epidemiology of staphylococcus infection. In: Fischetti VA, Novick RP, Ferretti JJ, Portnoy DA, Rood JI, eds. Gram-positive Pathogens. Washington, DC: American Society for Microbiology Press, 2000:414–21.
141 Ahrens P, Andresen LO. Cloning and sequence analysis of genes encoding *Staphylococcus hyicus* exfoliative toxin types A, B, C, and D. J Bacteriol 2004;186:1833–7.
142 Ladhani S. Recent developments in staphylococcal scalded skin syndrome. Clin Microbiol Infect 2001;7:301–7.
143 Yamasaki O, Tristan A, Yamaguchi T *et al*. Distribution of the exfoliative toxin D gene in clinical *Staphylococcus aureus* isolates in France. Clin Microbiol Infect 2006;12:585–8.
144 Melish ME, Glasgow LA. The staphylococcal scalded-skin syndrome. N Engl J Med 1970;282:1114–19.
145 Arbuthnott JP, Kent J, Lyell A, Gemmel CG. The role of extracellular products of 'phage group 2 staphylococci in toxic epidermal necrolysis. Contrib Microbiol Immunol 1973;1:434–40.
146 Kapral FA, Miller MM. Product of *Staphylococcus aureus* responsible for the scalded-skin syndrome. Infect Immun 1971;4:541–5.
147 Kondo I, Sakurai S, Sarai Y. Purification of exfoliatin produced by *Staphylococcus aureus* of bacteriophage group 2 and its physicochemical properties. Infect Immun 1973;8:156–64.
148 Kondo I, Sakurai S, Sarai Y. New type of exfoliatin obtained from staphylococcal strains, belonging to phage groups other than group II, isolated from patients with impetigo and Ritter's disease. Infect Immun 1974;10:851–61.
149 Melish ME, Glasgow LA, Turner MD. The staphylococcal scalded-skin syndrome: isolation and partial characterization of the exfoliative toxin. J Infect Dis 1972;125:129–40.
150 Lee CY, Schmidt JJ, Johnson-Winegar AD, Spero L, Iandolo JJ. Sequence determination and comparison of the exfoliative toxin A and toxin B genes from *Staphylococcus aureus*. J Bacteriol 1987;169:3904–9.
151 Yamaguchi T, Hayashi T, Takami H *et al*. Phage conversion of exfoliative toxin A production in *Staphylococcus aureus*. Mol Microbiol 2000;38:694–705.
152 Yamaguchi T, Hayashi T, Takami H *et al*. Complete nucleotide sequence of a *Staphylococcus aureus* exfoliative toxin B plasmid and identification of a novel ADP-ribosyltransferase, EDIN-C. Infect Immun 2001;69:7760–71.

153 de Azavedo JC, Bailey CJ, Arbuthnott JP. Purification of epidermolytic toxin of *Staphylococcus aureus*. Methods Enzymol 1988;165:32–6.
154 Vath GM, Earhart CA, Monie DD, Iandolo JJ, Schlievert PM, Ohlendorf DH. The crystal structure of exfoliative toxin B: a superantigen with enzymatic activity. Biochemistry 1999; 38:10239–46.
155 Vath GM, Earhart CA, Rago JV *et al*. The structure of the superantigen exfoliative toxin A suggests a novel regulation as a serine protease. Biochemistry 1997;36:1559–66.
156 Lillibridge CB, Melish ME, Glasgow LA. Site of action of exfoliative toxin in the staphylococcal scalded-skin syndrome. Pediatrics 1972;50:728–38.
157 Elias PM, Fritsch P, Dahl MV, Wolff K. Staphylococcal toxic epidermal necrolysis: pathogenesis and studies on the subcellular site of action of exfoliatin. J Invest Dermatol 1975; 65:501–12.
158 McLay AL, Arbuthnott JP, Lyell A. Action of staphylococcal epidermolytic toxin on mouse skin: an electron microscopic study. J Invest Dermatol 1975;65:423–8.
159 Wuepper KD, Dimond RL, Knutson DD. Studies of the mechanism of epidermal injury by a staphylococcal epidermolytic toxin. J Invest Dermatol 1975;65:191–200.
160 Baker DH, Dimond RL, Wuepper KD. The epidermolytic toxin of *Staphylococcus aureus*: its failure to bind to cells and its detection in blister fluids of patients with bullous impetigo. J Invest Dermatol 1978;71:274–5.
161 Rago JV, Vath GM, Bohach GA, Ohlendorf DH, Schlievert PM. Mutational analysis of the superantigen staphylococcal exfoliative toxin A (ETA). J Immunol 2000;164:2207–13.
162 Monday SR, Vath GM, Ferens WA *et al*. Unique superantigen activity of staphylococcal exfoliative toxins. J Immunol 1999; 162:4550–9.
163 Fleischer B, Bailey CJ. Recombinant epidermolytic (exfoliative) toxin A of *Staphylococcus aureus* is not a superantigen. Med Microbiol Immunol 1992;180:273–8.
164 Smith TP, John DA, Bailey CJ. The binding of epidermolytic toxin from *Staphylococcus aureus* to mouse epidermal tissue. Histochem J 1987;19:137–49.
165 Smith TP, John DA, Bailey CJ. Epidermolytic toxin binds to components in the epidermis of a resistant species. Eur J Cell Biol 1989;49:341–9.
166 Smith TP, Bailey CJ. Epidermolytic toxin from *Staphylococcus aureus* binds to filaggrins. FEBS Lett 1986;194:309–12.
167 Bailey CJ, Smith TP. The reactive serine residue of epidermolytic toxin A. Biochem J 1990;269:535–7.
168 Prevost G, Rifai S, Chaix ML, Piemont Y. Functional evidence that the Ser-195 residue of staphylococcal exfoliative toxin A is essential for biological activity. Infect Immun 1991;59:3337–9.
169 Rago JV, Vath GM, Tripp TJ, Bohach GA, Ohlendorf DH, Schlievert PM. Staphylococcal exfoliative toxins cleave alpha- and beta-melanocyte-stimulating hormones. Infect Immun 2000;68:2366–8.
170 Amagai M, Matsuyoshi N, Wang ZH, Andl C, Stanley JR. Toxin in bullous impetigo and staphylococcal scalded-skin syndrome targets desmoglein 1. Nat Med 2000;6:1275–7.
171 Hanakawa Y, Schechter NM, Lin C, Nishifuji K, Amagai M, Stanley JR. Enzymatic and molecular characteristics of the efficiency and specificity of exfoliative toxin cleavage of desmoglein 1. J Biol Chem 2004;279:5268–77.
172 Amagai M, Yamaguchi T, Hanakawa Y, Nishifuji K, Sugai M, Stanley JR. Staphylococcal exfoliative toxin B specifically cleaves desmoglein 1. J Invest Dermatol 2002;118:845–50.
173 Freer JH, Arbuthnott JP. Toxins of *Staphylococcus aureus*. Pharmacol Ther 1982;19:55–106.
174 Bhakdi S, Tranum-Jensen J. Alpha-toxin of *Staphylococcus aureus*. Microbiol Rev 1991;55:733–51.
175 Gray GS, Kehoe M. Primary sequence of the alpha-toxin gene from *Staphylococcus aureus* Wood 46. Infect Immun 1984;46:615–18.
176 O'Reilly M, Kreiswirth B, Foster TJ. Cryptic alpha-toxin gene in toxic shock syndrome and septicaemia strains of *Staphylococcus aureus*. Mol Microbiol 1990;4:1947–55.
177 Bernheimer AW, Schwartz LL. Isolation and composition of staphylococcal alpha toxin. J Gen Microbiol 1963;30:455–68.
178 Harshman S, Boquet P, Duflot E, Alouf JE, Montecucco C, Papini E. Staphylococcal alpha-toxin: a study of membrane penetration and pore formation. J Biol Chem 1989;264:14978–84.
179 Gouaux JE, Braha O, Hobaugh MR *et al*. Subunit stoichiometry of staphylococcal alpha-hemolysin in crystals and on membranes: a heptameric transmembrane pore. Proc Natl Acad Sci USA 1994;91:12828–31.
180 Bhakdi S, Muhly M, Fussle R. Correlation between toxin binding and hemolytic activity in membrane damage by staphylococcal alpha-toxin. Infect Immun 1984;46:318–23.
181 Bhakdi S, Valeva A, Walev I, Zitzer A, Palmer M. Pore-forming bacterial cytolysins. Symp Ser Soc Appl Microbiol 1998;27:15S–25S.
182 Hildebrand A, Pohl M, Bhakdi S. *Staphylococcus aureus* alpha-toxin. Dual mechanism of binding to target cells. J Biol Chem 1991;266:17195–200.
183 Cassidy P, Harshman S. Studies on the binding of staphylococcal 125I-labeled alpha-toxin to rabbit erythrocytes. Biochemistry 1976;15:2348–55.
184 Walev I, Martin E, Jonas D *et al*. Staphylococcal alpha-toxin kills human keratinocytes by permeabilizing the plasma membrane for monovalent ions. Infect Immun 1993;61:4972–9.
185 Jonas D, Walev I, Berger T, Liebetrau M, Palmer M, Bhakdi S. Novel path to apoptosis: small transmembrane pores created by staphylococcal alpha-toxin in T lymphocytes evoke internucleosomal DNA degradation. Infect Immun 1994;62:1304–12.
186 Walev I, Plamer M, Martin E *et al*. Recovery of human fibroblasts from attack by the pore-forming alpha-toxin of *Staphylococcus aureus*. Microb Pathog 1994;17:187–201.
187 Walker B, Krishnasastry M, Zorn L, Kasianowicz J, Bayley H. Functional expression of the alpha-hemolysin of *Staphylococcus aureus* in intact *Escherichia coli* and in cell lysates. Deletion of five C-terminal amino acids selectively impairs hemolytic activity. J Biol Chem 1992;267:10902–9.
188 Suttorp N, Seeger W, Dewein E, Bhakdi S, Roka L. Staphylococcal alpha-toxin-induced PGI2 production in endothelial cells: role of calcium. Am J Physiol 1985;248:C127–C134.
189 Suttorp N, Seeger W, Zucker-Reimann J, Roka L, Bhakdi S. Mechanism of leukotriene generation in polymorphonuclear leukocytes by staphylococcal alpha-toxin. Infect Immun 1987; 55:104–10.
190 Seeger W, Birkemeyer RG, Ermert L, Suttorp N, Bhakdi S, Duncker HR. Staphylococcal alpha-toxin-induced vascular

leakage in isolated perfused rabbit lungs. Lab Invest 1990;63: 341–9.

191 Glenny A, Stevens NF. Staphylococcal toxins and antitoxins. J Pathol Bacteriol 1935;40:201.

192 Coleman DC, Arbuthnott JP, Pomeroy HM, Birkbeck TH. Cloning and expression in *Escherichia coli* and *Staphylococcus aureus* of the beta-lysin determinant from *Staphylococcus aureus*: evidence that bacteriophage conversion of beta-lysin activity is caused by insertional inactivation of the beta-lysin determinant. Microb Pathog 1986;1:549–64.

193 Projan SJ, Kornblum J, Kreiswirth B, Moghazeh SL, Eisner W, Novick RP. Nucleotide sequence: the beta-hemolysin gene of *Staphylococcus aureus*. Nucleic Acids Res 1989;17:3305.

194 Doery HM, Magnusson BJ, Cheyne IM, Sulasekharam J. A phospholipase in staphylococcal toxin which hydrolyses sphingomyelin. Nature 1963;198:1091–2.

195 Huseby M, Shi K, Brown CK *et al.* Structure and biological activities of beta toxin from *Staphylococcus aureus*. J Bacteriol 2007;189:8719–26.

196 Low DK, Freer JH, Arbuthnott JP, Mollby R, Wadstrom T. Consequences of spingomyelin degradation in erythrocyte ghost membranes by staphylococcal beta-toxin (sphingomyelinase C). Toxicon 1974;12:279–85.

197 Marshall MJ, Bohach GA, Boehm DF. Characterization of *Staphylococcus aureus* beta-toxin induced leukotoxicity. J Nat Toxins 2000;9:125–38.

198 Woodin AM. Fractionation of a leucocidin from *Staphylococcus aureus*. Biochem J 1959;73:225–37.

199 Woodin AM. Purification of the two components of leucocidin from *Staphylococcus aureus*. Biochem J 1960;75:158–65.

200 Prévost G, Couppie P, Prévost P *et al.* Epidemiological data on *Staphylococcus aureus* strains producing synergohymenotropic toxins. J Med Microbiol 1995;42:237–45.

201 Barrio MB, Rainard P, Prévost G. LukM/LukF'-PV is the most active *Staphylococcus aureus* leukotoxin on bovine neutrophils. Microbes Infect 2006;8:2068–74.

202 Dalla Serra M, Coraiola M, Viero G *et al. Staphylococcus aureus* bicomponent gamma-hemolysins, HlgA, HlgB, and HlgC, can form mixed pores containing all components. J Chem Inf Model 2005;45:1539–45.

203 Bronner S, Monteil H, Prévost G. Regulation of virulence determinants in *Staphylococcus aureus*: complexity and applications. FEMS Microbiol Rev 2004;28:183–200.

204 Menestrina G, Serra MD, Prévost G. Mode of action of beta-barrel pore-forming toxins of the staphylococcal alpha-hemolysin family. Toxicon 2001;39:1661–72.

205 Prévost G, Mourey L, Colin DA, Menestrina G. Staphylococcal pore-forming toxins. Curr Top Microbiol Immunol 2001;257: 53–83.

206 Szmigielski S, Prevost G, Monteil H, Colin DA, Jeljaszewicz J. Leukocidal toxins of staphylococci. Zentralbl Bakteriol 1999; 289:185–201.

207 Szmigielski S, Sobiczewska E, Prévost G, Monteil H, Colin DA, Jeljaszewicz J. Effect of purified staphylococcal leukocidal toxins on isolated blood polymorphonuclear leukocytes and peritoneal macrophages in vitro. Zentralbl Bakteriol 1998;288:383–94.

208 Ferreras M, Höper F, Dalla Serra M, Colin DA, Prévost G, Menestrina G. The interaction of *Staphylococcus aureus* bi-component gamma-hemolysins and leucocidins with cells and lipid membranes. Biochim Biophys Acta 1998;1414:108–26.

209 Siqueira JA, Speeg-Schatz C, Freitas FI, Sahel J, Monteil H, Prévost G. Channel-forming leucotoxins from *Staphylococcus aureus* cause severe inflammatory reactions in a rabbit eye model. J Med Microbiol 1997;46:486–94.

210 Konig B, Prevost G, Konig W. Composition of staphylococcal bi-component toxins determines pathophysiological reactions. J Med Microbiol 1997;46:479–85.

211 Cooney J, Kienle Z, Foster TJ, O'Toole PW. The gamma-hemolysin locus of *Staphylococcus aureus* comprises three linked genes, two of which are identical to the genes for the F and S components of leukocidin. Infect Immun 1993;61:768–71.

212 Cooney J, Mulvey M, Arbuthnott JP, Foster TJ. Molecular cloning and genetic analysis of the determinant for gamma-lysin, a two-component toxin of *Staphylococcus aureus*. J Gen Microbiol 1988;134:2179–88.

213 Plommet M. Preparation and purification of gamma-hemolysin of staphylococci. Methods Enzymol 1988;165:8–16.

214 Prevost G, Cribier B, Couppié P *et al.* Panton–Valentine leucocidin and gamma-hemolysin from *Staphylococcus aureus* ATCC 49775 are encoded by distinct genetic loci and have different biological activities. Infect Immun 1995;63:4121–9.

215 Noda M, Kato I. Purification and crystallization of staphylococcal leukocidin. Methods Enzymol 1988;165:22–32.

216 Guillet V, Roblin P, Werner S *et al.* Crystal structure of leucotoxin S component: new insight into the staphylococcal beta-barrel pore-forming toxins. J Biol Chem 2004;279:41028–37.

217 Pedelacq JD, Maveyraud L, Prévost G *et al.* The structure of a *Staphylococcus aureus* leucocidin component (LukF-PV) reveals the fold of the water-soluble species of a family of transmembrane pore-forming toxins. Structure 1999;7:277–87.

218 Pedelacq JD, Prévost G, Monteil H, Mourey L, Samama JP. Crystal structure of the F component of the Panton–Valentine leucocidin. Int J Med Microbiol 2000;290:395–401.

219 Dufour P, Gillet Y, Bes M *et al.* Community-acquired methicillin-resistant *Staphylococcus aureus* infections in France: emergence of a single clone that produces Panton–Valentine leukocidin. Clin Infect Dis 2002;35:819–24.

220 Francis JS, Doherty MC, Lopatin U *et al.* Severe community-onset pneumonia in healthy adults caused by methicillin-resistant *Staphylococcus aureus* carrying the Panton–Valentine leukocidin genes. Clin Infect Dis 2005;40:100–7.

221 Naimi TS, LeDell KH, Boxrud DJ *et al.* Epidemiology and clonality of community-acquired methicillin-resistant *Staphylococcus aureus* in Minnesota, 1996–1998. Clin Infect Dis 2001;33:990–6.

222 Voyich JM, Otto M, Mathema B *et al.* Is Panton–Valentine leukocidin the major virulence determinant in community-associated methicillin-resistant *Staphylococcus aureus* disease? J Infect Dis 2006;194:1761–70.

223 Labandeira-Rey M, Couzon F, Boisset S *et al. Staphylococcus aureus* Panton–Valentine leukocidin causes necrotizing pneumonia. Science 2007;315:1130–3.

224 Wardenburg JB, Bae T, Otto M, DeLeo FR, Schneewind O. Poring over pores: alpha hemolysin and Panton Valentine leukocidin in *Staphylococcus aureus* pneumonia. Nat Med 2007;13:1405–6.

225 Centers for Disease Control and Prevention. Four pediatric deaths from community-acquired methicillin-resistant *Staphylococcus aureus*: Minnesota and North Dakota, 1997–1999. JAMA 1999; 282:1123–5.

226 Kravitz GR, Dries DJ, Peterson ML, Schlievert PM. Purpura fulminans due to *Staphylococcus aureus*. Clin Infect Dis 2005;40:941–7.
227 Fitton JE, Dell A, Shaw WV. The amino acid sequence of the delta haemolysin of *Staphylococcus aureus*. FEBS Lett 1980; 115:209–12.
228 Birkbeck TH, Freer JH. Purification and assay of staphylococcal delta-lysin. Methods Enzymol 1988;165:16–22.
229 Freer JH, Birkbeck TH. Possible conformation of delta-lysin, a membrane-damaging peptide of *Staphylococcus aureus*. J Theor Biol 1982;94:535–40.
230 Dhople VM, Nagaraj R. Delta-toxin, unlike melittin, has only hemolytic activity and no antimicrobial activity: rationalization of this specific biological activity. Biosci Rep 1993;13:245–50.
231 Lee KH, Fitton JE, Wuthrich K. Nuclear magnetic resonance investigation of the conformation of delta-haemolysin bound to dodecylphosphocholine micelles. Biochim Biophys Acta 1987;911:144–53.
232 Thelestam M, Mollby R. Determination of toxin-induced leakage of different-size nucleotides through the plasma membrane of human diploid fibroblasts. Infect Immun 1975;11:640–8.
233 Mellor IR, Thomas DH, Sansom MS. Properties of ion channels formed by *Staphylococcus aureus* delta-toxin. Biochim Biophys Acta 1988;942:280–94.

Chapter 7
Host Defense Against Staphylococcal Infection

Chapter 7a Mechanism of Host Defense

Hattie D. Gresham
New Mexico Veterens Affairs Health Care System, University of New Mexico, Albuquerque, NM, USA

Introduction

Host defense is an organism-specific response that involves coordination of evolutionarily driven effectors that are either innate or acquired upon exposure, and work in concert to provide infection control. For bacteria like the staphylococci that are primarily colonizers of humans but also opportunistic pathogens, the innate and acquired effectors that have evolved in the majority of hosts are sufficient to limit infection to minor superficial skin infections [1]. The redundancy in these effectors is exemplified by the number of staphylococci required to initiate infection in either normal human hosts or experimental animals (~ 10^6–10^7) [2,3], demonstrating that they represent an effective barrier against invasive infection. On the other side of the host–pathogen balance, staphylococci have evolved sensors and numerous virulence factors that signal the presence of particular host defense elements and impair their normal function [4] (see Chapter 7b). This bidirectional evolutionary pressure has created a host–pathogen equilibrium that limits persistent colonization to approximately 25–30% of the adult population, superficial skin and soft tissue infections to about 3% [1], and invasive disease to an even smaller number (< 0.1%) of hosts who commonly have chronic diseases, loss of barrier integrity by medical intervention or trauma, genetic or acquired immunodeficiencies, or impaired defense functions at the extremes of age [5]. Thus, the coordination and cooperation of both innate and acquired effectors is sufficient to provide infection control in the majority of human hosts.

The redundancy in host defense effectors also implies that gain or loss of one effector will not have a major impact on either susceptibility to infection or the severity of infection. This is exemplified by the number of proteins that have opsonic activity against staphylococci (about 10) and either directly or indirectly promote phagocyte uptake and clearance of these bacteria. For example, deficiency or genetically low levels of mannose-binding lectin (MBL) in adults is not associated with an increased risk of staphylococcal infection [6] whereas naive mice that are MBL deficient are more susceptible to infection especially if they lack the complement protein C3 [7]. Similarly, patients with the chronic lung disease cystic fibrosis are more likely to retain staphylococci within the lung if they have low levels of MBL [6]. Therefore, multiple defects in immunity are required to observe impaired host defense against staphylococci. Likewise, the addition of another opsonin, as with opsonic antibody following immunization, may have minimal impact given the presence of multiple functional opsonins. This fact makes the important therapeutic goal of enhancing host defense mechanisms in patients susceptible to invasive infection particularly daunting. Given an ocean of host defense effectors, providing an extra drop may have little effect unless one knows the precise drop to provide and when and where to provide it.

Coordination of innate and acquired effectors for clearance of extracellular bacterial pathogens

The explosion in knowledge regarding innate and adaptive immunity is thoroughly covered in several recent textbooks and review articles. Therefore, the goal of this chapter is to highlight both recent work that significantly extends knowledge beyond that in basic immunology texts and areas where our knowledge of defense against staphylococci, primarily *Staphylococcus aureus*, is lacking.

Staphylococci in Human Disease, 2nd edition. Edited by Kent B. Crossley, Kimberly K. Jefferson, Gordon Archer, Vance G. Fowler, Jr.

Table 7a.1 Characteristics of innate and adaptive immune responses.

Innate	Adaptive
What you are born with	Acquired with exposure
Action is immediate	Days to weeks to develop
Evolutionarily ancient (flies, worms)	Higher vertebrates and mammals
Recognition is encoded in germline	Recognition requires genetic recombination
Nonclonal recognition	Clonal recognition
No secondary memory	Secondary memory present
Nonspecific recognition	Specific recognition
Low threshold for activation	High threshold for activation
Terminated by inhibitory cytokines	Terminated by regulatory cells/cytokines

Barriers to infection

Host defense comprises three barriers that an extracellular pathogen must evade to gain access to privileged sites for replication: a primary barrier consisting of structural and physiological factors like the mucociliary elevator of the lung removes bacteria from the lower airway; a secondary barrier consisting of the acute inflammatory response constitutes the majority of innate immunity against extracellular bacteria like staphylococci; and a tertiary barrier is provided by the adaptive immune response that is activated on exposure to the pathogen and provides infection control and memory to prevent subsequent infection. A breach in one of these barriers is usually required to permit *S. aureus* the opportunity to cause invasive infection. However, the emergence of strains that cause lethal necrotizing pneumonia in seemingly healthy hosts [5,8] suggests either that the pathogen is evolving virulence strategies for which we lack defense or that previously unrecognized host elements are essential for defense against invasive infection by these emerging strains.

Innate and adaptive responses are discrete and teleologically separate but have a mutual interdependence (Table 7a.1). For example, opsonic antibody produced during an adaptive response is only effective when linked to an Fc receptor-bearing phagocyte produced during the acute inflammatory response. Likewise, activation of pattern recognition receptors (PRRs) of the innate immune system is essential for optimal dendritic cell presentation of antigen to T lymphocytes. Therefore, even though there are differences that discriminate between these responses (Table 7a.1), their concerted actions provide a sophisticated system of soluble molecules and cells that defend the host against infection.

Recognition, activation, and effector phases of innate and adaptive responses for clearance of extracellular bacterial pathogens

Both the innate and adaptive arms of the immune response have elements that recognize the presence of foreign invaders and/or injured tissue and which signal to induce transcriptional responses in specific cell types that lead to the generation of effectors capable of killing and clearing extracellular pathogens. For staphylococci, the primary effectors of defense are opsonization, phagocyte mobilization and activation, and direct killing by antimicrobial peptides. Innate immune recognition and signaling to generate this module of effectors is essential for host defense, and adaptive immune recognition and activation is not able to substitute for it [9,10]. Adaptive immunity, as studied thus far, primarily provides defense by antibody production to aid opsonization and phagocyte uptake and killing [11] and by antigen-specific CD4 Th1 lymphocytes and perhaps the Th17 subclass that provide interferon (IFN)-γ and interleukin (IL)-17 [12–14] for optimal activation of phagocyte killing and mobilization of neutrophils. However, the vast complexity of adaptive immunity and how it has evolved to enhance innate immune effectors for host defense has not been well studied for this pathogen. For example, antibody acquired by exposure can antagonize adhesive binding to epithelial surfaces and neutralize toxins produced during invasive infection [15]. To what extent antibody provides defense in humans by these mechanisms is unknown. In addition, given the importance of Th17 cells for defense against other extracellular bacterial infections [16,17], they may play a more regulatory role in control of staphylococcal infections. Therefore, there is much more to learn about how adaptive immune responses can enhance the opsonin–phagocyte–antimicrobial peptide module of the innate immune system for host defense.

Pattern recognition receptors and inflammasome-mediated recognition

The description of the Toll gene in *Drosophila* and its importance for recognition and defense against fungal pathogens has created a paradigm for how the inflammatory response is activated in the presence of microbial organisms that cause harm [18]. Biochemical structures expressed primarily by microbes but not by mammals ligate receptors which then signal for transcriptional responses that generate cytokines, chemokines, cell mobilization and maturation, activation of complement, and activation of coagulation. The microbial structures, called pathogen-associated molecular patterns (PAMPs), range from surface carbohydrates to nucleic acid signatures and these ligate PRRs that are expressed ubiquitously, including on

Table 7a.2 Staphylococcal pathogen-associated molecular patterns (PAMPs) and host pattern recognition receptors (PRRs).

PAMPs	PRRs
Lipoteichoic acid	TLR2
Peptidoglycan	NOD2, PGRP-S
Lipoprotein	TLR2/TLR1; TLR2/TLR6
Diacylglyceride	CD36/TLR2
Phenol soluble modulins	TLR2
Mannose	MBL; mannose receptor
CpG-DNA	TLR9
Formylated peptides	FPR
?Toxin; ?RNA	NALP3 (cryopyrin)

FPR, formylpeptide receptor; MBL, mannose-binding lectin; PGRP, peptidoglycan recognition protein; TLR, Toll-like receptor.

cell membranes, within organelles, in the cytosol, and as soluble proteins in the blood. For staphylococci, a number of PAMPs have been described along with the PRRs that they ligate (Table 7a.2) [19]; these are widely expressed on plasma membranes (Toll-like receptors or TLRs, CD36, mannose receptor), within organelles (peptidoglycan recognition protein, PGRP-S), blood (MBL), and in cytosol (NOD1/2, NALP3). Of these, two have emerged as truly essential for optimal host defense: TLR2 and its associated membrane-bound signaling molecules TLR1, TLR6 and CD36 [10,19–22]; and NALP3 (cryopyrin), a component of the inflammasome [9,23–25]. While both of these recognition receptors signal through the adaptor MyD88 to generate cytokines that promote neutrophil recruitment and activation, their location dictates at what point in the pathogenesis of the infection they provide defense. In both animal models and in humans, optimal TLR2 signaling appears to be essential for defense against bacteremia and the control of sepsis to prevent septic shock and death [10,18,21]. Moreover, additional signaling molecules associated with TLR2, like the scavenger receptor CD36, contribute to this defense [22]. TLR2 recognizes a broad array of PAMPs, including lipoproteins, diacylglyceride, phenol soluble modulins, and lipoteichoic acid (Table 7a.2). Because recognition of *S. aureus* in the bloodstream requires the synthesis of lipoproteins by this pathogen [26], the ability of TLR2 and its associated receptors to recognize nonlipoprotein PAMPs cannot substitute for control of bacteremia. Moreover, defense against cutaneous infection, while still requiring MyD88, is independent of TLR2 and instead requires recognition by a set of cytosolic proteins termed the *inflammasome* [9,27]. The inflammasome is a molecular platform for controlled activation of caspase-1 that regulates the processing and secretion of the IL-1 family of cytokines. NALP3, also known as cryopyrin, assembles the platform in response to either endogenous danger signals or molecular motifs from pathogens [24,25]. For staphylococci, the PAMP may be a toxin or hemolysin that escapes from an endosome or phagolysosome and gains entry to the cytosol. For defense against cutaneous infection, a bone marrow-derived cell is essential for signaling for IL-1 production, which then signals through an IL-1 receptor on a nonhematogenous cell to promote neutrophil recruitment [27]. In the case of TLR2 and its associated receptors, the essential cell(s) that express it and provide defense against bloodstream infection is currently not known. Importantly, neutrophils appear to be the major effector activated by each of these PAMP–PRR signaling pairs [26,27].

Defense against colonization

Defense against colonization remains one of the most poorly understood aspects of human interaction with staphylococci, particularly for *S. aureus*. Given the important relationship between colonization and susceptibility to some kinds of infection, understanding what constitutes fitness for person-to-person transmission and whether the same virulence factors that are important for mediating invasive infection also contribute to colonization [28] is essential in order to fully understand host elements that defend against colonization. The majority of newborns become colonized with *S. aureus* yet in adults this is limited to 25–30% of the population, indicating that some maturational process alters colonization. If this involves adaptive immunity and what its antigenic targets might be are currently not known. The polymicrobial community within the nasal mucosa in which *S. aureus* competes and survives is complex, and this environment is distinctly different from the ultraviolet (UV)-exposed desiccating environment of the skin. Thus, the bacterial factors that promote colonization and the host elements that defend against it may vary depending on the habitat in which the bacteria are persisting.

Mucosal immunity

Commensal microbes at mucosal surfaces maintain a steady-state low-level inflammation that induces constant surveillance by neutrophils and antimicrobial peptides [29]. Some colonizing microbes compete within this niche by promoting an inflammatory response that they can survive but which others cannot. For example, the inflammatory response promoted by *Streptococcus pneumoniae* at a mucosal surface can eliminate *S. aureus* strains that do not express catalase [30]. Moreover, nasal colonizing strains of *S. aureus* can suppress the kinetics of acute inflammation in the mucosa to promote their own persistence [31]. While neutrophils figure prominently in this controlled inflammation, adaptive immunity almost certainly contributes. For example, HIV-infected patients have a higher rate of nasal colonization, indicating that $CD4^{+}$ T lymphocytes have a role in controlling *S. aureus* colonization. Whether the Th17 subpopulation is important in this scenario and is critical for recruiting neutrophils is unknown. Another potential effector is antigen-specific IgA, produced by the nasal-associated lymphoid tissue within the submucosa of the nasal epithelium, which could antagonize adhesins necessary for attachment to nasal epithelium. If adaptive immunity does assist the innate response in eliminating colonizing staphylococci, it is essential to elucidate the reason why this is successful in some humans but not others in order to fully exploit adaptive immunity for prevention of colonization.

Antimicrobial defense of the skin

Keratinocytes in both the nasal epithelium and the skin play a key role in innate defense against staphylococci. Several elegant studies have begun to elucidate their complex biology and the fate of *S. aureus* on the keratinocyte surface and following internalization [32,33]. The skin represents a hostile environment for microbes in that it is UV-exposed, oxygen rich, acidic, dry, and bathed in fatty acids. While these have long been appreciated as important components of the physical barrier, recent work on the role of fatty acids as directly bactericidal and on the microbial virulence factors required to resist killing has highlighted their importance in control of staphylococcal colonization [32]. Intriguingly, the virulence factor required to resist fatty acid killing, IsdA, is upregulated by iron starvation and is important for defense against oxidant-mediated killing by neutrophils [34]. Moreover, a pharmacological preparation of a human skin fatty acid was successful in treating a systemic *S. aureus* infection, indicating that an effector important for control of colonization could provide a unique nonredundant mechanism for control of invasive infection. In addition, *S. aureus* infecting an organotypic culture of human keratinocytes was eliminated by activation of multiple antimicrobial peptides, including β-defensin 3 and NGAL (lipocalin) following sterile wounding and secretion and signaling of epidermal growth factor (EGF) [33]. These data indicate that as part of the wound healing response, signaling occurs that activates multiple antimicrobial peptides whose combined and cooperative action contributes to sterilization of the wounded tissue. Whether other growth factors also contribute to mobilization of host defense mechanisms is unknown but it is intriguing to speculate that other growth factors activated at sites of invasive infection could provide defense by mobilization of antimicrobial peptides.

Defense against invasive infection: killing, clearance, and targeting virulence

Phagocytes have long been regarded as essential for defense against invasive staphylococcal infections because patients with either genetic or acquired defects in phagocyte number or function are more susceptible to infection with this largely extracellular pathogen. In 1905, Ilya Metchnikoff made the initial observation that ameboid-like cells had the ability to ingest foreign material and suggested that this process could be important for host defense [35]. Although internalization and destruction of extracellular staphylococci are certainly critical host defense effector mechanisms, the role of professional phagocytes, including how they work within the multifaceted environment of acute inflammation and how they coordinate with the lymphoid system for induction of adaptive immunity, is far more complex [36]. As such, their function is highly regulated, both positively and negatively [35,36]. This regulatory control is of substantial benefit to the host because it augments phagocytic responses by stimulation with matrix and coagulation proteins, cytokines, and lipid mediators present at sites of infection while limiting the production of tissue-damaging products generated during ingestion of the pathogen to that site. In addition, negative regulatory signals essential for terminating pro-inflammatory signals and initiating wound healing can polarize phagocytes toward a nonbactericidal phenotype [37]. Therefore, the overall milieu in which phagocytes encounter staphylococci plays a substantial role in determining the outcome of the interaction.

Opsonization

The term "opsonization" derives from the Greek word *opsonein*, meaning to provide with food. In other words, an opsonin is made by the host to mark something desirable for ingestion. In addition to the well-known opsonins such as antibody and complement fragments, many host proteins have the ability to mark staphylococci for uptake and destruction by specific receptors expressed by phagocytes, including coagulation proteins like fibrinogen, matrix proteins like fibronectin and thrombospondin, and lectin-binding proteins like MBL [6,7,38]. Intriguingly, opsonins from the pentraxin family like C-reactive protein that mark other common colonizers capable of invasive infection such as streptococci and *Hemophilus* spp. do not appear to have a role in defense against staphylococci. Because pentraxins work primarily through Fcγ receptors, their failure to recognize staphylococci in conjunction with protein A expression by the pathogen appears to be yet an additional mechanism for subverting Fcγ receptor signaling for optimal activation of phagocyte killing mechanisms. Because of this, IgM antibodies activating via the complement system provide the most effective opsonization of these bacteria, a fact reflecting the importance of the expression of virulence factors by this pathogen that inhibit complement function [4]. While natural IgM antibodies have been best studied for their role in defense against *Streptococcus pneumoniae* [35], they may well have an important role in defense against staphylococci because animals deficient in B lymphocytes in the marginal zone of the spleen and the peritoneum have increased susceptibility to *S. aureus* infection [11]. Clearly, one mechanism for increasing antibody-dependent therapeutics for preventing and treating this infection would be to generate opsonic IgG3 antibodies capable of avoiding protein A while still able to engage activating Fcγ receptors for optimal phagocyte activation.

The complement system is a collection of approximately 20 soluble and cell-surface receptors that function as a regulated triggered enzyme cascade for the rapid production of mediators that both mobilize and recruit phagocytes and which mark pathogens for uptake and destruction [39]. There are three pathways for activation of the complement system (Figure 7a.1), the classical, lectin, and alternative pathways, with all three contributing to marking and clearance of staphylococci, reflecting the redundancy for optimal deposition of opsonins on the bacterial surface. Three recognition mechanisms work via cleavage of C4 either by serine proteases within C1q or by MASP (MBL-associated serine protease): (i) IgM deposition; (ii) recognition of capsular polysaccharides by a lectin receptor, SIGN R1, on marginal zone macrophages in the spleen; and (iii) recognition of mannose on the surface of the bacteria

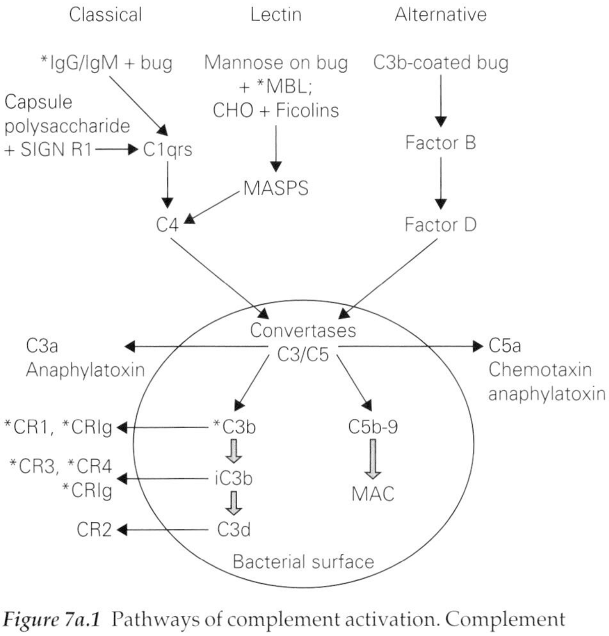

Figure 7a.1 Pathways of complement activation. Complement activation initiated by IgG or IgM opsonization of the bacterium, interaction of capsular polysaccharide with a lectin receptor SIGN R1, recognition of mannose residues on the bacterium by mannose-binding lectin (MBL), or by C3b deposition on the bacterium generates small fragments, C3a and C5a, that function as chemokines to recruit phagocytes and larger opsonic fragments that are covalently bound to the bacterium and ligate phagocytic receptors (CR1, CRIg, CR3, CR4) or receptors involved in promoting adaptive immunity (C3d). Deposition of C5b starts production of the lytic membrane attack complex. The asterisks indicate fragments/receptors with confirmed roles in host defense against staphylococci.

by MBL [40]. This cleavage step is essential for creating the multicomponent enzymes (convertases) that convert the large C3 and C5 proteins into fragments that are either covalently bound to the pathogen surface through a thioester bond (C3b) or which are soluble and interact with specific receptors on host cells to promote vasodilation for leukocyte and plasma extravasation (C3a) or are chemotactic for phagocytes (C5a). The cleavage of C5b initiates formation of the lytic membrane attack complex (MAC, C5b–C9). However, while the MAC is essential for defense against *Neisseria* spp., it plays little role in killing staphylococci. In contrast, the deposition of covalently bound C3b is central to optimal host defense and has multiple roles, including ligation of opsonic receptors, contributing to C5 enzymatic cleavage, providing an amplification mechanism for additional C3 cleavage via the alternative pathway, and producing ligands for additional receptors following enzymatic degradation [39]. Of the five receptors known to bind C3b or one of its cell-bound fragments, CR1, CR3 and the newly described CRIg [41] have been verified (experimentally or in humans with genetic defects) as essential for adequate host defense against *S. aureus* (Figure 7a.1).

Role of phagocytes

All professional phagocytes derive from a common myeloid precursor and include both blood-borne cells (neutrophils, eosinophils, basophils, and monocytes) and tissue-fixed cells (macrophages and dendritic cells). Following maturation induced by transcriptional programs stimulated by specific growth factors and matrix proteins, phagocytes occupy their various niches where they continuously sample and edit the extracellular environment. Once staphylococci have penetrated the epithelial barrier at the mucosal surfaces they colonize, the first phagocytes they encounter are a population of tissue-fixed macrophages within the lamina propria with a distinct surface phenotype (CX3CR1^{hi}, CCR2^{-}, Gr1^{-}) that derive from a monocyte subpopulation which traffics constitutively from the blood into tissues. In some mammals, these cells are able to differentiate into dendritic cells that can process the bacterium into small fragments, which they then deliver to local lymph nodes for presentation to lymphocytes to recruit the function of the adaptive immune system. Given the importance of these cells as sentinels for initiating both the acute inflammatory response and adaptive immunity, surprisingly little is known about the fate of staphylococci in either tissue macrophages or myeloid dendritic cells. One of these cells may well be the source of inflammasome-generated IL-1 and IL-18, whose production is essential for delivery of neutrophils for defense against *S. aureus* infection at cutaneous sites [27]. In addition, production of chemokines like IL-8 and cytokines like tumor necrosis factor (TNF)-α help to mobilize neutrophils and a short-lived population of inflammatory monocytes (CCR2^{+}, Gr1^{+}) from the vasculature that, along with select plasma elements, constitute

Table 7a.3 Neutrophil granules.

Granule	Exocytosis	Content
Secretory granule	++++	CR1, CR3, FPR, CD14, CD16
Gelatinase granule	+++	Gelatinase, lysozyme, PGRP-S
Specific (secondary) granule	++	Cytochrome b_{558}, lipocalin, lactoferrin, cathelicidin, collagenase
Azurophil (primary) granule	+	Myeloperoxidase, cathepsin G, defensins, elastase

FPR, formylpeptide receptor; PGRP, peptidoglycan recognition protein.

the acute inflammatory response. Whereas very little is known about this subpopulation of monocytes in control of invasive staphylococcal infection, a role for neutrophils has been clearly delineated and is increasing in complexity [36].

Neutrophils emerge from the bone marrow as short-lived cells after packaging more than 100 different proteins, representing various receptors, antimicrobial proteins, and proteases, into granules based on the timing of their respective biosynthesis [42]. Neutrophils rapidly undergo apoptosis, with removal by tissue-fixed macrophages in the spleen and the liver within a day or two of release from the bone marrow. A substantial literature has emerged on the signals present on the surface of apoptotic neutrophils and the receptors they engage for their uptake and removal [43]. In contrast, if neutrophils roll along the surface of endothelial cells overlying a tissue site of staphylococcal infection, they receive signals that stimulate a profound phenotypic change that alters their metabolic activity and shape and mobilizes cell surface receptors from within a secretory vesicle (Table 7a.3). These receptors ligate cytokines, chemokines, PAMPs, counter-adhesion molecules, and opsonins that permit rapid recognition of the pathogen and optimally activate signaling cascades that coordinate cytoskeletal remodeling with kinase activation and calcium mobilization necessary for cell migration and phagocytic uptake. The timing and magnitude of calcium mobilization dictates fusion of the three remaining granule types with either the plasma membrane or the forming phagosome, with the primary granule fusing last with the phagosomal membrane. The primary granule is a secretory lysosome and its fusion with the phagosome provides the effectors best known for killing and eliminating staphylococci (Table 7a.3). Fusion of the primary granule with the phagosome synchronizes with a phosphorylation cascade that assembles the components of a member of the NOX family of NADPH oxidases (NOX2) [44] on both the phagosomal and plasma membranes (Figure 7a.2). In oxygen-rich environments, this results in the consumption of molecular oxygen and its one-electron reduction to superoxide anion (Figure 7a.2). This "respiratory burst" has long been thought to provide reactive oxygen species (ROS) that directly kill internalized staphylococci by inducing permanent damage to key bacterial enzymes and DNA. However, NOX2 plays a critical role in host defense against staphylococci by working on multiple levels to control infection in both extracellular and intracellular locales [44,45]. Its newly described role in promoting killing of extracellular bacteria by neutrophil extracellular traps is discussed below. Within the milieu of the phagosome after fusion with the secretory and azurophil granules, the phagosome becomes protein rich, with high local concentrations of myeloperoxidase, multiple defensins, and proteases like cathepsin G. The bactericidal functions of these proteins appear to be promoted by increases in H^+ or K^+ that are actively transported through ion channels into the phagosome to counter the net negative charge following oxidase activation. In fact, treatment of neutrophils that have engulfed *S. aureus* with K^+ channel inhibitors prevents killing of these intracellular bacteria [46], suggesting that this cation transport is essential for optimal elimination of staphylococci. While this appears to challenge the more traditional paradigm involving production of ROS from hydrogen peroxide and myeloperoxidase, including the directly bactericidal HOCl and singlet oxygen (Figure 7a.3), in fact we know very little about the heterogeneity of neutrophil phagolysosomes and both of these mechanisms could be operative under differing conditions. In addition to promoting intracellular killing, ROS produced at the plasma membrane contribute to host defense by inactivating the autoinducing peptide pheromone (AIP) of *S. aureus* to limit production of secreted virulence factors like toxins and hemolysins [3]. In fact, multiple neutrophil effectors such as the cathepsins and other proteases could provide defense by targeting virulence factors for degradation [47]. Moreover, these functions are operative only under conditions where tissue oxygen concentrations exceed the K_m of the oxidase for binding molecular oxygen. Because sites of acute inflammation become rapidly hypoxic [48], neutrophil biology and physiology can change dramatically including reversal of their apoptotic death program in response to hypoxia [49]. Very little is known about the microbicidal ability of neutrophils in hypoxic tissues but because reversal of apoptosis is dependent on the transcription factor hypoxia inducible factor (HIF)-1α [49], it is intriguing to speculate that other HIF-1α-targeted genes, such as NOS2 or heme oxygenase

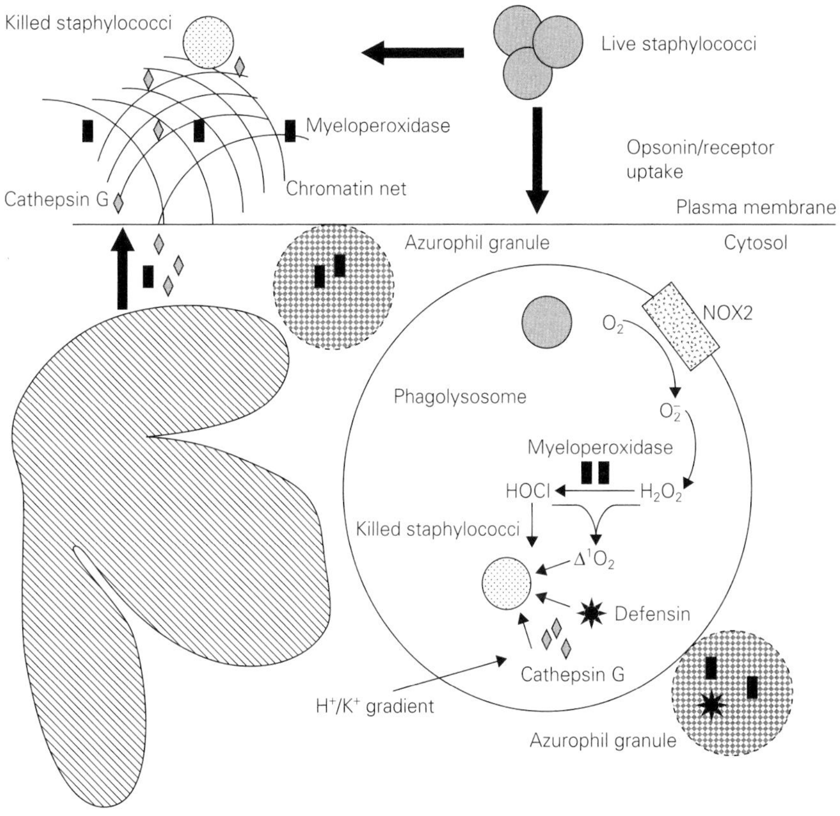

Figure 7a.2 Pathways of neutrophil killing. Neutrophils kill staphylococci in extracellular locales and those internalized into phagolysosomes. Neutrophils stimulated to undergo a novel cell death pathway release nuclear chromatin and the contents of azurophil granules to create extracellular nets for killing. Histones associated with disgorged nuclear chromatin are directly bactericidal. In oxygen-replete environments, neutrophils take up single or aggregated staphylococci into phagosomes that fuse first with secondary granules and ultimately with azurophil granules. IgG/FcR stimulation optimally recruits oxygen-dependent killing that begins with assembly of the phagocyte oxidase (NOX2) on the phagolysosomal membrane. The uptake of molecular oxygen by NOX generates reactive oxygen species that can be directly cidal. In addition, H^+/K^+ influx into the phagolysome activates proteases like cathepsin G for killing and acidifies the organelle for optimal defensin-dependent killing.

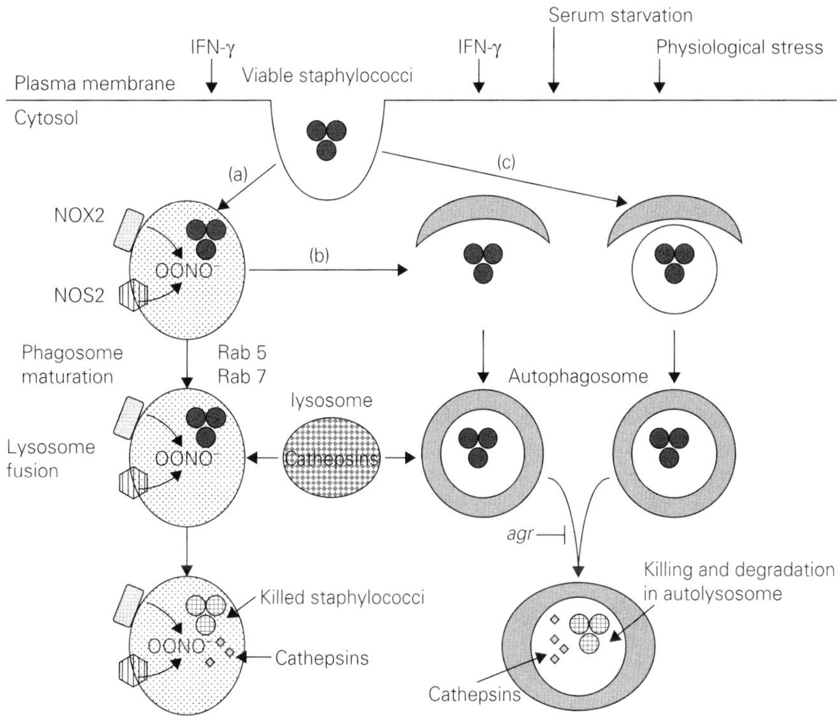

Figure 7a.3 Pathways of monocyte/macrophage killing. Monocytes/macrophages employ multiple killing strategies for internalized staphylococci following stimulation by optimal opsonin/receptor signaling, cytokine signaling, or stress responses. Interferon (IFN)-γ plays a critical role in promoting killing by either traditional phagolysosomal maturation (a) or autophagy-dependent mechanisms (b, c). In (a), assembly of both NOX2 and NOS2 on the phagolysosomal membrane generates reactive oxygen species and Reactive Nitrogen Intermediates that produce the most powerful cidal oxidant, peroxynitrite ($OONO^-$). Profound organelle acidification promotes cathepsin-dependent degradation. Staphylococci that escape the lysosome and reside in the cytosol (b) or which are in a conventional lysosome (c) can be surrounded by an autophagosomal membrane. Autophagosomes can fuse with lysosomes for acidification and cathepsin-dependent killing. Killing also involves nutrient restriction and interference with essential metabolism required for survival of the bacterium in this environment.

1, may be upregulated at these sites and provide either nitric oxide- or carbon monoxide-dependent killing.

If neutrophils and inflammatory monocytes are not able to limit infection to the lamina propria, *S. aureus* may invade across the endothelium into the bloodstream. At this point, specialized macrophages within the spleen and liver are primarily responsible for blood sterilization. In fact the novel opsonophagocytosis mechanisms used by macrophages within these organs do not contribute to the armamentarium of either monocytes or tissue-fixed macrophages, including a newly described member of the immunoglobulin receptor family, CRIg, which recognizes both C3b- and C3bi-opsonized staphylococci and plays a nonredundant role in bacterial clearance [41]. The specific signaling mechanism induced by this receptor is not presently known but its elucidation may provide great insight into the bactericidal mechanisms of organ-specific macrophages. Importantly, while we have learned much about the virulence factors that antagonize neutrophil function, we have no knowledge of the virulence factors that may impede the functioning of this clearance mechanism.

New ways of killing

Recently, some important observations have clearly demonstrated that the traditional paradigm of how *S. aureus* is killed and eliminated from sites of infection needs refining. The observations that *S. aureus* internalized by neutrophils is relatively resistant to killing [50,51] and that catalase production by this pathogen is essential at sites of colonization but not at acute inflammatory sites [30,32] suggest that the role of NOX2 and the oxidants it generates is more complex and goes beyond direct cidal activity for the control of invasive infection. All the newly described strategies for killing are optimal in the presence of ROS-dependent signaling, indicating that these more novel mechanisms for pathogen killing may contribute significantly to human host defense against staphylococci.

Neutrophil extracellular traps and serine proteases

The need for killing large or aggregated microorganisms has generated an evolutionary pressure for neutrophils and other granulocytes to develop mechanisms for extracellular killing. The elegant studies describing the formation of neutrophil extracellular traps (NETs), composed of chromatin threads with bound histones and specific proteins from neutrophil granules, have provided a novel paradigm for accomplishing this goal, including extracellular killing of *S. aureus* [52] (see Figure 7a.2). NET formation is induced following activation by chemokines, TLRs, and phagocytic receptors that result in a novel cell death pathway that is neither apoptosis nor necrosis. With the additional requirement of hydrogen peroxide, which may come from dismutation of superoxide anion, both the nuclear membrane and azurophil granule membranes dissolve leading to mixing of granular proteins with nuclear chromatin [45]. After cell rounding and contraction, the NETs are released extracellularly carrying antimicrobial proteases, myeloperoxidase for extracellular HOCl production for inactivation of AIP [3], enzymes that degrade virulence factors (cathepsin G) [47], and histones (see Figure 7a.2). The histone component is extremely interesting as it resurrects an observation published in 1958 that histone 2A has direct antimicrobial activity including against *S. aureus* [45]. Because *S. aureus* is present as large aggregates or as sheets within a biofilm in infected epithelial tissues, NET-dependent killing is likely a major mechanism for controlling infection in these more oxygen-rich environments. In addition, the invasion by staphylococci of epithelial cells present at the site, including sites of colonization [53], could then represent an effort to escape this extracellular killing mechanism [52]. The role of NETs in killing group A streptococci has been confirmed in a mouse model of skin infection but has not yet been confirmed for staphylococci *in vivo* [54]. Moreover, we know very little about virulence factors like DNase production in *S. aureus* that may limit NET-dependent killing [54].

Autophagy

In addition to killing by the classical paradigm of phagolysosome maturation in monocytes and macrophages, where generation of Reactive Nitrogen Intermediates and ROS cooperate for pathogen killing (see Figure 7a.3), autophagy-dependent killing of intracellular bacteria is increasingly being recognized as a major host defense mechanism [55]. In this fundamental cellular process, the machinery that removes damaged or surplus organelles as a stress response mechanism is used instead to remove intracellular bacterial pathogens which express virulence factors that limit traditional phagolysosomal killing and degradation [56]. In macrophages, autophagy can be induced by physiological stresses like serum starvation but also by the important host defense cytokine IFN-γ [55] and is promoted by TLR signaling during phagocytosis [57]. After induction, a double-membrane structure isolates the pathogen either within the cytosol or within a lysosome in response to unknown signals [55]. Following a multistep signaling cascade, the double membrane fuses and becomes competent for fusing with lysosomes for delivery of its cargo into a degradative organelle. The autophagosome-specific marker LC3 (microtubule-associated protein 1 light chain) associates with organelles destined for degradation in a manner dependent on this cascade and surprisingly can be found on traditional phagosomes after TLR signaling in macrophages [57]. These data suggest that professional phagocytes may use this degradative machinery to ramp up traditional phagocytic killing mechanisms. Given the dependence of blood clearance on TLR2 recognition [10], it is intriguing to speculate that TLR2 and CRIg signaling in splenic macrophages are essential for recruiting this more optimal degradative machinery. However, only two studies have addressed autophagy control of *S. aureus* intracellular survival [56,58] and both were conducted in epithelial cell lines and not in macrophages likely to be receiving additional signals like IFN-γ. In addition, these studies reached slightly different conclusions and depending on the bacterial strain, *S. aureus* can either be eliminated by autophagy [56] or use autophagy for intracellular replication and survival [58]. The potential for this process to be essential in the removal of staphylococci from the bloodstream and its emerging importance for control of other bacterial pathogens should make a more thorough study of autophagy-dependent control of staphylococcal infection a high priority.

Antimicrobial peptides

In humans, direct antimicrobial activity of mucus secretions, inflammatory exudates, blood, and leukocytes has been recognized since the 1950s with the description of the membranolytic activities of lysozyme, histones, and neutrophil granule content. Now with over 1000 different polypeptides described with direct cidal activity across the animal and plant kingdoms, it is clear that they posses phenomenal diversity in both structure and function and include not only cationic amphipathic antimicrobial peptides but also cytokines and chemokines, peptide hormones, fragments of proteolytic enzymes, nucleic acid-binding proteins, and metal-chelating proteins [59,60]. Moreover, while key aspects of their structure unite the ability of many of these polypeptides to insert into lipid bilayers to form pores by various mechanisms [60], others work by inhibiting key metabolic steps including cell wall synthesis, nucleic acid synthesis, protein synthesis, and enzymatic functions [59]. Thus, the mass action of all these polypeptides contributes to host defense at sites of infection. This diversity in killing mechanism and redundancy in numbers helps to explain why genetic deletion or mutation, either spontaneously in humans or intentionally in animal models, has not generated dramatic phenotypes of defective host defense against staphylococci. Moreover, membranolytic agents like group II phospholipase A2 synergize with oxidants derived from NOX2 to overcome the membrane modifications in *S. aureus* that resist phospholipase membranolytic activity [61,62], demonstrating that the sum total of all killing mechanisms contributes to defense against staphylococci.

Induction of killing activity is a key feature of most of these polypeptides independent of mechanism and demonstrates that upstream signaling events are essential for development of optimal antimicrobial activity [59,60]. This is best exemplified by the elegant studies of *S. aureus* eradication in organotypic cultures of human keratinocytes, where signaling downstream of the EGF receptor as a response to wound healing is required to generate three discrete antimicrobial peptides that combine to eliminate this pathogen [33]. In addition to synthesis of new proteins with antimicrobial activity, some antimicrobial function is not exposed until after the mature protein is proteolytically processed to reveal this new ability. Examples of this are lactoferrin [63] and cathepsin G [47], which are both components of neutrophil granules and are found in phagolysomes. In fact, the iron-binding function of lactoferrin may contribute little to defense against staphylococci while the protease function of a cleavage fragment may provide its major antibiotic activity [63]. In addition, cathepsin G acquires its antistaphylococcal function after proteolytic cleavage [47]. These data demonstrate that the milieu in which antimicrobial activity is induced is key to the development of efficacious intracellular and extracellular killing of staphylococci. Thus, defects in host defense may arise because of failure of the inflammatory response to provide the optimal milieu for the induction of potent antibiotic proteins by transcription, translation, or repurposing rather than by the absolute absence of antibiotic potential. What constitutes either an optimal or failed inflammatory response for induction of antibiotic activity is presently not known but certainly could involve genetic responses to hypoxia, negative signaling with chronic inflammation, and control of phagocyte activation. Moreover as with opsonins, because of the phenomenal redundancy in antibiotic peptide number and function, addition of a single therapeutic antibiotic peptide may have little effect especially if the inflammatory milieu does not support its optimal function.

Genetic defects that impair defense against staphylococcal infections

A number of both acquired and genetic defects in host defense contribute to increased susceptibility to staphylococcal infection. The study of some well-characterized genetic defects have contributed substantially to our understanding of host defense against particularly *S. aureus* infection, especially those involving neutrophil function and typified by chronic granulomatous disease (CGD), Job syndrome (hyper-IgE syndrome), leukocyte adhesion deficiency, and Chédiak–Higashi syndrome. In addition, genetic polymorphisms in genes that regulate responses to infection such as TLR2 may contribute to the pathological extent of infection such as the development of septic shock [21]. Of all these genetic causes, the best understood is CGD where the pattern of inheritance and the components of the phagocyte NADPH oxidase (NOX2) affected have been well described (Table 7a.4). Moreover, study of this oxidase has revealed the presence of other family members that are ubiquitously expressed and contribute oxidants for optimal intracellular signaling but also for defense at epithelial barriers [44,46,64]. NOX2 contributes to multiple steps in phagocyte-dependent defense including creation of NETs for extracellular killing [45], signaling

Table 7a.4 Genetic basis for chronic granulomatous disease.

Protein	Gene	Frequency
gp91^{phox} (NOX2)	*CYBB*	76%
p22^{phox}	*CYBA*	3%
p47^{phox}	*NCF1*	18%
p67^{phox}	*NCF2*	4%
Rac2	*RAC2*	Unknown

for autophagy-dependent clearance [55], modification of virulence protein expression by suppression of quorum sensing [3], resolution of acute inflammation [44], and full activation of the killing properties of the azurophil granule following fusion with the phagosome [46] (see Figures 7a.2 and 7a.3). In addition to NOX2, the recent elucidation of STAT3 as the genetic defect in hyper-IgE syndrome has provided another paradigm for investigating host defense against *S. aureus* infection [65]. For example, the transcription factor STAT3 is important in human airways for optimal activation of β-defensin 3 as well as important for production of Th17 lymphocytes that are known to play a critical role in *S. aureus* abscess formation [13] and in defense against other extracellular bacteria [16,17]. Thus, the study of STAT3 function at mucosal barriers may well help to elucidate the effectors essential for defense at these sites.

Summary

Multiple effectors contribute to host defense against staphylococcal infection and while traditional aspects of the opsonization–phagocyte–antimicrobial peptide module of innate immunity clearly contribute, novel mechanisms within this, such as killing by NETs, autophagy, and re-purposed proteins, are increasingly being recognized as important for defense. In contrast, knowledge of how adaptive immunity contributes to defense by this module is poorly understood and should be a focus of future studies in order to provide optimal vaccination-dependent defense.

References

1 McCaig LF, McDonald LC, Mandal S *et al.* *Staphylococcus aureus* associated skin and soft tissue infection in ambulatory care. Emerg Infect Dis 2006;12:1715–23.

2 Rogers DE, Melly MA. Speculations on the immunology of staphylococcal infections. Ann NY Acad Sci 1965;128:274–84.

3 Rothfork JM, Timmins GS, Harris M *et al.* Inactivation of a bacterial virulence pheromone by phagocyte-derived oxidants: new role for the NADPH oxidase in host defense. Proc Natl Acad Sci USA 2004;101:13867–72.

4 Nizet V. Understanding how leading bacterial pathogens subvert innate immunity to reveal novel therapeutic targets. J Allergy Clin Immunol 2007;120:13–22.

5 Klevens RM, Morrison MA, Nadle J *et al.* Invasive methicillin-resistant *Staphylococcus aureus* infections in the United States. JAMA 2007;298:1763–71.

6 Dommett RM, Klein N, Turner MW. Mannose-binding lectin in innate immunity: past, present, and future. Tissue Antigens 2006;68:193–209.

7 Takabashi K, Shi L, Gowda LD, Ezekowitz RA. Relative roles of complement factor 3 and mannose-binding lectin in host defense against infection. Infect Immun 2005;73:8188–93.

8 Frazee BW, Salz TO, Lambert L, Perdreau-Remington F. Fatal community acquired MRSA pneumonia in an immunocompetent young adult. Ann Emerg Med 2005;46:401–4.

9 Miller LS, O'Connell RM, Gutierrez MA *et al.* MyD88 mediates neutrophil recruitment initiated by IL-1R but not TLR2 activation in immunity against *Staphylococcus aureus*. Immunity 2006; 24:79–91.

10 Takeuchi O, Hoshino K, Akira S. Cutting edge: TLR2-deficient and MyD88-deficient mice are highly susceptible to *Staphylococcus aureus* infection. J Immunol 2000;165:5392–6.

11 Tanigaki J, Han H, Yamamoto N *et al.* Notch-RBP-J signaling is involved in cell fate determination of marginal zone B cells. Nat Immunol 2002;3:443–50.

12 Chung DR, Kasper DL, Panzo RJ *et al.* $CD4^+$ T cells mediate abscess formation in intra-abdominal sepsis by an IL-17-dependent mechanism. J Immunol 2003;170:1958–63.

13 McLoughlin RM, Solinga RM, Rich J *et al.* $CD4^+$ T cells and CXC chemokines modulate the pathogenesis of *Staphylococcus aureus* wound infections. Proc Natl Acad Sci USA 2006;103:10408–13.

14 Hultgren OH, Verdrengh M, Tarkowski A. T-box transcription factor-deficient mice display increased joint pathology and failure of infection control during staphylococcal arthritis. Microbes Infect 2004;6:529–35.

15 Dryla A, Prustomersky S, Gelbmann D *et al.* Comparison of antibody repertoires against *Staphylococcus aureus* in healthy individuals and in acutely infected patients. Clin Diagn Lab Immunol 2005;12:387–98.

16 Reiner SL. Development in motion: helper T cells at work. Cell 2007;129:33–6.

17 Annunziato F, Cosmi L, Santariasci V *et al.* Phenotypic and functional features of human Th17 cells. J Exp Med 2007; 204:1849–61.

18 Akira S, Uematsu S, Takeuchi O. Pathogen recognition and innate immunity. Cell 2006;124:783–801.

19 Fournier B, Philpott DJ. Recognition of *Staphylococcus aureus* by the innate immune system. Clin Microbiol Rev 2005;18:521–40.

20 Soong G, Reddy B, Sokol S *et al.* TLR2 is mobilized into an apical lipid raft receptor complex to signal infection in airway epithelial cells. J Clin Invest 2004;113:1482–9.

21 Lorenz E, Mira JP, Cornish KL *et al.* A novel polymorphism in the toll-like receptor 2 gene and its potential association with staphylococcal infection. Infect Immun 2005;68:6398–403.

22 Hoebe K, Georgel P, Rutschmann S *et al.* CD36 is a sensor of diacylglycerides. Nature 2005;433:523–7.

23 Chi H, Flavell RA. Immunology: sensing the enemy within. Nature 2007;448:423–6.

24 Mariathasan S, Weiss DS, Newton K *et al*. Cryopyrin activates the inflammasome in response to toxins and ATP. Nature 2006;440:228–33.

25 Mariathasan S, Monack DM. Inflammasome adaptors and sensors: intracellular regulators of infection and inflammation. Nat Rev Immunol 2007;7:31–8.

26 Wardenburg BJ, Williams WA, Missiakas D. Host defenses against *Staphylococcus aureus* infection require recognition of bacterial lipoproteins. Proc Natl Acad Sci USA 2006;103:1383–9.

27 Miller LS, Pietras EM, Uricchio LH *et al*. Inflammasome-mediated production of IL-1beta is required for neutrophil recruitment against *Staphylococcus aureus* in vivo. J Immunol 2007;179:6933–42.

28 Massey RC, Horsburgh MJ, Lina G *et al*. The evolution and maintenance of virulence in *Staphylococcus aureus*: a role for host-to-host transmission? Nat Rev Microbiol 2006;4:953–8.

29 Sansonetti PJ, Di Santo JP. Debugging how bacteria manipulate the immune response. Immunity 2007;26:149–61.

30 Park B, Nizet V, Liu GY. Role of *Staphylococcus aureus* catalase in niche competition against *Streptococcus pneumoniae*. J Bacteriol 2008;190:2275–8.

31 Quinn GA, Cole AM. Supression of innate immunity by a nasal carriage strain of *Staphylococcus aureus* increases its colonization on nasal epithelium. Immunology 2007;122:80–9.

32 Clarke S, Mohamed R, Bian L *et al*. The *Staphylococcus aureus* surface protein IsdA mediates resistance to innate defenses of human skin. Cell Host Microbe 2007;1:199–209.

33 Sorensen OE, Thapa DR, Roupe M *et al*. Injury-induced innate immune response in human skin mediated by transactivation of the epidermal growth factor receptor. J Clin Invest 2006; 116:1878–88.

34 Palazzolo-Ballance AM, Reniere ML, Braughton KR *et al*. Neutrophil microbicides induce a pathogen survival response in community-associated methicillin-resistant *Staphylococcus aureus*. J Immunol 2008;180:500–9.

35 Stuart LM, Ezekowitz RAB. Phagocytosis: elegant complexity. Immunity 2005;22:539–50.

36 Nathan C. Neutrophils and immunity: challenges and opportunities. Nat Rev Immunol 2006;6:173–93.

37 Tsuda Y, Takahashi H, Kobayashi M, Hanafusa T, Herndon D, Suzuki F. Three different neutrophil subsets exhibited in mice with different susceptibilities to infection by methicillin-resistant *Staphylococcus aureus*. Immunity 2004;21:215–26.

38 Flick MJ, Du X, Degen JL. Fibrin(ogen)-alpha M beta 2 interactions regulate leukocyte function and innate immunity. Exp Biol Med 2004;229:1105–12.

39 Roozendaal R, Carroll MC. Emerging patterns in complement-mediated pathogen recognition. Cell 2006;125:29–35.

40 Kang YS, Do Y, Lee HK *et al*. A dominant complement fixation pathway for pneumococcal polysaccharides initiated by SIGN-R1 interacting with C1q. Cell 2006;125:47–57.

41 Helmy KY, Katschke KJ, Gorgani N *et al*. CRIg: a macrophage complement receptor required for phagocytosis of circulating pathogens. Cell 2006;124:915–25.

42 Borregaard N, Sorensen OE, Theilgaard-Monch K. Neutrophil granules: a library of innate immunity proteins. Trends Immunol 2007;28:340–50.

43 Gardai SJ, McPhillips KA, Frasch SC *et al*. Cell-surface calreticulin initiates clearance of viable or apoptotic cells through transactivation of LRP on the phagocyte. Cell 2005;123:321–34.

44 Quinn M, Ammons MC, DeLeo FR. The expanding role of NADPH oxidases in health and disease: no longer just agents of death and destruction. Clin Sci 2006;111:1–20.

45 Brinkmann V, Zychlinsky A. Beneficial suicide: why neutrophils die to make NETs. Nat Rev Microbiol 2007;5:577–83.

46 Segal AW. How neutrophils kill microbes. Annu Rev Immunol 2005;23:197–223.

47 Pham CTN. Neutrophil serine proteases: specific regulators of inflammation. Nat Rev Immunol 2006;6:541–55.

48 Zinkernagel AS, Johnson RS, Nizet V. Hypoxia inducible factor (HIF) function in innate immunity and infection. J Mol Med 2007;85:1339–46.

49 Walmsley SR, Print C, Farahi N *et al*. Hypoxia-induced neutrophil survival is mediated by HIF-1 alpha-dependent NF-kappa B activity. J Exp Med 2005;201:105–15.

50 Gresham HD, Lowrance JH, Caver TE *et al*. Survival of *Staphylococcus aureus* inside neutrophils contributes to infection. J Immunol 2000;164:3713–22.

51 Voyich JM, Braughton KR, Sturdevant DE *et al*. Insights into mechanisms used by *Staphylococcus aureus* to avoid destruction by human neutrophils. J Immunol 2005;175:3907–12.

52 Brinkmann V, Reichard U, Goosmann C *et al*. Neutrophil extracellular traps kill bacteria. Science 2004;303:1532–5.

53 Clement S, Vaudaux P, Francois P *et al*. Evidence of an intracellular reservoir in the nasal mucosa of patients with recurrent *Staphylococcus aureus* rhinosinusitis. J Infect Dis 2005;192:1023–8.

54 Walker MJ, Hollands A, Sanderson-Smith ML *et al*. DNase Sda1 provides selection pressure for a switch to invasive group A streptococcal infection. Nat Med 2007;13:981–5.

55 Levine B, Deretic V. Unveiling the roles of autophagy in innate and adaptive immunity. Nat Rev Immunol 2007;7:767–77.

56 Amano A, Nakagawa I, Yoshimori T. Autophagy in innate immunity against intracellular bacteria. J Biochem 2006;140:161–74.

57 Sanjuan MA, Dillon CP, Tait SW *et al*. Toll-like receptor signaling in macrophages links the autophagy pathway to phagocytosis. Nature 2007;450:1253–7.

58 Schnaith A, Kashkar H, Leggio S *et al*. *Staphylococcus aureus* subvert autophagy for induction of caspase-independent host cell death. J Biol Chem 2007;282:2695–702.

59 Brogden KA. Antimicrobial peptides: pore formers or metabolic inhibitors in bacteria? Nat Rev Microbiol 2005;3:238–53.

60 Yeaman MR, Yount NY. Unifying themes in host defense effector polypeptides. Nat Rev Microbiol 2007;5:727–35.

61 Laine VJ, Grass D, Nevalainen TJ. Protection by group II phospholipase A2 against *Staphylococcus aureus*. J Immunol 1999; 162:7402–9.

62 Femling JK, Nauseef W, Weiss JP. Synergy between extracellular group IIA phospholipase A2 and phagocyte NADPH oxidase in digestion of phospholipids of *Staphylococcus aureus* ingested by human neutrophils. J Immunol 2005;175:4653–9.

63 Ward PP, Paz E, Conneely M. Multifunctional roles of lactoferrin: a critical overview. Cell Mol Life Sci 2005;62:2540–8.

64 Moskwa P, Larentzen D, Excoffon K *et al*. A novel host defense system of airways is defective in cystic fibrosis. Am J Respir Crit Care Med 2007;175:174–85.

65 Holland SM, DeLeo FR, Elloumi HZ *et al*. *STAT3* mutations in the hyper-IgE syndrome. N Engl J Med 2007;357:1608–19.

Chapter 7b Evasion of Host Defenses

Timothy J. Foster
Microbiology Department, Moyne Institute of Preventive Medicine, Trinity College, Dublin, Ireland

Introduction

There are more than 30 species in the genus *Staphylococcus* but only two, *Staphylococcus aureus* and *Staphylococcus epidermidis*, are responsible for the majority of infections in humans caused by this group of organisms. Both are primarily commensals and normally live in harmony with their hosts without causing symptoms. *Staphylococcus epidermidis* is a commensal of the skin and was rarely pathogenic before the advances in medical procedures involving implanted medical devices. In contrast, *S. aureus* is potentially much more pathogenic. Its primary habitats are the anterior nares and the throat [1,2]. The moist squamous epithelium of the anterior nares is defended by the nasal-associated lymphoid tissue (NALT), which involves both innate and induced immune responses. It has been argued that *S. epidermidis* lacks the complexity of *S. aureus* because it is adapted to exist on the skin surface where transmission from host to host is straightforward [3]. In contrast, in order for *S. aureus* to be transmitted from one host to another it must first be transferred from the nares to the skin of the donor, then to the skin of the recipient, and finally it must colonize the nares where it must overcome the NALT-controlled immune responses. Furthermore, not all hosts are available because only a proportion of humans can be permanently colonized and because of interference if the host is already colonized with an *S. aureus* strain from a different Agr group. It could therefore be argued that the virulence factors and immune avoidance mechanisms of *S. aureus* are mainly concerned with colonization of the hostile environment of the nares, which are protected by innate and induced immunity. Similarly for *S. epidermidis*, the primary function of factors that help it to infect susceptible hosts is to promote survival on skin.

The purpose of this chapter is to discuss how staphylococci avoid innate and induced immunity during both commensalism and infection. There is considerable overlap between the two so most of the discussion refers to disease pathogenesis with the exception of mechanisms that seem to be involved only in promoting survival externally. Immune evasion strategies are categorized according to whether they impede leukocyte migration, fixation of complement, recognition of opsonins by neutrophils, survival of bacteria within professional phagocytic cells, or the effective induction of antibodies and immunological memory.

Colonization

Adhesion

The ability of *S. aureus* to colonize the hostile environment of the anterior nares is likely to be determined by its ability to adhere to desquamated cells on the epithelial surface of the nasal vestibule. Two surface proteins have been shown to promote adhesion to squamous cells *in vitro*. Clumping factor (Clf)B is so named because its of ability to bind to fibrinogen [4,5]. The protein also binds to cytokeratin 10, a major surface component of squamous cells that likely provides a receptor for ClfB [6,7]. The nasal mucosa is an iron-restricted environment that stimulates expression of several iron-regulated surface determinant (Isd) proteins [8,9]. As well as being involved in iron acquisition and survival on skin [10], the IsdA protein also promotes bacterial adhesion to squames [11]. In experiments with bacteria lacking ClfB or IsdA that were grown in iron-restricted conditions, both surface proteins were shown to contribute significantly to bacterial adhesion to squamous cells. Furthermore, IsdA or ClfB mutants were defective in colonization of the nares of rodents [11,12] and, in the case of ClfB, human volunteers [13], showing that the proteins have a role *in vivo*. There is currently no information on the role of any *S. epidermidis* surface protein with regard to adherence to the squames of the epidermis.

Survival on skin

One of the unique features of the community-acquired methicillin-resistant *S. aureus* (CA-MRSA) strain USA300 is the presence of the arginine catabolic mobile element (ACME) [14]. ACME carries a cluster of genes encoding enzymes of the arginine deiminase pathway that converts arginine into carbon dioxide, ATP and ammonia. These genes occur in some strains of *S. epidermidis* but had not been detected before in *S. aureus*. It is postulated that production of ammonia aids pH homeostasis in the acid environment of the skin and could help bacterial survival. The possible acquisition of ACME by horizontal transfer from *S. epidermidis* might help explain why CA-MRSA strains have spread so rapidly in the community.

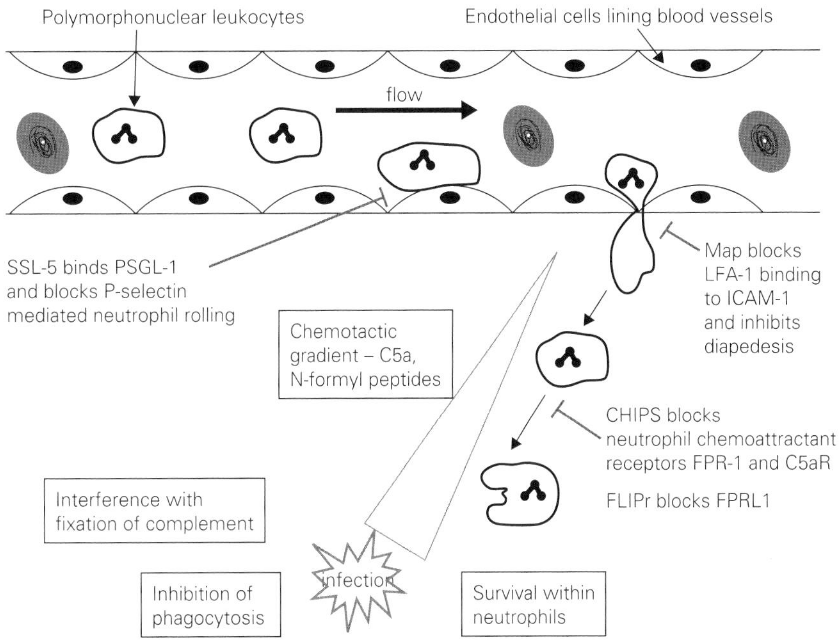

Figure 7b.1 Interference with neutrophil recruitment: *S. aureus* secretes a number of proteins that can obstruct different stages of the recruitment of neutrophils from the bloodstream to the site of infection. See text for definition of abbreviations.

Resistance to fatty acids

Fatty acids present in sebum are an important part of the antibacterial defenses of the skin and *cis*-6-hexadecanoic acid is the most potent bactericidal fatty acid against *S. aureus*. In order to defend against hydrophobic molecules the IsdA protein (mentioned above in the context of adhesion to squamous cells) makes the cell surface hydrophilic [10]. This is due to the amino acid composition of the C-terminal domain of the extended asymmetric protein, which is a major component of the surface of bacterial cells growing under iron-restricted conditions. An IsdA mutant was much more sensitive to killing *in vitro* by bactericidal lipids and the mutant survived poorly on the surface of human skin compared with the wild type. IsdA mutants are also more sensitive to cationic antimicrobial peptides (see below).

Resistance to defensin peptides

Resisting the bactericidal effects of both cationic and non-cationic antimicrobial peptides is likely to be of major importance in the ability of staphylococci to survive on skin. The mechanisms involved are discussed below in the context of survival within phagocytes.

Inhibition of neutrophil migration

As soon as *S. aureus* gains access to tissues in the body, several different chemoattractants are elaborated that stimulate the migration of neutrophils from the bloodstream to the site of infection. Two small peptides, C3a and C5a, are released during complement fixation by cleavage of C3 and C5 [15–17]. They diffuse away from the bacterial cell creating a concentration gradient. Also bacterial proteins are translated with formyl-methionine at their amino termini. Short formyl peptides are cleaved from newly synthesized bacterial proteins and are secreted, also creating a concentration gradient. Formyl peptides are not the only chemoattractant released by metabolizing bacteria. The supernatant of cultures of a formyltransferase mutant lacking the ability to formylate methionine still contained some chemoattractant activity, albeit less than the wild type [18]. The chemoattractants are recognized by G protein-coupled receptors on the neutrophil, which stimulate the process of migration when activated.

Several steps are involved in the recruitment of neutrophils [19] (Figure 7b.1). First, during inflammation, P-selectin is translocated to the surface of endothelial cells lining blood vessels. Its release from Weibel–Palade bodies is triggered by histamine and thrombin. The P-selectin glycoprotein ligand (PSGL)-1 on circulating neutrophils binds P-selectin and initiates the process of neutrophil rolling, which eventually captures the phagocytic cell allowing it to migrate into adjacent tissue.

Staphylococcal superantigen-like (SSL)5 is a small protein expressed by one of a family of *ssl* genes located in pathogenicity island 2. Different strains express between seven and eleven SSL proteins, which share 36–67% identity [20,21]. They have high structural similarity to enterotoxin superantigens but lack superantigenic activity because residues involved in binding major histocompatibility complex (MHC) class II to the T-cell receptor (TCR) are absent [22]. SSL5 specifically binds to PSGL-1 and inhibits binding to P-selectin *in vitro* and prevents neutrophil rolling on activated endothelial cells [23]. Thus SSL5 has the potential to stop the first step in neutrophil recruitment *in vivo*.

In order to migrate from the bloodstream, neutrophils must adhere firmly to endothelial cells. This is mediated by the β2 integrins Mac-1 and leukocyte function-associated antigen (LFA)-1 on leukocytes that interact with the counterreceptor intercellular adhesion molecule (ICAM)-1 on endothelial cells. The extracellular adherence protein (Eap), also known as MHC class II analog protein (Map), can bind to a multiplicity of ligands including ICAM-1. Binding to ICAM-1 blocks the interaction with LFA-1 and reduces diapedesis, the process of neutrophil attachment to and transmigration through endothelial cells [24]. *In vitro* studies were supported by a mouse peritonitis model in which an Eap mutant allowed recruitment of more neutrophils that the wild-type strain.

Migration from the blood vessels following diapedesis to the site of infection involves activation of several G protein-coupled receptors by chemoattractants [25]. *Staphylococcus aureus* can synthesize several small proteins that specifically and potently block receptors and inhibit leukocyte activation and migration. The chemotaxis inhibitory protein of staphylococci (CHIPS) binds to the formylpeptide receptor (FPR) and the C5a receptor (C5aR) [26]. This blocks the cognate agonist from binding. Two distinct domains on CHIPS bind to the N-terminal cytoplasmic domains of C5aR and FPR [27–29]. The formylpeptide receptor-like (FPRL)-1 is a lower-affinity receptor for formyl peptides than FPR and is more widely distributed on cells than FPR and C5aR. A protein with 28% identity to CHIPS called FLPR-1 inhibitory protein (FLIPr) binds to FPRL-1, impairing neutrophil responses to FPR-like agonists [30]. The gene encoding CHIPS is part of an immune evasion gene cluster present on a converting bacteriophage [31], whereas the *flr* gene encoding FLIPr is in a cluster of virulence genes encoding α-toxin and the extracellular fibrinogen-binding protein Efb [30].

Thus, *S. aureus* secretes a variety of proteins that can interfere with different stages of neutrophil recruitment during the earliest stages of an infection. It is very likely that more proteins will be discovered, for example among the SSL proteins of unknown function, which could contribute to this process.

Complement

Complement is a family of proteins and proteolytic fragments derived from them that have many roles in innate and acquired immunity [32]. Complement recruits effector molecules that label *S. aureus*, targeting the bacteria for destruction by immune effector cells, particularly neutrophils. The process of complement fixation occurs by three pathways (see Plate 7.1). The alternative and lectin pathways are components of innate immunity whereas the classical pathway requires specific interaction with antibodies that have bound to antigens on the surface of bacterial cells. One of the main purposes of complement fixation is opsonization, i.e., to promote phagocytosis by neutrophils and macrophages. The neutrophils recognize the Fc region of IgG by the specific receptor FcγRI and complement proteins bound to the bacterial cell surface by receptors CR1 and CR3. It is becoming apparent that *S. aureus* expresses several distinct mechanisms to interfere with complement by inactivation or sequestration of key components, and that this is crucial to the success of the pathogen.

Inactivation of complement

Assembly of C3 convertases on the surface of *S. aureus* is a prerequisite for complement activation (see Plate 7.1) [32,33]. The structurally and functionally related C4bC2a (classical and lectin pathways) and C3bBb (alternative pathway) carry out the essential function of cleaving C3, which results in the release of soluble C3a and covalent attachment of C3b to the bacterium. *Staphylococus aureus* secretes a small protein called staphylococcal complement inhibitor (SCIN) which binds to and stabilizes both C4bC2a and C3bBb resulting in inhibition of further C3b formation [34]. Normally C3 convertases are transiently active, with dissociation leaving the bound C4b and C3b to act as cofactors for further cleavage of C2 and factor B, respectively. Stabilization of the complexes by the secreted *S. aureus* protein SCIN blocks the crucial amplification loop and is a potent mechanism for preventing complement activation. SCIN has been shown to block phagocytosis and killing of *S. aureus* cells by human neutrophils [34].

Staphylococcus aureus has the ability to inactivate complement factor C3b and IgG molecules that are bound to the surface of opsonized bacterial cells. Host plasminogen can attach to the surface of *S. aureus* cells, where it is bound in 1 : 1 stoichiometry by staphylokinase, a plasminogen activator protein secreted by many strains of *S. aureus* [35]. The potent serine protease activity of plasminogen is activated in the staphylokinase–plasminogen complex and it is strategically placed to cleave surface-bound C3b and IgG molecules, resulting in reduced phagocytosis by neutrophils [36].

Complement factors I and H are natural downregulators of complement fixation that prevent uncontrolled activation [16,17]. Normally factor H binds to immobilized C3b and subsequently factor I binds and its protease function is activated and it cleaves C3b to iC3b. While both C3b and iC3b are recognized by specific receptors on neutrophils and therefore promote uptake, iC3b cannot activate the alternative pathway or the terminal cascade and is further degraded to C3d. *Staphylococcus aureus* can capture and activate factor I independently of factor H, which results in increased levels of iC3b on the cell surface, a decrease in total C3 fragments on cells, and a reduction in phagocytosis of bacteria by human neutrophils [37,38].

Binding complement components

The extracellular fibrinogen-binding protein Efb can also bind to complement factor C3 and block C3 deposition on the bacterial cell surface [39,40]. This prevents complement activation beyond C3b and inhibits phagocytosis. The structural basis of Efb–C3 interaction is understood from the X-ray crystal structure of the two proteins in complex [41]. Efb binds to the C3d domain and alters the conformation of C3 so that it cannot be processed to C3b and thus cannot become an opsonin. In addition, Efb binds to C3b with high affinity and induces a conformational change that blocks the thioester domain.

The iron-regulated surface determinant protein IsdH binds the haptoglobin–hemoglobin complex in order to remove hemoglobin at the beginning of the pathway to extract heme and transport it into the cytoplasm of the cell as a source of Fe^{3+} *in vivo* [9]. IsdH has been shown to bind C3 from serum in such a way that it is hinders opsonization and phagocytosis [42], possibly by preventing C3 from being converted to C3b. Binding of C3 occurs at the N-terminus of IsdH and involves a domain called NEAT1 and overlaps the site for haptoglobin–hemoglobin binding. Bacteria expressing IsdH are less susceptible to killing in whole blood compared with an IsdH mutant.

SSL7 has a similar three-dimensional structure to SSL5 and is also a product of pathogenicity island 2 [43]. It binds complement factor C5 and inhibits complement-mediated hemolysis (membrane attack complex formation) but does not prevent cleavage of C5 to C5b and C5a. SSL7 is specific for human C5 and therefore its *in vivo* significance cannot be studied in an animal model.

Resistance to phagocytosis

Staphylococus aureus expresses several surface-associated anti-opsonic proteins and a polysaccharide capsule that can both interfere with the deposition of antibodies and complement by classical and alternative pathways, or with their access to the neutrophil complement and Fc receptors. Efficient phagocytosis by neutrophils, which requires recognition of bound complement and antibody, is thus compromised.

Surface proteins

Protein A is a wall-anchored protein with four or five domains that can each bind to the Fc region of IgG [44]. Residues from helix I and helix II of the triple helical bundle required for binding IgG Fc are well known from the X-ray structure of the complex and from site-directed mutagenesis studies [45]. The interaction between protein A and IgG coats the surface of the cell with IgG molecules that are in the incorrect orientation to be recognized by the neutrophil Fc receptor and for activation of complement by the classical pathway. This explains the antiphagocytic effect of protein A *in vitro* [46] and why it is a virulence factor in several animal infection models [47,48].

ClfA is the major fibrinogen-binding protein expressed on the surface of cells during the stationary phase of growth [49,50]. The *clfA* gene is switched on by a sigma factor B-dependent promoter stimulating substantially higher levels in stationary phase compared with exponential phase when the gene is expressed from the weaker sigma 70-dependent promoter [51]. The N-terminal A domain of ClfA binds to the γ-chain of fibrinogen [52]. When cells are densely packed together in suspension the γ-chain C-termini located at either end of the elongated bivalent fibrinogen molecule can simultaneously bind two ClfA molecules on two different bacterial cells, which results in cell clumping. However, *in vivo* the density of cells is too low for clumping to occur. Instead bacterial cells are coated with fibrinogen molecules. ClfA is a virulence factor in a murine model of sepsis and arthritis [53]. Virulence is enhanced during the bacteremic phase. Cells become coated with fibrinogen, which likely results in impaired deposition and/or recognition of opsonins. *In vitro*, ClfA expression reduces opsonophagocytosis by human neutrophils in the presence of normal serum opsonins and this is due, in part, to the ability of the molecule to bind fibrinogen [51]. It seems possible that fibronectin-binding proteins and ClfB, which also bind fibrinogen [4,54,55], can protect bacteria in a similar way during the exponential phase of growth when these proteins are predominantly expressed.

Capsule

Most strains of *S. aureus* express a microcapsule that is composed of serotype 5, serotype 8 or serotype 336 capsular polysaccharide [56,57]. Expression of type 5 or type 8 capsule is associated with increased virulence in animal infection models [58–60]. *In vitro* the presence of capsule reduces uptake of bacterial cells by human neutrophils in the presence of normal serum opsonins, which indicates that the capsule is anti-opsonic [58,59]. Complement factors can assemble on the cell wall surface beneath the capsule but are inaccessible to complement receptors on the surface of neutrophils.

Many strains of *S. aureus* carry genes for the synthesis of the polysaccharide intercellular adhesin (PIA), also referred to as poly-*N*-acetylglucosamine, an extracellular polysaccharide that is of particular importance in *S. epidermidis* infections. The role of this surface polymer in biofilm formation and avoidance of phagocytosis is discussed in the section on *S. epidermidis* and in Chapter 5.

Toxins that kill leukocytes

Staphylococcus aureus can produce several toxins that damage the membranes of host cells. Cytolytic toxins that target leukocytes (leukotoxins) contribute to the development of abscesses by killing neutrophils that are attempting to engulf and kill bacteria. The archetypal toxin that forms β-barrel pores in the cytoplasmic membrane of target cells is α-toxin. It is secreted as a monomer that attaches to the membrane of cells. Monomers assemble into a heptamer in the membrane, with β-strands from each monomer forming a 14-stranded β-barrel that spans the membrane creating a pore [61]. The bicomponent leukotoxins comprise two subunits that are secreted separately and assemble into hexameric or heptameric oligomers in the membranes of leukocytes. There are four types of bicomponent leucotoxins: γ-toxin or γ-hemolysin, Panton–Valentine leukocidin (PVL), leukocidin E/D, and leukocidin M/F-PV-like. The γ-toxin lyses membranes of both erythrocytes and leukocytes whereas PVL is only toxic for leukocytes [62].

The *hlg* locus is present in the chromosome of the majority of *S. aureus* strains whereas the *pvl* genes encoding PVL are present in a converting bacteriophage that occurs only in 1–2% of strains [63,64]. There is a strong association between PVL and severe skin infections. Recently, CA-MRSA strains have emerged that cause severe necrotizing pneumonia and contagious severe skin infections in previously healthy individuals [65,66]. Evidence implicating PVL as a virulence factor has been demonstrated in an adult mouse model of pneumonia but whether it is truly an important virulence factor or simply a marker for virulent strains is still unclear [67,68]. Expression of PVL also causes dysregulation of expression of many other secreted and wall-associated proteins including protein A, which itself is a virulence factor in lung infections [67,69]. It is likely that CA-MRSA strains emerged by acquisition of a type IV or type V staphylococcal cassette chromosome (SCC*mec*) [14] encoding resistant to β-lactam antibiotics and became lysogenized with a *pvl*-converting phage [70].

Survival of *Staphylococcus aureus* in neutrophil phagosomes

If *S. aureus* is engulfed by neutrophils, it is well endowed with mechanisms that help it to survive in the phagosome. In *in vitro* phagocytosis assays with human neutrophils a significant fraction of engulfed bacterial cells survive killing mechanisms. In addition, *S. aureus* can survive for many days in primary human macrophages, which remain unaffected by the intracellular bacteria until eventually organisms start proliferating and the macrophages die [71]. This suggests that *S. aureus* can remain dormant in human macrophages as has been reported for mouse macrophages [72]. In mice, macrophage-carrying bacteria help disseminate the infecting organisms around the body.

Resistance to antimicrobial peptides

Modification of teichoic acids and of a membrane phospholipid result in an increase in positive charges on the cell surface that neutralize the negative charge of cationic antimicrobial defensin peptides that are secreted into the phagosome. The Dlt proteins result in D-alanine substitutions of ribitol teichoic acid and lipoteichoic acid [73], while the MprF protein adds an L-lysine residue to phosphatidylglycerol exposed on the outer face of the cytoplasmic membrane [74,75]. These modifications also protect bacteria from antimicrobial peptides on the surface of skin [10] as well as positively charged antimicrobial proteins in serum such as phospholipase A2 and lactoferrin. Mutants defective in Dlt and MprF are more susceptible to killing by cationic antimicrobial peptides *in vitro* and have markedly reduced virulence in several animal infection models [76–78].

Transcriptional profiling of *S. epidermidis* identified genes that were upregulated after treatment with human β-defensin, including a three-component regulatory system called the antimicrobial peptide sensor (Aps) [79]. As well as a typical histidine protein kinase sensory component (ApsS) and a response regulator (ApsR), the Aps system also includes a third protein component, ApsX, the function of which is not yet understood. The ApsS protein has two transmembrane segments with a short negatively charged loop on the external face of the cytoplasmic membrane that is involved in recognizing positively charged antimicrobial peptides. A wide variety of cationic peptides can activate this Aps system. Aps upregulates expression of the *dlt* operon that controls modification of teichoic acid and the *mprF* gene for modifying phospholipids, as well as a putative ABC transporter VraFG that could be involved in expelling antimicrobial peptides. The Aps regulatory system is well conserved among staphylococci so it is most likely that *S. aureus* responds to antimicrobial peptides in the same way as *S. epidermidis*.

The Aps system does not respond to noncationic antimicrobial peptides such as dermicidin that are also present on skin and epithelial surfaces and in neutrophil granules. Exposure of *S. epidermidis* to dermicidin stimulated upregulation of a metalloprotease SepA that is similar to aureolysin of *S. aureus* [80]. A SepA-defective mutant was more sensitive to dermicidin consistent with the protease being responsible for degrading the noncationic peptide. Dermicidin also stimulated upregulation of proteases in *S. aureus* so it is likely that proteases can protect against both cationic and noncationic peptides during infection by this organism.

Staphylococus aureus secretes proteins that can neutralize cationic peptides. Staphylokinase is a prothrombin activator that stimulates dissolution of fibrin clots and promotes cleavage of IgG and C3, but it also has a potent defensin-binding activity. It binds defensins with a stoichiometry of 1 : 6 and contributes to protection of bacteria *in vivo* [81,82]. In the infected lung cathelicidin is present on airway epithelial surfaces prior to inflammation. It binds to staphylokinase and stimulates staphylokinase-promoted fibrinolysis [83]. Thus *S. aureus* can utilize a host protease to promote bacterial dissemination and invasiveness. Furthermore, the metalloprotease aureolysin cleaves and inactivates human defensin peptide cathelicidin LL-37 and contributes significantly to resistance to the peptide *in vitro* [84].

Resistance to lysozyme

Lysozyme is an important component of innate defenses against bacterial infections. It is present in many body fluids and is expressed at enhanced levels in phagocytic cells that have been stimulated by proinflammatory signals during infection [85]. The biochemical basis of the resistance of *S. aureus* peptidoglycan to lysozyme degradation was recently attributed to a membrane-bound *O*-acetyltransferase that modifies the C-6 hydroxyl group of muramic acid [86]. A mutant in the *O*-acetyltransferase became sensitive to lysozyme whereas complementation with the wild-type gene restored acetylation and lysozyme resistance.

Survival in phagosomes

Staphylococcus aureus has several mechanisms that contribute to its innate resistance to phagocytic killing, including interference with endosome fusion and avoidance of the lethal effects of oxygen free radicals formed during the respiratory burst. It has been suggested that Toll-like receptor (TLR)2 on the membrane of the phagosome actually suppresses expression or activation of NADPH oxidase that results in reduced superoxide, but not nitrous oxide [87]. Thus *S. aureus* has a novel mechanism for hijacking an innate immune receptor to support its survival within phagocytes. Evidence came from uptake and survival of bacteria in murine macrophages derived from TLR2 knockout mice, which killed bacteria more effectively than macrophages from wild-type mice.

The yellow carotenoid pigment of *S. aureus*, staphyloxanthin, helps to scavenge oxygen free radicals. A mutant defective in synthesis of pigment was more susceptible to killing by neutrophils *in vitro* and was less virulent in a mouse subcutaneous abscess infection model [88]. Neutrophils from a patient with human chronic granulomatous disease (CGD), a disorder involving a defect in neutrophil respiratory burst, had a reduced ability to kill *S. aureus* compared with those from a normal individual. There was no difference in survival of the staphyloxanthin-deficient mutant in CGD neutrophils.

Staphylococcus aureus expresses two superoxide dismutases that remove superoxide. Mutants defective in these enzymes have reduced virulence in a murine abscess model, indicating a role in combating oxidative stress *in vivo* [89]. Manganese homeostasis is also an important defense against oxidative stress because of the cation's activity as a non-enzymatic superoxide dismutase [90]. Reactive oxygen compounds can damage proteins by oxidizing the sulfur atom of methionine to produce methionine sulfoxide. *Staphylococcus aureus* expresses three methionine sulfoxide reductases [91], one of which has been shown to be important for virulence in a mouse bacteremia infection model [92], indicating that it contributes to survival *in vivo*.

Staphylococcus aureus was once regarded as an exclusively extracellular pathogen but it is now abundantly evident that it can survive in neutrophils and macrophages as well being able to invade and survive within nonprofessional phagocytes such as endothelial and epithelial cells. Uptake into nonprofessional phagocytes is promoted by the fibronectin-binding protein forming a bridge with fibronectin to the α5β1 integrin on the host cell surface [93,94]. Intracellular survival allows *S. aureus* to escape host immunity until the cells are lysed by elaboration of membrane-damaging toxins. Intracellular survival is promoted by the small-colony variant phenotype, which is characterized by hemin or menadione auxotrophy, slow growth, and a lack of expression of the cytolytic toxins necessary to promote lysis from within [95]. Small-colony variants are discussed in greater detail in Chapter 5.

Avoidance of phagocytosis by *Staphylococcus epidermidis*

Staphylococcus epidermidis is a less aggressive pathogen than *S. aureus*. It has come to prominence because of its ability to colonize implanted medical devices and to form biofilm. Like *S. aureus* it has a number of mechanisms that allow it to survive on human skin and mucous surfaces, which also help protect it from host defenses within the body. The dominant virulence mechanism of *S. epidermidis* is the ability to form a biofilm [96,97], a multilayered dense structure that protects bacteria from antibiotics and the host immune system.

Biofilm formation is initiated when bacteria adhere to the biomaterial by surface-associated proteins such as the major autolysin AtlE [98] or the fibrinogen-binding protein Fbe/SdrG [99,100]. Cells in a typical multilayered biofilm are held together by PIA, a charged polymer comprising β-1,6-linked *N*-acetylglucosamine [101]. PIA can also contribute directly to avoidance of innate immunity by promoting resistance to both cationic and noncationic antimicrobial peptides as well as reducing neutrophil uptake and killing [102].

Some clinical isolates of *S. epidermidis* from device-associated infections form biofilm *in vitro* but do not express PIA. In some strains biofilm was promoted by the accumulation-associated protein (Aap) [103,104]. The full-length protein is cleaved by a protease to remove the N-terminal A domain and exposing the more distal repeated region, which promotes cell–cell binding presumably by homophilic protein–protein interactions.

A homolog of Aap expressed by *S. aureus* called SasG can also promote biofilm formation independently of PIA

[105]. The length of the SasG protein is crucial for biofilm formation: cells expressing SasG with fewer than five B repeats were biofilm negative. It is unclear if proteolytic cleavage of SasG is necessary. Clinical isolates of *S. aureus*, including some MRSA strains, can form biofilm *in vitro* that is independent of PIA [106].

Staphylococcus epidermidis also expresses a poly-γ-DL-glutamic acid (PGA) surface macromolecule [107]. PGA forms the capsule of *Bacillus anthracis* that is essential for virulence [108]. A PGA-defective mutant of *S. epidermidis* grew poorly in NaCl compared with the parental strain, indicating that PGA aids survival in high-osmolyte environments such as on the surface of the skin. Expression of PGA did not influence the ability of *S. epidermidis* to form biofilm *in vitro* but did contribute to resistance to killing by antimicrobial peptides and resistance to opsonophagocytosis by human neutrophils [107].

Immunomodulation

Protein A

Protein A is a potent immunomodulatory molecule because it can bind to the V_H3 region adjacent to the antigen-binding domain of IgM molecules exposed on the surface of B lymphocytes [109,110]. Cells bearing V_H3 IgM are stimulated to proliferate and undergo apoptosis, leading to depletion of a significant proportion of the repertoire of potential antibody-secreting B cells in the spleen and bone marrow [109]. The structural basis of the interaction is known. Helices II and III of the three-helix bundle that makes up each domain of protein A provide the residues that contact IgM [110–112], in contrast to the binding region for IgG, tumor necrosis factor receptor-1 and von Willebrand factor A1 domain which involve residues on the helix I–II face [69,113].

Enterotoxins and toxic shock syndrome toxin 1

Some strains of *S. aureus* can secrete enterotoxins, which exhibit superantigen activity when expressed systemically and elicit an emetic response when ingested. The superantigen activity of the protein is specified by a domain that is distinct from the domain determining the emetic response. Some strains also express the nonemetic superantigenic toxic shock syndrome toxin (TSST)-1, which was first associated with toxic shock syndrome caused by use of super-absorbent tampons. Superantigens bind to MHC class II protein on the surface of antigen-presenting cells and link it to the TCR on the surface of T helper cells. Binding occurs outside the antigen-binding cleft, circumventing the need for an antigenic peptide to be presented to a suitable TCR. Each type of enterotoxin recognizes a specific subset of variable Vβ chains of TCRs and therefore has a characteristic Vβ signature. Also there are different binding site specificities on the MHC class II protein family. Up to 30% of T cells can become activated in extreme cases leading to activation, proliferation and expression of high levels of cytokines causing toxic shock syndrome.

Expression of superantigens during infection also prevents development of a normal immune response. Antigen-specific T cells fail to proliferate in response to antigens that are presented normally by MHC class II, leading to a phenomenon called anergy. This causes immunosuppression due to failure to induce an appropriate immune response and a lack of immunological memory and prevents development of antibodies to the superantigen toxins themselves. Lack of antibody to superantigens is a common characteristic of patients with toxic shock syndrome. Superantigens are discussed further in Chapter 6.

The MHC class II analog protein Map (also called Eap, see above) comprises six repeated domains of 110 residues, each containing a 30-residue motif with strong homology to the peptide-binding groove of the MHC class II β-chain. Map can bind to the TCR on T cells resulting in alteration of T-cell function, causing a reduction in T-cell proliferation. It also causes a shift from a Th1 response to a Th2 response, which affects cell-mediated immunity and might explain the more rapid clearance of a Map-deficient mutant compared with the wild-type strain from internal abscesses in infected mice. Map also shows two different effects on peripheral blood mononuclear cells (PBMCs). At low concentrations it stimulates proliferation of PBMCs but at high concentrations it inhibits the proliferative effect of the superantigen TSST-1 and stimulates apoptosis of B and T cells. The mechanism by which Map elicits this effect on PBMCs is not known.

In vivo regulation of antiphagocytic virulence factors

Staphylococcus aureus has a two-component signal transduction system (HssRS) that can sense the concentration of heme. When heme is present a nearby operon is induced which encodes an ATP-binding cassette efflux pump called the heme-regulated transport system (HrtAB). This pumps surplus cytoplasmic heme from the cells that have been transported in by the Fur-regulated Isd heme-uptake system. When injected intravenously in mice, both HrtA- and HssR-defective mutants of strain Newman were hypervirulent, with increased bacterial loads in the liver [113]. Mutant bacteria grown in iron-restricted medium, which mimics *in vivo* growth conditions, expressed higher levels of several secreted proteins that are involved in immune evasion, including SSL5, Map-W, Efb, FLIPr and Eap. There were reduced numbers of phagocytic cells in the infected tissue, which could have been due to reduced influx, increased destruction, or both. It is proposed that increased intracellular Fe^{3+} induces stress responses that lead to upregulation of genes encoding secreted virulence factors.

Subversion of the humoral immune response

Staphylococcus aureus can bind to resting platelets and stimulate their activation. Platelet activation and subsequent aggregation is important in the pathogenesis of endovascular infections leading to infectious endocarditis. *Staphylococcus aureus* is now the leading cause of infectious endocarditis. Bacteria grow in platelet fibrin thrombi where they escape the attention of neutrophils. The fibronectin-binding proteins are the major surface proteins causing platelet activation on bacterial cells in exponential growth, and ClfA is the dominant component on the surface of cells from the stationary phase of growth. In both cases contact with resting platelets is made through a bridge to the nascent low-affinity GPIIb/IIIa integrin provided by fibrinogen or fibronectin. For activation to occur the binding of antibodies specific to the surface protein is required. Bound IgG engages the FcγRIIa receptor on the platelet surface. This causes clustering of Fc receptors and stimulation of intracellular signaling leading to activation and aggregation. Almost all individuals have low levels of antibodies to surface proteins of *S. aureus* sufficient to trigger platelet activation and disease pathogenesis. Thus *S. aureus* exploits the humoral response to previous exposures to the organism in order to promote disease pathogenesis.

Concluding remarks

Staphylococcus aureus has a multiplicity of mechanisms to thwart innate and induced immunity. It is particularly instructive to compare *S. aureus* with its close relative *S. epidermidis*, which essentially relies on surface polymers and its ability to form biofilm to survive in the host. This is likely to be a reflection of the different sites in the human body where the organisms reside in the commensal state [3]. *Staphylococcus epidermidis* is a commensal of the human skin, whereas the primary habitat of *S. aureus* is the moist squamous epithelium of the anterior nares where it encounters both innate and induced immunity.

In the post-genomic era, it is possible that novel mechanisms of immune evasion will be discovered. Previously unknown surface and secreted proteins have been identified from genome sequences and searches for functions have revealed that some are involved in avoiding host immune systems [23,42,43]. It seems reasonable to predict that other members of the SSL [20] and Sas [114,115] protein families, for example, might also have immune evasion functions.

There are indications that the dogma concerning expression of secreted and surface proteins is oversimplistic. It is widely believed that cell wall-associated proteins are expressed early in the exponential phase of growth to allow *S. aureus* to adhere to substrates early in infection and that extracellular proteins such as toxins and proteases are secreted in postexponential growth to facilitate bacterial invasion by degrading host tissues and cells [116]. However, several small secreted proteins are induced in the early exponential phase of growth to provide immediate protection against the early immune response to infection [117]. Conversely, the archetypal surface protein ClfA is expressed at a low level in the exponential phase but is induced from a sigma factor B-dependent promoter in the stationary phase [49]. Thus regulation of expression of virulence factors is undoubtedly more complicated than originally proposed.

References

1 Peacock SJ, de Silva I, Lowy FD. What determines nasal carriage of *Staphylococcus aureus*? Trends Microbiol 2001;9:605–10.

2 Nilsson P, Ripa T. *Staphylococcus aureus* throat colonization is more frequent than colonization in the anterior nares. J Clin Microbiol 2006;44:3334–9.

3 Massey RC, Horsburgh MJ, Lina G, Hook M, Recker M. The evolution and maintenance of virulence in *Staphylococcus aureus*: a role for host-to-host transmission? Nat Rev Microbiol 2006;4:953–8.

4 Ni Eidhin D, Perkins S, Francois P, Vaudaux P, Hook M, Foster TJ. Clumping factor B (ClfB), a new surface-located fibrinogen-binding adhesin of *Staphylococcus aureus*. Mol Microbiol 1998; 30:245–57.

5 Perkins S, Walsh EJ, Deivanayagam CC, Narayana SV, Foster TJ, Hook M. Structural organization of the fibrinogen-binding region of the clumping factor B MSCRAMM of *Staphylococcus aureus*. J Biol Chem 2001;276:44721–8.

6 Walsh EJ, O'Brien LM, Liang X, Hook M, Foster TJ. Clumping factor B, a fibrinogen-binding MSCRAMM (microbial surface components recognizing adhesive matrix molecules) adhesin of *Staphylococcus aureus*, also binds to the tail region of type I cytokeratin 10. J Biol Chem 2004;279:50691–9.

7 O'Brien LM, Walsh EJ, Massey RC, Peacock SJ, Foster TJ. *Staphylococcus aureus* clumping factor B (ClfB) promotes adherence to human type I cytokeratin 10: implications for nasal colonization. Cell Microbiol 2002;4:759–70.

8 Clarke SR, Wiltshire MD, Foster SJ. IsdA of *Staphylococcus aureus* is a broad spectrum, iron-regulated adhesin. Mol Microbiol 2004;51:1509–19.

9 Skaar EP, Schneewind O. Iron-regulated surface determinants (Isd) of *Staphylococcus aureus*: stealing iron from heme. Microbes Infect 2004;6:390–7.

10 Clarke SR, Mohamed R, Bian L *et al*. The *Staphylococcus aureus* surface protein IsdA mediates resistance to innate defenses of human skin. *Cell Host Microbe* 2007;1:199–212.

11 Clarke SR, Brummell KJ, Horsburgh MJ *et al*. Identification of in vivo-expressed antigens of *Staphylococcus aureus* and their

use in vaccinations for protection against nasal carriage. J Infect Dis 2006;193:1098–108.
12 Schaffer AC, Solinga RM, Cocchiaro *et al*. Immunization with *Staphylococcus aureus* clumping factor B, a major determinant in nasal carriage, reduces nasal colonization in a murine model. Infect Immun 2006;74:2145–53.
13 Wertheim HF, Walsh E, Choudhurry R *et al*. Key role for clumping factor B in *Staphylococcus aureus* nasal colonization of humans. PloS Med 2008;5:e17.
14 Diep BA, Gill SR, Chang RF *et al*. Complete genome sequence of USA300, an epidemic clone of community-acquired meticillin-resistant *Staphylococcus aureus*. Lancet 2006;367:731–9.
15 Gasque P. Complement: a unique innate immune sensor for danger signals. Mol Immunol 2004;41:1089–98.
16 Walport MJ. Complement. Second of two parts. N Engl J Med 2001;344:1140–4.
17 Walport MJ. Complement. First of two parts. N Engl J Med 2001;344:1058–66.
18 Durr MC, Kristian SA, Otto M *et al*. Neutrophil chemotaxis by pathogen-associated molecular patterns: formylated peptides are crucial but not the sole neutrophil attractants produced by *Staphylococcus aureus*. Cell Microbiol 2006;8:207–17.
19 Ley K. Integration of inflammatory signals by rolling neutrophils. Immunol Rev 2002;186:8–18.
20 Williams RJ, Ward JM, Henderson B *et al*. Identification of a novel gene cluster encoding staphylococcal exotoxin-like proteins: characterization of the prototypic gene and its protein product, SET1. Infect Immun 2000;68:4407–15.
21 Fitzgerald JR, Reid SD, Ruotsalainen E *et al*. Genome diversification in *Staphylococcus aureus*: molecular evolution of a highly variable chromosomal region encoding the staphylococcal exotoxin-like family of proteins. Infect Immun 2003; 71:2827–38.
22 Arcus VL, Langley R, Proft T, Fraser JD, Baker EN. The three-dimensional structure of a superantigen-like protein, SET3, from a pathogenicity island of the *Staphylococcus aureus* genome. J Biol Chem 2002;277:32274–81.
23 Bestebroer J, Poppelier MJ, Ulfman LH *et al*. Staphylococcal superantigen-like 5 binds PSGL-1 and inhibits P-selectin-mediated neutrophil rolling. Blood 2007;109:2936–43.
24 Chavakis T, Hussain M, Kanse SM *et al*. *Staphylococcus aureus* extracellular adherence protein serves as anti-inflammatory factor by inhibiting the recruitment of host leukocytes. Nat Med 2002;8:687–93.
25 Murdoch C, Finn A. Chemokine receptors and their role in inflammation and infectious diseases. Blood 2000;95:3032–43.
26 de Haas CJ, Veldkamp KE, Peschel A *et al*. Chemotaxis inhibitory protein of *Staphylococcus aureus*, a bacterial anti-inflammatory agent. J Exp Med 2004;199:687–95.
27 Haas PJ, de Haas CJ, Kleibeuker W *et al*. N-terminal residues of the chemotaxis inhibitory protein of *Staphylococcus aureus* are essential for blocking formylated peptide receptor but not C5a receptor. J Immunol 2004;173:5704–11.
28 Postma B, Kleibeuker W, Poppelier MJ *et al*. Residues 10–18 within the C5a receptor N terminus compose a binding domain for chemotaxis inhibitory protein of *Staphylococcus aureus*. J Biol Chem 2005;280:2020–7.
29 Postma B, Poppelier MJ, van Galen JC *et al*. Chemotaxis inhibitory protein of *Staphylococcus aureus* binds specifically to the C5a and formylated peptide receptor. J Immunol 2004;172:6994–7001.
30 Prat C, Bestebroer J, de Haas CJ, van Strijp JA, van Kessel KP. A new staphylococcal anti-inflammatory protein that antagonizes the formyl peptide receptor-like 1. J Immunol 2006;177:8017–26.
31 van Wamel WJ, Rooijakkers SH, Ruyken M, van Kessel KP, van Strijp JA. The innate immune modulators staphylococcal complement inhibitor and chemotaxis inhibitory protein of *Staphylococcus aureus* are located on β-hemolysin-converting bacteriophages. J Bacteriol 2006;188:1310–15.
32 Moore F. Complement. In: Pier GB, Lyczak JB, Wetzler LM, eds. *Immunology, Infection, and Immunity*. Washington, DC: ASM Press, 2004:85–109.
33 Fujita T. Evolution of the lectin-complement pathway and its role in innate immunity. Nat Rev Immunol 2002;2:346–53.
34 Rooijakkers SH, Ruyken M, Roos A *et al*. Immune evasion by a staphylococcal complement inhibitor that acts on C3 convertases. Nat Immunol 2005;6:920–7.
35 Bokarewa MI, Jin T, Tarkowski A. *Staphylococcus aureus*: staphylokinase. Int J Biochem Cell Biol 2006;38:504–9.
36 Rooijakkers SH, van Wamel WJ, Ruyken M, van Kessel KP, van Strijp JA. Anti-opsonic properties of staphylokinase. Microbes Infect 2005;7:476–84.
37 Cunnion KM, Buescher ES, Hair PS. Serum complement factor I decreases *Staphylococcus aureus* phagocytosis. J Lab Clin Med 2005;146:279–86.
38 Cunnion KM, Hair PS, Buescher ES. Cleavage of complement C3b to iC3b on the surface of *Staphylococcus aureus* is mediated by serum complement factor I. Infect Immun 2004;72:2858–63.
39 Lee LY, Hook M, Haviland D *et al*. Inhibition of complement activation by a secreted *Staphylococcus aureus* protein. J Infect Dis 2004;190:571–9.
40 Lee LY, Liang X, Hook M, Brown EL. Identification and characterization of the C3 binding domain of the *Staphylococcus aureus* extracellular fibrinogen-binding protein (Efb). J Biol Chem 2004;279:50710–16.
41 Hammel M, Sfyroera G, Ricklin D, Magotti P, Lambris JD, Geisbrecht BV. A structural basis for complement inhibition by *Staphylococcus aureus*. Nat Immunol 2007;8:430–7.
42 Visai L, Yanagisawa N, Josefsson E, Tarkowski A, Pezzali I, Rooijakkers SH, Foster TJ, Speziale P. Immune evasion *by Staphylococcus aureus conferred by iron-regulated surface determinant protein IsdH. Microbiology*. 2009 Mar; 155 (Pt 3):667–79.
43 Wines BD, Willoughby N, Fraser JD, Hogarth PM. A competitive mechanism for staphylococcal toxin SSL7 inhibiting the leukocyte IgA receptor, Fc alphaRI, is revealed by SSL7 binding at the C alpha2/C alpha3 interface of IgA. J Biol Chem 2006;281:1389–93.
44 Uhlen M, Guss B, Nilsson B, Gatenbeck S, Philipson L, Lindberg M. Complete sequence of the staphylococcal gene encoding protein A. A gene evolved through multiple duplications. J Biol Chem 1984;259:1695–702.
45 Cedergren L, Andersson R, Jansson B, Uhlen M, Nilsson B. Mutational analysis of the interaction between staphylococcal protein A and human IgG1. Protein Eng 1993;6:441–8.
46 Gemmell C, Tree R, Patel A, O'Reilly M, Foster TJ. Susceptibility to opsonophagocytosis of protein A, alpha-haemolysin and beta-toxin deficient mutants of *Staphylococcus aureus* isolated by allele-replacement. *Zentralbl Bakteriol* 1991;(suppl 21):273–7.
47 Palmqvist N, Foster T, Tarkowski A, Josefsson E. Protein A is a virulence factor in *Staphylococcus aureus* arthritis and septic death. Microb Pathog 2002;33:239–49.

48 Patel AH, Nowlan P, Weavers ED, Foster T. Virulence of protein A-deficient and alpha-toxin-deficient mutants of *Staphylococcus aureus* isolated by allele replacement. Infect Immun 1987; 55:3103–10.

49 Bischoff M, Dunman P, Kormanec J *et al*. Microarray-based analysis of the *Staphylococcus aureus* σB regulon. J Bacteriol 2004;186:4085–99.

50 O'Brien L, Kerrigan SW, Kaw G *et al*. Multiple mechanisms for the activation of human platelet aggregation by *Staphylococcus aureus*: roles for the clumping factors ClfA and ClfB, the serine-aspartate repeat protein SdrE and protein A. Mol Microbiol 2002;44:1033–44.

51 Higgins J, Loughman A, van Kessel KP, van Strijp JA, Foster TJ. Clumping factor A of *Staphylococcus aureus* inhibits phagocytosis by human polymorphonuclear leucocytes. FEMS Microbiol Lett 2006;258:290–6.

52 McDevitt D, Nanavaty T, House-Pompeo K *et al*. Characterization of the interaction between the *Staphylococcus aureus* clumping factor (ClfA) and fibrinogen. Eur J Biochem 1997; 247:416–24.

53 Josefsson E, Hartford O, O'Brien L, Patti JM, Foster T. Protection against experimental *Staphylococcus aureus* arthritis by vaccination with clumping factor A, a novel virulence determinant. J Infect Dis 2001;184:1572–80.

54 Wann ER, Gurusiddappa S, Hook M. The fibronectin-binding MSCRAMM FnbpA of *Staphylococcus aureus* is a bifunctional protein that also binds to fibrinogen. J Biol Chem 2000; 275:13863–71.

55 Keane FM, Loughman A, Valtulina V, Brennan M, Speziale P, Foster TJ. Fibrinogen and elastin bind to the same region within the A domain of fibronectin binding protein A, an MSCRAMM of *Staphylococcus aureus*. Mol Microbiol 2007;63:711–23.

56 Roghmann M, Taylor KL, Gupte A *et al*. Epidemiology of capsular and surface polysaccharide in *Staphylococcus aureus* infections complicated by bacteraemia. J Hosp Infect 2005;59:27–32.

57 O'Riordan K, Lee JC. *Staphylococcus aureus* capsular polysaccharides. Clin Microbiol Rev 2004;17:218–34.

58 Nilsson IM, Lee JC, Bremell T, Ryden C, Tarkowski A. The role of staphylococcal polysaccharide microcapsule expression in septicemia and septic arthritis. Infect Immun 1997;65:4216–21.

59 Thakker M, Park JS, Carey V, Lee JC. *Staphylococcus aureus* serotype 5 capsular polysaccharide is antiphagocytic and enhances bacterial virulence in a murine bacteremia model. Infect Immun 1998;66:5183–9.

60 Luong TT, Lee CY. Overproduction of type 8 capsular polysaccharide augments *Staphylococcus aureus* virulence. Infect Immun 2002;70:3389–95.

61 Montoya M, Gouaux E. Beta-barrel membrane protein folding and structure viewed through the lens of α-hemolysin. Biochim Biophys Acta 2003;1609:19–27.

62 Menestrina G, Dalla Serra M, Comai M *et al*. Ion channels and bacterial infection: the case of beta-barrel pore-forming protein toxins of *Staphylococcus aureus*. FEBS Lett 2003;552:54–60.

63 Peacock SJ, Moore CE, Justice A *et al*. Virulent combinations of adhesin and toxin genes in natural populations of *Staphylococcus aureus*. Infect Immun 2002;70:4987–96.

64 Prevost G, Cribier B, Couppie P *et al*. Panton–Valentine leucocidin and γ-hemolysin from *Staphylococcus aureus* ATCC 49775 are encoded by distinct genetic loci and have different biological activities. Infect Immun 1995;63:4121–9.

65 Gillet Y, Issartel B, Vanhems P *et al*. Association between *Staphylococcus aureus* strains carrying gene for Panton–Valentine leukocidin and highly lethal necrotising pneumonia in young immunocompetent patients. Lancet 2002;359:753–9.

66 Lina G, Piémont Y, Godail-Gamot F *et al*. Involvement of Panton–Valentine leukocidin-producing *Staphylococcus aureus* in primary skin infections and pneumonia. Clin Infect Dis 1999;29:1128–32.

67 Labandeira-Rey M, Couzon F, Boisset S *et al*. *Staphylococcus aureus* Panton–Valentine leukocidin causes necrotizing pneumonia. Science 2007;315:1130–3.

68 Voyich JM, Otto M, Mathema B *et al*. Is Panton–Valentine leukocidin the major virulence determinant in community-associated methicillin-resistant *Staphylococcus aureus* disease? J Infect Dis 2006;194:1761–70.

69 Gomez MI, O'Seaghdha M, Magargee M, Foster TJ, Prince AS. *Staphylococcus aureus* protein A activates TNFR1 signaling through conserved IgG binding domains. J Biol Chem 2006; 281:20190–6.

70 Narita S, Kaneko J, Chiba J *et al*. Phage conversion of Panton–Valentine leukocidin in *Staphylococcus aureus*: molecular analysis of a PVL-converting phage, phiSLT. Gene 2001;268:195–206.

71 Kubica M, Guzik K, Koziel J *et al*. A potential new pathway for *Staphylococcus aureus* dissemination: the silent survival and intracellular proliferation of *S. aureus* phagocytosed by human monocyte-derived macrophages. PLoS ONE 2007;3:e1409.

72 Gresham HD, Lowrance JH, Caver TE, Wilson BS, Cheung AL, Lindberg FP. Survival of *Staphylococcus aureus* inside neutrophils contributes to infection. J Immunol 2000;164:3713–22.

73 Peschel A, Otto M, Jack RW, Kalbacher H, Jung G, Gotz F. Inactivation of the *dlt* operon in *Staphylococcus aureus* confers sensitivity to defensins, protegrins, and other antimicrobial peptides. J Biol Chem 1999;274:8405–10.

74 Peschel A, Jack RW, Otto M *et al*. *Staphylococcus aureus* resistance to human defensins and evasion of neutrophil killing via the novel virulence factor MprF is based on modification of membrane lipids with l-lysine. J Exp Med 2001;193:1067–76.

75 Staubitz P, Neumann H, Schneider T, Wiedemann I, Peschel A. MprF-mediated biosynthesis of lysylphosphatidylglycerol, an important determinant in staphylococcal defensin resistance. FEMS Microbiol Lett 2004;231:67–71.

76 Kristian SA, Durr M, van Strijp JA, Neumeister B, Peschel A. MprF-mediated lysinylation of phospholipids in *Staphylococcus aureus* leads to protection against oxygen-independent neutrophil killing. Infect Immun 2003;71:546–9.

77 Kristian SA, Lauth X, Nizet V *et al*. Alanylation of teichoic acids protects *Staphylococcus aureus* against Toll-like receptor 2-dependent host defense in a mouse tissue cage infection model. J Infect Dis 2003;188:414–23.

78 Collins LV, Kristian SA, Weidenmaier C *et al*. *Staphylococcus aureus* strains lacking D-alanine modifications of teichoic acids are highly susceptible to human neutrophil killing and are virulence attenuated in mice. J Infect Dis 2002;186:214–19.

79 Li M, Lai Y, Villaruz AE, Cha DJ, Sturdevant DE, Otto M. Gram-positive three-component antimicrobial peptide-sensing system. Proc Natl Acad Sci USA 2007;104:9469–74.

80 Lai Y, Villaruz AE, Li M, Cha DJ, Sturdevant DE, Otto M. The human anionic antimicrobial peptide dermcidin induces proteolytic defence mechanisms in staphylococci. Mol Microbiol 2007;63:497–506.

81 Bokarewa M, Tarkowski A. Human alpha-defensins neutralize fibrinolytic activity exerted by staphylokinase. Thromb Haemost 2004;91:991–9.

82 Jin T, Bokarewa M, Foster T, Mitchell J, Higgins J, Tarkowski A. *Staphylococcus aureus* resists human defensins by production of staphylokinase, a novel bacterial evasion mechanism. J Immunol 2004;172:1169–76.

83 Braff MH, Jones AL, Skerrett SJ, Rubens CE. *Staphylococcus aureus* exploits cathelicidin antimicrobial peptides produced during early pneumonia to promote staphylokinase-dependent fibrinolysis. J Infect Dis 2007;195:1365–72.

84 Sieprawska-Lupa M, Mydel P, Krawczyk K *et al*. Degradation of human antimicrobial peptide LL-37 by *Staphylococcus aureus*-derived proteinases. Antimicrob Agents Chemother 2004;48:4673–9.

85 Keshav S, Chung P, Milon G, Gordon S. Lysozyme is an inducible marker of macrophage activation in murine tissues as demonstrated by in situ hybridization. J Exp Med 1991; 174:1049–58.

86 Bera A, Herbert S, Jakob A, Vollmer W, Götz F. Why are pathogenic staphylococci so lysozyme resistant? The peptidoglycan *O*-acetyltransferase OatA is the major determinant for lysozyme resistance of *Staphylococcus aureus*. Mol Microbiol 2005;55:778–87.

87 Watanabe I, Ichiki M, Shiratsuchi A, Nakanishi Y. TLR2-mediated survival of *Staphylococcus aureus* in macrophages: a novel bacterial strategy against host innate immunity. J Immunol 2007;178:4917–25.

88 Liu GY, Essex A, Buchanan JT *et al*. *Staphylococcus aureus* golden pigment impairs neutrophil killing and promotes virulence through its antioxidant activity. J Exp Med 2005;202:209–15.

89 Karavolos MH, Horsburgh MJ, Ingham E, Foster SJ. Role and regulation of the superoxide dismutases of *Staphylococcus aureus*. Microbiology 2003;149:2749–58.

90 Horsburgh MJ, Wharton SJ, Cox AG, Ingham E, Peacock S, Foster SJ. MntR modulates expression of the PerR regulon and superoxide resistance in *Staphylococcus aureus* through control of manganese uptake. Mol Microbiol 2002;44:1269–86.

91 Singh VK, Moskovitz J. Multiple methionine sulfoxide reductase genes in *Staphylococcus aureus*: expression of activity and roles in tolerance of oxidative stress. Microbiology 2003; 149:2739–47.

92 Mei JM, Nourbakhsh F, Ford CW, Holden DW. Identification of *Staphylococcus aureus* virulence genes in a murine model of bacteraemia using signature-tagged mutagenesis. Mol Microbiol 1997;26:399–407.

93 Schwarz-Linek U, Werner JM, Pickford AR *et al*. Pathogenic bacteria attach to human fibronectin through a tandem beta-zipper. Nature 2003;423:177–81.

94 Peacock SJ, Foster TJ, Cameron BJ, Berendt AR. Bacterial fibronectin-binding proteins and endothelial cell surface fibronectin mediate adherence of *Staphylococcus aureus* to resting human endothelial cells. Microbiology 1999;145:3477–86.

95 Proctor RA, von Eiff C, Kahl BC *et al*. Small colony variants: a pathogenic form of bacteria that facilitates persistent and recurrent infections. Nat Rev Microbiol 2006;4:295–305.

96 Mack D. Molecular mechanisms of *Staphylococcus epidermidis* biofilm formation. J Hosp Infect 1999;43(suppl):S113–S125.

97 Mack D, Becker P, Chatterjee I *et al*. Mechanisms of biofilm formation in *Staphylococcus epidermidis* and *Staphylococcus aureus*: functional molecules, regulatory circuits, and adaptive responses. Int J Med Microbiol 2004;294:203–12.

98 Heilmann C, Hussain M, Peters G, Götz F. Evidence for autolysin-mediated primary attachment of *Staphylococcus epidermidis* to a polystyrene surface. Mol Microbiol 1997;24:1013–24.

99 Hartford O, O'Brien L, Schofield K, Wells J, Foster TJ. The Fbe (SdrG) protein of *Staphylococcus epidermidis* HB promotes bacterial adherence to fibrinogen. Microbiology 2001;147:2545–52.

100 Nilsson M, Frykberg L, Flock JI, Pei L, Lindberg M, Guss B. A fibrinogen-binding protein of *Staphylococcus epidermidis*. Infect Immun 1998;66:2666–73.

101 Mack D, Fischer W, Krokotsch A *et al*. The intercellular adhesin involved in biofilm accumulation of *Staphylococcus epidermidis* is a linear β-1,6-linked glucosaminoglycan: purification and structural analysis. J Bacteriol 1996;178:175–83.

102 Vuong C, Voyich JM, Fischer ER *et al*. Polysaccharide intercellular adhesin (PIA) protects *Staphylococcus epidermidis* against major components of the human innate immune system. Cell Microbiol 2004;6:269–75.

103 Hennig S, Nyunt Wai S, Ziebuhr W. Spontaneous switch to PIA-independent biofilm formation in an ica-positive *Staphylococcus epidermidis* isolate. Int J Med Microbiol 2007;297:117–22.

104 Rohde H, Burdelski C, Bartscht K *et al*. Induction of *Staphylococcus epidermidis* biofilm formation via proteolytic processing of the accumulation-associated protein by staphylococcal and host proteases. Mol Microbiol 2005;55:1883–95.

105 Corrigan RM, Rigby D, Handley P, Foster TJ. The role of *Staphylococcus aureus* surface protein SasG in adherence and biofilm formation. Microbiology 2007;153:2435–46.

106 O'Gara JP. *ica* and beyond: biofilm mechanisms and regulation in *Staphylococcus epidermidis* and *Staphylococcus aureus*. FEMS Microbiol Lett 2007;270:179–88.

107 Kocianova S, Vuong C, Yao Y *et al*. Key role of poly-gamma-DL-glutamic acid in immune evasion and virulence of *Staphylococcus epidermidis*. J Clin Invest 2005;115:688–94.

108 Little SF, Ivins BE. Molecular pathogenesis of *Bacillus anthracis* infection. Microbes Infect 1999;1:131–9.

109 Goodyear CS, Silverman GJ. Staphylococcal toxin induced preferential and prolonged in vivo deletion of innate-like B lymphocytes. Proc Natl Acad Sci USA 2004;101:11392–7.

110 Graille M, Stura EA, Corper AL *et al*. Crystal structure of a *Staphylococcus aureus* protein A domain complexed with the Fab fragment of a human IgM antibody: structural basis for recognition of B-cell receptors and superantigen activity. Proc Natl Acad Sci USA 2000;97:5399–404.

111 Silverman GJ, Cary S, Graille M *et al*. A B-cell superantigen that targets B-1 lymphocytes. Curr Top Microbiol Immunol 2000;252:251–63.

112 Silverman GJ, Goodyear CS. A model B-cell superantigen and the immunobiology of B lymphocytes. Clin Immunol 2002;102:117–34.

113 O'Seaghdha M, van Schooten CJ, Kerrigan SW *et al*. *Staphylococcus aureus* protein A binding to von Willebrand factor A1 domain is mediated by conserved IgG binding regions. *FEBS J* 2006;273:4831–41.

114 Roche FM, Massey R, Peacock SJ *et al*. Characterization of novel LPXTG-containing proteins of *Staphylococcus aureus* identified from genome sequences. Microbiology 2003;149:643–54.

115 Mazmanian SK, Ton-That H, Schneewind O. Sortase-catalysed anchoring of surface proteins to the cell wall of *Staphylococcus aureus*. Mol Microbiol 2001;40:1049–57.

116 Cheung AL, Bayer AS, Zhang G, Gresham H, Xiong YQ. Regulation of virulence determinants in vitro and in vivo in *Staphylococcus aureus*. FEMS Immunol Med Microbiol 2004;40:1–9.

117 Rooijakkers SH, Ruyken M, van Roon J, van Kessel KP, van Strijp JA, van Wamel WJ. Early expression of SCIN and CHIPS drives instant immune evasion by *Staphylococcus aureus*. Cell Microbiol 2006;8:1282–93.

Antimicrobial Resistance in Staphylococci

Chapter 8 Resistance to β-Lactam Antibiotics

Brigitte Berger-Bächi, Maria Magdalena Senn, Miriam Ender, Kati Seidl, Judith Hübscher, Bettina Schulthess, Roni Heusser, Patricia Stutzmann Meier and Nadine McCallum

Institute of Medical Microbiology, University of Zürich, Zürich, Switzerland

Introduction

The rapid evolution of drug resistance in bacteria, which started in 1940, is driven by the increasing use of antibiotics in the clinical environment, animal husbandry, and agriculture. Bacteria easily acquire resistance by mutation of their genome. Due to their large number and a spontaneous mutation rate around 10^{-8}, mutants with decreased drug susceptibility were present within bacterial populations even before antibiotic use. Such first-step mutants, sometimes not reaching clinically relevant resistance levels, are selected by antibiotic treatment and are the breeding ground for increased resistance during further selection steps, leading finally to therapy failure. Additionally, bacteria have very efficient means of intraspecies and interspecies gene exchange by transduction, transformation, and conjugation by which they share DNA elements carrying resistance determinants. The pool of resistance determinants increases proportionately with antibiotic use. In addition to acquiring genetically defined resistance mechanisms, bacteria can also be phenotypically refractory to drugs depending on their metabolic status [1].

The speed with which pathogens can adapt to the introduction of antibiotics into clinical use is best reflected by *Staphylococcus aureus*, which has demonstrated a remarkable ability to rapidly develop resistance against any new drug. Resistance to β-lactam drugs in *S. aureus* is principally conferred by two mechanisms, one based on the inactivation of the drug by penicillinases, causing resistance to penicillins, the second and more important based on the acquisition of a new insensitive target molecule, the low-affinity penicillin-binding protein (PBP)2a/PBP2′. PBP2a extends the resistance to all penicillinase-resistant penicillins and their derivatives in methicillin-resistant *S. aureus* (MRSA). There is also a third, much less frequent and currently not well understood mechanism that gives rise to borderline oxacillin-resistant *S. aureus* (BORSA) that is based on mutational changes in the genome, mainly affecting the production and affinity of endogenous PBPs [2].

Evolution of β-lactam resistance in *Staphylococcus aureus*

In the 1940s, when penicillin was introduced into clinical practice, the number of penicillinase-producing *S. aureus* was very low. However, within a few years their prevalence rose rapidly [3,4], mainly due to a phage type 80/81 penicillinase-producing clone that appeared in the 1950s and began spreading all over the world, causing hospital- and community-acquired infections [5]. Besides clonal spreading, the fact that staphylococcal penicillinases are located on transposable elements and are generally plasmid borne [6,7] has contributed to the wide dissemination of penicillin resistance in clinical *S. aureus* isolates.

The selective pressure changed in 1959 with the introduction of methicillin, the first semisynthetic penicillinase-resistant β-lactam, and 1961 saw the appearance of the first MRSA strains, which were resistant to virtually all β-lactams and their derivatives, [8]. They first spread throughout the UK, then to other European countries, and finally to all other parts of the world. MRSA first established themselves in hospitals and places of high antibiotic use. Within a short time, they acquired additional resistance to all commonly used antibiotics, resulting in typical hospital-acquired multidrug-resistant MRSA (HA-MRSA) strains. MRSA have since developed into a worldwide

Staphylococci in Human Disease, 2nd edition. Edited by Kent B. Crossley, Kimberly K. Jefferson, Gordon Archer, Vance G. Fowler, Jr.
 ISBN 978-14051-6332-3.

health problem, the threat of which is still increasing. According to Centers for Disease Control (CDC) data, in 1974, MRSA infections accounted for 2% of the total number of staphylococcal infections, in 1995 for 22%, and in 2004 for 63%. A similar trend was observed in the 1999–2005 surveillance study by the European Antimicrobial Surveillance System (EARSS) (http://www.earss.rivm.nl) which showed increasing MRSA prevalence in most European countries. Today, MRSA are no longer confined to hospitals. Recent reports show the emergence of distinctive MRSA, with apparently higher fitness and altered resistance patterns, in the community (CA-MRSA) [3,9]. These new strains are bound to enter hospitals [10] and adapt to the higher antibiotic use. The evolution of β-lactam resistance in staphylococci is thus an ongoing dynamic process, triggered by selective pressure for fitness and antibiotic resistance [11].

Mechanism of β-lactam action

The β-lactams and their derivatives form the largest class of antibiotics. This class of antibiotics interferes with cell wall biosynthesis. Their structure mimics the D-Ala-D-Ala terminus of the muropeptide, which takes part in cross-linking two neighboring peptidoglycan strands during cell wall synthesis. This transpeptidase reaction is catalyzed by the PBPs [12]. β-Lactams acylate the active site serine of the PBP transpeptidase domain, which undergoes only very slow deacylation, and thus block their access to the true substrate. This leads to a rapid decline in cross-linking of the cell wall peptidoglycan, to inhibition of new septum initiation, and to activation of the cell's autolytic enzymes. The exact mechanism of penicillin-induced death, which can be divided into two distinct processes, namely lytic and nonlytic death, is still poorly understood [13]. The effect of penicillin is concentration dependent. Low concentrations of the drug cause growth retardation, higher concentrations above the minimum inhibitory concentration (MIC) cause growth inhibition and lysis, and at very high concentrations nonlytic death occurs. Peptidoglycan precursor synthesis continues in the presence of inhibitory concentrations of penicillin, but the material is no longer cross-linked and is deposited as amorphous material in the septal plane. The cell can still perform one-cell separation through the existing septum, and lyses at the onset of the following cell separation [14]. β-Lactams therefore disconnect cell wall synthesis from autolytic activities.

Besides inhibiting cell wall synthesis, β-lactams have also been shown to affect other staphylococcal properties. Subinhibitory concentrations have been shown to induce the expression of virulence factors such as coagulase, hemolysins, nuclease, and fibronectin-binding protein by the SaeRS two-component sensor transducer [15,16]. Higher, inhibitory concentrations induce the cell wall stress response [17,18] by the VraSR two-component system, which senses the disturbance of cell wall synthesis [19]. This system controls a set of genes, some of which may contribute to antibiotic resistance in general ways [20]. The β-lactams are also known to induce the SOS response, which in turn induces phages and promotes the transfer of virulence determinants [21].

Gene rearrangements may sometimes cause unusual effects. A fusion of a truncated *blaZ* gene with the bifunctional 6′-aminoglycoside-*N*-acetyltransferase/2″-aminoglycoside phosphotransferase gene AAC(6′)-APH(2″), identified in a clinical MRSA isolate [22], resulted in antagonism between aminoglycosides and β-lactams, due to the β-lactam-inducible aminoglycoside resistance.

Penicillinases

The most widespread β-lactam resistance mechanism involves inactivation of the drug by β-lactamases. Serine β-lactamases have evolved from ancestral PBPs. Unlike PBPs which readily form acyl-enzyme complexes but are inefficient at turning over β-lactams and thus are almost irreversibly blocked, β-lactamases hydrolyze the drug. Penicillinases were present in staphylococci long before the antibiotic era, though only in a few strains. The wide use of penicillins in therapy triggered a rapid spread of the penicillinases among staphylococci. Penicillin-resistant *S. aureus* first appeared in hospitals but they are now also prevalent in the community. In contrast to Gram-negative bacteria, penicillinases in staphylococci are membrane-anchored lipoproteins that can also be liberated into the growth medium on induction [23]. Interestingly, the membrane anchor of the penicillinase, and not the penicillinase activity itself, was shown to increase susceptibility of *S. aureus* to linoleic acid. This unsaturated fatty acid inhibits growth by depolarizing membranes, suggesting that the membrane anchoring of the penicillinase may alter membrane properties or the interaction of the membrane with linoleic acid [24].

Regulation of *blaZ* transcription

The penicillinase operon consists of *blaZ*, coding for the penicillinase structural gene, and the divergently transcribed *blaR1-blaI* genes, which code for the transmembrane β-lactam sensor transducer BlaR1 and the repressor BlaI, respectively. Under uninduced conditions, two BlaI dimers bind to the *bla* operator region, thereby preventing transcription of both *blaR1-blaI* and *blaZ* [25]. BlaR1 acts as a β-lactam sensor and is required for the induction of the *bla* operon by β-lactams. The β-lactam-sensing domain in the C-terminus is exposed on the cell surface and is separated by a transmembrane segment from a Zn peptidase domain facing the cytosol that is followed by three

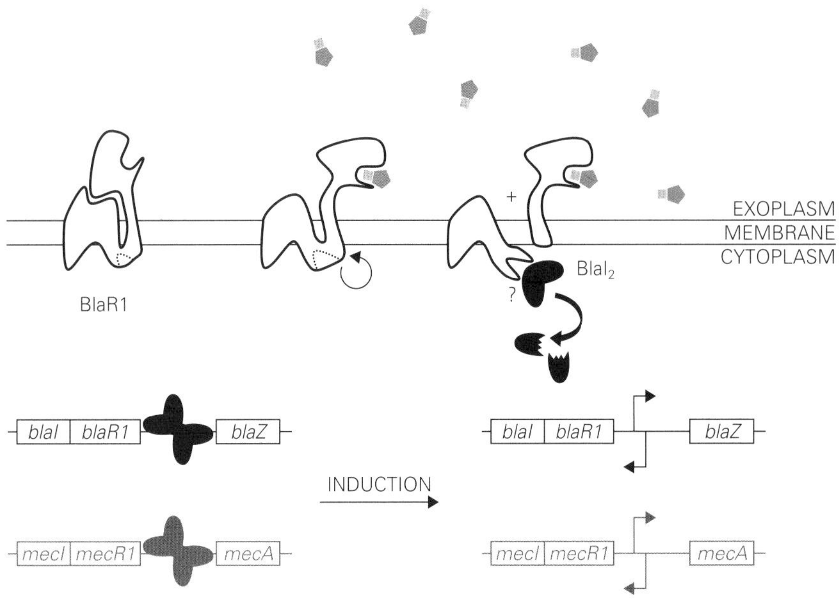

Figure 8.1 Regulation of the *bla* and *mec* operons. Under noninduced conditions, both the *bla* and *mec* operator regions are bound by two dimers of the BlaI or MecI repressor. In the presence of β-lactams, the sensors BlaR1 and MecR1 undergo a conformational change on binding of the antibiotic. Thereby, their cytoplasmic protease domain (indicated by dashed lines) becomes activated and autocleavage follows. Directly or indirectly, activated BlaR1 and MecR1 lead to the degradation of their cognate repressors (only BlaR1/BlaI is shown), allowing synthesis of the sensor (BlaR1; MecR1), repressor (BlaI; MecI), the β-lactamase BlaZ, and PBP2a.

transmembrane N-terminal domains [26]. The structures of the acyl-enzyme complex with benzylpenicillin and ceftazidime have been solved independently using X-ray crystallography [26,27]. On interaction with a β-lactam, BlaR1 is acylated and transmits a signal to the cytoplasmic side by conformational changes, in an as yet poorly understood way, leading to activation of the cytoplasmic Zn protease and the autocatalytic cleavage of BlaR1 (Figure 8.1). The molecular events have been reviewed by Fuda *et al.* [28]. The metalloprotease then either directly cleaves BlaI or promotes, in concert with other factors, BlaI degradation. This prevents the formation of the BlaI dimer and its binding to the promoter region, derepressing the transcription of *blaZ* and *blaR1-blaI* [29–31]. The transmembrane sensor transducer BlaR1 is inactivated by the cleavage and has to be resynthesized. Additional factors are postulated to be involved in the control of *blaZ* transcription, but have yet to be characterized. Cohen and Sweeney [32] identified a chromosomal locus termed *R2* involved in the regulation of penicillinase production. $R2^-$ mutants were constitutive penicillinase producers; however, penicillinase production in these mutants was temperature sensitive, being higher at 30°C than at 42°C. Penicillinase production was derepressed variably, depending on whether *blaZ* was on a plasmid or chromosomal, leading the authors to suggest a positional effect [33]. However, this locus has not yet been identified, nor is the nature of the regulatory mechanism known.

Interestingly, although penicillinases are now widely spread among staphylococci, they have never evolved to a similar extent as β-lactamases in Gram-negative bacteria, which by mutation have greatly broadened their spectrum of activity. Staphylococci, like other Gram-positive pathogens such as enterococci and streptococci, rather escape β-lactams by modification of the β-lactam target, namely the PBPs.

Methicillin resistance

Methicillin-susceptible *S. aureus* (MSSA) possess four PBPs: three high-molecular-mass PBPs, namely PBP1 (approximately 185 copies per cell), PBP2 (460 copies per cell), and PBP3 (150 copies per cell); and a low-molecular-mass PBP4 (285 copies per cell) [34]. The lethal targets are PBP1, an essential monofunctional class B PBP, which is involved in the cell division process [35,36], and PBP2, the only bifunctional class A PBP, harboring both transpeptidase and β-lactam-insensitive transglycosylase activities [37]. The class B PBP3, and the low-molecular-mass PBP4, which is involved in secondary cross-linking of the peptidoglycan [38,39], are not essential for growth. Inactivation of PBP3 is accompanied by reduced autolysis, and its function is postulated to be taken over by PBP1 [40]. In growing cells, PBPs localize through substrate recognition at the site of new cell wall synthesis in the septal plane. Blocking of the active sites of PBP2, as well as masking or modifying the peptidoglycan precursor, was shown to cause dislocation of PBP2 from the septal plane to the cell surface [41] (Figure 8.2). MRSA express an additional PBP, PBP2a/PBP2′, which is encoded by the gene *mecA*. PBP2a has a lower affinity to the penicillinase-stable penicillins than the cell's own PBPs, and it is thought to function as a transpeptidase when the native staphylococcal PBPs are acylated by β-lactams, allowing survival and growth in the presence of otherwise inhibitory concentrations of β-lactams.

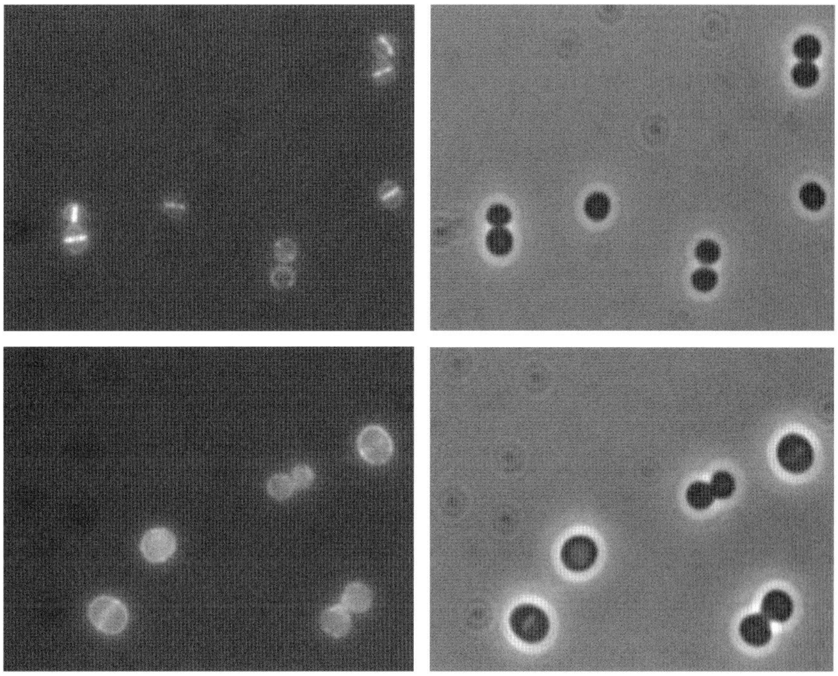

Figure 8.2 Effect of the addition of oxacillin to the localization of PBP2 using an N-terminal GFP fusion. (*Left*) Fluorescence images; (*right*) phase contrast images. (*Top*) In the absence of antibiotic, PBP2 is concentrated at the septum; (*bottom*) in the presence of inhibitory concentrations of oxacillin, PBP2 localization is lost and the protein becomes dispersed over the entire surface of the cell. (Images kindly provided by M. Pinho.)

SCC*mec*

Methicillin resistance is due to the acquisition of a resistance island, the staphylococcal chromosomal cassette *mec* (SCC*mec*), in which the *mecA* gene is embedded. The *mecA* gene is a prerequisite for methicillin resistance, as it codes for the additional PBP2a. It is not only the large resistance spectrum to β-lactams that renders MRSA a threat to hospitalized patients, but also the potential of the SCC element to capture and collect additional nonrelated resistance determinants, leading to the accumulation of multiple resistances in MRSA [42]. Initially, in 1960, MRSA spread from a single clone with low-level oxacillin resistance, which was presumably the ancestor of the European MRSA [43]. Today's worldwide spread of MRSA is still mainly restricted to a few successful epidemic clones [44].

SCC*mec* is a mobile chromosomal element ranging in size from 21 kb up to more than 64 kb, which integrates site-specifically into the 3′ end of *orfX*, an open reading frame of unknown function close to the origin of replication. A characteristic feature of SCC*mec* is a set of direct and inverted repeat sequences framing the element at its chromosomal junctions. Only a small fraction of the element, the 2-kb long *mecA* gene, is responsible for methicillin resistance. The *mec* complex forms a divergon consisting of the *mecA* gene and the regulatory genes *mecR1-mecI*. It is noteworthy that the *mecA* gene is transcribed counterclockwise to the direction of replication, an orientation usually common to poorly expressed genes. Several additional features are associated with the *mec* complex: the *ugpQ* gene, coding for an *sn*-glycerophosphoryl diester phosphodiesterase; a variable region of direct repeats (*dru*); and the insertion sequence IS*431*$_{\text{mec}}$ [45]. The *mec* complex can be truncated by various IS elements that remove *mecI* and part of *mecR1*. As long as the *mecA* gene remains functional, the strain is considered to be an MRSA. Besides the *mec* complex, all other genes located on the SCC*mec* generally do not appear to contribute to methicillin resistance and vary depending on the element type. In addition, many genes seem to have degenerated. Common to all elements, but differing in sequence, are the recombinases of the *ccr* complex, which are involved in the precise excision and integration of the element into the chromosome. SCC*mec* elements are divided into different types according to the organization of the *mec* complex, the allotypes of the *ccr* complex, and the genes and plasmids localized in the so-called J (junkyard) regions. Six major SCC*mec* types have been identified so far [46]. The smaller SCC*mec* types IV, V and VI, often found in CA-MRSA, are associated with more diverse staphylococcal lineages and are thought to be more mobile than the larger HA-MRSA associated types I, II and III [11,47]. Discussion among staphylococcal researchers on a consensus for defining SCC*mec* element types is ongoing [46,48].

Even though the *mecA* gene in SCC*mec* type V is flanked by two IS*431* elements, making it potentially transposable, the *mecA* gene has never been found on a plasmid in clinical isolates. However, there has been one report of a transient association of *mecA* with a penicillinase plasmid in a transduction experiment [49]. Unfortunately, this experiment could never be confirmed.

With improved molecular methods and more detailed analyses, new combinations of SCC*mec* elements are constantly being identified. This suggests that multiple rearrangement and insertion/deletion events take place within SCC*mec*, making it a dynamic structure with considerable genetic plasticity [50–52].

Generally, increasing numbers of insertion sequences within an element make it more prone to rearrangements or deletions [53]. Selection for glycopeptide resistance can trigger loss of parts of SCC*mec* [54], sometimes including *mecA* [55]. Deletions originating within SCC*mec* may encompass the right-end SCC*mec* junction (J_R) and reach far into the staphylococcal genome. Observations have suggested that a greater than 60-kb genomic region distal to J_R is dispensable with no major consequences for *S. aureus* [54,56], whereas the sequences left of J_L, toward the origin of replication, harbor essential genes.

The origin of the SCC*mec* element is not known. However, coagulase-negative *Staphylococcus epidermidis*, which is much more frequently methicillin resistant and harbors a much higher diversity of SCC*mec* elements than *S. aureus* [57,58], is postulated to be the source for horizontal SCC*mec* transfer to *S. aureus* [59–61], although the mechanism of the interspecies transfer has not yet been reconstructed experimentally [62].

Regulation of *mecA* transcription

The *mec* operon is thought to have arisen by recombination of a PBP structural gene with the regulatory elements of a penicillinase [63]. The *mecA* regulatory elements MecR1 and MecI show substantial similarity to the BlaR1 and BlaI elements of the penicillinase, and they function in a similar fashion. The extracellular penicillin-binding domain of MecR1, the sensor transducer required for induction, reacts with β-lactams. β-Lactams acylate the active site serine and trigger an autocatalytic cleavage of MecR1 by the cytosolic metalloprotease. Cleavage of MecI is postulated to be catalyzed by an unknown enzyme that is activated by the MecR1 protease [64]. This autoproteolytic switch is irreversible and its members have to be constantly replenished. However, induction by the MecR1-controlled system is much slower than that via the BlaR1-controlled system [65,66]. Although MecI and BlaI can both repress the *mecA* and *blaZ* operons, induction only occurs over their cognate membrane sensor transducer [67]. In the absence of an inducer, *mecA* is strongly repressed by MecI. This tight control and slow induction of *mecA* through its own regulatory elements is sometimes not rapid enough to prevent β-lactam-induced death. MRSA with slow PBP2a induction often display low oxacillin MICs. Many clinical MRSA isolates are mutants with a constitutive or more rapid PBP2a induction. They carry either a nonfunctional repressor or deletions removing parts of or the entire regulatory *mecR1-mecI* region, resulting in either constitutive PBP2a production or, if harboring a penicillinase, rapid induction by the faster reacting BlaR1-BlaI control. The observation that in some MRSA penicillinases seem to be required for the stability of the *mecA* gene when grown in the absence of penicillin [68,69] may indicate that constitutive PBP2a production is deleterious. This suggests that the control of *mecA* is required in the absence of antibiotics.

The *mecA* gene is highly conserved within different MRSA and SCC*mec* types according to the published sequences in freely accessible databases. Recently, though, new *mecA* variants have been identified in methicillin-resistant *Staphylococcus* spp. other than *S. aureus* that were isolated from horses before hospitalization [70]. The variant *mecA* and the corresponding PBP2a sequences showed 91% nucleotide sequence identity and 90% amino acid sequence identity to the *S. aureus mecA* and PBP2a, respectively. Through contact with human staphylococcal strains it may be just a matter of time before we see transfer of new *mecA* variants into MRSA.

The origin of the *mecA* gene is unknown. The closest PBP homolog to PBP2a is a native *Staphylococcus sciuri* PBP [71,72] with 88% similarity to the *S. aureus* PBP2a. The *S. sciuri mecA*, when overexpressed, can confer methicillin resistance in its natural host as well as in *S. aureus* [73,74]. This finding, and the fact that an *ugpQ* gene is found downstream of the native *S. sciuri mecA* gene [75], suggests that it may be a potential evolutionary precursor of the *S. aureus mecA*.

PBP2a

Lim and Strynadka [76] resolved the crystal structure of PBP2a at 0.18 nm resolution and investigated the structure of the acyl-PBP complexes of PBP2a with different β-lactams. It was found that the bulky substitutions, rendering penicillin derivatives resistant to penicillinase, prevent their access to and acylation of the PBP2a active site, which has a rather closed conformation; penicillin and nitrocefin acylate PBP2a with a slightly higher efficiency [77,78]. It has been proposed that on contact with the polymeric peptidoglycan substrate, surface interactions stimulate a conformational change in PBP2a, making its active site accessible to its natural substrate, whereas the small-molecule β-lactams are unable to elicit such interactions [79]. Although PBP2a acts as a transpeptidase and can seemingly substitute for all native PBPs, it is dependent on a functional transglycosylase module of the native PBP2 in media containing β-lactams [80]. PBP2 that is dispersed over the cell surface on inhibition by β-lactams is redirected to the septal site by PBP2a through substrate recognition [41,81,82] (see Figure 8.2). This suggests that there may be a physical interaction between PBP2a and PBP2. On depletion of PBP2 in an MRSA strain, by placing the PBP2-encoding gene *pbpB* under the IPTG-controllable *spac* promoter, *mecA* transcription decreases, resuming again on addition of isopropyl-beta-D-thiogalactopyranosid (IPTG). No changes in the expression of the other native PBPs were observed [83]. Based on this observation, a hypothesis has been put forward that the transcription of *pbpB* and *mecA* may be linked by some regulatory signal.

PBP2a compatibility in *Staphylococcus aureus*

SCC*mec* appears to have entered different lineages of susceptible *S. aureus* on several different occasions. The fact that relatively few distinct genetic clusters carry SCC*mec*, and that HA-MRSA initially spread rather clonally, suggests that SCC*mec* transfer among *S. aureus* is not such a frequent event as the transfer of penicillinases. This could be due in part to the large size of SCC*mec* types I, II, and III in HA-MRSA. The smaller SCC*mec* types IV, V, and VI generally found in CA-MRSA seem to be present in more diverse genetic backgrounds, suggesting that they may be more mobile. Alternatively, the low methicillin resistance often accompanying type IV SCC*mec* may be of a lesser burden to the susceptible recipient strain. The natural transfer mechanism that SCC*mec* uses to enter a new host strain has not yet been identified. The exchange of SCC*mec* elements between staphylococcal species is so far only based on epidemiological observations. SCC*mec* type I can be transduced experimentally by transducing phages, although at extremely low frequencies ($< 10^{-9}$) [84]. Earlier studies showed that susceptible recipient strains needed to harbor a penicillinase plasmid and a functional penicillinase to acquire SCC*mec* by transduction [85]. Of note, a transduction also functioned shortly after experimental curing of such a strain from the penicillinase plasmid [86]. This theme was taken up again in 2003, when the observation was made that the introduction of the *mecA* gene into a naive *S. aureus* was difficult. Attempts to electroporate a plasmid with a constitutive *mecA* gene into various susceptible strains, with selection for the plasmid marker, showed that naive susceptible *S. aureus* that had never harbored an SCC*mec* or a penicillinase plasmid before selected against the expression of PBP2a. This was in contrast to strains that had previously contained *mecA*, which readily allowed PBP2a production and could express methicillin resistance [39]. Presence of a penicillinase plasmid facilitated the acceptance of *mecA* and the expression of resistance. This suggests the existence of a barrier, preventing introduction of PBP2a into susceptible strains. By downregulation of *mecA* at the first encounter, staphylococci may therefore gain time to adapt to the new PBP. Constitutive expression of *mecA* can lead to the accumulation of about twice as many copies of the protein (825) than any resident PBP (150–460) [34]. It is likely that such a high number may disturb the cell wall synthesis complex, especially in the absence of β-lactams, when PBP2a does not seem to contribute to cell wall synthesis [87]. Katayma *et al.* [88] found that susceptible *S. aureus* belonging to genetic lineages that correspond to major MRSA lineages more easily accepted, maintained, and expressed PBP2a than other strains. This suggests that specific genetic backgrounds may be responsible for the apparent barrier encountered during *mecA* acquisition. One possible explanation could be the mode of integration of PBP2a into the cell wall synthesis complex. Successful accommodation may be crucial for its functionality and vary according to the degree of interaction compatibility with the endogeneous cell envelope proteins and peptidoglycan precursor.

Carriage of SCC*mec* in *S. epidermidis* is much more frequent than in *S. aureus*, and the SCC*mec* elements of methicillin-resistant *S. epidermidis* (MRSE) are more diverse [58]. Hovever, oxacillin resistance is generally lower in MRSE than in MRSA. To date, the reasons for these differences are unknown. *Staphylococcus epidermidis* may be more permissive for the incorporation of the additional PBP2a into the cell wall synthesis complex than *S. aureus*, or it may benefit in an unknown way from the acquisition of an SCC*mec* element. For instance, biofilm formation is known to be an important virulence factor of *S. epidermidis*. A positive correlation between levels of oxacillin resistance and biofilm formation was observed in MRSE [89]. Some insertions of Tn*917* in the *S. epidermidis* genome, which reduced transcription of the *ica* operon and therefore biofilm formation, also affected methicillin resistance in MRSE, suggesting a connection of the two phenotypes through a structural factor or a regulatory mechanism [90].

Heterogeneity of methicillin resistance

MRSA exhibit a wide range of oxacillin resistance levels, from very highly resistant strains with oxacillin MICs far above 500 μg/mL, to strains with oxacillin MICs as low as those of susceptible strains (MSSA) around or even below 1 μg/mL. The latter are accordingly difficult to detect by phenotypic methods. CA-MRSA, in particular, tend to exhibit extremely low oxacillin MICs [91,92] and therapy failures have occurred due to the misinterpretation of such phenotypically "susceptible MRSA" as MSSA. The reason behind this is the resistance heterogeneity expressed by MRSA. This phenomenon is strongly dependent on the genetic background of the strain lineage into which SCC*mec* has entered [93]. As long as *S. aureus* strains, including phenotypically "susceptible MRSA," carry a functional *mecA* gene that can produce PBP2a, they have to be regarded and treated as MRSA. This is based on the fact that in the presence of β-lactams they can segregate highly resistant subclones (Figure 8.3).

β-Lactam concentrations above the MIC kill the major fraction of an MRSA culture. The size of the subpopulation that survives these inhibitory concentrations is a characteristic of the strain's genetic background [93]. Once selected, these higher-resistance variants generally retain their high resistance levels even in the absence of antibiotic pressure, suggesting that they may be mutants. Moreover, the frequency of highly resistant clones formed can be quite high, several logs above the spontaneous mutation rate. The mechanism leading to such an extraordinary frequency of conversion to high resistance is unknown.

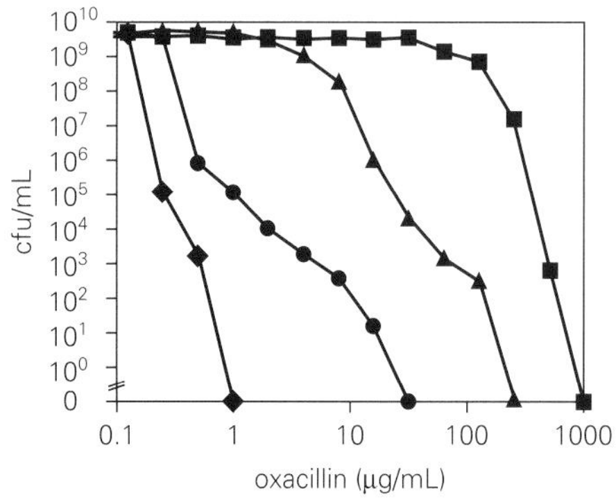

	Strain	Oxacillin MIC [μg/mL]	Doubling time [min]
●	cMRSA	1.5	22
◆	cMRSA ΔSCC*mec*	0.38	22
▲	cMRSA 1st step	32	35
■	cMRSA 2nd step	>256	35

Figure 8.3 Population analysis profile on oxacillin. Overnight cultures were plated on increasing concentrations of oxacillin and the colony-forming units (cfu)/mL were recorded after 48 hours of incubation.

It could be due to a single locus subject to an elevated frequency switch, such as slippage in a mononucleotide run, as previously observed for the *agr* locus [94]. Alternatively, multiple different mutations each leading to high-level resistance might add to the resulting high conversion frequency.

Methicillin resistance depends primarily on the functional *mecA* gene and its PBP2a production. A plasmid-borne *mecA* gene is sufficient to produce a typical methicillin resistance phenotype when introduced into an MSSA, thereby indicating that the surrounding SCC*mec*-associated sequences are dispensable [95]. The ability to form high and homogeneous methicillin resistance is dependent on the strain's genetic background [96]. Thus a mutation(s) *chr** within the chromosome was postulated that allows the strain to express high homogeneous resistance [95]. Multiple independent research groups have repeatedly observed that the amount of PBP2a does not correlate with the resistance level, since MRSA were found to contain comparable amounts of PBP2a [97] irrespective of their MICs. Again these findings point to an involvement of the staphylococcal genome in modulating resistance levels. High methicillin resistance is thus determined by chromosomal genes. Methicillin resistance levels can also be modulated by external factors, such as osmolarity, pH, temperature, and growth medium [98,99].

Methicillin resistance and fitness

An inverse correlation between resistance levels and growth rate is commonly observed. Transformation of an MSSA strain with SCC*mec* type I resulted in both heterogeneously resistant and highly homogeneously resistant transformants. The lower-level heterogeneously resistant transformants had a similar growth rate to the parent MSSA, whereas the highly resistant variants grew significantly slower. In growth competition experiments against the MSSA parent, the original highly resistant MRSA were eliminated but gave rise to faster-growing variants. Interestingly, these faster-growing variants had lost their high-level resistance and became heterogeneously resistant. Therefore, high-level oxacillin resistance does not seem to be compatible with rapid growth, suggesting that high resistance carries a fitness cost [100]. The rapidly growing but low-level resistant CA-MRSA seem to be an example for this correlation in the clinical setting. High resistance may be fixed mutationally in established highly resistant MRSA. When measuring fitness costs of isogenic MRSA, differing only in their SCC*mec* type, by using identical continuous culture conditions and thus forcing upon the strains an identical growth rate, type I showed increased glucose consumption and ATP demand per gram of cells synthesized and had decreased cell yields compared with those of the parent strain. In contrast, a type IV SCC*mec* element had no adverse energetic effects [101]. The cause and genetic basis for this different efficiency still needs to be analysed.

Chromosomal genes modulating methicillin resistance

The mystery of high-level resistance lies within the staphylococcal genome. Using transposon-mediated random insertional inactivation of MRSA and screening for altered levels of methicillin resistance, multiple genes have been identified that influence methicillin resistance levels (Table 8.1). Apparently they often do not affect *mecA* expression. This method does not allow the inactivation of essential genes. However, in some cases inserts in the non-translated mRNA or truncation of the C-terminus have been observed, which attenuate gene expression allowing some residual protein activity. A similar approach, using controlled downregulation of essential genes fused to the IPTG-controlled *spac* promoter, was used to follow the events occurring in the time-span of depletion and resynthesis of essential proteins in MRSA. It is clear that translation of such experimental data into the real world of clinical isolates is difficult, and does not necessarily explain hetero-resistance. Nevertheless, these findings have contributed to a better understanding of staphylococcal metabolism and regulation. They have revealed the high complexity and redundancy of staphylococcal cell wall synthesis, and demonstrated the plasticity of the staphylococcal genome and its amazing ability to compensate for the inactivation of single genes.

Table 8.1 Factors encoded by the *S. aureus* genome that affect methicillin resistance.

Gene ID number[1]	Gene, synonym	Gene description	Relevant function in β-lactam resistance	Reference
SA0104	*norG*	GntR-like transcriptional regulator of multidrug transporters	NorG, a repressor of *abcA*, modulates resistance to quinolones and β-lactams. Inactivation of *norG* enhances resistance to β-lactams	175
SA0250 SA0251	*lytSR*	Two-component sensor histidine kinase, response regulator	LytRS regulates the activity of the cell wall-associated murein hydrolase through regulation of *lrgA* and *lrgB*	142, 221
SA0252 SA0253	*lrgA* *lrgB*	Antiholin-like proteins	Involved in modulation of murein hydrolase activity and penicillin tolerance. LrgA inhibits the expression or activity of extracellular murein hydrolases by interacting, possibly together with LrgB, with the holin-like proteins CidA and/or CidB. The LrgAB and CidAB proteins may also affect the protonmotive force	221
SA0455–SA0456	*yabJ-spoVG*	*sigB*-dependent regulatory operon	Inactivation of the *spoVG* operon reduces methicillin resistance	164, 165
SA0573	*sarA*	Staphylococcal accessory regulator A	Inactivation of SarA reduces methicillin resistance	167
SA0598	*pbpD*	PBP4	PBP4 seems to be essential for β-lactam resistance in CA-MRSA	133
SA0599	*abcA*	ATP-dependent transporter	AbcA is involved in cell autolysis, is regulated by *agr*, repressed by NorG, and induced by methicillin. AbcA overexpression enhances resistance to more the lipophilic β-lactam drugs (nafcillin, benzylpenicillin)	174, 175
SA0614 SA0615	*graR* *graS*	Two-component sensor transducer system	GraRS regulates the downstream *vraFG* (ABC ATP-cassette transporter) and positively regulates the *dlt* operon. Overexpression of GraR reduces oxacillin resistance	151, 152
SA0641	*rat, mgrA*	Regulator of autolytic activity	MgrA binds to *lytRS* and *arlRS* promoters, is a negative regulator of *lytM* and *lytN* and a direct activator of *abcA*. Inactivation increases sensitivity to Triton X-100 and penicillin; overexpression enhances methicillin resistance	175, 222
SA0702	*llm, tagO*	Lipophilic protein, undecaprenyl-phosphate-α-*N*-acetylglucosaminyl-1-phosphate transferase	A *tagO* mutant produces no teichoic acids. Inactivation increases bacterial lysis rates and decreases methicillin resistance	155, 157–159
SA0793–6	*dlt* operon	D-Alanyl-lipoteichoic acid synthesis operon	D-Alanine esterification of teichoic acids confers a positive net charge to the bacterial surface. *dltB* inactivation raises methicillin resistance	149, 150
SA0876	*murE*	UDP-*N*-acetyl tripeptide synthetase	Inactivation of *murE* causes accumulation of UDP-muramyl-dipeptides, preventing cell wall cross-linking, and reduces methicillin resistance	113
SA0909	*fmtA*	UDP-*N*-acetylglucosamine transferase	Autolysis and methicillin resistance related protein; *fmtA* mutants are unable to form wall teichoic acids, do not form biofilm, and have reduced methicillin resistance	19, 153, 155
SA1075	*hmrB, acpP*	Acylcarrier protein	*hmrB* is involved in fatty acid synthesis. Overexpression enhances methicillin resistance	181
SA1149–SA1150	*glnRA*	Glutamine synthetase operon	Inactivation of *glnR* reduces the amount of the glutamine synthetase GlnA and thus the cellular gutamine pool, resulting in reduced amidation of the peptidoglycan iD-glutamate and reduced methicillin resistance	116
SA1193	*mprF, fmtC*	Lysylphosphatidylglycerol synthetase	MprF catalyzes the lysinylation of membrane phospholipids, and thus confers an increased positive charge to the cell surface. Inactivation of *mprF/fmtC* reduces methicillin resistance	223–225
SA1194	*msrA2*	Methionine sulfoxide reductase	Inactivation of *msrA2* has no effect on methicillin resistance MIC, but overexpression enhances methicillin resistance	152, 177
SA1195	*msrR*	Membrane protein with extracellular LytR-CpsA-Psr domain	Protein of unknown function. *msrR* inactivation reduces methicillin resistance and virulence	178, 180

Table 8.1 (*cont'd*)

Gene ID number[1]	Gene, synonym	Gene description	Relevant function in β-lactam resistance	Reference
SA1206	*femA*	Nonribosomal peptidyltransferase aminoacyltransferase	FemA adds glycines 2 and 3 of the pentaglycine bridge, using glycyl-tRNA(Gly) as the donor. Inactivation of *femA* completely abolishes methicillin resistance, and confers hypersusceptibility to other classes of drugs	122, 226
SA1207	*femB*	Nonribosomal peptidyltransferase aminoacyltransferase	FemB adds glycines 4 and 5 of the pentaglycine bridge, using glycyl-tRNA(Gly) as the donor. Inactivation of *femB* severely reduces methicillin resistance	123
SA1249	*sa1249*	Hypothetical protein	Inactivation of *sa1249*, which appears to form an operon with *murG* (undecaprenyl-PP-MurNAc-pentapeptide-UDPGlcNAc GlcNAc transferase), is accompanied by decreased oxacillin resistance	115
SA1283	*pbpB*	Bifunctional transpeptidase–transglycosylase	PBP2 is essential for PBP2a-mediated methicillin resistance	80
SA1458	*lytH*	*N*-Acetyl-muramoyl amidase	Deletion of *lytH* increases methicillin resistance	139
SA1557	*ccpA*	Carbon catabolite control protein	CcpA is a regulator of carbon metabolism. It affects expression of methicillin resistance and virulence factors, and acts as a repressor of the *cap* operon	103, 171
SA1665		DNA-binding protein	Inactivation of *sa1665* enhances methicillin resistance in heterogeneously resistant MRSA in a PBP2a-independent manner	173
SA1701–SA1700	*vraSR* operon	Two-component sensor transducer system mediating the cell wall stress stimulon	*vraSR* inactivation abrogates methicillin resistance	227
SAS065, SA1842–4	*agr* operon	Accessory gene regulator	Inactivation of the *agr* operon reduces methicillin resistance	167
SA1869	*sigB*	Alternative, stress inducible sigma factor B	Inactivation of *sigB* reduces methicillin resistance	163
SA1886	*murF*	UDP-*N*-acetylmuramyl-pentapeptide synthetase	Inactivation of *murF* reduces methicillin resistance and *mecA* transcription	114
SA1935	*hmrA*	Similar to amidase	HmrA overexpression enhances methicillin resistance	181
SA1959	*glmS*	Glucosamine-fructose-6-phosphate aminotransferase	GlmS occupies a central position between cell wall synthesis and glycolysis; *glmS* inactivation reduces methicillin resistance	109
SA1964	*fmtB*, *mrp*, *sasB*	Cell envelope protein with LPXTG-motif, function unknown, truncated in some MRSA strains	Inactivation of *fmtB* reduces methicillin resistance. The mutation cannot be complemented by *fmtB* in *trans*, but by *glmM* overexpression or by supplementing the growth medium with *N*-acetylglucosamine or glucosamine	110, 111
SA1965	*glmM*, *femD*, *femR315*	Phosphoglucosamine mutase	GlmM inactivation reduces methicillin resistance and increases teicoplanin resistance	106, 108
SA2057	*fmhB*, *femX*	Nonribosomal peptidyltransferase aminoacyltransferase	*fmhB* is an essential gene. It adds glycine 1 of the pentaglycine bridge, using glycyl-tRNA(Gly) as donor	125
SA2062	*sarV*	Transcriptional regulator	*sarV* is repressed by SarA and MgrA. A *sarV* mutant was more resistant to Triton X-100 and penicillin-induced lysis and had decreased extracellular murein hydrolase activity	228
SA2329–SA2328	*cidA-cidB*	Holin-like protein	Increases the activity of extracellular murein hydrolases, possibly by mediating their export via hole formation. Inhibited by the antiholin-like proteins LrgAB. LrgAB products probably inhibit the function of the CidAB proteins. Inactivation of *cidAB* decreases susceptibility to penicillin killing	144
SAS030	*graF*	Protein with a bipartite nuclear targeting domain	Overexpression of GraF enhances methicillin resistance, and is postulated to repress the nitrite/nitrate assimilation system	177

[1] Gene ID numbers correspond to those of the *S. aureus* N315 genome.

The genes identified by insertional inactivation were initially termed *fem* (*f*actors *e*ssential for *m*ethicillin resistance) [102], *aux* (auxiliary factors) [103,104], *fmt* [105], or *hmr* (*h*igh *m*ethicillin *r*esistance) and were renamed when their sequence or potential function became known. A general picture has emerged in that most genes that affect resistance levels to β-lactams are directly or indirectly involved in the synthesis of the peptidoglycan precursor, in cell wall synthesis and turnover, or envelope biogenesis. Cell wall biosynthesis occurs in three compartments. Starting in the cytoplasm with the assembly of constituents of the peptidoglycan precursor, it is followed by membrane-bound steps leading to the synthesis of lipid II, and ends with extracellular steps which cross-link the peptidoglycan precursor to the nascent cell wall. Cell wall turnover and degradation of the cell wall constitute additional, essential processes taking place outside the cell. The attenuation of the genes encoding enzymes involved in these various steps of cell wall biosynthesis affects methicillin resistance. Conversely, inactivation of autolytic activities, involved in cell separation and peptidoglycan turnover, seem to protect against penicillin-induced death, increasing methicillin resistance. Regulatory elements and external conditions, which control the expression of these genes and modulate their activity, consequently also influence methicillin resistance. Several genes identified by insertional inactivation are still of unknown function.

Interestingly, many mutants with inactivated *fem* factors are still able to produce a higher resistant subpopulation, demonstrating that *S. aureus* has multiple ways to compensate for defects. Identification and characterization of these compensatory mutations are expected to reveal further important factors affecting resistance.

Peptidoglycan precursor formation

Slowed production of cell wall precursors and/or altered chemical composition of the muropeptide were found to have a negative impact on methicillin resistance. PBP2a does not seem to be very flexible and appears to require an optimized supply and defined chemical composition of the muropeptide precursor to fulfil its protective function against β-lactams.

glmM

Phosphoglucosamine mutase, an essential enzyme in *Escherichia coli* [106], converts glucosamine 6-phosphate to glucosamine 1-phosphate, the initial step in the formation of the nucleotide sugar UDP-*N*-acetylglucosamine which is involved in peptidoglycan synthesis. Disruption of *glmM* in MRSA decreases methicillin resistance and causes teicoplanin hypersusceptibility without affecting the synthesis of PBP2a and endogenous PBPs. A 5% decrease in peptidoglycan cross-linking and a reduction of the minor component alanyl-tetraglycine instead of the pentaglycine at the ε-L-lysine of the muropeptide was observed in *glmM* mutants [107]. Suppressor mutants selected for growth on methicillin remained *glmM* negative, showed reduced autolytic activity, and interestingly remained teicoplanin hypersusceptible. Since the inactivation of GlmM is tolerated in *S. aureus*, there may exist alternative ways to synthesize glucosamine 1-phosphate in staphylococci [108].

glmS

The glutamine-fructose-6-phosphate aminotransferase GlmS, producing glucosamine 6-phosphate, occupies a central position between cell wall synthesis and glycolysis. Inactivation of GlmS results in poor growth and decreases oxacillin and teicoplanin MICs [109].

fmtB (synonyms *mrp*, *sasB*)

Downstream of *glmM* is a gene coding for a cell wall-anchored envelope protein of unknown function, FmtB [110], with multiple tandem 75-amino-acid repeats, which is also called Mrp [111] or SasB [112]. It seems to contain an uncharacterized sugar-binding domain possibly recognizing *N*-acetylglucosamine as a substrate. Inactivation of FmtB is linked with reduced methicillin resistance. Remarkably, complementation with a functional GlmM, but not with FmtB, restored methicillin resistance, as did the external addition of *N*-acetylglucosamine or glucosamine. Apparently, *fmtB* inactivation has an indirect effect on methicillin resistance, which can be relieved by increasing the production of the cell wall precursor glucosamine 1-phosphate [110].

murE, *murF*

The controlled downregulation of *murE* (UDP-*N*-acetyl-muramyl-tripeptide synthetase) [113], or of *murF* (UDP-*N*-acetyl-muramyl-pentapeptide synthetase) [114], leads to the accumulation of unfinished peptidoglycan precursor in the cytoplasm and of aberrant muropeptide components in the cell wall. Results are a decreased degree of cross-linking and a specific reduction in methicillin resistance but not of other antibiotics, such as glycopeptides. A parallel reduction in *pbpB* and *mecA* transcription is observed in *murE* and *murF* mutants, suggesting that the resulting reduced amounts of PBP2 and PBP2a may be the cause for the reduction in methicillin resistance [113,114]. A subpopulation of the cells, presumably suppressor mutants, showed parental-type resistance levels with increased *mecA* transcription but with aberrant cell walls identical to the mutants [114]. A genetic link coordinating *murE* and *murF* activity with *pbpB* and *mecA* synthesis has been postulated, but this effect could also be a consequence of reduced growth rate.

sa1249

Inactivation of *sa1249*, a putative gene, which appears to form an operon with the gene *murG*, was accompanied by a decrease in oxacillin resistance from 25 to 0.75 μg/mL

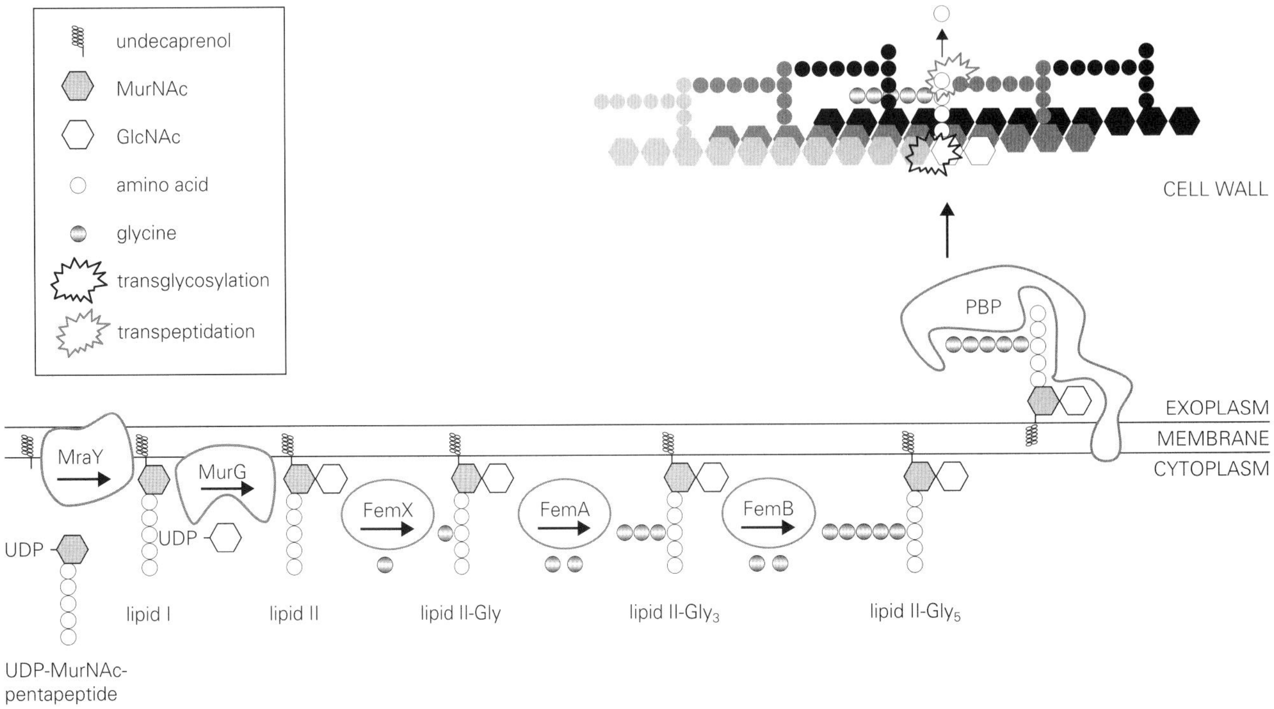

Figure 8.4 Schematic representation of membrane-bound steps in *S. aureus* peptidoglycan synthesis. The soluble product of MurF, UDP-MurNAc-pentapeptide, is prenylated by the translocase MraY to yield lipid I. UDP-GlcNAc is then added by the transferase MurG to produce the FemX substrate lipid II. The FemABX factors synthesize specific parts of the pentaglycine chain as indicated. Once finished, the peptidoglycan precursor lipid II-Gly$_5$ is flipped by an unknown mechanism to the outside of the bacterium. Incorporation into the cell wall through transglycosylation and transpeptidation is catalyzed by the PBPs. The last amino acid of the stem peptide is cleaved off during cross-linking of adjacent peptidoglycan strands. MurNAc, *N*-acetylmuramic acid; GlcNAc, *N*-acetylglucosamine.

and an increase in vancomycin resistance. While MurG is known to be involved in cell wall synthesis, the role of SA1249 has not yet been determined [115].

glnR (synonym *femC*)

The staphylococcal muropeptide iD-glutamate is amidated, although the enzyme catalyzing the amidation is not known. Reduction of the amidation of the iD-glutamate strongly reduces methicillin resistance, as observed on insertional inactivation of the glutamine synthetase operon *glnRA*, which reduces glutamine availability in the cells [116]. The amidation has been implicated in peptidoglycan cross-linking efficiency [117]. Interestingly, suppressor mutants could be selected on high concentrations of methicillin, which had regained methicillin resistance but still showed reduced amidation and carried the insert in *glnR* [118].

femX (synonym *fmhB*), *femA*, *femB*

Staphylococcus aureus peptidoglycan possesses a characteristic pentaglycine interpeptide branching off the ε-L-lysine of the stem peptide. This long and flexible bridge allows a high degree of cross-linking (80–90%) between the peptidoglycan strands. Moreover, the pentaglycine bridge functions as the anchor for cell surface proteins [119]. Shortening the length of the pentaglycine bridge reduces cell wall cross-linking and prevents the expression of methicillin resistance. The synthesis of the pentaglycine bridge is catalyzed in a sequential fashion by proteins belonging to the FemABX family of nonribosomal peptidyltransferases [120] using glycyl-tRNA as the glycine donor and lipid II as the acceptor [121]. FemX attaches the first glycine, FemA the second and third glycine, and FemB the last two glycines [121–125] (Figure 8.4). The FemA structure has been resolved at 0.21 nm resolution by X-ray crystallography, revealing a certain similarity with the Gcn5-related *N*-acetyltransferase (GNAT) superfamily, which generally catalyzes the transfer of an acyl group [126]. Although performing a similar reaction, FemA, FemB, and FemX cannot substitute for each other. Inactivation of *femA* alone or of the *femAB* operon results in a peptidoglycan with a monoglycine interpeptide and drastically reduces methicillin resistance and cell wall cross-linking, impairs growth, and renders *S. aureus* hypersusceptible to not only methicillin but also multiple other unrelated antibiotic classes [124]. Survival of cells with a monoglycine interpeptide requires a compensatory mutation(s) [127]. FemX inactivation is lethal [125]. The staphylococcal cell possesses no means to compensate for the loss of FemA activity, since mutants with a monoglycine bridge are completely unable to form methicillin-resistant suppressor mutants. The FemABX family of proteins is thus a potential target for drugs that could be used in combination to restore β-lactam efficacy in MRSA and increase susceptibility to other antibiotics. Interestingly, there seems to be a correlation between amount of *femA* transcript and levels of methicillin resistance in *S. aureus* [128].

pbpB

The endogenous PBP2 is the only bifunctional staphylococcal PBP with transpeptidase and transglycosylase activity [129,130]. PBP2 is part of the cell wall stress stimulon, being upregulated by inhibitory concentrations of cell wall-damaging agents [19]. PBP2 is maintained at the division site by binding to its substrate [82]. Acylation of PBP2 by β-lactams or elimination of its natural substrate causes its dislocation from the septum to the cell surface. PBP2 plays an important role in methicillin resistance. Its transglycosylase activity is essential and required by PBP2a to confer methicillin resistance [80]. In MRSA, addition of oxacillin does not result in delocalization of PBP2, indicating that the acylated PBP2 is recruited to the septum by the functional PBP2a [82].

pbpD

PBP4 is a nonessential secondary transpeptidase that contributes to increased cell wall cross-linking and cooperates with PBP2 and PBP2a in staphylococcal cell wall biosynthesis [131]. Disruption of the *pbp4* gene in the highly resistant strain COLn only had a minor effect on methicillin resistance [132], although loss of *pbpD* has been shown to severely reduce methicillin resistance in CA-MRSA [133].

Murein hydrolysis

Cell wall synthesis in *S. aureus* initiates at the mid-cell with the development of a ring-like structure to form the septum where the cell wall synthesis machinery – FtsZ, the PBPs, and hydrolases – are thought to assemble [41]. Autolysins are involved in multiple biological processes such as cell wall synthesis and turnover and daughter cell separation [134]. Atl, one of the major autolysins, localizes at the periphery of the septum on the cell surface in a ring-like structure, at the site of future cell separation [134], and is, according to the model of Giesbrecht *et al.* [135], organized in distinct murosomes along the septal periphery. Deregulation of cell wall synthesis by β-lactams prevents new septum formation. After the addition of β-lactams, the cells continue to grow for approximately one generation and can separate through the preexisting septum. However, at the time-point of the next division round, the autolysins, located along the periphery of the missing septum, perforate the cell wall releasing the high internal pressure, which leads to cell lysis [14,136]. The expression of autolysins is tightly regulated on the transcriptional, translational, and posttranslational level. Regulatory elements and physiological conditions that influence the activity of murein hydrolases are therefore likely to modulate the cell response to β-lactams.

atl

Inactivation of Atl, the major bifunctional autolysin, which has glucosaminidase and amidase activity, suppresses detergent- and antibiotic-induced lysis and reduces cell wall turnover rates, but does not increase methicillin resistance in a methicillin-sensitive background and causes a minor decrease in methicillin resistance in an MRSA background [137,138].

lytH

Deletion of *lytH*, an *N*-acetylmuramoyl-L-alanine-amidase [139,140], turns heterogeneously resistant MRSA into highly homogeneously resistant but slow-growing MRSA. However, mutations in the *lytH* region were only found in 0.74% of the highly resistant subpopulation of the parent MRSA, suggesting that LytH inactivation is one of several factors that may cause high methicillin resistance.

lytSR, lrgAB, cidABC

The two-component system LytSR, thought to sense a decrease in membrane potential [141], has been shown to affect murein hydrolase activities and tolerance to penicillin [142]. LytSR controls the downstream genes *lrgA-lrgB*, which act as an antiholin, reducing extracellular murein hydrolase activities [143]. The antiholin Lrg together with the holin Cid, which is encoded by the distant *cidABC* operon [144], control murein hydrolases and are postulated to constitute the molecular components of cell death in response to environmental stimuli [145]. A *cidA* mutant was shown to be less susceptible to penicillin killing, whereas *lrg* inactivation causes increased hydrolase activities. This holin–antiholin system affects murein hydrolase activity, stationary phase survival, and tolerance to β-lactams. Its effects in a methicillin-resistant background have not yet been measured, nor is it known if this system is a discriminator between high-level and low-level methicillin resistance.

Teichoic acid synthesis and modulation of murein hydrolase activities

Teichoic acids are important constituents of the staphylococcal cell wall, playing a role in cation homeostasis; trafficking of ions, nutrients, proteins, and antibiotics; regulation of autolysins; and presentation of envelope proteins [146]. Wall teichoic acids are linked to the cell wall peptidoglycan and consist of ribitol-phosphate polymers, while lipoteichoic acids are polymers of glycerol-phosphate attached to glycolipids that are intercalated in the membrane. Both are modified with D-alanyl esters and *N*-acetylglucosamine residues. The positively charged D-alanyl esters provide a means of changing the net anionic charge of the cell envelope, determining the binding capacity for positively charged molecules and modulating autolytic activities [147]. Certain growth conditions such as high salt concentrations reduce D-alanine substitution of teichoic acids, resulting in increased anionic charge and inhibition of autolytic activities [148]. Posttranslational modulation of autolytic activities by teichoic acids was found to play an important role in methicillin resistance. Several genes involved in the synthesis or modification of teichoic acids have been shown to affect methicillin resistance.

dlt operon

The *dlt* operon is responsible for the D-alanine esterification of teichoic acids and thus confers a more positive net charge to the bacterial surface. Inactivation of *dltB* in the *dlt* operon was found to raise methicillin resistance [149] due to a lack of D-alanine substitution of teichoic acids, and the resulting increased negative charge of these polymers that is inhibitory to autolytic activities [150]. Overexpression of the putative regulator GraR, which is postulated to positively regulate the *dlt* operon [151], reduced oxacillin resistance [152], confirming the important role of teichoic acid alanylation in modulating methicillin resistance.

fmtA

FmtA localizes in the cell wall fraction and has two of the three conserved motifs found in PBPs [153]. It was recently shown to bind with low affinity to β-lactams and peptidoglycan [154]. Transcription of *fmtA* is induced by high concentrations of β-lactam antibiotics and cell wall synthesis inhibitors, and *fmtA* is therefore part of the cell wall stress stimulon [19]. The function of FmtA is unclear, but *fmtA*-inactivation mutants were reported to produce no wall teichoic acid and to have reduced capacity to form biofilm [155]. Inactivation of *fmtA* was shown to reduce methicillin resistance levels and cause cells to lyse more rapidly in the presence of Triton X-100 [153,156].

tagO (synonym *llm*)

Inactivation of *tagO*, coding for an undecaprenyl-phosphate-α-*N*-acetylglucosaminyl-1-phosphate transferase, results in mutants lacking teichoic acids [157]. TagO was initially identified as a lipophilic membrane protein named Llm [158]. Its inactivation, by a transposon insert in the 3′ terminal region, reduced methicillin resistance with a concomitant increase in Triton X-100-induced autolysis rate. Resistant revertants obtained from *llm* mutants were shown to have increased *llm* expression due to the insertion of IS*256* forming a new promoter [159].

Global regulators

The genome of *S. aureus* possesses a complex global regulatory network controlling the growth phase- and environment-dependent expression of virulence factors, thus enabling rapid adaptation to the varying conditions encountered during infection [160]. It comprises two-component sensor transducers, transcription factors, and alternative sigma factors. Since methicillin resistance is influenced by multiple factors involved in cell envelope biogenesis and turnover, it is not surprising that global regulators controlling these factors also interfere with methicillin resistance levels.

sigB

The alternative sigma factor SigB is involved in the general stress response and controls a large regulon, including virulence genes and global regulators [161]. In addition, SigB is also involved in basic cellular processes such as cell envelope composition, membrane transport, and intermediary metabolism [162]. Inactivation of *sigB* was shown to reduce methicillin resistance [163]. The genes or systems controlled by SigB, and relevant for the decrease in methicillin resistance, have not yet been identified. However, we recently demonstrated that the effect of SigB on methicillin resistance is mediated indirectly over the SigB-controlled regulatory system YabJ-SpoVG [164,165], and therefore may comprise genes not preceded by a characteristic Sigma B promoter consensus sequence.

agr, sarA

The quorum sensor and regulator of cell wall-associated and excreted virulence factors, *agr*, is the most prominent representative of all known *S. aureus* two-component systems [166]. On the other hand, SarA is the best-studied regulator of the large family of SarA-related transcription factors. Inactivation of both *sarA* and the *agr* operon were shown to decrease the ability of heterogeneously resistant MRSA to segregate highly resistant variants [167]. The amount of PBP2a was not altered but a reduction in PBP1 and PBP3 was observed. The effect was small but should be reevaluated in highly resistant MRSA. It is conceivable that the *agr* operon, whose activity can change rapidly due to slipped mispairing [94], may contribute to methicillin resistance heterogeneity.

ccpA

The preferential use of glucose as a carbon source in Gram-positive organisms is controlled by the carbon catabolite protein CcpA [168]. CcpA was one of a series of identified *aux* factors found to reduce methicillin resistance on inactivation [103]. Recently, *ccpA* allelic replacement revealed that CcpA functions not only in carbon metabolism but also in the regulation of virulence factors [169], biofilm formation [170], and resistance to cell wall antibiotics such as methicillin and teicoplanin [171]. Methicillin resistance is thus linked to carbon metabolism, as has also been indicated by the effect of *glmS* inactivation [109].

vraSR

High inhibitory concentrations of β-lactams induce the so-called cell wall stress stimulon [18] through a two-component sensor transducing system, VraS-VraR [19], which is itself induced by cell wall stress [20]. A large number of genes, including several that encode proteins involved in cell wall metabolism (such as *pbpB*, *murZ*, *fmtA*) or in stress responses, are thus upregulated [17,172]. This cell wall stress stimulon resembles an inherent defense mechanism against cell wall damage. Some of the genes involved in this stress response may contribute to resistance, since inactivation of *vraSR* in MRSA abrogates methicillin resistance [19,172]. One of the VraSR regulated genes is *pbpB*, encoding the bifunctional transpeptidase transglycosylase PBP2, which is essential in PBP2a-mediated methicillin resistance. Whether high-level resistance is paired with constant activation of members of the *vraSR* regulon is unknown. The events occurring within the cell on β-lactam stress possibly hint toward the ongoing processes that may contribute to high-level resistance.

sa1665

Deletion of the DNA-binding protein SA1665 increases methicillin resistance in heterogeneously resistant MRSA in a *mecA*- and PBP2a-independent fashion, presumably by controlling chromosomal genes contributing to methicillin resistance. The extent of the impact of SA1665 on methicillin resistance is strain-dependent [173].

Other genes reported to affect oxacillin resistance

Overexpression of some genes can also enhance methicillin resistance. However, their natural contribution to high methicillin resistance in clinical isolates has yet to be proven.

abcA

AbcA is an ATP-dependent transporter involved in cell autolysis, and is thought to have an indirect function in the control of autolytic activities [174]. The gene *abcA* shares an overlapping promoter region with the divergently transcribed *pbp4* (*pbpD*), but is independently regulated. *abcA* expression is *agr* dependent, induced by methicillin and repressed by NorG, a member of the family of GntR-like transcriptional regulators. Disruption of *norG* caused overexpression of AbcA, which was found to lead to increased resistance against β-lactams. This was also confirmed by overexpressing *abcA* on a plasmid [175]. MgrA is a transcriptional regulator belonging to the MarR family. As a direct activator of *abcA*, MgrA enhances methicillin resistance when overexpressed [175]. Furthermore, MgrA overexpression was also found to enhance glycopeptide resistance [152].

Multidrug efflux pump

The efflux pump inhibitor reserpine reduces methicillin resistance in highly resistant MRSA, suggesting that multidrug exporters may contribute to methicillin resistance, although the pump involved has not yet been identified [176].

msrA2

Staphylococcus aureus contains three genes encoding MsrA-specific methionine sulfoxide reductase (Msr) activity (*msrA1*, *msrA2* and *msrA3*) [177]. Inactivation of *msrA2* had no effect on the oxacillin MIC of MRSA, but overexpression was found to increase glycopeptide and methicillin resistance and to result in a thickened cell wall [152].

msrR

MsrR belongs to the so-called LytR-CpsA-Psr family of cell envelope-associated transcriptional attenuators, which are found in Gram-positive bacteria [178]. It is a membrane protein, with a small intracellular part, one transmembrane segment, and a large extracellular domain. MsrR affects surface characteristics of the staphylococcal envelope and plays a role in cell separation and virulence [179]. Inactivation of *msrR* decreases oxacillin resistance levels [180]. MsrR also belongs to the cell wall stress stimulon as its transcription is induced by cell wall-active antibiotics [180] via the VraSR two-component system (unpublished results). Although members of this protein family have been reported to function as transcriptional attenuators, transcriptomic analysis of an *msrR* mutant did not reveal a distinct regulon [179].

hmrA

Overexpression of *hmrA*, which has homology to amino-hydrolases, was found to produce tolerance to high concentrations of methicillin [181]. The finding of high expression levels of *hmrA* in two of ten homogeneously resistant MRSA strains may indicate a possible role in methicillin resistance.

hmrB

Tolerance to high concentrations of methicillin was conferred by overexpression of *hmrB*, coding for an acyl carrier protein involved in fatty acid synthesis [181].

graF

Overexpression of GraF, a hypothetical protein containing a bipartite nuclear targeting domain, enhanced both methicillin and glycopeptide resistance and thickened the cell wall by over 20% [152]. The genes regulated by GraF are unknown, but a nitrite/nitrate assimilation system was postulated to be repressed by GraF [152].

Borderline methicillin resistance in the absence of *mecA*

Clinical *S. aureus* isolates that lack the *mecA* gene but which display "borderline" methicillin or oxacillin resistance are called BORSA. BORSA have a reduced susceptibility to penicillinase-resistant penicillins, with MICs around the breakpoint. They are isolated occasionally, but are of lesser clinical relevance and cannot compete against MRSA.

BORSA isolates can be divided into two main groups according to their phenotype and resistance mechanism: strains with penicillinase overproduction and strains with modifications of their own PBPs.

Penicillinase hyperproducers

Borderline resistance was observed in clinical isolates with penicillinase hyperproduction in 1986 [182]. This massive penicillinase overproduction, thought to slowly inactivate penicillinase-stable penicillins, was initially postulated to be the reason for the borderline resistance but could not be confirmed [183]. Later, a membrane-bound methicillinase-like activity was identified that hydrolyzed penicillinase-resistant penicillins [184,185], although this activity has not yet been attributed to any gene. Interestingly, the penicillinase-overproducing borderline-resistant strains were found to form a rather homogeneous group belonging to phage group 94/96 and to harbor a specific plasmid pBW15, coding for a penicillinase A. Upon curing the penicillinase plasmid, these strains still showed a slightly higher resistance to penicillinase-resistant penicillins compared with other susceptible strains [186], suggesting that they had some inherent resistance due to chromosomal genes. The penicillinase plasmid pBW15, when transferred into unrelated staphylococcal lineages, was unable to confer borderline resistance despite production of the penicillinase [187]. However, on introduction into penicillinase-free phage type 94/96 isolates, it produced borderline resistance [186]. These observations strongly suggest that the specific genetic background of phage group 94/96 contributes to the borderline phenotype.

PBP-based non-*mecA* borderline resistance

A second group of clinical borderline resistant isolates that lack the *mecA* gene presumably arises from susceptible *S. aureus* by antibiotic pressure and selection in the patient. This results in strains with low-level resistance against penicillinase-resistant penicillins that is neither associated with penicillinase hyperproduction nor with *mecA*, but with changes in their normal set of PBPs. Such borderline-resistant *S. aureus*, also termed MODSA due to their modified PBPs, were shown to have increased amounts of PBP4, and mutations in PBP1 and PBP2, which lowered their affinity to the drug [188–190]. In contrast to the typical heterogeneous resistance of MRSA, they possess homogeneous low-level resistance [188]. Strains with a similar borderline resistance and changes in their PBP2 and PBP4 content or drug affinity can be obtained from susceptible *S. aureus* by *in vitro* selection for growth on increasing concentrations of β-lactams [191] or by PBP4 overproduction [192]. Although they can reach quite high levels of methicillin resistance, *in vitro* selected strains may not be competitive in nature, since increased resistance is accompanied by a reduction in growth rate. However, in clinical isolates, additional selection pressure may apply. Recently, a *mecA*-negative strain with a high methicillin MIC of 64 μg/mL has been described, with highly increased PBP2 activity and a thick rough cell wall [193]. This strain had initially been isolated in 1961, but on further subcultivation *in vitro* lost its resistance phenotype. This observation is not uncommon. A decrease in resistance to cell wall antibiotics on repeated subcultivation of fresh clinical isolates coming directly from the patient seems to be a frequent phenomenon, since on agar plates and in liquid medium, selection favors faster-growing variants.

Small-colony variants

Small-colony variants are usually isolated from chronic infections or following antibiotic therapy. This slow-growing subpopulation can cause persistent and relapsing infections due to an increased capacity to invade cells [194] and to remain intracellular by regulating virulence factors differently [195]. They form minute colonies, have unusual biochemical characteristics, and are often impaired in electron transport [196]. The latter results in a reduced transmembrane potential, which makes small-colony variants more resistant than their wild-type counterparts to cationic antibiotics [197], while the effectiveness of cell wall antibiotics is thought to be reduced due to their slow growth [198]. The reason for reduced susceptibility of some small-colony variants to β-lactam antibiotics has not yet been elucidated, and this phenomenon is independent of the presence of the *mecA* gene (unpublished results).

Surface adherence and methicillin resistance

Staphylococcus aureus adhering to surfaces or residing in biofilms have different metabolic characteristics than their planktonic counterparts [199–201]. Biofilm cells express a decreased susceptibility to different antibiotics including oxacillin [202] and are more refractory to antibiotic treatment than planktonic bacteria [203], as are detached biofilm clumps [204]. This might be due to slower growth, altered physiological status of the cells, altered membrane permeability [205], selection of more resistant variants by adhesion, or the nature of the material forming the biofilm [206]. In addition to immobilization, biofilm formation facilitates bacterial escape from the immune system. Their resistance is possibly due less to a barrier function of the biofilm and restricted penetration of drugs, but rather to the altered metabolic activities and slower growth of the immobilized bacteria in the biofilm and expression of biofilm-specific genes contributing to resistance.

There seems to be a difference in the nature of biofilm produced by MSSA and MRSA. In a selection of clinical isolates, MSSA frequently produced an *ica*-dependent polysaccharide biofilm in the presence of NaCl and glucose, whereas biofilm production in MRSA was not induced by NaCl and was associated with *ica*-independent protein-adhesin production in the presence of glucose [207]. The genetic basis behind this observation is unknown. In *S. epidermidis*, which are generally good slime producers, a positive correlation between *mecA* transcription and slime production has been described [208,209].

Methicillin versus glycopeptide resistance

Several publications have reported a form of mutual exclusion between methicillin and glycopeptide resistance, whereby methicillin resistance is lost or severely decreased as a consequence of increased intrinsic glycopeptide resistance. In many cases the acquisition of increased glycopeptide resistance triggered, or at least coincided with, loss or inactivation of the *mecA* gene [54,55,210,211]. Reintroduction of an intact *mecA* into one of these strains partially restored oxacillin resistance, but at the cost of a corresponding drop in vancomycin resistance, showing a reciprocal antagonistic effect. Conversely, increasing oxacillin resistance can trigger a decrease in glycopeptide resistance [212]. In other cases the genetic mechanism promoting the loss of β-lactam resistance is unknown [115,211,213], but could result from mutations or alterations in the expression of genes influencing the resistance phenotypes.

However, such an antagonistic relationship is not always observed. No alterations in oxacillin MICs have also been reported during *in vitro* passage selection of glycopeptide intermediate-resistant *S. aureus* (GISA) strains [214], or between apparently isogenic GISA and non-GISA isolates [215,216]. The resistance exclusion is also specific for intrinsic GISA-type glycopeptide resistance, as high-level vancomycin-resistant strains characterized so far have maintained high-level methicillin resistance [217,218].

However, the model of antagonism between β-lactam and glycopeptide resistance phenotypes could explain reports regarding synergistic effects of β-lactams and vancomycin against GISA-MRSA strains, where neither β-lactams nor vancomycin was effective alone [219]. A combination of β-lactams and vancomycin was shown to have an antagonistic effect at concentrations below their MICs but showed synergism at methicillin concentrations near the MIC, when used against vancomycin-intermediate and vancomycin-hetero-intermediate resistant strains. High concentrations of methicillin were also proposed to cause inhibition of the synthesis of proteins essential for the expression of vancomycin resistance, thereby producing synergy [220]. Climo *et al.* [219] suggested that the synergism may be related to the substrate specificity of PBP2a for monomeric peptidoglycan units, and an inability to cross-link to oligomeric muropeptides found in high proportion in the GISA cell wall.

Interestingly, although it was shown that acquisition of VanA-mediated vancomycin resistance did not affect oxacillin MICs, it was found that the presence of oxacillin inhibited vancomycin resistance expression and that the presence of vancomycin had a mutually inhibitory effect on oxacillin resistance in strain COLVA. This *S. aureus* strain was constructed by introducing the VanA-containing plasmid from VRSA strain HIP11714 into the highly oxacillin-resistant strain COL [217]. Decreased expression of vancomycin resistance by oxacillin was thought to be the result of PBP2a, the only transpeptidase still active in the presence of oxacillin, being unable to effectively recognize depsipeptide cell wall precursors present in VRSA [217].

The antagonism between β-lactams and glycopeptides probably lies in the different requirements of the corresponding resistance mechanisms for optimal expression. PBP2a needs an ordered and well-balanced synthesis of the cell wall precursor, while vancomycin-intermediate resistance, which is accompanied by the upregulation of cell wall synthesis, is counterproductive to methicillin resistance.

Acknowledgments

We thank M. Pinho (Portugal) for providing Figure 8.2, and the Swiss National Science Foundation grants 31-117707 to B.B.B., PMPDB-114323 to P.S., Forschungskredit der Universität Zürich to N.M. and Bonizzi Theler Stiftung to M.M.S.

References

1 Levin BR, Rozen DE. Non-inherited antibiotic resistance. Nat Rev Microbiol 2006;4:556–62.
2 de Lencastre H, Sa Figueiredo AM, Urban C, Rahal J, Tomasz A. Multiple mechanisms of methicillin resistance and improved methods for detection in clinical isolates of *Staphylococcus aureus*. Antimicrob Agents Chemother 1991;35:632–9.
3 Chambers HF. The changing epidemiology of *Staphylococcus aureus*? Emerg Infect Dis 2001;7:178–82.
4 Livermore DM. Antibiotic resistance in staphylococci. Int J Antimicrob Agents 2001;16(suppl 1):3–10.
5 Robinson DA, Kearns AM, Holmes A *et al*. Re-emergence of early pandemic *Staphylococcus aureus* as a community-acquired meticillin-resistant clone. Lancet 2005;365:1256–8.
6 Dyke KGH, Richmond MH. Occurrence of various types of penicillinase plasmid among "hospital" staphylococci. J Clin Pathol 1967;20:75–9.
7 Rowland SJ, Dyke KG. Characterization of the staphylococcal beta-lactamase transposon Tn*552*. EMBO J 1989;8:2761–73.
8 Jevons MP, Coe AW, Parker MT. Methicillin resistance in staphylococci. Lancet 1963;i:904–7.

9 Chambers HF. Community-associated MRSA: resistance and virulence converge. N Engl J Med 2005;352:1485–7.

10 Huang YH, Tseng SP, Hu JM, Tsai JC, Hsueh PR, Teng LJ. Clonal spread of SCC*mec* type IV methicillin-resistant *Staphylococcus aureus* between community and hospital. Clin Microbiol Infect 2007;13:717–24.

11 Deurenberg RH, Vink C, Kalenic S, Friedrich AW, Bruggeman CA, Stobberingh EE. The molecular evolution of methicillin-resistant *Staphylococcus aureus*. Clin Microbiol Infect 2007; 13:222–35.

12 Goffin C, Ghuysen J-M. Multimodular penicillin-binding proteins: an enigmatic family of orthologs and paralogs. Microbiol Mol Biol Rev 1998;62:1079–93.

13 Giesbrecht P, Kersten T, Maidhof H, Wecke J. Staphylococcal cell wall: morphogenesis and fatal variations in the presence of penicillin. Microbiol Mol Biol Rev 1998;62:1371–414.

14 Maidhof H, Johannsen L, Labischinski H, Giesbrecht P. Onset of penicillin-induced bacteriolysis in staphylococci is cell cycle dependent. J Bacteriol 1989;171:2252–7.

15 Kuroda H, Kuroda M, Cui L, Hiramatsu K. Subinhibitory concentrations of beta-lactam induce haemolytic activity in *Staphylococcus aureus* through the SaeRS two-component system. FEMS Microbiol Lett 2007;268:98–105.

16 Ohlsen K, Ziebuhr W, Koller K-P, Hell W, Wichelhaus TA, Hacker J. Effects of subinhibitory concentrations of antibiotics on alpha-toxin (*hla*) gene expression of methicillin-sensitive and methicillin-resistant *Staphylococcus aureus* isolates. Antimicrob Agents Chemother 1998;42:2817–23.

17 Utaida S, Dunman PM, Macapagal D *et al*. Genome-wide transcriptional profiling of the response of *Staphylococcus aureus* to cell-wall-active antibiotics reveals a cell-wall-stress stimulon. Microbiology 2003;149:2719–32.

18 McCallum N, Spehar G, Bischoff M, Berger-Bachi B. Strain dependence of the cell wall-damage induced stimulon in *Staphylococcus aureus*. Biochim Biophys Acta 2006;1760:1475–81.

19 Kuroda M, Kuroda H, Oshima T, Takeuchi F, Mori H, Hiramatsu K. Two-component system VraSR positively modulates the regulation of cell-wall biosynthesis pathway in *Staphylococcus aureus*. Mol Microbiol 2003;49:807–21.

20 Yin S, Daum RS, Boyle-Vavra S. VraSR two-component regulatory system and its role in induction of *pbp2* and *vraSR* expression by cell wall antimicrobials in *Staphylococcus aureus*. Antimicrob Agents Chemother 2006;50:336–43.

21 Maiques E, Ubeda C, Campoy S *et al*. Beta-lactam antibiotics induce the SOS response and horizontal transfer of virulence factors in *Staphylococcus aureus*. J Bacteriol 2006;188:2726–9.

22 Ida T, Okamoto R, Nonoyama M, Irinoda K, Kurazono M, Inoue M. Antagonism between aminoglycosides and beta-lactams in a methicillin-resistant *Staphylococcus aureus* isolate involves induction of an aminoglycoside-modifying enzyme. Antimicrob Agents Chemother 2002;46:1516–21.

23 Nielsen J, Lampen J. Membrane-bound penicillinases in Gram-positive bacteria. J Biol Chem 1982;257:4490–5.

24 Greenway DL, Dyke KG. The effect of membrane-bound beta-lactamase on linoleic acid sensitivity in *Staphylococcus aureus*. J Gen Microbiol 1983;129:2457–65.

25 Safo MK, Zhao Q, Ko T-P *et al*. Crystal structures of the BlaI repressor from *Staphylococcus aureus* and its complex with DNA: insights into transcriptional regulation of the *bla* and *mec* operons. J Bacteriol 2005;187:1833–44.

26 Wilke MS, Hills TL, Zhang H-Z, Chambers HF, Strynadka NCJ. Crystal structures of the apo and penicillin-acylated forms of the BlaR1 beta-lactam sensor of *Staphylococcus aureus*. J Biol Chem 2004;279:47278–87.

27 Birck C, Cha JY, Cross J *et al*. X-ray crystal structure of the acylated beta-lactam sensor domain of BlaR1 from *Staphylococcus aureus* and the mechanism of receptor activation for signal transduction. J Am Chem Soc 2004;126:13945–7.

28 Fuda C, Fisher JF, Mobashery S. Beta-lactam resistance in *Staphylococcus aureus*: the adaptive resistance of a plastic genome. Cell Mol Life Sci 2005;62:2617–33.

29 Zhang HZ, Hackbarth CJ, Chansky KM, Chambers HF. A proteolytic transmembrane signaling pathway and resistance to beta-lactams in staphylococci. Science 2001;291:1962–5.

30 Golemi-Kotra D, Cha JY, Meroueh SO, Vakulenko SB, Mobashery S. Resistance to beta-lactam antibiotics and its mediation by the sensor domain of the transmembrane BlaR signaling pathway in *Staphylococcus aureus*. J Biol Chem 2003; 278:18419–25.

31 Thumanu K, Cha J, Fisher JF, Perrins R, Mobashery S, Wharton C. Discrete steps in sensing of beta-lactam antibiotics by the BlaR1 protein of the methicillin-resistant *Staphylococcus aureus* bacterium. Proc Natl Acad Sci USA 2006;103:10630–5.

32 Cohen S, Sweeney HM. Constitutive penicillinase formation in *Staphylococcus aureus* owing to a mutation unlinked to the penicillinase plasmid. J Bacteriol 1968;95:1368–74.

33 Cohen S, Vernon EG, Sweeney HM. Differential depression of staphylococcal plasmid and chromosomal penicillinase genes by a class of unlinked chromosomal mutations ($R2^-$). J Bacteriol 1970;103:616–21.

34 Pucci MJ, Dougherty TJ. Direct quantitation of the numbers of individual penicillin-binding proteins per cell in *Staphylococcus aureus*. J Bacteriol 2002;184:588–91.

35 Wada A, Watanabe H. Penicillin-binding protein 1 of *Staphylococcus aureus* is essential for growth. J Bacteriol 1998;180:2759–65.

36 Pereira SFF, Henriques AO, Pinho MG, de Lencastre H, Tomasz A. Role of PBP1 in cell division of *Staphylococcus aureus*. J Bacteriol 2007;189:3525–31.

37 Lovering AL, de Castro LH, Lim D, Strynadka NCJ. Structural insight into the transglycosylation step of bacterial cell-wall biosynthesis. Science 2007;315:1402–5.

38 Wyke AW, Ward JB, Hayes MV, Curtis NA. A role *in vivo* for penicillin-binding protein-4 of *Staphylococcus aureus*. Eur J Biochem 1981;119:389–93.

39 Katayama Y, Zhang H-Z, Hong D, Chambers HF. Jumping the barrier to beta-lactam resistance in *Staphylococcus aureus*. J Bacteriol 2003;185:5465–72.

40 Pinho MG, de Lencastre H, Tomasz A. Cloning, characterization, and inactivation of the gene *pbpC*, encoding penicillin-binding protein 3 of *Staphylococcus aureus*. J Bacteriol 2000; 182:1074–9.

41 Scheffers D-J, Pinho MG. Bacterial cell wall synthesis: new insights from localization studies. Microbiol Mol Biol Rev 2005;69:585–607.

42 Hiramatsu K, Cui L, Kuroda M, Ito T. The emergence and evolution of methicillin-resistant *Staphylococcus aureus*. Trends Microbiol 2001;9:486–93.

43 de Lencastre H, Chung M, Westh H. Archaic strains of methicillin-resistant *Staphylococcus aureus*: molecular and microbiological properties of isolates from 1960 in Denmark. Microb Drug Resist 2000;6:1–10.

44 Robinson DA, Enright MC. Multilocus sequence typing and the evolution of methicillin-resistant *Staphylococcus aureus*. Clin Microbiol Infect 2004;10:92–7.

45 Ryffel C, Bucher R, Kayser FH, Berger-Bachi B. The *Staphylococcus aureus mec* determinant comprises an unusual cluster of direct repeats and codes for a gene product similar to the *Escherichia coli sn*-glycerophosphoryl diester phosphodiesterase. J Bacteriol 1991;173:7416–22.

46 Kondo Y, Ito T, Ma XX *et al*. Combination of multiplex PCRs for staphylococcal cassette chromosome *mec* type assignment: rapid identification system for *mec*, *ccr*, and major differences in junkyard regions. Antimicrob Agents Chemother 2007;51:264–74.

47 Enright MC, Robinson DA, Randle G, Feil EJ, Grundmann H, Spratt BG. The evolutionary history of methicillin-resistant *Staphylococcus aureus* (MRSA). Proc Natl Acad Sci USA 2002; 99:7687–92.

48 Chongtrakool P, Ito T, Ma XX *et al*. Staphylococcal cassette chromosome *mec* (SCC*mec*) typing of methicillin-resistant *Staphylococcus aureus* strains isolated in 11 Asian countries: a proposal for a new nomenclature for SCC*mec* elements. Antimicrob Agents Chemother 2006;50:1001–12.

49 Trees DL, Iandolo JJ. Identification of a *Staphylococcus aureus* transposon (Tn*4291*) that carries the methicillin resistance gene(s). J Bacteriol 1988;170:149–54.

50 Qi W, Ender M, O'Brien F *et al*. Molecular epidemiology of methicillin-resistant *Staphylococcus aureus* in Zurich, Switzerland (2003): prevalence of type IV SCC*mec* and a new SCC*mec* element associated with isolates from intravenous drug users. J Clin Microbiol 2005;43:5164–70.

51 Heusser R, Ender M, Berger-Bachi B, McCallum N. Mosaic staphylococcal cassette chromosome *mec* containing two recombinase loci and a new *mec*-complex, B2. Antimicrob Agents Chemother 2007;51:390–3.

52 Stephens AJ, Huygens F, Giffard PM. Systematic derivation of marker sets for staphylococcal cassette chromosome *mec* typing. Antimicrob Agents Chemother 2007;51:2954–64.

53 Deplano A, Tassios PT, Glupczynski Y, Godfroid E, Struelens MJ. *In vivo* deletion of the methicillin resistance *mec* region from the chromosome of *Staphylococcus aureus* strains. J Antimicrob Chemother 2000;46:617–20.

54 Reipert A, Ehlert K, Kast T, Bierbaum G. Morphological and genetic differences in two isogenic *Staphylococcus aureus* strains with decreased susceptibilities to vancomycin. Antimicrob Agents Chemother 2003;47:568–76.

55 Adhikari RP, Scales GC, Kobayashi K, Smith JMB, Berger-Bachi B, Cook GM. Vancomycin-induced deletion of the methicillin resistance gene *mecA* in *Staphylococcus aureus*. J Antimicrob Chemother 2004;54:360–3.

56 Wada A, Katayama Y, Hiramatsu K, Yokota T. Southern hybridization analysis of the *mecA* deletion from methicillin-resistant *Staphylococcus aureus*. Biochem Biophy Res Commun 1991;176:1319–25.

57 Miragaia M, Couto I, de Lencastre H. Genetic diversity among methicillin-resistant *Staphylococcus epidermidis* (MRSE). Microb Drug Res 2005;11:83–93.

58 Miragaia M, Thomas JC, Couto I, Enright MC, de Lencastre H. Inferring a population structure for *Staphylococcus epidermidis* from multilocus sequence typing data. J Bacteriol 2007;189: 2540–52.

59 Suzuki E, Kuwahara-Arai K, Richardson JF, Hiramatsu K. Distribution of *mec* regulator genes in methicillin-resistant *Staphylococcus* clinical strains. Antimicrob Agents Chemother 1993;37:1219–26.

60 Archer GL, Niemeyer DM. Origin and evolution of DNA associated with resistance to methicillin in staphylococci. Trends Microbiol 1994;2:343–7.

61 Hanssen A-M, Kjeldsen G, Sollid JUE. Local variants of staphylococcal cassette chromosome *mec* in sporadic methicillin-resistant *Staphylococcus aureus* and methicillin-resistant coagulase-negative staphylococci: evidence of horizontal gene transfer? Antimicrob Agents Chemother 2004;48:285–96.

62 Hanssen A-M, Ericson Sollid JU. SCC*mec* in staphylococci: genes on the move. FEMS Immunol Med Microbiol 2006;46:8–20.

63 Song MD, Wachi M, Doi M, Ishino F, Matsuhashi M. Evolution of an inducible penicillin-target protein in methicillin-resistant *Staphylococcus aureus* by gene fusion. FEBS Lett 1987;221:167–71.

64 Marrero A, Mallorqui-Fernandez G, Guevara T, Garcia-Castellanos R, Gomis-Ruth FX. Unbound and acylated structures of the MecR1 extracellular antibiotic-sensor domain provide insights into the signal-transduction system that triggers methicillin resistance. J Mol Biol 2006;361:506–21.

65 Ryffel C, Kayser FH, Berger-Bachi B. Correlation between regulation of *mecA* transcription and expression of methicillin resistance in staphylococci. Antimicrob Agents Chemother 1992;36:25–31.

66 Cha J, Vakulenko SB, Mobashery S. Characterization of the beta-lactam antibotic sensor domain of the MecR1 signal sensor/transducer in methicillin-resistant *Staphylococcus aureus*. Biochemistry 2007;46:7822–31.

67 McKinney TK, Sharma VK, Craig WA, Archer GL. Transcription of the gene mediating methicillin resistance in *Staphylococcus aureus* (*mecA*) is corepressed but not coinduced by cognate *mecA* and beta-lactamase regulators. J Bacteriol 2001; 183:6862–8.

68 Hiramatsu K, Suzuki E, Takayama H, Katayama Y, Yokota T. Role of penicillinase plasmids in the stability of the *mecA* gene in methicillin-resistant *Staphylococcus aureus*. Antimicrob Agents Chemother 1990;34:600–4.

69 Rosato AE, Kreiswirth BN, Craig WA, Eisner W, Climo MW, Archer GL. *mecA-blaZ* corepressors in clinical *Staphylococcus aureus* isolates. Antimicrob Agents Chemother 2003;47:1460–3.

70 Schnellmann C, Gerber V, Rossano A *et al*. Presence of new *mecA* and *mph(C)* variants conferring antibiotic resistance in *Staphylococcus* spp. isolated from the skin of horses before and after clinic admission. J Clin Microbiol 2006;44:4444–54.

71 Couto I, de Lencastre H, Severina E *et al*. Ubiquitous presence of a *mecA* homologue in natural isolates of *Staphylococcus sciuri*. Microb Drug Resist 1996;2:377–91.

72 Fuda C, Suvorov M, Shi Q, Hesek D, Lee M, Mobashery S. Shared functional attributes between the *mecA* gene product of *Staphylococcus sciuri* and penicillin-binding protein 2a of methicillin-resistant *Staphylococcus aureus*. Biochemistry 2007; 46:8050–7.

73 Severin A, Wu SW, Tabei K, Tomasz A. High-level beta-lactam resistance and cell wall synthesis catalyzed by the *mecA* homologue of *Staphylococcus sciuri* introduced into *Staphylococcus aureus*. J Bacteriol 2005;187:6651–8.

74 Wu SW, de Lencastre H, Tomasz A. Recruitment of the *mecA* gene homologue of *Staphylococcus sciuri* into a resistance determinant and expression of the resistant phenotype in *Staphylococcus aureus*. J Bacteriol 2001;183:2417–24.

75 Wu S, de Lencastre H, Tomasz A. Genetic organization of the *mecA* region in methicillin-susceptible and methicillin-resistant strains of *Staphylococcus sciuri*. J Bacteriol 1998;180:236–42.

76 Lim D, Strynadka NCJ. Structural basis for the beta-lactam resistance of PBP2a from methicillin-resistant *Staphylococcus aureus*. Nat Struct Biol 2002;9:870–6.

77 Fuda C, Suvorov M, Vakulenko SB, Mobashery S. The basis for resistance to beta-lactam antibiotics by penicillin-binding protein 2a of methicillin-resistant *Staphylococcus aureus*. J Biol Chem 2004;279:40802–6.

78 Lu W-P, Sun Y, Bauer MD, Paule S, Koenigs PM, Kraft WG. Penicillin-binding protein 2a from methicillin-resistant *Staphylococcus aureus*: kinetic characterization of its interactions with beta-lactams using electrospray mass spectrometry. Biochemistry 1999;38:6537–46.

79 Fuda C, Hesek D, Lee M, Morio K-I, Nowak T, Mobashery S. Activation for catalysis of penicillin-binding protein 2a from methicillin-resistant *Staphylococcus aureus* by bacterial cell wall. J Am Chem Soc 2005;127:2056–7.

80 Pinho MG, de Lencastre H, Tomasz A. An acquired and a native penicillin-binding protein cooperate in building the cell wall of drug-resistant staphylococci. Proc Natl Acad Sci USA 2001;98:10886–91.

81 Pinho MG, Filipe SR, de Lencastre H, Tomasz A. Complementation of the essential peptidoglycan transpeptidase function of penicillin-binding protein 2 (PBP2) by the drug resistance protein PBP2A in *Staphylococcus aureus*. J Bacteriol 2001;183:6525–31.

82 Pinho MG, Errington J. Recruitment of penicillin-binding protein PBP2 to the division site of *Staphylococcus aureus* is dependent on its transpeptidation substrates. Mol Microbiol 2005;55:799–807.

83 Gardete S, de Lencastre H, Tomasz A. A link in transcription between the native *pbpB* and the acquired *mecA* gene in a strain of *Staphylococcus aureus*. Microbiology 2006;152:2549–58.

84 Cohen S, Sweeney HM. Effect of the prophage and penicillinase plasmid of the recipient strain upon the transduction and the stability of methicillin resistance in *Staphylococcus aureus*. J Bacteriol 1973;116:803–11.

85 Stewart GC, Rosenblum ED. Transduction of methicillin resistance in *Staphylococcus aureus*: recipient effectiveness and beta-lactamase production. Antimicrob Agents Chemother 1980;18:424–32.

86 Beck WD, Berger-Bachi B, Kayser FH. Additional DNA in methicillin-resistant *Staphylococcus aureus* and molecular cloning of *mec*-specific DNA. J Bacteriol 1986;165:373–8.

87 de Jonge B, Chang Y, Gage D, Tomasz A. Peptidoglycan composition of a highly methicillin-resistant *Staphylococcus aureus* strain. The role of penicillin binding protein 2A. J Biol Chem 1992;267:11248–54.

88 Katayama Y, Robinson DA, Enright MC, Chambers HF. Genetic background affects stability of *mecA* in *Staphylococcus aureus*. J Clin Microbiol 2005;43:2380–3.

89 Christensen GD, Baddour LM, Madison BM *et al*. Colonial morphology of staphylococci on Memphis agar: phase variation of slime porduction, resistance to beta-lactam antibiotics, and virulence. J Infect Dis 1990;161:1153–69.

90 Mack D, Sabottke A, Dobinsky S, Rohde H, Horstkotte MA, Knobloch JK-M. Differential expression of methicillin resistance by different biofilm-negative *Staphylococcus epidermidis* transposon mutant classes. Antimicrob Agents Chemother 2002;46:178–83.

91 Hososaka Y, Hanaki H, Endo H *et al*. Characterization of oxacillin-susceptible *mecA*-positive *Staphylococcus aureus*: a new type of MRSA. J Infect Chemother 2007;13:79–86.

92 Witte W, Pasemann B, Cuny C. Detection of low-level oxacillin resistance in *mecA*-positive *Staphylococcus aureus*. Clin Microbiol Infect 2007;13:408–12.

93 de Lencastre H, Figueiredo AM, Tomasz A. Genetic control of population structure in heterogeneous strains of methicillin resistant *Staphylococcus aureus*. Eur J Clin Microbiol Infect Dis 1993;12(suppl 1):S13–S18.

94 Traber K, Novick R. A slipped-mispairing mutation in *agrA* of laboratory strains and clinical isolates results in delayed activation of *agr* and failure to translate delta- and alpha-haemolysins. Mol Microbiol 2006;59:1519–30.

95 Ryffel C, Strassle A, Kayser FH, Berger-Bachi B. Mechanisms of heteroresistance in methicillin-resistant *Staphylococcus aureus*. Antimicrob Agents Chemother 1994;38:724–8.

96 Ender M, McCallum N, Berger-Bächi B. Impact of mecA promoter mutations on *mecA* expression and β-lactam resistance levels. Int J Med Microbiol 2008;298:607–17.

97 de Lencastre H, de Jonge BL, Matthews PR, Tomasz A. Molecular aspects of methicillin resistance in *Staphylococcus aureus*. J Antimicrob Chemother 1994;33:7–24.

98 Madiraju MV, Brunner DP, Wilkinson BJ. Effects of temperature, NaCl, and methicillin on penicillin-binding proteins, growth, peptidoglycan synthesis, and autolysis in methicillin-resistant *Staphylococcus aureus*. Antimicrob Agents Chemother 1987;31:1727–33.

99 Brown DFJ, Kothari D. The reliability of methicillin sensitivity tests on four culture media. J Clin Pathol 1974;27:420–6.

100 Ender M, McCallum N, Adhikari R, Berger-Bachi B. Fitness cost of SCC*mec* and methicillin resistance levels in *Staphylococcus aureus*. Antimicrob Agents Chemother 2004;48:2295–7.

101 Lee SM, Ender M, Adhikari R, Smith JMB, Berger-Bachi B, Cook GM. Fitness cost of staphylococcal cassette chromosome *mec* in methicillin-resistant *Staphylococcus aureus* by way of continuous culture. Antimicrob Agents Chemother 2007;51: 1497–9.

102 Berger-Bachi B, Strassle A, Gustafson JE, Kayser FH. Mapping and characterization of multiple chromosomal factors involved in methicillin resistance in *Staphylococcus aureus*. Antimicrob Agents Chemother 1992;36:1367–73.

103 de Lencastre H, Wu SW, Pinho MG *et al*. Antibiotic resistance as a stress response: complete sequencing of a large number of chromosomal loci in *Staphylococcus aureus* strain COL that impact on the expression of resistance to oxacillin. Microb Drug Resist 1999;5:163–75.

104 de Lencastre H, Tomasz A. Reassessment of the number of auxiliary genes essential for expression of high-level methicillin resistance in *Staphylococcus aureus*. Antimicrob Agents Chemother 1994;38:2590–8.

105 Suzuki J, Komatsuzawa H, Sugai M *et al*. Effects of various types of Triton X on the susceptibilities of methicillin-resistant staphylococci to oxacillin. FEMS Microbiol Lett 1997;153:327–31.

106 Jolly L, Wu S, van Heijenoort J, de Lencastre H, Mengin-Lecreulx D, Tomasz A. The *femR315* gene from *Staphylococcus aureus*, the interruption of which results in reduced methicillin

resistance, encodes a phosphoglucosamine mutase. J Bacteriol 1997;179:5321–5.

107 Roos MHH. Das Murein von *Staphylococcus aureus*. Untersuchung des Einflusses von Antibiotikaresistenzdeterminanten auf die Feinstruktur des Peptidoglycan von *Staphylococcus aureus*. Thesis, Freie Universität Berlin, Germany, 1995.

108 Glanzmann P, Gustafson J, Komatsuzawa H, Ohta K, Berger-Bachi B. *glmM* operon and methicillin-resistant *glmM* suppressor mutants in *Staphylococcus aureus*. Antimicrob Agents Chemother 1999;43:240–5.

109 Komatsuzawa H, Fujiwara T, Nishi H *et al*. The gate controlling cell wall synthesis in *Staphylococcus aureus*. Mol Microbiol 2004;53:1221–31.

110 Komatsuzawa H, Ohta K, Sugai M *et al*. Tn*551*-mediated insertional inactivation of the *fmtB* gene encoding a cell wall-associated protein abolishes methicillin resistance in *Staphylococcus aureus*. J Antimicrob Chemother 2000;45:421–31.

111 Wu SW, de Lencastre H. Mrp: a new auxiliary gene essential for optimal expression of methicillin resistance in *Staphylococcus aureus*. Microb Drug Resist 1999;5:9–18.

112 Gill SR, Fouts DE, Archer GL *et al*. Insights on evolution of virulence and resistance from the complete genome analysis of an early methicillin-resistant *Staphylococcus aureus* strain and a biofilm-producing methicillin-resistant *Staphylococcus epidermidis* strain. J Bacteriol 2005;187:2426–38.

113 Gardete S, Ludovice AM, Sobral RG, Filipe SR, de Lencastre H, Tomasz A. Role of *murE* in the expression of beta-lactam antibiotic resistance in *Staphylococcus aureus*. J Bacteriol 2004; 186:1705–13.

114 Sobral RG, Ludovice AM, Gardete S, Tabei K, de Lencastre H, Tomasz A. Normally functioning *murF* is essential for the optimal expression of methicillin resistance in *Staphylococcus aureus*. Microb Drug Resist 2003;9:231–41.

115 Mwangi MM, Wu SW, Zhou Y *et al*. Tracking the in vivo evolution of multidrug resistance in *Staphylococcus aureus* by whole-genome sequencing. Proc Natl Acad Sci USA 2007;104:9451–6.

116 Gustafson J, Strassle A, Hachler H, Kayser FH, Berger-Bachi B. The *femC* locus of *Staphylococcus aureus* required for methicillin resistance includes the glutamine synthetase operon. J Bacteriol 1994;176:1460–7.

117 Sinha RK, Neuhaus FC. Biosynthesis of peptidoglycan in *Gaffkya homari*: on the target(s) of benzylpenicillin. Antimicrob Agents Chemother 1991;35:1753–9.

118 Stranden A, Roos M, Berger-Bachi B. Glutamine synthetase and heteroresistance in methicillin-resistant *Staphylococcus aureus*. Microb Drug Resist 1996;2:201–7.

119 Mazmanian SK, Ton-That H, Schneewind O. Sortase-catalysed anchoring of surface proteins to the cell wall of *Staphylococcus aureus*. Mol Microbiol 2001;40:1049–57.

120 Hegde SS, Shrader TE. FemABX family members are novel nonribosomal peptidyltransferases and important pathogen-specific drug targets. J Biol Chem 2001;276:6998–7003.

121 Schneider T, Senn MM, Berger-Bachi B, Tossi A, Sahl H-G, Wiedemann I. In vitro assembly of a complete, pentaglycine interpeptide bridge containing cell wall precursor (lipid II-Gly5) of *Staphylococcus aureus*. Mol Microbiol 2004;53:675–85.

122 Maidhof H, Reinicke B, Blumel P, Berger-Bachi B, Labischinski H. *femA*, which encodes a factor essential for expression of methicillin resistance, affects glycine content of peptidoglycan in methicillin-resistant and methicillin-susceptible *Staphylococcus aureus* strains. J Bacteriol 1991;173:3507–13.

123 Henze U, Sidow T, Wecke J, Labischinski H, Berger-Bachi B. Influence of *femB* on methicillin resistance and peptidoglycan metabolism in *Staphylococcus aureus*. J Bacteriol 1993;175:1612–20.

124 Stranden A, Ehlert K, Labischinski H, Berger-Bachi B. Cell wall monoglycine cross-bridges and methicillin hypersusceptibility in a *femAB* null mutant of methicillin-resistant *Staphylococcus aureus*. J Bacteriol 1997;179:9–16.

125 Rohrer S, Ehlert K, Tschierske M, Labischinski H, Berger-Bachi B. The essential *Staphylococcus aureus* gene *fmhB* is involved in the first step of peptidoglycan pentaglycine interpeptide formation. Proc Natl Acad Sci USA 1999;96:9351–6.

126 Vetting MW, S. de Carvalho LP, Yu M *et al*. Structure and functions of the GNAT superfamily of acetyltransferases. Arch Biochem Biophys 2005;433:212–26.

127 Ling B, Berger-Bachi B. Increased overall antibiotic susceptibility in *Staphylococcus aureus femAB* null mutants. Antimicrob Agents Chemother 1998;42:936–8.

128 Xiong YL, Fan XJ, Zhang L *et al*. Study on the correlation between resistance phaenotype and expression level of *femA* of *Staphylococcus aureus*. Sichuan Da Xue Xue Bao Yi Xue Ban 2007;38:268–71.

129 Terrak M, Nguyen-Disteche M. Kinetic characterization of the monofunctional glycosyltransferase from *Staphylococcus aureus*. J Bacteriol 2006;188:2528–32.

130 Barrett D, Leimkuhler C, Chen L, Walker D, Kahne D, Walker S. Kinetic characterization of the glycosyltransferase module of *Staphylococcus aureus* PBP2. J Bacteriol 2005;187:2215–17.

131 Leski TA, Tomasz A. Role of penicillin-binding protein 2 (PBP2) in the antibiotic susceptibility and cell wall cross-linking of *Staphylococcus aureus*: evidence for the cooperative functioning of PBP2, PBP4, and PBP2A. J Bacteriol 2005;187:1815–24.

132 Katayama Y, Zhang H-Z, Chambers HF. Effect of disruption of *Staphylococcus aureus* PBP4 gene on resistance to beta-lactam antibiotics. Microb Drug Resist 2003;9:329–36.

133 Memmi G, Filipe SR, Pinho MG, Fu Z, Cheung A. *Staphylococcus aureus* PBP4 is essential for β-lactam resistance in community-acquired methicillin-resistant strains. Antimicrob Agents Chemother 2008;52:3955–66.

134 Yamada S, Sugai M, Komatsuzawa H *et al*. An autolysin ring associated with cell separation of *Staphylococcus aureus*. J Bacteriol 1996;178:1565–71.

135 Giesbrecht P, Labischinski H, Wecke J. A special morphogenetic defect and the subsequent activity of "murosomes" as the very reason for penicillin-induced bacteriolysis. Arch Microbiol 1985;141:315–24.

136 Sugai M, Yamada S, Nakashima S *et al*. Localized perforation of the cell wall by a major autolysin: *atl* gene products and the onset of penicillin-induced lysis of *Staphylococcus aureus*. J Bacteriol 1997;179:2958–62.

137 Oshida T, Tomasz A. Isolation and characterization of a Tn*551*-autolysis mutant of *Staphylococcus aureus*. J Bacteriol 1992;174:4952–9.

138 Takahashi J, Komatsuzawa H, Yamada S *et al*. Molecular characterization of an *atl* null mutant of *Staphylococcus aureus*. Microbiol Immunol 2002;46:601–12.

139 Fujimura T, Murakami K. Increase of methicillin resistance in *Staphylococcus aureus* caused by deletion of a gene whose product is homologous to lytic enzymes. J Bacteriol 1997;179:6294–301.

140 Fujimura T, Murakami K. *Staphylococcus aureus* clinical isolate with high-level methicillin resistance with an *lytH* mutation caused by IS1182 insertion. Antimicrob Agents Chemother 2008;52:643–7.
141 Patton TG, Yang S-J, Bayles KW. The role of proton motive force in expression of the *Staphylococcus aureus cid* and *lrg* operons. Mol Microbiol 2006;59:1395–404.
142 Brunskill E, Bayles K. Identification and molecular characterization of a putative regulatory locus that affects autolysis in *Staphylococcus aureus*. J Bacteriol 1996;178:611–18.
143 Bayles KW. The bactericidal action of penicillin: new clues to an unsolved mystery. Trends Microbiol 2000;8:274–8.
144 Rice KC, Firek BA, Nelson JB, Yang S-J, Patton TG, Bayles KW. The *Staphylococcus aureus cidAB* operon: evaluation of its role in regulation of murein hydrolase activity and penicillin tolerance. J Bacteriol 2003;185:2635–43.
145 Yang S-J, Dunman PM, Projan SJ, Bayles KW. Characterization of the *Staphylococcus aureus* CidR regulon: elucidation of a novel role for acetoin metabolism in cell death and lysis. Mol Microbiol 2006;60:458–68.
146 Neuhaus FC, Baddiley J. A continuum of anionic charge: structures and functions of D-alanyl-teichoic acids in Gram-positive bacteria. Microbiol Mol Biol Rev 2003;67:686–723.
147 Fischer W, Rosel P, Koch HU. Effect of alanine ester substitution and other structural features of lipoteichoic acids on their inhibitory activity against autolysins of *Staphylococcus aureus*. J Bacteriol 1981;146:467–75.
148 Koch HU, Doker R, Fischer W. Maintenance of D-alanine ester substitution of lipoteichoic acid by reesterification in *Staphylococcus aureus*. J Bacteriol 1985;164:1211–17.
149 Nakao A, Imai S-I, Takano T. Transposon-mediated insertional mutagenesis of the D-alanyl-lipoteichoic acid (*dlt*) operon raises methicillin resistance in *Staphylococcus aureus*. Res Microbiol 2000;151:823–9.
150 O'Brien MJ, Kuhl SA, Starzyk MJ. Correlation of teichoic acid D-alanyl esterification with the expression of methicillin resistance in *Staphylococcus aureus*. Microbios 1955;83:119–37.
151 Meehl M, Herbert S, Gotz F, Cheung A. Interaction of the GraRS two-component system with the VraFG ABC-transporter to support vancomycin-intermediate resistance in *Staphylococcus aureus*. Antimicrob Agents Chemother 2007;51:2679–89.
152 Cui L, Lian J-Q, Neoh H-M, Reyes E, Hiramatsu K. DNA microarray-based identification of genes associated with glycopeptide resistance in *Staphylococcus aureus*. Antimicrob Agents Chemother 2005;49:3404–13.
153 Komatsuzawa H, Ohta K, Labischinski H, Sugai M, Suginaka H. Characterization of *fmtA*, a gene that modulates the expression of methicillin resistance in *Staphylococcus aureus*. Antimicrob Agents Chemother 1999;43:2121–5.
154 Fan X, Liu Y, Smith D, Konermann L, Siu KWM, Golemi-Kotra D. Diversity of penicillin-binding proteins: resistance factor FmtA of *Staphylococcus aureus*. J Biol Chem 2007;282:35143–52.
155 Tu Quoc PH, Genevaux P, Pajunen M *et al*. Isolation and characterization of biofilm formation-defective mutants of *Staphylococcus aureus*. Infect Immun 2007;75:1079–88.
156 Komatsuzawa H, Sugai M, Ohta K *et al*. Cloning and characterization of the *fmt* gene which affects the methicillin resistance level and autolysis in the presence of triton X-100 in methicillin-resistant *Staphylococcus aureus*. Antimicrob Agents Chemother 1997;41:2355–61.
157 Weidenmaier C, Kokai-Kun JF, Kristian SA *et al*. Role of teichoic acids in *Staphylococcus aureus* nasal colonization, a major risk factor in nosocomial infections. Nat Med 2004;10:243–5.
158 Maki H, Yamaguchi T, Murakami K. Cloning and characterization of a gene affecting the methicillin resistance level and the autolysis rate in *Staphylococcus aureus*. J Bacteriol 1994;176:4993–5000.
159 Maki H, Murakami K. Formation of potent hybrid promoters of the mutant *llm* gene by IS*256* transposition in methicillin-resistant *Staphylococcus aureus*. J Bacteriol 1997;179:6944–8.
160 Novick RP. Autoinduction and signal transduction in the regulation of staphylococcal virulence. Mol Microbiol 2003; 48:1429–49.
161 Bischoff M, Dunman P, Kormanec J *et al*. Microarray-based analysis of the *Staphylococcus aureus* sigmaB regulon. J Bacteriol 2004;186:4085–99.
162 Pane-Farre J, Jonas B, Forstner K, Engelmann S, Hecker M. The sigmaB regulon in *Staphylococcus aureus* and its regulation. Int J Med Microbiol 2006;296:237–58.
163 Wu S, de Lencastre H, Tomasz A. Sigma-B, a putative operon encoding alternate sigma factor of *Staphylococcus aureus* RNA polymerase: molecular cloning and DNA sequencing. J Bacteriol 1996;178:6036–42.
164 Meier S, Goerke C, Wolz C *et al*. sigmaB and the sigmaB-dependent *arlRS* and *yabJ-spoVG* loci affect capsule formation in *Staphylococcus aureus*. Infect Immun 2007;75:4562–71.
165 Schulthess B, Meier S, Homerova D *et al*. Functional characterization of the SigB-dependent *yabJ-spoVG* operon in *Staphylococcus aureus*: role in methicillin and glycopeptide resistance. Antimicrob Agents Chemother 2009;53:1832–9.
166 Novick RP, Projan SJ, Kornblum J *et al*. The *agr* P2 operon: an autocatalytic sensory transduction system in *Staphyoloccus aureus*. Mol Gen Genet 1995;248:446–58.
167 Piriz Duran S, Kayser FH, Berger-Bachi B. Impact of *sar* and *agr* on methicillin resistance in *Staphylococcus aureus*. FEMS Microbiol Lett 1996;141:255–60.
168 Titgemeyer F, Hillen W. Global control of sugar metabolism: a Gram-positive solution. Antonie van Leeuwenhoek 2002; 82:59–71.
169 Seidl K, Bischoff M, Berger-Bachi B. CcpA mediates the catabolite repression of *tst* in *Staphylococcus aureus*. Infect Immun 2008;76:5093–9.
170 Seidl K, Goerke C, Wolz C, Mack D, Berger-Bachi B, Bischoff M. *Staphylococcus aureus* CcpA affects biofilm formation. Infect Immun 2008;76:2044–50.
171 Seidl K, Stucki M, Ruegg M *et al*. *Staphylococcus aureus* CcpA affects virulence determinant production and antibiotic resistance. Antimicrob Agents Chemother 2006;50:1183–94.
172 Gardete S, Wu SW, Gill S, Tomasz A. Role of VraSR in antibiotic resistance and antibiotic-induced stress response in *Staphylococcus aureus*. Antimicrob Agents Chemother 2006;50:3424–34.
173 Ender M, Berger-Bachi B, McCallum N. A novel DNA binding protein modulating methicillin resistance in *Staphylococcus aureus*. BMC Microbiol 2009;9:15.
174 Schrader-Fischer G, Berger-Bachi B. The AbcA transporter of *Staphylococcus aureus* affects cell autolysis. Antimicrob Agents Chemother 2001;45:407–12.
175 Truong-Bolduc QC, Hooper DC. The transcriptional regulators NorG and MgrA modulate resistance to both quinolones and

beta-lactams in *Staphylococcus aureus*. J Bacteriol 2007;189:2996–3005.

176 Kristiansen MM, Leandro C, Ordway D *et al*. Thioridazine reduces resistance of methicillin-resistant *Stapyhlococcus aureus* by inhibiting a reserpine-sensitive efflux pump. In Vivo 2006; 20:361–6.

177 Singh VK, Moskovitz J. Multiple methionine sulfoxide reductase genes in *Staphylococcus aureus*: expression of activity and roles in tolerance of oxidative stress. Microbiology 2003;149:2739–47.

178 Hübscher J, Lüthy L, Berger-Bachi B, Stutzmann Meier P. Phylogenetic distribution and membrane topology of the LytR-CpsA-Psr protein family. BMC Genomics 2008;9:617.

179 Hübscher J, McCallum N, Sifri CD *et al*. MsrR contributes to cell surface characteristics and virulence in *Staphylococcus aureus*. FEMS Microbiol Lett [in press].

180 Rossi J, Bischoff M, Wada A, Berger-Bachi B. MsrR, a putative cell envelope-associated element involved in *Staphylococcus aureus sarA* attenuation. Antimicrob Agents Chemother 2003; 47:2558–64.

181 Kondo N, Kuwahara-Arai K, Kuroda-Murakami H, Tateda-Suzuki E, Hiramatsu K. Eagle-type methicillin resistance: new phenotype of high methicillin resistance under *mec* regulator gene control. Antimicrob Agents Chemother 2001;45:815–24.

182 McDougal LK, Thornsberry C. The role of beta-lactamase in staphylococcal resistance to penicillinase-resistant penicillins and cephalosporins. J Clin Microbiol 1986;23:832–9.

183 Massidda O, Montanari MP, Mingoia M, Varaldo P. Cloning and expression of the penicillinase from a borderline methicillin-susceptible *Staphylococcus aureus* in *Escherichia coli*. FEMS Microbiol Lett 1994;119:263–9.

184 Massidda O, Montanari M, Mingoia M, Varaldo P. Borderline methicillin-susceptible *Staphylococcus aureus* strains have more in common than reduced susceptibility to penicillinase-resistant penicillins. Antimicrob Agents Chemother 1996;40:2769–74.

185 Gal Z, Kovacs F, Herndi F *et al*. Investigation of oxacillin-hydrolyzing beta-lactamase in borderline methicillin-resistant clinical isolates of *Staphylococcus aureus*. Chemotherapy 2001; 47:233–8.

186 Barg N, Chambers H, Kernodle D. Borderline susceptibility to antistaphylococcal penicillins is not conferred exclusively by the hyperproduction of beta-lactamase. Antimicrob Agents Chemother 1991;35:1975–9.

187 Massidda O, Mingoia M, Fadda D, Whalen MB, Montanari MP, Varaldo PE. Analysis of the beta-lactamase plasmid of borderline methicillin-susceptible *Staphylococcus aureus*: focus on *bla* complex genes and cadmium resistance determinants *cadD* and *cadX*. Plasmid 2006;55:114–27.

188 Tomasz A, Drugeon HB, de Lencastre HM, Jabes D, McDougall L, Bille J. New mechanism for methicillin resistance in *Staphylococcus aureus*: clinical isolates that lack the PBP 2a gene and contain normal penicillin-binding proteins with modified penicillin-binding capacity. Antimicrob Agents Chemother 1989;33:1869–74.

189 Hackbarth C, Kocagoz T, Kocagoz S, Chambers H. Point mutations in *Staphylococcus aureus* PBP 2 gene affect penicillin-binding kinetics and are associated with resistance. Antimicrob Agents Chemother 1995;39:103–6.

190 Nadarajah J, Lee MJS, Louie L *et al*. Identification of different clonal complexes and diverse amino acid substitutions in penicillin-binding protein 2 (PBP2) associated with borderline oxacillin resistance in Canadian *Staphylococcus aureus* isolates. J Med Microbiol 2006;55:1675–83.

191 Berger-Bachi B, Strassle A, Kayser FH. Natural methicillin resistance in comparison with that selected by in-vitro drug exposure in *Staphylococcus aureus*. J Antimicrob Chemother 1989;23:179–88.

192 Henze U, Berger-Bachi B. Penicillin-binding protein 4 overproduction increases beta-lactam resistance in *Staphylococcus aureus*. Antimicrob Agents Chemother 1996;40:2121–5.

193 Yoshida R, Kuwahara-Arai K, Baba T, Cui L, Richardson JF, Hiramatsu K. Physiological and molecular analysis of a *mecA*-negative *Staphylococcus aureus* clinical strain that expresses heterogeneous methicillin resistance. J Antimicrob Chemother 2003;51:247–55.

194 Vaudaux P, Francois P, Bisognano C *et al*. Increased expression of clumping factor and fibronectin-binding proteins by *hemB* mutants of *Staphylococcus aureus* expressing small colony variant phenotypes. Infect Immun 2002;70:5428–37.

195 Senn MM, Bischoff M, von Eiff C, Berger-Bachi B. sigma B activity in a *Staphylococcus aureus hemB* mutant. J Bacteriol 2005;187:7397–406.

196 Proctor RA, von Eiff C, Kahl BC *et al*. Small colony variants: a pathogenic form of bacteria that facilitates persistent and recurrent infections. Nat Rev Microbiol 2006;4:295–305.

197 Baumert N, von Eiff C, Schaaff F, Peters G, Proctor RA, Sahl H-G. Physiology and antibiotic susceptibility of *Staphylococcus aureus* small colony variants. Microb Drug Resist 2002;8:253–60.

198 Looney WJ. Small-colony variants of *Staphylococcus aureus*. Br J Biomed Sci 2000;57:317–22.

199 Beenken KE, Dunman PM, McAleese F *et al*. Global gene expression in *Staphylococcus aureus* biofilms. J Bacteriol 2004; 186:4665–84.

200 Resch A, Rosenstein R, Nerz C, Gotz F. Differential gene expression profiling of *Staphylococcus aureus* cultivated under biofilm and planktonic conditions. Appl Environ Microbiol 2005;71:2663–76.

201 Resch A, Leicht S, Saric M *et al*. Comparative proteome analysis of *Staphylococcus aureus* biofilm and planktonic cells and correlation with transcriptome profiling. Proteomics 2006;6: 1867–77.

202 Saginur R, St Denis M, Ferris W *et al*. Multiple combination bactericidal testing of staphylococcal biofilms from implant-associated infections. Antimicrob Agents Chemother 2006;50:55–61.

203 Hola V, Ruzicka F, Votava M. Differences in antibiotic susceptibility in biofilm-positive and biofilm-negative *Staphylococcus epidermidis* isolates. Epidemiol Mikrobiol Imunol 2004;53:66–9.

204 Fux CA, Wilson S, Stoodley P. Detachment characteristics and oxacillin resistance of *Staphyloccocus aureus* biofilm emboli in an *in vitro* catheter infection model. J Bacteriol 2004;186:4486–91.

205 Williams I, Venables W, Lloyd D, Paul F, Critchley I. The effects of adherence to silicone surfaces on antibiotic susceptibility in *Staphylococcus aureus*. Microbiology 1997;143:2407–13.

206 Arciola CR, Campoccia D, Montanaro L. Effects on antibiotic resistance of *Staphylococcus epidermidis* following adhesion to polymethylmethacrylate and to silicone surfaces. Biomaterials 2002;23:1495–502.

207 O'Neill E, Pozzi C, Houston P *et al*. Association between methicillin susceptibility and biofilm regulation in *Staphylococcus*

aureus isolates from device-related infections. J Clin Microbiol 2007;45:1379–88.

208 Mempel M, Feucht H, Ziebuhr W, Endres M, Laufs R, Gruter L. Lack of *mecA* transcription in slime-negative phase variants of methicillin-resistant *Staphylococcus epidermidis*. Antimicrob Agents Chemother 1994;38:1251–5.

209 Mempel M, Muller E, Hoffmann R, Feucht H, Laufs R, Gruter L. Variable degree of slime production is linked to different levels of beta-lactam susceptibility in *Staphylococcus epidermidis* phase variants. Med Microbiol Immunol 1995;184:109–13.

210 Sieradzki K, Tomasz A. Gradual alterations in cell wall structure and metabolism in vancomycin-resistant mutants of *Staphylococcus aureus*. J Bacteriol 1999;181:7566–70.

211 Bhateja P, Purnapatre K, Dube S, Fatma T, Rattan A. Characterisation of laboratory-generated vancomycin intermediate resistant *Staphylococcus aureus* strains. Int J Antimicrob Agents 2006;27:201–11.

212 Sieradzki K, Wu SW, Tomasz A. Inactivation of the methicillin resistance gene *mecA* in vancomycin-resistant *Staphylococcus aureus*. Microb Drug Resist 1999;5:253–7.

213 Naimi TS, Anderson D, O'Boyle C *et al.* Vancomycin-intermediate *Staphylococcus aureus* with phenotypic susceptibility to methicillin in a patient with recurrent bacteremia. Clin Infect Dis 2003;36:1609–12.

214 Pfeltz RF, Singh VK, Schmidt JL *et al.* Characterization of passage-selected vancomycin-resistant *Staphylococcus aureus* strains of diverse parental backgrounds. Antimicrob Agents Chemother 2000;44:294–303.

215 Howden BP, Johnson PD, Ward PB, Stinear TP, Davies JK. Isolates with low-level vancomycin resistance associated with persistent methicillin-resistant *Staphylococcus aureus* bacteremia. Antimicrob Agents Chemother 2006;50:3039–47.

216 Boyle-Vavra S, Carey RB, Daum RS. Development of vancomycin and lysostaphin resistance in a methicillin-resistant *Staphylococcus aureus* isolate. J Antimicrob Chemother 2001; 48:617–25.

217 Severin A, Tabei K, Tenover F, Chung M, Clarke N, Tomasz A. High level oxacillin and vancomycin resistance and altered cell wall composition in *Staphylococcus aureus* carrying the staphylococcal *mecA* and the enterococcal *vanA* gene complex. J Biol Chem 2004;279:3398–407.

218 Weigel LM, Clewell DB, Gill SR *et al.* Genetic analysis of a high-level vancomycin-resistant isolate of *Staphylococcus aureus*. Science 2003;302:1569–71.

219 Climo MW, Patron RL, Archer GL. Combinations of vancomycin and beta-lactams are synergistic against staphylococci with reduced susceptibilities to vancomycin. Antimicrob Agents Chemother 1999;43:1747–53.

220 Howe RA, Wootton M, Bennett PM, MacGowan AP, Walsh TR. Interactions between methicillin and vancomycin in methicillin-resistant *Staphylococcus aureus* strains displaying different phenotypes of vancomycin susceptibility. J Clin Microbiol 1999;37:3068–71.

221 Groicher KH, Firek BA, Fujimoto DF, Bayles KW. The *Staphylococcus aureus lrgAB* operon modulates murein hydrolase activity and penicillin tolerance. J Bacteriol 2000;182:1794–801.

222 Ingavale SS, Van Wamel W, Cheung AL. Characterization of RAT, an autolysis regulator in *Staphylococcus aureus*. Mol Microbiol 2003;48:1451–66.

223 Peschel A, Jack RW, Otto M *et al. Staphylococcus aureus* resistance to human defensins and evasion of neutrophil killing via the novel virulence factor MprF is based on modification of membrane lipids with L-lysine. J Exp Med 2001;193:1067–76.

224 Staubitz P, Neumann H, Schneider T, Wiedemann I, Peschel A. MprF-mediated biosynthesis of lysylphosphatidylglycerol, an important determinant in staphylococcal defensin resistance. FEMS Microbiol Lett 2004;231:67–71.

225 Komatsuzawa H, Ohta K, Fujiwara T, Choi GH, Labischinski H, Sugai M. Cloning and sequencing of the gene, *fmtC*, which affects oxacillin resistance in methicillin-resistant *Staphylococcus aureus*. FEMS Microbiol Lett 2001;203:49–54.

226 Berger-Bachi B, Barberis-Maino L, Strässle A, Kayser FH. FemA, a host-mediated factor essential for methicillin resistance in *Staphylococcus aureus*: moleuclar cloning and characterization. Mol Gen Genet 1989;219:263–9.

227 Boyle-Vavra S, Yin S, Daum RS. The VraS/VraR two-component regulatory system required for oxacillin resistance in community-acquired methicillin-resistant *Staphylococcus aureus*. FEMS Microbiol Lett 2006;262:163–71.

228 Manna AC, Ingavale SS, Maloney M, van Wamel W, Cheung AL. Identification of sarV (SA2062), a new transcriptional regulator, is repressed by SarA and MgrA (SA0641) and involved in the regulation of autolysis in *Staphylococcus aureus*. J Bacteriol 2004;186:5267–80.

Chapter 9
Resistance to Glycopeptides

Keiichi Hiramatsu
Department of Bacteriology, Juntendo University, Tokyo, Japan

Global historical perspective on vancomycin resistance in staphylococci

Staphylococcus aureus did not easily become resistant to vancomycin

Vancomycin was introduced into clinical use in 1956. Initially its use was limited because of high renal toxicity and the availability of other potent β-lactam antibiotics with activity against *Staphylococcus aureus*. However, when methicillin-resistant *S. aureus* (MRSA), first reported in 1961 [1], became prevalent as a hospital pathogen in the 1970s, vancomycin gained its profile as a reliable antibiotic against MRSA. Improvements in the purification method made vancomycin less toxic, which further accelerated its use as the last-resort antibiotic against MRSA infection. Despite the fact that vancomycin has been in use since the early days of antibiotic history, it remained effective against MRSA for almost 40 years before the appearance of vancomycin-intermediate *S. aureus* (VISA) in 1996 [2].

Initial studies conducted before 1996 revealed that vancomycin resistance does not develop readily on repeated exposure of *S. aureus* and MRSA clinical strains to vancomycin *in vitro* [3]. This indicated that the accumulation of a small collection of single mutations would not make *S. aureus* cells resistant to vancomycin unlike other antibiotics such as rifampin and quinolone. Watanakunakorn [4] considered that the difficulty was due to the multiple actions of vancomycin against bacterial cells, including inhibition of not only cell wall synthesis but also RNA synthesis and integrity of the cytoplasmic membrane. However, recent studies on telavancin, a semisynthetic derivative of vancomycin, have revealed that vancomycin does not affect membrane integrity as appreciably as telavancin does [5]. Telavancin possesses a hydrophobic fatty acid side chain that seems to affect membrane integrity and increase membrane permeability [5]. However, vancomycin also exerts inhibitory effects on diverse macromolecular pathways including peptidoglycan, RNA, fatty acid, and protein synthesis [5]. Telavancin inhibits synthesis of peptidoglycan, RNA and fatty acids, but not protein synthesis.

While glycopeptide antibiotics appear to target multiple macromolecular synthetic pathways, the vital target of vancomycin is the D-alanyl-D-alanine residue situated at the terminus of the murein-monomer precursor *N*-acetylglucosamine (GlcNAc)-*N*-acetylmuramic acid (MurNAc) decapeptide. It is present as lipid II in the outer surface of the cytoplasmic membrane. As expected, the inhibitory activity of vancomycin and telavancin on peptidoglycan synthesis is antagonized by the presence of a competitive ligand, *N*,*N*-diacetyl-L-Lys-D-Ala-D-Ala (dKAA) [5]. Intriguingly, not only the binding of telavancin to the cytoplasmic membrane (where the target molecule lipid II is present) but also the increase in membrane permeability is inhibited by dKAA. This suggests that D-alanyl-D-alanine is the main target of vancomycin and related compounds including telavancin. That D-alanyl-D-alanine is the main target is also supported by the mechanism of resistance in vancomycin-resistant enterococci (VRE). In VRE, the D-alanyl-D-alanine residue of the murein monomer precursor is replaced by a depsipeptide D-alanyl-D-lactate, to which vancomycin cannot bind with high affinity and it is subsequently totally inactive against these strains, even at concentrations as high as 1000 mg/L [6].

In light of these findings, it is likely that delayed development of vancomycin resistance in *S. aureus* was due to the complexity involved in preventing binding of the glycopeptide to D-alanyl-D-alanine within the cell wall. Historically, *S. aureus* has been exceptionally versatile with respect to the acquisition of antibiotic resistance. It acquired methicillin resistance in 1960, the same year that methicillin was successfully launched for clinical use [1]. The methicillin resistance gene *mecA* was found on the staphylococcal cassette chromosome (SCC) integrated in the *S. aureus* chromosome near the origin of replication [7,8]. The mobile genetic element SCC is unique to *Staphylococcus* species and is considered to be a versatile interspecies gene transfer system that *S. aureus* utilizes for better survival in the human host [9]. Genes for capsule formation, superantigen production, and resistance to various antiseptics or antibiotics have been identified in SCCs

Staphylococci in Human Disease, 2nd edition. Edited by Kent B. Crossley, Kimberly K. Jefferson, Gordon Archer, Vance G. Fowler, Jr.
 ISBN 978-14051-6332-3.

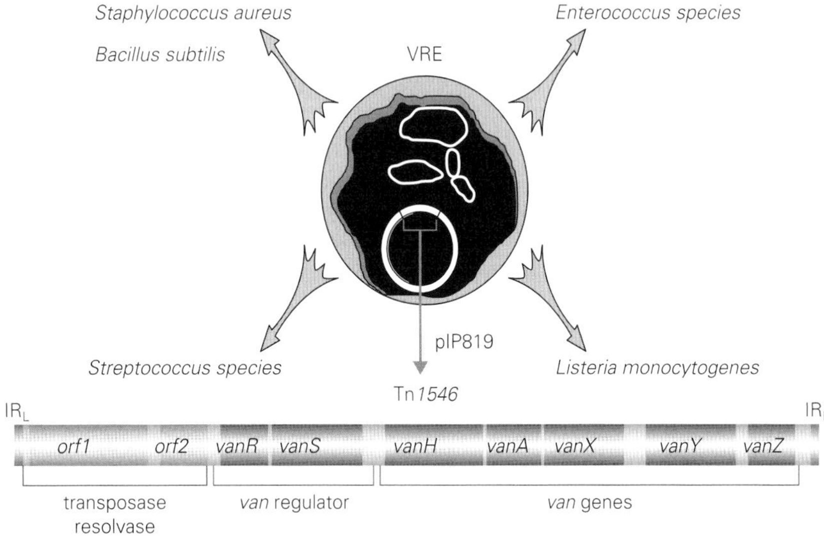

Figure 9.1 Vancomycin resistance of vancomycin-resistant enterococci (VRE) can be actively transmitted to a variety of Gram-positive bacteria via a conjugative plasmid. The transposon that harbors the *vanA* gene complex, Tn*1546*, is carried by a conjugative plasmid and is highly transmissible to various bacterial species such as *Listeria monocytogenes*, *Streptococcus sanguis*, *Streptococcus lactis*, *Streptococcus pyogenes* [77] and even to *Staphylococcus aureus* [14].

of clinical *S. aureus* strains [10]. Despite the apparent versatility of the SCC gene transfer system, no SCCs that carry the genes conferring vancomycin resistance (*vanA* or *vanB*) have been found. The *vanA* genes were introduced into MRSA clinical strains by the conjugative plasmid of a VRE strain in 2002, half a century after the introduction of vancomycin in 1956 [11,12]. This late occurrence of *van* gene transfer to *S. aureus* might mean that the microorganisms harboring the *van* gene system (probably glycopeptide-producing organisms) did not come into contact with staphylococci frequently, and therefore *van* genes were beyond the reach of the SCC gene transfer system.

Figure 9.1 illustrates the conjugative plasmid in a VRE cell on which the *vanA* genes are aligned on a transposon, Tn*1546* [13]. The plasmid bears the *tra* gene and is capable of intergeneric transfer to various Gram-positive genera such as *Bacillus*, *Enterococcus*, *Streptococcus*, and *Listeria*. In 1992, Noble *et al.* [14] achieved successful experimental transfer of the plasmid carrying the *vanA* transposon from *Enterococcus faecium* to *S. aureus*. Therefore, in the early 1990s, it was a general feeling of researchers that if *S. aureus* were to acquire vancomycin resistance it would be through the acquisition of the *vanA* gene transposon. It was considered a matter of time before transformation of an *S. aureus* clinical isolate with a *vanA* gene plasmid occurred. Contrary to our expectations of early emergence of vancomycin-resistant *S. aureus* (VRSA), it took 16 years before the prevalence of VRE in the human community expanded to the extent that these organisms finally came into close enough contact with MRSA cells and transferred its resistance plasmid to them.

Emergence of VISA and VRSA

Since the emergence of VRSA had been feared by researchers after Noble *et al.*'s *van* gene transfer experiment in 1992, our report of VISA clinical strain Mu50 from an infection refractory to vancomycin therapy caused worldwide terror in 1997 [2]. We referred to Mu50 as "vancomycin resistant" based on the refractory nature of the infection it caused. It was not resolved even after prolonged vancomycin therapy (45 mg/kg daily for 29 days) [15]. However, Mu50 was negative for *vanA* or any other *van* gene homologs.

Now, clinical VRSA strains are divided into two categories based on minimum inhibitory concentration (MIC) of vancomycin: strains with an MIC of 4–8 mg/L are referred to as VISA; those with an MIC of 16 mg/L or greater are referred to as VRSA [16]. However, nomenclature reflects underlying genetic mechanisms: spontaneous mutations lead to VISA, while *van* gene transfer leads to VRSA. It should be noted that there are some VISA strains with MICs of 16 mg/L, and some VRSA strains with MICs less than 16 mg/L (because of masked expression of *van* gene phenotype).

Figure 9.2 shows the temporal change in frequency of VISA (defined as those with vancomycin MICs ≥ 4 mg/L) among MRSA, that of vancomycin-intermediate *S. epidermidis* (VISE) among methicillin-resistant *S. epidermidis*, and that of vancomycin-intermediate *S. haemolyticus* (VISH) among methicillin-resistant *S. haemolyticus* clinical isolates from Juntendo University Hospital (JUH). It should be noted that the injectable form of vancomycin was not available in Japan until 1991 (see below). It is interesting that the vancomycin-intermediate phenoptype was much more frequent in *S. haemolyticus* than in *S. epidermidis* and *S. aureus*. This is coincidental with the historical order of emergence of vancomycin resistance in staphylococcal species [15]: a clinical isolate of *S. haemolyticus* with vancomycin MIC of 8 mg/L was identified in 1987 [17], followed by *S. epidermidis* with vancomycin MIC of 16 mg/L in 1991 [18], before the discovery of VISA in 1996. *Staphylococcus haemolyticus* was also the first staphylococcal

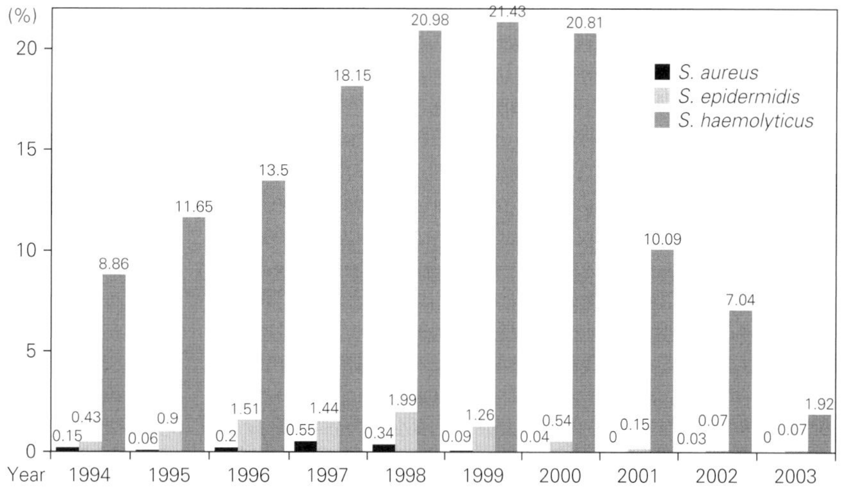

Total of strains	1994	1995	1996	1997	1998	1999	2000	2001	2002	2003
(Staphylococci)	3800	4633	4400	4375	4062	3687	3892	3966	4427	4616
S. aureus	2627	3100	2942	2703	2664	2219	2411	2447	2880	3148
S. epidermidis	936	1224	1258	1391	1255	1272	1308	1301	1405	1364
S. haemolyticus	237	309	200	281	143	196	173	218	142	104

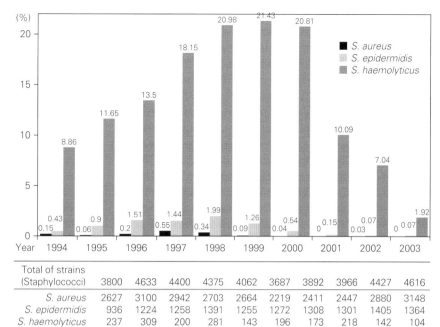

Figure 9.2 Emergence and decline of vancomycin-intermediate staphylococci at Juntendo University Hospital. *Staphylococcus haemolyticus* is more likely to acquire vancomycin resistance than other staphylococcal species. Note that after the clinical introduction of vancomycin in 1991, vancomycin-intermediate staphylococci started to be detected and reached peak prevalence around 1997; however, a rapid decline in these organisms was observed thereafter.

species to acquire teicoplanin resistance in 1986 [19]. This ability seems to be associated with the extraordinarily high flexibility of the *S. haemolyticus* genome due to the presence of multiple active insertion sequence (IS) copies scattered throughout its chromosome [20,21]. Figure 9.2 shows that the rate of VISA isolation was highest in 1997, then declined quickly, and we have found VISA only occasionally at JUH in the 2000s. Surprisingly this decline of vancomycin-intermediate staphylococci was not correlated with annual vancomycin consumption in JUH. This subject is addressed in the section Unique experience in Japan.

Subsequent to our report of Mu50, VISA strains with vancomycin MICs of 8 mg/L were isolated from various geographical areas such as the USA, Europe, Africa (South Africa), and South America (Brazil) [22,23]. Despite their low MICs, the infection caused by VISA was invariably refractory to vancomycin therapy. This is explained by the extremely low tissue concentrations achievable by regular drip-infusion vancomycin therapy. Injection of vancomycin at a daily dose of 2 g does not raise tissue concentrations above 2–3 mg/L in the lung or 5 mg/L in the skin and soft tissue [24]. A clinical study conducted by the Centers for Disease Control in the USA demonstrated that even MRSA strains with vancomycin MICs of 4 mg/L are equally refractory to vancomycin therapy as MRSA strains with MICs of 8 mg/L [25]. This finding finally changed the Clinical and Laboratory Standards Institute MIC breakpoints for the vancomycin susceptibility test [16]. Today, the vancomycin MIC breakpoints are as follows: susceptible, ≤ 2 mg/L; intermediate, 4–8 mg/L; resistant, ≥ 16 mg/L. A fault of this definition is that strains with "intermediate" MICs of 4 and 8 mg/L are clinically "resistant" to vancomycin therapy. Although the naming of VRSA was reserved for strains harboring *van* genes, it should be noted that an MIC of 16 mg/L is also achievable by mutational mechanisms. We found that one of the VISA strains, MI, had an MIC of 16 mg/L (unpublished observations). Although it is convenient to use the terms VISA and VRSA for the two distinct resistance mechanisms in order to avoid confusion, it should be kept in mind that MIC values are variable in individual VISA and VRSA strains.

Finally, the emergence of VRSA was confirmed in 2002 when two vancomycin-resistant isolates of *S. aureus* (MIC 32 mg/L) harboring *vanA* gene plasmids were identified from clinical cases [11,12]; VRE and MRSA seemed to have jointly colonized the necrotic tissue of the diabetic patients. This signaled the fulfillment of Noble's prophecy, and again caused worldwide alarm. However, having discovered the limitations of vancomycin pharmacokinetics, the emergence of VRSA in the USA may be no more ominous than the ubiquitous distribution of VISA elsewhere in the world.

Historical perspective on vancomycin resistance in Japan

Despite the slowness and difficulty with which *S. aureus* became "resistant" to vancomycin (including the intermediate status of MIC 8 mg/L), it was found that resistance to vancomycin 8 mg/L could be easily selected from Japanese hospital-associated MRSA strains [26]. As a matter of fact, VISA were found to be spontaneously generated at high frequency in populations of certain Japanese MRSA strains [26]. Such MRSA strains (designated "hetero-VISA") have vancomycin MICs ranging from 0.5 to 2 mg/L and yet spontaneously generate VISA in their cell populations with a frequency greater than 1 in 10^6. These strains were found to constitute 9.3% of 129 isolates from seven university hospitals and 1.3% of 950 isolates from 195 nonuniversity hospitals or clinics in 1996 [24]. Initially we designated them "hetero-VRSA" since they were the direct progenitors of VRSA (which we designated Mu50 initially). The name was changed after the discovery of VRSA harboring the *vanA* gene plasmid and an MIC of 32 mg/L or above; accordingly, Mu50 was renamed VISA. Figure 9.3 shows a population analysis of vancomycin-susceptible *S. aureus* (VSSA), VISA, and hetero-VISA. This demonstrates the relative proportions of the total cell population that exhibit different levels of vancomycin resistance. About 10^7 cfu (colony-forming units) of each strain were analyzed. All cells of the VSSA strain are inhibited from growth by vancomycin 1 or 2 mg/L, whereas VISA cells grow in vancomycin 4 mg/L. Since expression of vancomycin resistance is more pronounced in strains grown on BHI, we have been using BHI-agar plates for population analysis. In this experimental condition, most VISA strains grow in vancomycin 4 mg/L. They appear less resistant to vancomycin when using Mueller-Hinton (MH) broth or agar; with MH, we usually see colonies in vancomycin 2 mg/L but not in vancomycin 4 mg/L. Figure 9.3 clearly shows that the hetero-VISA population contains VISA cells (that

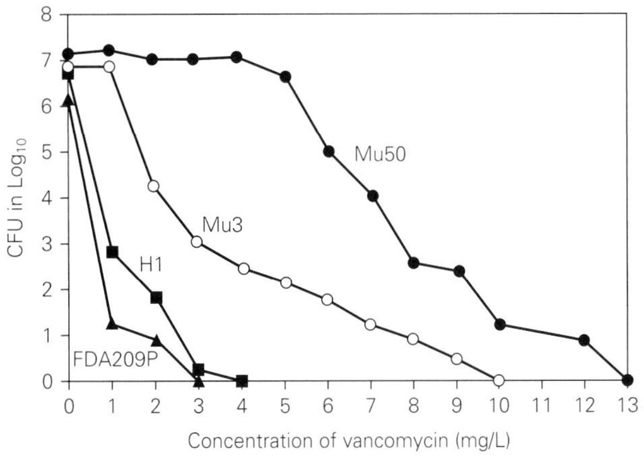

Figure 9.3 Population analysis of vancomycin-susceptible *S. aureus* (VSSA), vancomycin-intermediate *S. aureus* (VISA), and hetero-VISA. About 10^7 cfu (colony-forming units) of Mu3 cells were spread onto agar plates containing various concentrations of vancomycin. As illustrated, growth of more than 99.99% of the cell population was inhibited on plates containing vancomycin 4 mg/L, indicating that the majority of the cells were susceptible to this concentration of vancomycin (MIC ≤ 4 mg/L). However, growth in the presence of vancomycin 4 mg/L resulted in homotypic vancomycin resistance comparable with that of VISA strain Mu50. Vancomycin completely inhibited growth of VSSA cells at a concentration of less than 4 mg/L.

can grow in vancomycin 4 mg/L). The distribution of hetero-VISA in Japanese hospitals was unexpected considering the initial observation that vancomycin-resistant mutants were difficult to obtain from clinical *S. aureus* strains. Selection of vancomycin resistance *in vitro* might not have been detected in earlier studies because the changes in MIC are very subtle and a twofold to fourfold increase in MIC may not have been considered clinically significant if the researchers were not cognizant of the fact that the concentration of vancomycin remains low in tissues. Another consideration is that there are certain genotypes from which intermediate vancomycin resistance appears to be more readily derived. Among them is clonotype II-A, one of the MRSA genotypes possessing SCC*mec* type IIa and multilocus sequence type (MLST) 5 [27], also referred to as NewYork/Japanese clone [28]. Most of the VISA strains in the world were derived from this genotype. Clonotype II-A MRSA is predominantly distributed in the USA, Korea, and Japan, the countries where VISA and hetero-VISA are found relatively frequently [29]. MRSA with distinct genotype designated "British Empire" strain (SCC*mec* type 3A and MLST 239) is distributed in England and Southeast Asian countries, where VISA strains have been less frequently isolated [30]. Strict comparative analysis using various MRSA clonotypes has not yet been performed to determine the rate of emergence of hetero-VISA. However, we have observed that clonotype II-A Japanese MRSA clinical strains generate mutants with the VISA phenotype through two-step selection: (i) VSSA to hetero-VISA is achieved by first-step vancomycin selection and (ii) hetero-VISA to VISA conversion is achieved by second-step vancomycin selection [31]. In Japan, clonotype II-A MRSA has dominated hospital MRSA isolates since the mid-1980s [32]. We found a considerable proportion (9.3%) of hetero-VISA strains among clonotype II-A MRSA strains in Japanese university hospitals in 1996 [24]. Since VISA spontaneously emerges at high frequency among cell populations of hetero-VISA, early emergence of VISA in Japan was a natural consequence of the unique Japanese MRSA epidemiology in the 1990s.

Clonal expansion of homo-MRSA of clonotype II-A in Japanese hospitals

In Japanese hospitals, an explosion of MRSA occurred around 1980 [32]. The initial reports by Japanese clinicians describing the historical upsurge of MRSA in the early 1980s have been reviewed elsewhere [32]. However, clinical introduction of injectable forms of vancomycin was delayed, and Japanese clinicians were unable to use vancomycin against MRSA infection until 1991. This void in MRSA chemotherapy brought about a unique historical event in Japanese MRSA epidemiology, which led to the early emergence of VISA in 1996 only 5 years after the clinical introduction of vancomycin. Plate 9.1 shows the degree of methicillin resistance of MRSA isolates in the University of Tokyo Hospital in 1982 and 1992. In 1982, the MRSA strains possessed MICs that ranged from susceptible to moderate levels of resistance. Population analysis showed that they were heterogeneously resistant to methicillin (and also to other potent β-lactam antibiotics such as imipenem and oxacillin), and hence designated "hetero-MRSA" [33–35]. Coagulase typing of the strains shown in Plate 9.1 reveals that they were composed of strains of various genotypes. On the other hand, in 1992 all the MRSA strains isolated in the University of Tokyo Hospital possessed coagulase type 2, which turned out to be the clonal expansion of clonotype II-A MRSA [27]. Almost all the clonotype II-A MRSA strains were homogeneously highly resistant to methicillin, i.e., "homo-MRSA" strains [33]. This significant change in MRSA epidemiology in Japanese hospitals is considered the result of unique anti-MRSA chemotherapy. Since vancomycin was not available until 1991, Japanese clinicians used imipenem (introduced in 1987) or cephalosporins such as cefmetazole to treat MRSA infection. Subsequently, most of the MRSA genoytypes prevalent in the early 1980s disappeared and only one genotype, clonotype II-A, remained with its elevated level of methicillin resistance [32]. Note in Plate 9.1 that only two clonotype II-A strains remained that were susceptible and moderately resistant to methicillin. Therefore, the significant feature of MRSA with clonotype II-A genotype is the ability to acquire homogeneously high methicillin resistance on exposure to potent β-lactam antibiotics. The rapid spread of homo-MRSA strains in hospitals was a unique situation with regard to MRSA epidemiology when vancomycin was first introduced into clinical use in 1991.

Figure 9.4 shows the annual amount of vancomycin (in defined daily dose) sold in Japan by Shionogi & Company. This pharmaceutical company was the only one selling vancomycin until 2002, and vancomycin was the only glycopeptide antibiotic until 1998, the year teicoplanin was introduced for clinical use. Therefore, the amount sold by the company corresponds with the national consumption of vancomycin from 1991 to 1998. The steep rise in the graph reflects the explosive use of vancomycin for MRSA infection during those years. When compared with the annual detection rate of VISA among MRSA in JUH (see Figure 9.2), it is noticeable that the VISA rate increased with the introduction of vancomycin but its decline was disproportionate to the national trend of vancomycin consumption (vancomycin consumption curve in JUH 1995–2002 is practically parallel to the national consumption curve; S. Hori *et al.*, unpublished data). This indicates that the use of vancomycin alone does not cause increase in VISA. This is an intriguing phenomenon that reveals the unique characteristics of Japanese MRSA strains (homo-MRSA with clonotype II-A) in the early 1990s. It is speculated that a number of hetero-VISA strains already existed among homo-MRSA strains irrespective of the introduction of vancomycin.

Figure 9.5 illustrates an *in vitro* experiment simulating the unique Japanese experience prior to vancomycin introduction in 1991. N315ΔIP, representing Japanese hetero-MRSA strain of clonotype II-A, was exposed to selective concentrations of imipenem. Among 50 derivative strains with elevated methicillin resistance (with homo-MRSA phenotype), one strain designated N315ΔIP-H14 showed heterogeneous vancomycin resistance in addition to high methicillin resistance. It is speculated that such hetero-VISA strains present among the homo-MRSA strains were exposed to vancomycin, yielding VISA strains in the early 1990s.

The disproportionate decline in VISA relative to the decrease in vancomycin consumption after 1997 was quite unexpected, but can be explained by the nature of the VISA phenotype. First, resistance to vancomycin carries a high fitness cost and the number of bacteria exhibiting intermediate resistance in a bacterial population tends to decline during competitive proliferation with susceptible counterparts in many generations under no selective pressure [36]. Second, hetero-VISA may not be selected by vancomycin as effectively as by β-lactam antibiotics. Clearly, the treatment of MRSA infection by β-lactam antibiotics in

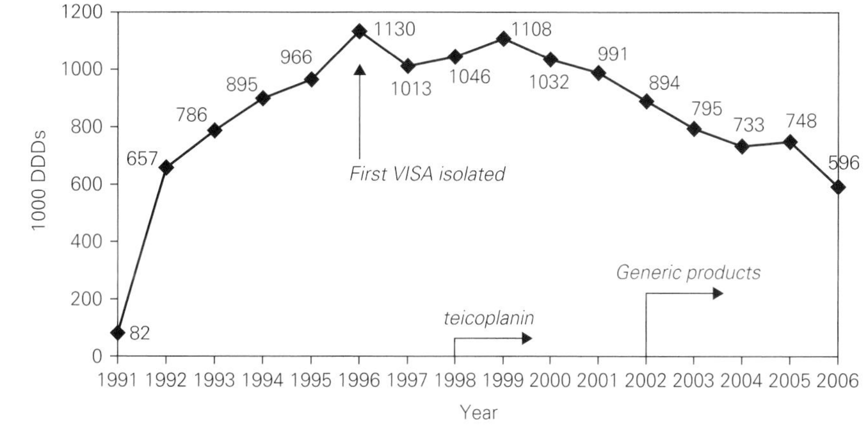

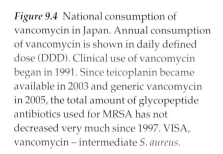

Figure 9.4 National consumption of vancomycin in Japan. Annual consumption of vancomycin is shown in daily defined dose (DDD). Clinical use of vancomycin began in 1991. Since teicoplanin became available in 2003 and generic vancomycin in 2005, the total amount of glycopeptide antibiotics used for MRSA has not decreased very much since 1997. VISA, vancomycin – intermediate *S. aureus*.

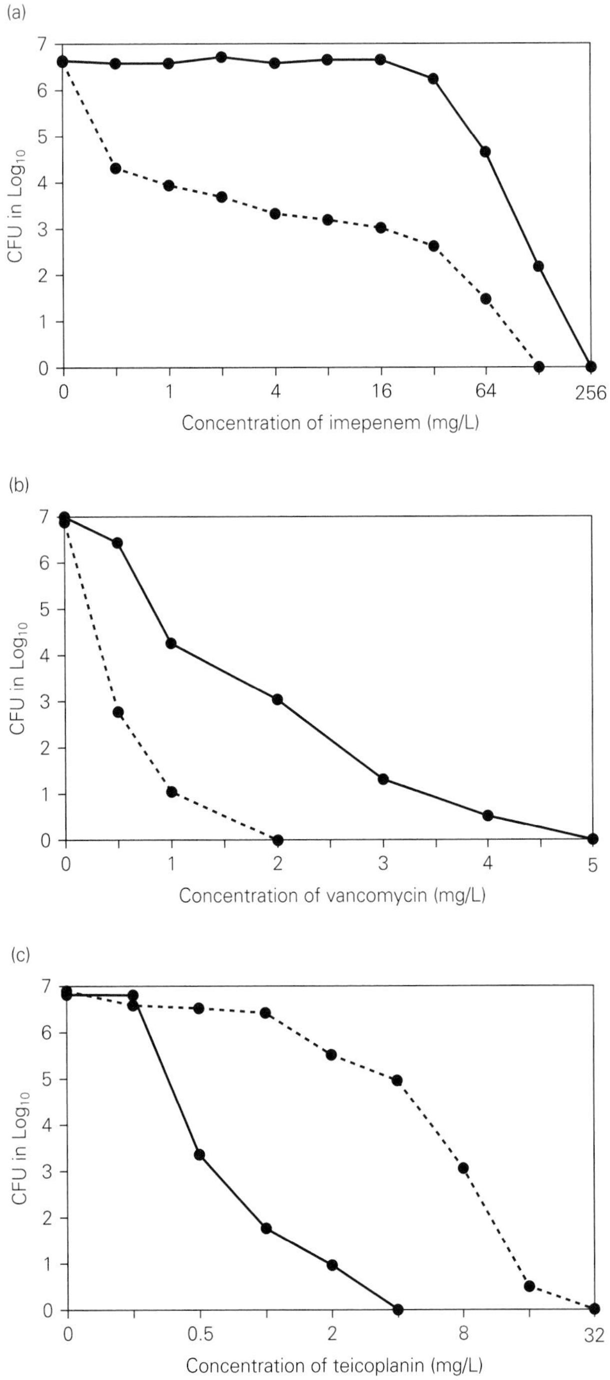

Figure 9.5 *In vitro* selection of clonotype II-A MRSA with imipenem generates hetero-VISA in the absence of vancomycin exposure. N315ΔIP was exposed to imipenem and derivative strains with increased methicillin resistance were isolated. One of the imipenem-selected homo-MRSA mutants turned out to be hetero-VISA. Analysis of resistant cell subpopulations (population analysis) of N315 (black circles) and its imipenem-selected mutant strain N315ΔIP-H14 (gray circles) is presented. The following antibiotics were tested: (a) imipenem; (b) vancomycin; (c) teicoplanin. The mutant N315ΔIP-H14 possessed a missense mutation in *vraS*, a sensor–transducer regulating cell wall synthesis (see text for details). (From Hiramatsu [36] with permission.)

the 1980s must have become less common with the availability of vancomycin after 1991. Thus, generation of hetero-VISA by β-lactam selection should have declined gradually in the 1990s. Since vancomycin consumption did not decrease significantly after 1997 and clonotype II-A MRSA continued to prevail, appropriate therapeutic use of vancomycin may not provide enough selective pressure on MRSA to yield hetero-VISA. In contrast, VRSA may have the potential to become a great threat in the future because it may retain resistance to vancomycin in the absence of continuous selective pressure [31]. In any case, the unique Japanese history of anti-MRSA chemotherapy now explains why VISA was first isolated in Japan. It also implies that VISA strains in Japan may also have unique genetic mechanisms of resistance compared with those of other countries where vancomycin has been in use since 1956.

Clinical significance of hetero-VISA

VISA is generated within cell populations of hetero-VISA. When VISA is repeatedly passaged in drug-free medium it tends to lose vancomycin resistance and reverts to hetero-VISA [37]. Subsequent exposure of hetero-VISA to vancomycin again selects out VISA at a greater efficiency of 10^{-3}–10^{-5} [37]. Thus, VISA is considered a subpopulation of hetero-VISA, and it appears in clinical settings when hetero-VISA-infected patients are treated with vancomycin. In fact, a closer look at clinical cases reveals that hetero-VISA precedes the clinical course and VISA is finally isolated several days after initiation of vancomycin therapy [38]. Therefore, we have to be aware that the prevalence of hetero-VISA in the hospital is an index of VISA prevalence, and vice versa [36].

Typical clinical case of hetero-VISA infection

The first hetero-VISA strain, Mu3, was isolated from an MRSA pneumonia case. About 6 months before the isolation of VISA strain Mu50, we encountered an unusual clinical case of MRSA pneumonia. The patient was treated with vancomycin for 11 days. Initially, the shadow on the chest radiograph became smaller, and fever subsided. However, from the seventh day, the shadow became denser and fever rose again despite continued drip infusion of vancomycin [24]. The patient was successfully treated with arbekacin (an aminoglycoside introduced in Japan in 1990) and ampicillin/sulbactam [15]. The MRSA strain isolated from the patient was hetero-VISA Mu3; the population analysis curve of this strain is illustrated in Figure 9.3. This figure shows that about 100 of 10^7 cfu were able to grow in the presence of vancomycin 4 mg/L (MIC > 4 mg/L), indicating that the Mu3 cell population contains VISA cells at a frequency of 1 in 100 000 cfu. It also contains a subpopulation of cells with much higher vancomycin resistance at a lower frequency (Figure 9.3). Some of the colonies that formed on plates containing vancomycin 4–9 mg/L exhibited intermediate vancomycin MICs

Table 9.1 Site of infection and clinical outcome of patients infected with hetero-VISA compared with those infected with VSSA.

Patient	Site of infection	No. of patients (%)			
		Total	Died or failure	Recovered	Not evaluable
Infected with hetero-VISA	Respiratory tract	7	4 (57.1)	3 (42.9)	
	Skin and soft tissue	3		3	
	Local abdomen	1		1	
	Overall	11	4 (36.4)	7 (63.6)	
Infected with VSSA	Surgical wound	36	3 (8.8)	31 (91.2)	2
	Skin and soft tissue	32	6 (20.7)	23 (79.3)	3
	Respiratory tract	19	6 (33.3)	12 (66.7)	1
	Bacteremia	13	5 (41.7)	7 (58.3)	1
	Urinary tract	7	1 (14.3)	6 (85.7)	
	Local abdomen	3	2 (66.7)	1 (33.3)	
	Peritonium	2	2		
	Eye	1		1	
	Overall	113	25 (23.6)	81 (76.4)	7

VISA, vancomycin-intermediate *S. aureus*; VSSA, vancomycin-susceptible *S. aureus*.

(8 mg/L) when tested again by population analysis [24]. This prompted us to search for VISA clinical isolates among the MRSA samples of JUH inpatients. We found that Mu50 isolated from an infant patient with surgical site infection 6 months after the isolation of Mu3 was the VISA strain with vancomycin MIC 8 mg/L [2]. The infant had undergone heart surgery and was infected with MRSA at the surgical site; 29 days of vancomycin therapy failed to resolve the infection. The patient was cured subsequently by combination therapy with sulbactam/ampicillin and arbekacin [15].

Mu50 and Mu3 were indistinguishable on pulsed-field gel electrophoresis (PFGE) and antibiogram except that Mu50 was additionally resistant to rifampin. The frequency of hetero-VISA in JUH in 1996 was 20% [24]. Since the rate of VISA in the same year was 0.2% (see Figure 9.2), the ratio of VISA to hetero-VISA was 1 : 100. Therefore, VISA is only the tip of the iceberg; the major source of resistance is submerged in the ocean as hetero-VISA.

Prospective study of hetero-VISA infection

To evaluate the clinical significance of hetero-VISA, we conducted a prospective study in collaboration with the Infection Control Team in Mahidol University Hospital, which enrolled a total of 124 MRSA-infected patients during the period 1999–2001. Screening for hetero-VISA strains was performed by spreading the overnight culture (10^7 cfu) onto BHI agar plates containing vancomycin 4 mg/L. Those strains yielding colonies were subsequently analyzed by population analysis. The procedure identified a total of 11 hetero-VISA strains among 124 MRSA strains (each strain representing one patient).

Table 9.1 shows the sites of MRSA infection and the prognosis of the patients. This shows that most of the hetero-VISA strains (7 of 11, 63.6%) were isolated from lower respiratory tract infections. In contrast, VSSA strains rarely caused pneumonia (19 of 113, 16.8%). Therefore, a predilection for lower respiratory tract infection is an important clinical feature of hetero-VISA. Since MRSA strains with various genotypes, including the 11 hetero-VISA strains, caused lower respiratory tract infection, the preference of hetero-VISA for the respiratory tract was considered to be due to the vancomycin resistance phenotype rather than to the genetically determined affinity of the clone for lung tissue. The tissue concentration of vancomycin in the lung is as low as 2–3 mg/L [24]. Therefore, hetero-VISA with resistant subpopulations with MICs of 2–4 mg/L would be perfectly suited to survive vancomycin therapy. Hetero-VISA pneumonia caused more deaths than VSSA pneumonia (57.1% vs. 33.3%). This is probably associated with the limitations on tissue penetration of vancomycin rather than the greater virulence of hetero-VISA. Prolonged vancomycin therapy (> 14 days) was associated with 87.5% of hetero-VISA cases as compared with 41.2% of VSSA cases.

The MRSA strains in this hospital belonged to MLST 239 of clonal complex (CC)8 [30]. However, it was noted that 10 of 11 hetero-VISA strains had an identical pattern on PFGE, whereas the VSSA strains exhibited 14 pulsotypes including the type of the hetero-VISA strains. This again supports the view that hetero-VISA status is not easily achieved by all MRSA genotypes on exposure to vancomycin, and that an established hetero-VISA clone tends to transmit from patient to patient. It was also discovered that one of the 11 hetero-VISA strains had a unique genotype among the Thai MRSA strains. Remarkably, the pulsotype was closely associated with that of Mu3 and Mu50 (clonotype II-A), the most prevalent genotype of VISA strains throughout the world.

Detection of hetero-VISA

Development of a method to detect hetero-VISA was an important task, especially in hospitals where advanced medical practice such as cancer chemotherapy and organ transplantation are frequently performed. A disproportionate number of immunocompromised patients are treated in such institutions, and elevated consumption of antibiotics is unavoidable. The gold standard of hetero-VISA detection is population analysis [39]. However, this is a time-consuming method and not suitable for routine screening of many clinical strains. A simplified one-point population analysis can be performed for screening hundreds of clinical strains, and this was successfully used to survey the prevalence of hetero-VISA in several publications [24,29,40]. Antagonism between β-lactam and vancomycin against Mu3 [41] has been exploited as a disk diffusion method to detect hetero-VISA strains [3]. Although these are useful methods, they still require confirmation using population analysis.

It is reported that the E-test macro-method can be successfully used to detect hetero-VISA [42]. The cost-effectiveness for large-scale use may be the question for the E-test. For practical purposes, at JUH regular MIC tests have been used for the detection of at least some hetero-VISA strains in routine vancomycin susceptibility tests. Instead of reading the results only after 24 hours of incubation, results are also read 48 hours after incubation. This is an easy way to detect at least some proportions of hetero-VISA and VISA without any additional resources or labor. This practice is based on our observation of colony size variation of hetero-VISA strain Mu3 [43]. The VISA phenotype is closely associated with increased cell wall thickness and decreased doubling time (i.e., growth rate) of the strains [37]. Slow growth of VISA has been experienced in the clinical laboratory as well [44]. Therefore we can speculate that VISA cells spontaneously generated within the population of hetero-VISA grow more slowly than the major cell population. Mu3 will form at least five distinct colony size classes on drug-free BHI agar plates: regular-sized colony (RC), small colony (SC), pinpoint colony (PC), colony formed after 48 hours (C2), and colony formed after 72 hours (C3) [43]. The latter two may be regarded as small-colony variants with as yet unknown alterations in metabolic pathway(s). PC strains have relatively higher vancomycin resistance than those belonging to the other colony size classes [43]. Consequently, the MIC of hetero-VISA judged after 48 hours tends to be greater than the MIC value after 24 hours.

The colony size variation of Mu3 appears to correlate with the underlying genetic mechanism of the conversion of hetero-VISA to VISA (discussed later). Cells forming smaller colonies within the hetero-VISA cell population may have an unfavorable metabolic status as a "side effect" of a mutation responsible for vancomycin resistance expression. This perturbed metabolic status may be resolved after the incorporation of additional mutations that would serve to stabilize cell physiology. If a certain degree of improvement in relative fitness is achieved without loss of vancomycin resistance, then the population would be recognized as VISA during the course of vancomycin therapy. However, premature VISA with unstable physiology first generated in cell populations of hetero-VISA may not become stabilized with the VISA phenotype. Instead it might suffer a critical defect in the gene responsible for vancomycin resistance and revert to VSSA. We have identified an illustrative strain Mu50Ω representing this phenomenon. Strain Mu50Ω (vancomycin MIC 1 mg/L) was isolated 1 year later from the patient from whom Mu50 (MIC 8 mg/L) was isolated [45]. The strain was vancomycin susceptible, because the *vraS* gene was inactivated by incorporation of a nonsense mutation within the coding region (L. Cui *et al.*, 2009). Regardless of the stability of VISA cells generated in cell populations of hetero-VISA, a retarded growth rate is likely to be associated with increased vancomycin resistance. Therefore, if the bacteriology laboratory in the hospital is using an automated MIC detection system such as Walkaway, evaluation of MIC values should include readings at 48 or even 72 hours after incubation in addition to 24 hours after incubation to enhance the detection of hetero-VISA. If the isolate showed an MIC of 4 mg/L at 48 hours or later, it is very likely that the strain is hetero-VISA. Since this method does not require any additional labor for clinical technologists or any additional resources, we recommend this for routine use. The same method was successfully used to detect *vanB*-positive VRE, which showed susceptible vancomycin MICs at 24 hours but intermediate MICs at 48 hours (M. Ikeda *et al.*, published in Japanese). Using this information, we could detect the nonsymptomatic spread of VRE within a ward at JUH, and could implement measures to prevent an outbreak of VRE infection.

Mechanisms of vancomycin resistance

VRSA

van gene-mediated resistance

VRE was discovered in 1986, and its extraordinary mechanisms of vancomycin resistance elucidated by the early 1990s. Resistance is due to a complete change in the

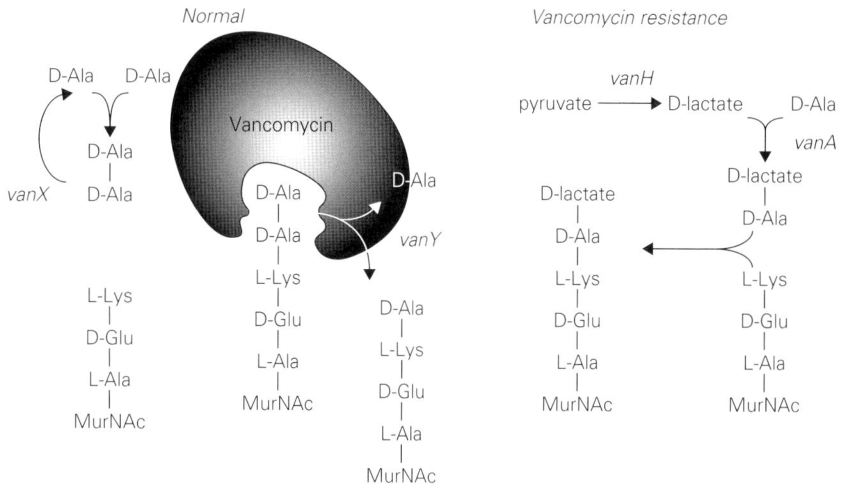

Figure 9.6 Four *van* gene products work together to attain full expression of vancomycin resistance in VRSA. VanH dehydrogenase reduces pyruvate to D-lactate (D-Lac). Then VanA ligates D-lactate with D-alanine and the resulting depsipeptide D-Ala-D-Lac is ligated to MurNAc-L-Ala-D-Glu-L-Lys by the host cell enzyme to produce muramyl pentadepsipeptide. To prevent any incorporation of the normal muramyl pentapeptide, VanX dipeptidase hydrolyzes D-alanyl-D-alanine before it is ligated to the muramyl tripeptide, and VanY D,D-carboxypeptidase cleaves between D-alanyl-D-alanine residues of the completed murein monomer precursor. As a result, normal muramyl pentapeptide is completely replaced by the muramyl pentadepsipeptide when the four gene products cooperate in vancomycin-resistant enterococci.

chemical structure of cell wall peptidoglycan precursor molecules such that the binding site for vancomycin (D-alanyl-D-alanine residue) is missing from the cell surface of VRE. This drastic change was brought about as a result of cooperative expression of at least four genes, *vanA*, *vanH*, *vanX*, and *vanY* found on Tn*1546* [6]. Figure 9.6 illustrates how the four *van* genes on the *vanA* gene plasmid work together to replace normal murein monomer precursor of the host cell with the altered structure. First, VanH dehydrogenase reduces pyruvate to D-lactate (D-Lac). Then VanA ligates D-lactate with D-alanine. The depsipeptide D-Ala-D-Lac thus produced is ligated to MurNAc-L-Ala-D-Glu-L-Lys by the host cell enzyme, thus providing muramyl pentadepsipeptide. However, the host cell also provides muramyl pentapeptide containing D-Ala-D-Ala dipeptide at its terminus. If the cell produced a considerable proportion of the normal murein monomer precursors, vancomycin would still bind to them and exert antimicrobial activity. However, VanX dipeptidase hydrolyzes D-alanyl-D-alanine before it is ligated to the muramyl tripeptide and, furthermore, VanY D,D-carboxypeptidase cleaves between D-alanyl-D-alanine residues of the completed murein monomer precursor. As a result, normal muramyl pentapeptide is completely replaced by the muramyl pentadepsipeptide when the four genes work together in the VRE cell. The same change of flow in the peptidoglycan synthesis pathway is expected to occur in VRSA cells. Tomasz's group demonstrated that this is the case by introducing the *vanA* gene-carrying *S. aureus* plasmid of a VRSA strain into MRSA strain COL [46].

vanA and *mecA*

As of August 2007, only seven VRSA strains have been isolated, all in the USA. The resistance mechanism is identical to that in VRE, namely alteration of cell wall peptidoglycan structure. A set of genes carried by a transposon on the plasmid replaces the target structure of vancomycin, D-alanyl-D-alanine of peptidoglycan, to D-alanyl-D-lactate to which vancomycin cannot bind. The mechanism is inducible by exposure to vancomycin, and is repressed by a two-component regulatory system *vanSR*, which is also a component of Tn*1546* [47]. The fitness cost associated with resistance is not as great as with VISA resistance because the resistance mechanism is not expressed in the absence of vancomycin. It is highly likely that VRSA, once generated, can persist without frequent exposure to vancomycin [31]. However, acquisition of *vanA* resistance may be a great disadvantage to the host MRSA strain. Figure 9.7 shows checkerboard susceptibility tests using vancomycin and oxacillin. It was noted that combination of the two antibiotics exerts synergistic antimicrobial activity against VRSA strains. The synergy of oxacillin and vancomycin was observed with all the seven strains so far analyzed (A. Tomiyama, unpublished observation). This is a curious phenomenon that is probably caused by the substrate-binding preference of *mecA*-encoded penicillin-binding protein (PBP)2′ (or PBP2a) [46]. Methicillin resistance is expressed because PBP2′ recognizes D-alanyl-D-alanine residues of murein in a transpeptidation reaction that cross-links nascent peptidoglycan chain to the preexisting peptidoglycan layers [48]. Since β-lactam antibiotics including methicillin are structural homologs of the

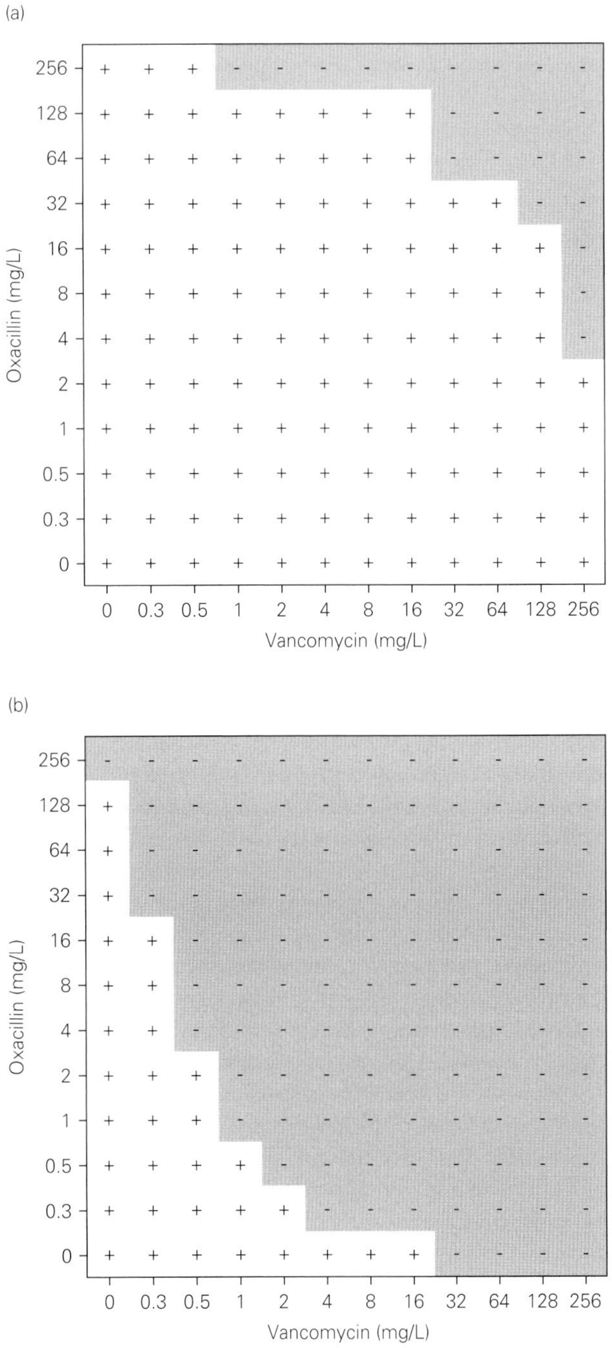

Figure 9.7 Oxacillin and vancomycin combination against two VRSA strains. (a) VRSA1 and (b) VRSA2 were cultured in various concentrations of oxacillin and vancomycin. Note that there is strong synergy between the two antibiotics. However, there is a subpopulation of VRSA1 that is capable of growth in clinically relevant concentrations of both antibiotics.

D-alanyl-D-alanine residue, they can covalently bind to the D-alanyl-D-alanine-binding pockets of *S. aureus* PBPs (there are four inherent PBPs, PBP1–4, in *S. aureus*), thus preventing the PBPs from performing cross-linking of the peptidoglycans. However, the binding pocket of PBP2′ has low binding affinities to β-lactam antibiotics while retaining the binding affinity to D-alanyl-D-alanine residues of peptidoglycan. Therefore, MRSA can continue synthesizing peptidoglycan in the presence of high concentrations of β-lactam antibiotics [36]. This logically leads to a critical question about whether PBP2′, despite its extraordinarily fastidious binding specificity, is able to recognize the D-alanyl-D-lactate residues with sufficiently high affinity. Tomasz's group observed that D-alanyl-D-lactate does not serve as an efficient substrate for transpeptidation by PBP2′ [46]. This incompatibility between *vanA*- and *mecA*-mediated resistance phenotype reflects in the strong synergistic effect of oxacillin and vancomycin (Figure 9.7). This synergy was utilized successfully in the treatment of experimental endocarditis caused by VRSA with a combination of vancomycin and β-lactam antibiotics [49]. However, as Figure 9.7a shows, some colonies grow in the presence of vancomycin 64 mg/L and oxacillin 32 mg/L. Whether these colonies contain certain mutations that could tolerate the combination therapy of vancomycin and β-lactam is a critical question that affects future anti-VRSA chemotherapy.

VISA and hetero-VISA

Accelerated cell wall peptidoglycan synthesis

Vancomycin binds to D-alanyl-D-alanine residues of murein monomers on the cytoplasmic membrane (lipid II). Murein monomers are the substrate for the peptidoglycan synthesis enzyme, glycosyltransferase, which polymerizes them into nascent peptidoglycan chains. However, the enzyme cannot utilize vancomycin-bound murein monomers and therefore peptidoglycan synthesis stops in the presence of vancomycin. An initial study of ours on peptidoglycan synthesis in VISA strain Mu50 and hetero-VISA strain Mu3 showed that both exhibited increased cell wall synthesis relative to control VSSA strains [50]. There was a threefold to fivefold increase in expression of PBP2 and PBP2′, a fourfold to eightfold greater amount of cytoplasmic murein monomer precursor pool, a threefold to 20-fold increase in incorporation of GlcNAc into cell wall peptidoglycan, and increased turnover of cell wall material into culture medium as compared with control strains [50]. Therefore, hetero-VISA Mu3 was very different from VSSA strains and shared the abnormal physiological features with VISA strain Mu50. However, compared with Mu3, the cell wall of Mu50 had increased amounts of glutamine nonamidated muropeptides and decreased cross-linking of peptidoglycan [51]. Since glutamine nonamidated murein monomers serve as a poor substrate for PBP-mediated transpeptidation, the cell wall peptidoglycan of Mu50 is under-cross-linked and a large number of D-Ala-D-Ala residues are present in the peptidoglycan [52]. As a result, a unit weight of peptidoglycan of Mu50 binds 1.4 times more vancomycin molecules than that of Mu3. Since the peptidoglycan layers of Mu50 are about twice as thick as Mu3, a single Mu50 cell is estimated to bind 2.8 times (2 × 1.4) more vancomycin molecules than a single Mu3 cell. Moreover, vancomycin binds to glutamine nonamidated muropeptide with higher affinity than to amidated muropeptide [51]. Therefore, the cell wall of Mu50 adsorbs far more vancomycin molecules than Mu3 and VSSA cells. Since the vancomycin-binding sites in the cell-wall peptidoglycan layers are not the real targets of vancomcyin action (i.e., pseudotargets [3]), a large number of vancomycin molecules are sequestered in the peptidoglycan layers of Mu50 without exerting antimicrobial activity. The adsorption of vancomycin to the cell wall of Mu50 leads not only to a decrease in effective concentration of vancomycin in infected tissue but also to a decrease in vancomycin diffusion to the real target (lipid II) on the cytoplasmic membrane, as explained below.

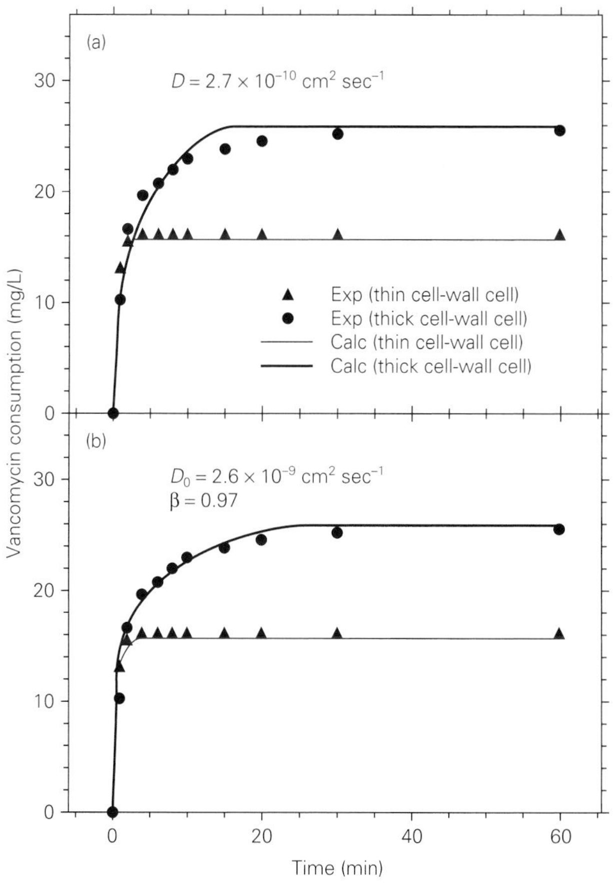

Figure 9.8 Consumption of vancomycin by the thick-cell-wall and thin-cell-wall cells of Mu50. (a) Vancomycin consumption curves for cells with thin and thick cell walls calculated using a standard reaction–diffusion equation with diffusion constant D and compared with experimental data. (b) Vancomycin consumption curves for cells with thin and thick cell walls calcluated using a clogging model according to equation 3 (see text) and compared with experimental data. (From Cui *et al.* [53] with permission.)

Clogging of peptidoglycan mesh of the thickened cell wall

Besides the adsorption of vancomycin, the thick cell wall of a VISA cell serves as an obstacle for vancomycin, delaying penetration of vancomycin molecules to the cytoplasmic membrane. All VISA strains so far tested have unusually thickened cell walls as a common feature [37]. Figure 9.8 illustrates the time-course of vancomycin consumption from the culture supernatant of Mu50 cells with thick and thin cell walls prepared experimentally in a defined medium (resting medium) with and without glucose, respectively [53]. The prolonged consumption of vancomycin observed with thick-cell-wall Mu50 cells signifies the delay in complete saturation with vancomycin at D-Ala-D-Ala residues present in both cell-wall peptidoglycan layers and lipid II in the cytoplasmic membrane. In contrast, consumption of vancomycin by thin-cell-wall cells quickly reached plateau within a few minutes. Calculation was performed using two mathematical models and the results compared with the experimental data. Competition between the diffusion (penetration) of vancomycin through the peptidoglycan layers and the binding reactions with their D-Ala-D-Ala residues is formulated into the following one-dimensional coupled equations:

$$\frac{\partial \upsilon(x,t)}{\partial t} = \frac{\partial}{\partial x}\left[D(x,t)\frac{\partial \upsilon(x,t)}{\partial x} \right] - k\upsilon(x,t)[M_0 - \nu(x,t)] \quad (1)$$

$$\frac{\partial (x,t)}{\partial t} = k\upsilon(x,t)[M_0 - (x,t)] \quad (2)$$

where $\upsilon(x,t)$ and $\nu(x,t)$ represent the concentrations of free and bound vancomycin respectively, M_0 the concentration of D-Ala-D-Ala residues at the initial time in the cell wall, and k the reaction rate for the binding of vancomycin and D-Ala-D-Ala residues. The diffusion coefficient $D(x,t)$ is a function of position (x) from the bacterial cell surface and time (t). Vancomycin consumption curves in Figure 9.8a for cells with thin and thick cell walls were calculated using the above formulae assuming that the diffusion coefficient D is constant throughout the course of vancomycin diffusion. It should be noted that the curve and experimental data are discrepant. In Figure 9.8b, the consumption curves were calculated using the assumption that the diffusion constant decreases with time, as shown in equation 3:

$$D(x,t) = D_0\left\{1 - \beta\frac{\nu(x,t)}{M_0}\right\} \quad (3)$$

The curve matches best with the experimental data when diffusion constant D_0 and clogging parameter β were determined as the best-fit values for these data. Therefore, clogging of the peptidoglycan mesh occurs in the thick-cell-wall peptidoglycan of VISA strains [53].

In the peptidoglycan clogging model, diminution of diffusion rate for vancomycin through the peptidoglycan layers causes the delay in timing of the vancomycin mediated inhibition of cell wall synthesis to occur after the blocking of lipid II by bound vancomycin molecules in the timing of inhibition of cell wall synthesis mediated by the blocking of all lipid II molecules by vancomycin. In the clinically infected tissues of patients, the available concentration of vancomycin is limited (< 5 mg/L). In such conditions, mathematical modeling predicts that the delay in timing would be greater than 15 min. This is a large delay compared with less than 1 min for VSSA strains with thin cell walls. VISA cells would continue growing by producing more peptidoglycan before vancomycin reaches the cytoplasmic membrane and blocks all the lipid II molecules there [53].

Genetic basis for vancomycin resistance in hetero-VISA

To explore the genetic basis for VISA phenotype, we analyzed the gene transcription profiles of VISA strain Mu50, hetero-VISA strain Mu3, and VSSA strain Mu50Ω. Strain Mu50Ω was isolated from the same patient from whom Mu50 was isolated. The patient visited JUH with a relapse of infection 1 year after discharge. The strain was isolated from a mediastinal drain together with VISA strain Mu50. Mu50Ω had an identical pattern on PFGE as Mu50 but was sensitive to vancomycin, with an MIC of 1 mg/L. Mu3, though isolated from a different patient, exhibited the same pattern on PFGE as Mu50 and Mu50Ω. Using differential hybridization, 11 novel genes whose transcription was upregulated in Mu50 compared with Mu50Ω were identified [45]. Among them, seven were found upregulated in Mu3 as well. This corresponds to our previous observation that Mu3 and Mu50 have similar physiological features associated with increased cell wall synthesis [50]. The other four genes consisted of two sets of ABC transporter genes, designated *vraDE* and *vraFG* (see next section). The most significant of the 11 upregulated genes was *vraR*, which encodes a response regulator of the two-component regulatory system *vraSR* [54]. VraSR turned out to be a positive regulator of cell wall synthesis. The sensor transducer VraS is a membrane protein and responds to the exposure of cells to various antibiotics acting on peptidoglycan synthesis, such as β-lactams, vancomycin, teicoplanin, bacitracin, and fosfomycin [54]. Later it was shown that *vraSR* also responds to an experimentally manipulated condition where the cell-wall synthesis enzyme PBP2 was underexpressed [55]. Thus, signal transducer protein VraS seems to sense the inhibition of smooth cell wall synthesis or perturbation of cell metabolism as a consequence of inhibited cell wall synthesis. Activated VraS then phosphorylates VraR, converting it to the active form, which then upregulates at least 50 genes encoding known or as yet unknown functions [54]. Among these regulated genes are those encoding enzymes involved in cell wall peptidoglycan synthesis such as PBP2 (*pbp2*), UDP-*N*-acetylglucosamine enolpyruvyltransferase (*murZ*), and monofunctional glycosyltransferase (*sgtB*) [54]. Overexpression of the *vraR* gene confers upon *S. aureus* resistance to most cell-wall synthesis inhibitor antibiotics such as β-lactams, teicoplanin, vancomycin, fosfomycin, and bacitracin [54]. Furthermore, overexpression of the *vraS* gene was demonstrated in the laboratory-derived strain N315ΔIP-H14. This strain (described on p. 197) was found among the homo-MRSA strains generated *in vitro* by selecting hetero-MRSA strain N315ΔIP with imipenem. As shown in Table 9.2, H14 exhibited resistance to multiple cell-wall synthesis inhibitor antibiotics besides β-lactams. N315ΔIP-H14 also shows a typical hetero-VISA phenotype (see Figure 9.5). The strain harbored a mutation in *vraS*. The mutated *vraS* gene, *vraSH14*, was then introduced into N315ΔIP by gene replacement. The resultant strain N315ΔIP-*vraSH14* showed an identical resistance profile to that of N315ΔIP-H14 (Table 9.2). The transcription of *vraR* is enhanced in N315ΔIP-*vraSH14*, showing that the mutation in *vraS* is responsible for the increased transcription of *vraR* and upregulation of cell wall synthesis (Y. Katayama *et al.*, submitted (now modified, will be accepted soon.)). This explains why hetero-VISA strains were already prevalent in Japan in 1996 only 5 years after the introduction of vancomycin (see Figure 9.2).

When compared with that of N315, the *vraS* genes of Mu3 and Mu50 suffered a common mutation. Although the position of the mutation differs from that found in N315ΔIP-H14, the mutated gene also caused heterogeneous

Table 9.2 Antibiotic susceptibility of N315ΔIP and its derivative strains.

Strain	Ampicillin MIC (mg/L)	Oxacillin MIC (mg/L)	Imipenem MIC (mg/L)	Vancomycin MIC (mg/L)	Teicoplanin MIC (mg/L)	Fosfomycin MIC (mg/L)	Bacitracin MIC (mg/L)	Daptomycin MIC (mg/L)	Gentamicin MIC (mg/L)
N315ΔIP	2	6	0.75	1	1	1	32	0.75	0.75
N315ΔIP-H14	12	> 256	> 32	2	8	96	96	1.75	0.75
N315ΔIP-*vraSH14*	12	> 256	> 32	2	8	96	96	1.75	0.75
Mu3	16	> 256	> 32	3	24	> 1024	256	2	384

vancomycin resistance when introduced into N315ΔIP (Y. Katayama, unpublished observation).

Conversion of hetero-VISA to VISA

Whole-genome sequencing of strains Mu50 and Mu3 was performed to identify the genetic alterations underlying the phenotypic conversion from hetero-VISA to VISA [56]. A total of 16 single nucleotide polymorphisms (SNPs) and three mismatches were found [56]. Among them, there was a missense mutation in *graSR*, another two-component system present in the *S. aureus* genome (there are a total of 17 two-component systems in the genome). Unlike *vraSR*, however, the mutation was identified in the response regulator gene *graR*. The mutated *graR* of Mu50, designated *graR**, had previously been observed to raise vancomycin MICs slightly when introduced into N315 using the multicopy plasmid pYT3 [57]. We then found that introduction of *graR** into hetero-VISA strain Mu3 raised its vancomycin MIC to a level comparable with that of VISA strain Mu50 [56]. Transcription of *graSR* is not induced by vancomycin. However, deletion of the *graSR* operon of Mu3 decreased vancomycin MIC from 2 to 1 mg/L and teicoplanin MIC from 32 to 8 mg/L. Thus, it seems that *graSR*, at its natural level of expression, is already contributing to some extent to glycopeptide resistance in hetero-VISA. Complementation of glycopeptide resistance does occur by the introduction of *graR** alone in Mu3Δ*graRS*, a derivative strain deleted for both *graR* and *graS* genes. Therefore, GraR* seems to be functional without the activating signal from the putative signal transducer protein GraS. This implies that the mutated response regulator GraR* is already in an active form able to induce (or repress) effector genes involved in elevated glycopeptide resistance [56]. Expression of *graR** in Mu3 enhances the transcription of several genes whose transcription is also increased in Mu50 relative to Mu3. Among them are two sets of ABC transporters, *vraDE* and *vraFG*, and *mprF* (or *fmtC*). Transposon-mediated disruption of *mprF* is reported to cause increased vancomycin binding to the cytoplasmic membrane and increased susceptibility to vancomycin [58]. The *mprF* gene encodes lysylphosphatidylglycerol synthase [59], which modifies anionic phosphatidylglycerol with positively charged L-lysine, resulting in repulsion of cationic antibiotics from the cell surface [59]. Therefore, increased activity of *mprF* induced by *graR** expression might make the cell surface more positively charged and vancomycin molecules (positively charged) might be repulsed from the outer surface of the cytoplasmic membrane where its targets of action exist.

Introduction of *graR** (on high copy-number plasmid pYT3) into Mu3 caused thickening of the cell wall, decreased autolysis, and reduced growth rate [56]. Therefore, introduction of the *graR** gene was found to convert hetero-VISA Mu3 into a VISA strain whose biological properties were very similar to Mu50 [56].

Why are mutations in regulators required for VISA?

We have just started to learn the genetic mechanism of VISA, and we expect more diverse genetic mechanisms will be found in the future. However, it is also clear that the expected physiological outcome of the genetic alterations underlying the VISA phenotype is a thickened cell-wall peptidoglycan layer on the cell surface that prevents the access of vancomycin to its target in the cytoplasmic membrane. In this sense, we expect to find different combinations of mutations that would lead to this common phenotypic feature. A considerable number of separate mutations would likely be required to endow a VSSA strain with this phenotype. For example, the number of mutations required for activation of all the genes of the cell wall synthesis pathway would be enormous. Furthermore, the enzymes must be produced at a balanced rate so that efficient production of cell wall is guaranteed. To achieve VISA status with only a small number of mutations it would be necessary to take advantage of regulator genes. If enhancement of cell wall synthesis is achieved by a single mutation in *vraS*, and if reduction of cell wall turnover and accumulation of excess amounts of cell wall peptidoglycan are achieved by a single mutation in *graR*, VISA might be generated even within the cell population of a VSSA strain in the body of a patient. This may be the advantage of "regulator-gene mutations" as an efficient strategy for survival of bacteria [60]. Since single mutations in *vraSR* and *graRS* would alter the expression of more than 100 genes, extreme perturbation of cellular function would be brought about. Several complementary mutations would be generated spontaneously. A dozen of the SNPs observed between Mu3 and Mu50 might correspond to such complementary mutations. The cell population of the regulator-mutated *S. aureus* would become a mixture of a huge number of mutants with a heterogeneous profile of vancomycin susceptibility. This would correspond to the phenotype of "hetero-VISA." The most stable mutant cell would be selected out from this chaotic melting pot by vancomycin and established as a VISA strain.

Other genes of interest associated with vancomycin resistance

Besides *vraSR* and *graRS* underlying the expression of vancomycin resistance in the Mu3/Mu50 lineage, other genetic mechanisms have been implicated as contributing to vancomycin resistance in *S. aureus*. They may represent other mechanisms for the generation of VISA under different selective pressures from those under which Mu3 and Mu50 were generated (see p. 197 for discussion) or they may augment vancomycin resistance beyond the level attained by mutations in *vraSR* and *graRS*. With a thick peptidoglycan layer, the cell could afford to decrease cross-linking and subsequently increase the number of vancomycin-binding sites (D-Ala-D-Ala residues) without sacrificing the strength of its cell wall. Cross-linking can be decreased by repressing expression of PBP4, known as a secondary transpeptidase [61]. Reportedly, cell wall thickening is also induced by the overexpression of the alternative sigma factor SigB, which could also contribute to resistance [62].

Electronic repulsion of positively charged vancomycin molecules from the cell surface is implicated upon altered expression of the *dltABCD* operon, which is responsible for the D-alanine transfer into teichoic acids on the cell surface [63]. Since D-alanine esters introduce positively charged amino groups into negatively charged teichoic acids, disruption of the operon makes the cell adsorb more vancomycin molecules and thus makes cells more susceptible to vancomycin. Another gene of interest is *mprF* (*fmtC*). As mentioned above, inactivation of *mprF* by transposon insertion causes significant increase in the binding of vancomycin, and increased susceptibility to vancomycin, likely by reducing the overall positive charge associated with the cell surface [58]. Transcription of *mprF* is enhanced in Mu50 and Mu3 (p*graR**) but not in Mu3, indicating that this mechanism might be at work in VISA strain Mu50 [56]. The *lysC* gene, encoding aspartokinase II, involved in the biosynthesis of lysine from aspartic acid, is also reported to influence vancomycin susceptibility [64].

The *tcaA* gene, encoding putative membrane protein with a metal-binding motif, is reported to mediate teicoplanin susceptibility [65]. The gene is truncated in VISA strain MI, and complementation with intact *tcaA* gene recovered its susceptibility to teicoplanin [66]. It is speculated that TcaA may interact with teicoplanin in the outer surface of the cytoplasmic membrane [66].

In addition to the above genes, there is a list of *S. aureus* genes whose introduction into VSSA strain N315 increases its vancomycin MIC [57]. The list includes such genes as *mgrA* [67], *msrA2* [68], and *msrR* [69]. However, it remains to be investigated whether these genes really are involved in clinically isolated VISA or hetero-VISA strains.

Finally, destruction of the accessory gene regulator (*agr*) two-component system is frequently seen in VISA clinical strains [70]. It has also been pointed out that *agr* group II is dominant in VISA and hetero-VISA [71]; Mu3 and Mu50 belong to *agr* group II.

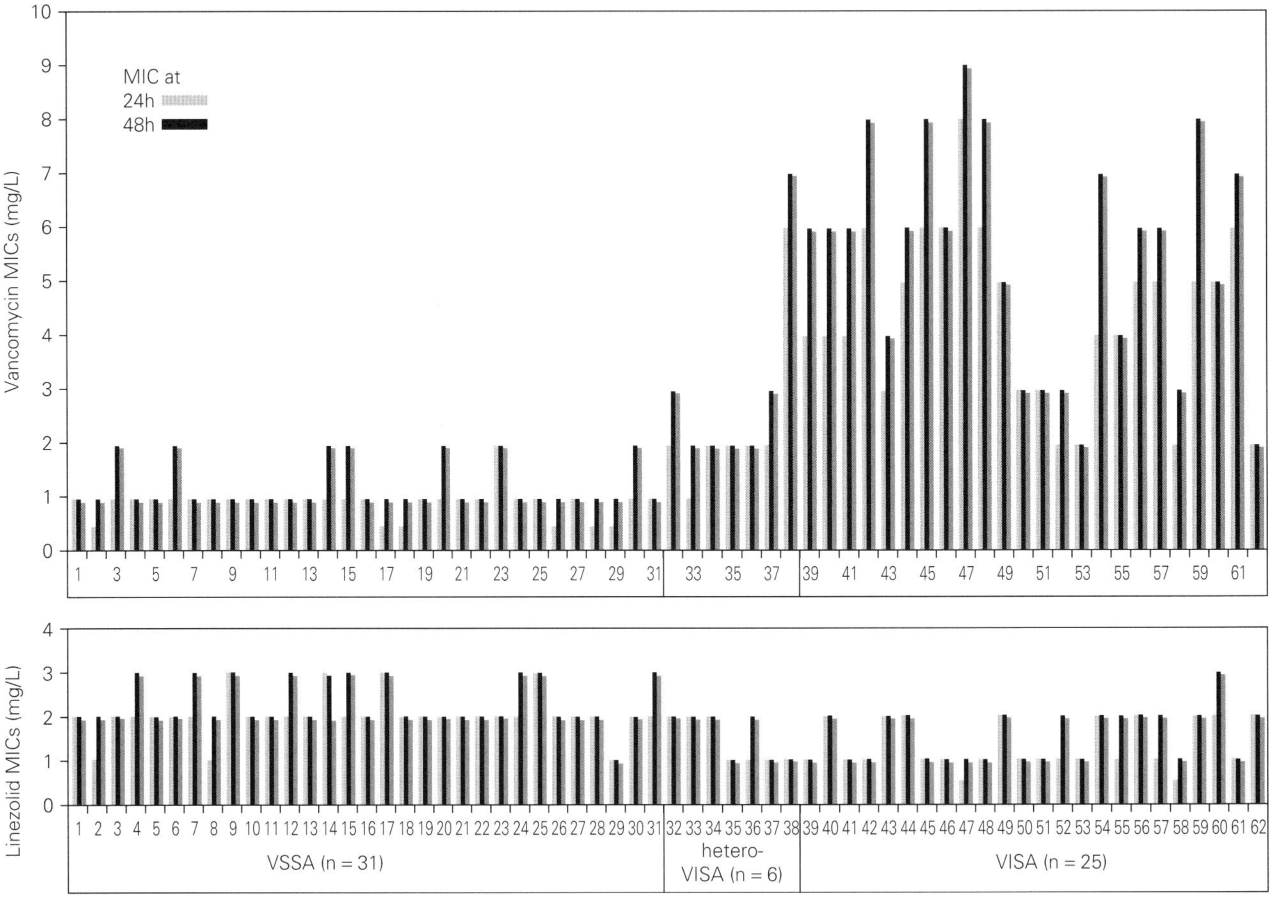

Figure 9.9 Inverse correlation between MICs of vancomycin and linezolid. The vertical axis represents the MIC of each strain measured at 24 and 48 hours after incubation. Note that vancomycin MICs of VISA strains tend to increase significantly after prolonged incubation (see text for discussion). Linezolid MICs of VISA strains are lower than those of VSSA strains.

Altered susceptibilities of VISA strains to other antibiotics

Most of the hetero-VISA strains so far analyzed have raised teicoplanin MICs (8–16 mg/L) compared with VSSA (≤ 4 mg/L). Shlaes and Shlaes [72] published a notable observation that teicoplanin resistance could be easily acquired by VSSA, and that the resultant teicoplanin-resistant derivatives were cross-resistant to vancomycin. As a matter of fact, before the clinical emergence of hetero-VISA and VISA in 1996, teicoplanin resistance was detected in some clinical *S. aureus* strains [60,73]. Intermediate teicoplanin resistance can be easily obtained *in vitro*. Introduction of high copies of the *pbp2* gene can raise the teicoplanin MIC of N315 from 1 to 8 mg/L without appreciably raising the vancomycin MIC [50]. Overproduction of PBP2 has also been reported in clinical strains [74], and it is speculated that the large number of PBP2 molecules in such strains compete with teicoplanin for binding to lipid II. As we have described above, the *pbp2* gene is listed among the genes upregulated by *vraSR* [54]. Therefore, these teicoplanin-resistant clinical strains might have been hetero-VISA, which may have been overlooked because of the relatively low-level increase in vancomycin MIC. It was only after our experience of clinical failure of therapy of a pneumonia patient that strains such as Mu3, with vancomycin MICs in the "susceptible" range, could be categorized as clinically "resistant" to vancomycin therapy [3]. Since certain hetero-VISA and VISA strains have activated *vraS*, it is not surprising that they tend to have greater resistance to most of the cell-wall synthesis inhibitor antibiotics such as β-lactams, teicoplanin, bacitracin, and fosfomycin [54]. In addition to the cell-wall synthesis inhibitor antibiotics, VISA strains are also cross-resistant to daptomycin [75]. Our data show that expression of *graR** also increases daptomycin MIC. However, the mechanism for the cross-resistance is not known at present.

Figure 9.9 shows a curious phenomenon regarding the susceptibilities of vancomycin and linezolid, one of the potent anti-MRSA chemotherapeutics. Unlike other antibiotics, linezolid tends to have better activity against VISA than VSSA (MRSA) strains [76]. Although the mechanism is unknown, this makes linezolid a unique agent for VISA infection. Since hetero-VISA infection is more frequent in pneumonia cases and vancomycin achieves limited tissue concentration in lung tissues, linezolid, which achieves high lung tissue concentrations, may be an ideal therapeutic for MRSA pneumonia caused by hetero-VISA (and VISA).

Acknowledgments

I thank all my colleagues in Juntendo University, especially Drs Teruyo Ito, Kyoko Kuwahara, Tadashi Baba, Longzhu Cui, Yuki Katayama, Miki Matsuo, Mayumi Aminaka, and Satoshi Hori, for data presentation and discussion. I also thank Dr Ayako Nakamura and Toyoko Oguri for the precious data of the Clinical Microbiology Laboratory in Juntendo Hospital and Prof. Somwang Danchaivijitr, Division of Infectious Disease, Department of Medicine Siriraj Hospital, Mahidol University for the data of the hetero VISA prospective study. I appreciate the cooperation of Shionogi & Company for the vancomycin consumption data.

References

1 Jevons M. Celbenin-resistant staphylococci. BMJ 1961;1:124–5.
2 Hiramatsu K, Hanaki H, Ino T, Yabuta K, Oguri T, Tenover FC. Methicillin-resistant *Staphylococcus aureus* clinical strain with reduced vancomycin susceptibility. J Antimicrob Chemother 1997;40:135–6.
3 Hiramatsu K. Vancomycin resistance in staphylococci. Drug Resist Updat 1998;1:135–50.
4 Watanakunakorn C. Mode of action and in-vitro activity of vancomycin. J Antimicrob Chemother 1984;14(suppl D):7–18.
5 Higgins DL, Chang R, Debabov DV *et al.* Telavancin, a multifunctional lipoglycopeptide, disrupts both cell wall synthesis and cell membrane integrity in methicillin-resistant *Staphylococcus aureus*. Antimicrob Agents Chemother 2005;49:1127–34.
6 Arthur M, Reynolds PE, Depardieu F *et al.* Mechanisms of glycopeptide resistance in enterococci. J Infect 1996;32:11–16.
7 Ito T, Katayama Y, Hiramatsu K. Cloning and nucleotide sequence determination of the entire mec DNA of pre-methicillin-resistant *Staphylococcus aureus* N315. Antimicrob Agents Chemother 1999;43:1449–58.
8 Kuroda M, Ohta T, Uchiyama I *et al.* Whole genome sequencing of meticillin-resistant *Staphylococcus aureus*. Lancet 2001; 357:1225–40.
9 Katayama Y, Ito T, Hiramatsu K. A new class of genetic element, staphylococcus cassette chromosome mec, encodes methicillin resistance in *Staphylococcus aureus*. Antimicrob Agents Chemother 2000;44:1549–55.
10 Ito T, Okuma K, Ma XX, Yuzawa H, Hiramatsu K. Insights on antibiotic resistance of *Staphylococcus aureus* from its whole genome: genomic island SCC. Drug Resist Updat 2003;6:41–52.
11 Centers for Disease Control. Vancomycin-resistant *Staphylococcus aureus*: Pennsylvania, 2002. MMWR 2002;51:902.
12 Centers for Disease Control. *Staphylococcus aureus* resistant to vancomycin: United States, 2002. MMWR 2002;51:565–7.
13 Arthur M, Depardieu F, Reynolds P, Courvalin P. Quantitative analysis of the metabolism of soluble cytoplasmic peptidoglycan precursors of glycopeptide-resistant enterococci. Mol Microbiol 1996;21:33–44.
14 Noble WC, Virani Z, Cree RG. Co-transfer of vancomycin and other resistance genes from *Enterococcus faecalis* NCTC 12201 to *Staphylococcus aureus*. FEMS Microbiol Lett 1992;72:195–8.
15 Clinical and Laboratory Standards Institute. Performance Standards for Antimicrobial Susceptibility Testing, 15th Informational Supplement M100-S15. Wayne, PA: Clinical and Laboratory Standards Institute, 2005.

16 Hiramatsu K. The emergence of *Staphylococcus aureus* with reduced susceptibility to vancomycin in Japan. Am J Med 1998;104:7S–10S.
17 Schwalbe RS, Stapleton JT, Gilligan PH. Emergence of vancomycin resistance in coagulase-negative staphylococci. N Engl J Med 1987;316:927–31.
18 Sanyal D, Johnson AP, George RC, Cookson BD, Williams AJ. Peritonitis due to vancomycin-resistant *Staphylococcus epidermidis*. Lancet 1991;337:54.
19 Wilson AP, O'Hare MD, Felmingham D, Gruneberg RN. Teicoplanin-resistant coagulase-negative staphylococcus. Lancet 1986;ii:973.
20 Takeuchi F, Watanabe S, Baba T *et al.* Whole-genome sequencing of *Staphylococcus haemolyticus* uncovers the extreme plasticity of its genome and the evolution of human-colonizing staphylococcal species. J Bacteriol 2005;187:7292–308.
21 Watanabe S, Ito T, Morimoto Y, Takeuchi F, Hiramatsu K. Precise excision and self-integration of a composite transposon as a model for spontaneous large-scale chromosome inversion/deletion of the *Staphylococcus haemolyticus* clinical strain JCSC1435. J Bacteriol 2007;189:2921–5.
22 Hiramatsu K, Kapi M, Tajima Y, Cui L, Trakulsomboon S, Ito T. Advances in vancomycin resistance: research in *Staphylococcus aureus*. In: White DG, Alekshun MN, McDermott PF, eds. Frontiers in Antimicrobial Resistance: a Tribute to Stuart B. Levy. Washington, DC: ASM Press, 2005:289–98.
23 Walsh TR, Howe RA. The prevalence and mechanisms of vancomycin resistance in *Staphylococcus aureus*. Annu Rev Microbiol 2002;56:657–75.
24 Hiramatsu K, Aritaka N, Hanaki H *et al.* Dissemination in Japanese hospitals of strains of *Staphylococcus aureus* heterogeneously resistant to vancomycin. Lancet 1997;350:1670–3.
25 Fridkin SK, Hageman J, McDougal LK *et al.* Epidemiological and microbiological characterization of infections caused by *Staphylococcus aureus* with reduced susceptibility to vancomycin, United States, 1997–2001. Clin Infect Dis 2003;36:429–39.
26 Hiramatsu K, Cui L, Kuroda M, Ito T. The emergence and evolution of methicillin-resistant *Staphylococcus aureus*. Trends Microbiol 2001;9:486–93.
27 Hiramatsu K, Kondo N, Ito T. Genetic basis for molecular epidemiology of MRSA. J Infect Chemother 1996;2:117–29.
28 Oliveira DC, Tomasz A, de Lencastre H. The evolution of pandemic clones of methicillin-resistant *Staphylococcus aureus*: identification of two ancestral genetic backgrounds and the associated mec elements. Microb Drug Resist 2001;7:349–61.
29 Song JH, Hiramatsu K, Suh JY *et al.* Emergence in Asian countries of *Staphylococcus aureus* with reduced susceptibility to vancomycin. Antimicrob Agents Chemother 2004;48:4926–8.
30 Chongtrakool P, Ito T, Ma XX *et al.* Staphylococcal cassette chromosome mec (SCCmec) typing of methicillin-resistant *Staphylococcus aureus* strains isolated in 11 Asian countries: a proposal for a new nomenclature for SCCmec elements. Antimicrob Agents Chemother 2006;50:1001–12.
31 Hiramatsu K, Cui L, Kuwahara-Arai K. Has vancomycin-resistant *Staphylococcus aureus* started going it alone? Lancet 2004;364:565–6.
32 Tanaka T, Okuzumi K, Iwamoto A, Hiramatsu K. A retrospective study on methicillin-resistant *Staphylococcus aureus* clinical strains in Tokyo University Hospital. J Infect Chemother 1995; 1:42–51.
33 Hiramatsu K. Molecular evolution of MRSA. Microbiol Immunol 1995;39:531–43.
34 Sabath LD, Wallace SJ. Factors influencing methicillin resistance in staphylococci. Ann NY Acad Sci 1971;182:258–66.
35 Matthews PR, Stewart PR. Resistance heterogeneity in methicillin-resistant *Staphylococcus aureus*. FEMS Microbiol Lett 1984;22:161–6.
36 Hiramatsu K. Vancomycin-resistant *Staphylococcus aureus*: a new model of antibiotic resistance. Lancet Infect Dis 2001;1:147–55.
37 Cui L, Ma X, Sato K *et al.* Cell wall thickening is a common feature of vancomycin resistance in *Staphylococcus aureus*. J Clin Microbiol 2003;41:5–14.
38 Haraga I, Nomura S, Fukamachi S *et al.* Emergence of vancomycin resistance during therapy against methicillin-resistant *Staphylococcus aureus* in a burn patient: importance of low-level resistance to vancomycin. Int J Infect Dis 2002;6:302–8.
39 Hanaki H, Nomura S, Akagi H, Hiramatsu K. Improvement of water-soluble cephalosporin derivatives having antibacterial activity against methicillin-resistant *Staphylococcus aureus*. Chemotherapy 2001;47:170–6.
40 Trakulsomboon S, Danchaivijitr S, Rongrungruang Y *et al.* First report of methicillin-resistant *Staphylococcus aureus* with reduced susceptibility to vancomycin in Thailand. J Clin Microbiol 2001;39:591–5.
41 Aritaka N, Hanaki H, Cui L, Hiramatsu K. Combination effect of vancomycin and beta-lactams against a *Staphylococcus aureus* strain, Mu3, with heterogeneous resistance to vancomycin. Antimicrob Agents Chemother 2001;45:1292–4.
42 Voss A, Mouton JW, Elzakker EP *et al.* A multi-center blinded study on the efficiency of phenotypic screening methods to detect glycopeptide intermediately susceptible *Staphylococcus aureus* (GISA) and heterogeneous GISA (h-GISA). Ann Clin Microbiol Antimicrob 2007;6:9.
43 Hiramatsu K, Watanabe S, Takeuchi F, Ito T, Baba T. Genetic characterization of methicillin-resistant *Staphylococcus aureus*. Vaccine 2004;22(suppl 1):S5–S8.
44 Marlowe EM, Cohen MD, Hindler JF, Ward KW, Bruckner DA. Practical strategies for detecting and confirming vancomycin-intermediate *Staphylococcus aureus*: a tertiary-care hospital laboratory's experience. J Clin Microbiol 2001;39:2637–9.
45 Kuroda M, Kuwahara-Arai K, Hiramatsu K. Identification of the up- and down-regulated genes in vancomycin-resistant *Staphylococcus aureus* strains Mu3 and Mu50 by cDNA differential hybridization method. Biochem Biophys Res Commun 2000;269:485–90.
46 Severin A, Tabei K, Tenover F, Chung M, Clarke N, Tomasz A. High level oxacillin and vancomycin resistance and altered cell wall composition in *Staphylococcus aureus* carrying the staphylococcal mecA and the enterococcal vanA gene complex. J Biol Chem 2004;279:3398–407.
47 Weigel LM, Clewell DB, Gill SR *et al.* Genetic analysis of a high-level vancomycin-resistant isolate of *Staphylococcus aureus*. Science 2003;302:1569–71.
48 Pinho MG, Filipe SR, de Lencastre H, Tomasz A. Complementation of the essential peptidoglycan transpeptidase function of penicillin-binding protein 2 (PBP2) by the drug resistance protein PBP2A in *Staphylococcus aureus*. J Bacteriol 2001;183: 6525–31.
49 Fox PM, Lampen RJ, Stumpf KS, Archer GL, Climo MW. Successful therapy of experimental endocarditis caused by

vancomycin-resistant *Staphylococcus aureus* with a combination of vancomycin and beta-lactam antibiotics. Antimicrob Agents Chemother 2006;50:2951–6.

50 Hanaki H, Kuwahara-Arai K, Boyle-Vavra S, Daum RS, Labischinski H, Hiramatsu K. Activated cell-wall synthesis is associated with vancomycin resistance in methicillin-resistant *Staphylococcus aureus* clinical strains Mu3 and Mu50. J Antimicrob Chemother 1998;42:199–209.

51 Hanaki H, Labischinski H, Inaba Y, Kondo N, Murakami H, Hiramatsu K. Increase in glutamine-non-amidated muropeptides in the peptidoglycan of vancomycin-resistant *Staphylococcus aureus* strain Mu50. J Antimicrob Chemother 1998;42:315–20.

52 Stranden AM, Roos M, Berger-Bachi B. Glutamine synthetase and heteroresistance in methicillin-resistant *Staphylococcus aureus*. Microb Drug Resist 1996;2:201–7.

53 Cui L, Iwamoto A, Lian JQ *et al.* Novel mechanism of antibiotic resistance originating in vancomycin-intermediate *Staphylococcus aureus*. Antimicrob Agents Chemother 2006;50:428–38.

54 Kuroda M, Kuroda H, Oshima T, Takeuchi F, Mori H, Hiramatsu K. Two-component system VraSR positively modulates the regulation of cell-wall biosynthesis pathway in *Staphylococcus aureus*. Mol Microbiol 2003;49:807–21.

55 Gardete S, Wu SW, Gill S, Tomasz A. Role of VraSR in antibiotic resistance and antibiotic-induced stress response in *Staphylococcus aureus*. Antimicrob Agents Chemother 2006;50:3424–34.

56 Neoh H-M, Cui L, Yuzawa H, Takeuchi F, Hiramatsu K. Mutated response-regulator *graR* is responsible for hetero-VISA to VISA phenotypic conversion of vancomycin resistance in *Staphylococcus aureus*. Antimicrob Agents Chemother 2007;52:45–53.

57 Cui L, Lian JQ, Neoh HM, Reyes E, Hiramatsu K. DNA microarray-based identification of genes associated with glycopeptide resistance in *Staphylococcus aureus*. Antimicrob Agents Chemother 2005;49:3404–13.

58 Ruzin A, Severin A, Moghazeh SL *et al.* Inactivation of mprF affects vancomycin susceptibility in *Staphylococcus aureus*. Biochim Biophys Acta 2003;1621:117–21.

59 Staubitz P, Neumann H, Schneider T, Wiedemann I, Peschel A. MprF-mediated biosynthesis of lysylphosphatidylglycerol, an important determinant in staphylococcal defensin resistance. FEMS Microbiol Lett 2004;231:67–71.

60 Hiramatsu K, Hanaki H. Glycopeptide resistance in staphylococci. Curr Opin Infect Dis 1998;11:653–8.

61 Sieradzki K, Pinho MG, Tomasz A. Inactivated pbp4 in highly glycopeptide-resistant laboratory mutants of *Staphylococcus aureus*. J Biol Chem 1999;274:18942–6.

62 Morikawa K, Maruyama A, Inose Y, Higashide M, Hayashi H, Ohta T. Overexpression of sigma factor, sigma(B), urges *Staphylococcus aureus* to thicken the cell wall and to resist beta-lactams. Biochem Biophys Res Commun 2001;288:385–9.

63 Peschel A, Vuong C, Otto M, Götz F. The D-alanine residues of *Staphylococcus aureus* teichoic acids alter the susceptibility to vancomycin and the activity of autolytic enzymes. Antimicrob Agents Chemother 2000;44:2845–7.

64 Nishi H, Komatsuzawa H, Fujiwara T, McCallum N, Sugai M. Reduced content of lysyl-phosphatidylglycerol in the cytoplasmic membrane affects susceptibility to moenomycin, as well as vancomycin, gentamicin, and antimicrobial peptides, in *Staphylococcus aureus*. Antimicrob Agents Chemother 2004;48:4800–7.

65 Brandenberger M, Tschierske M, Giachino P, Wada A, Berger-Bachi B. Inactivation of a novel three-cistronic operon *tcaR-tcaA-tcaB* increases teicoplanin resistance in *Staphylococcus aureus*. Biochim Biophys Acta 2000;1523:135–9.

66 Maki H, McCallum N, Bischoff M, Wada A, Berger-Bachi B. *tcaA* inactivation increases glycopeptide resistance in *Staphylococcus aureus*. Antimicrob Agents Chemother 2004;48:1953–9.

67 Kaatz GW, Thyagarajan RV, Seo SM. Effect of promoter region mutations and *mgrA* overexpression on transcription of *norA*, which encodes a *Staphylococcus aureus* multidrug efflux transporter. Antimicrob Agents Chemother 2005;49:161–9.

68 Singh VK, Moskovitz J. Multiple methionine sulfoxide reductase genes in *Staphylococcus aureus*: expression of activity and roles in tolerance of oxidative stress. Microbiology 2003;149:2739–47.

69 Rossi J, Bischoff M, Wada A, Berger-Bachi B. MsrR, a putative cell envelope-associated element involved in *Staphylococcus aureus sarA* attenuation. Antimicrob Agents Chemother 2003;47:2558–64.

70 Sakoulas G, Eliopoulos GM, Fowler VG Jr *et al.* Reduced susceptibility of *Staphylococcus aureus* to vancomycin and platelet microbicidal protein correlates with defective autolysis and loss of accessory gene regulator (*agr*) function. Antimicrob Agents Chemother 2005;49:2687–92.

71 Sakoulas G, Eliopoulos GM, Moellering RC Jr *et al.* Accessory gene regulator (*agr*) locus in geographically diverse *Staphylococcus aureus* isolates with reduced susceptibility to vancomycin. Antimicrob Agents Chemother 2002;46:1492–502.

72 Shlaes DM, Shlaes JH. Teicoplanin selects for *Staphylococcus aureus* that is resistant to vancomycin. Clin Infect Dis 1995;20:1071–3.

73 Kaatz GW, Seo SM, Dorman NJ, Lerner SA. Emergence of teicoplanin resistance during therapy of *Staphylococcus aureus* endocarditis. J Infect Dis 1990;162:103–8.

74 Shlaes DM, Shlaes JH, Vincent S, Etter L, Fey PD, Goering RV. Teicoplanin-resistant *Staphylococcus aureus* expresses a novel membrane protein and increases expression of penicillin-binding protein 2 complex. Antimicrob Agents Chemother 1993;37:2432–7.

75 Cui L, Tominaga E, Neoh HM, Hiramatsu K. Correlation between reduced daptomycin susceptibility and vancomycin resistance in vancomycin-intermediate *Staphylococcus aureus*. Antimicrob Agents Chemother 2006;50:1079–82.

76 Tajima Y, Komatsu M, Ito T, Hiramatsu K. Rapid detection of *Staphylococcus aureus* strains having reduced susceptibility to vancomycin using a chemiluminescence-based drug-susceptibility test. J Microbiol Methods 2007;70:434–41.

77 Leclercq R, Derlot E, Weber M, Duval J, Courvalin P. Transferable vancomycin and teicoplanin resistance in *Enterococcus faecium*. Antimicrob Agents Chemother 1989;33:10–15.

78 Cui L, Neoh HM, Shoji M, Hiramatsu K. Contribution of vraSR and graSR Point Mutations to Vancomycin Resistance in Vancomycin-intermediate *Staphylococcus aureus*. Antimicrob Agents Chemother 2009 Mar; 53(3):1231–4.

Chapter 10
Resistance to Other Agents

Jacob Strahilevitz[1] *and David C. Hooper*[2]
[1] Department of Clinical Microbiology and Infectious Diseases, Hebrew University, Jerusalem, Israel
[2] Division of Infectious Diseases, Massachusetts General Hospital, Boston, Massachusetts, USA

Introduction

In addition to β-lactams and glycopeptides, which have been the mainstay of antistaphylococcal antimicrobial therapy, a number of other antistaphylococcal agents have been increasingly used or newly developed, partly in response to emerging β-lactam and glycopeptide resistance. As with resistance to β-lactams and glycopeptides, resistance to other agents has also emerged, albeit to varying degrees and with a diversity of mechanisms as addressed in this chapter.

Mechanisms of resistance

Macrolides, ketolides, clindamycin, and streptogramins

Erythromycin, the first macrolide isolated in 1952 from a strain of *Saccharopolyspora erythraea*, was followed around 40 years later by the semisynthetic macrolide derivatives clarithromycin and roxithromycin (the latter not in use in the USA), the azalide azithromycin, and more recently by the ketolides telithromycin and cethromycin (ABT 773), which has been under clinical development [1]. The macrolides (and newer derivatives) are safe antibiotics useful as an alternative in patients with hypersensitivity to penicillins and other β-lactams. Among the macrolides, the activity of clarithromycin against methicillin-sensitive *Staphylococcus aureus* (MSSA) and methicillin-resistant *S. aureus* (MRSA) was slightly better (twofold) than those of other macrolides [2,3]. Telithromycin had at least a fourfold lower minimum inhibitory concentration (MIC) than that of the macrolides against macrolide-susceptible *S. aureus* strains [3,4] and manifested a pharmacodynamic activity similar to that of clarithromycin against *S. aureus* [5]. In general, because ketolides are weak inducers of ribosomal methylase (see below), they remain active against *S. aureus* strains carrying inducible MLS_B resistance (see next section) [6]. Clindamycin, a lincosamide, shares similar mechanisms of action and resistance with erythromycin but is chemically unrelated. Because the overall activity of clindamycin against *S. aureus* is better than that of erythromycin [7,8], clindamycin is often used as an alternative for patients with suspected staphylococcal infections, particularly those involving skin and soft tissues. However, increasing resistance in some MRSA strains has limited its utility [9,10]. The streptogramin antibiotics were discovered in the 1960s and have been used extensively in animal feed or as a therapeutic agent. Some, like pristinamycin, which is given orally and is available in Europe, and the more recently developed parenteral compound quinupristin/dalfopristin are effective drugs against MRSA [11–13].

All macrolides (and derivatives), clindamycin, and chloramphenicol (which is not discussed further in this chapter) interact with the 23S ribosomal RNA at the peptidyltransferase center and do not interact with ribosomal proteins. They are thus potentially subject to similar mechanisms of resistance [14]. The macrolides are thought to bind nucleotides at domain V of rRNA, located at the upper part of the ribosomal peptide exit tunnel, at a distance from the peptidyltransferase center. By this means they block the tunnel that channels the nascent peptides away from the peptidyltransferase center [15], allowing the formation of six to eight peptide bonds before the nascent protein chain reaches the bound macrolide and dissociation of peptidyl-tRNA occurs [14]. Although ketolides bind to a similar region of the ribosome as do macrolides, they also possess a second site of interaction with the ribosome at domain II on the 23S rRNA of the 50S ribosomal subunit and thereby have substantially higher binding affinity that allows binding to erythromycin-resistant ribosomes [16].

The lincosamides interact with both the acceptor A and donor P sites of the ribosome. Clindamycin interferes with the positioning of the aminoacyl group at the A site and the peptidyl group at the P site while also sterically blocking the progression of the nascent peptide toward the tunnel, thereby physically hindering the path of the growing peptide chain. This hinderance induces dissociation of peptidyl-tRNAs containing only two to four amino acid

Staphylococci in Human Disease, 2nd edition. Edited by Kent B. Crossley, Kimberly K. Jefferson, Gordon Archer, Vance G. Fowler, Jr.
ISBN 978-14051-6332-3.

residues [14,17]. Thus, the primary effect of the lincosamide drugs is to inhibit the formation of peptide bonds, whereas the main effect of macrolides is to block the passage of the newly synthesized peptide chain through the exit tunnel.

The streptogramins are unique among the ribosome-targeting antibiotics because they consist of two components, type A streptogramins (S_A) and type B streptogramins (S_B), which together act synergistically [18]. Dalfopristin, a type A streptogramin, interferes with positioning of both the A-site and P-site substrates but not in the case of ribosomes actively engaged in protein synthesis. Quinupristin, a type B streptogramin, functions at a later stage of protein synthesis than dalfopristin by binding and occupying the same space in the 23S rRNA as the macrolides [19,20]. The synergistic inhibitory activity of type A and type B streptogramins is attributable to the strong hydrophobic interactions between them that lead to a reduction of their solvent accessible surface and to increases in the conformational changes in the universally conserved nucleotide U2585 in the 50S ribosomal subunit that are induced by the attachment of the type A streptogramin. In addition, type A and B streptogramins inhibit the early and late stages respectively of protein synthesis [19,20].

The two main mechanisms of macrolide resistance in *S. aureus* are ribosomal modification by methylation and drug efflux, which confer high- and low-level resistance respectively. Additional mechanisms include drug modification.

MLS_B ribosomal methylation

The N^6-dimethylation of a highly conserved adenine residue A2058 (*Escherichia coli* numbering) in the 23S rRNA [21] is effected by a ribosomal methylase encoded by the *erm* (*e*rythromycin *r*ibosomal *m*ethylase) genes and leads to a conformational change in the ribosome that prevents binding of erythromycin, other macrolides, lincosamides, and type B streptogramins. This modification protects the ribosome from these several drug classes and effects a resistance phenotype known as MLS_B (macrolide lincosamide streptogramin B) [14,22]. The prototype genes of this class of mechanism of resistance, which is prevalent among many taxa, were initially discovered in *S. aureus* [23]. Several distinct methylase genes have been detected in staphylococci, including *ermA*, *ermB* (also named *ermAM*), *ermC* [24–26], and more recently *ermF* [27] and *ermY* (originally designated *ermGM*) [28]. Expression of MLS_B resistance in staphylococci may be constitutive or inducible. When expression is constitutive, the strains are resistant to all macrolides, ketolides [29], lincosamides, and type B streptogramin antibiotics. When expression is inducible, the strains are resistant to the 14-membered (erythromycin, roxithromycin, and often oleandomycin) and 15-membered (azithromycin) macrolides only. The 16-membered macrolides (spiramycin, josamycin, miocamycin, and midecamycin), the ketolides, the lincosamides, and the streptogramin antibiotics remain active. This dissociated resistance is due to differences in the inducing abilities of MLS antibiotics; only 14- and 15-membered macrolides are effective inducers of methylase synthesis [30]. In agar disk diffusion tests, D-shaped zones of inhibition around disks impregnated with a noninducing macrolide, a lincosamide, or a type B streptogramin can be observed if a disk of erythromycin is placed nearby [30,31]. Although treatment of infections caused by *S. aureus* strains that demonstrate inducible MLS_B resistance with clindamycin should not usually select for resistance to clindamycin, a few treatment failures have been reported [32], and changes in induction specificity have been reported in mutants of *S. aureus* obtained *in vitro* by selection with lincosamides [33,34]. These effects have led the Clinical Laboratory Standards Institute (formerly the National Committee for Clinical Laboratory Standards) to recommend that clindamycin-susceptible MLS_B-positive strains be reported as resistant by the laboratory with the following comment: "this isolate is presumed to be resistant based on detection of inducible clindamycin resistance. Clindamycin may still be effective in some patients." The ketolides, telithromycin and cethromycin (ABT 773), were also able to select for constitutive *ermA* mutants, in a mechanism similar to that of other macrolides [34] (see below). The inducible or constitutive character of resistance is not related to the class of *erm* determinant but depends on the DNA sequence of the regulatory region upstream from the structural gene for the methylase. The regulation of expression of the *ermC* determinant from staphylococcal plasmid pE194 has been extensively studied and is explained by a translation attenuation mechanism of an mRNA leader sequence [21,35]. In the absence of erythromycin, the mRNA is in an inactive conformation due to a sequestered Shine–Dalgarno sequence, preventing efficient initiation of translation of the *erm* transcripts. In the presence of erythromycin, an antibiotic-bound ribosome is thought to stall while translating the 19-amino-acid leader peptide located upstream from the methylase coding region [36]. Deletions, duplications, and multiple or single point mutations in the *erm* regulatory region can change inducible MLS_B phenotype into a constitutive MLS_B phenotype, with added resistance to all MLS_B antibiotics, including clindamycin and quinupristin [30]. Expression of *ermA* and *ermY* has always been inducible by erythromycin, whereas *ermB* is expressed constitutively in staphylococci, and the expression of *ermC* may be either inducible or constitutive [28,37]. Inducible strains predominated in the 1960s and 1970s. Today, however, it is more common in many geographical areas to find isolates that constitutively produce the rRNA methylase without preexposure to antibiotics [25]. Many of the *erm* genes are associated with conjugative or nonconjugative transposons, which tend to reside on the chromosome but have on occasion been found on plasmids. The *erm* genes are often associated with other antibiotic resistance genes, especially tetracycline resistance genes [25]. *ermA* is most often harbored on transposon Tn*554*, which also encodes resistance to the aminoglycoside spectinomycin. In epidemiological studies of erythromycin-resistant clinical isolates of *S. aureus*, recovered from patients hospitalized in Denmark and the USA from 1958 to 1969, *ermA* was found at varying locations on the chromosome, suggesting that transposons carrying *ermA* were acquired by *S. aureus* on multiple occasions [38,39]. *ermB* is often associated with transposon Tn*551* and the penicillinase plasmid, pI258, and was rare among human isolates of *S. aureus* [37,39]. The *ermC* gene, which appears to be rare in strains isolated prior to 1970 [39], has become more prevalent in recent years [38,40] and is normally located on small nonconjugative multicopy plasmids ranging in size from 2.4 to 5 kb [30]. *ermY*, encoding an inducible MLS_B phenotype, carried on plasmid pMS97, was found in a clinical isolate of *S. aureus* that also harbors *msrA* and *mphC*, genes that encode an efflux mechanism and a putative phosphorylase, respectively [28].

Other ribosomal modification mechanisms

In addition to resistance to macrolides via ribosomal modification in *trans* by the *erm* genes, modification can also be achieved in *cis*, via mutations of 23S rRNA (encoded by the *rrl* genes) and ribosomal proteins L4/L22, located near the macrolide-binding site of the ribosome, encoded by the *rplD* and *rplV* genes, respectively [26]. The latter resistance mechanism, which is most frequently associated with the A2058G mutation, the same residue methylated by Erm, has rarely been reported in organisms with more than two copies of 23 rRNA genes, such as *Streptococcus pneumoniae* (four copies) [41,42]. *Staphylococus aureus* carries five or six copies of rRNA genes and thus uncommonly carries mutational resistance to MLS_B antibiotics. In select settings, however, mutational macrolide resistance has been reported in *S. aureus*. Cystic fibrosis patients are chronically colonized with *S. aureus* and are commonly treated with antibiotics, thus leading to a state favoring hypermutability. A recent study of 20 erythromycin-resistant *S. aureus* isolates from nine patients with cystic fibrosis revealed that these strains were hypermutable and had various mutations in *rrl*, *rplD*, and *rplV* [43]. As in *Streptococcus pneumoniae* [41,42], the A2058G mutation did not necessarily confer resistance to clindamycin and quinupristin [43].

Drug inactivation

Enterobacteriaceae can inactivate erythromycin and other macrolides by esterase and phosphotransferase enzymes, but these mechanisms of resistance have rarely been described in *S. aureus*. Wondrack *et al.* [44] described an *S. aureus* strain that possessed weak esterase activity that hydrolyzed 14- and 16-membered macrolides (including erythromycin and clarithromycin), although a later report from the same group that screened isolates for resistance determinants did not identify the esterase-encoding genes *ereA* and *ereB* in that strain [45]. More recently, these genes were found in a few erythromycin-resistant *S. aureus* blood culture isolates [46]. Although a phosphotransferase encoded by *mphB* could also inactivate erythromycin in *S. aureus* [47], this gene has not yet been described in clinical isolates.

Lincosamide inactivation is more common than macrolide inactivation in *S. aureus* [24]. The gene *linA'*, located on pP856, a 2.6-kb nonconjugative plasmid, encodes 3-lincomycin 4-clindamycin *O*-nucleotidyltransferase that catalyzes the nucleotidylation of the hydroxyl group in position 4 of clindamycin [48]. Although clindamycin was inactivated in cell-free extracts of this strain, and it exhibited impaired bactericidal activity and decreased activity with high inocula of this strain, a resistance phenotype was not detected by routine methods of susceptibility testing [49], thus potentially leading to an erroneous report of susceptibility [50].

Resistance to streptogramin antibiotics by modification of both type A and type B components was first described in 1975 in *S. aureus* [24]. Type A streptogramins can be enzymatically inactivated by acetyltransferases, the most prevalent resistance mechanism for these agents. The virginiamycin acetyltransferases (Vat) can transfer an acetyl group from acetyl-CoA onto the secondary hydroxyl of a type A streptogramin. This hydroxyl, which is present in dalfopristin, forms a hydrogen bond with G2505 of the 23S rRNA, and acetylation prohibits drug binding to the ribosome by steric hindrance [20]. Genes *vat* [51] and the related *vatB* [52] encode such acetyltransferases and are flanked by two copies of the insertion sequence IS*257* and are located on conjugative plasmids. *vat* and *vatB* are frequently encountered in food animal strains of staphylococci and enterococci, probably reflecting the widespread use of the streptogramin virginiamycin as a growth promoter in animal husbandry [53]. Resistance to type A streptogramins and combinations of types A and B streptogramins (quinupristin/dalfopristin) in staphylococci is usually associated with the presence of multiple genes, such as *vat* in conjunction with *vga*, and *vgaB*, which encode drug efflux mechanisms, and *erm* encoding ribosomal methylases [54,55] (see below). The *vat* gene, which was initially cloned from plasmid pIP680, was shown to be contiguous to a *vgb* gene [51]. The other streptogramin inactivation mechanism associated with pathogenic bacteria is due to Vgb lyase, which inactivates type B streptogramins. Vgb was first described in a clinical isolate of *S. aureus* in 1977 [56]. The lyase activity encoded by *vgb*, which was originally found on a plasmid in *S. aureus* [57], linearizes the peptide at the ester linkage, generating an inactive antibiotic in a reaction facilitated by Mg^{2+} [56,58].

Drug efflux

Efflux is the other common mechanism of resistance to macrolides, clindamycin, and streptogramins in *S. aureus*. Hassan *et al.* [59] provide a recent review of the various types of transporters in *S. aureus*.

Msr(A)

The *msrA* determinant was first identified on an *S. epidermidis* macrolide-resistance plasmid and encodes a 488-amino-acid protein, Msr(A), an ATP-binding cassette (ABC) type of transporter [60]. In *S. aureus* it confers resistance to erythromycin, 14- and 15-membered ring macrolides, ketolides, and type B streptogramins in a dose-dependent erythromycin-inducible manner [61]. In a recent study in Europe, *msrA* was found only among MSSA [47], whereas it was responsible for erythromycin resistance in USA300, an important strain of community-acquired MRSA currently circulating in the USA [62].

VgaA/VgaAv and VgaB

The other ABC-type efflux pumps that mediate drug resistance in *S. aureus* are the VgaA and VgaB proteins. *vgaA* was initially found on the *S. aureus* plasmid pIP680 and displays 35% amino acid sequence identity with MsrA [51]. The plasmid-encoded VgaB protein [63] and chromosomally encoded VgaA variant (VgaAv) [64] display 48% and 81% amino acid sequence identity with VgaA, respectively. Although MsrA and VgaA exhibit structural similarities, they have distinct drug specificities; VgaA, VgaAv, and VgaB mediate resistance to type A streptogramins and clindamycin to varying degrees but not to macrolides [59]. The MIC of pristinamycin in an isogenic strain of *S. aureus* transformed with plasmids expressing the various genes increased 4–32-fold relative to that with a plasmid without these genes, whereas the MIC of clindamycin increased only twofold [65]. The *vga* genes have not been found alone in resistant *S. aureus* clinical isolates [55].

MdeA

MdeA (multidrug efflux A) belongs to the major facilitator superfamily (MFS) of efflux pumps [66]. There are limited data on the effect of this pump on the MICs of the MLS group of antibiotics. The MIC of virginiamycin (type A streptogramin) increased 16-fold when the chromosomally encoded *mdeA* was overexpressed from a plasmid in *S. aureus* [66]. However, *S. aureus* harboring mutations at the promoter region of *mdeA*, and expression of a homolog from *S. haemolyticus* in *B. subtilis*, yielded efflux activity against type A streptogramins as well as erythromycin and lincomycin [66]. In a recent study of clinical *S. aureus* isolates, a 10-fold increase in *mdeA* expression was found in 11% of the strains [67]. Thus, additional information is needed to assess the role of *mdeA* in resistance to the MLS antibiotics.

Tetracyclines

Tetracyclines reversibly inhibit bacterial protein synthesis by disrupting the interaction of aminoacyl-tRNA with the ribosome [68]. Tetracyclines bind to a high-affinity site on the 30S ribosomal subunit, although low-affinity sites have been identified on both 30S and 50S subunits. Binding appears to involve the S7 ribosomal protein, but other ribosomal proteins such as S3, S8, S14, and S19 appear to contribute to an optimal drug-binding conformation [69–71]. Drug binding is also thought to be in proximity to the 16S rRNA component of the ribosome.

Ribosomal protection

Target protection without modification is one of the two principal mechanisms of resistance to tetracyclines. Tetracycline resistance determinants TetM, TetO, and OtrA are proteins that interact with ribosomes to protect them from the action of tetracycline, and the structurally similar TetS, TetT, TetQ, TetB(P), TetW, Tet(32), and Tet(36) are thought to function in the same way. These resistance determinants are found on plasmids and transposons and have been identified in Gram-positive and Gram-negative bacteria [72–76]. Best studied of these determinants is *tetM* encoding the TetM protein in streptococci, and a related resistance determinant, *tetA*(M), is found on the chromosome of some strains of *S. aureus* [77]. There was 92% nucleotide and amino acid sequence similarity between staphylococcal *tetA*(M) and streptococcal *tetM* [77]. Thus, much of what is understood from *tetM* likely applies to the staphylococcal gene and protein as well. Ribosomes isolated from *tetM*-containing cells are resistant to tetracycline in *in vitro* translation systems if extracted under low-salt but not high-salt conditions, and purified TetM protein confers tetracycline resistance on ribosomes isolated from tetracycline-susceptible cells [78]. However, binding of tetracycline to the ribosome is not altered by TetM, and resistance occurs even when ribosomes are in substantial excess of TetM *in vitro*, suggesting that TetM acts catalytically [79]. TetM and TetO have structural similarities to elongation factors EF-Tu and EF-G, which bind ribosomes and also have GTPase activity. TetM mediates the release of tetracycline from the ribosome in a GTP-dependent manner [80], and TetM and EF-G compete for binding to the ribosome [81].

Host factors also appear to be important in that chromosomal *miaA* mutations, which cause defects in Δ^2-isopentenylpyrophosphate transferase, an enzyme that modifies adenosine at position 37 of tRNA, had partial loss of tetracycline resistance in *tetM* cells [79], and *rpsL* mutations causing streptomycin resistance by alteration in the S12 protein also reduce *tetM*- and *tetO*-mediated tetracycline resistance [82]. Modification of base A37 of tRNA is important for accuracy of translation, but it is uncertain if the effects of *miaA* mutations on tetracycline resistance reflect a direct or indirect effect on tetracycline interaction with

Table 10.1 Mechanisms of resistance to different antibiotics.

Antibiotic	Antibiotic target	Mechanism of resistance	Gene involved
Macrolides (erythromycin, clarithromycin, roxithromycin, azithromycin, telithromycin[1], cethromycin[1])	23S rRNA. Blocks passage of peptide chain through exit tunnel of the ribosome	Target modification: methylation of 23S rRNA	Erythromycin ribosomal methylase (*ermA, ermB, ermC, ermF, ermY*)
		Target modification	Mutations within gene for 23S rRNA (*rrl* genes)
		Target modification	Mutations within genes for ribosomal proteins
		Drug inactivation by hydrolysis	Esterases (*ereA, ereB*)
		Efflux	*msrA, mdeA*
Lincosamides (clindamycin)	Inhibits formation of peptide bonds	Target modification: methylation of 23S rRNA	Constitutive and induced *erm* genes
		Drug modification by nucleotidylation	*linA'*
		Efflux	*vgaA, vgaAv, vgaB, mdeA*
Streptogramins (pristinamycin, quinupristin/dalfopristin)	Cooperative inhibition of peptide synthesis: type A inhibits formation of peptide bonds; type B blocks passage of peptide chain through exit tunnel of the ribosome	Drug modification	Constitutive and induced *erm* genes Virginiamycin acetyltransferase (*vat, vatB*) Vgb lyase (*vgb*)
		Efflux	*msrA, vgaA, vgaAv, vgaB* Multidrug efflux (*mdeA*)
Tetracyclines (tetracycline, minocycline, doxycycline)	30S ribosomal proteins. Blocks interaction of aminoacyl-tRNA with the ribosome	A protein binds to the ribosome and interferes with binding of tetracycline	*tetM, tetO, otrA, tetS, tetT, tetQ, tetB, tetW, tet*
Glycylcycline (tigecycline)		Efflux	*tetK, tetL, tet38, mepA*
Aminoglycosides (arbekacin, amikacin, gentamicin, tobramycin, streptomycin, kanamycin)	30S ribosomal subunit	Drug modification	Acetyl CoA-dependent *N*-acetylation (*aac(6')*) ATP-dependent *O*-phosphorylation (*aph(2"), aph(3')-III*) ATP-dependent *O*-adenylation (*ant(4')(4")-Ia*)
		Entry inhibition	Defects in electron transport in small-colony variants
Rifamycins (rifampin, rifabutin, rifapentene, refaximin)	β-subunit of DNA-dependent RNA polymerase	Target modification	Mutations in *rpoB*
Mupirocin	Isoleucyl-tRNA synthetase (protein synthesis)	Acquisition of gene for resistant isoleucyl-tRNA synthetase	*ileS2* (*mupA*)
		Target modification: mutations within native gene for isoleucyl-tRNA synthetase	*ileS*
Quinolones (norfloxacin, ciprofloxacin, levofloxacin, moxifloxacin, gemifloxacin, garenoxacin, DC-159a)	DNA gyrase and topoisomerase IV (DNA replication)	Target modification: mutations within type II topoisomerase genes	Quinolone resistance-determining regions: *parC, gyrA, gyrB, parE*
		Drug efflux	*norA, norB, norC, sdrM, mepA*
Trimethoprim (TMP) and sulfamethoxazole (SMX)	Inhibition of folic acid metabolism: SMX inhibits dihydropteroate synthetase (DHPS); TMP inhibits dihydrofolate reductase (DHFR)	Target modification: mutations within DHFR and DHPS, additional plasmid-encoded copies of DHFR	Mutant form of DHFR (*dfrA, dfrB, dfrG*)
Oxazolidinones (linezolid)	Block ribosome assembly	Target modification: mutations within multiple genes for 23S rRNA	*rrl* genes
		Target modification: methylation of 23S rRNA	RNA methyltransferase (*cfr*)
Daptomycin	Bacterial membrane; causes membrane depolarization	Target modification: alterations in membrane phospholipids and membrane charge	Step1: mutation 5' to a putative acetate-CoA ligase/acetyl-CoA synthetase Step2: lysylphosphatidylglycerol synthetase (*mprF*) Step 3: sensor histidine kinase (*yycG*), RNA polymerase (*rpoB, rpoC*)

[1] Does not induce *erm* genes.

the ribosome [83]. Current hypotheses about the exact mechanism of ribosome protection include an interaction between TetM and the ribosome that eliminates the binding of tetracycline specifically to ribosomes that are actively engaged in protein synthesis or which allows aminoacyl-tRNA to enter the A site on the ribosome in the presence of tetracycline [84,85].

Expression of tetracycline resistance by *tetM* and *tetA*(M), like expression of *erm*-mediated resistance to macrolides, is inducible and, in the case of *tetM*, has been shown to be regulated by transcriptional and translational attenuation [77,86]. Upstream of *tetM* is an open reading frame (ORF) that encodes two regions of GC-rich RNA inverted repeats flanked by a series of uracil (U) residues, promoting formation of hairpin secondary structures, which cause RNA polymerase to pause. The series of U residues downstream also produces an unstable RNA/DNA hybrid that facilitates destabilization of binding of RNA polymerase. In the absence of tetracycline, translation of the ORF is thought to be retarded because five of the first eight codons require rare aminoacyl-tRNAs. Read-through transcription of *tetM* is more likely to occur if the translating ribosome is in proximity to the transcription complex, thereby destabilizing the hairpin structures that would otherwise terminate transcription [87]. In this model, in the presence of tetracycline as an inducer, the A and P sites on the ribosome are occupied by drug. Transcription and translation are thus delayed and availability of aminoacyl-tRNAs is increased, allowing proximity of the ribosome to the transcribing RNA polymerase and subsequent transcription and translation of *tetM*.

Active efflux of tetracyclines

Multiple tetracycline resistance determinants encoding drug efflux proteins have been described in many species of bacteria [88], and in staphylococci the *tetK* (*S. aureus*) and *tetL* (*S. hyicus*) determinants on plasmids and the chromosomal *tet38* (*S. aureus*) determinant have been characterized [89–91]. The Tet pumps are members of MFS and contain either 12 or 14 membrane-spanning segments [92]. They are secondary transporters that utilize the proton gradient or, in the case of TetL, the sodium gradient across the membrane to drive the extrusion of cation-complexed tetracyclines in antiport [93,94]. The Tet pumps have relatively narrow substrate profiles, being limited to members of the tetracycline class of antimicrobials and with some variation in the level of resistance they confer for different tetracycline derivatives. For example, *tetK* confers a greater than 256-fold increase in the MIC of tetracycline but only a fourfold increase in the MIC of minocycline. The extent to which these differences reflect the substrate properties of the Tet pumps, the ability of different compounds to induce pump expression, or both is not clear. Most recently tigecycline, a glycylcycline derivative of minocycline, has been released for clinical use. Tigecycline remains active against strains containing *tetM*- or *tetK*-mediated tetracycline resistance with little or no change in its MIC in the presence and absence of these resistance genes [95–97]. TetK and TetL have been shown to transport tetracycline in everted membrane vesicles with a dependence on the presence of divalent cations [93,94,98], similar to what was found with other related Tet pumps [99].

tetK has been found on plasmids pT181 and pNS1 [100,101] and in some strains is located on the chromosome due to IS*257*-mediated integration of a pT181-like plasmid [102]. *tetL* in *S. hyicus* has been described on plasmid pSTE1 [91]. *tet38* was found on the chromosome of an *S. aureus* 8325 strain, and Tet38 had 49% amino acid similarity to TetK [90]. The expression of *tet38* is indirectly negatively regulated by MgrA, a broad transcriptional regulator of genes encoding other efflux pumps, autolysins, and proteins involved in capsule synthesis [103–105]. Overexpression of *tet38* confers resistance to tetracycline but not minocycline. MepA, a member of the multidrug and toxin extrusion (MATE) family of efflux proteins, confers resistance to tigecycline and other structurally distinct compounds [106] (see below). The *mepA* gene is located on the *S. aureus* chromosome, and its expression is regulated at least in part by the *mepR* gene.

Aminoglycosides

The aminoglycosides have broad-spectrum antibacterial activity, including against *S. aureus*. Yet, with the exception of arbekacin, which is regarded as a first-line drug in the treatment of MRSA infections in Japan, they are seldom used as primary treatment in staphylococcal infections, but are used more frequently as a synergistic or additive combination with β-lactams or glycopeptides for the treatment of *S. aureus* infective endocarditis (see below) [107].

Aminoglycoside antibiotics possess a range of pleiotropic effects, including tight binding to the 30S subunit of prokaryotic ribosomes at the mRNA decoding site and mistranslation of the genetic code. This mechanism of action has been confirmed by the demonstration that point mutations in ribosomal components that reduce aminoglycoside binding to the ribosome can confer high-level resistance in bacteria. However, the processes that lead to bactericidal effect are controversial [108,109].

Drug modification

Although mutations at the 16S rRNA could result in resistance, these are rare and have not been found in *S. aureus*. Aminoglycoside resistance in the clinic is primarily due to the presence of enzymes that catalyze drug modification of hydroxy or amino groups through one or more of three routes: ATP-dependent *O*-phosphorylation by phosphotransferases (Aph); ATP-dependent *O*-adenylation by nucleotidyltransferases (Ant); and acetyl CoA-dependent

N-acetylation by acetyltransferases (Aac) [110]. Modified aminoglycosides bind poorly to the ribosome, allowing bacteria to survive in the presence of the drug [110,111].

Resistance to aminoglycosides in staphylococci is usually mediated by a bifunctional enzyme, encoded by *aac(6′)Ie-aph(2″)* [112,113], that modifies these drugs by acetylation (Aac(6′)) and phosphorylation (Aph(2″)) [114,115]. The aminoglycoside acetyltransferase activity is located in the N-terminal domain and the aminoglycoside kinase activity in the C-terminal domain, with the two domains operating independently [116]. The drugs affected by this enzyme are gentamicin, tobramycin, and kanamycin [117], with a variable effect on amikacin and no effect on arbekacin [118]. More recently, a deletion in the promoter region of *aacA-aphD* that created a strong promoter and overexpression of the bifunctional enzyme [119], and a Gly80Asp mutation with subsequent replacement of Aac(6′)-Aph(2″) with a truncated protein named Aac(4‴) [120], were each associated with extension of the resistance pattern to encompass amikacin and arbekacin. *aac(6′)Ie-aph(2″)* is encoded on a composite transposon Tn*4001*; Tn*4001*-like elements are widely distributed in *S. aureus* and may be located on plasmids or the chromosome. In isolates from the USA, the gene is usually found on large structurally related plasmids that are predominantly conjugative [113,121], whereas resistance genes in isolates from Europe and Australia are located either on smaller nonconjugative plasmids or in the chromosome [122,123]. As mentioned above, the combination of a β-lactam with an aminoglycoside is considered synergistic against staphylococci. Recently, an MRSA strain in Japan manifested increased Aac(6′)-Aph(2″) activity and a fourfold to eightfold increased MIC of arbekacin, gentamicin and netilmicin when induced by exposure to various β-lactams [124]. The mechanism of induction is believed to be a rearrangement of a *blaZ* promoter upstream of *aac(6′)Ie-aph(2″)* [124].

Ant(4′)(4″)-Ia modifies aminoglycosides by transferring AMP to their hydroxyl groups at the 4′ and 4″ positions and produces resistance to tobramycin, kanamycin, and amikacin but not to gentamicin [125,126]. The *ant(4′)(4″)-Ia* genes (often referred to as *aadD*) are often carried on small plasmids, and then integrated into larger conjugative plasmids, such as pSK41 [127], and subsequently into the staphylococcal cassette chromosome (SCC)*mec* (that encodes for methicillin resistance) region of the chromosome of some *S. aureus* isolates [128], probably as a result of IS*257*-mediated recombination events [129]. It is the predominant mechanism of aminoglycoside resistance in Japan among strains of *S. aureus* that produce aminoglycoside-modifying enzymes [130] and has been identified alone or in combination with other enzymes in more then 50% of MRSA in Europe [112]. Because the frequency of *ant(4′)(4″)-Ia* differs among *S. aureus* strains isolated from different countries [131], the determinant genes and phenotype of aminoglycoside resistance among clones of MRSA may vary.

In addition to Aph(2″), an ATP-dependent phosphotransferase in *S. aureus* is also encoded by *aph(3′)-III* [115,132,133]. This enzyme confers resistance to kanamycin, amikacin, and gentamicin B, but not gentamicin C [134]. *aph(3′)-III* is the least common of the three aminoglycoside-modifying enzymes [112,130].

ant(9)-Ia is a rare gene that encodes a spectinomycin adenyltransferase, Aad(9), and had been reported in Tn*554* of *S. aureus* [135]. However, spectinomycin is not used for the treatment of *S. aureus* infections.

Alterations in aminoglycoside transport

Resistance to aminoglycosides can also be mediated by entry inhibition. Small-colony variants (SCVs) of *S. aureus* are slow-growing morphological variants that have been implicated in persistent, relapsing, and antibiotic-resistant infections [136]. The altered phenotype of SCVs in most strains has been attributed to defects in electron transport due to mutations in hemin or menadione biosynthesis and this phenotype can be reversed by supplementation with these substances (for a more detailed discussion, refer to Chapter 5 and for a recent review see Proctor and Peters [137]). The defects in electron transport, by affecting the electrochemical gradient across the bacterial membrane, reduce the penetration of aminoglycosides into cells, thereby leading to resistance to gentamicin and other aminoglycosides [109,138,139]. Methyltransferases that can modify G1405 of the 16S rRNA molecule and cause resistance to all aminoglycosides have been found in Gram-negative bacteria but not yet in staphylococci [140]. Similarly, multidrug efflux pumps that can confer resistance to aminoglycosides such as that found in *Pseudomonas aeruginosa* have not been described in staphylococci [141].

Rifampin

Rifampin and the related rifamycins, rifabutin, rifapentene, and rifaximin, are inhibitors of the essential bacterial enzyme DNA-dependent RNA polymerase and have been used for treatment of staphylococcal and other bacterial infections or colonizations. RNA polymerase appears to be the sole target of rifampin action. Core RNA polymerase is composed of three subunits, β, β′, and α. Core polymerase combines with one of several σ subunits to enable specific binding to promoters and initiation of transcription. Rifampin forms a 1 : 1 complex with RNA polymerase and blocks the initiation of transcription [142,143].

Resistance to rifampin has been most studied in *E. coli* and occurs by mutations in the *rpoB* gene that encode amino acid changes in the β subunit of RNA polymerase [144]. These mutations are clustered in three highly conserved regions of *rpoB* in the midportion of the gene (cluster I, codons 507–511 and 513–533; cluster II, codons 563–564 and 572; cluster III, codon 687) [144]. These regions appear to be involved in the polymerase antitermination process, because most resistance mutations affected the polymerase read-through of termination signals, although the importance of this occurrence for the fitness of rifampin-resistant mutants *in vivo* is uncertain [145]. It is presumed that these changes reduce the affinity of RNA polymerase for rifampin, although direct binding studies have not been reported. Although most of the work on mechanisms of rifampin resistance has been done in *E. coli*, there have been similar findings on resistance selection [146] and mutations in similar regions of *rpoB* in *S. aureus* [147,148], and single mutations in *S. aureus* selected *in vitro* and *in vivo* have been associated with both high and low levels of resistance depending on the nature of the amino acid change [147,148]. Some clinical isolates of *S. aureus* have been found to have multiple mutations in the cluster regions [149]. Strains that are resistant to rifampin are generally also resistant to other related rifamycins [150]. In surveys of clinical isolates of staphylococci, the occurrence of established rifampin resistance varies with the clinical setting, and methicillin-resistant strains may have higher percentages of rifampin resistance than methicillin-susceptible strains [151], possibly due to the known ability of methicillin-resistant strains to spread in healthcare settings.

The ability of single spontaneous mutations to confer high-level rifampin resistance in the laboratory correlates with clinical observations that resistance develops rapidly in clinical settings when rifampin is used alone for therapy of established staphylococcal infections in which there may initially be a large population of bacteria within which resistant mutants may exist at a frequency of 10^{-6}–10^{-8} [146,152]. Thus, rifampin is used for therapy almost exclusively in combination with other antistaphylococcal agents to reduce the likelihood of selection for rifampin resistance.

Mupirocin

Mupirocin (pseudomonic acid) is an antibiotic derived from cultures of *Pseudomonas fluorescens* that inhibits isoleucyl tRNA synthetase, encoded by *ileS*, and thus indirectly inhibits bacterial protein synthesis by depriving the cell of the ability to incorporate a common amino acid into protein. Mupirocin is used in topical preparations to eradicate nasal colonization with *S. aureus* and for treatment of certain staphylococcal skin infections or colonizations. Resistant strains have been shown to emerge by plasmid transfer, clonal spread, and selection of low-level resistance mutations.

High-level resistance

High-level resistance to mupirocin in *S. aureus* has been found to be encoded on a variety of transferable plasmids [153–155]. Two isoleucyl tRNA synthetase activities have been isolated from high-level resistant strains. One was also found in susceptible strains and those with low-level resistance. The other was found only in high-level resistant strains, and it had substantially reduced sensitivity to mupirocin [156,157]. A gene, *ileS2* (originally termed *mupA*), encoding a mupirocin-resistant isoleucyl tRNA synthase was identified on resistance plasmids and found to encode a protein with 57% identity and 30% similarity in amino acid sequence to the native IleS protein [158]. The origin of the *ileS2* gene is uncertain, but it has been found on plasmids in both *S. aureus* and coagulase-negative staphylococci and has also been found in a chromosomal location in some strains of *S. aureus* [159,160]. High-level mupirocin resistance has been transferred between coagulase-negative staphylococci and *S. aureus* on plasmids [161,162]. On some plasmids *ileS2* is flanked by direct repeats of the insertion sequence IS*257* [163], suggesting that it is located on a transposable element. In one case, the acquisition of the mupirocin resistance determinant was found on a variant of an established multidrug resistance conjugative plasmid, pGO1, flanked with two direct copies of IS*431*/*257* and associated with loss of several other resistance determinants [154]. A frameshift mutation in *ileS2* was associated with loss of mupirocin resistance, but reversion to wild-type allele occurred with high frequency [164].

Low-level resistance

Low-level mupirocin resistance can occur on exposure of *S. aureus* to mupirocin by selection of mutations in the native *ileS* gene. A mutation changing valine at position 588 to phenylalanine is common and appears to confer little fitness cost [159,165]. Further selections for higher-level resistance have been associated with additional mutations in *ileS*, some of which have apparent fitness costs, but compensatory mutations are able to mitigate these costs [166]. In *Salmonella typhimurium*, additional low-level resistance mutations selected in the laboratory include tryptophan to arginine at position 443, histidine to tyrosine at position 594, phenylalanine to leucine at position 596, and tryptophan–valine at positions 630–631 to leucine [167]. These mutations are localized in the Ile-AMP/mupirocin binding pocket, and all conferred a fitness cost, although to varying degrees. Compensatory mutations in *ileRS* or additional gene dosage of mutant *ileRS* were able to restore defects in cell growth and aminoacylation kinetics of IleS associated with these mutations [167]. In addition, some strains of *S. aureus* with low levels of mupirocin resistance also appear to contain the usually plasmid-encoded *ile2* gene on the chromosome [155,160,168,169].

Thus, an acquired resistant isoleucyl tRNA synthetase that bypasses the sensitive native enzyme allows protein synthesis to proceed in the presence of mupirocin. That the level of resistance to mupirocin is higher when the gene encoding this enzyme is located on plasmids relative to the chromosome suggests that differences in gene expression due to either plasmid copy number or differences in promoter strength or regulation of expression in the two locations may be responsible for the different levels of resistance.

Quinolones

The introduction of fluoroquinolones was followed soon after by reports of emerging drug resistance, particularly among Gram-positive pathogens [170]. Newer fluoroquinolones retain *in vitro* activity against ciprofloxacin-resistant staphylococci [171]. However, using these drugs in the background of prior fluoroquinolone exposure may facilitate selection of even more highly resistant mutants [172,173]. In addition, in the nosocomial setting, treatment with levofloxacin or ciprofloxacin was associated with subsequent isolation of MRSA but not MSSA [174].

Quinolones target two bacterial type II topoisomerases, DNA gyrase and topoisomerase IV. DNA topoisomerases are essential enzymes that regulate the conformational changes in DNA topology by catalyzing the concerted breakage and rejoining of DNA strands during normal cellular growth [175]. DNA gyrase and topoisomerase IV are A_2B_2 heterotetrameric enzymes; gyrase is encoded by *gyrA* and *gyrB*, and topoisomerase IV by *parC* and *parE*. The central event in the interaction between the quinolones and gyrase or topoisomerase IV is formation of a reaction intermediate that contains quinolone, enzyme, and broken DNA. The topoisomerase-mediated DNA cleavage reaction consists of a pair of single-stranded scissions occurring on opposite sides of the DNA duplex, staggered by four base pairs. These nicks function as the gate through which the other DNA segment can pass [175]. Quinolones stabilize this "cleavable" complex, and addition of a protein denaturant, such as sodium dodecyl sulfate, releases DNA ends (cleavage complexes) [176,177]. The resulting ternary complex blocks DNA replication and triggers additional, incompletely defined events that lead to cell death [178]. In Gram-negative bacteria, such as *E. coli*, first-step resistance mutations map in the genes encoding gyrase subunits [176,177], usually *gyrA*, implying that gyrase is the primary target *in vivo* and is more sensitive than topoisomerase IV to fluoroquinolone-mediated attack. In contrast, in *S. aureus*, *parC* and *parE* mutants selected with many fluoroquinolones are sufficient alone to cause resistance in a *gyrA*$^+$ background [179], and *gyrA* mutations alone are silent [180], contributing incrementally to fluoroquinolone resistance only in the presence of *parC* or *parE* mutations. Catalytic and noncatalytic assays using purified enzymes corroborate these results for the older fluoroquinolones. Whereas the sensitivity of topoisomerase IV in *E. coli* and *S. aureus* (using the same DNA substrate) to many fluoroquinolones is similar, *S. aureus* gyrase appears to have substantially reduced intrinsic sensitivity to quinolones compared with *E. coli*, reversing the relative sensitivities of the two enzymes (in comparison with Gram-negative bacteria) and explaining why topoisomerase IV is the primary fluoroquinolone target in *S. aureus* [181]. The reduced sensitivity of *S. aureus* gyrase to fluoroquinolones was related to structural differences from *E. coli* in the extended $\alpha 4$ domain of GyrA, and this effect was modulated by K^+-glutamate [182]. Hence, fluoroquinolones are less active in attacking gyrase in *S. aureus* and in interrupting its pivotal role in the cell cycle.

Target modification

The main mechanism of quinolone resistance is by mutations in topoisomerase IV and DNA gyrase. Topoisomerase-based resistance to the quinolones occurs stepwise, with moderate levels of resistance arising from single mutations in the primary target of the drug (topoisomerase IV or gyrase). Once reduced sensitivity to the drug arises from the first mutation, higher levels of resistance may occur from additional mutations in both the primary and secondary enzyme targets [178]. Therefore, to limit the emergence of resistance, fluoroquinolones should possess similarly potent dual targeting properties [183,184]. The mutations associated with quinolone resistance have classically been clustered in distinct regions of gyrase and topoisomerase IV, named the quinolone resistance-determining regions (QRDRs), which are located at the 5′ terminus of *gyrA* and *parC* and midportions of *gyrB* and *parE* [178], and are thought to be the quinolone-binding domain [178,185, 186]. Mutations in this region of *gyrA* of *E. coli* have been shown to reduce drug binding affinity for the enzyme [187] and presumably other mutations have in most cases similar effects on drug binding to the target enzyme.

Newer fluoroquinolones in clinical use, such as moxifloxacin [171], gemifloxacin [188], those under development such as garenoxacin [173,189], WCK 771 [190] and DC-159a [191], and those no longer marketed or under development such as gatifloxacin [192] and DX-119 [172], possess better pharmacokinetic and pharmacodynamic properties than older quinolones, like norfloxacin and ciprofloxacin, against *S. aureus* [193,194], and some have balanced activity against the two target enzymes, thereby reducing the likelihood of emergence of resistance under treatment. The newer fluoroquinolones frequently select for mutations outside the classical QRDR [171,172,188,189]. A structure of topoisomerase IV or gyrase with bound quinolone has not yet been solved, and the molecular mechanisms of fluoroquinolone resistance for these novel mutations remain to be determined. It is possible that the novel mutations affect the catalytic activity and structure of the topoisomerases such that the mutant enzymes form unstable or reduced levels of drug–enzyme–DNA complexes [192].

Unlike other classes of antibiotics, such as the macrolides, for which resistance is usually by the acquisition of resistance genes, resistance to fluoroquinolones occurs most commonly through spontaneous mutations that were present as small subpopulations before treatment or which can occur under treatment with the fluoroquinolone [195]. Consequently, resistant populations can appear concurrently with the eradication of susceptible cells. Moreover, fluoroquinolones, probably through their mechanism of action, may increase the probability of emerging subpopulations resistant to the fluoroquinolones themselves. Ciprofloxacin induces double-stranded DNA breaks and stalled replication forks, both of which are processed to single-stranded DNA [177]. In response to this DNA damage, RecA protein forms filaments on the single-stranded (ss)DNA, and these nucleoprotein filaments facilitate recombinational repair as well as bind the SOS gene repressor LexA, stimulating its autoproteolysis. This proteolysis inactivates the LexA repressor and results in the induction of the SOS genes. The SOS response, among other effects [196], also induces a hypermutable state through error-prone DNA repair [197]. Thus, by inducing repair pathways that involve RecA-ssDNA filament formation, ciprofloxacin promotes the mutations that confer resistance to itself [198]. These same phenomena have also been shown in *S. aureus* with rifamycins [199], trimethoprim [200], and β-lactams [201].

Drug efflux

The complete genome of *S. aureus* N315 is 2.81 Mb in length and contains 210 genes predicted to encode transporters; 67 of these transporters are predicted to be ATP-dependent, representing 31% of the total. The majority of the ATP-dependent transporters belong to the ABC family (63 ABC transporters, or 94% of the total of 67). Among the 114 (54%) secondary transporters energized by ion gradients across the membrane, there are 28 efflux pumps (25%) belonging to MFS and fewer that are members of other families [202]. A similar distribution is found in the genomes of *S. aureus* strains COL, Mu50, and NCTC 8325. Of those efflux transporters that were analyzed, some extrude Qs, including NorA [203], NorB [90], NorC [204], and SdrM [205] that belong to the MFS transporters, and MepA, a multidrug resistance pump belonging to the MATE family [206]. These transporters are responsible for decreases in susceptibility to hydrophilic (norfloxacin and ciprofloxacin) and hydrophobic (moxifloxacin and sparfloxacin) quinolones. The structural features of a quinolone that determine whether it is affected by an efflux system are not fully defined but correlate with hydrophilicity for the NorA pump of *S. aureus* [203].

The level of resistance conferred by the various transporters depends on their capacity and level of expression. For example, the wild-type level of expression of *norB* (as inferred from a *norB* knockout mutant) was insufficient to affect drug susceptibility, but when overexpressed in the same wild-type strain (ISP794) it increased the MIC of moxifloxacin fourfold to 0.25 μg/mL [90]. Baseline expression of *norC* in the same wild-type strain increased the MIC of moxifloxacin twofold relative to ISP794, but when overexpressed the MIC of moxifloxacin increased to the same level as with NorB [204]. A complex picture of expression of various transporters is emerging, and it is likely that regulation of transporter expression is controlled at a number of levels. The regulation of expression of the chromosomally encoded NorA efflux pump depends on at least two systems, the two-component regulatory system ArlRS and the global regulator MgrA (formerly NorR), which binds the *norA* promoter and when overexpressed from a plasmid causes increased expression of *norA*. Mutations in either regulator or the promoter region of *norA* and in the coding region of *norA* can affect quinolone resistance [103,207,208]. In addition to its role in regulation of *norA* expression, MgrA downregulates expression of *norB* and *norC*; its effect on *norB*, like that on *norA*, is direct whereas its effect on *norC* is indirect [90,204]. Since the MgrA and ArlRS regulators are known to have effects on multiple other cellular processes [209,210], it is likely that they play a key role in integrating efflux pump expression with other cellular processes and in coordinating cellular responses to various environmental stresses.

More recently, a new positive regulator of *norB* has been found. The protein, NorG, belongs to the gluconate regulatory protein family of regulators, binds to the promoter region of *norB*, and directly activates *norB* expression. To add to the complexity, MgrA acts as an indirect repressor of *norG* [211]. Similar to the MFS pumps operating in *S. aureus*, the expression of MepA, which is encoded on the *mepRAB* operon, is under regulation of MepR [206]. MepR, which has strong homology with the transcriptional regulator of *E. coli* MarR, is an autoregulatory repressor, repressing the expression of its own gene as well as that of *mepA* [212].

Trimethoprim–sulfamethoxazole

The first sulfonamide of clinical importance, prontosil rubrum, was first used in 1935, although its mode of action was not initially clear [213]. Boils caused by *S. aureus* that were treated with surgical intervention were then cured with sulfa drugs, and sulfapyridine was sometimes effective in staphylococcal septicemia. Trimethoprim (TMP) was synthesized in 1956 [214] and became available in a mixture with sulfamethoxazole (SMX). Despite bactericidal activity against *S. aureus*, irrespective of its methicillin susceptibility, the combination of TMP and SMX has not become a first-line antibiotic against this bacterium because of studies suggesting inferiority to other drugs in the treatment of invasive diseases [215] and because of resistance [216].

The antibacterial drug combination of TMP–SMX inhibits two steps in the enzymatic pathway of bacterial folate synthesis. Dihydropteroate synthetase (DHPS) catalyzes the formation of dihydrofolate from para-aminobenzoic acid (PABA). Sulfonamides are structural analogs of PABA and act as alternative substrates for DHPS. The reaction results in sulfa-containing pteroate derivatives, sulfapterines, that cannot be used in the subsequent steps of the biosynthetic pathway, thus depleting the folate-cofactor pool. In the subsequent step of the pathway, TMP, by its structural similarity, inhibits dihydrofolate reductase (DHFR), which is chromosomally encoded by *dfrB* and catalyzes the formation of tetrahydrofolate from dihydrofolate. The combination of TMP and SMX is synergistic against *S. aureus* [217].

Different mechanisms mediate bacterial resistance to TMP and to sulfonamides. Resistance to TMP can be conferred by a single amino acid substitution, phenylalanine to tyrosine at position 98, located in the active site of DHFR that disrupts the hydrogen bond between the 4-amino group of the enzyme and TMP, leading to reduced affinity of TMP for the enzyme. However, this mutation in *dfrB* results in only low-level resistance to TMP [218]. Plasmid-mediated production of additional DHFRs that are TMP-resistant by virtue of the same phenylalanine to tyrosine replacement at position 98 is required for elevated resistance. The mutant enzyme can function in place of the susceptible chromosomal enzyme. S1 DHFR, encoded by *dfrA*, was initially found on conjugative plasmids in *S. aureus* [219–221]. Plasmid-encoded *dfr* leads to high-level resistance to TMP that is associated with overproduction of DHFR mediated by changes in the promoter region and transcription level of the mutant *dfr* [218,222,223]. *dfrA* is flanked by insertion sequence IS*257* and is carried on Tn*4003* [224], supporting its dissemination among strains of *S. aureus*. Interestingly, a novel gene, *dfrG*, encoding a protein that is only 41% similar to wild-type *S. aureus* DHFR, was found in *S. aureus* isolates from Thailand and Japan. *dfrG* was flanked by an insertion sequence, suggesting that it may also have been acquired by recombination. The precise location of *dfrG* is unclear; although it was detected by Southern blotting on fragments of genomic DNA and was not transferable, suggesting a chromosomal location, it did not replace *dfrB*.

Resistance to sulfonamides in *S. aureus*, similar to that in *Streptococcus pyogenes* [225], has only been found to be mediated by chromosomal mutations [226]. According to the crystallographic structure of *S. aureus* DHPS, the amino acid mutations associated with resistance were widely distributed over the surface of the enzyme with no mutation common to all clinical isolates with an altered DHPS, making a simple structural explanation for the resistance mechanism difficult [227]. It has also been suggested that *S. aureus* can become resistant to sulfonamides by synthesizing PABA in excess, to overcome the competition with the drug. This synthesis is constitutive and occurs in both the absence and the presence of sulfonamides [228,229].

Oxazolidinones

Oxazolidinones inhibit bacterial protein synthesis by interacting with the ribosome and interrupting the formation of the initiation complex of mRNA and the 30S and 50S ribosomal subunits. Linezolid is currently the only oxazolidinone antimicrobial in clinical use, and it has indications for the treatment of infections due to vancomycin-resistant enterococci (VRE) and MRSA.

Mutation in ribosomal RNA genes

Most human pathogens have multiple genomic copies of the *rrl* genes encoding 23S rRNA, and staphylococci have five to six copies. Thus, resistance caused by mutations in *rrl* genes requires that multiple gene copies be altered, thereby reducing the likelihood of mutational resistance. Linezolid-resistant strains of VRE have been reported to emerge in patients treated with and without extended courses of linezolid [230–232] and by nosocomial transmission [233]. Similarly, but in lesser numbers, clinical strains of linezolid-resistant MRSA [234–236] and coagulase-negative staphylococci [237,238] have also been identified. Linezolid-resistant coagulase-negative staphylococci have also been shown to spread clonally in a healthcare setting [238]. In both *S. aureus* and enterococci, mutations changing G to U at position 2576 in domain V of 23S rRNA have been found in the resistant clinical isolates [234,235, 239,240]. In one *S. aureus* isolate, all five copies of the 23S rRNA gene had the G2576T mutation, and the resistance phenotype was stable on passage in the absence of linezolid [241]. However, other isolates with this mutation have shown reductions in the number of mutant genes and the resistance level on passage without antibiotics [242]. A T2500A mutation, also in domain V, was also linked with linezolid resistance emerging during therapy and was unstable in the absence of linezolid selection [236]. In another report, resistance and mutation emerged with linezolid treatment, reverted when linezolid was stopped, and reemerged with resumption of linezolid therapy [243]. Increasing resistance has been associated both with increasing numbers of *rrl* genes mutated [235] and with loss of a single copy of an *rrl* gene [236]. It is not yet clear the extent to which sequential mutations in *rrl* genes occurring under selective pressure and/or duplication of the initial mutation in other gene copies by gene conversion contribute to multiple mutated gene copies.

Laboratory-selected linezolid-resistant mutants of enterococci, *E. coli*, and *Halobacterium halobium* have also revealed additional resistance mutations in the central region of domain V of 23S rRNA, suggesting the specific site of linezolid interaction with the ribosome [244–246]. Low-level resistance to linezolid has also been associated with small deletions in riboprotein L4 in *Streptococcus pneumoniae* [247].

As with any acquired resistance mechanism, the prevalence of resistant strains can be amplified by transmission of resistant strains from patient to patient along with continued selective pressure from antimicrobial use [233,238].

Ribosomal modification

Most recently, a Cfr rRNA methyltransferase was found among chloramphenicol-resistant animal isolates of several staphylococcal species (*Staphylococcus hyicus*, *Staphylococcus warneri*, *Staphylococcus sciuri*, and *Staphylococcus simulans*) [248,249]. This enzyme was initially shown to modify A2503 of 23S rRNA [250] and to confer resistance to chloramphenicol, lincosamides, and streptogramin A antibiotics [251]. It was also later found in a human clinical isolate of MRSA, CM05, and shown to confer low-level resistance to linezolid [252]. The *cfr* gene was located on plasmids in animal isolates of staphylococci but was found on the chromosome of *S. aureus* CM05 in association with IS*21–558*, other plasmid DNA sequences, and *ermB*, with which it appeared to share an operon structure, resulting in coordinated expression of *ermB* and *cfr* and modification of both A2058 (by ErmB) and A2053 (by Cfr). These two rRNA modifications resulted in resistance to all clinically available ribosome-targeting antibiotics [252]. Although the original source of the *cfr* gene is not certain, IS*21–558* has been associated with mobilization of *cfr* on plasmids [249]. Thus, it appears that *cfr* in *S. aureus* CM05 may have been mobilized from a plasmid and integrated into the CM05 chromosome. Should the *cfr* gene become mobilized more widely on plasmids or to the chromosomes of additional *S. aureus* isolates, the clinical utility of linezolid could be substantially compromised. The mechanistic linkage of *cfr* with other antibiotic resistances also poses the risk that use of other antibiotics will provide selection pressures in addition to that with linezolid use.

Daptomycin

Daptomycin is a cyclic lipopeptide antimicrobial recently released for clinical use. Its activity is limited to Gram-positive bacteria, and it has equivalent activity against methicillin-sensitive and methicillin-resistant strains of *S. aureus* [253,254]. Daptomycin is bactericidal and acts by binding to and inserting into Gram-positive bacterial membranes, resulting in membrane depolarization and leakage of potassium ions from the cell [255]. Antibacterial activity is dependent on the presence of calcium ions in the medium. Recent transcriptional profiling of *S. aureus* cells exposed to daptomycin generated a complex pattern of changes in gene expression, including overlap with patterns seen with exposure to inhibitors of cell wall synthesis and to *m*-chlorophenylhydrazone, a proton ionophore that collapses the membrane pH gradient [256]. Thus, daptomycin might act on cell wall synthesis in addition to its effects on membrane depolarization, but the molecular mechanisms of these effects remain to be delineated.

Laboratory selection of single-step mutants of *S. aureus* with resistance to daptomycin occurs at exceedingly low frequency ($< 1 \times 10^{-10}$) [257]. However, serial passage of *S. aureus* in sub-MIC concentrations of daptomycin results in fourfold to 27-fold increases in MIC, and such mutants accumulate, first, mutations 5′ to a putative acetate-CoA ligase/acetyl-CoA synthetase (MW2528), then in *mprF*, followed in varying order by mutations in *yycG*, *rpoB*, and *rpoC* [258]. Notably, mutations in *mprF* were found in all three post-therapy daptomycin nonsusceptible clinical isolates studied and an additional mutation in *yycG* was also found in one of them. *mprF* encodes a lysylphosphatidylglycerol synthetase, *yycG* a sensor histidine kinase, and *rpoB* and *rpoC* subunits of RNA polymerase. The *mprF* mutation is the first in the series that is associated with an increase in MIC of daptomycin. MprF adds lysine to membrane phosphatidylglycerol, and thus mutants in this enzyme likely have alterations in membrane phospholipids and membrane charge that could affect daptomycin binding to the membrane. The *mprF* mutation in the daptomycin-resistant strains may represent a gain-of-function mutation, since *mprF* null mutants exhibit increased susceptibility to daptomycin [259]. YycG has regulatory functions and has been shown to affect fatty acid biosynthesis and membrane composition, and thus it too might be postulated to affect daptomycin binding to the membrane [260]. However, how mutant RpoB and RpoC might contribute to increased daptomycin resistance is as yet undefined. The mutations in RpoB are in a domain distinct from that involved in rifampin resistance.

Recently, daptomycin-resistant clinical isolates (compared with their initially susceptible pretreatment parental strains) were shown to exhibit increased membrane fluidity, increased translocation of lysylphosphatidylglycerol to the outer membrane leaflet, and increased net positive surface charge that correlated with reduced surface binding of daptomycin and reduced daptomycin-induced membrane depolarization [259]. Interestingly, and perhaps not unexpectedly, these membrane changes were also associated with resistance to cationic antimicrobial peptides. A serially passaged daptomycin-resistant laboratory mutant has also been shown to exhibit reduced daptomycin binding to whole cells and cell membranes [261].

Somewhat unexpectedly, some strains of *S. aureus* that have acquired intermediate resistance to vancomycin following vancomycin exposure and without exposure to daptomycin have also developed reduced susceptibility to daptomycin [262–267]. Such a change in daptomycin susceptibility occurred in some strains in the absence of an *mprF* mutation [262] and was correlated with the degree of increase in cell wall thickness that has been seen in strains with intermediate susceptibility to vancomycin, suggesting that a thickened cell wall might provide a barrier to daptomycin action [264]. With whole-genome sequencing of *S. aureus* mutants that emerged from a patient with persistently positive cultures on vancomycin therapy, the emergence of increases in daptomycin MIC coincided with the appearance of *rpoC* and *yycH* mutations [265]. Daptomycin-resistant strains have also emerged in patients treated with vancomycin followed by daptomycin [268,269]. The complexity of the changes in membrane and cell wall structure associated with resistance to daptomycin requires further study to provide a fully coherent genetic and mechanistic explanation.

Spread of resistance and multidrug resistance

The ability of *S. aureus* and coagulase-negative staphylococci to colonize skin and some mucous membranes of humans efficiently and their ability to survive and persist on environmental surfaces enable the establishment of reservoirs of bacteria that can be spread by human activities involving person-to-person contact or shared contact with contaminated objects. Animals may also provide reservoirs of staphylococci that can be spread to humans by contact. Among the most dramatic examples of this facility for spread in human populations is the emergence of penicillin-resistant and later methicillin-resistant staphylococci by oligoclonal spread worldwide [270] and more recently by the clonal dissemination of the community-associated (CA)-MRSA strain USA300 in the USA, Canada, and Europe [9,271,272]. Although another CA-MRSA strain, USA400, was the first to be recognized in the USA, it was later supplanted by strain USA300, which became the dominant CA-MRSA strain in the USA. The bacterial factors that determine which staphylococcal clones will be most successful in spread are as yet poorly defined. Although virulence factors and resistance determinants may contribute to the ability of strains to spread, it is likely that there are distinct biological determinants of the ability to spread as well [273,274].

Although resistant (as well as susceptible) staphylococci can spread between persons who are not receiving antimicrobials [275], spread of resistant strains is amplified by antimicrobial use due to the selective advantage for growth or persistence provided to resistant cells in the presence of antimicrobials. This effect can act at several levels depending on the mechanisms of resistance to a particular antimicrobial. For example, quinolone treatment of persons without infection or with appropriately susceptible nonstaphylococcal infections can result in the selection of multiclonal quinolone-resistant coagulase-negative staphylococci that colonize skin and may be shared with other persons [276]. In this instance, quinolone use acts both to select the small numbers of quinolone-resistant mutants in a large otherwise susceptible population of staphylococci and to promote the acquisition of established resistant strains from others.

Such dual effects of antimicrobial exposure on resistance are most likely to occur with those antimicrobials for which selection of single resistance mutations provides a robust resistance phenotype and thus occurs readily; quinolones and rifampin are in this category of antimicrobials for staphylococci. Mupirocin resistance via single mutation also occurs, but single mutations confer only small incremental increase in MIC. Resistance to macrolides, clindamycin, streptogramins, and linezolid can occur by mutation but are less likely to be selected *de novo* because of the multiple genomic copies of the rRNA genes in staphylococci, a substantial proportion of which need to be mutated for a resistance phenotype to occur [235]. Mutational resistance or reduced susceptibility to daptomycin, as with reduced susceptibility to vancomycin, appears to require multiple mutations in distinct loci and thus most often emerges after prolonged antimicrobial exposure in patients with sites of infection (e.g., undrained abscesses or infection in the presence of foreign bodies) where bacterial reservoirs can persist.

Resistance due to acquired genes affects the largest number of antimicrobial classes used for treatment of staphylococcal infections, including (in addition to β-lactams) tetracyclines, trimethoprim, aminoglycosides, macrolides, clindamycin, streptogramins, and mupirocin. All of these antibiotics are natural products, and resistance determinants likely emerged either from the antibiotic-producer organisms themselves or from other organisms living in the same natural environment. For such resistance mechanisms, spread of established resistant strains between persons and spread of resistance determinants (if present on mobile genetic elements) into other bacterial strains are the primary means by which resistance disseminates. Mobility of resistance determinants in staphylococci can be mediated by any of a large number of plasmids, transposons, insertion sequences, conjugative transposons, and integrating conjugative elements, the details of which are beyond the scope of this chapter [277–280].

Multidrug resistance (MDR) is common in hospital-associated strains of MRSA [281]. These additional resistances are in many cases due to the acquisition of other resistance determinants within the *mec* gene cassette. For example, the staphylococcal chromosome cassettes associated with *mec* elements (SCC*mec*) in various hospital clones include the additional integrated resistance determinants plasmid pUB110, which contains the *ant(4')* gene encoding resistance to kanamycin and tobramycin (in SCC*mec* type II); Tn*554*, which contains *ermA* encoding inducible resistance to macrolides, clindamycin, and streptogramins (in SCC*mec* types II and III); plasmid pI258, which encodes resistance to penicillin and heavy metals (in SCC*mec* type III); and pT181, which encodes tetracycline resistance (SCC*mec* type III) [281]. Additional acquired resistance genes can occur by independent acquisition of resistance plasmids, which themselves may have multiple resistance determinants, or by integration of other resistance determinants into other sites on the chromosome mediated by insertion sequences and transposons. Quinolone resistance due to topoisomerase mutations emerged rapidly in hospital MRSA isolates and to a lesser extent in MSSA isolates in a number of medical centers [282].

CA-MRSA strains were initially susceptible to a number of non-β-lactam antimicrobials, in part because their smaller SCC*mec* type IV element contained no resistance elements other than the *mec* genes. However, such strains have begun to acquire additional resistance to macrolides, clindamycin, and mupirocin due to acquisition of *ermC* and *mupA* on a large conjugative plasmid, pUSA03 [283], to macrolides, clindamycin, and tetracycline due to acquisition of *ermC* and *tetK* likely on a plasmid(s) [284], and to quinolones due to topoisomerase mutations [284,285]. Community-associated strains have also begun to intermix epidemiologically with traditional hospital-associated strains as a cause of hospital infections [286,287].

Independent acquisition of plasmids containing multiple antibiotic resistance genes is well described as a cause of MDR in staphylococci, as reviewed by Paulsen *et al.* [280]. Small class I plasmids (1–5 kb), such as pT181 and pC194, typically carry a single resistance determinant [100,288]. In contrast, class II MDR plasmids are generally larger (15–40 kb) and have lower copy numbers than class I plasmids. Class II plasmids include the β-lactamase/heavy metal resistance families; the pSK1 family, members of which often contain *qacA*, which encodes resistance to antiseptics and disinfectants [289], and variously either alone or in combination Tn*4001*, Tn*4002*, or Tn*4003* encoding resistance to aminoglycosides, penicillin, or trimethoprim, respectively [224,290,291]; and several miscellaneous MDR plasmids, including pSTE1 [91].

Conjugative class III plasmids (30–60 kb) are larger than class II plasmids and also typically have multiple resistance determinants in addition to genes involved in the plasmid conjugation machinery [280]. The pSK41 family of class III plasmids, such as pGO1, a well-studied example [292], often contains the *qacC* gene encoding antiseptic and disinfectant resistance, several genes encoding aminoglycoside-modifying enzymes, and *dfrA* encoding trimethoprim resistance or *blaZ* β-lactamase encoding penicillin resistance. Other class III plasmids, such as pJ3358, carry *tetA(K)* and *mupA* genes encoding tetracycline and mupirocin resistance, respectively [163]. MDR can also occur from ribosomal modification when the sites modified are involved in the action of different classes of protein synthesis inhibitors, such as resistance to linezolid and chloramphenicol from the actions of Cfr methylase [252].

Broad-spectrum or MDR efflux pumps may alone cause resistance to a number of drugs that are within their substrate profile [293]. The genes encoding such pumps can be on plasmids or the chromosome. In the latter case, they may be part of the native genome, rather than acquired from other sources, with the native function of the encoded pumps likely being to remove natural environmental toxins, which could include natural product antibiotics. The expression of many such MDR pumps is regulated, with substrate and other environmental signals as inducers resulting in increased expression associated with increased resistance. The details of the regulatory pathways for expression of various efflux pumps is beyond the scope of this chapter but have been reviewed recently [294]. Since that time additional global regulatory genes, *arlRS*, *mgrA*, and *norG*, which are involved variously in the regulation of expression of the *norA*, *norB*, *norC*, *tet38*, and *abcA* genes encoding efflux pumps [90,204,208,211], and *mepR*, which regulates expression of the *mepA* efflux pump gene [106], have also been identified on the *S. aureus* chromosome. Mutations in regulatory elements or the promoter/operator regions of pump genes usually underlie stable increased expression of pump structural genes [103,207,208,211,295]. However, apart from substrate induction identified in some cases [212,296], the natural physiological signals that trigger changes in expression of MDR efflux pumps remain undefined in many cases. Thus, differences in susceptibility to a broad range of antimicrobials in different growth environments may be mediated in part by physiological changes in pump expression.

In *S. aureus* the most studied MDR pumps have been members of MFS, as are the narrow-spectrum Tet pumps (TetK and Tet38) discussed above. MFS pumps are energized by the proton gradient across the cell membrane. The Qac MDR pumps, which are located on plasmids and have been found on chromosomes, confer resistance to structurally diverse antiseptics, disinfectants, and dyes, which are organic cations, but not to antimicrobials used in humans. QacA confers resistance to monovalent cations such as benzalkonium and cetrimide and to divalent cations such as chlorhexidine [297]. QacB confers resistance principally to monovalent organic cations as a result of an amino acid change, aspartic acid to alanine at position 323, from QacA [297,298]. QacC (also referred to as Smr) confers resistance to quarternary ammonium disinfectants [299]. The chromosomal *norA* and *norB* genes when overexpressed from plasmids confer increased resistance to quinolones, cetrimide, and the dyes tetraphenylphosphonium (TPP) and ethidium bromide (EtBr) [90,300].

Other classes of MDR pumps have also been identified in *S. aureus*. AbcA is a member of the ABC pump family, members of which are energized by ATP hydrolysis. The chromosomal *abcA* gene encodes AbcA and when overexpressed from a plasmid confers resistance to a range of β-lactams, TPP, and EtBr [211]. MepA, a member of the MATE pump family, is also energized by the membrane proton gradient. Overexpression of *mepA* confers resistance to tigecycline, other glycylcyclines, norfloxacin, cetrimide, TPP, EtBr, and chlorhexidine [106,206]. MsrA overexpression confers resistance to macrolides, ketolides, and type B streptogramins [61], and VgaA and VgaB expression can cause resistance to clindamycin and type B streptogramins [59].

Given the substantial number of putative efflux transporters identified by sequencing of *S. aureus* genomes [301], it is likely that other pumps that affect antimicrobial susceptibility will be identified in the future. Understanding how the expression of such a complex array of drug efflux pumps is integrated into the physiology of staphylococcal cells will be important for optimizing the effectiveness of antimicrobials against staphylococci and other bacteria present in a variety of growth environments.

Resistance to antimicrobials in biofilms

Staphylococcus aureus can persist and can frequently cause recurrent infections, particularly among patients with indwelling medical devices. Critical to the establishment of these infections is the ability of staphylococci first to adhere to a surface and then to form a mucoid biofilm, previously referred to as "slime." Biofilms are sophisticated communities of exopolysaccharide matrix-encased, surface-attached multilayered bacterial clusters that exhibit a distinct phenotype [167] (for a detailed discussion of biofilms, refer to Chapter 5). Bacterial biofilms are inherently resistant to antimicrobial agents. It is likely that biofilms evade antimicrobial challenges by multiple mechanisms including diffusion limitation, altered metabolic activity, and phenotypic and genotypic distinct states of biofilm cells [302].

One mechanism of biofilm resistance to antimicrobial agents is the failure of an agent to penetrate the full depth of the biofilm. The extracellular polymeric substances that make up the matrix of a biofilm are composed mainly of water (up to 95–99%), but also include bacterial polysaccharides, extracellular protein, and DNA as well as excreted host cellular products such as mucopolysaccharides, fibrin, and collagen. The exopolysaccharide matrix of *S. aureus*, composed primarily of a polymer of β-1-6-linked *N*-acetylglucosamine, can retard but probably not prevent the diffusion of antibiotics [303], or can help to concentrate enzymes that inactivate antibiotics within the biofilm [304]. Delayed penetration was observed for aminoglycosides and, in some studies, for β-lactam antibiotics [303]. Recent work on the diffusion of vancomycin through *S. aureus*-formed and synthetic biofilms showed that the diffusion of the drug into the depth of the biofilm was retarded but that this mechanism alone could not explain the increased tolerance demonstrated by *S. aureus* in viscous media [305,306].

A second hypothesis to explain reduced biofilm susceptibility to antibiotics posits that at least some of the cells in a biofilm experience nutrient limitation and therefore exist in a slow-growing or starved state [302]. SCVs constitute a slow-growing subpopulation of bacteria [307]. It was shown that small-colony *P. aeruginosa* produced biofilm [308]. Similarly, a stable small-colony coagulase-negative staphylococcal mutant was able to form a biofilm [309]. The association of biofilm formation by *S. aureus* SCVs that manifest decreased susceptibility to antibiotic killing (see section on aminoglycoside resistance) awaits further study. Inherent to the mechanism of action of some antimicrobials, such as the β-lactams, is a requirement for cell growth for bactericidal activity; slow growth reduces bacterial killing relative to rapidly growing cells [310]. Aminoglycosides and quinolones can kill nongrowing cells, but they are distinctly more effective in killing rapidly dividing cells [302,311]. Thus, the slow-growth phenotype in a biofilm contributes to antibiotic resistance.

A third mechanism of reduced biofilm susceptibility, which is more speculative than the preceding hypotheses, is that at least some of the cells in a biofilm adopt a distinct and protected biofilm phenotype [302,303]. The persistence of bacteria within a biofilm requires an adaptive response appropriate for the sessile lifestyle. A comparison of gene expression in a mature *S. aureus* biofilm and planktonic cultures identified 48 genes whose expression was increased at least twofold and 84 genes whose expression was decreased at least twofold. Among the genes identified to have increased expression in biofilms, several encode transporters, including ABC transporters [312] that could thus potentially extrude antimicrobials. In addition, biofilm development is under the regulation of several loci [313]; some, like the staphylococcal accessory regulator *sarA* [314], affect antibiotic resistance [103,315].

Cell-to-cell contact occurs naturally in microbial biofilms, and biofilms can be polymicrobial [303], thereby serving as a niche for genetic exchange of antimicrobial resistance determinants between bacteria. In this respect it is worth noting that the first clinical isolate of vancomycin-resistant *S. aureus* (VRSA) that was isolated in 2002 from a dialysis catheter [316] acquired the resistance encoding gene *vanA* from a vancomycin-resistant *Enterococcus faecalis* [317]. More recently the *vanA* gene was localized to a plasmid in VRSA and *E. faecium* isolates from a biofilm on an infected nephrostomy tube [318]. In addition in theory in a mixed bacterial biofilm population the ability of one species to inactivate or sequester an antibiotic could confer resistance on another otherwise susceptible species within the biofilm.

References

1 Cethromycin: A-195773, A-195773-0, A-1957730, Abbott-195773, ABT 773. *Drugs R D* 2007;8:95–102.
2 Fernandes PB, Bailer R, Swanson R *et al.* In vitro and in vivo evaluation of A-56268 (TE-031), a new macrolide. Antimicrob Agents Chemother 1986;30:865–73.
3 Nilius AM, Bui MH, Almer L *et al.* Comparative in vitro activity of ABT-773, a novel antibacterial ketolide. Antimicrob Agents Chemother 2001;45:2163–8.
4 Canton R, Loza E, Morosini MI, Baquero F. Antimicrobial resistance amongst isolates of *Streptococcus pyogenes* and *Staphylococcus aureus* in the PROTEKT antimicrobial surveillance programme during 1999–2000. J Antimicrob Chemother 2002;50(suppl S1):9–24.
5 Alferova IV, Vostrov SN, Portnoy YA, Lubenko IY, Zinner SH, Firsov AA. Comparative pharmacodynamics of telithromycin and clarithromycin with *Streptococcus pneumoniae* and

Staphylococcus aureus in an in vitro dynamic model: focus on clinically achievable antibiotic concentrations. Int J Antimicrob Agents 2005;26:197–204.

6 Clarebout G, Leclercq R. Fluorescence assay for studying the ability of macrolides to induce production of ribosomal methylase. Antimicrob Agents Chemother 2002;46:2269–72.

7 Fritsche TR, Sader HS, Jones RN. Comparative activity and spectrum of broad-spectrum beta-lactams (cefepime, ceftazidime, ceftriaxone, piperacillin/tazobactam) tested against 12 295 staphylococci and streptococci: report from the SENTRY antimicrobial surveillance program (North America: 2001–2002). Diagn Microbiol Infect Dis 2003;47:435–40.

8 Singh KV, Malathum K, Murray BE. In vitro activities of a new ketolide, ABT-773, against multidrug-resistant gram-positive cocci. Antimicrob Agents Chemother 2001;45:3640–3.

9 Moran GJ, Krishnadasan A, Gorwitz RJ *et al.* Methicillin-resistant *S. aureus* infections among patients in the emergency department. N Engl J Med 2006;355:666–74.

10 Szumowski JD, Cohen DE, Kanaya F, Mayer KH. Treatment and outcomes of infections by methicillin-resistant *Staphylococcus aureus* at an ambulatory clinic. Antimicrob Agents Chemother 2007;51:423–8.

11 Dancer SJ, Robb A, Crawford A, Morrison D. Oral streptogramins in the management of patients with methicillin-resistant *Staphylococcus aureus* (MRSA) infections. J Antimicrob Chemother 2003;51:731–5.

12 Rybak MJ, Hershberger E, Moldovan T, Grucz RG. In vitro activities of daptomycin, vancomycin, linezolid, and quinupristin-dalfopristin against staphylococci and enterococci, including vancomycin-intermediate and -resistant strains. Antimicrob Agents Chemother 2000;44:1062–6.

13 Low DE, Nadler HL. A review of in-vitro antibacterial activity of quinupristin/dalfopristin against methicillin-susceptible and -resistant *Staphylococcus aureus*. J Antimicrob Chemother 1997;39:53–8.

14 Schlunzen F, Zarivach R, Harms J *et al.* Structural basis for the interaction of antibiotics with the peptidyl transferase centre in eubacteria. Nature 2001;413:814–21.

15 Nissen P, Hansen J, Ban N, Moore PB, Steitz TA. The structural basis of ribosome activity in peptide bond synthesis. Science 2000;289:920–30.

16 Berisio R, Harms J, Schluenzen F *et al.* Structural insight into the antibiotic action of telithromycin against resistant mutants. J Bacteriol 2003;185:4276–9.

17 Tenson T, Lovmar M, Ehrenberg M. The mechanism of action of macrolides, lincosamides and streptogramin B reveals the nascent peptide exit path in the ribosome. J Mol Biol 2003;330:1005–14.

18 Cocito C. Antibiotics of the virginiamycin family, inhibitors which contain synergistic components. Microbiol Rev 1979; 43:145–92.

19 Cocito C, Di GM, Nyssen E, Vannuffel P. Inhibition of protein synthesis by streptogramins and related antibiotics. J Antimicrob Chemother 1997;39(suppl A):7–13.

20 Harms JM, Schlunzen F, Fucini P, Bartels H, Yonath A. Alterations at the peptidyl transferase centre of the ribosome induced by the synergistic action of the streptogramins dalfopristin and quinupristin. BMC Biol 2004;2:4.

21 Lai CJ, Weisblum B. Altered methylation of ribosomal RNA in an erythromycin-resistant strain of *Staphylococcus aureus*. Proc Natl Acad Sci USA 1971;68:856–60.

22 Weaver JR, Pattee PA. Inducible resistance to erythromycin in *Staphylococcus aureus*. J Bacteriol 1964;88:574–80.

23 Murphy E. Nucleotide sequence of *ermA*, a macrolide-lincosamide-streptogramin B determinant in *Staphylococcus aureus*. J Bacteriol 1985;162:633–40.

24 Leclercq R, Courvalin P. Intrinsic and unusual resistance to macrolide, lincosamide, and streptogramin antibiotics in bacteria. Antimicrob Agents Chemother 1991;35:1273–6.

25 Roberts MC, Sutcliffe J, Courvalin P, Jensen LB, Rood J, Seppala H. Nomenclature for macrolide and macrolide-lincosamide-streptogramin B resistance determinants. Antimicrob Agents Chemother 1999;43:2823–30.

26 Weisblum B. Erythromycin resistance by ribosome modification. Antimicrob Agents Chemother 1995;39:577–85.

27 Chung WO, Werckenthin C, Schwarz S, Roberts MC. Host range of the *ermF* rRNA methylase gene in bacteria of human and animal origin. J Antimicrob Chemother 1999;43:5–14.

28 Matsuoka M, Inoue M, Nakajima Y, Endo Y. New *erm* gene in *Staphylococcus aureus* clinical isolates. Antimicrob Agents Chemother 2002;46:211–15.

29 Shortridge VD, Zhong P, Cao ZS *et al.* Comparison of in vitro activities of ABT-773 and telithromycin against macrolide-susceptible and -resistant streptococci and staphylococci. Antimicrob Agents Chemother 2002;46:783–6.

30 Leclercq R, Courvalin P. Bacterial resistance to macrolide, lincosamide, and streptogramin antibiotics by target modification. Antimicrob Agents Chemother 1991;35:1267–72.

31 Davis KA, Crawford SA, Fiebelkorn KR, Jorgensen JH. Induction of telithromycin resistance by erythromycin in isolates of macrolide-resistant *Staphylococcus* spp. Antimicrob Agents Chemother 2005;49:3059–61.

32 Lewis JS, Jorgensen JH. Inducible clindamycin resistance in staphylococci: should clinicians and microbiologists be concerned? Clin Infect Dis 2005;40:280–5.

33 Tanaka T, Weisblum B. Mutant of *Staphylococcus aureus* with lincomycin- and carbomycin-inducible resistance to erythromycin. Antimicrob Agents Chemother 1974;5:538–40.

34 Schmitz FJ, Petridou J, Jagusch H, Astfalk N, Scheuring S, Schwarz S. Molecular characterization of ketolide-resistant *erm*(A)-carrying *Staphylococcus aureus* isolates selected *in vitro* by telithromycin, ABT-773, quinupristin and clindamycin. J Antimicrob Chemother 2002;49:611–17.

35 Gryczan TJ, Grandi G, Hahn J, Grandi R, Dubnau D. Conformational alteration of mRNA structure and the post-transcriptional regulation of erythromycin-induced drug resistance. Nucleic Acids Res 1980;8:6081–97.

36 Mayford M, Weisblum B. Conformational alterations in the *ermC* transcript in vivo during induction. EMBO J 1989;8:4307–14.

37 Eady EA, Ross JI, Tipper JL, Walters CE, Cove JH, Noble WC. Distribution of genes encoding erythromycin ribosomal methylases and an erythromycin efflux pump in epidemiologically distinct groups of staphylococci. J Antimicrob Chemother 1993;31:211–17.

38 Westh H, Hougaard DM, Vuust J, Rosdahl VT. Prevalence of *erm* gene classes in erythromycin-resistant *Staphylococcus aureus* strains isolated between 1959 and 1988. Antimicrob Agents Chemother 1995;39:369–73.

39 Nicola FG, McDougal LK, Biddle JW, Tenover FC. Characterization of erythromycin-resistant isolates of *Staphylococcus*

aureus recovered in the United States from 1958 through 1969. Antimicrob Agents Chemother 1998;42:3024–7.
40 Schmitz FJ, Petridou J, Fluit AC *et al*. Distribution of macrolide-resistance genes in *Staphylococcus aureus* blood-culture isolates from fifteen German university hospitals. Eur J Clin Microbiol Infect Dis 2000;19:385–7.
41 Tait-Kamradt A, Davies T, Cronan M, Jacobs MR, Appelbaum PC, Sutcliffe J. Mutations in 23S rRNA and ribosomal protein L4 account for resistance in pneumococcal strains selected in vitro by macrolide passage. Antimicrob Agents Chemother 2000;44:2118–25.
42 Farrell DJ, Douthwaite S, Morrissey I *et al*. Macrolide resistance by ribosomal mutation in clinical isolates of *Streptococcus pneumoniae* from the PROTEKT 1999–2000 study. Antimicrob Agents Chemother 2003;47:1777–83.
43 Prunier AL, Malbruny B, Tandé D, Picard B, Leclercq R. Clinical isolates of *Staphylococcus aureus* with ribosomal mutations conferring resistance to macrolides. Antimicrob Agents Chemother 2002;46:3054–6.
44 Wondrack L, Massa M, Yang BV, Sutcliffe J. Clinical strain of *Staphylococcus aureus* inactivates and causes efflux of macrolides. Antimicrob Agents Chemother 1996;40:992–8.
45 Sutcliffe J, Grebe T, Tait-Kamradt A, Wondrack L. Detection of erythromycin-resistant determinants by PCR. Antimicrob Agents Chemother 1996;40:2562–6.
46 Schmitz FJ, Sadurski R, Kray A *et al*. Prevalence of macrolide-resistance genes in *Staphylococcus aureus* and *Enterococcus faecium* isolates from 24 European university hospitals. J Antimicrob Chemother 2000;45:891–4.
47 Noguchi N, Tamura Y, Katayama J, Narui K. Expression of the *mphB* gene for macrolide 2′-phosphotransferase II from *Escherichia coli* in *Staphylococcus aureus*. FEMS Microbiol Lett 1998;159:337–42.
48 Brisson-Noel A, Delrieu P, Samain D, Courvalin P. Inactivation of lincosaminide antibiotics in *Staphylococcus*. Identification of lincosaminide O-nucleotidyltransferases and comparison of the corresponding resistance genes. J Biol Chem 1988;263: 15880–7.
49 Leclercq R, Brisson-Noel A, Duval J, Courvalin P. Phenotypic expression and genetic heterogeneity of lincosamide inactivation in *Staphylococcus* spp. Antimicrob Agents Chemother 1987;31:1887–91.
50 Barcs I. Different kinetic of enzymatic inactivation of lincomycin and clindamycin in *Staphylococcus aureus*. J Chemother 1993;5:215–22.
51 Allignet J, Loncle V, Simenel C, Delepierre M, el Solh N. Sequence of a staphylococcal gene, *vat*, encoding an acetyltransferase inactivating the A-type compounds of virginiamycin-like antibiotics. Gene 1993;130:91–8.
52 Allignet J, el Solh N. Diversity among the gram-positive acetyltransferases inactivating streptogramin A and structurally related compounds and characterization of a new staphylococcal determinant, *vatB*. Antimicrob Agents Chemother 1995;39:2027–36.
53 Thal LA, Zervos MJ. Occurrence and epidemiology of resistance to virginiamycin and streptogramins. J Antimicrob Chemother 1999;43:171–6.
54 Liassine N, Allignet J, Morvan A, Aubert S, el Solh N. Multiplicity of the genes and plasmids conferring resistance to pristinamycin in staphylococci selected in an Algerian hospital. Zentralbl Bakteriol 1997;286:389–99.
55 Lina G, Quaglia A, Reverdy ME, Leclercq R, Vandenesch F, Etienne J. Distribution of genes encoding resistance to macrolides, lincosamides, and streptogramins among staphylococci. Antimicrob Agents Chemother 1999;43:1062–6.
56 Korczynska M, Mukhtar TA, Wright GD, Berghuis AM. Structural basis for streptogramin B resistance in *Staphylococcus aureus* by virginiamycin B lyase. Proc Natl Acad Sci USA 2007;104:10388–93.
57 Bouanchaud DH, Fouace JM, Bieth G. Physical studies of a *Staphylococcus aureus* plasmid mediating resistance to streptogramins, lincosamins and aminoglycosides. Ann Microbiol (Paris) 1977;128B:431–7.
58 Mukhtar TA, Koteva KP, Hughes DW, Wright GD. Vgb from *Staphylococcus aureus* inactivates streptogramin B antibiotics by an elimination mechanism not hydrolysis. Biochemistry 2001;40:8877–86.
59 Hassan KA, Skurray RA, Brown MH. Active export proteins mediating drug resistance in staphylococci. J Mol Microbiol Biotechnol 2007;12:180–96.
60 Ross JI, Eady EA, Cove JH, Cunliffe WJ, Baumberg S, Wootton JC. Inducible erythromycin resistance in staphylococci is encoded by a member of the ATP-binding transport supergene family. Mol Microbiol 1990;4:1207–14.
61 Reynolds ED, Cove JH. Resistance to telithromycin is conferred by *msr(A)*, *msrC* and *msr(D)* in *Staphylococcus aureus*. J Antimicrob Chemother 2005;56:1179–80.
62 Tenover FC, McDougal LK, Goering RV *et al*. Characterization of a strain of community-associated methicillin-resistant *Staphylococcus aureus* widely disseminated in the United States. J Clin Microbiol 2006;44:108–18.
63 Allignet J, el Solh N. Characterization of a new staphylococcal gene, *vgaB*, encoding a putative ABC transporter conferring resistance to streptogramin A and related compounds. Gene 1997;202:133–8.
64 Haroche J, Allignet J, Buchrieser C, el Solh N. Characterization of a variant of *vga*(A) conferring resistance to streptogramin A and related compounds. Antimicrob Agents Chemother 2000; 44:2271–5.
65 Chesneau O, Ligeret H, Hosan-Aghaie N, Morvan A, Dassa E. Molecular analysis of resistance to streptogramin A compounds conferred by the Vga proteins of staphylococci. Antimicrob Agents Chemother 2005;49:973–80.
66 Huang J, O'Toole PW, Shen W *et al*. Novel chromosomally encoded multidrug efflux transporter MdeA in *Staphylococcus aureus*. Antimicrob Agents Chemother 2004;48:909–17.
67 DeMarco CE, Cushing LA, Frempong-Manso E, Seo SM, Jaravaza TA, Kaatz GW. Efflux-related resistance to norfloxacin, dyes, and biocides in bloodstream isolates of *Staphylococcus aureus*. Antimicrob Agents Chemother 2007;51: 3235–9.
68 Epe B, Wooley P, Hornig H. Competition between tetracycline and tRNA at both P and A sites of the ribosome of *Escherichia coli*. FEBS Lett 1987;213:443–7.
69 Goldman RA, Hasan T, Hall CC, Strycharz WA, Cooperman BS. Photoincorporation of tetracycline into *Escherichia coli* ribosomes. Identification of the major proteins photolabeled by native tetracycline and tetracycline photoproducts and implications for the inhibitory action of tetracycline on protein synthesis. Biochemistry 1983;22:359–68.
70 Buck MA, Cooperman BS. Single protein omission reconstitu-

tion studies of tetracycline binding to the 30S subunit of *Escherichia coli* ribosomes. Biochemistry 1990;29:5374–9.

71 Arbuck SG, Takimoto CH. An overview of topoisomerase I-targeting agents. Semin Hematol 1998;35:3–12.

72 Martin P, Tieu-Cuot P, Courvalin P. Nucleotide sequence of the *tetM* tetracycline resistance determinant of the streptococcal conjugative shuttle transposon Tn*1545*. Nucleic Acids Res 1986;14:7047–58.

73 LeBlanc DJ, Lee LN, Titmas BM, Smith CJ, Tenover FC. Nucleotide sequence analysis of tetracycline resistance gene *tetO* from *Streptococcus mutans* DL5. J Bacteriol 1988;170: 3618–26.

74 Taylor DE. Plasmid-mediated tetracycline resistance in *Campylobacter jejuni*: expression in *Escherichia coli* and identification of homology with streptococcal class M determinant. J Bacteriol 1986;165:1037–9.

75 Atkinson BA, Abu-Al-Jaibat A, LeBlanc DJ. Antibiotic resistance among enterococci isolated from clinical specimens between 1953 and 1954. Antimicrob Agents Chemother 1997;41: 1598–600.

76 Ahmed M, Borsch CM, Taylor SS, Vazquez-Laslop N, Neyfakh AA. A protein that activates expression of a multidrug efflux transporter upon binding the transporter substrates. J Biol Chem 1994;269:28506–13.

77 Nesin M, Svec P, Lupski JR *et al.* Cloning and nucleotide sequence of a chromosomally encoded tetracycline resistance determinant, *tetA*(M), from a pathogenic, methicillin-resistant strain of *Staphylococcus aureus*. Antimicrob Agents Chemother 1990;34:2273–6.

78 Burdett V. Purification and characterization of Tet(M), a protein that renders ribosomes resistant to tetracycline. J Biol Chem 1991;266:2872–7.

79 Burdett V. tRNA modification activity is necessary for Tet(M)-mediated tetracycline resistance. J Bacteriol 1993;175:7209–15.

80 Burdett V. Tet(M)-promoted release of tetracycline from ribosomes is GTP-dependent. J Bacteriol 1996;178:3246–51.

81 Dantley KA, Dannelly HK, Burdett V. Binding interaction between Tet(M) and the ribosome: requirements for binding. J Bacteriol 1998;180:4089–92.

82 Taylor DE, Trieber CA, Trescher G, Bekkering M. Host mutations (*miaA* and *rpsL*) reduce tetracycline resistance mediated by Tet(O) and Tet(M). Antimicrob Agents Chemother 1998; 42:59–64.

83 Schnappinger D, Hillen W. Tetracyclines: antibiotic action, uptake, and resistance mechanisms. Arch Microbiol 1996; 165:359–69.

84 Taylor DE, Chau A. Tetracycline resistance mediated by ribosomal protection. Antimicrob Agents Chemother 1996;40: 1–5.

85 Connell SR, Tracz DM, Nierhaus KH, Taylor DE. Ribosomal protection proteins and their mechanism of tetracycline resistance. Antimicrob Agents Chemother 2003;47:3675–81.

86 Widdowson CA, Klugman KP. The molecular mechanisms of tetracycline resistance in the pneumococcus. Microb Drug Resist 1998;4:79–84.

87 Su YA, He P, Clewell DB. Characterization of the *tet*(M) determinant of Tn*916*: evidence for regulation by transcriptional attenuation. Antimicrob Agents Chemother 1992;36:769–78.

88 Roberts MC. Update on acquired tetracycline resistance genes. FEMS Microbiol Lett 2005;245:195–203.

89 Speer BS, Shoemaker NB, Salyers AA. Bacterial resistance to tetracycline: mechanisms, transfer, and clinical significance. Clin Microbiol Rev 1992;5:387–99.

90 Truong-Bolduc QC, Dunman PM, Strahilevitz J, Projan SJ, Hooper DC. MgrA is a multiple regulator of two new efflux pumps in *Staphylococcus aureus*. J Bacteriol 2005;187:2395–405.

91 Schwarz S, Cardoso M, Wegener HC. Nucleotide sequence and phylogeny of the *tet(L)* tetracycline resistance determinant encoded by plasmid pSTE1 from *Staphylococcus hyicus*. Antimicrob Agents Chemother 1992;36:580–8.

92 Pao SS, Paulsen IT, Saier MH Jr. Major facilitator superfamily. Microbiol Mol Biol Rev 1998;62:1–34.

93 Yamaguchi A, Shiina Y, Fujihira E, Sawai T, Noguchi N, Sasatsu M. The tetracycline efflux protein encoded by the *tet(K)* gene from *Staphylococcus aureus* is a metal-tetracycline/H^+ antiporter. FEBS Lett 1995;365:193–7.

94 Guffanti AA, Krulwich TA. Tetracycline/H^+ antiport and Na^+/H^+ antiport catalyzed by the *Bacillus subtilis* TetA(L) transporter expressed in *Escherichia coli*. J Bacteriol 1995; 177:4557–61.

95 Rasmussen BA, Gluzman Y, Tally FP. Inhibition of protein synthesis occurring on tetracycline-resistant TetM-protected ribosomes by a novel class of tetracyclines, the glycylcyclines. Antimicrob Agents Chemother 1994;38:1658–60.

96 Bergeron J, Ammirati M, Danley D *et al.* Glycylcyclines bind to the high-affinity tetracycline ribosomal binding site and evade Tet(M)- and Tet(O)-mediated ribosomal protection. Antimicrob Agents Chemother 1996;40:2226–8.

97 Petersen PJ, Jacobus NV, Weiss WJ, Sum PE, Testa RT. In vitro and in vivo antibacterial activities of a novel glycylcycline, the 9-t-butylglycylamido derivative of minocycline (GAR-936). Antimicrob Agents Chemother 1999;43:738–44.

98 McMurry LM, Park BH, Burdett V, Levy SB. Energy-dependent efflux mediated by class L (*tetL*) tetracycline resistance determinant from streptococci. Antimicrob Agents Chemother 1987;31:1648–50.

99 McMurry L, Petrucci RE Jr, Levy SB. Active efflux of tetracycline encoded by four genetically different tetracycline resistance determinants in *Escherichia coli*. Proc Natl Acad Sci USA 1980;77:3974–7.

100 Mojumdar M, Khan SA. Characterization of the tetracycline resistance gene of plasmid pT181 of *Staphylococcus aureus*. J Bacteriol 1988;170:5522–8.

101 Noguchi N, Hase M, Kitta M, Sasatsu M, Deguchi K, Kono M. Antiseptic susceptibility and distribution of antiseptic-resistance genes in methicillin-resistant *Staphylococcus aureus*. FEMS Microbiol Lett 1999;172:247–53.

102 Gillespie MT, May JW, Skurray RA. Detection of an integrated tetracycline resistance plasmid in the chromosome of methicillin-resistant *Staphylococcus aureus*. J Gen Microbiol 1986;132:1723–8.

103 Truong-Bolduc QC, Zhang X, Hooper DC. Characterization of NorR protein, a multifunctional regulator of *norA* expression in *Staphylococcus aureus*. J Bacteriol 2003;185:3127–38.

104 Luong TT, Newell SW, Lee CY. *mgr*, a novel global regulator in *Staphylococcus aureus*. J Bacteriol 2003;185:3703–10.

105 Ingavale SS, Van Wamel W, Cheung AL. Characterization of RAT, an autolysis regulator in *Staphylococcus aureus*. Mol Microbiol 2003;48:1451–66.

106 McAleese F, Petersen P, Ruzin A *et al.* A novel MATE family efflux pump contributes to the reduced susceptibility of laboratory-derived *Staphylococcus aureus* mutants to tigecycline. Antimicrob Agents Chemother 2005;49:1865–71.
107 Le T, Bayer AS. Combination antibiotic therapy for infective endocarditis. Clin Infect Dis 2003;36:615–21.
108 Yoshizawa S, Fourmy D, Puglisi JD. Structural origins of gentamicin antibiotic action. EMBO J 1998;17:6437–48.
109 Hancock RE. Aminoglycoside uptake and mode of action with special reference to streptomycin and gentamicin. II. Effects of aminoglycosides on cells. J Antimicrob Chemother 1981;8: 429–45.
110 Davies J, Wright GD. Bacterial resistance to aminoglycoside antibiotics. Trends Microbiol 1997;5:234–40.
111 Llano-Sotelo B, Azucena EF Jr, Kotra LP, Mobashery S, Chow CS. Aminoglycosides modified by resistance enzymes display diminished binding to the bacterial ribosomal aminoacyl-tRNA site. Chem Biol 2002;9:455–63.
112 Schmitz FJ, Fluit AC, Gondolf M *et al.* The prevalence of aminoglycoside resistance and corresponding resistance genes in clinical isolates of staphylococci from 19 European hospitals. J Antimicrob Chemother 1999;43:253–9.
113 Thomas WD Jr, Archer GL. Mobility of gentamicin resistance genes from staphylococci isolated in the United States: identification of Tn*4031*, a gentamicin resistance transposon from *Staphylococcus epidermidis*. Antimicrob Agents Chemother 1989; 33:1335–41.
114 Dowding JE. Mechanisms of gentamicin resistance in *Staphylococcus aureus*. Antimicrob Agents Chemother 1977;11:47–50.
115 Ubukata K, Yamashita N, Gotoh A, Konno M. Purification and characterization of aminoglycoside-modifying enzymes from *Staphylococcus aureus* and *Staphylococcus epidermidis*. Antimicrob Agents Chemother 1984;25:754–9.
116 Boehr DD, Daigle DM, Wright GD. Domain–domain interactions in the aminoglycoside antibiotic resistance enzyme AAC(6′)-APH(2″). Biochemistry 2004;43:9846–55.
117 Shannon K, Phillips I. Mechanisms of resistance to aminoglycosides in clinical isolates. J Antimicrob Chemother 1982; 9:91–102.
118 Vakulenko SB, Mobashery S. Versatility of aminoglycosides and prospects for their future. Clin Microbiol Rev 2003;16: 430–50.
119 Matsuo H, Kobayashi M, Kumagai T, Kuwabara M, Sugiyama M. Molecular mechanism for the enhancement of arbekacin resistance in a methicillin-resistant *Staphylococcus aureus*. FEBS Lett 2003;546:401–6.
120 Fujimura S, Tokue Y, Takahashi H *et al.* Novel arbekacin- and amikacin-modifying enzyme of methicillin-resistant *Staphylococcus aureus*. FEMS Microbiol Lett 2000;190:299–303.
121 Byrne ME, Gillespie MT, Skurray RA. Molecular analysis of a gentamicin resistance transposonlike element on plasmids isolated from North American *Staphylococcus aureus* strains. Antimicrob Agents Chemother 1990;34:2106–13.
122 Storrs MJ, Courvalin P, Foster TJ. Genetic analysis of gentamicin resistance in methicillin- and gentamicin-resistant strains of *Staphylococcus aureus* isolated in Dublin hospitals. Antimicrob Agents Chemother 1988;32:1174–81.
123 Gillespie MT, Lyon BR, Messerotti LJ, Skurray RA. Chromosome- and plasmid-mediated gentamicin resistance in *Staphylococcus aureus* encoded by Tn*4001*. J Med Microbiol 1987;24:139–44.
124 Ida T, Okamoto R, Nonoyama M, Irinoda K, Kurazono M, Inoue M. Antagonism between aminoglycosides and β-lactams in a methicillin-resistant *Staphylococcus aureus* isolate involves induction of an aminoglycoside-modifying enzyme. Antimicrob Agents Chemother 2002;46:1516–21.
125 Santanam P, Kayser FH. Purification and characterization of an aminoglycoside inactivating enzyme from *Staphylococcus epidermidis* FK109 that nucleotidylates the 4′- and 4″-hydroxyl groups of the aminoglycoside antibiotics. J Antibiot (Tokyo) 1978;31:343–51.
126 Le GF, Martel A, Capmau ML *et al.* New plasmid-mediated nucleotidylation of aminoglycoside antibiotics in *Staphylococcus aureus*. Antimicrob Agents Chemother 1976;10:258–64.
127 Berg T, Firth N, Apisiridej S, Hettiaratchi A, Leelaporn A, Skurray RA. Complete nucleotide sequence of pSK41: evolution of staphylococcal conjugative multiresistance plasmids. J Bacteriol 1998;180:4350–9.
128 Ito T, Katayama Y, Hiramatsu K. Cloning and nucleotide sequence determination of the entire *mec* DNA of pre-methicillin-resistant *Staphylococcus aureus* N315. Antimicrob Agents Chemother 1999;43:1449–58.
129 Byrne ME, Gillespie MT, Skurray RA. 4′,4″-Adenyltransferase activity on conjugative plasmids isolated from *Staphylococcus aureus* is encoded on an integrated copy of pUB110. Plasmid 1991;25:70–5.
130 Ida T, Okamoto R, Shimauchi C, Okubo T, Kuga A, Inoue M. Identification of aminoglycoside-modifying enzymes by susceptibility testing: epidemiology of methicillin-resistant *Staphylococcus aureus* in Japan. J Clin Microbiol 2001;39:3115–21.
131 Chongtrakool P, Ito T, Ma XX *et al.* Staphylococcal cassette chromosome mec (SCCmec) typing of methicillin-resistant *Staphylococcus aureus* strains isolated in 11 Asian countries: a proposal for a new nomenclature for SCCmec elements. Antimicrob Agents Chemother 2006;50:1001–12.
132 Courvalin P, Fiandt M. Aminoglycoside-modifying enzymes of *Staphylococcus aureus*: expression in *Escherichia coli*. Gene 1980;9:247–69.
133 Gray GS, Fitch WM. Evolution of antibiotic resistance genes: the DNA sequence of a kanamycin resistance gene from *Staphylococcus aureus*. Mol Biol Evol 1983;1:57–66.
134 Wright GD, Thompson PR. Aminoglycoside phosphotransferases: proteins, structure, and mechanism. Front Biosci 1999; 4:D9–D21.
135 Murphy E. Nucleotide sequence of a spectinomycin adenyltransferase AAD(9) determinant from *Staphylococcus aureus* and its relationship to AAD(3″) (9). Mol Gen Genet 1985; 200:33–9.
136 Proctor RA, van Langevelde P, Kristjansson M, Maslow JN, Arbeit RD. Persistent and relapsing infections associated with small-colony variants of *Staphylococcus aureus*. Clin Infect Dis 1995;20:95–102.
137 Proctor RA, Peters G. Small colony variants in staphylococcal infections: diagnostic and therapeutic implications. Clin Infect Dis 1998;27:419–22.
138 Proctor RA, Kahl B, Von Eiff C, Vaudaux PE, Lew DP, Peters G. Staphylococcal small colony variants have novel mechanisms for antibiotic resistance. Clin Infect Dis 1998;27:S68–S74.

139 Miller MH, Edberg SC, Mandel LJ, Behar CF, Steigbigel NH. Gentamicin uptake in wild-type and aminoglycoside-resistant small-colony mutants of *Staphylococcus aureus*. Antimicrob Agents Chemother 1980;18:722–9.

140 Galimand M, Courvalin P, Lambert T. Plasmid-mediated high-level resistance to aminoglycosides in *Enterobacteriaceae* due to 16S rRNA methylation. Antimicrob Agents Chemother 2003;47:2565–71.

141 Sobel ML, McKay GA, Poole K. Contribution of the MexXY multidrug transporter to aminoglycoside resistance in *Pseudomonas aeruginosa* clinical isolates. Antimicrob Agents Chemother 2003;47:3202–7.

142 Kumar KP, Chatterji D. Differential inhibition of abortive transcription initiation at different promoters catalysed by *E. coli* RNA polymerase. Effect of rifampicin on purine or pyramidine-initiated phosphodiester synthesis. FEBS Lett 1992;306:46–50.

143 Kumar KP, Reddy PS, Chatterji D. Proximity relationship between the active site of *Escherichia coli* RNA polymerase and rifampicin binding domain: a resonance energy-transfer study. Biochemistry 1992;31:7519–26.

144 Jin DJ, Gross CA. Mapping and sequencing of mutations in the *Escherichia coli rpoB* gene that lead to rifampicin resistance. J Mol Biol 1988;202:45–58.

145 Jin DJ, Cashel M, Friedman DI, Nakamura Y, Walter WA, Gross CA. Effects of rifampicin resistant *rpoB* mutations on antitermination and interaction with *nusA* in *Escherichia coli*. J Mol Biol 1988;204:247–61.

146 Morrow TO, Harmon SA. Genetic analysis of *Staphylococcus aureus* RNA polymerase mutants. J Bacteriol 1979;137:374–83.

147 Wichelhaus TA, Schäfer V, Brade V, Böddinghaus B. Molecular characterization of *rpoB* mutations conferring cross-resistance to rifamycins on methicillin-resistant *Staphylococcus aureus*. Antimicrob Agents Chemother 1999;43:2813–16.

148 Aubry-Damon H, Soussy CJ, Courvalin P. Characterization of mutations in the *rpoB* gene that confer rifampin resistance in *Staphylococcus aureus*. Antimicrob Agents Chemother 1998; 42:2590–4.

149 Padayachee T, Klugman KP. Molecular basis of rifampin resistance in *Streptococcus pneumoniae*. Antimicrob Agents Chemother 1999;43:2361–5.

150 Varaldo PE, Debbia E, Schito GC. In vitro activities of rifapentine and rifampin, alone and in combination with six other antibiotics, against methicillin-susceptible and methicillin-resistant staphylococci of different species. Antimicrob Agents Chemother 1985;27:615–18.

151 Varaldo PE, Cipriani P, Foca A *et al*. Identification, clinical distribution, and susceptibility to methicillin and 18 additional antibiotics of clinical *Staphylococcus* isolates: nationwide investigation in Italy. J Clin Microbiol 1984;19:838–43.

152 Archer GL, Climo MW. Antimicrobial susceptibility of coagulase-negative staphylococci. Antimicrob Agents Chemother 1994;38:2231–7.

153 Cookson BD. The emergence of mupirocin resistance: a challenge to infection control and antibiotic prescribing practice. J Antimicrob Chemother 1998;41:11–18.

154 Morton TM, Johnston JL, Patterson J, Archer GL. Characterization of a conjugative staphylococcal mupirocin resistance plasmid. Antimicrob Agents Chemother 1995;39:1272–80.

155 Bradley SF, Ramsey MA, Morton TM, Kauffman CA. Mupirocin resistance: clinical and molecular epidemiology. Infect Control Hosp Epidemiol 1995;16:354–8.

156 Farmer TH, Gilbart J, Elson SW. Biochemical basis of mupirocin resistance in strains of *Staphylococcus aureus*. J Antimicrob Chemother 1992;30:587–96.

157 Gilbart J, Perry CR, Slocombe B. High-level mupirocin resistance in *Staphylococcus aureus*: evidence for two distinct isoleucyl-tRNA synthetases. Antimicrob Agents Chemother 1993;37:32–8.

158 Hodgson JE, Curnock SP, Dyke KGH, Morris R, Sylvester DR, Gross MS. Molecular characterization of the gene encoding high-level mupirocin resistance in *Staphylococcus aureus* J2870. Antimicrob Agents Chemother 1994;38:1205–8.

159 Yun HJ, Lee SW, Yoon GM *et al*. Prevalence and mechanisms of low- and high-level mupirocin resistance in staphylococci isolated from a Korean hospital. J Antimicrob Chemother 2003;51:619–23.

160 Udo EE, Al-Sweih N, Noronha BC. A chromosomal location of the *mupA* gene in *Staphylococcus aureus* expressing high-level mupirocin resistance. J Antimicrob Chemother 2003;51:1283–6.

161 Janssen DA, Zarins LT, Schaberg DR, Bradley SF, Terpenning MS, Kauffman CA. Detection and characterization of mupirocin resistance in *Staphylococcus aureus*. Antimicrob Agents Chemother 1993;37:2003–6.

162 Hurdle JG, O'Neill AJ, Mody L, Chopra I, Bradley SF. In vivo transfer of high-level mupirocin resistance from *Staphylococcus epidermidis* to methicillin-resistant *Staphylococcus aureus* associated with failure of mupirocin prophylaxis. J Antimicrob Chemother 2005;56:1166–8.

163 Needham C, Rahman M, Dyke KG, Noble WC. An investigation of plasmids from *Staphylococcus aureus* that mediate resistance to mupirocin and tetracycline. Microbiology 1994;140:2577–83.

164 Driscoll DG, Young CL, Ochsner UA. Transient loss of high-level mupirocin resistance in *Staphylococcus aureus* due to MupA polymorphism. Antimicrob Agents Chemother 2007;51:2247–8.

165 Hurdle JG, O'Neill AJ, Chopra I. The isoleucyl-tRNA synthetase mutation V588F conferring mupirocin resistance in glycopeptide-intermediate *Staphylococcus aureus* is not associated with a significant fitness burden. J Antimicrob Chemother 2004;53:102–4.

166 Hurdle JG, O'Neill AJ, Ingham E, Fishwick C, Chopra I. Analysis of mupirocin resistance and fitness in *Staphylococcus aureus* by molecular genetic and structural modeling techniques. Antimicrob Agents Chemother 2004;48:4366–76.

167 Paulander W, Maisnier-Patin S, Andersson DI. Multiple mechanisms to ameliorate the fitness burden of mupirocin resistance in *Salmonella typhimurium*. Mol Microbiol 2007;64:1038–48.

168 Ramsey MA, Bradley SF, Kauffman CA, Morton TM. Identification of chromosomal location of *mupA* gene, encoding low-level mupirocin resistance in staphylococcal isolates. Antimicrob Agents Chemother 1996;40:2820–3.

169 Bonilla HF, Zarins LT, Bradley SF, Kauffman CA. Susceptibility of ciprofloxacin-resistant staphylococci and enterococci to trovafloxacin. Diagn Microbiol Infect Dis 1996;26:17–21.

170 Ball P. Quinolone generations: natural history or natural selection? J Antimicrob Chemother 2000;46:17–24.

171 Ince D, Zhang X, Hooper DC. Activity of and resistance to moxifloxacin in *Staphylococcus aureus*. Antimicrob Agents Chemother 2003;47:1410–15.

172 Strahilevitz J, Truong-Bolduc QC, Hooper DC. DX-619, a novel des-fluoro(6)-quinolone manifesting low frequency of selection of resistant mutants in *Staphylococcus aureus*: quinolone resistance beyond attack of type II topoisomerases. Antimicrob Agents Chemother 2005;49:5069–75.
173 Zhao XL, Eisner W, Perl-Rosenthal N, Kreiswirth B, Drlica K. Mutant prevention concentration of garenoxacin (BMS-284756) for ciprofloxacin-susceptible or -resistant *Staphylococcus aureus*. Antimicrob Agents Chemother 2003;47:1023–7.
174 Weber SG, Gold HS, Hooper DC, Karchmer AW, Carmeli Y. Fluoroquinolones and the risk for methicillin-resistant *Staphylococcus aureus* in hospitalized patients. Emerg Infect Dis 2003;9:1415–22.
175 Wang JC. DNA topoisomerases. Annu Rev Biochem 1996; 65:635–92.
176 Gellert M, Mizuuchi K, O'Dea MH, Itoh T, Tomizawa JI. Nalidixic acid resistance: a second genetic character involved in DNA gyrase activity. Proc Natl Acad Sci USA 1977;74:4772–6.
177 Sugino A, Peebles CL, Kreuzer KN, Cozzarelli NR. Mechanism of action of nalidixic acid: purification of *Escherichia coli nalA* gene product and its relationship to DNA gyrase and a novel nicking-closing enzyme. Proc Natl Acad Sci USA 1977;74: 4767–71.
178 Hooper DC. Mechanisms of quinolone resistance. In: Hooper DC, Rubinstein E, eds. Quinolone Antimicrobial Agents. Washington, DC: ASM Press, 2003:41–67.
179 Trucksis M, Wolfson JS, Hooper DC. A novel locus conferring fluoroquinolone resistance in *Staphylococcus aureus*. J Bacteriol 1991;173:5854–60.
180 Ng EY, Trucksis M, Hooper DC. Quinolone resistance mutations in topoisomerase IV: relationship of the *flqA* locus and genetic evidence that topoisomerase IV is the primary target and DNA gyrase the secondary target of fluoroquinolones in *Staphylococcus aureus*. Antimicrob Agents Chemother 1996; 40:1881–8.
181 Blanche F, Cameron B, Bernard FX *et al.* Differential behaviors of *Staphylococcus aureus* and *Escherichia coli* type II DNA topoisomerases. Antimicrob Agents Chemother 1996;40:2714–20.
182 Strahilevitz J, Robicsek A, Hooper DC. Role of the extended alpha4 domain of *Staphylococcus aureus* gyrase A protein in determining low sensitivity to quinolones. Antimicrob Agents Chemother 2006;50:600–6.
183 Zhao X, Xu C, Domagala J, Drlica K. DNA topoisomerase targets of the fluoroquinolones: a strategy for avoiding bacterial resistance. Proc Natl Acad Sci USA 1997;94:13991–6.
184 Strahilevitz J, Hooper DC. Dual targeting of topoisomerase IV and gyrase to reduce mutant selection: direct testing of the paradigm by using WCK-1734, a new fluoroquinolone, and ciprofloxacin. Antimicrob Agents Chemother 2005;49:1949–56.
185 Barnard FM, Maxwell A. Interaction between DNA gyrase and quinolones: effects of alanine mutations at GyrA subunit residues Ser^{83} and Asp^{87}. Antimicrob Agents Chemother 2001; 45:1994–2000.
186 Morais Cabral JH, Jackson AP, Smith CV, Shikotra N, Maxwell A, Liddington RC. Crystal structure of the breakage-reunion domain of DNA gyrase. Nature 1997;388:903–6.
187 Willmott CJ, Maxwell A. A single point mutation in the DNA gyrase A protein greatly reduces binding of fluoroquinolones to the gyrase–DNA complex. Antimicrob Agents Chemother 1993;37:126–7.
188 Ince D, Zhang X, Silver LC, Hooper DC. Topoisomerase targeting with and resistance to gemifloxacin in *Staphylococcus aureus*. Antimicrob Agents Chemother 2003;47:274–82.
189 Ince D, Zhang X, Silver LC, Hooper DC. Dual targeting of DNA gyrase and topoisomerase IV: target interactions of garenoxacin (BMS-284756, T3811ME), a new desfluoroquinolone. Antimicrob Agents Chemother 2002;46:3370–80.
190 Jacobs MR, Bajaksouzian S, Windau A *et al.* In vitro activity of the new quinolone WCK 771 against staphylococci. Antimicrob Agents Chemother 2004;48:3338–42.
191 Hoshino K, Inoue K, Murakami Y *et al.* In vitro and in vivo antibacterial activities of DC-159a, a new fluoroquinolone. Antimicrob Agents Chemother 2008;52:65–76.
192 Ince D, Hooper DC. Mechanisms and frequency of resistance to gatifloxacin in comparison to AM-1121 and ciprofloxacin in *Staphylococcus aureus*. Antimicrob Agents Chemother 2001; 45:2755–64.
193 Firsov AA, Lubenko IY, Vostrov SN, Portnoy YA, Zinner SH. Antistaphylococcal effect related to the area under the curve/MIC ratio in an in vitro dynamic model: predicted breakpoints versus clinically achievable values for seven fluoroquinolones. Antimicrob Agents Chemother 2005;49:2642–7.
194 Metzler K, Hansen GM, Hedlin P, Harding E, Drlica K, Blondeau JM. Comparison of minimal inhibitory and mutant prevention drug concentrations of 4 fluoroquinolones against clinical isolates of methicillin-susceptible and -resistant *Staphylococcus aureus*. Int J Antimicrob Agents 2004;24:161–7.
195 Lipsitch M, Levin BR. The population dynamics of antimicrobial chemotherapy. Antimicrob Agents Chemother 1997;41:363–73.
196 Ubeda C, Maiques E, Knecht E, Lasa I, Novick RP, Penades JR. Antibiotic-induced SOS response promotes horizontal dissemination of pathogenicity island-encoded virulence factors in staphylococci. Mol Microbiol 2005;56:836–44.
197 McKenzie GJ, Harris RS, Lee PL, Rosenberg SM. The SOS response regulates adaptive mutation. Proc Natl Acad Sci USA 2000;97:6646–51.
198 Cirz RT, Jones MB, Gingles NA *et al.* Complete and SOS-mediated response of *Staphylococcus aureus* to the antibiotic ciprofloxacin. J Bacteriol 2007;189:531–9.
199 Cirz RT, Chin JK, Andes DR, de Crecy-Lagard V, Craig WA, Romesberg FE. Inhibition of mutation and combating the evolution of antibiotic resistance. PLoS Biol 2005;3:e176.
200 Lewin CS, Amyes SG. The role of the SOS response in bacteria exposed to zidovudine or trimethoprim. J Med Microbiol 1991;34:329–32.
201 Maiques E, Ubeda C, Campoy S *et al.* Beta-lactam antibiotics induce the SOS response and horizontal transfer of virulence factors in *Staphylococcus aureus*. J Bacteriol 2006;188:2726–9.
202 Ren Q, Kang KH, Paulsen IT. TransportDB: a relational database of cellular membrane transport systems. Nucleic Acids Res 2004;32:D284–D288.
203 Yoshida H, Bogaki M, Nakamura S, Ubukata K, Konno M. Nucleotide sequence and characterization of the *Staphylococcus aureus norA* gene, which confers resistance to quinolones. J Bacteriol 1990;172:6942–9.
204 Truong-Bolduc QC, Strahilevitz J, Hooper DC. NorC, a new efflux pump regulated by MgrA of *Staphylococcus aureus*. Antimicrob Agents Chemother 2006;50:1104–7.
205 Yamada Y, Hideka K, Shiota S, Kuroda T, Tsuchiya T. Gene cloning and characterization of SdrM, a chromosomally-

encoded multidrug efflux pump, from *Staphylococcus aureus*. Biol Pharm Bull 2006;29:554–6.

206 Kaatz GW, McAleese F, Seo SM. Multidrug resistance in *Staphylococcus aureus* due to overexpression of a novel multidrug and toxin extrusion (MATE) transport protein. Antimicrob Agents Chemother 2005;49:1857–64.

207 Fournier B, Truong-Bolduc QC, Zhang X, Hooper DC. A mutation in the 5′ untranslated region increases stability of *norA* mRNA, encoding a multidrug resistance transporter of *Staphylococcus aureus*. J Bacteriol 2001;183:2367–71.

208 Fournier B, Aras R, Hooper DC. Expression of the multidrug resistance transporter NorA from *Staphylococcus aureus* is modified by a two-component regulatory system. J Bacteriol 2000;182:664–71.

209 Ingavale S, van Wamel W, Luong TT, Lee CY, Cheung AL. Rat/MgrA, a regulator of autolysis, is a regulator of virulence genes in *Staphylococcus aureus*. Infect Immun 2005;73:1423–31.

210 Fournier B, Klier A. Protein A gene expression is regulated by DNA supercoiling which is modified by the ArlS-ArlR two-component system of *Staphylococcus aureus*. Microbiology 2004;150:3807–19.

211 Truong-Bolduc QC, Hooper DC. Transcriptional regulators NorG and MgrA modulate resistance to both quinolones and β-lactams in *Staphylococcus aureus*. J Bacteriol 2007;189:2996–3005.

212 Kaatz GW, DeMarco CE, Seo SM. MepR, a repressor of the *Staphylococcus aureus* MATE family multidrug efflux pump MepA, is a substrate-responsive regulatory protein. Antimicrob Agents Chemother 2006;50:1276–81.

213 Finkelstein R, Birkeland JM. The mode of action of sulfanilamide and prontosil. Science 1938;87:441–2.

214 Roth B, Falco EA, Hitchings GH, Bushby SR. 5-Benzyl-2,4-diaminopyrimidines as antibacterial agents. I. Synthesis and antibacterial activity in vitro. J Med Pharm Chem 1962;91: 1103–23.

215 Markowitz N, Quinn EL, Saravolatz LD. Trimethoprim–sulfamethoxazole compared with vancomycin for the treatment of *Staphylococcus aureus* infection. Ann Intern Med 1992;117:390–8.

216 Huovinen P, Sundstrom L, Swedberg G, Sköld O. Trimethoprim and sulfonamide resistance. Antimicrob Agents Chemother 1995;39:279–89.

217 Bushby SR. Synergy of trimethoprim–sulfamethoxazole. Can Med Assoc J 1975;112:63–6.

218 Dale GE, Broger C, D'Arcy A *et al.* A single amino acid substitution in *Staphylococcus aureus* dihydrofolate reductase determines trimethoprim resistance. J Mol Biol 1997;266:23–30.

219 Coughter JP, Johnston JL, Archer GL. Characterization of a staphylococcal trimethoprim resistance gene and its product. Antimicrob Agents Chemother 1987;31:1027–32.

220 Young HK, Skurray RA, Amyes SG. Plasmid-mediated trimethoprim-resistance in *Staphylococcus aureus*. Characterization of the first gram-positive plasmid dihydrofolate reductase (type S1). Biochem J 1987;243:309–12.

221 Tennent JM, Young HK, Lyon BR, Amyes SG, Skurray RA. Trimethoprim resistance determinants encoding a dihydrofolate reductase in clinical isolates of *Staphylococcus aureus* and coagulase-negative staphylococci. J Med Microbiol 1988; 26:67–73.

222 Leelaporn A, Firth N, Paulsen IT, Skurray RA. IS257-mediated cointegration in the evolution of a family of staphylococcal trimethoprim resistance plasmids. J Bacteriol 1996;178:6070–3.

223 Leelaporn A, Firth N, Byrne ME, Roper E, Skurray RA. Possible role of insertion sequence IS*257* in dissemination and expression of high- and low-level trimethoprim resistance in staphylococci. Antimicrob Agents Chemother 1994;38:2238–44.

224 Rouch DA, Messerotti LJ, Loo LS, Jackson CA, Skurray RA. Trimethoprim resistance transposon Tn*4003* from *Staphylococcus aureus* encodes genes for a dihydrofolate reductase and thymidylate synthetase flanked by three copies of IS*257*. Mol Microbiol 1989;3:161–75.

225 Swedberg G, Ringertz S, Skold O. Sulfonamide resistance in *Streptococcus pyogenes* is associated with differences in the amino acid sequence of its chromosomal dihydropteroate synthase. Antimicrob Agents Chemother 1998;42:1062–7.

226 Then RL, Kohl I, Burdeska A. Frequency and transferability of trimethoprim and sulfonamide resistance in methicillin-resistant *Staphylococcus aureus* and *Staphylococcus epidermidis*. J Chemother 1992;4:67–71.

227 Hampele IC, D'Arcy A, Dale GE *et al.* Structure and function of the dihydropteroate synthase from *Staphylococcus aureus*. J Mol Biol 1997;268:21–30.

228 Landy M, Larkum NW, Oswald EJ, Streightoff F. Increased synthesis of p-aminobenzoic acid associated with the development of sulfonamide resistance in *Staphylococcus aureus*. Science 1943;97:265–7.

229 Lewis EL, Lacey RW. Present significance of resistance to trimethoprim and sulphonamides in coliforms, *Staphylococcus aureus*, and *Streptococcus faecalis*. J Clin Pathol 1973;26:175–80.

230 Gonzales RD, Schreckenberger PC, Graham MB, Kelkar S, DenBesten K, Quinn JP. Infections due to vancomycin-resistant *Enterococcus faecium* resistant to linezolid. Lancet 2001;357:1179.

231 Burleson BS, Ritchie DJ, Micek ST, Dunne WM. *Enterococcus faecalis* resistant to linezolid: case series and review of the literature. Pharmacotherapy 2004;24:1225–31.

232 Jones RN, Della-Latta P, Lee LV, Biedenbach DJ. Linezolid-resistant *Enterococcus faecium* isolated from a patient without prior exposure to an oxazolidinone: report from the SENTRY Antimicrobial Surveillance Program. Diagn Microbiol Infect Dis 2002;42:137–9.

233 Herrero IA, Issa NC, Patel R. Nosocomial spread of linezolid-resistant, vancomycin-resistant *Enterococcus faecium*. N Engl J Med 2002;346:867–9.

234 Tsiodras S, Gold HS, Sakoulas G *et al.* Linezolid resistance in a clinical isolate of *Staphylococcus aureus*. Lancet 2001;358:207–8.

235 Wilson P, Andrews JA, Charlesworth R *et al.* Linezolid resistance in clinical isolates of *Staphylococcus aureus*. J Antimicrob Chemother 2003;51:186–7.

236 Meka VG, Pillai SK, Sakoulas G *et al.* Linezolid resistance in sequential *Staphylococcus aureus* isolates associated with a T2500A mutation in the 23S rRNA gene and loss of a single copy of rRNA. J Infect Dis 2004;190:311–17.

237 Cieloszyk K, Modio-Groton M, Saeed M, Coyle CM. Linezolid resistance in three isolates of coagulase-negative staphylococci. Ann Pharmacother 2007;41:526–7.

238 Potoski BA, Adams J, Clarke L *et al.* Epidemiological profile of linezolid-resistant coagulase-negative staphylococci. Clin Infect Dis 2006;43:165–71.

239 Swaney SM, Aoki H, Ganoza MC, Shinabarger DL. The oxazolidinone linezolid inhibits initiation of protein synthesis in bacteria. Antimicrob Agents Chemother 1998;42:3251–5.

240 Meka VG, Gold HS. Antimicrobial resistance to linezolid. Clin Infect Dis 2004;39:1010–15.

241 Pillai SK, Sakoulas G, Wennersten C *et al.* Linezolid resistance in *Staphylococcus aureus*: characterization and stability of resistant phenotype. J Infect Dis 2002;186:1603–7.

242 Meka VG, Gold HS, Cooke A *et al.* Reversion to susceptibility in a linezolid-resistant clinical isolate of *Staphylococcus aureus*. J Antimicrob Chemother 2004;54:818–20.

243 Swoboda S, Fritz S, Martignoni ME *et al.* Varying linezolid susceptibility of vancomycin-resistant *Enterococcus faecium* isolates during therapy: a case report. J Antimicrob Chemother 2005;56:787–9.

244 Xiong LQ, Kloss P, Douthwaite S *et al.* Oxazolidinone resistance mutations in 23S rRNA of *Escherichia coli* reveal the central region of domain V as the primary site of drug action. J Bacteriol 2000;182:5325–31.

245 Kloss P, Xiong L, Shinabarger DL, Mankin AS. Resistance mutations in 23S rRNA identify the site of action of the protein synthesis inhibitor linezolid in the ribosomal peptidyl transferase center. J Mol Biol 1999;294:93–101.

246 Prystowsky J, Siddiqui F, Chosay J *et al.* Resistance to linezolid: characterization of mutations in rRNA and comparison of their occurrences in vancomycin-resistant enterococci. Antimicrob Agents Chemother 2001;45:2154–6.

247 Wolter N, Smith AM, Farrell DJ *et al.* Novel mechanism of resistance to oxazolidinones, macrolides, and chloramphenicol in ribosomal protein L4 of the pneumococcus. Antimicrob Agents Chemother 2005;49:3554–7.

248 Kehrenberg C, Schwarz S. Distribution of florfenicol resistance genes *fexA* and *cfr* among chloramphenicol-resistant *Staphylococcus* isolates. Antimicrob Agents Chemother 2006;50:1156–63.

249 Kehrenberg C, Aarestrup FM, Schwarz S. IS21–558 insertion sequences are involved in the mobility of the multiresistance gene *cfr*. Antimicrob Agents Chemother 2007;51:483–7.

250 Kehrenberg C, Schwarz S, Jacobsen L, Hansen LH, Vester B. A new mechanism for chloramphenicol, florfenicol and clindamycin resistance: methylation of 23S ribosomal RNA at A2503. Mol Microbiol 2005;57:1064–73.

251 Long KS, Poehlsgaard J, Kehrenberg C, Schwarz S, Vester B. The Cfr rRNA methyltransferase confers resistance to phenicols, lincosamides, oxazolidinones, pleuromutilins, and streptogramin A antibiotics. Antimicrob Agents Chemother 2006; 50:2500–5.

252 Toh SM, Xiong L, Arias CA *et al.* Acquisition of a natural resistance gene renders a clinical strain of methicillin-resistant *Staphylococcus aureus* resistant to the synthetic antibiotic linezolid. Mol Microbiol 2007;64:1506–14.

253 Sader HS, Streit JM, Fritsche TR, Jones RN. Antimicrobial susceptibility of gram-positive bacteria isolated from European medical centres: results of the Daptomycin Surveillance Programme (2002–2004). Clin Microbiol Infect 2006;12:844–52.

254 Pfaller MA, Sader HS, Jones RN. Evaluation of the in vitro activity of daptomycin against 19615 clinical isolates of Gram-positive cocci collected in North American hospitals (2002–2005). Diagn Microbiol Infect Dis 2007;57:459–65.

255 Silverman JA, Perlmutter NG, Shapiro HM. Correlation of daptomycin bactericidal activity and membrane depolarization in *Staphylococcus aureus*. Antimicrob Agents Chemother 2003; 47:2538–44.

256 Muthaiyan A, Silverman JA, Jayaswal RK, Wilkinson BJ. Transcriptional profiling reveals that daptomycin induces the *Staphylococcus aureus* cell wall stress stimulon and genes responsive to membrane depolarization. Antimicrob Agents Chemother 2008;52:980–90.

257 Silverman JA, Oliver N, Andrew T, Li T. Resistance studies with daptomycin. Antimicrob Agents Chemother 2001;45:1799–802.

258 Friedman L, Alder JD, Silverman JA. Genetic changes that correlate with reduced susceptibility to daptomycin in *Staphylococcus aureus*. Antimicrob Agents Chemother 2006;50:2137–45.

259 Jones T, Yeaman MR, Sakoulas G *et al.* Failures in clinical treatment of *Staphylococcus aureus* infection with daptomycin are associated with alterations in surface charge, membrane phospholipid asymmetry, and drug binding. Antimicrob Agents Chemother 2008;52:269–78.

260 Mohedano ML, Overweg K, de la Fuente A *et al.* Evidence that the essential response regulator YycF in *Streptococcus pneumoniae* modulates expression of fatty acid biosynthesis genes and alters membrane composition. J Bacteriol 2005;187:2357–67.

261 Kaatz GW, Lundstrom TS, Seo SM. Mechanisms of daptomycin resistance in *Staphylococcus aureus*. Int J Antimicrob Agents 2006;28:280–7.

262 Pillai SK, Gold HS, Sakoulas G, Wennersten C, Moellering RC Jr, Eliopoulos GM. Daptomycin nonsusceptibility in *Staphylococcus aureus* with reduced vancomycin susceptibility is independent of alterations in MprF. Antimicrob Agents Chemother 2007;51:2223–5.

263 Sakoulas G, Alder J, Thauvin-Eliopoulos C, Moellering RC Jr, Eliopoulos GM. Induction of daptomycin heterogeneous susceptibility in *Staphylococcus aureus* by exposure to vancomycin. Antimicrob Agents Chemother 2006;50:1581–5.

264 Cui L, Tominaga E, Neoh HM, Hiramatsu K. Correlation between reduced daptomycin susceptibility and vancomycin resistance in vancomycin-intermediate *Staphylococcus aureus*. Antimicrob Agents Chemother 2006;50:1079–82.

265 Mwangi MM, Wu SW, Zhou Y *et al.* Tracking the in vivo evolution of multidrug resistance in *Staphylococcus aureus* by whole-genome sequencing. Proc Natl Acad Sci USA 2007; 104:9451–6.

266 Patel JB, Jevitt LA, Hageman J, McDonald LC, Tenover FC. An association between reduced susceptibility to daptomycin and reduced susceptibility to vancomycin in *Staphylococcus aureus*. Clin Infect Dis 2006;42:1652–3.

267 Boucher HW, Sakoulas G. Antimicrobial resistance: perspectives on daptomycin resistance, with emphasis on resistance in *Staphylococcus aureus*. Clin Infect Dis 2007;45:601–8.

268 Bennett JW, Murray CK, Holmes RL, Patterson JE, Jorgensen JH. Diminished vancomycin and daptomycin susceptibility during prolonged bacteremia with methicillin-resistant *Staphylococcus aureus*. Diagn Microbiol Infect Dis 2008;60:437–40.

269 Mariani PG, Sader HS, Jones RN. Development of decreased susceptibility to daptomycin and vancomycin in a *Staphylococcus aureus* strain during prolonged therapy. J Antimicrob Chemother 2006;58:481–3.

270 Kreiswirth B, Kornblum J, Arbeit RD *et al.* Evidence for a clonal origin of methicillin resistance in *Staphylococcus aureus*. Science 1993;259:227–30.

271 Gilbert M, MacDonald J, Gregson D *et al.* Outbreak in Alberta of community-acquired (USA300) methicillin-resistant *Staphylococcus aureus* in people with a history of drug use, homelessness or incarceration. Can Med Assoc J 2006;175:149–54.

272 Larsen A, Stegger M, Goering R, Sørum M, Skov R. Emergence and dissemination of the methicillin resistant *Staphylococcus aureus* USA300 clone in Denmark (2000–2005). Euro Surveillance 2007;12.

273 De Silva GDI, Justice A, Wilkinson AR *et al.* Genetic population structure of coagulase-negative staphylococci associated with carriage and disease in preterm infants. Clin Infect Dis 2001;33:1520–8.

274 Peacock SJ, De Silva I, Lowy FD. What determines nasal carriage of *Staphylococcus aureus*? Trends Microbiol 2001;9:605–10.

275 Gorak EJ, Yamada SM, Brown JD. Community-acquired methicillin-resistant *Staphylococcus aureus* in hospitalized adults and children without known risk factors. Clin Infect Dis 1999;29:797–800.

276 Høiby N, Jarlov JO, Kemp M *et al.* Excretion of ciprofloxacin in sweat and multiresistant *Staphylococcus epidermidis*. Lancet 1997;349:167–9.

277 Ito T, Okuma K, Ma XX, Yuzawa H, Hiramatsu K. Insights on antibiotic resistance of *Staphylococcus aureus* from its whole genome: genomic island SCC. Drug Resist Updat 2003;6:41–52.

278 Novick RP. Staphylococcal plasmids and their replication. Annu Rev Microbiol 1989;43:537–63.

279 Burrus V, Waldor MK. Shaping bacterial genomes with integrative and conjugative elements. Res Microbiol 2004;155:376–86.

280 Paulsen IT, Firth N, Skurray RA. Resistance to antimicrobial agents other than β-lactams. In: Crossley K, Archer GL, eds. The Staphylococci in Human Diseases. New York: Churchill Livingstone, 1997:175–203.

281 Deurenberg RH, Vink C, Kalenic S, Friedrich AW, Bruggeman CA, Stobberingh EE. The molecular evolution of methicillin-resistant *Staphylococcus aureus*. Clin Microbiol Infect 2007; 13:222–35.

282 Blumberg HM, Rimland D, Carroll DJ, Terry P, Wachsmuth IK. Rapid development of ciprofloxacin resistance in methicillin-susceptible and -resistant *Staphylococcus aureus*. J Infect Dis 1991;163:1279–85.

283 Diep BA, Chambers HF, Graber CJ *et al.* Emergence of multidrug-resistant, community-associated, methicillin-resistant *Staphylococcus aureus* clone USA300 in men who have sex with men. Ann Intern Med 2008;148:249–57.

284 Han LL, McDougal LK, Gorwitz RJ *et al.* High frequencies of clindamycin and tetracycline resistance in methicillin-resistant *Staphylococcus aureus* pulsed-field type USA300 isolates collected at a Boston ambulatory health center. J Clin Microbiol 2007;45:1350–2.

285 Diep BA, Gill SR, Chang RF *et al.* Complete genome sequence of USA300, an epidemic clone of community-acquired meticillin-resistant *Staphylococcus aureus*. Lancet 2006;367:731–9.

286 Seybold U, Kourbatova EV, Johnson JG *et al.* Emergence of community-associated methicillin-resistant *Staphylococcus aureus* USA300 genotype as a major cause of health care-associated blood stream infections. Clin Infect Dis 2006;42:647–56.

287 Huang YH, Tseng SP, Hu JM, Tsai JC, Hsueh PR, Teng LJ. Clonal spread of SCCmec type IV methicillin-resistant *Staphylococcus aureus* between community and hospital. Clin Microbiol Infect 2007;13:717–24.

288 Horinouchi S, Weisblum B. Nucleotide sequence and functional map of pC194, a plasmid that specifies inducible chloramphenicol resistance. J Bacteriol 1982;150:815–25.

289 Tennent JM, Lyon BR, Midgley M, Jones IG, Purewal AS, Skurray RA. Physical and biochemical characterization of the *qacA* gene encoding antiseptic and disinfectant resistance in *Staphylococcus aureus*. J Gen Microbiol 1989;135:1–10.

290 Rouch DA, Byrne ME, Kong YC, Skurray RA. The *aacA-aphD* gentamicin and kanamycin resistance determinant of Tn*4001* from *Staphylococcus aureus*: expression and nucleotide sequence analysis. J Gen Microbiol 1987;133:3039–52.

291 Gillespie MT, Lyon BR, Skurray RA. Structural and evolutionary relationships of beta-lactamase transposons from *Staphylococcus aureus*. J Gen Microbiol 1988;134:2857–66.

292 Archer GL, Coughter JP, Johnston JL. Plasmid-encoded trimethoprim resistance in staphylococci. Antimicrob Agents Chemother 1986;29:733–40.

293 Saidijam M, Benedetti G, Ren Q *et al.* Microbial drug efflux proteins of the major facilitator superfamily. Curr Drug Targets 2006;7:793–811.

294 Grkovic S, Brown MH, Skurray RA. Regulation of bacterial drug export systems. Microbiol Mol Biol Rev 2002;66:671–701.

295 Kaatz GW, Seo SM, Foster TJ. Introduction of a *norA* promoter region mutation into the chromosome of a fluoroquinolone-susceptible strain of *Staphylococcus aureus* using plasmid integration. Antimicrob Agents Chemother 1999;43:2222–4.

296 Grkovic S, Hardie KM, Brown MH, Skurray RA. Interactions of the QacR multidrug-binding protein with structurally diverse ligands: implications for the evolution of the binding pocket. Biochemistry 2003;42:15226–36.

297 Mitchell BA, Brown MH, Skurray RA. QacA multidrug efflux pump from *Staphylococcus aureus*: comparative analysis of resistance to diamidines, biguanidines, and guanylhydrazones. Antimicrob Agents Chemother 1998;42:475–7.

298 Paulsen IT, Brown MH, Littlejohn TG, Mitchell BA, Skurray RA. Multidrug resistance proteins QacA and QacB from *Staphylococcus aureus*: membrane topology and identification of residues involved in substrate specificity. Proc Natl Acad Sci USA 1996;93:3630–5.

299 Leelaporn A, Paulsen IT, Tennent JM, Littlejohn TG, Skurray RA. Multidrug resistance to antiseptics and disinfectants in coagulase-negative staphylococci. J Med Microbiol 1994;40:214–20.

300 Neyfakh AA, Borsch CM, Kaatz GW. Fluoroquinolone resistance protein NorA of *Staphylococcus aureus* is a multidrug efflux transporter. Antimicrob Agents Chemother 1993;37:128–9.

301 Ren Q, Paulsen IT. Large-scale comparative genomic analyses of cytoplasmic membrane transport systems in prokaryotes. J Mol Microbiol Biotechnol 2007;12:165–79.

302 Costerton JW, Stewart PS, Greenberg EP. Bacterial biofilms: a common cause of persistent infections. Science 1999;284:1318–22.

303 Donlan RM, Costerton JW. Biofilms: survival mechanisms of clinically relevant microorganisms. Clin Microbiol Rev 2002;15:167–93.

304 Stewart PS. Theoretical aspects of antibiotic diffusion into microbial biofilms. Antimicrob Agents Chemother 1996;40:2517–22.

305 Kostenko V, Ceri H, Martinuzzi RJ. Increased tolerance of *Staphylococcus aureus* to vancomycin in viscous media. FEMS Immunol Med Microbiol 2007;51:277–88.

306 Jefferson KK, Goldmann DA, Pier GB. Use of confocal microscopy to analyze the rate of vancomycin penetration through *Staphylococcus aureus* biofilms. Antimicrob Agents Chemother 49:2467–73.

307 Proctor RA, von Eiff C, Kahl BC *et al.* Small colony variants: a pathogenic form of bacteria that facilitates persistent and recurrent infections. Nat Rev Microbiol 2006;4:295–305.

308 Deziel E, Comeau Y, Villemur R. Initiation of biofilm formation by *Pseudomonas aeruginosa* 57RP correlates with emergence of hyperpiliated and highly adherent phenotypic variants deficient in swimming, swarming, and twitching motilities. J Bacteriol 2001;183:1195–204.

309 Al Laham N, Rohde H, Sander G *et al.* Augmented expression of polysaccharide intercellular adhesin in a defined *Staphylococcus epidermidis* mutant with the small-colony-variant phenotype. J Bacteriol 2007;189:4494–501.

310 Tipper DJ. Mode of action of beta-lactam antibiotics. Pharmacol Ther 1985;27:1–35.

311 Lewis K. Riddle of biofilm resistance. Antimicrob Agents Chemother 2001;45:999–1007.

312 Beenken KE, Dunman PM, McAleese F *et al.* Global gene expression in *Staphylococcus aureus* biofilms. J Bacteriol 2004; 186:4665–84.

313 O'Gara JP. *ica* and beyond: biofilm mechanisms and regulation in *Staphylococcus epidermidis* and *Staphylococcus aureus*. FEMS Microbiol Lett 2007;270:179–88.

314 Valle J, Toledo-Arana A, Berasain C *et al.* SarA and not σ^B is essential for biofilm development by *Staphylococcus aureus*. Mol Microbiol 2003;48:1075–87.

315 Riordan JT, O'Leary JO, Gustafson JE. Contributions of *sigB* and *sarA* to distinct multiple antimicrobial resistance mechanisms of *Staphylococcus aureus*. Int J Antimicrob Agents 2006;28:54–61.

316 Chang S, Sievert DM, Hageman JC *et al.* Infection with vancomycin-resistant *Staphylococcus aureus* containing the *vanA* resistance gene. N Engl J Med 2003;348:1342–7.

317 Weigel LM, Clewell DB, Gill SR *et al.* Genetic analysis of a high-level vancomycin-resistant isolate of *Staphylococcus aureus*. Science 2003;302:1569–71.

318 Weigel LM, Donlan RM, Shin DH *et al.* High-level vancomycin-resistant *Staphylococcus aureus* isolates associated with a polymicrobial biofilm. Antimicrob Agents Chemother 2007;51:231–8.

Laboratory Studies

Chapter 11
Issues in the Identification and Susceptibility Testing of Staphylococci

Betty A. Forbes
Department of Pathology, Virginia Commonwealth University School of Medicine, Richmond, Virginia, USA

Introduction

In North America and in other parts of the world, the last three decades have witnessed the emerging clinical importance of staphylococci, with an expansion of the number of staphylococcal subspecies coupled with the parallel increase in resistance among these organisms. *Staphylococcus aureus* is currently the most common cause of nosocomial and community-based infections. Of significance, treatment of infections caused by *S. aureus* has become even more problematic in recent years since the development of antimicrobial resistance, particularly resistance to methicillin. Similarly, coagulase-negative staphylococci (CoNS) have also shown an increased rate of resistance to antimicrobials including ceftazidime, oxacillin, norfloxacin, ciprofloxacin, fusidic acid, and cefoxitin, with invasive CoNS being more resistant than noninvasive isolates to most antibiotics [1]. Furthermore, recent reports confirm that CoNS remain important causes of bacteremia in hospitalized patients in addition to their association with the presence of foreign bodies. Members of the genus *Staphylococcus* present significant challenges to the clinical microbiology laboratory with respect to accurate identification and detection of antimicrobial resistance. This chapter reviews issues associated with identification and susceptibility testing of staphylococci, as well as those associated with strain typing.

Identification of staphylococci

The clinical laboratory must be able to separate *S. aureus* from CoNS. Examination of colony morphology for pigment (staphyloxanthin) production and hemolysis on routine blood agar is generally followed by one or more of a variety of tests for *S. aureus*-specific factors including production of protein A, cell-associated clumping factor, extracellular coagulase, and heat-stable nuclease. In addition to phenotypic tests, molecular methods have been developed.

The circumstances that warrant speciation of CoNS clinical isolates remain a matter of debate. CoNS are common culture contaminants and it can be difficult to distinguish between a true positive and a contaminated culture taken from a patient with clinical features of infection [2]. Thus, it is often helpful to identify the species under these circumstances, and also when there is a mixed population in a clinically significant sample or when samples from different sites or serial samples are positive. Although the antibiogram is often used as a surrogate marker for the presence of the same or different species, this is not 100% reliable. Species-level identification rarely leads to an intervention or change in therapy, and no compelling clinical reason is apparent to identify to the species level. However, the recent emergence of CoNS as significant pathogens in the last two decades, coupled with newly developed molecular-based assays for accurate and timely speciation of CoNS, has put increasing pressure on laboratories to consider speciation. It is felt that speciation of CoNS has become medically important in order to define their clinical significance, carry out epidemiological surveillance, and to manage patients with CoNS infections [3]. For example, routine speciation of certain CoNS is important to define their clinical significance with certain infections, namely *Staphylococcus lugdunensis* with endocarditis and *Staphylococcus saprophyticus* with urinary tract infections. Unfortunately, many manual and instrument-based methods for identifying CoNS based on phenotypic characteristics, which are variable in their expression, have high error rates and thus have significant limitations [4–6]. Considerable progress has been made using nucleic acid-based methods for the identification of not only

Staphylococci in Human Disease, 2nd edition. Edited by Kent B. Crossley, Kimberly K. Jefferson, Gordon Archer, Vance G. Fowler, Jr.
 ISBN 978-14051-6332-3.

S. aureus but also CoNS. These methods are discussed in the following section.

Phenotypic methods

Coagulase/nuclease

The tube coagulase measures the production of free (extracellular) coagulase, staphylocoagulase. The tube coagulase test with citrated rabbit plasma and subsequent examination of tubes for clot formation after 4 hours and 24 hours of incubation is the standard test for routine identification of *S. aureus* and is considered the gold standard [2,7]; any degree of clotting is considered a positive test. If incubation exceeds 4 hours, the following must be considered: (i) staphylokinase produced by some strains might lyse the fibrin clot yielding a false-negative result; (ii) false-negative or false-positive results may occur if the plasma is not sterile; and (iii) if a colony selected for testing is not pure, false results may occur after prolonged incubation [8]. Other species of staphylococci, including *Staphylococcus schleiferi*, *Staphylococcus intermedius*, *Staphylococcus lutrae*, *Staphylococcus delphini*, and *Staphylococcus pseudointermedius*, may also give positive results but are uncommon isolates from human specimens.

A slide coagulase test detects clumping factor, a cell wall-associated protein that binds to fibrinogen. Slides must be read quickly (within 10 s) or false-positive results may occur. Moreover, colonies should not be selected from high salt-containing media such as mannitol salt agar because autoagglutination and false-positive results can occur. As a consequence of the time involved with a tube coagulase, rapid test kits that employ latex particles and/or sensitized sheep erythrocytes to detect the presence of clumping factor, protein A, and/or other specific surface antigens are widely used for identification of *S. aureus* [7–9]. In general, any test including clumping factor may give false-positive results with *S. lugdunensis* and *S. schleiferi* [8,10,11]. Similarly, false-negative results with methicillin-resistant *S. aureus* (MRSA) isolates using commercially available latex agglutination tests have been reported [12,13] and is purported to be due to changes in various surface components, such as capsular polysaccharides or clumping factor [14,15].

Finally, most strains of *S. aureus*, *S. schleiferi*, *S. intermedius*, and *S. hyicus* produce a heat-stable staphylococcal nuclease that has endonucleolytic and exonucleolytic properties and can cleave DNA and RNA [8]. The presence of this enzyme can be detected by a metachromatic-agar diffusion method and DNA-toluidine blue agar.

Commercial biochemical tests

There is a variety of commercial kits and automated instruments that include identification of *S. aureus* [16–18]. Although performance of these methods may be acceptable, in general they require more technical time, are more expensive, and are slower than tests such as the coagulase and/or latex agglutination. For the most part, the identification of *S. aureus* isolates is uncomplicated. However, the commonly used tests such as those for staphylocoagulase, protein A and clumping factor may give false-positive or false-negative results. A combination of a slide or latex agglutination and a thermonuclease test should recognize the majority of *S. aureus* isolates. If there is disagreement between the results of these tests or colony features, another phenotypic means of identification (Table 11.1) or a molecular method should be used.

With respect to CoNS, there are also a number of commercial kits and automated systems for species-level identification. Since their introduction, some of these systems

Table 11.1 Some commercially available methods/systems for the identification of *S. aureus* and coagulase-negative staphylococci (CoNS).

System	Manufacturer	Features
RAPIDEC Staph	BioMérieux	Identifies *S. aureus*, *S. epidermidis*, and *S. saprophyticus*
API Staph	BioMérieux	Overnight conventional identification of staphylococci and micrococci
VITEK 1 and VITEK 2	BioMérieux	Automated identification and susceptibility system
MicroScan Pos ID panel	Dade MicroScan, Inc., West Sacramento, CA	Can be read manually or by automation
BD Phoenix	Becton Dickinson	Automated identification and susceptibility system
MIDI Sherlock identification system	MIDI, Newark, DE	Automates microbial identification by combining cellular fatty acid analysis with computerized high-resolution chromatography
RiboPrinter microbial characterization system	Qualicon Inc., Wilmington, DE	Ribotype pattern analysis
AccuProbe culture identification	Gen-Probe, Inc., San Diego, CA	DNA probe assay directed against rRNA for *S. aureus* identification
BD BBL Crystal Identification Systems; Gram-positive ID kit	Becton Dickinson	Miniaturized identification method employing modified conventional, fluorogenic and chromogenic substrates. Identifies *S. aureus* and a number of CoNS

have been improved for increased accuracy in identification of CoNS. However, in general, methods based on phenotypic characteristics are often hampered by the fact that they depend on the expression of metabolic activities and/or morphological features. Table 11.1 shows some of the methods for identifying both *S. aureus* and CoNS. One limitation of some of these identification systems is that the databases may not be current. Limitations of these are discussed further in the sections on molecular methods of identification. Studies have also been published using simplified approaches for speciation of those CoNS commonly isolated from clinical specimens using phenotypic methods [19,20]. However, results should be viewed as presumptive since only a limited number of species were identified and results were compared with reference methods using only phenotypic analysis.

Molecular methods for identifying *Staphylococcus aureus*

With respect to molecular methods for identification of *S. aureus*, and more specifically MRSA strains, considerable progress has been made using nucleic acid-based methods; most have been based on polymerase chain reaction (PCR). Currently, a range of primers designed to amplify species-specific targets have been developed and include such targets as the nuclease (*nuc*), coagulase (*coa*), protein A (*spa*), *femA* and *femB*, *sa442*, 16S rRNA, and surface-associated fibrinogen-binding protein genes [21–27]. For the most part, these *S. aureus*-specific gene targets are useful when occasional isolates of *S. aureus* give equivocal results in coagulase or other biochemical tests and there is a need to confirm identity by an alternative method.

Molecular methods for speciating CoNS

The enlargement of the genus *Staphylococcus* to 37 validated species, including 21 subspecies [28], is a particular challenge for clinical laboratories attempting to speciate staphylococci. Numerous studies evaluating various phenotypic methods, including commercially available kits and automated identification systems, have been published. However, it is becoming apparent that despite seemingly good performance when compared with other phenotypic methods, these very same methods when compared with results obtained using molecular methods are not superior and are, in some instances, inadequate [3,5,6,29]. In general, molecular methods employ PCR using consensus primers in conjunction with either restriction fragment length polymorphism (RFLP) or sequencing for speciation. A number of targets have been used such as 16S rRNA, elongation factor Tu (*tuf*), glyceraldehyde 3-phosphate dehydrogenase (*gap*), superoxide dismutase A (*sodA*), and RNA polymerase B (*rpoB*) genes [3,5,6,29–31]. Finally, Tang *et al.* [32] evaluated a commercial system, StaphPlex (Genaco Biomedical Products, Inc., Huntsville, AL), that speciated staphylococci and detected genes encoding Panton–Valentine leukocidin and antimicrobial resistance determinants using a unique target-enriched multiplex PCR method in conjunction with a Luminex 100 suspension array. Although promising, based on their results, further improvements in assay performance are needed.

Susceptibility testing

The clinical microbiology laboratory is responsible for providing susceptibility testing information that contributes to the efficacious use of antimicrobial agents to therapeutically manage staphylococcal infections. However, meeting this responsibility has become more difficult because of the increasing complexities of bacterial resistance among these organisms. Accurate detection of resistance in staphylococci has mandated the addition of methods beyond the more conventional methods of antimicrobial susceptibility testing. In addition, the "traditional" bimodal distribution of very susceptible and very resistant organisms is not as well delineated and newer resistance patterns have become more subtle. Thus, the unpredictable nature of any clinical isolate of staphylococci requires that testing be done as a guide to therapy. The Clinical Laboratory Standards Institute (CLSI; formerly known as the National Committee for Clinical Laboratory Standards, NCCLS) provides guidelines for the antimicrobial agents to be tested, the methods (including manual and commercial instrument-based methods) to detect antimicrobial resistance, guidelines for interpreting results, and criteria outlining quality control test criteria [33,34]; these documents are published every 3 years with annual informational supplements [35]. Although susceptibility testing of staphylococci is generally accurate, reproducible, and predictable of clinical outcome, there are certain caveats, which are addressed in the following discussion.

Detection of β-lactamase

The two major mechanisms of staphylococcal resistance to β-lactam antibiotics are (i) the production of β-lactamase and (ii) the production of an altered target penicillin-binding protein (PBP), PBP2a [36]. The β-lactamase is encoded by the *blaZ* gene, which is generally plasmid borne, and is an inducible narrow-spectrum penicillinase that inactivates benzylpenicillin and structurally related penicillins [37]. Expression of *blaZ* is regulated by two genes, *blaR1* and *blaI*. CLSI recommends that staphylococci be tested for penicillin resistance by dilution or disk diffusion methods [33,34]. Although a penicillin minimum inhibitory concentration (MIC) of 0.03 μg/mL or less usually implies lack of β-lactamase production and MICs of 0.25 μg/mL or more indicate resistance, staphylococci with penicillin MICs between 0.06 and 0.12 μg/mL may or may not produce β-lactamase. An induced β-lactamase test can clarify these MICs. For those laboratories using commercial susceptibility testing systems, the manufacturer's recommendations for guidance in this situation should be followed.

A variety of β-lactamase assays are available and include acidometric, iodometric, and chromogenic methods; a positive result indicates resistance to all penicillinase-labile penicillins, including amoxicillin, ampicillin, azlocillin, carbenicillin, mezlocillin, piperacillin, and ticarcillin [38]. Acidometric and iodometric methods use a colorimetric indicator to detect the presence of penicilloic acid in the reaction tube following β-lactamase hydrolysis of penicillin. Chromogenic assays, in either a test tube or incorporated into a filter paper-type disk or strip formats, detect an electron shift that results in a colored product as the chromogenic cephalosporin, nitrocefin, is hydrolyzed. Regardless of the method employed, if staphylococci produce a positive β-lactamase without induction, results can be reported. However, if no β-lactamase is detected, the test should then be performed with cells that have been grown in the presence of subinhibitory concentrations of a β-lactam antibiotic such as oxacillin or cefoxitin. Because a positive result may take longer to develop in staphylococci than in other organisms, the test should not be interpreted as negative until it has been allowed to react for at least 60 min [38].

Methicillin (oxacillin) resistance

Complications with the detection of methicillin resistance

The β-lactam antibiotics act by inhibiting enzymes involved in assembling the bacterial cell wall; these enzymes catalyze the cross-linking reaction between the peptidoglycan polymers. Many of these enzymes covalently bind β-lactam antibiotics at their active site and are termed PBPs. Methicillin resistance in staphylococci is associated with production of a unique PBP, referred to as either PBP2a or PBP2′. The gene for this PBP, *mecA*, is not present in susceptible staphylococci. This additional PBP has a low binding affinity for β-lactam antibiotics, thereby conferring broad resistance to the entire β-lactam class (termed methicillin or oxacillin resistant). The *mecA* gene, like β-lactamase, is also inducible by β-lactam antibiotics and is located on a mobile genetic element, the staphylococcal cassette chromosome (SCC)*mec*, which is horizontally transferable among staphylococcal species. SCC*mec* also carries *ccr* genes for precise integration into and excision from the *S. aureus* genome [39]. To date, five different types of SCC*mec* (I–V) have been defined by the combination of the *ccr* and *mec* complexes; SCC*mec* types I, IV, and V do not contain any antibiotic resistance genes in addition to *mecA*, whereas types II and III do [40,41].

Although methicillin is no longer used in treatment, it was the first penicillinase-resistant penicillin to be used in the 1960s and at that time was considered the most reliable agent for routine susceptibility testing. Subsequently, resistant strains were termed MRSA. Later use of oxacillin as a more stable and more sensitive alternative to methicillin for susceptibility testing led to the term "oxacillin-resistant *S. aureus*" (ORSA); thus these designations are synonymous.

Accurate prediction of *mecA*-mediated resistance in *Staphylococcus* species has been and continues to be a challenge for the clinical microbiologist since the discovery of methicillin resistance. Methicillin resistance is genetically and biochemically complex. Staphylococci that possess *mecA* are either heterotypic or homotypic in their expression of resistance. With homotypic methicillin resistance, virtually all cells express resistance when tested by standard susceptibility testing methods. In contrast, although all cells within a heterotypic strain may carry the genetic information for methicillin resistance, only rare cells, perhaps as few as 1 in 10^8, express the resistant phenotype under *in vitro* test conditions. The majority of cells in a heterotypic MRSA population will be killed by low concentrations of oxacillin, while only a small subpopulation of cells (usually 0.1–0.01%) are resistant to more than 10 μg/mL of oxacillin [42]. This complex mode of phenotypic expression, referred to as heterotypic resistance, is strain-specific and is under genetic control. The genetic basis for this phenotype is not completely understood, but chromosomal elements are known to influence the expression of the methicillin resistance phenotype (for a detailed discussion refer to Chapter 8). Upstream from *mecA* are two genes, *mecR1* and *mecI*, which are homologs of *blaR1-blaI*; their respective products repress *mecA* as well as *blaZ* transcription [43]. *mecA* is regulated by the repressor MecI and the transmembrane β-lactam-sensing signal transducer MecRI [44].

While expression of both *blaZ* and *mecA* are inducible, the kinetics of induction differ, with MecR1 induction of *mecA* expression taking hours, while *blaZ* expression by BlaR1 requires only minutes [45]. This is yet another factor contributing to the difficulty in detecting methicillin resistance in staphylococci using *in vitro* laboratory methods. These regulatory genes may also help to stabilize *mecA* and possibly facilitate its dissemination among methicillin-susceptible *S. aureus* (MSSA) isolates [36]. Some MRSA strains select against the expression of PBP2a, presumably due to a fitness cost posing a barrier to the stability and maintenance of *mecA*. Thus, genetic background contributes to both the phenotype and genotype of methicillin resistance with stabilization of *mecA* by *mec* and *bla* regulatory elements [36,46]. Finally, although *mecR1* and *mecI* largely control the expression of *mecA*, additional genes may also regulate its expression [47]. Thus, any mutation in the *mec* complex that may affect the function of these genes would be expected to affect expression of methicillin resistance as well. A number of mutations in *mecI* and *mecA* as well as the *mecA* promoter from clinical isolates have been previously described [47,48]. These phenomena, coupled with the usually slower growth of the resistant subpopulation compared with the susceptible subpopulation, are why heteroresistant strains may be missed during laboratory testing.

Finally, methicillin resistance that is not dependent on the presence of the *mecA* gene and thus is genetically distinct from MRSA has been reported [49–51]. These staphylococcal isolates have MICs that are close to the resistant breakpoints and do not possess the *mecA* gene. The mechanisms delineating this resistance are thought to be due to either alterations to existing PBPs or increased levels of β-lactamase production [49,51–54]; these strains are often referred to as borderline oxacillin-resistant *S. aureus* (BORSA). However, animal model experiments indicate that their clinical significance is doubtful and to date there are no reports of treatment failure with penicillinase-resistant penicillins in infections with such isolates [50]. Of note, many of the earlier observations regarding these strains were made without determining the presence or absence of the *mecA* gene, so the prevalence of strains with non-*mecA*-dependent mechanisms may have been overestimated. Studies to determine the prevalence of these isolates have not been done, but it is assumed that these mechanisms occur only rarely and their clinical significance remains unclear.

Phenotypic methods to detect methicillin resistance

Since virtually all cells in the population express high-level methicillin resistance, detection of clinical isolates with homogeneous resistance presents little or no problem for laboratories. The challenge for laboratories in detecting methicillin resides in those isolates with heterogeneous resistance. Initially, the accuracy of phenotypic testing methods for the detection of oxacillin resistance in staphylococci was traditionally assessed by the oxacillin MIC determined by a dilution method. Conflicting data arose in the earlier published literature as it became apparent that the test antimicrobial, media components, inoculum size, and length and temperature of incubation can all affect the detection of oxacillin resistance in heterogeneously resistant strains of staphylococci. Thus, evaluations of phenotypic tests presented in earlier published literature may not accurately reflect the true performance in detecting methicillin resistance.

For the most part, successful detection of heteroresistant strains using phenotypic tests rests largely on promoting the growth of the resistant subpopulations, which is favored by cooler temperatures (30–35°C), larger inocula, increased osmotic strength in the growth media (2–4% NaCl), longer incubation times, and growth in a neutral pH [38]. Of note, while these factors may help augment the expression of resistance, they can vary in their effect and can also impact the accuracy of the test. For example, the effect of osmolarity on resistance expression depends not only on the NaCl concentration but on the basal medium, inoculum size, and incubation temperature used in the test [56]. Swenson *et al.* [55] found that oxacillin MICs for 16 of 36 *mecA*-negative strains increased from 0.25–4 μg/mL (obtained by broth microdilution using 2% NaCl) to 4–8 μg/mL when testing by agar dilution with 4% salt (the conditions used in the oxacillin agar screen method). Similarly, Witte *et al.* [57] evaluated the performance of several phenotypic assays for detecting oxacillin resistance in 74 low-level MRSA strains (oxacillin MIC ≤ 1 μg/mL), 46 MRSA strains (oxacillin MIC ≥ 2 μg/mL), and 117 MSSA strains. All strains were tested by microbroth dilution assays using CLSI recommendations and disk diffusion tests using oxacillin 1-μg disks, oxacillin 5-μg disks, cefoxitin 10-μg disks, and cefoxitin 30-μg disks with different inoculum sizes and agars. Screening for detection of MRSA was performed using oxacillin–salt agar plates [Mueller–Hinton (MH) agar containing 4% NaCl and oxacillin 6 μg/mL], oxacillin-salt-sulbactam tube test and Chromagar MRSA. With this group of challenge organisms, 25% of *mecA*-positive isolates were determined to be oxacillin susceptible using the CLSI breakpoint for oxacillin resistance (≥ 4 μg/mL) but this decreased to only 3.6% using the Deutsches Institut für Normung, Medizinische Mikrobiologie (DIN) breakpoint (≥ 2 μg/mL). In contrast, the oxacillin 1-μg disk had a sensitivity and specificity of 92% and 95%, respectively, using the CLSI standard (confluent growth on MH agar), while the oxacillin 5-μg disk had a sensitivity of only 8.6% using the DIN and Swedish Reference Group for Antibiotics (SRGA; 5-μg disk, semiconfluent inoculum). Thus, optimal conditions for detection of resistance can vary among strains, and no single set of test conditions is necessarily suitable for the phenotypic detection of all resistant strains. Finally, the type of media employed for susceptibility testing, i.e., MH agar versus PDM blood agar, will render varying methicillin results, as well as the same media type from different commercial sources [58–60].

Another factor contributing to conflicting results among various phenotypic methods is the isolates/strains used to evaluate assay performance. Although published studies evaluating test performance include different clinical isolates, isolates from one study compared with another may vary markedly in their degree of heterogeneity, and therefore behave differently under identical test conditions. In other words, the overall performance of a particular test might appear to have high accuracy if the majority of isolates have homotypic oxacillin resistance, while another study, using the same test parameters, might have significantly less accuracy if a greater proportion of strains tested happen to have very low-level oxacillin resistance. For example, many studies showed that the oxacillin screen test performed well for detection of *S. aureus* strains that contained the *mecA* gene [57,58,61,62], while other studies that included strains whose resistance was heterogeneous found that the test performed less well [63,64]. For these reasons, Swenson *et al.* [65,66] used a group of challenge *S. aureus* isolates that included several borderline oxacillin-resistant *mecA*-positive strains as well as *mecA*-negative strains that might be falsely detected as resistant in order to evaluate several methods for detecting oxacillin resistance. Using this challenge set of organisms and performing the agglutination reaction for the MRSA-Screen latex agglutination test (Denka Seiken Co. Ltd, Tokyo, Japan) according to the manufacturer's instructions, the sensitivity of this assay was 90% in contrast to other studies reporting a sensitivity of 97% or more [63,67–69]. In a similar fashion, Witte *et al.* [57] evaluated the performance of several phenotypic assays to detect oxacillin resistance with strains belonging to clonal lineage ST80, a widely disseminated, community MRSA lineage in Europe that exhibits pronounced heteroresistance. These investigators found sensitivities less than previously reported for some phenotypic assays including microbroth dilution MICs for oxacillin.

There are a large number of phenotypic assays for detecting methicillin resistance; some of these methods are listed in Table 11.2. Additional information regarding some of these assays is shown in Table 11.3. As previously mentioned, the appearance of *S. aureus* strains with very low-level heterotypic resistance has presented particular challenges for the clinical microbiology laboratory. In a 2004 document, CLSI first approved a 30-μg cefoxitin disk test for predicting *mecA*-mediated resistance in staphylococci based on its high sensitivity and specificity, particularly for CoNS [56,70]. Of significance, cefoxitin disk diffusion tests were also easier to interpret and did not require transmitted light to identify resistance compared with oxacillin disk diffusion. In 2005, CLSI made the cefoxitin disk test a surrogate for oxacillin susceptibility and the description "screening test" was removed since a confirmatory test was determined to be unnecessary [71]. Moreover, in this same document, *S. lugdunensis* interpretative criteria for both oxacillin and cefoxitin, using either disk diffusion testing or broth microdilution, were grouped with *S. aureus* rather than with the CoNS. A recent study of 135 *S. aureus* isolates with either borderline resistant MICs to oxacillin by a non-*mecA*-mediated mechanism (1–4 μg/mL, i.e., BORSA strains) or low-level heteroresistant *S. aureus* isolates that were *mecA* positive were tested using the oxacillin and cefoxitin disk tests, oxacillin agar screen plate, reference broth dilution, automated susceptibility testing systems (VITEK Legacy, VITEK-2, MicroScan, and Phoenix systems) and results were compared to *mecA* PCR [72]. Results of this study indicate that a cefoxitin test might be used alone to predict *mecA*-mediated resistance (Table 11.4). With the possible replacement of oxacillin by cefoxitin for susceptibility testing, a potential caveat would be the elimination of finding non-*mecA*-mediated resistance. Thus, a crucial question that remains to be answered is whether there is a clinical significance for strains that are phenotypically resistant to penicillinase-stable penicillins but which are *mecA* negative. Also, there is concern that *mecA*-negative *S. aureus* isolates with higher, clinically significant oxacillin MICs (> 16 μg/mL) may emerge [73]. Finally, there might be other potential limitations with the cefoxitin disk diffusion test. Witte *et al.* [57] found that the 30-μg cefoxitin disk diffusion test had a sensitivity of 96% when *S. aureus* strains with low-level oxacillin resistance, particularly community MRSA strains belonging to clonal lineage ST80, were evaluated. This group also raised concerns about the possibility of having large inhibition zones with the 30-μg cefoxitin disk that could interfere with those of adjacent disks. In an evaluation of a 10-μg cefoxitin disk using the different criteria of Skov *et al.* [74], Witte *et al.* achieved a

Table 11.2 Phenotypic assays for detecting methicillin resistance.

Phenotypic test	Manufacturer
Dilution methods: agar dilution, broth microdilution	
Commercial, automated methods	BioMérieux, St Louis, MO
Vitek 1 and Vitek 2	BD Diagnostics Systems, Sparks, MD
BD Phoenix System	Dade Behring, Inc./MicroScan Inc., West
MicroScan	Sacramento, CA
Sensititre	TREK Diagnostic Systems, Cleveland, OH
E-test method	AB Biodisk, Solna, Sweden
Agar screening method (recommended for confirmation of suspect resistance in disk diffusion tests)	
Oxacillin disk diffusion	
Latex agglutination: detection of PBP2a	
MRSA Screen Test (FDA cleared)	Denka-Seikin Co. Ltd, Tokyo, Japan
PBP2′ Latex Agglutination Test (FDA cleared)	Oxoid Ltd, Basingstoke, Hampshire, UK
Mastalex test	Mast Diagnostics, Bootle, UK
Slidex MRSA Detection	BioMérieux, Maroy L'Étoile, France

Table 11.3 Phenotypic methods for detecting *mecA*-dependent methicillin resistance: CLSI guidelines.

Method	Interpretation	Additional comments about method	Limitations
Cefoxitin disk diffusion (30-μg disk)	*S. aureus* and *S. lugdunesis*: ≤ 19 mm, ox^R; ≥ 20 mm, ox^S CoNS: ≤ 24 mm, ox^R; ≥ 25 mm, ox^S	Read with reflected light	Fails to detect *mecA*-positive *S. simulans* Equal sensitivity but greater specificity compared with CoNS oxacillin disk diffusion, therefore preferred method
Cefoxitin agar dilution screen		Detects borderline resistance caused by *mecA*	Classifies BORSA strains not containing *mecA* as susceptible
Reference dilution methods			
Broth (oxacillin)	*S. aureus* and *S. lugdunensis*: ≤ 2 μg/mL, ox^S; ≥ 2 μg/mL, ox^R	MH broth with 2% NaCl Inoculum: 5 × 10^5 cfu/mL 33–35°C for 24 hours	Optimal only for *S. epidermidis*, *S. haemolyticus*, and possibly *S. hominis*
Agar (oxacillin)	*S. aureus* and *S. lugdunensis*: ≤ 2 μg/mL, ox^S; ≥ 4 μg/mL, ox^R	MH broth with 2% NaCl agar Inoculum: 10^4 cfu/mL 33–35°C for 24 hours	99% sensitivity and 100% specificity compared with *mecA* PCR
Oxacillin–salt agar screening test: MH agar supplemented with 4% NaCl and oxacillin 6 μg/mL	Growth of more than 1 colony indicates ox^R	Select colonies from overnight growth on nonselective media Inoculum: 0.5 McFarland standard Inoculate screening plate using a cotton swab or 1-μL loop Incubate 24 hours at 35°C	Not recommended for CoNS
Oxacillin disk diffusion (1-μg disk)	*S. aureus*: ≤ 10 mm, ox^R; 11–12 mm, ox^I; ≥ 13 mm, ox^S CoNS except *S. lugdunensis*: ≤ 17 mm, ox^R; ≥ 18 mm, ox^S	Read for light growth within the zone of inhibition using transmitted light	Cefoxitin disk diffusion is preferred method for testing CoNS May overcall resistance in CoNS excepting *S. lugdunensis*
Detection of PBP2a			
MRSA Screen Test (Denka-Seikin Co. Ltd): FDA cleared		Induction required for CoNS with cefoxitin or oxacillin	Cleared only for *S. aureus*
PBP2′ Latex Agglutination Test (Oxoid Ltd): FDA cleared		Direct testing from blood cultures	Cleared for *S. aureus* and CoNS
Mastalex test (Mast Diagnostics, Bootle, UK)			
Slidex MRSA Detection Test (BioMérieux, Maroy L'Etoile, France)			

BORSA, borderline oxacillin-resistant *S. aureus*; CoNS, coagulase-negative staphylococci; MH, Mueller–Hinton; ox^S, oxacillin sensitive; ox^R, oxacillin resistant; ox^I, oxacillin intermediate.

Table 11.4 Summary of results of phenotypic methods for detecting *mecA*-mediated resistance in a collection of *S. aureus* expressing borderline oxacillin MICs [72].

Drug	Method	Sensitivity (%)	Specificity (%)
Cefoxitin	Disk diffusion (30-μg disk)	99	100
	E-test (≤ 6 μg/mL as susceptible)	99	98
	Phoenix MIC (≤ 4 μg/mL as susceptible)	98	100
	Reference broth microdilution (≤ 6 μg/mL as susceptible)	98	100
	Reference agar dilution (≤ 6 μg/mL as susceptible)	98	100
Oxacillin	Oxacillin–salt agar screen	80–85	50–86
	Disk diffusion (1-μg disk)	91	59
	Reference broth microdilution (≤ 2 μg/mL as susceptible)	85	88
	Commercial automated susceptibility systems		
	MicroScan system	89	96
	VITEK Legacy	82	93
	VITEK 2	91	73
	Phoenix	67	96

sensitivity and specificity of 97% and 98%, respectively. Based on their findings in a recent evaluation of *mecA*-positive and *mecA*-negative *S. aureus* strains, Skov *et al.* [75] proposed that the CLSI breakpoint interpretation for cefoxitin disk diffusion be adjusted from 19 mm to 21 mm for resistance.

Detection of oxacillin resistance in CoNS

Detection of oxacillin resistance in CoNS deserves additional comment. All the antibiotic resistance mechanisms described for *S. aureus* have also been found in CoNS, including penicillinase production and production of the additional PBP2a encoded by the *mecA* gene. Like *S. aureus*, because of the inducible character of oxacillin resistance in CoNS and its heterogeneous expression, detection of oxacillin resistance is challenging for the clinical laboratory [76]. Hussain *et al.* [77] evaluated slide latex agglutination for PBP2a, oxacillin disk diffusion as described by CLSI [33,35], and the Vitek system for their ability to detect methicillin resistance in CoNS; PCR was used as the gold standard. Of all methods evaluated, detection of PBP2a by latex agglutination following overnight induction with an oxacillin 1-μg disk was the most sensitive and specific when compared with PCR. Some studies have increased sensitivity with this test by either increasing inoculum size or time for agglutination [77,78]. The French Committee for Antibiotic Susceptibility Testing of the French Society of Microbiology (CA-SFM) presently recommends the use of three β-lactams, i.e., oxacillin, cefoxitin and moxalactam, for determination of oxacillin resistance in CoNS. Although oxacillin MICs are defined by the CA-SFM (susceptible, ≤ 0.25 μg/mL; resistant, > 2 μg/mL) as well as CLSI (susceptible, ≤ 0.25 μg/mL; resistant, ≥ 0.5 μg/mL), no breakpoints for cefoxitin or moxalactam MICs have been proposed. The CA-SFM introduced the cefoxitin and moxalactam disks in 2004 and 2005, respectively [79,80]; the moxalactam disk was slightly better for *mecA*-positive strains compared with cefoxitin. Similar results were found in which moxalactam was a better drug as an indicator of methicillin resistance in CoNS in an evaluation of moxalactam with the BD Phoenix system [81].

Genotypic methods for detecting methicillin resistance

The accuracy with which various phenotype testing methods detect methicillin resistance is now largely determined by PCR assays that detect the presence of *mecA* in staphylococcal strains. As previously mentioned, a large number of real-time PCR methods have been developed for detecting the *mecA* gene in conjunction with *S. aureus*-specific genome fragments such as *nuc*, *sa442*, *chaperonin 60* and *sodM* [21,22,82,83]. However, there can be some discrepancies between the *mecA* genotype and results of tests recommended by CLSI or other phenotypic assays to detect oxacillin resistance. For example, occasional oxacillin-susceptible *S. aureus* strains carrying a nonfunctional or nonexpressed *mecA* will be detected; the incidence of phenotypically susceptible *mecA*-positive strains is unknown. Discrepant results can also arise if an endemic strain is present in a particular geographic location that lacks the target sequence. Thus, any molecular assay used to detect the presence of the *mecA* gene must be validated by each institution.

Screening (surveillance) for methicillin resistance and direct detection

Because infections caused by MRSA increase the length of hospital stays, play a role in rising healthcare costs, and have a high attributable mortality, reliable detection of MRSA carriage is becoming an essential part of epidemiological investigations and for prompt implementation of barrier isolation of colonized patients [84]. There are a large number of publications describing methods for detecting the presence of MRSA in screening samples. More conventional approaches include solid agar media with or without enrichment. Most media contain an indicator system (a carbohydrate such as mannitol and a pH indicator) to distinguish *S. aureus* from other organisms and oxacillin, methicillin or cefoxitin to select for methicillin-resistant strains. However, the interpretation of results is challenging because of a number of factors:

- varying incubation conditions;
- possible bias in results due to the prevalence of a particular local strain;
- study design, with some studies using only pure isolates and others using nasal swabs, yet other studies using multiple media but using only one nasal swab;
- use of enrichment broths and then subsequent plating to selective agars;
- comparators employed to evaluate the performance of the various media;
- the swabs employed for sampling (e.g., rayon, unmoistened, dry, charcoal).

Some studies have reported enhanced sensitivity for detection of MRSA with preenrichment of the specimen in salt-containing tryptic soy broth for 24 hours before plating on solid media [85,86]. However, the concentration of salt in the broth has varied widely in the different studies; too high a concentration may inhibit growth of MRSA while too low a concentration may result in overgrowth of Gram-negative bacteria [84]. Also, studies vary as to the selective agents employed and indicator systems. Most recently, chromogenic indicators have been used. There are several recently marketed chromogenic media containing cefoxitin (Table 11.5) for which manufacturers claim good performance. A recent study compared the performance of the MRSA ID, MRSA*Select* and CHROMagar MRSA with two molecular methods (IDI-MRSA and GenoType MRSA Direct PCR) to detect MRSA directly in

Table 11.5 Chromogenic agars containing cefoxitin used to screen for MRSA in clinical specimens.

Chromogenic media	Manufacturer
MRSA Select	Bio-Rad Laboratories, Marnes-la-Coquette, France
CHROMagar MRSA	CHROMagar Microbiology, Paris, France
MRSA ID	BioMérieux

swabs from the nares, groin or axilla [87]. The specificities for all assays were high (95–99%), while the sensitivities with nasal swabs ranged from 68 to 75% using the selective media and from 70 to 94% for the molecular assays. In an attempt to increase the sensitivity of the screening agars, plates were incubated an additional 24 hours and then read. Although additional incubation increased the detection of MRSA, there was a corresponding significant decrease in specificity. Thus, although many different microbiological media and techniques have been studied for the recovery of MRSA from clinical specimens and for screening, no consensus exists as to the most sensitive and accurate method. The reader is referred to the review by Brown *et al.* [88] for an excellent summary of these methods.

A Food and Drug Administration (FDA)-cleared commercial assay, the IDI-MRSA (Becton Dickinson), is able to rapidly detect MRSA directly in nasal swab samples [89]. This assay couples PCR primers that are specific for *mecA* and the *S. aureus*-specific gene *orfX*, a highly conserved open reading frame, with detection by complementary molecular beacon probes to account for variants of the SCC*mec* elements [90]. Warren *et al.* [91] compared results of this assay with direct plating to mannitol salt agar plates and an enrichment broth (TSB with 6.5% NaCl) culture method. The sensitivity, specificity, and positive and negative predictive values were 91.7%, 93.5%, 82.5% and 97.1%, respectively. A concern for this assay is that although the assay has excellent sensitivity and a high negative predictive value, it appears to have a low positive predictive value due to false-positive results [91–95]. A possible complete or partial loss of the SCC*mec* genetic element has been reported such that the IDI-MRSA assay is positive, but the organism is methicillin susceptible [92]. Donnio *et al.* [96] described MSSA isolates from French hospitals negative for both *mecA* and the *ccrAB* loci but positive for the IS*431*::pUB110::IS*431*::*dcs* structure. Thus, these MSSA strains containing SCC*mec* elements may pose some problems in laboratories that use real-time amplification assays of the *dcs*::*orfX* junction for SCC*mec* to detect MRSA. Another commercial assay recently cleared by the FDA is the Xpert TM MRSA Test (Cepheid, Sunnyvale, CA). Another PCR-based test for rapid detection of MRSA, this assay is more expensive than the Becton Dickinson assay, yet is more amenable to performing "on demand" because of faster sample processing. Because of similar primers and probe design, complete or partial loss of the SCC*mec* element can also occur as with the Becton Dickinson assay. Mehta *et al.* [97] compared the performance of the Becton Dickinson and Cepheid assays with culture; no difference was noted between the performance of the two systems in terms of sensitivity, specificity, and negative and positive predictive values.

Van Hal *et al.* [87] evaluated the performance of the IDI-MRSA assay with another commercially available molecular assay, the GenoType MRSA Direct (Hain Lifescience, Nehren, Germany), for detecting MRSA in screening swab samples from three different sites (nares, axilla and groin). The GenoType MRSA Direct amplifies SCC*mec* I–IV as its target. Sensitivity of the IDI-MRSA assay (90%) for detection of MRSA in nasal swab specimens was comparable to previously reported rates [90,91]. Although more expensive, the IDI-MRSA assay was rapid and more sensitive, regardless of the swab site, compared with the GenoType MRSA Direct. Of note, the GenoType MRSA Direct was significantly less sensitive (69%), independent of the swab site. This result was lower than the published rate of 95% [98]. The test had a noticeable inability to detect MRSA that were susceptible to two or more non-β-lactam antibiotics; the reason for this lower sensitivity remains unanswered. Finally, another system not yet cleared by the FDA is the BacLite system for MRSA (3M Medical Diagnostics Clinical Lab Products, St Paul, MN). This culture test, available now in Europe, delivers same-day results and can confirm a negative result within 5 hours and a positive result within 24 hours by measuring adenylate kinase activity, an essential housekeeping enzyme found in all cells. By supplying purified ADP *in vitro*, the amplified levels of ATP produced can be measured using bioluminescence when the organism is grown in the presence of oxacillin.

There are other issues surrounding the implementation of molecular assays for screening from the laboratory perspective. First, because infection control is usually poorly reimbursed and molecular methods cost approximately five to six times more per test than agar-based methods, cost remains an issue [87,93]. Also, there are similar issues as previously described for solid agar media. And regardless of the type of format employed for MRSA screening, i.e., solid agar or molecular methods, the optimum method for sampling in order to detect MRSA colonization remains an issue. The best site for sampling (nares, axilla, throat, groin, or rectal), the type of swab employed, how to sample (e.g., how many times to roll the swab about the site), and the acceptability of pooling specimens all remain to be delineated [99–104].

Finally, molecular and phenotypic assays have been used for the direct identification of *S. aureus* as well as MRSA in positive blood cultures [105–107]. Another molecular method evaluated in these studies besides real-time amplification included peptide nucleic acid fluorescence *in situ* hybridization (FISH; AdvanDx, BioMérieux). Both real-time amplification and FISH had excellent sensitivity and specificity. Phenotypic assays for direct identification included the tube coagulase test and API RAPIDECstaph (BioMérieux). The tube coagulase test had sensitivities of 65–82%, while the sensitivity of the API RAPIDECstaph was 96%; both tests had very high specificities.

Vancomycin resistance

In recent years, vancomycin (glycopeptide)-resistant *S. aureus* (VRSA) and both homogeneous vancomycin (glycopeptide)-intermediate *S. aureus* (VISA) and heterogeneous VISA (hetero-VISA) have been reported with increasing frequency [108–111] (see Chapter 9 for a detailed discussion of vancomycin resistance). In detecting these clinical isolates with varying degrees of susceptibility to vancomycin, the clinical microbiology laboratory faces many of the same issues as those associated with detecting oxacillin resistance. For example, VRSA strains exhibit vancomycin MICs of 32 µg/mL or more, having acquired *vanA* from *Enterococcus facecalis/Enterococcus faecium* [108,112]. Although identification of such strains is presumed to be straightforward using standard protocols, their identification with automated systems is reported to be questionable [113]; only three of six automated methods reliably detected VRSA. Some manufacturers subsequently optimized their systems and these are thus considered validated for VRSA detection. Like the growth rate of MRSA strains compared with oxacillin-susceptible isolates, VISA strains have a slower growth rate than do vancomycin-susceptible *S. aureus* isolates [114]. In addition, these strains include modestly heterogeneous subpopulations that have vancomycin MICs of 5–14 µg/mL, such that VISA exhibit MICs of 4–8 µg/mL; thus, similar to detection of oxacillin resistance, detection of VISA is another challenge for the clinical laboratory. Recently, infections caused by MRSA with reduced susceptibility to vancomycin have seemingly emerged. These hetero-VISA strains appear to be susceptible on routine MIC determinations (MIC 1–4 µg/mL), but possess low-number subpopulations of vancomycin-intermediate cells. Under selective pressure, these strains can exhibit overt intermediate resistance to vancomycin and cause persistent infection in the face of appropriately dosed vancomycin [115,116]. However, controversy remains as to the significance of hetero-VISA and whether vancomycin "MIC creep" is an emerging phenomenon. Analysis of surveillance studies of staphylococci isolated from blood during an 11-year period failed to detect evidence of vancomycin MIC creep [110]; similar findings for staphylococci have been reported for 1986–2002 on a national level in Spain [117]. In contrast, other studies have reported decreased susceptibility to vancomycin and teicoplanin antibiotics in MRSA [118,119].

Table 11.6 Methods for detecting vancomycin-resistant *S. aureus* (VRSA) and vancomycin-intermediate *S. aureus* (VISA) [120].[1]

Strain	Method	Vancomycin MIC (µg/mL)[2]
VRSA	Reference broth microdilution	≥ 16
	Reference agar dilution	
	E-test	
	Overnight MicroScan	
	Synergies plus	
	BD Phoenix system	
	Disk diffusion[3]	
	BHI with 6 µg/mL[4]	
VISA	Reference broth microdilution	4–8
	Reference agar dilution	
	E-test	

[1] To date, all tests use a direct colony suspension adjusted to a 0.5 McFarland standard, incubation at 35°C in ambient air for a full 24 hours. If using a non-FDA-cleared automated system or disk diffusion to determine vancomycin susceptibility, a vancomycin screen agar plate should be used for enhanced detection.
[2] CLSI breakpoints (see ref. 35).
[3] All staphylococcal isolates for which vancomycin zone diameters are 14 mm or less should be tested by a reference MIC method [35].
[4] A 10-µL inoculum is spotted onto the agar using a micropipette or a swab dipped in the suspension, excess liquid expressed and used to inoculate the plate; growth of greater than one colony is considered positive. Any isolate that grows should be confirmed by testing using an FDA-cleared MIC.

Methods that detect VRSA and VISA are listed in Table 11.6. As previously mentioned, not all susceptibility methods detect VISA and VRSA isolates. It is important that if an automated system does not have FDA clearance for VRSA detection, laboratories should include a vancomycin agar screen plate for enhanced detection of VRSA for all staphylococci. Laboratories may opt to only screen MRSA isolates since nearly all VISA and all VRSA reported to date have been MRSA. Laboratories using disk diffusion to determine vancomycin susceptibility should consider adding a second method for VISA detection such as a vancomycin agar screen plate [120]. The Centers for Disease Control and Prevention have a VISA/VRSA testing algorithm that presents a strategy for confirming VISA and VRSA using appropriate test methods (Figure 11.1).

As previously mentioned, there is still controversy regarding the clinical significance of low-level vancomycin resistance in *S. aureus* as well as the definition of such strains [110,121]. Much of the uncertainty arises from the difficulties in laboratory detection of hetero-VISA, which has been beset by problems due to unreliable methods [122–124]. Again, test antimicrobials, media components, inoculum size, and length and temperature of incubation can all affect the detection of vancomycin resistance

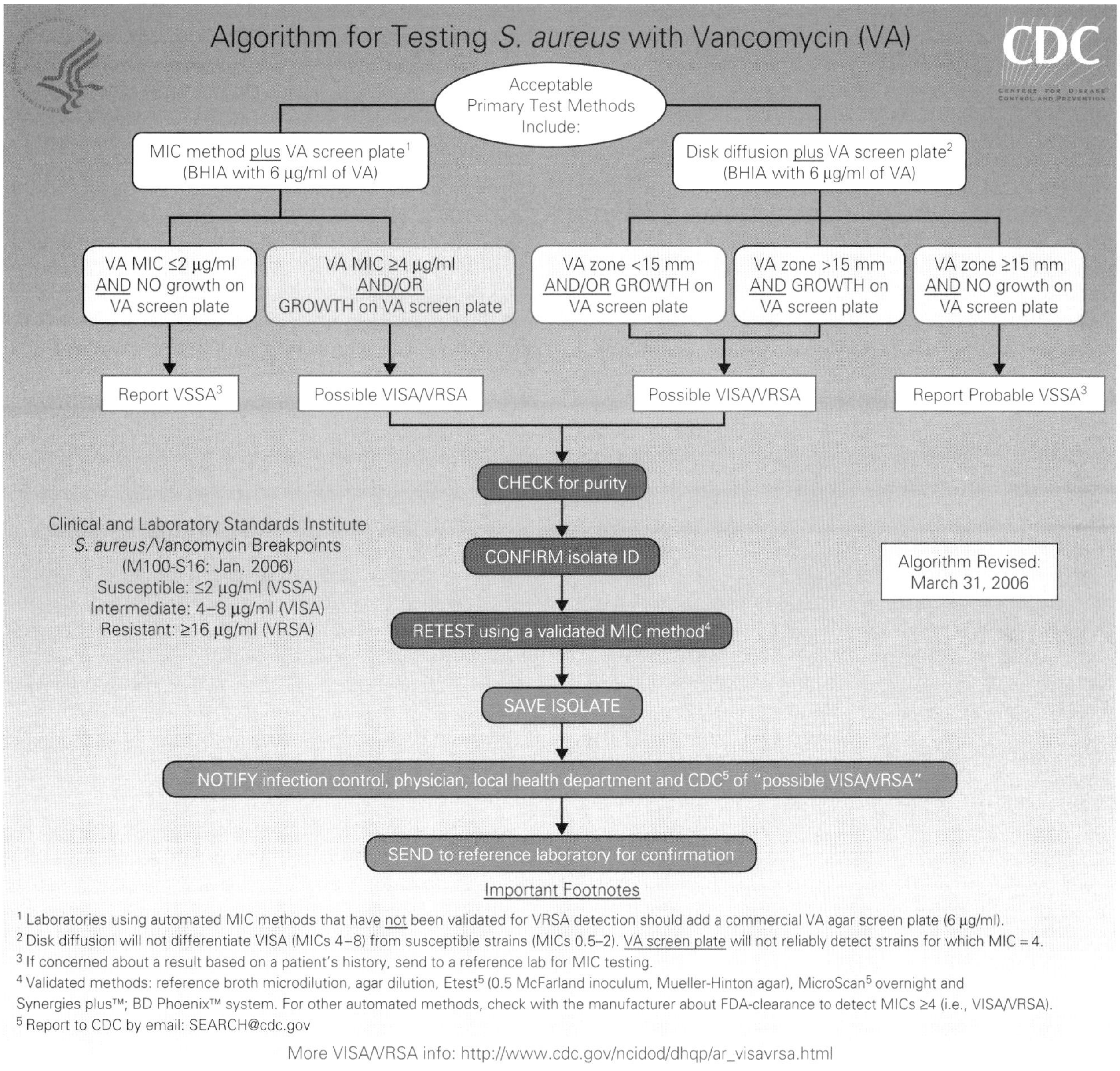

Figure 11.1 CDC algorithm for testing *S. aureus* with vancomycin.

in heterogeneously resistant strains of staphylococci. Currently, the most reliable method for definitive identification of hetero-VISA (as well as VISA) is the population analysis profile–area under the curve method (PAP-AUC) [125]. In this method, suspected hetero-VISA strains are compared with the hetero-VISA control strain Mu3 (ATCC 700698). An AUC ratio of 0.9 or more has been used to define hetero-VISA [125]. The procedure involves making serial dilutions of an overnight broth culture and inoculating these various dilutions onto agar plates with various concentrations of vancomycin. After 48 hours of incubation, the number of colony-forming units per milliliter is calculated and plotted against the vancomycin concentration. The AUC is then calculated and the ratio of the test to Mu3 is used to calculate the PAP-AUC ratio. Unfortunately, this method is very labor-intensive and is beyond the resources of most routine clinical laboratories.

A recent study evaluated three of the most commonly used and recommended screening methodologies for detection of *S. aureus* strains with reduced susceptibility to glycopeptide antibiotics in a multicenter multinational comparison using the PAP-AUC method as the gold standard [126]. The three methods evaluated were brain–heart infusion agar containing vancomycin 6 µg/mL (BHIA6V), macrodilution method Etest (MET) for teicoplanin and vancomycin, and Mueller–Hinton agar containing teicoplanin 5 µg/mL (MHA5T); for both the MET and MHA5T tests, an inoculum with an equivalent turbidity to a #2 McFarland was used. In this study, BHIA6V lacked sensitivity (35.16%) and showed the greatest variation among laboratories. MHA5T was slightly better at predicting glycopeptide susceptibility, but less accurate at predicting intermediate glycopeptide resistance. MET produced fewer false-positive results. Based on false-negative and false-positive results for MHA5T and MET, Wootton *et al.* [126] proposed that diagnostic laboratories assess the relative benefits of the MET and MHA5T methods with respect to screening costs and the costs for confirmatory testing. A recent study using a chemiluminescent method measuring metabolic activity of *S. aureus* strains grown in the presence of varying vancomycin concentrations might be useful for screening hetero-VISA and VISA strains [127]. Thus, optimal methods for detection of VISA and hetero-VISA remain to be delineated.

Macrolide resistance and other resistance in staphylococci

Macrolides, lincosamides, and streptogramins are referred to as the MLS group of antimicrobial agents. Although chemically quite distinct, their mechanism of action (inhibition of protein synthesis by binding to the 50S ribosomal subunit) and mechanisms of resistance are similar. In staphylococci, resistance to MLS antibiotics is acquired and resistance is via target modification or active efflux of the antibiotic. Target modification confers resistance to macrolides, lincosamides, and streptogramin B agents (MLS_B phenotype), while antibiotic efflux confers resistance to macrolides only (designated M-type for macrolide) and is mediated by the *msrA* gene. With respect to the MLS_B phenotype, modification of the target site by methylation of an adenine nucleotide of rRNA causes cross-resistance to these drugs because their binding sites overlap. Ribosomal methylation via a methylase is mediated in staphylococci by an *erm* gene; in staphylococci three methylase genes have been detected [128]. Of significance, the MLS_B phenotype can be either inducible or constitutive. If inducible, the isolate will be resistant to erythromycin and appears susceptible to clindamycin when tested using routine susceptibility methods unless it is induced by a macrolide. If an isolate has M-type resistance, it will be resistant to erythromycin but susceptible to clindamycin even following induction by a macrolide. Thus if clindamycin is being considered for therapy, it is important that the laboratory determine if inducible resistance to clindamycin exists. Detection of inducible clindamycin resistance is accomplished by using a disk diffusion procedure, referred to as the D zone test, in which a 15-µg erythromycin disk is placed 15–26 mm apart from a 2-µg clindamycin disk. After overnight incubation, plates are examined for the presence (or absence) of a flattening of the clindamycin zone, which looks like the letter D. By placing the disks 15–20 mm apart, test results may be easier to interpret. If flattening is observed, the isolate is clindamycin resistant by means of an *erm* gene, but if not observed the isolate is therefore clindamycin susceptible and an efflux gene is present. If the laboratory routinely performs antibiotic susceptibility testing by methods other than disk diffusion, testing should be available by request where clindamycin is being considered for therapy. Two other comments regarding the D zone test must be made. First, although this test can be performed on a standard blood agar plate used for purity checks [129], a later study determined that the BBL Prompt system (Becton Dickinson, Sparks, MD) should not be used to directly inoculate the purity plate [130]. Subsequently, Hindler and Bruckner [131] showed that transferring an inoculum for testing directly from the Prompt reservoir tray using a 10-µL loop and streaking one-third of the purity plate to obtain confluent growth was acceptable. Second, there is some controversy as to whether laboratories should report isolates that are D zone test-positive as clindamycin resistant since clindamycin has been effective in some situations despite demonstrating clindamycin-inducible resistance [132]. It has been suggested by CLSI that clindamycin resistance be reported and to include a statement for these inducibly clindamycin-resistant strains which qualifies that the drug could still be effective in some patients [35].

Finally, some SCC*mec* types carry additional genetic elements such as pT181, which encodes tetracycline resistance but can confer resistance to additional antibiotic classes. In addition, staphylococci can have varying susceptibility to trimethoprim–sulfamethoxazole and ciprofloxacin. A three-dimensional microarray system described by Nagaoka *et al.* [133] appeared to have a 10-fold greater sensitivity than that of standard PCR for simultaneously detecting resistance to levofloxacin and the presence of the *mecA* gene in *S. aureus*. As previously discussed, when using currently available systems and adhering to CLSI guidelines, the clinical laboratory is able to accurately and reproducibly provide susceptibility results that are predictive of clinical outcome.

Typing of staphylococci

Typing of staphylococci, particularly MRSA, is used in the clinical setting to investigate the relationship between strains associated with a cluster of infections or to track the spread of strains among units, hospitals, or even countries. Such information is essential for effective infection control in terms of outbreak intervention and prevention strategies as well as understanding the changing epidemiology of MRSA infections [134]. Typing may also be used for patients with recurrent staphylococcal infections to determine whether these infections represent independent episodes or relapse. Typing of CoNS is often used to determine whether two or more strains from a patient represent contamination or infection. For a detailed discussion of typing methods, refer to Chapter 3.

For the most part, major emphasis for typing has been with MRSA including both hospital and community-onset strains. A typing system must be able to characterize all strains tested, be reproducible, and be able to discriminate between unrelated isolates. Many different genotyping methods are currently in use, but the most widely used is pulsed field gel electrophoresis (PFGE) of *Sma*I-digested genomic DNA [135] to determine the relatedness of isolates for epidemiological purposes. Although invaluable in investigations of nosocomial outbreaks, initially there were difficulties in reproducibility and interlaboratory reliability until electrophoresis conditions were standardized and normalization and analysis software were developed [136,137].

Although PFGE is still considered the reference standard for typing MRSA isolates, there are limitations in terms of its turn-around time, costs for analysis, lack of a common nomenclature on an international level, and need for specialized training for performance and interpretation [138]. Thus, other techniques have been developed including ribotyping and PCR-based methods, such as repetitive-element PCR, amplified RFLP typing and, more recently, DNA sequencing approaches [134,139–145]. Multilocus sequence typing (MLST) is another typing method for investigating the clonal evolution of MRSA [138,146]. This method is based on sequence analysis of 0.5-kb fragments from seven *S. aureus* housekeeping genes: *arcC*, *aroE*, *glpF*, *gmk*, *pta*, *tpi*, and *yqiL*. Different sequences are assigned distinct alleles of each housekeeping gene, and each isolate is defined by the alleles of the seven genes; this results in an allelic profile or sequence type (ST). However, like PFGE, a disadvantage of MLST is its labor-intensiveness. A single-locus sequence typing method for *S. aureus* using sequences of the polymorphic region X of the *S. aureus spa* gene has been introduced and, in contrast to MLST, both molecular evolution and hospital outbreaks of MRSA can be investigated [147]. Another advantage of *spa* typing over MLST is its simplicity since only a single locus is sequenced. Other typing methods characterize SCC*mec* using a variety of methods involving PCR and parts of the *mec* complex and *ccr* genes [138,140,145]. Finally, a DNA microarray with gene-specific oligonucleotide probes that detect important *S. aureus* genes as well as types of genomic islands including SCC*mec* has been recently developed to genotype MRSA isolates [148].

References

1 Laverdière M, Weiss K, Rivest R, Delorme J. Trends in antibiotic resistance of staphylococci over an eight-year period: difference in the emergence of resistance between coagulase positive and coagulase-negative staphylococci. Microb Drug Resist 1998;4:119–22.

2 Kloos WE, Musselwhite MS. Distribution and persistence of *Staphylococcus* and *Micrococcus* species and other aerobic bacteria on skin. Appl Microbiol 1975;30:381–95.

3 Alexopuoulou K, Foka A, Petinaki E, Jelastopulu E, Dimitracopoulos G, Spiliopoulou I. Comparison of two commercial methods with PCR restriction fragment length polymorphism of the *tuf* gene in the identification of coagulase-negative staphylococci. Lett Appl Microbiol 2006;43:450–4.

4 De Paulis AN, Predari SC, Chazarreta CD, Santoianni JE. Five-test scheme for species-level identification of clinically significant coagulase-negative staphylococci. J Clin Microbiol 2003;41:1219–24.

5 Heikens E, Fleer A, Paauw A, Florijn A, Fluit AC. Comparison of genotypic and phenotypic methods for species-level identification of clinical isolates of coagulase-negative staphylococci. J Clin Microbiol 2005;43:2286–90.

6 Layer F, Ghebremedhin B, Moder KA, König W, König B. Comparative study using various methods for identification of *Staphylococcus* species in clinical specimens. J Clin Microbiol 2006;44:2824–30.

7 Wichelhaus TA, Kern S, Schäfer V, Brade V, Hunfeld KP. Evaluation of modern agglutination tests for identification of methicillin-susceptible and methicillin-resistant *Staphylococcus aureus*. Eur J Clin Microbiol Infect Dis 1999;8:756–8.

8 Bannerman TL, Peacock SJ. *Staphylococcus*, *Micrococcus*, and other catalase-positive cocci. In: Murray PR, Baron EJ, Jorgensen JH, Landry ML, Pfaller MA, eds. Manual of Clinical Microbiology, 9th edn. Washington, DC: ASM Press, 2007, pp. 390–411.

9 Davies S. Detection of methicillin-resistant *Staphylococcus aureus*: the evaluation of rapid agglutination methods. Br J Biomed Sci 1997;54:13–15.

10 Peacock SJ, Lina G, Etienne J, Foster TJ. *Staphylococcus schleiferi* subsp. *schleiferi* expresses a fibronectin-binding protein. J Clin Microbiol 1999;67:4272–5.

11 Leung MJ, Nuttall N, Mazur M, Taddel TL, McComish M, Pearman JW. Case of *Staphylococcus schleiferi* endocarditis and a simple scheme to identify clumping factor-positive staphylococci. J Clin Microbiol 1999;37:3353–6.

12 Weist K, Cimbal A-K, Lecke C, Kampf G, Rüden H, Vonberg R-P. Evaluation of six agglutination tests for *Staphylococcus aureus* identification depending upon local prevalence of methicillin-resistant *S. aureus*. J Med Microbiol 56, 283–90, 2006.

13 Brakstad OG, Tveten Y, Nato F, Fournier JM. Comparison of various methods and reagents for species identification of *Staphylococcus aureus* positive or negative for the mecA gene. APMIS 1993;101:651–4.

14 Fournier JM, Bouvet A, Boutonnier A *et al.* Predominance of capsular polysaccharide type 5 among oxacillin-resistant *Staphylococcus aureus*. J Clin Microbiol 1987;25:1932–3.

15 Kuusela P, Hilden P, Savolainen K, Vuento M, Lyytikainen O, Vuopio-Varika J. Rapid detection of methicillin-resistant *Staphylococcus aureus* strains not identified by slide agglutination tests. J Clin Microbiol 1994;32:143–7.

16 Spanu T, Sanguinetti M, D'Inzeo A *et al.* Identification of methicillin-resistant isolates of *Staphylococcus aureus* and coagulase-negative staphylococci responsible for bloodstream infections with the Phoenix system. Diag Microbiol Infect Dis 2004;48:221–7.

17 Spanu T, Sanguinetti M, Ciccaglione D, Romano L, Leone F, Fadda G. Use of the VITEK 2 system for rapid identification of clinical isolates of staphylococci from blood stream infections. J Clin Microbiol 2003;4:4259–63.
18 Ligozzi M, Bernini C, Bonora MG, Defatima M, Zuliani J, Fontana R. Evaluation of the VITEK 2 system for identification and antimicrobial susceptibility testing of medically relevant gram-positive cocci. J Clin Microbiol 2002;40:1681–6.
19 Iorio NLP, Ferreira RBR, Schuenck RP *et al.* Simplified and reliable scheme for species-level identification of *Staphylococcus* clinical isolates. J Clin Microbiol 2007;45:2564–9.
20 DePaulis AN, Predari SC, Chazarreta CD, Santoianni JE. Five-test simple scheme for species-level identification of clinically significant coagulase-negative staphylococci. J Clin Microbiol 2003;41:1219–24.
21 Elsayed S, Chow BL, Hamilton NL, Gregson DB, Pitout JD, Church DL. Development and validation of a molecular beacon probe-based real time polymerase chain reaction assay for rapid detection of methicillin resistance in *Staphylococcus aureus*. Arch Pathol Lab Med 2003;127:845–9.
22 Reischl U, Linde H-J, Metz M, Leppmeier B, Lehn N. Rapid identification of methicillin-resistant *Staphylococcus aureus* and simultaneous species confirmation using real-time fluorescence PCR. J Clin Microbiol 2000;38:2429–33.
23 Mason WJ, Blevins JS, Beenken K, Wibowo N, Ojha N, Smeltzer MS. Multiplex PCR protocol for the diagnosis of staphylococcal infection. J Clin Microbiol 2001;39:3332–8.
24 Perez-Roth E, Claverie-Martin F, Villar J, Mendez-Alvarez S. Multiplex PCR for simultaneous identification of *Staphylococcus aureus* and detection of methicillin and mupirocin resistance. J Clin Microbiol 2001;39:4037–41.
25 Vannuffel P, Gigi J, Ezzedine H *et al.* Specific detection of methicillin-resistant *Staphylococcus* species by multiplex PCR. J Clin Microbiol 1995;33:2864–7.
26 Levi K, Bailey C, Bennett A, Marsh P, Cardy DL, Towner KJ. Evaluation of an isothermal signal amplification method for rapid detection of methicillin-resistant *Staphylococcus aureus* from patient-screening swabs. J Clin Microbiol 2003;41:3187–91.
27 Misawa A, Yoshida A, Saito R *et al.* Application of loop-mediated isothermal amplification technique to rapid and direct detection of methicillin-resistant *Staphylococcus aureus* (MRSA) in blood cultures. J Infect Chemother 2007;13:134–40.
28 Euzéby JP. List of bacterial names with standing in nomenclature: a folder available on the Internet. Int J Syst Bacteriol 1997;47:590–2.
29 Becker K, Harmsen D, Mellmann A *et al.* Development and evaluation of a quality-controlled ribosomal sequence database for 16S ribosomal DNA-based identification of *Staphylococcus* species. J Clin Microbiol 2004;42:4988–95.
30 Poyart C, Quesne G, Boumaila C, Trieus-Cuot P. Rapid and accurate species-level identification of coagulase-negative staphylococci by using the *sodA* gene as target. J Clin Microbiol 2001;39:4296–301.
31 Mellmann A, Becker K, von Eiff C, Keckevoet U, Schumann P, Harmsen, D. Sequencing and staphylococci identification. Emerg Infect Dis 2006;12:333–6.
32 Tang Y-W, Kilic A, Yang Q *et al.* StaphPlex system for rapid and simultaneous identification of antibiotic resistance determinants and Panton–Valentine leukocidin detection of staphylococci from positive blood cultures. J Clin Microbiol 2007;45:1867–73.
33 Clinical Laboratory Standards Institute. Performance standards for antimicrobial disk susceptibility tests. Approved standard M2-A9, 9th edn. Wayne, PA: Clinical Laboratory Standards Institute, 2006.
34 Clinical Laboratory Standards Institute. Methods for dilution antimicrobial susceptibility tests for bacteria that grow aerobically. Approved standard M7-A7, 7th edn. Wayne, PA: Clinical Laboratory Standards Institute, 2006.
35 Clinical Laboratory Standards Institute. Performance standards for antimicrobial susceptibility testing. Seventeenth Informational Supplement M100-S17. Wayne, PA: Clinical Laboratory Standards Institute, 2007.
36 Katayama Y, Zhang H-Z, Hong D, Chambers HF. Jumping the barrier to β-lactam resistance in *Staphylococcus aureus*. J Bacteriol 2003;185:5465–72.
37 Asheshov EH, Dyke KG. Regulation of the synthesis of penicillinase in diploids of *Staphylococcus aureus*. Biochem Biophys Res Commun 1968;30:213–18.
38 Swenson JM, Patel JB, Jorgensen JH. Special phenotypic methods for detecting antibacterial resistance. In: Murray PR, Baron EJ, Jorgensen JH, Landry ML, Pfaller MA, eds. Manual of Clinical Microbiology, 9th edn. Washington, DC: ASM Press, 2007:1173–92.
39 Ito T, Katayama Y, Asada K *et al.* Structural comparison of three types of staphylococcal cassette chromosome *mec* integrated in the chromosome in methicillin-resistant *Staphylococcus aureus*. Antimicrob Agents Chemother 2001;45:1323–36.
40 Hanssen A-M, Sollid UE. SCCmec in staphylococci: genes on the move. FEMS Immunol Med Microbiol 2006;46:8–20.
41 Tomasz A, Nachman S, Leaf H. Stable classes of phenotypic expression in methicillin-resistant clinical isolates of staphylococci. Antimicrob Agents Chemother 1991;35:124–9.
42 Finan JE, Rosato AE, Dickinson TM, Ko D, Archer GL. Conversion of oxacillin-resistant staphylococci from heterotypic to homotypic resistance expression. Antimicrob Agents Chemother 2002;46:24–30.
43 McKinney TK, Sharma VK, Craig WA, Archer GL. Transcription of the gene mediating methicillin resistance in *Staphylococcus aureus* (*mecA*) is corepressed but not coinduced by cognate *mecA* and β-lactamase regulators. J Bacteriol 2001;183:6862–8.
44 Hiramatsu K. Elucidation of the mechanism of antibiotic resistance acquisition of methicillin-resistant *Staphylococcus aureus* (MRSA) and determination of its whole genome nucleotide sequence. Jpn Med Assoc J 2004;47:153–9.
45 Archer GL, Bosilevec JM. Signaling antibiotic resistance in staphylococci. Science 2001;291:1915–16.
46 Katayama Y, Robinson DA, Enright MC, Chambers HF. Genetic background affects stability of *mecA* in *Staphylococcus aureus*. J Clin Microbiol 2005;43:2380–3.
47 Shukla SK, Ramaswamy SV, Conradt J *et al.* Novel polymorphisms in *mec* genes and a new *mec* complex type in methicillin-resistant *Staphylococcus aureus* isolates obtained in rural Wisconsin. Antimicrob Agents Chemother 2004;48:3080–5.
48 Rosato AE, Craig WA, Archer GL. Quantitation of *mecA* transcription in oxacillin-resistant *Staphylococcus aureus* clinical isolates. J Bacteriol 2003;185:3446–52.

49 Chambers HF, Archer G, Matsuhashi M. Low-level methicillin resistance in strains of *Staphylococcus aureus*. Antimicrob Agents Chemother 1989;33:424–8.

50 Thauvin-Eliopoulos C, Rice LB, Eliopoulos GM, Moellering RC. Efficacy of oxacillin and ampicillin–sulbactam combination in experimental endocarditis caused by β-lactamase-hyperproducing *Staphylococcus aureus*. Antimicrob Agents Chemother 1990;37:728–32.

51 Massidda O, Montanari MP, Varaldo PE. Evidence for a methicillin-hydrolyzing β-lactamase in *Staphylococcus aureus* strains with borderline susceptibility to this drug. FEMS Microbiol Lett 1992;92:223–7.

52 Tomasz A, Drugeon HB, de Lencastre HM, Jabes D, McDougal L, Bille J. New mechanism for methicillin-resistance in *Staphylococcus aureus*: clinical isolates that lack the PBP 2a gene and contain normal penicillin-binding proteins with modified penicillin-binding capacity. Antimicrob Agents Chemother 1989;33:1869–74.

53 Henze UU, Berger-Bächi B. *Staphylococcus aureus* penicillin-binding protein 4 and intrinsic β-lactam resistance. Antimicrob Agents Chemother 1995;39:2415–22.

54 Chambers HF. Methicillin resistance in staphylococci: molecular and biochemical basis and clinical implications. Clin Microbiol Rev 1997;10:781–91.

55 Brown DF, Yates VS. Methicillin susceptibility testing of *Staphylococcus aureus* on media containing five percent sodium hydroxide. Eur J Clin Microbiol 1986;5:726–8.

56 Swenson JM, Tenover FC and the Cefoxitin Disk Study Group. Results of disk diffusion testing with cefoxitin correlate with presence of *mecA* in *Staphylococcus* spp. J Clin Microbiol 2005; 43:3818–23.

57 Witte W, Pasemann B, Cuny C. Detection of low-level oxacillin resistance in *mecA*-positive *Staphylococcus aureus*. Clin Microbiol Infect 2007;13:408–12.

58 Monsen T, Persson S, Edebro H, Granstrom S, Wistrom J. Mueller-Hinton agar is superior to PDM blood agar for detection of methicillin-resistant *Staphylococcus aureus*. Clin Microbiol Infect 2003;9:61–4.

59 Hindler JA, Warner NL. Effect of source of Mueller-Hinton agar on detection of oxacillin resistance in *Staphylococcus aureus* using a screening methodology. J Clin Microbiol 1987;25:734–5.

60 Hindler JA, Inderlied CB. Effect of the source of Mueller-Hinton agar and resistance frequency on the detection of methicillin-resistant *Staphylococcus aureus*. J Clin Microbiol 1985;21:205–10.

61 Kobayashi Y, Kizaki M, Kawakami K, Uchida H, Ikeda Y. Assessment of oxacillin salt agar for detection of MRSA identified by presence of the *mecA* gene. J Hosp Infect 1993;23:279–85.

62 Unal S, Werner K, DeGirolami P, Barsanti F, Eliopoulos G. Comparison of tests for detection of methicillin-resistant *Staphylococcus aureus* in a clinical microbiology laboratory setting. Antimicrob Agents Chemother 1994;38:345–7.

63 Cavassini M, Wenger A, Jaton K, Blanc DS, Bille J. Evaluation of MRSA-Screen, a simple anti-PBP2a slide latex agglutination kit for rapid detection of methicillin resistance in *Staphylococcus aureus*. J Clin Microbiol 1999;37:1591–4.

64 Resende CA, Figueiredo AM. Discrimination of methicillin-resistant *Staphylococcus aureus* from borderline-resistant and susceptible isolates by different methods. J Med Microbiol 1997;46:145–9.

65 Swenson JM, Williams PP, Killgore G, O'Hara CM, Tenover FC. Performance of eight methods, including two new rapid methods, for detection of oxacillin resistance in a challenge set of *Staphylococcus aureus* organisms. J Clin Microbiol 2001; 39:3785–8.

66 Swenson JA, Spargon J, Tenover FC, Ferraro MJ. Optimal inoculation methods and quality control for the NCCLS oxacillin agar screen test for detection of oxacillin resistance in *Staphylococcus aureus*. J Clin Microbiol 2001;39:3781–4.

67 Sakoulas G, Gold HS, Venkataraman L, DeGirolami PC, Eliopoulos GM, Qian Q. Methicillin-resistant *Staphylococcus aureus*: comparison of susceptibility testing methods and analysis of *mecA*-positive susceptible strains. J Clin Microbiol 2001; 39:3946–51.

68 Udo EE, Mokadas EM, Al-Haddad A, Mathew B, Jacob LE, Sanyal SC. Rapid detection of methicillin resistance in staphylococci using a slide latex agglutination kit. Int J Antimicrob Agents 2000;15:19–24.

69 Jafri AK, Reisner BS, Woods GL. Evaluation of a latex agglutination assay for rapid detection of oxacillin resistant *Staphylococcus aureus*. Diagn Microbiol Infect Dis 2000;36:57–9.

70 NCCLS/Clinical Laboratory Standards Institute. Performance standards for antimicrobial susceptibility testing. Fourteenth Informational Supplement M100-S14. Wayne, PA: Clinical Laboratory Standards Institute, 2004.

71 Clinical Laboratory Standards Institute. Performance standards for antimicrobial susceptibility testing. Fifteenth Informational Supplement M100-S15. Wayne, PA: Clinical Laboratory Standards Institute, 2005.

72 Swenson JM, Lonsway D, McAllister S *et al*. Detection of mecA-mediated resistance using reference commercial testing methods in a collection of *Staphylococcus aureus* expression borderline oxacillin MICs. Diagn Microbiol Infect Dis 2007;58:33–9.

73 Skov RL, Pallesen LV, Poulsen RL, Espersen F. Evaluation of a new 3-h hybridization method for detecting the *mecA* gene in *Staphylococcus aureus* and comparison with existing genotypic and phenotypic susceptibility testing methods. J Antimicrob Chemother 1999;43:467–75.

74 Skov R, Smyth R, Larsen AR, Frimodt-Moller N, Kahlmeter G. Evaluation of cefoxitin 5 and 10 μg discs for the detection of methicillin resistance in staphylococci. J Antimicrob Chemother 2005;55:157–61.

75 Skov R, Smyth R, Larsen AR *et al*. Phenotypic detection of methicillin resistance in *Staphylococcus aureus* by disk diffusion testing and Etest on Mueller-Hinton agar. J Clin Microbiol 2006;44:4395–9.

76 Kobayashi N, Taniguchi K, Urasawa S. Analysis of diversity of mutations in the *mecI* gene and *mecA* promoter/operator region of methicillin-resistant *Staphylococcus aureus* and *Staphylococcus epidermidis*. Antimicrob Agents Chemother 1998;42:717–20.

77 Hussain Z, Stoakes L, Garrow S, Longo S, Fitzgerald V, Lannigan R. Rapid detection of mecA-positive and mecA-negative coagulase negative staphylococci by an anti-penicillin binding protein 2a slide latex agglutination test. J Clin Microbiol 2000;38:2051–4.

78 Horstkotte MA, Knobloch JK-M, Rohde H, Mack D. Rapid detection of methicillin resistance in coagulase-negative staphylococci by a penicillin-binding protein 2a-specific latex agglutination test. J Clin Microbiol 2001;39:3700–2.

79 Soussy CJ. Communiqué 2004. Commité de l'Antibiogramme de la Societé Française de Microbiologie, Paris, France, 2004.
80 Soussy CJ. Communiqué 2005. Commité de l'Antibiogramme de la Societé Française de Microbiologie, Paris, France, 2005.
81 Pupin H, Renaudin H, Join-Lambert O, Bébéar C, Mégraud F, Lehours P. Evaluation of moxalactam with the BD Phoenix System for detection of methicillin resistance in coagulase-negative staphylococci. J Clin Microbiol 2007;45:2005–8.
82 Valderas MW, Gatson JW, Wreyford N, Hart ME. The superoxide dismutase gene *sodM* is unique to *Staphylococcus aureus*: absence of *sodM* in coagulase-negative staphylococci. J Bacteriol 2002;184:2465–72.
83 Goh SH, Santucci Z, Kloos WE *et al.* Identification of *Staphylococcus* species and subspecies by the chaperonin 60 gene identification method and reverse checkerboard hybridization. J Clin Microbiol 1997;35:3116–21.
84 Safdar N, Narans L, Gordon B, Maki DG. Comparison of culture screening methods for detection of nasal carriage of methicillin-resistant *Staphylococcus aureus*: a prospective study comparing 32 methods. J Clin Microbiol 2003;41:3163–6.
85 Gardam M, Brunton J, Willey B, McGreer A, Low D, Conly J. A blinded comparison of three laboratory protocols for the identification of patients colonized with methicillin-resistant *Staphylococcus aureus*. Infect Control Hosp Epidemiol 2001; 22:152–6.
86 Davies S, Zadik PM. Comparison of methods for the isolation of methicillin-resistant *Staphylococcus aureus*. J Clin Pathol 1997;50:257–8.
87 van Hal SJ, Stark D, Lockwood B, Marriott D, Harkness J. Methicillin-resistant *Staphylococcus aureus* (MRSA) detection: comparison of two molecular methods (IDI-MRSA PCR assay and GenoType MRSA Direct PCR assay) with three selective MRSA agars (MRSA ID, MRSASelect, and CHROMagar MRSA) for use with infection-control swabs. J Clin Microbiol 2007;45:2486–90.
88 Brown DFJ, Edwards DI, Hawkey *et al*. On behalf of the Joint Working Party of the British Society for Antimicrobial Chemotherapy, Hospital Infection Society and Infection Control Nurses Association: guidelines for the laboratory diagnosis and susceptibility testing of methicillin-resistant *Staphylococcus aureus* (MRSA). J Antimicrob Chemother 2005;56:1000–18.
89 Huletsky A, Giroux R, Rossbach V *et al.* New real-time PCR assay for rapid detection of methicillin-resistant *Staphylococcus aureus* directly from specimens containing a mixture of staphylococci. J Clin Microbiol 2004;42:1875–84.
90 Huletsky A, Lebel P, Picard FJ, Bernier M, Gagnon M, Boucher N. Identification of methicillin-resistant *Staphylococcus aureus* carriage in less than 1 hour during a hospital surveillance program. Clin Infect Dis 2005;40:976–81.
91 Warren DK, Liao RS, Merz LR, Eveland M, Dunne WM. Detection of methicillin-resistant *Staphylococcus aureus* directly from nasal swab specimens by a real-time PCR assay. J Clin Microbiol 2004;42:5578–81.
92 Desjardins M, Guibord C, Lalonde B, Toye B, Ramotar K. Evaluation of the IDI-MRSA assay for detection of methicillin-resistant *Staphylococcus aureus* from nasal and rectal specimens pooled in a selective broth. J Clin Microbiol 2006;44:1219–23.
93 Bishop EJ, Grabsch EA, Ballard SA *et al.* Concurrent analysis of nose and groin swab specimens by the IDI-MRSA PCR assay is comparable to analysis by individual-specimen PCR and routine culture assays for detection of colonization by methicillin-resistant *Staphylococcus aureus*. J Clin Microbiol 2006;44:2904–8.
94 Oberdorfer K, Pohl S, Frey M, Heeg K, Wendt C. Evaluation of a single-locus real-time polymerase chain reaction as a screening test for specific detection of methicillin-resistant *Staphylococcus aureus* in ICU patients. Eur J Clin Microbiol Infect Dis 2006;25:657–63.
95 Paule SM, Hacek DM, Kufner B *et al.* Performance of the BD GeneOhm methicillin-resistant *Staphylococcus aureus* test before and during high-volume clinical use. J Clin Microbiol 2007;45:2993–8.
96 Donnio PY, Oliviera DC, Faria NA, Wilhelm N, Le Coustumier A, de Lencastre H. Partial excision of the chromosomal cassette containing the methicillin resistance determinant results in methicillin-susceptible *Staphylococcus aureus*. J Clin Microbiol 2005;43:4191–3.
97 Mehta M, Gonzalsies T, Hacek D, Bursdall D, Ng C, Peterson L. Performance of two FDA-cleared PCR tests for MRSA compared to microbiological cultures. Abstract D-880. Presented at the 47th ICAAC Meeting, Chicago, IL, October 2007.
98 Holfelder M, Eigner U, Turnwald AM, Witte W, Weizenegger M, Fahr A. Direct detection of methicillin-resistant *Staphylococcus aureus* in clinical specimens by a nucleic acid-based hybridisation assay. Clin Microbiol Infect 2006;12:1163–7.
99 Zhang SX, Drews SJ, Tomassi J, Katz KC. Comparison of two versions of the IDI-MRSA assay using charcoal swabs for prospective nasal and nonnasal surveillance samples. J Clin Microbiol 2007;45:2278–80.
100 Rosenthal A, White D, Churilla S, Brodie S, Katz KC. Optimal surveillance culture sites for detection of methicillin-resistant *Staphylococcus aureus* in newborns. J Clin Microbiol 2006; 44:4234–6.
101 Nilsson P, Ripa T. *Staphylococcus aureus* throat colonization is more frequent than colonization in the anterior nares. J Clin Microbiol 2006;44:3334–9.
102 Bourbeau PP, Riley JA, Shoemaker BC, Jones KS. Use of CultureSwab Plus swabs with Amies gel agar for testing of naris specimens with the GeneOhm MRSA assay. J Clin Microbiol 2007;45:2281–3.
103 Lee YL, Cesario T, Gupta G *et al.* Surveillance of colonization and infection with *Staphylococcus aureus* susceptible or resistant to methicillin in a community skilled-nursing facility. Am J Infect Control 1997;25:312–21.
104 Singh K, Gavin PJ, Vescio T *et al.* Microbiologic surveillance using nasal cultures alone is sufficient for detection of methicillin-resistant *Staphylococcus aureus* isolates in neonates. J Clin Microbiol 2003;41:2755–7.
105 Stamper PD, Cai M, Howard T, Speser S, Carroll KC. Clinical validation of the Molecular BD GeneOhm StaphySR assay for direct detection of *Staphylococcus aureus* and methicillin-resistant *Staphylococcus aureus* in positive blood cultures. J Clin Microbiol 2007;45:2191–6.
106 Chapin K, Musgnug M. Evaluation of three rapid methods for the direct identification of *Staphylococcus aureus* from positive blood cultures. J Clin Microbiol 2003;41:4324–7.
107 Qian Q, Eichelberger K, Kirby JE. Rapid identification of *Staphylococcus aureus* in blood cultures by use of the direct tube coagulase test. J Clin Microbiol 2003;45:2267–9.
108 Centers for Disease Control and Prevention. Vancomycin-resistant *Staphylococcus aureus*: Pennsylvania. MMWR 2002;51:902.

109 Walsh TR, Howe RA. The prevalence and mechanisms of vancomycin resistance in *Staphylococcus aureus*. Annu Rev Microbiol 2002;56:657–75.

110 Jones RN. Microbiological features of vancomycin in the 21st century: minimum inhibitory concentration creep, bactericidal/static activity, and applied breakpoints to predict clinical outcomes or detect resistant strains. Clin Infect Dis 2006;42:S13–S24.

111 Hiramatsu K, Hanaki H. Glycopeptide resistance in staphylococci. Curr Opin Infect Dis 1998;11:653–8.

112 Chang SD, Sievert DM, Hageman JC *et al.* Infection with vancomycin-resistant *Staphylococcus aureus* containing the *vanA* resistance gene. N Engl J Med 2003;348:1342–7.

113 Tenover FC, Weigel LM, Appelbaum PC *et al.* Vancomycin-resistant *Staphylococcus aureus* isolate from a patient in Pennsylvania. Antimicrob Agents Chemother 2004;48:275–80.

114 Liu C, Chambers HF. *Staphylococcus aureus* with heterogeneous resistance to vancomycin: epidemiology, clinical significance, and critical assessment of diagnostic methods. Antimicrob Agents Chemother 2003;47:3040–5.

115 Khosrovaneh A, Riederer K, Saeed S *et al.* Frequency of reduced vancomycin susceptibility and heterogeneous subpopulation in persistent or recurrent methicillin-resistant *Staphylococcus aureus* bacteremia. Clin Infect Dis 2004;38:1328–30.

116 Howden BP, Ward PB, Charles PG *et al.* Treatment outcomes for serious infections caused by methicillin-resistant *Staphylococcus aureus* with reduced vancomycin susceptibility. Clin Infect Dis 2004;38:521–8.

117 Cuevas O, Cercenado E, Vindel A *et al.* Evolution of the antimicrobial resistance in *Staphylococcus* spp. in Spain: five nationwide prevalence studies, 1986 to 2002. Antimicrob Agents Chemother 2004;48:4240–5.

118 Robert J, Bismuth R, Jarlier V. Decreased susceptibility to glycopeptides in methicillin-resistant *Staphylococcus aureus*: a 20 year study in a large French teaching hospital, 1983–2002. J Antimicrob Chemother 2006;57:506–10.

119 Wang G, Hindler JF, Ward KW, Bruckner DA. Increased vancomycin MICs for *Staphylococcus aureus* clinical isolates from a university hospital during a 5-year period. J Clin Microbiol 2006;44:3883–6.

120 Centers for Disease Control and Prevention. Laboratory detection of vancomycin-intermediate/resistant *Staphylococcus aureus*. Available at http://www.cdc.gov/ncidod/dhqp/ar_visavrsa_algo_html. Accessed April 2009.

121 Wootton M, Walsh TR, MacGowan AP. Evidence for reduction in breakpoints used to determine vancomycin susceptibility in *Staphylococcus aureus*. Antimicrob Agents Chemother 2005; 49:3982–3.

122 Tenover FC, Lancaster MV, Hill BC *et al.* Characterization of staphylococci with reduced susceptibility to vancomycin and other glycopeptides. J Clin Microbiol 1998;36:1020–7.

123 Kralovic SM, Danko LH, Roselle GA. Laboratory reporting of *Staphylococcus aureus* with reduced susceptibility to vancomycin in United States Department of Veterans Affairs facilities. Emerg Infect Dis 2002;8:402–7.

124 Walsh TR, Bolmström A, Quarnstrom A *et al.* Evaluation of current methods of detecting vancomycin resistance and hetero-resistance in *Staphylococcus aureus* and other staphylococci. J Clin Microbiol 2001;39:2439–44.

125 Wootton M, Howe RA, Hillman R, Walsh TR, Bennett PM, MacGowan AP. A modified population analysis profile (PAP) method to detect hetero-resistance in vancomycin in *Staphylococcus aureus* in a UK hospital. J Antimicrob Chemother 2001;47:399–403.

126 Wootton M, MacGowan AP, Walsh TR, Howe RA. A multicenter study evaluating the current strategies for isolating *Staphylococcus aureus* strains with reduced susceptibility to glycopeptides. J Clin Microbiol 2007;45:329–32.

127 Tajima Y, Komatsu M, Ito T, Hiramatsu K. Rapid detection of *Staphylococcus aureus* strains having reduced susceptibility to vancomycin using a chemiluminescence-based drug-susceptibility test. J Microbiol Methods 2007;70:434–41.

128 LeClercq R, Courvalin P. Bacterial resistance to macrolide, lincosamide, and streptogramin antibiotics by target modification. Antimicrob Agents Chemother 1991;35:1267–72.

129 Jorgensen JH, Crawford SA, McElmeel ML, Feibelkorn KR. Detection of inducible clindamycin resistance of staphylococci in correlation with performance of automated broth susceptibility testing. J Clin Microbiol 2004;42:1800–2.

130 Zelazny AM, Ferraro MJ, Glennen A *et al.* Selection of strains for quality assessment of the disk induction method for detection of inducible clindamycin resistance in staphylococci: a CLSI collaborative study. J Clin Microbiol 2005;43:2613–15.

131 Hindler JF, Bruckner DA. Abstract C-325. Presented at the 105th General Meeting of the American Society of Microbiology, June 5–9, 2005.

132 Lewis JS II, Jorgensen JH. Inducible clindamycin resistance in staphylococci: should clinicians and microbiologists be concerned? Clin Infect Dis 2005;40:280–5.

133 Nagaoka T, Horii T, Satoh T *et al.* Use of a three-dimensional microarray system for detection of levofloxacin resistance and the *mecA* gene in *Staphylococcus aureus*. J Clin Microbiol 2005;43:5187–94.

134 Tenover FC, Vaugh RR, McDougal LK, Fosheim GE, McGowan JE. Multiple-locus variable-number tandem-repeat assay analysis of methicillin-resistant *Staphylococcus aureus* strains. J Clin Microbiol 2007;45:2215–19.

135 Maslow R, Slutsky AM, Arbeit RD. Application of pulsed-field gel electrophoresis in molecular epidemiology. In: White TJ, ed. Diagnostic Molecular Microbiology: Principles and Applications. Washington, DC: ASM Press, 1993:563–72.

136 Chung M, de Lencastre P, Matthews P *et al.* Molecular typing of methicillin-resistant *Staphylococcus aureus* by pulsed field gel electrophoresis: a comparison of results obtained in a multilaboratory effort using identical protocols and MRSA strains. Microb Drug Resist 2000;6:189–98.

137 Duck WM, Steward CD, Banerjee SN, McGowan JE Jr, Tenover FC. Optimization of computer software settings improves accuracy of pulsed field gel electrophoresis macrorestriction fragment pattern analysis. J Clin Microbiol 2003;41:3035–42.

138 Deurenberg RH, Vink C, Kalenic S, Friedrich AW, Bruggeman CA, Stobberingh EE. The molecular evolution of methicillin-resistant *Staphylococcus aureus*. Clin Microbiol Infect 2007; 13:222–35.

139 Deplano A, Schuermans A, Van-Eldere J *et al.* Multicenter evaluation of epidemiological typing of methicillin-resistant *Staphylococcus aureus* strains by repetitive-element PCR analysis. J Clin Microbiol 2000;38:3527–33.

140 Shopsin B, Gomez M, Montgomery SO *et al.* Evaluation of protein A gene polymorphic region DNA sequencing for typing of *Staphylococcus aureus* strains. J Clin Microbiol 1999;37:3556–63.

141 Preheim L, Pitcher D, Owen R, Cookson B. Typing of methicillin-resistant and susceptible *Staphylococcus aureus* strains by ribosomal RNA gene restriction patterns using a biotinylated probe. Eur J Clin Microbiol Infect Dis 1991;10:428–36.
142 Hookey JV, Edwards V, Patel S, Richardson JF, Cookson BD. Use of fluorescent amplified fragment length polymorphism (FAELP) to characterize methicillin-resistant *Staphylococcus aureus*. J Microbiol Methods 1999;37:7–15.
143 Shopsin B, Gomez M, Waddington M, Riehman M, Kreiswirth BN. Use of coagulase gene (*coa*) repeat region nucleotide sequencing for typing of methicillin-resistant *Staphylococcus aureus* strains. J Clin Microbiol 2000;38:3453–6.
144 Robinson DA, Enright MC. Evolutionary models of the emergence of methicillin-resistant *Staphylococcus aureus*. Antimicrob Agents Chemother 2003;47:3926–34.
145 Oliveira DC, de Lencastre H. Multiplex PCR strategy for rapid identification of structural type and variants of the *mec* element in methicillin-resistant *Staphylococcus aureus*. Antimicrob Agents Chemother 2002;46:2155–61.
146 Enright MC, Day NP, Davies CE, Peacock SJ, Spratt BG. Multilocus sequence typing for characterization of methicillin-resistant and methicillin-susceptible clones of *Staphylococcus aureus*. J Clin Microbiol 2000;38:1008–15.
147 Frénay HM, Bunschoten AE, Schouls LM *et al.* Molecular typing of methicillin-resistant *Staphylococcus aureus* on the basis of protein A gene polymorphism. Eur J Clin Microbiol Infect Dis 1996;15:60–4.
148 Otsuka J, Kondoh Y, Amemiya T *et al.* Development and validation of microarray-based assay for epidemiological study of MRSA. Mol Cell Probes 2008;22:1–13.

Section II
Epidemiology of Staphylococcal Infection

Chapter 12
Colonization with *Staphylococcus aureus* and the Role of Colonization in Causing Infection

Henri A. Verbrugh
Erasmus University Medical Center, Rotterdam, Netherlands

Introduction

Colonization with *Staphylococcus aureus* occurs early in life and persists throughout life in a significant proportion of the population. Those colonized are called *S. aureus* carriers. The anterior nares, the throat, and the perineum are the niches from which *S. aureus* can be cultured. The nose is the site most frequently found to yield staphylococci and it is generally accepted that the nose is the principal site of growth of *S. aureus*. Attention was first drawn to this point in 1935 by Chris Dolman [1].

> *A pure or almost pure culture of haemolytic staphylococcus obtained by direct inoculation of a blood-agar plate with a nose or throat swab is a finding which should neither be ignored as due to "contamination" nor dismissed as of no pathological significance; particularly when swabs taken at intervals yield consistently the same growth. In a healthy person such a finding indicates a potential source of staphylococcal infection to himself and others, while in a patient with existing symptoms of infection of the nose and throat, the probable causal micro-organism is thus made evident.*

However, independent colonization of the throat and the perineum also occurs, albeit at a much lower frequency [2–4]. The skin of the hands and forearms of carriers are typically also culture-positive but these are considered sites of secondary seeding and not sites where *S. aureus* may persist and multiply independently over time [5]. Other carriage sites, including the gastrointestinal tract, the vagina and axillae, harbor *S. aureus* much less frequently (Figure 12.1).

The localization of nasal *S. aureus* has been studied in some detail. Initial observations found *S. aureus* to be present more commonly in the anterior nares, the vestibulum

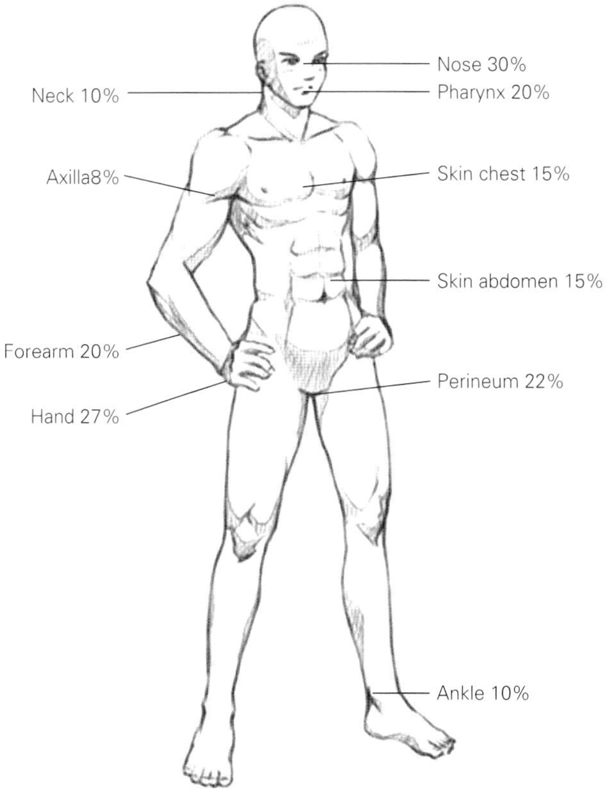

Figure 12.1 Carriage rates of *S. aureus* according to body site in adults in the general population.

nasi, compared with sampling of the more inner or proximal mucous parts of the nose [2]. The vestibulum nasi is limited laterally by the interior of the wing of the nostril and medially by a mucous fold termed limen nasi, behind which the nasal cavity with its mucosal linings begins [6]. The inner wall of the nostril is covered by fully keratinized squamous epithelium containing follicles of the nose hairs (vibrissae), sebaceous glands, and apocrine sweat glands. More detailed topological sampling of the vestibulum nasi revealed that the highest number of *S. aureus* can be cultured from the moist squamous epithelium of the septum

Staphylococci in Human Disease, 2nd edition. Edited by Kent B. Crossley, Kimberly K. Jefferson, Gordon Archer, Vance G. Fowler, Jr.

adjacent to the ostium nasi and from the deeper hairless areas of the lateral wall of the vestibulum; vibrissae and the hair-covered areas of the lateral wall carry much lower numbers of *S. aureus* [7]. In patients with chronic sinusitis, *S. aureus* has been recovered from mucosal lesions, including polyps, in the middle meatus, and the bacteria apparently reside within the columnar epithelial lining cells and cells of mucous glands [8]. The tonsils are the sites where *S. aureus* preferentially resides in the throat, especially in long-term throat carriers of *S. aureus* [9]. There the bacteria can be found in the deep crypts of the tonsils.

Carriers of *S. aureus* have an increased risk of developing staphylococcal infections caused by the strain they carry. Such infections have variously been labeled "self-infections," "autoinfections," or "endogenous infections" [2]. However, *S. aureus* carriers are usually healthy and do not suffer from staphylococcal infection, but may develop endogenous infections when their natural barriers against *S. aureus* infection are breached. In particular, (micro)trauma of the skin and mucous membranes provides opportunities for staphylococci to invade the tissues of its host and cause infection. In addition to endogenous infections, *S. aureus* carriers may also cause "cross-infections" when their strain is transmitted and infects individuals free from *S. aureus*. Endogenous infections, transmission of strains, and cross-infections occur frequently in hospitals where crowding of patients and personnel, combined with multiple invasive diagnostic and therapeutic procedures, provide many opportunities for *S. aureus* to become an invasive pathogen. However, similar circumstances may occur outside the healthcare setting especially where crowding of people is combined with activities, including those associated with sport and employment, that yield abrasions or other (micro)traumas of the skin [10]. The carrier state is therefore key in the epidemiology of both community- and healthcare-associated infections due to *S. aureus*. This chapter reviews the natural history of *S. aureus* carriage and discusses the genetic and environmental determinants of normal healthy carriage and its association with staphylococcal disease when healthy carriage transforms into harmful carriage of *S. aureus*.

Staphylococcus aureus is also carried naturally by, and causes disease in, several animal species including domestic cattle, farm pigs, chickens, dairy sheep and goats, hares, and a few other species. The strains carried by animal species tend to belong to *S. aureus* clones or genetic lineages not normally present on humans. These biotypes or biovars of *S. aureus* can be distinguished to some extent by simple biochemical tests [11] but are better differentiated when phage typing and genetic typing systems are employed [12,13]. This chapter does not discuss carriage of *S. aureus* among domestic animals except where relevant for human carriage and diseases. Pet animals such as dogs and cats living in the household may play a role in *S. aureus* carriage in humans [14].

Healthy carriage of *S. aureus*

Epidemiology

Although staphylococci have been studied since their discovery in 1888, carriage of *S. aureus* by healthy humans was appreciated only after the introduction of the coagulase test in the 1930s [2,15]. For the first time, by using this test, one could reliably distinguish between pathogenic and nonpathogenic species of *Staphylococcus*. Carriage of *S. aureus*, especially nasal colonization, was found to be common but not universal. Cross-sectional point prevalence studies categorized individuals into those carrying *S. aureus* and those not at a given point in time. Early point prevalence studies in the 1940s and 1950s using nasal swabs in populations of healthy adults outside hospitals yielded carriage rates of 20–50% [16]. The large variation in observed rates is partly due to differences in the quality of sampling and of culture methods employed in these studies. Cross-sectional studies performed more recently have generally reported nasal carriage rates of less than 30%, a decline that remains largely unexplained but which may be due to reduced exposure to *S. aureus* as a consequence of better living conditions and improved hygienic precautions [16]. Also, the rate of carriage may be lower in tropical countries. Carriage rates among the general population reported recently from developing countries vary widely, from 10% in Indonesia [17], 14.8% in Pakistan [18], 21% in Saudi Arabia (Hajj pilgrims) [19], 23% in Malaysia [20], 25% in Taiwan [21], to 29% in India [22]. Ethnicity, socioeconomic circumstances, and prior exposure to antimicrobial agents are likely to be involved since rates may differ between ethnic groups in a given country (see below) [2,23]. However, a 2001–2002 national survey of 9622 individuals representative of the population of the USA revealed a rate of nasal carriage of *S. aureus* of 32.4% [24]. The rates of *S. aureus* carriers among healthcare workers are similar to those found among adults in the general public [16], although some early studies found nurses to have higher rates [2]. Also, physicians may have higher rates compared with other professionals in society [25]. Among adult patients at the time of admission or presentation to a hospital, the rates of *S. aureus* carriage are also comparable to those found in the general population (Table 12.1). This is also true for pediatric patient populations, although rates tend to be higher among children compared with adults (Table 12.1) [33,35,36]. Again, children living in underdeveloped countries may have lower carriage rates compared with children in the developed world [34].

When individuals are studied longitudinally, i.e., cultured repeatedly over time, only about 20% (range 10–30%) of the population always carry *S. aureus* and they are labeled "persistent carriers." In addition, longitudinal studies show that approximately 20% (range 6–38%) of the population never carry *S. aureus* (persistent noncarriers) and that the remaining 60% (range 28–70%) are intermittently positive

Table 12.1 Carriage rates for *S. aureus* recently observed among adult and pediatric patients at the time of admission to hospital.

Age class	Patients admitted to	Country	No. of patients screened	No. *S. aureus* positive (%)	Reference
Adults	Nonsurgical wards	Netherlands	17 529	4479 (26%)	26
Adults	Surgical wards	Netherlands	6512	1999 (31%)	27
Adults	Cardiac surgery	USA	6334	1342 (21%)	28
Adults	Surgical wards	USA	3864	891 (23%)	29
Adults	Acute care wards, patients > 75 years old	Switzerland	797	212 (27%)	30
Adults	All wards except psychiatry and burn unit	USA	726	172 (24%)	31
Adults	Tertiary care hospital, wards not specified	USA	387	96 (25%)	32
Children	All admissions, mean age 6.1 years	Switzerland	1337	562 (41%)	33
Children	Admitted for respiratory disease or meningitis, age < 5 years	Brazil	686	93 (14%)	34
Children	"Convenience" sample of admissions to a general pediatric ward, mean age 4.7 years	USA	350	125 (36%)	35
Children	Predominantly healthy children visiting the clinic, mean age 5 years	USA	275	96 (35%)	36

when cultured for *S. aureus* [2]. Persistent carriers have significantly higher numbers of staphylococci in their nares (10^3–10^6 cfu) compared with intermittent carriers ($\leq 10^3$ cfu) [5,37,38], resulting in increased dispersal of staphylococci in the environment [5]. In addition, persistent carriers tend to carry a single phage type or genotype of *S. aureus* over long periods, up to 10 years, whereas intermittent carriers serially harbor different genotypes [39]. When volunteers are first made free of *S. aureus* and are subsequently artificially inoculated with a mixture of *S. aureus* strains, those volunteers who were persistent carriers before will select their original strain from the inoculation mixture and become carriers again, whereas the noncarriers quickly eliminate all *S. aureus* cells from their nares [40]. These observations have led to the hypothesis that persistent *S. aureus* carriers are biologically different from individuals who do not carry *S. aureus* or do so only intermittently [41]. In this concept, intermittent carriers and noncarriers are biologically similar since they are essentially intolerant of *S. aureus* and will eliminate staphylococcal cells that have adhered to their nasal epithelial surfaces, albeit at variable rates: noncarriers rapidly eliminate *S. aureus* (within hours or a few days and are therefore culture-negative when screened), whereas intermittent carriers require weeks or months to do so (and are therefore intermittently culture-positive when screened repeatedly). The more nasal cultures analyzed over increasing lengths of time, the higher the chance of identifying an intermittent carrier among previously negative persons.

The level and frequency of exposure to sources of *S. aureus* will of course also determine the chance of temporary carriage. Prospective nasal carriage studies in small groups of men totally isolated in Antarctica for 1 year have confirmed the existence of individuals who persistently carry a single strain of *S. aureus* as opposed to the other group members who remain culture-negative or only intermittently culture-positive [42,43]. Lack of new sources of staphylococci yields rather stable carriage patterns in such secluded populations, with persistent carriers being the dominant source of strains that induce temporary carriage in other individuals in the community. Thus, many variables influence the actual number of carriers, including the population sampled, the frequency of sampling, duration of follow-up, and the technique of sampling and culture. A typical distribution of carrier states in a population is depicted in Figure 12.2.

Important variables in sampling and culture technique include the number of body sites sampled, the type of swabs used for sampling, the use of enrichment broth and selective media in the laboratory, and the duration of incubation [39,44]. To reliably screen for *S. aureus* carriers, including carriers of methicillin-resistant *S. aureus* (MRSA),

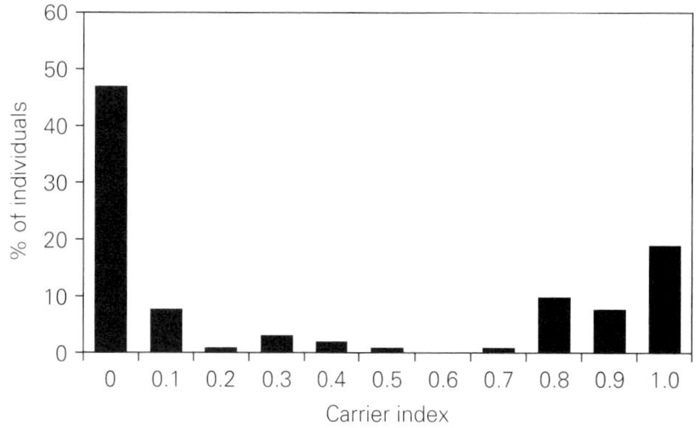

Figure 12.2 Distribution of *S. aureus* nasal carrier indices among 91 healthy adults repeatedly cultured over a 10–12 week period. The carrier index is defined as the proportion of cultures yielding *S. aureus* for a given individual (From VandenBergh *et al.* [39] with permission.)

it is recommended to culture at least both nares, the throat, and the perineum using dry rayon or charcoal-coated rayon swabs, and to incubate the swabs in enrichment broth for 24 hours prior to plating onto selective media for a further 48 hours of incubation [45]. Rectal swabs are better compared with stool culture [46]. The recent introduction of chromogenic media and polymerase chain reaction (PCR)-based technologies has further facilitated the detection of *S. aureus* and its methicillin-resistant variants [47,48]. A simple culture rule, based on two quantitative nasal cultures taken 1 week apart, has been proposed for reliably identifying persistent *S. aureus* carriers in the population and discriminating them from intermittent carriers or noncarriers of *S. aureus* [38].

Carriage rates vary significantly by age category. Newborn babies are highly susceptible to colonization and 50–70% of newborns become *S. aureus* positive within days to a few weeks after birth. The umbilical stump is commonly colonized as well as the nares of the newborn [49]. The mother is the usual source of the strain colonizing the newborn, but other members of the household (or hospital personnel) may also be a source. Newborns tend to carry this same strain during the first 6 months of life. Breast-feeding promotes *S. aureus* carriage. However, after approximately 8 weeks, carriage rates tend to fall to about 20% at the age of 6 months and to 10–15% at 1 year [49,50]. The determinants of the fall in *S. aureus* carriage rates in the first year of life have yet to be elucidated. However, bacterial interference (especially with *Streptococcus pneumoniae*, which interferes with the growth of *S. aureus* and vice versa), host genetics, and immune responses may all be involved (see below). Carriage of *S. aureus* at 2–8 weeks predicts carrier status at 6 months but not later in life.

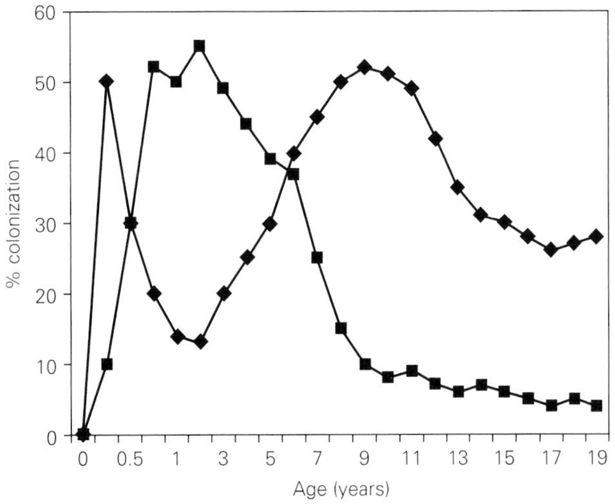

Figure 12.3 Rates of nasopharyngeal carriage of *S. aureus* (◆) and *Streptococcus pneumoniae* (■) in children according to age. (Based on data from references 49–51.)

From the age of approximately 1 year onwards the rate of *S. aureus* nasopharyngeal carriage increases again to reach a peak at the age of approximately 10 years (Figure 12.3). There is a transition from persistent carriage to intermittent carriage during adolescence. Again, epidemiological data support the concept of bacterial interference between *S. aureus* and *Streptococcus pneumoniae* in the nasopharyngeal niche [51]. The rate of *S. aureus* carriage during adulthood remains rather stable, with males consistently showing higher rates compared with females [52]. Among the elderly, *S. aureus* carriage rates slowly decline with advanced age [10,16,52].

Diseases associated with increased carriage rates of *S. aureus*

Patients with diabetes mellitus are well known to suffer from *S. aureus* infections more frequently than healthy persons and such infections may precipitate a crisis in the course of their disease. This observation led Smith and O'Connor [53] in 1966 to screen insulin-dependent children, insulin-dependent adults, and noninsulin-dependent adults for nasal *S. aureus*. Compared with age controls, the prevalence of *S. aureus* nasal carriage was much higher among the insulin-dependent diabetic children (76% vs. 44%) and insulin-dependent adults (53% vs. 34%) but not among the noninsulin-dependent diabetics (35%). This finding has since been confirmed [54–60]. When blood glucose concentration was taken as an indicator of diabetes control, an increased rate was found in those with the poorest control [55]. The mechanism underlying the increased rate of *S. aureus* carriage in insulin-dependent diabetics remains to be elucidated. One possibility is that repeated injections with insulin somehow promotes *S. aureus* carriage since other diseases and conditions similarly associated with repeated punctures of the skin by needles or catheters also are associated with higher rates of *S. aureus* carriage (see below). However, an alternative, more attractive hypothesis is that the increased concentration of glucose in the blood results in higher availability of glucose in the skin and on mucosal surfaces and that this may promote the local growth of *S. aureus* [61]. Indeed fasting glucose levels, even in the normal range, have been observed in a large-scale population-based study to be directly correlated to the risk of being a persistent *S. aureus* nasal carrier (Figure 12.4) [52].

Patients with end-stage renal disease on chronic dialysis are also more likely to be carriers of *S. aureus*. Patients on hemodialysis as well as those on chronic ambulatory peritoneal dialysis have increased carriage rates [10,62]. This increase in carriage is not due to confounding by diabetes mellitus as the underlying cause of their end-stage renal disease [63]. The increased rate of nasal and skin carriage remains unexplained apart from the hypothesis that

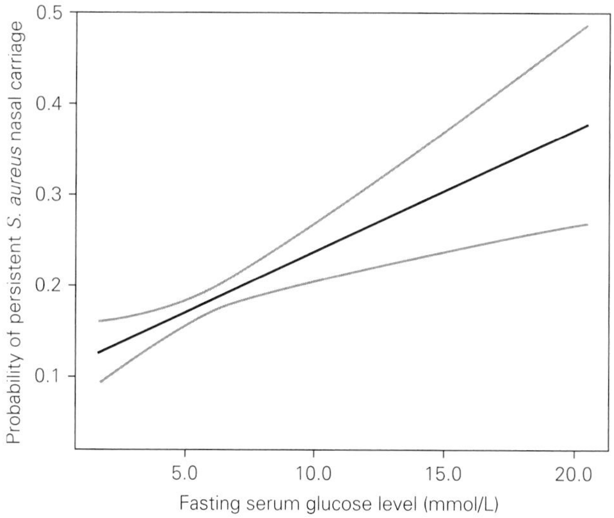

Figure 12.4 Correlation between fasting blood glucose concentration and probability of persistent *S. aureus* nasal carriage. Graph shows line of interaction with 95% confidence intervals. (From Nouwen [52] with permission.)

these patients have frequent healthcare contacts, repeated breaches of their skin, and may have acquired an immune disorder relevant for staphylococcal carriage. The same determinants may also underlie the increased *S. aureus* carriage rates observed in patients with HIV infection [10,16], in those with end-stage liver disease [64], and in intravenous drug abusers [10,65]. However, chronic liver infection with hepatitis B virus is not associated with increased rates of *S. aureus* carriage [66].

Higher rates of *S. aureus* nasal carriage have been found in patients with certain chronic skin diseases, including psoriasis [67] and atopic dermatitis [16,68–70]. Several reports suggest that patients with allergic rhinitis, either perennial or due to dust mites, have higher rates of *S. aureus* carriage especially when treated with allergen injections [71–74]. However, other factors than the regular use of needles, in particular abnormalities related to the atopic constitution of these patients, may predispose them for *S. aureus* carriage [75]. In contrast, chronic rhinosinusitis is not associated with increased rates of *S. aureus* carriage [76], although the disease itself may be caused by this species [77].

Nasal anatomical abnormalities, even minor ones, have been associated with increased carriage of *S. aureus* [78] as has the habit of nose-picking [79]. Nasal mucosal abnormalities are also present in patients with Wegener granulomatosis and, in this form of autoimmune vasculitis, *S. aureus* carriage rates are high and associated with the relapse rate of the vasculitis. The increased carriage may be due to the frequent presence of mucosal lesions in the nose, but has also been ascribed to the immunosuppressive therapy given to these patients [80]. Other autoimmune-mediated diseases, including Behçet disease, myasthenia gravis and rheumatoid arthritis, have not been consistently associated with increased rates of *S. aureus* carriage [81–84], although oral carriage may be higher among patients with rheumatoid arthritis [85]. Among patients with advanced cancer and xerostomia, 28% have also been noted to carry *S. aureus* in their oral cavity but these studies did not include control subjects [86,87]. Healthy subjects may carry oral *S. aureus* at similar rates [85]. Obesity and a history of stroke have also been added to the list of factors associated with higher *S. aureus* nasal carriage rates among patients screened preoperatively [88]. The underlying mechanisms for these latter associations are not clear.

Environmental determinants of carriage

Staphylococcus aureus is acquired from sources in the environment. In newborns it is predominantly the mother and closely associated carers who are the sources of *S. aureus*. Infants born in the hospital may acquire their strain from the hospital and, at a later date, induce mastitis in the mother [2,89]. Although human carriers of *S. aureus* are undoubtedly the most important reservoirs from which strains are transmitted, environmental reservoirs of *S. aureus* may also be involved since *S. aureus* is dispersed from carriers onto innate surfaces in the environment. *Staphylococcus aureus* can readily be cultured from dust, and will survive on most types of surfaces for weeks or months. Persistent nasal and perineal carriers of *S. aureus* disperse more colony-forming units compared with intermittent carriers or carriers who only have *S. aureus* in their throats [5]. Males disperse more colony-forming units compared with female carriers, and intercurrent viral respiratory infection in a carrier may temporarily increase dispersion significantly ("cloud" healthcare workers) [90].

Environmental sources likely to become heavily contaminated by carriers include bedding, clothes, bath tubs, dust, and various appliances commonly used by persistent *S. aureus* carriers in household settings. In hospitals, diagnostic, therapeutic and monitoring instruments, computer keyboards, telephone handles, wound dressings, and surgical gowns are additional potential reservoirs of *S. aureus* [2,15]. Again, persistent carriers among patients and hospital personnel are the origin from which the environment is contaminated, with patients having *S. aureus*-infected skin lesions posing a special risk [5]. Hands are the main vector for the transmission of staphylococci from a reservoir to the nasal niche [5]. *Staphylococcus aureus* also appears in the air in the vicinity of *S. aureus* dispersers, or when environmental reservoirs of *S. aureus* are disturbed. Thus, *S. aureus* colony-forming units per cubic meter of air may attain very high numbers during bed-making in a hospital ward. Therefore, airborne transmission of *S. aureus*

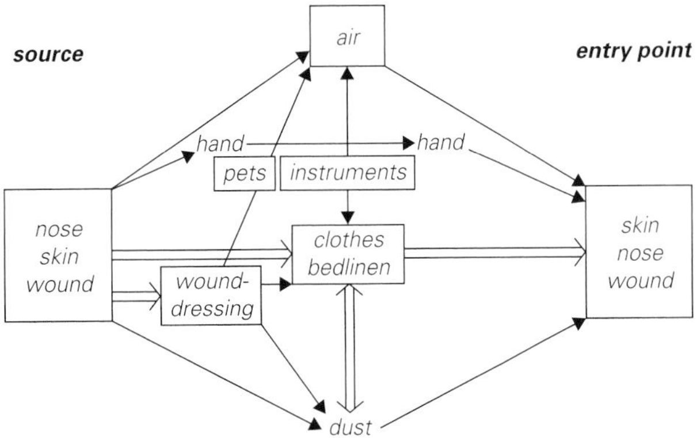

Figure 12.5 Transmission routes of *S. aureus*.

is another distinct possibility, although more difficult to evaluate separately from the other modes of transmission [5] (Figure 12.5).

Exposure to sources of *S. aureus* is an important determinant of carriage, especially for intermittent carriage. The level of crowding in households and hospitals, and the level of hygiene maintained in these settings, are directly associated with the rate of transmission [2]. Hospitalization itself may be a risk factor for the acquisition of new strains of *S. aureus* [91], most evident when patients are exposed to hospitals with endemic antibiotic-resistant strains of *S. aureus* (nosocomial MRSA). Indeed, in countries with endemic nosocomial MRSA, previous hospitalization is the most important risk factor for MRSA carriage at the time of admission to hospital [30,92–96]. Patients receiving antimicrobial agents during hospital stay have an increased risk of acquiring a hospital strain of *S. aureus* [97].

Nursing homes are now also recognized as important reservoirs of MRSA-positive individuals in the community [98,99]. In households where carriers and noncarriers of *S. aureus* live closely together, transmission occurs between those who carry *S. aureus* persistently and those who do not. In these circumstances carrier states become shared between the household members [52]. Up to 65% of individuals with positive cultures living within one household share the same genotypic strain. Virulent or antibiotic-resistant strains of *S. aureus*, including MRSA, may be introduced from healthcare settings into households and passed on to family members by healthcare workers who have picked up such strains during their work in their institution [100,101]. Domestic pets and companion animals in the household may become part of the chain of transmission [102,103]. Conditions in prisons, public housing projects, military barracks, and daycare centers are also known to favor the transmission of *S. aureus* [104–108].

Activities leading leading to repeated (minor) skin lesions may further promote the spread and acquisition of *S. aureus*. These include sports [109,110] and job-related activities [111–114]. Poverty and lower socioeconomic class in general are associated with *S. aureus* infections, probably reflecting in part the effects of crowding and repeated injuries [114–117].

In summary, *S. aureus* transmission and acquisition occurs in several niches in healthcare settings as well as in households and other settings in the community where people live together or have close physical contact (Figure 12.6). There is no relation between carriage rate and seasonality, temperature, or humidity [2,118,119]. However, active smoking is inversely related with *S. aureus* carriage and is thought to be due to a protective effect resulting

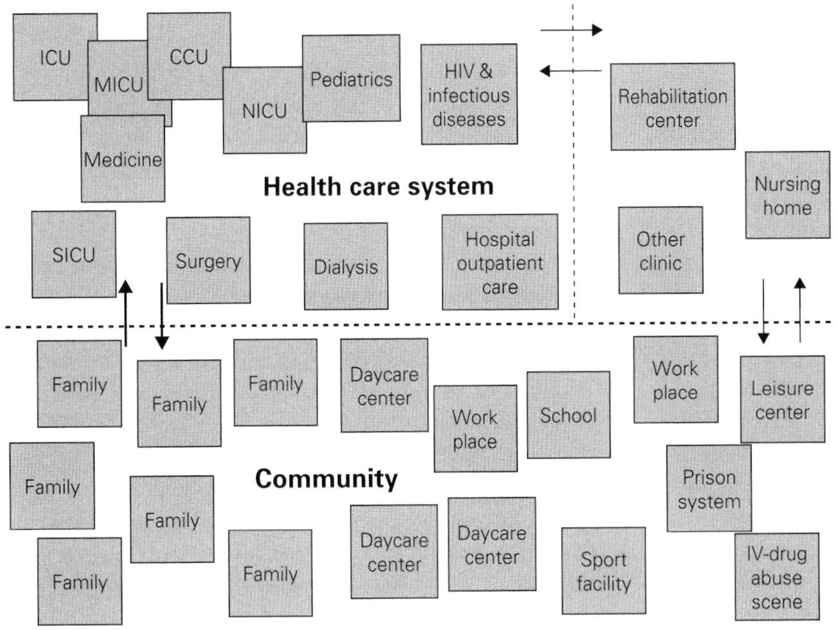

Figure 12.6 Niches in healthcare and the community considered "hotspots" for transmission and acquisition of *S. aureus*. CCU, coronary care unit; ICU, intensive care unit; MICU, medical intensive care unit; NICU, neonatal intensive care unit; SICU, surgical intensive care unit.

from the chronic low-grade inflammation in the respiratory tract induced by smoking [51,52,88].

Nasal microbial ecology and bacterial interference

Although the total microbial community living in the anterior nares has not been studied systematically (i.e., no meta-genomic data have been presented for this niche), the nasal flora of healthy subjects consists of lipophilic and nonlipophilic aerobic diphtheroids, propionibacteria, and different staphylococcal species. Other bacteria, including coliforms, and yeasts are found only occasionally [120]. It was already noted in 1951 that carriage of one strain of *S. aureus* appeared to act as some protection against the acquisition of another strain from the hospital environment [121]. The presence of *S. aureus* was related to diminished numbers of other staphylococcal species and propionibacteria [120]. In a more recent observation, nasal carriage of a methicillin-sensitive *S. aureus* (MSSA) seemed to protect against the acquisition of MRSA [122]. Apparently one bacterial strain can interfere with the growth of other strains in a particular niche. This phenomenon, later termed "bacterial interference," was shown to cross species barriers and has been exploited in the past to protect infants from hospital acquisition of virulent strains of *S. aureus* [123,124]. In particular, persistent carriers seem to be protected from acquiring new strains of *S. aureus*, e.g., during hospitalization. This barrier or colonization resistance is reduced when carriers are treated with antibiotics [118].

In infancy and childhood there is a significant negative association between nasopharyngeal *S. aureus* and other species of bacteria, notably *Streptococcus pneumoniae* (see Figure 12.3) [49,51,125,126]. Although the interfering effect was limited to vaccine-type strains of *Streptococcus pneumoniae*, there were no differences between the various clones of *S. aureus* in their capacity to compete with *Streptococcus pneumoniae* [127]. A competing strain of a *Corynebacterium* species (API profile 5100304), isolated from volunteers, was shown in Japan to be able to replace *S. aureus* in the majority of carriers [128]. The mechanism underlying the phenomenon of bacterial interference remains to be elucidated. Candidate mechanisms include competition for binding sites or nutrients, release of bacteriophages, production of bacteriocins, release of inhibitory quorum-sensing molecules, and release of metabolites including hydrogen peroxide, ammonia or free fatty acids. Recently it was suggested that it is hydrogen peroxide produced by *Streptococcus pneumoniae* that is driving its bacterial interfering activity [125]. However, cross-inhibition of the expression of adhesion and other virulence factors by small signaling peptide products of gene regulatory systems of *S. aureus* may be the mechanism by which one strain of *S. aureus* prevents colonization with another [129,130]. The validity of this suggestion has been questioned [131]. It is likely that multiple mechanisms are at play in balancing the microbial community of the nasal vestibulum.

The niche itself influences the nasal microflora. Nasal secretions have a prominent role in the innate defense of the host against infection. Components of nasal secretions that may influence the microflora include IgA and IgG, lysozyme, lactoferrin, and antimicrobial peptides [132]. It has been postulated that *S. aureus* carriers have defects in their local innate defenses. Carriers, as opposed to non-carriers, of *S. aureus* tend to have raised levels of proteins in their nasal secretions, including albumin, immunoglobulins, α-defensins, and β-defensins, which typifies an exudate compatible with the presence of a localized chronic, albeit subclinical, inflammatory response [133]. However, these secretions from carriers were not bactericidal for *S. aureus in vitro*, and were therefore postulated to be defective. Alternatively, *S. aureus* has been shown to be intrinsically rather resistant to lysozyme [134] and defensin molecules [135–137], and its primary niche, the vestibulum nasi, may not be within reach of nasal secretions containing antimicrobial peptides. Whether resistance of *S. aureus* to human defensins and other cationic peptides is a determinant of *S. aureus* nasal carriage remains to be further elucidated. Cathelicidin can act synergistically with defensins to exert a bactericidal effect on *S. aureus* [135]. Adult human serum contains immunoglobulins that (cross)react with a wide range of cellular and extracellular products of *S. aureus*, including antibodies against its major cell wall components peptidoglycan and ribitol teichoic acid and against the dominant exotoxin, α-toxin [138]. These antibodies appear early in life and are functional, i.e., they (help) opsonize the bacteria [139] and neutralize its toxins [140]. Antibody titers increase significantly, albeit temporarily, during acute invasive infections but not in the case of superficial or chronic indolent infections [138]. Although they may be boosted by the carrier state, these antibodies do not interfere with the carrier state. Thus, the influence of an acquired humoral immune response on the carrier state is probably small or even nonexistent.

Molecular and genetic determinants of *S. aureus* carriage

Although many environmental factors influence the risk of becoming an *S. aureus* carrier, much research has been focused on the genetic determinants and molecular mechanisms of carriage. From the bacterial perspective the question remains as to which bacterial ligand(s) or adhesins are involved in the adherence and subsequent colonization of the anterior nares. Many candidate surface-exposed structures and moieties of the bacterium may play a role in a typical redundant fashion. There is no consensus about the surface components of *S. aureus* that mediate binding in the nasal niche. The target for adherence would be the squamous keratinized epithelium lining the vestibulum nasi, but nasal secretions, containing mucins, may also play an intermediary role [141,142]. Adherence of *S. aureus* may also be nonspecific: it may not depend on classical ligand–receptor interactions but rather be mediated partly by hydrophobic interactions and other physicochemical forces [140,143,144]. *In vitro* studies have shown that *S. aureus* will adhere to desquamated and mucous nasal epithelial cells, especially to those derived from carriers [145,146]. One adhesin likely to be involved is the *S. aureus* surface protein G (SasG), which has sequence similarity with the proteins Pls (plasmin sensitive) of *S. aureus* and Aap (accumulation-associated protein) of *Staphylococcus epidermidis* [147]. The same group showed previously that *S. aureus* adheres to desquamated epithelial cells and that clumping factor (Clf)B, a surface-located MSCRAMM (*m*icrobial *s*urface *c*omponents *r*ecognizing *a*dhesive *m*atrix *m*olecules) known for its ability to bind to the α-chain of fibrinogen, is partly responsible [148]. ClfB also binds directly to human type 10 cytokeratin present in nasal squames [149], and immunization with ClfB reduces nasal colonization in a murine model [150]. A third candidate adhesin is the iron-responsive surface determinant A (IsdA) of *S. aureus*. IsdA had previously been shown to adhere to many serum and extracellular matrix proteins. It also adheres to desquamated human nasal cells and was needed for colonization in a cotton rat model [151]. A final candidate adhesin is cell wall teichoic acid. It has been suggested that wall teichoic acid (WTA), a surface-exposed staphylococcal polymer, is essential for nasal colonization and mediates the interaction with human nasal epithelial cells. Free teichoic acid was shown to block the binding of staphylococci to keratinized cells; the staphylococci adhered better to fully keratinized cells than to granular or spinous cells present deeper in the epidermis [152]. WTA-deficient mutants were later shown to be impaired in their adherence to nasal cells, and unable to colonize cotton rat nares [153]. However, the exclusivity of WTA in mediating adherence to squamous epithelia has been challenged [154]. It seems more likely that the binding of *S. aureus* is multifactorial and that several surface moieties of the bacterium are involved. In a human volunteer model of nasal carriage, the significant contribution of ClfB was recently confirmed [155].

Environmental factors, i.e., exposure to staphylococci, alone cannot explain the existence of various carrier states among humans. A human genetic component in determining the (persistent) carrier state seems likely and has been explored for many years. An early study pointed out that there is concordance in the carrier state among monozygotic twins [156]. A second study did not find a significant concordance between identical twins and non-identical twins or pairs of unrelated children [157]. In another early study, *S. aureus* carriage was associated with human leukocyte antigen (HLA) class II. HLA-DR3 was associated with carriage whereas several other HLA types were associated with lack of carriage [158]. However, the design of the study did not control for confounding by the underlying diseases of the patients included. More robust, population-based screening of large cohorts of healthy adults have recently allowed the study of the association between *S. aureus* carriage and polymorphisms in several human genes deemed important in host defense (Table 12.2).

Table 12.2 Human genes studied for the association between single nucleotide polymorphisms (SNPs) and *S. aureus* nasal carriage.

Human gene	Polymorphisms studied	Risk for *S. aureus* carriage	Reference
Vitamin D receptor	Cdx2, *Fok*I and *Bsm*I–*Apa*I–*Taq*I	Not affected by SNPs	163
C1 inhibitor	Valine-480 → methionine	Val/Val genotype: less risk	160
Glucocorticoid receptor	Bcl1, 9β, N363S, ER22/23EK	GG homozygotes of 9β (haplotype 1) indicates 68% less risk; haplotype combination 1+5 indicates 80% increased risk	159
α-Defensin	G-1623-T	Not affected by SNPs	162
β-Defensin	C-1748-T	Not affected by SNPs	
Mannose-binding lectin (MBL)	A-3′UTR-G G-5′UTR-C GGC-codon 54 exon 1-GAC GGA-codon 57 exon 1-GAA G-promotor-221-C	MBL haplotype A: increased risk	
Interleukin 4	C-524-T	T allele: less risk C/C type: increased risk	161
C-reactive protein	1184C/T, 2042 C/T, 2911 C/G	Not affected by individual SNPs, but C-C-C haplotype indicates less risk and C-C-G haplotype increased risk	
TNF-α	A-863-C	Not affected by this SNP	
Complement factor H	C-402-T	Not affected by this SNP	

Associations were found between persistent *S. aureus* nasal carriage and single nucleotide polymorphisms (SNPs) in the glucocorticoid receptor gene [159], in the serine protease inhibitor gene of human complement component C1 [160], in interleukin-4 and C-reactive protein genes [161], and with haplotype A of the human mannose-binding lectin [162], but not with SNPs in the vitamin D receptor [163], human defensins [162], complement factor H, and tumor necrosis factor (TNF)-α genes [161].

Although the mechanisms by which the observed polymorphisms may influence the susceptibility of the host to nasal carriage with *S. aureus* cannot be deduced directly from these observations, the contribution of some parts of the innate host defenses to the risk of staphylococcal carriage has become more certain. Results from genome-wide screening for 500 000 SNPs potentially associated with *S. aureus* nasal carriage are underway and are expected to provide a more comprehensive and coherent understanding of the variability in susceptibility of humans to persistent nasal carriage with *S. aureus* in the near future.

Harmful carriage of *S. aureus*

Individuals who carry *S. aureus* have an increased risk of infection by their own strain, i.e., endogenous infections. It is then when healthy carriage turns into harmful carriage. Virtually all major classes of *S. aureus* infections, those acquired in the community as well as those acquired in healthcare settings, have been associated with prior nasal carriage (Table 12.3). The first associations were based on the observation that most patients with infections were found to also carry the same *S. aureus* in their nose, and that patients with recurrent infection harbor the same phage type of *S. aureus* in their nose for prolonged periods regardless of whether they have lesions [2]. These early investigators also observed that recurrence of skin lesions can be prevented by elimination of the nasal staphylococci [187].

More recent observations include patients undergoing transplantation or cardiac surgery, patients being admitted to intensive care units, and MRSA-carrying residents in nursing homes. Overall there is now evidence that *S. aureus* carriage is associated with increased risk of all major types of staphylococcal disease, whether occurring in the community or associated with healthcare settings, or whether caused by methicillin-susceptible or methicillin-resistant strains of *S. aureus*. In the community, carriage has been linked to increased risk for skin and respiratory infections and with osteomyelitis and endocarditis. Vaginal carriage with toxic shock syndrome toxin (TSST)-1-producing *S. aureus* has been associated with an increased risk of developing toxic shock syndrome, and for nursing home residents carriage of MRSA increases their 6-month mortality rate (Table 12.3). In healthcare settings, *S. aureus* carriage has been shown to increase the risk of invasive staphylococcal infections associated with certain procedures or interventions (surgery, use of intravenous devices), in certain patient groups (post liver transplantation, HIV infection, end-stage renal disease, disabled elderly), and with certain services (intensive care unit, long-term care facilities).

The exact mode of endogenous infection remains to be studied in most of these infections, but it seems likely that the high density of nasal carriage and the extensive secondary colonization of multiple body sites (on the skin, in the gut) associated with the persistent nasal carriage phenotype predisposes these individuals to staphylococcal invasion once the mechanical barrier of the skin or mucosa is breached at a given body site by (surgical) trauma. Persistent carriers are therefore especially at risk, whereas the risk of such opportunistic infection may be not be elevated for individuals who carry *S. aureus* only intermittently [188]. In HIV-infected patients the risk of staphylococcal infection is higher in those who are neutropenic [178], indicating that this part of the innate host defenses is important in controlling *S. aureus* invasion. MRSA strains may be more likely to cause infections compared with MSSA strains in diverse healthcare settings [158,160,179,182]. This may not be due to the intrinsic virulence of MRSA strains but rather to the increased ability of MRSA, as compared with MSSA, to survive in clinical environments, including the intensive care unit, where the density of antibiotic use is very high.

In intensive-care settings, nasal carriage has also been shown to lead to frequent cross-infections [189]. Importantly, cross-infections have been traced to *S. aureus* or MRSA carriers among hospital staff [101,190–195]. Hospital personnel may spread their own *S. aureus* strain or strains, including MRSA, that they have picked up from patients or from contaminated surfaces or instruments in the environment during work [196,197]. Compliance with standard infection control practices, especially hand disinfection, may limit such spread [198].

Prevention

Prevention of *S. aureus* infections is discussed in depth in Chapter 30. In general, prevention of infection targets endogenous infections as well as exogenous infections or cross-infections by *S. aureus*. The central role played by the *S. aureus* carrier state in both types of infection should encourage clinicians to direct prevention efforts at modulating the carrier state, either temporarily or more permanently [199]. Elimination of *S. aureus* from the body eliminates the risk of endogenous infection, and by eliminating a source from which *S. aureus* spreads also reduces the risk of cross-infection for those who reside in the

Table 12.3 Infections and other risks associated with nasal carriage of *S. aureus*.

Infection type	Acquired in	Association with (nasal) carriage of *S. aureus*	No. of individuals in study	Reference
Community settings				
"Skin sepsis"	Military setting	RR 1.7	3512	164
"Beat disorders" (cellulitis, bursitis)	Coal mining	RR 2.2 times higher	112	165
Toxic shock syndrome	Community	With vaginal carriage of TSST-1-producing strains	495	166
Endocarditis	Intravenous drug abusers in community	Same phage type in blood and on skin	10	167
Osteomyelitis	Community	Nasal carriage more common in children with previous osteomyelitis than in age- and sex-matched controls	104	168
Six-month mortality	Nursing home residents	RR 2.3 for those carrying MRSA	447	169
Chronic rhinosinusitis	Community	Intracellular carriage in mucosal cells	39	74
Healthcare settings				
Intravenous device bacteremia	Various healthcare settings	RR 6.3–12.4	Two studies including 101 and 488 patients respectively	10 (1990–1996 data summarized)
Bacteremia	Hospital acquired, surgery department	OR 4.0	288	170
Exit site and peritonitis	CAPD patients	RR 2.1–13.4 for exit site RR 4.0–14 for peritonitis	Six studies including 30–167 patients	10 (1982–1993 data summarized)
All types	Due to MRSA in long-term care	RR 5.5	197	171
All types	Among liver transplant recipients	RR 1.9 All infections due to MRSA	30	172
All types	Hospitalized patients with liver cirrhosis	RR 5.7	84	173
All types	Due to MRSA in ICU	RR 20.2	484	174
All types	Patients admitted to ICU	RR 59.6	752	175
All types	Patients on hemodialysis or peritoneal dialysis	RR 2.8	297	176
CAPD-related infections	Patients on CAPD	RR 2.6 for exit site RR 3.3 for peritonitis	146	177
Bacteremia	HIV-infected patients	RR not applicable because 8/72 carriers vs. 0/64 noncarriers became bacteremic	136	178
All types	Patients receiving liver transplantation	RR 3.9 for MSSA carriage RR 8.7 for MRSA carriage	87	179
Postoperative wound infection	Hospital settings	RR 1.8 in period 1959–1970 RR 7.1 in period 1970–1996	19 studies including 125–3056 patients per study	10 (1959–1996 data summarized)
Surgical site infection	Patients receiving CABG or other cardiac surgery	RR 2.1	376	180
Surgical site infection	Patients receiving orthopedic surgery	RR 8.9	272	181
Postoperative intraabdominal infection	Patients in surgical ICU	RR 4.0	73	182
Sepsis due to MRSA	Following liver transplantation	RR 3.4 for MRSA carriers	157	183
All types	Surgical intensive care and transplant unit	RR 9.4	204	184
Intravenous device bacteremia	Diabetes type II on hemodialysis	RR 3.2	208	185
Bacteremia and urinary tract infections	Cirrhotic patients in hospital	RR 5.4 for MSSA RR 7.4 for MRSA	551	186

CABG, coronary artery bypass graft; CAPD, continuous ambulatory peritoneal dialysis; ICU, intensive care unit; MRSA, methicillin-resistant *S. aureus*; MSSA, methicillin-sensitive *S. aureus*; OR, odds ratio; RR, relative risk; TSST, toxic shock syndrome toxin.

vicinity of the original carrier and would otherwise be exposed to a source of *S. aureus*. Elimination can be achieved by treating carriers topically with nasal cream containing antimicrobial agents (e.g., mupirocin) or disinfectants (e.g., chlorhexidine) combined with total body washes using medicated soaps or shampoos (e.g., containing chlorhexidine or hexachlorophenes) [200–203]. Oral therapy with combinations of systemic antimicrobial agents may also be effective [204,205]. A 3–5 day course usually suffices to eliminate *S. aureus* from healthy carriers. However, recolonization will occur thereafter and within months affects a sizeable proportion of those treated [206]. Although such treatments are thus only temporarily effective in eradicating *S. aureus*, they may be worthwhile when the objective is to reduce risk of *S. aureus* infection only temporarily. For example, this strategy would counteract the temporarily increased risk of endogenous *S. aureus* infection associated with admission to an acute care hospital. In this way endogenously acquired nosocomial *S. aureus* infections can, theoretically, be avoided [29]. A metaanalysis of several inconclusive studies addressing this issue showed that such a strategy may be beneficial [207]. A large prospective multicenter trial recently provided robust evidence that rapid screening for, and elimination of, the *S. aureus* carrier state in patients being admitted to hospitals for surgical procedures will largely prevent endogenous *S. aureus* surgical-site infection [27].

Patients with underlying conditions, including those with end-stage renal diseases on chronic dialysis who have an increased risk of endogenous *S. aureus* disease more or less permanently, would require long-lasting elimination of *S. aureus* from their nose and other body sites. Such can be achieved by repeated prophylactic treatment with nasal mupirocin [208,209], although there is then a risk of resistance developing over time against the prophylactic agent used. Another, ecologically more attractive option would be to use the principle of bacterial interference discussed above, essentially replacing the wild-type virulent strain of *S. aureus* carried by the patient with an avirulent variant strain of *S. aureus*. Bacterial interference has been used in the past rather successfully [210], and one could today reapply this concept more successfully, especially by engineering strains that will effectively colonize humans but not cause disease due to removal of essential virulence factors.

Finally, *S. aureus* cross-infection still occurs in hospitals and other settings with (over)crowding, and these cross-infections seem to be more lethal compared with endogenous infection [211]. Thus, prevention of transmission of virulent (and often multiresistant) strains of *S. aureus* in such settings can be reduced by infection control measures. These control measures should take into account the multiple sources, including environmental ones, and the multiple routes of transmission available to *S. aureus* that are discussed above.

Conclusion

Carriage of *S. aureus* by humans is a natural phenomenon associated with health and disease. One in five to ten individuals carries *S. aureus* for many years, even life, and they are at increased risk of developing *S. aureus* infections with their own strain (self-infection or endogenous infection). Carriers of *S. aureus* are the primary source for cross-infections to individuals who do not normally have this bacterium in their commensal microflora. Individuals normally free from *S. aureus* may have less immunity against the lethal consequences of *S. aureus* infections compared with those who are persistent carriers of the species and suffer from endogenous infections. Environmental sources also play a role in carriage, spread of *S. aureus*, and disease occurrence. The determinants of carriage are multiple and include a genetic predisposition of the host. However, repeated or prolonged exposure to *S. aureus* sources is also important and should be taken into account when designing strategies to prevent *S. aureus* infections.

References

1 Dolman CE. Clinical uses of *Staphylococcus* toxoid. Lancet 1935;i:306–13.

2 Williams REO. Healthy carriage of *Staphylococcus*: its prevalence and importance. Bacteriol Rev 1963;27:56–71.

3 Nilsson P, Ripa T. *Staphylococcus aureus* throat colonization is more frequent than colonization in the anterior nares. J Clin Microbiol 2006;44:3334–9.

4 Mertz D, Frei R, Jaussi B *et al*. Throat swabs are necessary to reliably detect carriers of *Staphylococcus aureus*. Clin Infect Dis 2007;45:475–7.

5 Solberg CO. Spread *of Staphylococcus aureus* in hospitals: causes and prevention. Scand J Infect Dis 2000;32:587–95.

6 Krstic RV. Human Microscopic Anatomy. An Atlas for Students of Medicine and Biology. Heidelberg: Springer Verlag, 1991.

7 Cole AM, Tahk S, Oren A *et al*. Determinants of *Staphylococcus aureus* nasal carriage. Clin Diagn Lab Immunol 2001;8:1064–9.

8 Clement S, Vaudaux P, Francois P *et al*. Evidence of an intracellular reservoir in the nasal mucosa of patients with recurrent *Staphylococcus aureus* rhinosinusitis. J Infect Dis 2005;192:1023–8.

9 Leenders AC, Renders NR, Pelk M, Janssen M. Tonsilectomy for treatment of persistent methicillin-resistant *Staphylococcus aureus* throat carriage. J Hosp Infect 2005;59:266–7.

10 Kluytmans J, van Belkum A, Verbrugh H. Nasal carriage of *Staphylococcus aureus*: epidemiology, underlying mechanisms, and associated risks. Clin Microbiol Rev 1997;10:505–20.

11 DeVriese LA. A simplified system for biotyping *Staphylococcus aureus* strains isolated from different animal species. J Appl Bacteriol 1984;56:215–30.

12 Van Leeuwen WB, Melles DC, Alaida A *et al*. Host- and tissue-specific pathogenic traits of *Staphylococcus aureus*. J Bacteriol 2005;187:4584–91.

13 Zadoks RN, van Leeuwen WB, Kreft D *et al*. Comparison of *Staphylococcus aureus* isolates from bovine and human skin,

milking equipment, and bovine milk by phage typing, electrophoresis, and binary typing. J Clin Microbiol 2002;40:3894–902.

14 Boost MV, O'Donoghue MM, James A. Prevalence of *Staphylococcus aureus* carriage among dogs and their owners. Epidemiol Infect 2008;136:953–64.

15 Dolman CE. The *Staphylococcus*: seven decades of research (1885–1955). Can J Med 1956;2:189–200.

16 Wertheim HFL, Melles DC, Vos MC, van Leeuwen W, Verbrugh HA, van Belkum A. The role of nasal carriage in *Staphylococcus aureus* infections. Lancet Infect Dis 2005;5:751–62.

17 Lestari ES, Severin JA, Filius PM *et al*. Antimicrobial resistance among commensal isolates of *Escherichia coli* and *Staphylococcus aureus* in the Indonesian population inside and outside hospitals. Eur J Clin Microbiol Infect Dis 2008;27:45–51.

18 Anwar MS, Jaffery G, Rehman Bhatti KU, Tayyib M, Bokhari SR. *Staphylococcus aureus* and MRSA nasal carriage in the general population. J Coll Physicians Surg Pak 2004;14:661–4.

19 Memish ZA, Balkhy H, Almuneef M, Al-Haj-Hussein B, Osaba A. Carriage of *Staphylococcus aureus* between Hajj pilgrims. Saudi Med J 2006;27:1367–72.

20 Choi CS, Yin CS, Bakar AA *et al*. Nasal carriage of *Staphylococcus aureus* among healthy adults. J Microbiol Immunol Infect 2006;39:458–64.

21 Lu PL, Chin LC, Peng CF *et al*. Risk factors and molecular analysis of community methicillin-resistant Staphylococcus aureus carriage. J Clin Microbiol 2005;43:132–9.

22 Saxena S, Singh K, Talwar V. Methicillin-resistant *Staphylococcus aureus* prevalence in the community in the East Delhi area. Jpn J Infect Dis 2003;56:54–6.

23 Block CS, Carmichael M. Community versus hospital *Staphylococcus aureus*. Antimicrobial susceptibilities and some features of nasal carriage and acquisition. S Afr Med J 1978;54:225–9.

24 Gorwitz RJ, Kruszon-Moran D, McAllister SK *et al*. Changes in the prevalence of nasal colonization with *Staphylococcus aureus* in the United States, 2001–2004. J Infect Dis 2008;197:1226–34.

25 Nulens E, Gould I, MacKenzie F *et al*. *Staphylococcus aureus* carriage among participants at the 13th European Congress of Clinical Microbiology and Infectious Diseases. Eur J Clin Microbiol Infect Dis 2005;24:145–8.

26 Wertheim HF, Vos MC, Ott A *et al*. Mupirocin prophylaxis against nosocomial *Staphylococcus aureus* infections in nonsurgical patients: a randomized study. Ann Intern Med 2004;140:419–25.

27 Bode LGM, Kluytmans JAJW, Wertheim HFL *et al*. A randomized trial of admission screening and decolonization of *Staphylococcus aureus* carriers to prevent nosocomial *S. aureus* infections. Abstract K-1711. Abstracts of the 48th Annual Interscience Conference on Antimicrobial Agents and Chemotherapy, Washington, DC, 2008.

28 Shrestha NK, Banbury MK, Weber M *et al*. Safety of targeted perioperative mupirocin treatment for preventing infections after cardiac surgery. Ann Thorac Surg 2006;81:2183–8.

29 Perl TM, Cullen JJ, Wenzel RP *et al*. Intranasal mupirocin to prevent postoperative *Staphylococcus aureus* infections. N Engl J Med 2002;346:1871–7.

30 Lucet JC, Grenet K, Armand-Lefevre L *et al*. High prevalence of carriage of methicillin-resistant *Staphylococcus aureus* at hospital admission in elderly patients: implications for infection control strategies. Infect Control Hosp Epidemiol 2005;26:121–6.

31 Hidron AI, Kourbatova EV, Halvosa JS *et al*. Risk factors for colonization with methicillin-resistant *Staphylococcus aureus* (MRSA) in patients admitted to an urban hospital: emergence of community-acquired MRSA nasal carriage. Clin Infect Dis 2005;41:159–66.

32 Troillet N, Carmeli Y, Samore MH *et al*. Carriage of methicillin-resistant *Staphylococcus aureus* at hospital admission. Infect Control Hosp Epidemiol 1998;19:181–5.

33 Heininger U, Datta F, Gervaix A *et al*. Prevalence of nasal colonization with methicillin-resistant *Staphylococcus aureus* (MRSA) in children: a multicenter cross-sectional study. Pediatr Infect Dis J 2007;26:544–6.

34 Lamaro-Cardoso J, Castanheira M, de Oliveira RM *et al*. Carriage of methicillin-resistant *Staphylococcus aureus* in children in Brazil. Diagn Microbiol Infect Dis 2007;57:467–70.

35 Alfaro C, Masher-Denen M, Fergie J, Purcell K. Prevalence of methicillin-resistant *Staphylococcus aureus* nasal carriage in patients admitted to Driscoll Children's hospital. Pediatr Infect Dis J 2006;25:459–61.

36 Shopsin B, Mathema B, Martinez J *et al*. Prevalence of methicillin-resistant and methicillin-susceptible *Staphylococcus aureus* in the community. J Infect Dis 2000;182:359–62.

37 Solberg CO. A study of carriers of *Staphylococcus aureus* with special regard to quantitative bacterial estimations. Acta Med Scand Suppl 1965;436:1–96.

38 Nouwen JL, Ott A, Kluytmans-VandenBergh MF *et al*. Predicting the *Staphylococcus aureus* nasal carrier state: derivation and validation of a "culture rule." Clin Infect Dis 2004;39:806–11.

39 VandenBergh MFQ, Yzerman EPF, van Belkum A, Boelens HAM, Sijmons M, Verbrugh HA. Follow-up of *Staphylococcus aureus* nasal carriage after 8 years: redefining the persistent carrier state. J Clin Microbiol 1999;37:3133–40.

40 Nouwen J, Boelens H, van Belkum A, Verbrugh H. Human factor in *Staphylococcus aureus* nasal carriage. Infect Immun 2004;72:6685–8.

41 van Belkum A, Melles DC, Nouwen J *et al*. Co-evolutionary aspects of human colonisation and infection by *Staphylococcus aureus*. Infect Genet Evol 2009;9:32–47.

42 Hadley MDM. Nasal carriage of staphylococci in an Antarctic community. In: Macdonald M, Smith G, eds. The Staphylococci. Aberdeen: Aberdeen University Press, 1981:239–54.

43 Krikler SJ. *Staphylococcus aureus* in Antartica: carriage and attempted eradication. J Hyg 1986;97:427–44.

44 Eriksen NH, Espersen F, Rosdahl VT, Jensen K. Carriage of *Staphylococcus aureus* among 104 healthy persons during a 19-month period. Epidemiol Infect 1995;115:51–60.

45 Safdar N, Narans L, Gordon B, Maki DG. Comparison of culture screening methods for detection of nasal carriage of methicillin-resistant *Staphylococcus aureus*: a prospective study comparing 32 methods. J Clin Microbiol 2003;41:3163–6.

46 Crossley K, Solliday J. Comparison of rectal swabs and stool cultures for the detection of gastrointestinal carriage *of Staphylococcus aureus*. J Clin Microbiol 1980;11:433–4.

47 Compernolle V, Verschraegen G, Claeys G. Combined use of Pastorex Staph-Plus and either of two new chromogenic agars, MRSA ID and CHROMagar MRSA, for detection of methicillin-resistant *Staphylococcus aureus*. J Clin Microbiol 2007;45:154–8.

48 Paule SM, Hacek DM, Kufner B *et al*. Performance of the BD GeneOhm methicillin-resistant *Staphylococcus aureus* test before and during high-volume clinical use. J Clin Microbiol 2007; 45:2993–8.
49 Lebon A, Labout JA, Verbrugh HA *et al*. Dynamics and determinants of *Staphylococcus aureus* carriage in infancy: the Generation R Study. J Clin Microbiol 2008;46:3517–21.
50 Harrison LM, Morris JA, Telford DR, Brown SM, Jones K. The nasopharyngeal bacterial flora in infancy: effects of age, gender, season, viral upper respiratory infection and sleeping position. FEMS Immunol Med Microbiol 1999;25:19–28.
51 Bogaert D, van Belkum A, Sluijter M *et al*. Colonisation by *Streptococcus pneumoniae* and *Staphylococcus aureus* in healthy children. Lancet 2004;363:1871–2.
52 Nouwen JL. Determinants, risks and dynamics of *Staphylococcus aureus* nasal carriage. Thesis, Erasmus University, Rotterdam, Netherlands, 2004.
53 Smith JA, O'Connor JJ. Nasal carriage of *Staphylococcus aureus* in diabetes mellitus. Lancet 1966;ii:776–7.
54 Tuazon CU, Perez A, Kishaba T, Sheagren JN. *Staphylococcus aureus* among insulin-injecting diabetic patients. An increased carrier rate. JAMA 1975;231:1272.
55 Chandler PT, Chandler SD. Pathogenic carrier rate in diabetes mellitus. Am J Med Sci 1977;273:259–65.
56 Lipsky BA, Pecoraro RE, Chen MS, Koepsell TD. Factors affecting staphylococcal colonization among NIDDM outpatients. Diabetes Care 1987;10:483–6.
57 Berman DS, Schaefler S, Simberkoff MS, Rahal JJ. *Staphylococcus aureus* colonization in intravenous drug abusers, dialysis patients, and diabetics. J Infect Dis 1987;155:829–31.
58 Boyko EJ, Lipsky BA, Sandoval R *et al*. NIDDM and prevalence of nasal *Staphylococcus aureus* colonization. San Luis Valley Diabetes Study. Diabetes Care 1989;12:189–92.
59 Mey A, Gille Y, Thivolet CH. Carriage of *Staphylococcus aureus* and local infections in diabetic outpatients treated with insulin pen. Diabetes Care 1990;13:451–2.
60 Tamer A, Karabay O, Ekerbicer H. *Staphylococcus aureus* nasal carriage and associated factors in type 2 diabetic patients. Jpn J Infect Dis 2006;59:10–14.
61 Philips BJ, Redman J, Brennan A *et al*. Glucose in bronchial aspirates increases the risk of respiratory MRSA in intubated patients. Thorax 2005;60:761–4.
62 Johnson LB, Jose J, Yousif F *et al*. Prevalence of colonization with community-associated methicillin-resistant *Staphylococcus aureus* among end-stage renal disease patients and healthcare workers. Infect Control Hosp Epidemiol 2009;30: 4–8.
63 Duran N, Ocak S, Eskiocak AF. *Staphylococcus aureus* nasal carriage among the diabetic and non-diabetic haemodialysis patients. Int J Clin Pract 2006;60:1204–9.
64 Chapoutot C, Pageaux GP, Perrigault PF *et al*. *Staphylococcus aureus*, nasal carriage in 104 cirrhotic and control patients: a prospective study. J Hepatol 1999;30:249–53.
65 Al-Rawahi GN, Schreader AG, Porter SD *et al*. Methicillin-resistant *Staphylococcus aureus* nasal carriage among injection drug users: six years later. J Clin Microbiol 2008;46:477–9.
66 Karbay O, Tamer A, Sahin I, Celebi H. Does chronic hepatitis B increase *Staphylococcus* nasal carriage? Ethiop Med J 2006;44: 121–4.
67 Singh G, Rao DJ. Bacteriology of psoriatic plaques. Dermatologica 1978;157:21–7.
68 Gilani SJ, Gonzalez M, Hussain I, Finlay AY, Patel GK. *Staphylococcus aureus* re-colonization in atopic dermatitis: beyond the skin. Clin Exp Dermatol 2005;30:10–13.
69 Falanga V, Campbell DE, Leyden JJ, Douglas SD. Nasal carriage of *Staphylococcus aureus* and antistaphylococcal immunoglobulin E antibodies in atopic dermatitis. J Clin Microbiol 1985;22:452–4.
70 Goh CL, Wong JS, Giam YC. Skin colonization of *Staphylococcus aureus* in atopic dermatitis patients seen at the National Skin Centre, Singapore. Int J Dermatol 1997;36:653–7.
71 Kirmani N, Tuazon CU, Alling D. Carriage rate of *Staphylococcus aureus* among patients receiving allergy injections. Ann Allergy 1980;45:235–7.
72 Shiomori T, Yoshida S, Miyamoto H, Makishima K. Relationship of nasal carriage of *Staphylococcus aureus* to pathogenesis of perennial allergic rhinitis. J Allergy Clin Immunol 2000; 105:449–54.
73 Baysoy G, Arslan S, Karabay O, Uyan A. Nasal carriage of *Staphylococcus aureus* in children with allergic rhinitis and the effect of intranasal fluticasone propionate treatment on carriage status. Int J Pediatr Otorhinolaryngol 2007;71:205–9.
74 Riechelmann H, Essig A, Rau A, Rothermel B, Weschta M. Nasal carriage of *Staphylococcus aureus* in house dust mite allergic patients and healthy controls. Allergy 2005;60:1418–23.
75 Bassetti S, Dunagan DP, d'Agostino RB Jr, Sherertz RJ. Nasal carriage of *Staphylococcus aureus* among patients receiving allergen-injection immunotherapy: associated factors and quantitative nasal cultures. Infect Control Hosp Epidemiol 2001;22:741–5.
76 Damm M, Quante G, Jurk T, Sauer J. Nasal colonization with *Staphylococcus aureus* is not associated with the severity of symptoms or the extent of the disease in chronic rhinosinusitis. Otolaryngol Head Neck Surg 2004;131:200–6.
77 Clement S, Vaudaux P, Francois P *et al*. Evidence of an intracellular reservoir in the nasal mucosa of patients with recurrent *Staphylococcus aureus* rhinosinusitis. J Infect Dis 2005;192:1023–8.
78 Jacobs SI, Williamson GM, Willis AT. Nasal abnormality and the carrier rate of *Staphylococcus aureus*. J Clin Pathol 1961;14:519–21.
79 Wertheim HF, van Kleef M, Vos MC, Ott A, Verbrugh HA, Fokkens W. Nose picking and nasal carriage of *Staphylococcus aureus*. Infect Control Hosp Epidemiol 2006;27:863–7.
80 Stegeman CA, Tervaert JWC, Sluiter WJ, Manson WL, de Jong PE, Kallenberg CGM. Association of chronic nasal carriage of *Staphylococcus aureus* and higher relapse rates in Wegener granulomatosis. Ann Intern Med 1994;120:12–17.
81 Keser G, Erdogan M, Aydemir S *et al*. Nasal *Staphylococcus aureus* carriage is not increased in Behçet's disease. Rheumatol Int 2005;25:567–8.
82 Johnson RB, Muder RR, Kominos SD, Nasca TJ. Staphylococcal carriage and infection in myasthenia gravis patients receiving therapeutic apheresis. J Clin Apheresis 1988;4:155–7.
83 Bassetti S, Wasmer S, Hasler P *et al*. *Staphylococcus aureus* in patients with rheumatoid arthritis under conventional and anti-tumor necrosis factor-alpha treatment. J Rheumatol 2005; 32:2125–9.
84 Tabarya D, Hoffman WL. *Staphylococcus aureus* nasal carriage in rheumatoid arthritis: antibody response to toxic shock syndrome toxin-1. Ann Rheum Dis 1996;55:823–8.

85 Jackson MS, Bagg J, Gupta MN, Sturrock RD. Oral carriage of staphylococci in patients with rheumatoid arthritis. Rheumatology (Oxford) 1999;38:572–5.
86 Jobbins J, Bagg J, Parsons K, Finlay I, Addy M, Newcombe RG. Oral carriage of yeasts, coliforms and staphylococci in patients with advanced malignant disease. Oral Pathol Med 1992; 21:305–8.
87 Sweeney MP, Bag J, Baxter WP, Aitchison TC. Oral disease in terminally ill cancer patients with xerostomia. Oral Oncol 1998;34:123–6.
88 Herwaldt LA, Cullen JJ, French P *et al*. Preoperative risk factors for nasal carriage of *Staphylococcus aureus*. Infect Control Epidemiol 2004;25:481–4.
89 Amir LH, Garland SM, Lumley J. A case-control study of mastitis: nasal carriage of *Staphylococcus aureus*. BMC Fam Pract 2006;7:57.
90 Sheretz RJ. "Cloud" health-care workers. Emerg Infect Dis 2001;7:241–4.
91 Goslings WR, Buchli K. Nasal carrier rate of antibiotic-resistant staphylococci: influence of hospitalization on carrier rate in patients, and their household contacts. Arch Intern Med 1958;102:691–715.
92 Samad A, Banerjee D, Carnbarns N, Ghosh S. Prevalence of methicillin-resistant *Staphylococcus aureus* colonization in surgical patients, on admission to a Welsh hospital. J Hosp Infect 2002;51:43–6.
93 Lucet JC, Chevret S, Durand-Zaleski I, Chastang C, Regnier B. Prevalence and risk factors for carriage of methicillin-resistant *Staphylococcus aureus* at admission to the intensive care unit: results of a multicenter study. Arch Intern Med 2003;163:181–8.
94 Fukuda M, Tanaka H, Kajiwara Y *et al*. High-risk populations for nasal carriage of methicillin-resistant *Staphylococcus aureus*. J Infect Chemother 2004;10:189–91.
95 Haley CC, Mittal D, Laviolette A, Jannapureddy S, Parvez N, Haley RW. Methicillin-resistant *Staphylococcus aureus* infection or colonization present at hospital admission: multivariable risk factor screening to increase efficiency of surveillance culturing. J Clin Microbiol 2007;45:3031–8.
96 Gopal Rao G, Michalczyk P, Nayeem N, Walker G, Wigmore L. Prevalence and risk factors for methicillin-resistant *Staphylococcus aureus* in adult emergency admissions: a case for screening all patients? J Hosp Infect 2007;66:15–21.
97 Berntsen CA, McDermott W. Increased transmissibility of staphylococci to patients receiving an antimicrobial drug. N Engl J Med 1960;262:637–42.
98 Barr B, Wilcox MH, Brady A, Parnell P, Darby B, Tompkins D. Prevalence of methicillin-resistant *Staphylococcus aureus* colonization among older residents of care homes in the United Kingdom. Infect Control Hosp Epidemiol 2007;28:853–9.
99 Kreman T, Hu J, Pottinger J, Herwaldt LA. Survey of long-term-care facilities in Iowa for policies and practices regarding residents with methicillin-resistant *Staphylococcus aureus* or vancomycin-resistant enterococci. Infect Control Hosp Epidemiol. 2005;26:811–15.
100 Eveillard M, Martin Y, Hidri N, Boussougant Y, Joly-Guillou ML. Carriage of methicillin-resistant *Staphylococcus aureus* among hospital employees: prevalence, duration, and transmission to households. Infect Control Hosp Epidemiol 2004;25:114–20.
101 Reboli AC, John IF Jr, Platt CG, Cantey JR. Methicillin-resistant *Staphylococcus aureus* outbreak at a Veterans Affairs Medical Center: importance of carriage of the organism by hospital personnel. Infect Control Hosp Epidemiol 1990;11:291–6.
102 Simoons-Smit AM, Savelkoul PH, Stoof J, Starink TM, Vandenbroucke-Grauls CM. Transmission of *Staphylococcus aureus* between humans and domestic animals in a household. Eur J Clin Microbiol Infect Dis 2000;19:150–2.
103 Weese JS, Dick H, Willey BM *et al*. Suspected transmission of methicillin-resistant *Staphylococcus aureus* between domestic pets and humans in veterinary clinics and in the household. Vet Microbiol 2006;115:148–55.
104 Hota B, Ellenbogen C, Hayden MK, Aroutcheva A, Rice TW, Weinstein RA. Community-associated methicillin-resistant *Staphylococcus aureus* skin and soft tissue infections at a public hospital: do public housing and incarceration amplify transmission? Arch Intern Med 2007;167:1026–33.
105 Aiello AE, Lowy FD, Wright LN, Larson EL. Methicillin-resistant *Staphylococcus aureus* among US prisoners and military personnel: review and recommendations for future studies. Lancet Infect Dis 2006;6:335–41.
106 Adcock PM, Pastor P, Medley F, Patterson JE, Murphy TV. Methicillin-resistant *Staphylococcus aureus* in two child care centers. J Infect Dis 1998;178:577–80.
107 Jensen JU, Jensen ET, Larsen AR *et al*. Control of a methicillin-resistant *Staphylococcus aureus* (MRSA) outbreak in a day-care institution. J Hosp Infect 2006;63:84–92.
108 Pagac BB, Reiland RW, Bolesh DT, Swanson DL. Skin lesions in barracks: consider community-acquired methicillin-resistant *Staphylococcus aureus* infection instead of spider bites. Milit Med 2006;171:830–2.
109 Reinberg J, Ailor SK, Dyer JA. Common sports-related dermatologic infections. Mod Med 2007;104:119–23.
110 Kazakova SV, Hageman JC, Matava M *et al*. A clone of methicillin-resistant *Staphylococcus aureus* among professional football players. N Engl J Med 2005;352:468–75.
111 Barnham M, Kerby J. A profile of skin sepsis in meat handlers. J Infect 1984;9:43–50.
112 Decker MD, Lybarger JA, Vaughn WK, Hutcheson RH Jr, Schaffner W. An outbreak of staphylococcal skin infections among river rafting guides. Am J Epidemiol 1986;124:969–76.
113 Armand-Lefevre L, Ruimy R, Andremont A. Clonal comparison of of *Staphylococcus aureus* isolates from healthy pig farmers, human controls, and pigs. Emerg Infect Dis 2005;11:711–14.
114 Mahdi SE, Ahmed AO, Boelens H *et al*. An epidemiological study on the occurrence of *Staphylococcus aureus* in superficial abscesses of patients presenting for surgery in a teaching hospital in Khartoum, Sudan. FEMS Immunol Med Microbiol 2000;29:155–62.
115 Agarwal AK, Sethi A, Sethi D, Mrig S, Chopra S. Role of socioeconomic factors in deep neck abscess: a prospective study of 120 patients. Br J Oral Maxillofac Surg 2007;45:553–5.
116 Nickerson EK, Wuthiekanun V, Day NP, Chaowagul W, Peacock SJ. Methicillin-resistant *Staphylococcus aureus* in rural Asia. Lancet Infect Dis 2006;6:70–1.
117 Bagger JP, Zindrou D, Taylor KM. Postoperative infection with methicillin-resistant *Staphylococcus aureus* and socioeconomic background. Lancet 2004;363:706–8.
118 Noble WC, Williams RE, Jevons MP, Shooter RA. Some aspects of nasal carriage of staphylococci. J Clin Pathol 1964;17:79–83.

119 Miles AA, Williams REO, Clayton-Cooper B. The carriage of *Staphylococcus (pyogenes) aureus* in man and its relation to wound infection. J Pathol Bacteriol 1944;56:513–56.

120 Heczko PB, Hoffler U, Kasprowicz A, Pulverer G. Quantitative studies of the flora of the nasal vestibule in relation to nasal carriage of *Staphylococcus aureus*. J Med Microbiol 1981;14:233–41.

121 Rountree PM, Barbour RG. Nasal carrier rates of *Staphylococcus pyogenes* in hospital nurses. J Pathol Bacteriol 1951;63:313–24.

122 Dall'Antonia M, Coen PG, Wilks M, Whiley A, Millar M. Competition between methicillin-sensitive and -resistant *Staphylococcus aureus* in the anterior nares. J Hosp Infect 2005;61:62–7.

123 Shinefield HR, Wilsey JD, Ribble JC, Boris M, Eichenwald HF, Dittmar CI. Interactions of staphylococcal colonization. Influence of normal nasal flora and antimicrobials on inoculated *Staphylococcus aureus* strain 502A. Am J Dis Child 1966;111: 11–21.

124 Aly R, Maibach HI, Shinefield HR, Mandel A, Strauss WG. Bacterial interference among strains of *Staphylococcus aureus* in man. J Infect Dis 1974;129:720–4.

125 Regev-Yochay G, Trzcinski K, Thompson CM, Malley R, Lipsitch M. Interference between *Streptococcus pneumoniae* and *Staphylococcus aureus*: in vitro hydrogen peroxide-mediated killing by *Streptococcus pneumoniae*. J Bacteriol 2006;188:4996–5001.

126 Watson K, Carville K, Bowman J *et al*. Upper respiratory tract bacterial carriage in Aboriginal and non-Aboriginal children in a semi-arid area of Western Australia. Pediatr Infect Dis J 2006;25:782–90.

127 Melles DC, Bogaert D, Gorkink RF *et al*. Nasopharyngeal co-colonization with *Staphylococcus aureus* and *Streptococcus pneumoniae* in children is bacterial genotype independent. Microbiology 2007;153:386–92.

128 Uehara Y, Nakama H, Agematsu K *et al*. Bacterial interference among nasal inhabitants: eradication of *Staphylococcus aureus* from nasal cavities by artificial implantation of *Corynebacterium* sp. J Hosp Infect 2000;44:127–33.

129 Ji G, Beavis R, Novick RP. Bacterial interference caused by autoinducing peptide variants. Science 1997;276:2027–30.

130 Lina G, Boutite F, Tristan A, Bes M, Etienne J, Vandenesch F. Bacterial competition for human nasal cavity colonization: role of staphylococcal agr alleles. Appl Environ Microbiol 2003;69:18–23.

131 van Leeuwen W, van Nieuwenhuizen W, Gijzen C, Verbrugh H, van Belkum A. Population studies of methicillin-resistant and -sensitive *Staphylococcus aureus* strains reveal a lack of variability in the agrD gene, encoding a staphylococcal autoinducer peptide. J Bacteriol 2000;182:5721–9.

132 Kaliner MA. Human nasal respiratory secretions and host defense. Am Rev Respir Dis 1991;144:S52–S56.

133 Cole AM, Dewan P, Ganz T. Innate antimicrobial activity of nasal secretions. Infect Immun 1999;67:326–75.

134 Bera A, Herbert S, Jakob A, Vollmer W, Gotz F. Why are pathogenic staphylococci so lysozyme resistant? The peptidoglycan *O*-acetyltransferase OatA is the major determinant for lysozyme resistance of *Staphylococcus aureus*. Mol Microbiol 2005;55:778–87.

135 Nagaoka I, Hirota S, Yomogida S, Ohwada A, Hirata M. Synergistic actions of antibacterial neutrophil defensins and cathelicidins. Inflamm Res 2000;49:73–9.

136 Ong PY, Ohtake T, Brandt C *et al*. Endogenous antimicrobial peptides and skin infections in atopic dermatitis. N Engl J Med 2002;347:1151–60.

137 Peschel A, Jack RW, Otto M *et al*. *Staphylococcus aureus* resistance to human defensins and evasion of neutrophil killing via the novel virulence factor MprF is based on modification of membrane lipids with L-lysine. J Exp Med 2001;193:1067–76.

138 Verbrugh HA, Peters R, Goessens WH, Michel MF. Distinguishing complicated from uncomplicated bacteremia caused by *Staphylococcus aureus*: the value of "new" and "old" serological tests. J Immunol 1986;153:109–15.

139 Verbrugh HA, Peterson PK, Nguyen BY, Sisson SP, Kim Y. Opsonization of encapsulated *Staphylococcus aureus*: the role of specific antibody and complement. J Immunol 1982;129:1681–7.

140 Lee JC. The prospects for developing a vaccine against *Staphylococcus aureus*. Trends Microbiol 1996;4:162–6.

141 Sanford BA, Thomas VL, Ramsay MA. Binding of staphylococci to mucus in vivo and in vitro. Infect Immun 1989;57:3735–42.

142 Shuter J, Hatcher VB, Lowy FD. *Staphylococcus aureus* binding to human nasal mucin. Infect Immun 1996;64:310–18.

143 Carruthers MM, Kabat WJ. Mediation of staphylococcal adherence to mucosal cells by lipoteichoic acid. Infect Immun 1983;40:444–6.

144 Schwab UE, Wold AE, Carson JL *et al*. Increased adherence of *Staphylococcus aureus* from cystic fibrosis lungs to airway epithelial cells. Am Rev Respir Dis 1993;148:365–9.

145 Bibel DJ, Aly R, Shinefield HR, Maibach HI, Strauss WG. Importance of the keratinized epithelial cell in bacterial adherence. J Invest Dermatol 1982;79:250–3.

146 Aly R, Shinefield HI, Strauss WG, Maibach HI. Bacterial adherence to nasal mucosal cells. Infect Immun 1977;17:546–9.

147 Corrigan RM, Rigby D, Handley P, Foster TJ. The role of *Staphylococcus aureus* surface protein SasG in adherence and biofilm formation. Microbiology 2007;153:2435–46.

148 Walsh EJ, O'Brien LM, Liang X, Hook M, Foster TJ. Clumping factor B, a fibrinogen-binding MSCRAMM (microbial surface components recognizing adhesive matrix molecules) adhesin of *Staphylococcus aureus*, also binds to the tail region of type I cytokeratin 10. J Biol Chem 2004;279:50691–9.

149 O'Brien LM, Walsh EJ, Massey RC, Peacock SJ, Foster TJ. *Staphylococcus aureus* clumping factor B (ClfB) promotes adherence to human type I cytokeratin 10: implications for nasal colonization. Cell Microbiol 2002;4:759–70.

150 Schaffer AC, Solinga RM, Cocchiaro J *et al*. Immunization with *Staphylococcus aureus* clumping factor B, a major determinant in nasal carriage, reduces nasal colonization in a murine model. Infect Immun 2006;74:2145–53.

151 Clarke SR, Brummell KJ, Horsburgh MJ *et al*. Identification of in vivo-expressed antigens of *Staphylococcus aureus* and their use in vaccinations for protection against nasal carriage. J Infect Dis 2006;193:1098–108.

152 Aly R, Levit S. Adherence of *Staphylococcus aureus* to squamous epithelium: role of fibronectin and teichoic acid. Rev Infect Dis 1987;9(suppl 4):S341–S350.

153 Weidemaier C, Kokai-Fun JF, Kristian SA *et al*. Role of teichoic acids in *Staphylococcus aureus* nasal colonization, a major risk factor in nosocomial infections. Nat Med 2004;10:243–5.

154 Foster TJ. Nasal colonization by *Staphylococcus aureus*. Nat Med 2004;10:447.
155 Wertheim HFL, Walsh E, Choudhurry R *et al*. Key role for clumping factor B in *Staphylococcus aureus* nasal colonization of humans. PLoS Med 2008;5:e17.
156 Hoeksma A, Winkler KC. The normal flora of the nose in twins. Acta Leidensia 1963;32:123–33.
157 Aly R, Maibach HI, Shinefield HR, Mandel AD. *Staphylococcus aureus* carriage in twins. Am J Dis Child 1974;127:486–8.
158 Kinsman OS, McKenna R, Noble WC. Association between histocompatability antigens (HLA) and nasal carriage of *Staphylococcus aureus*. J Med Microbiol 1983;16:215–20.
159 van den Akker EL, Nouwen JL, Melles DC *et al*. *Staphylococcus aureus* nasal carriage is associated with glucocorticoid receptor gene polymorphisms. J Infect Dis 2006;194:814–18.
160 Emonts M, de Jongh CE, Houwing-Duistermaat JJ *et al*. Association between nasal carriage of *Staphylococcus aureus* and the human complement cascade activator serine protease C1 inhibitor (C1INH) valine vs. methionine polymorphism at amino acid position 480. FEMS Immunol Med Microbiol 2007;50:330–2.
161 Emonts M, Uitterlinden AG, Nouwen JL *et al*. Host polymorphisms in interleukin 4, complement factor H and C-reactive protein associated with nasal carriage of *Staphylococcus aureus* and occurrence of boils. J Infect Dis 2008;197:1244–53.
162 van Belkum A, Emonts M, Wertheim H *et al*. The role of human innate immune factors in nasal colonization by *Staphylococcus aureus*. Microbes Infect 2007;9:1471–7.
163 Claassen M, Nouwen J, Fang Y *et al*. *Staphylococcus aureus* nasal carriage is not associated with known polymorphism in the vitamin D receptor gene. FEMS Immunol Med Microbiol 2005;43:173–6.
164 Miller DL, McDonald JC, Jevons MP, Williams REO. Staphylococcal disease and nasal carriage in the Royal Air Force. J Hyg 1962;60:451–65.
165 Atkins JB, Marks J. The role of staphylococcal infection in beat disorders of miners. Br J Ind Med 1952;9:296–302.
166 Chow AW, Bartlett KH, Percival-Smith R, Morrison BJ. Vaginal colonization with *Staphylococcus aureus*, positive for toxic-shock marker protein, and *Escherichia coli* in healthy women. J Infect Dis 1984;150:80–4.
167 Tuazon CU, Sheagren JN. Staphylococcal endocarditis in parenteral drug abusers: source of the organism. Ann Intern Med 1975;82:788–90.
168 Gillespie WJ, Haywood-Farmer M, Fong R, Harding SM. Aspects of the microbe–host relationship in staphylococcal hematogenous osteomyelitis. Orthopedics 1987;10:475–80.
169 Niclaes L, Buntinx F, Banuro F, Lesaffre E, Heyrman J. Consequences of MRSA carriage in nursing home residents. Epidemiol Infect 1999;122:235–9.
170 Jensen AG, Wachmann CH, Poulsen KB *et al*. Risk factors for hospital-acquired *Staphylococcus aureus* bacteremia. Arch Intern Med 1999;159:1437–44.
171 Muder RR, Brennen C, Wagener MM *et al*. Methicillin-resistant staphylococcal colonization and infection in a long-term care facility. Ann Intern Med 1991;114:107–12.
172 Chang FY, Singh N, Gayowski T, Drenning SD, Wagener MM, Marino IR. Staphylococcus aureus nasal colonization and association with infection in liver transplantation recipients. Transplantation 1998;65:1169–72.
173 Chang FY, Singh N, Gayowski T, Wagener MM, Marino IR. *Staphylococcus aureus* nasal colonization in patients with cirrhosis: prospective assessment of association with infection. Infect Control Hosp Epidemiol 1998;19:328–32.
174 Mest DR, Wong DH, Shimoda KJ, Mulligan ME, Wilson SE. Nasal colonization with methicillin-resistant *Staphylococcus aureus* on admission to the surgical intensive care unit increases the risk of infection. Anesth Analg 1994;78:644–50.
175 Corbella X, Dominguez MA, Pujol M *et al*. *Staphylococcus aureus* nasal carriage as a marker for subsequent staphylococcal infections in intensive care unit patients. Eur J Clin Microbiol Infect Dis 1997;16:351–7.
176 Zimakoff J, Pedersen FB, Bergen L *et al*. *Staphylococcus aureus* carriage and infections among patients in four haemo- and peritoneal dialysis centres in Denmark. J Hosp Infect 1996; 33:289–300.
177 Lye WC, Leong SO, van der Straaten J, Lee EJC. *Staphylococcus aureus* CAPD related infections are associated with nasal carriage. Adv Perit Dial 1994;10:163–5.
178 Weinke T, Schiller R, Fehrenbach FJ, Pohle HD. Association between *Staphylococcus aureus* nasopharyngeal colonization and septicemia in patients infected with the human immunodeficiency virus. Eur J Clin Microbiol Infect Dis 1992;11:985–9.
179 Bert F, Galdbart J-O, Zarrouk V *et al*. Association between nasal carriage of *Staphylococcus aureus* and infection in liver transplant recipients. Clin Infect Dis 2000;31:1295–9.
180 Jakob HG, Borneff-Lipp M, Bach A *et al*. The endogenous pathway is a major route for deep sternal wound infection. Eur J Cardiothorac Surg 2000;17:154–60.
181 Kalmeijer MD, van Nieuwland-Bollen E, Bogaers-Hofman D, de Baere GA. Nasal carriage of *Staphylococcus aureus* is a major risk factor for surgical-site infections in orthopedic surgery. Infect Control Hosp Epidemiol 2000;21:319–23.
182 Fierobe L, Decré D, Mùller C *et al*. Methicillin-resistant *Staphylococcus aureus* as a causative agent of postoperative intra-abdominal infection: relation to nasal colonization. Clin Infect Dis 1999;29:1231–8.
183 Desai D, Desai N, Nightingale P, Elliott T, Neuberger J. Carriage of MRSA is associated with an increased risk of infection after liver transplantation. Liver Transpl 2003;9:754–9.
184 Squier C, Rihs JD, Risa KJ *et al*. *Staphylococcus aureus* rectal carriage and its association with infections in patients in a surgical intensive care unit and a liver transplant unit. Infect Control Hosp Epidemiol 2002;23:495–501.
185 Saxena AK, Panhotra BR, Venkateshappa CK, Sundaram DS, Uzzaman NM, Al Mulhim K. The impact of nasal carriage of methicillin-resistant and methicillin-susceptible *Staphylococcus aureus* (MRSA and MSSA) on vascular access-related septicemia among patients with type-II diabetes on dialysis. Ren Fail 2002;24:763–77.
186 Dupeyron C, Campillo SB, Mangeney N, Richardet JP, Leluan G. Carriage of *Staphylococcus aureus* and of gram-negative bacilli resistant to third-generation cephalosporins in cirrhotic patients: a prospective assessment of hospital-acquired infections. Infect Control Hosp Epidemiol 2001;22:427–33.
187 Tulloch LG, Alder VG, Gillespie WA. Treatment of chronic furunculosis. BMJ 1960;2:354–6.
188 Nouwen JL, Fieren MW, Snijders S, Verbrugh HA, van Belkum A. Persistent (not intermittent) nasal carriage of *Staphylococcus*

aureus is the determinant of CPD-related infections. Kidney Int 2005;67:1084–93.

189 Talon D, Rouget C, Cailleaux V *et al*. Nasal carriage of *Staphylococcus aureus* and cross-contamination in a surgical intensive care unit: efficacy of mupirocin ointment. J Hosp Infect 1995;30:39–49.

190 Gawler DM, Royle JP, Tosolini FA. Intractable nasal carriage of methicillin-resistant *Staphylococcus aureus*. Med J Aust 1980; 11:607–8.

191 Mitsuda T, Arai K, Ibe M, Imagawa T, Tomono N, Yokota S. The influence of methicillin-resistant *Staphylococcus aureus* (MRSA) carriers in a nursery and transmission of MRSA to their households. J Hosp Infect 1999;42:45–51.

192 Cetinkaya Y, Kocagoz S, Hayran M *et al*. Analysis of a mini-outbreak of methicillin-resistant *Staphylococcus aureus* in a surgical ward by using arbitrarily primed-polymerase chain reaction. J Chemother 2000;12:138–44.

193 Fascia P, Martin I, Mallaval FO *et al*. Possible implication of student nurses in the transmission of methicillin-resistant *Staphylococcus aureus* during a nosocomial outbreak. Pathol Biol 2003;51:479–82.

194 Cookson B, Peters B, Webster M, Phillips I, Rahman M, Noble W. Staff carriage of epidemic methicillin-resistant *Staphylococcus aureus*. J Clin Microbiol 1989;27:1471–6.

195 Ben-David D, Mermel LA, Parenteau S. Methicillin-resistant *Staphylococcus aureus* transmission: the possible importance of unrecognized health care worker carriage. Am J Infect Control 2008;36:93–7.

196 Cespedes C, Miller M, Quagliarello B, Vavagiakis P, Klein RS, Lowy FD. Differences between *Staphylococcus aureus* isolates from medical and nonmedical hospital personnel. J Clin Microbiol 2002;40:2594–7.

197 Tammelin A, Klotz F, Hambraeus A, Stahle E, Ransjo U. Nasal and hand carriage of *Staphylococcus aureus* in staff at a department for thoracic and cardiovascular surgery: endogenous or exogenous source? Infect Control Hosp Epidemiol 2003;24:686–9.

198 Sowirka O, Carron A, Perri M, Zervos M, Hyde K, Maddens M. Prevalence of *Staphylococcus aureus* carriage among asymptomatic nursing home personnel: a pilot study. J Am Med Dir Assoc 2000;1:159–63.

199 Kluytmans JA, Wertheim HF. Nasal carriage of *Staphylococcus aureus* and prevention of nosocomial infections. Infection 2005;33:3–8.

200 Doebbeling BN. Nasal and hand carriage of *Staphylococcus aureus* in healthcare workers. J Chemother 1994;6(suppl 2):11–17.

201 Watanakunakorn C, Axelson C, Bota B, Stahl C. Mupirocin ointment with and without chlorhexidine baths in the eradication of *Staphylococcus aureus* nasal carriage in nursing home residents. Am J Infect Control 1995;23:306–9.

202 Mupirocin Study Group. Nasal mupirocin prevents *Staphylococcus aureus* exit-site infection during peritoneal dialysis. J Am Soc Nephrol 1996;7:2403–8.

203 Segers P, Speekenbrink RG, Ubbink DT, van Ogtrop ML, de Mol BA. Prevention of nosocomial infection in cardiac surgery by decontamination of the nasopharynx and oropharynx with chlorhexidine gluconate: a randomized controlled trial. JAMA 2006;297:1059–60.

204 McAnally TP, Lewis MR, Brown DR. Effect of rifampin and bacitracin on nasal carriers of *Staphylococcus aureus*. Antimicrob Agents Chemother 1984;25:422–6.

205 Yu VL, Goetz A, Wagener M *et al*. *Staphylococcus aureus* nasal carriage and infection in patients on hemodialysis. Efficacy of antibiotic prophylaxis. N Engl J Med 1986;315:91–6.

206 Mody L, Kauffman CA, McNeil SA, Galecki AT, Bradley SF. Mupirocin-based decolonization of *Staphylococcus aureus* carriers in residents of two long-term care facilities: a randomized, double-blind, placebo-controlled trial. Clin Infect Dis 2003;37: 1467–74.

207 van Rijen M, Bonten M, Wenzel R, Kluytmans J. Intranasal mupirocin for reduction of *S. aureus* infections in surgical patients with nasal carriage. J Antimicrob Chemother 2008;61:254–61.

208 Boelaert JR, Van Landuyt HW, Godard CA *et al*. Intranasal mupirocin to prevent postoperative *Staphylococcus aureus* infections. Nephrol Dial Transplant 1993;8:235–9.

209 Boelaert JR, Van Landuyt HW, Gordts BZ, De Baere YA, Messer SA, Herwaldt LA. Nasal and cutaneous carriage of *Staphylococcus aureus* in hemodialysis patients: the effect of nasal mupirocin. Infect Control Hosp Epidemiol 1996;17:809–11.

210 Shinefield HR, Ribble JC, Boris M, Eichenwald H, Aly R, Maibach H. Bacterial interference between strains of *S. aureus*. Ann NY Acad Sci 1974;236:444–55.

211 Wertheim HF, Vos MC, Ott A *et al*. Risk and outcome of nosocomial *Staphylococcus aureus* bacteraemia in nasal carriers versus non-carriers. Lancet 2004;364:703–5.

Chapter 13
Epidemiology of Community-associated *Staphylococcus aureus* Infections

Rachel J. Gorwitz and John A. Jernigan
Division of Healthcare Quality Promotion, National Center for Preparedness, Detection, and Control of Infectious Diseases, Centers for Disease Control and Prevention, Atlanta, Georgia, USA

Background

Staphylococcus aureus has long been recognized as a predominant cause of localized and invasive infections and syndromes in the community, with a disease spectrum encompassing skin and soft tissue infections (SSTIs), muscle and visceral abscesses, septic arthritis, osteomyelitis, pneumonia, pleural empyema, bloodstream infections, endocarditis, and toxin-mediated syndromes including toxic shock syndrome (TSS), scalded skin syndrome, and food poisoning [1–4].

More recently, methicillin-resistant *S. aureus* (MRSA), previously seen almost exclusively in persons with significant healthcare exposure [5], has emerged as a community pathogen. The first reported outbreak of MRSA in a community setting occurred among intravenous drug users in Detroit in 1980 [6]. In this outbreak, MRSA infection among intravenous drug users was significantly associated with recent cephalosporin use [7]. Subsequently, two single-center reports published in the 1980s described MRSA infections among healthy Midwestern children without identifiable risk factors for healthcare-associated (HA) infections [8,9]. The MRSA isolates described in both of these pediatric case series had nonmultiresistant susceptibility profiles distinct from those of MRSA strains circulating in healthcare settings. Almost a decade later, the emergence of MRSA as a community pathogen on a broader scale, both in the USA [10–12] and elsewhere in the world [13,14], became apparent. Transmission of MRSA in community settings has now been described in most regions of the world [15–18].

Staphylococci in Human Disease, 2nd edition. Edited by Kent B. Crossley, Kimberly K. Jefferson, Gordon Archer, Vance G. Fowler, Jr.
 ISBN 978-14051-6332-3

Definitions and terminology

Most definitions of community-associated (CA)-MRSA have included the elements of disease onset in the community (or within the initial days of a hospital admission) and absence of risk factors that would suggest the patient initially acquired MRSA colonization in a healthcare setting [12,19,20]. However, specific criteria have varied somewhat from study to study. In multistate active surveillance for MRSA infection sponsored by the Centers for Disease Control and Prevention (CDC), infections are classified as HA-MRSA if (i) MRSA is isolated from a culture obtained 48 hours or more after a patient is hospitalized, (ii) the patient has a history of hospitalization, surgery, dialysis, or residence in a long-term care facility within 1 year before the MRSA culture date, (iii) the patient has an indwelling device at the time of culture, or (iv) the patient has a previous history of MRSA infection or colonization; these healthcare-associated infections are further classified as "hospital-onset" (≥ 48 hours after hospital admission) or "community-onset" [19,21]. In some reports, the term "community-acquired MRSA" is used to describe community-onset MRSA infections in patients lacking established HA-MRSA risk factors. However, it is generally not possible to determine with certainty where MRSA was initially acquired.

The term CA-MRSA has also been used to refer to MRSA strains with bacteriological characteristics (e.g., genotype, antimicrobial susceptibility profile) typical of isolates obtained from patients with CA-MRSA infections [22]. Initially, these characteristics were distinct from characteristics of isolates obtained from patients with HA-MRSA infections, suggesting the new strains emerged *de novo* in the community via acquisition of methicillin-resistance genes by circulating strains of methicillin-susceptible *S. aureus* (MSSA) [23]. However, epidemiological case classifications (e.g., CA-MRSA) and strain characteristics are becoming less closely linked over time. For example, several reports have documented healthcare-associated infections

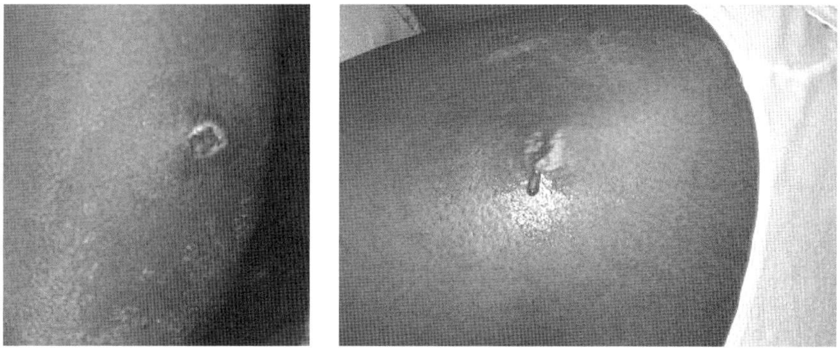

Figure 13.1 Methicillin-resistant *S. aureus* (MRSA) skin infection. MRSA skin lesions may begin as small papules and then develop into larger pustules or abscesses with areas of necrosis and surrounding erythema. Lesions are often confused with spider bites. (Courtesy of P. Hicks, Children's Medical Center of Dallas.)

caused by MRSA strains initially identified in community settings [24–28].

Disease spectrum

SSTIs, including impetigo, folliculitis, furuncles (abscessed hair follicles or "boils"), carbuncles (coalesced masses of furuncles), cutaneous abscesses, and cellulitis, are the most common manifestation of *S. aureus* infection in the community. Bullous impetigo is invariably caused by toxin-producing *S. aureus*. While β-hemolytic streptococci were previously the leading cause of the more common nonbullous impetigo, *S. aureus* subsequently replaced β-hemolytic streptococci as the most common cause of these infections [29,30]. Data about outpatient visits from the National Ambulatory Medical Care Survey in which a diagnosis code for impetigo was assigned decreased significantly between 1992–1994 and 2001–2003, while outpatient visits for abscess and cellulitis increased [31]. While pathogen information was frequently not available for these visits, the increase in abscess and cellulitis visits may reflect the emergence of CA-MRSA, which has most frequently been associated with furuncles, carbuncles, and cutaneous abscesses (Figure 13.1) [19,32]. The role of CA-MRSA in pure cellulitis without focal purulence is less clear, because cultures are not frequently obtained from these lesions. CA-MRSA skin lesions have frequently been confused with spider bites by both patients and clinicians, even in areas of the country where spiders capable of causing necrotic skin lesions are not endemic [33]. This may reflect the spontaneous appearance of a painful red lesion at a site where the patient recalls no obvious preceding trauma. The lesions also often have a necrotic-appearing center, which clinicians may associate with venomous spider bites [34]. The severity of *S. aureus* SSTIs varies from mild superficial infections to deeper soft-tissue abscesses. Deeper abscesses frequently require emergency department care or hospital admission for surgical drainage and parenteral antibacterial agents [35,36]. The proportion of patients with culture-confirmed *S. aureus* SSTIs who are hospitalized for treatment has ranged from 20 to 25% in several published studies [36–38]. A common presentation of *S. aureus* skin infection in otherwise healthy newborns is pustulosis in the groin, upper thigh, and sacral regions (areas covered by the diaper), which has been described in association with both MRSA and MSSA [39,40]. This manifestation has been reported to be relatively mild, but sometimes results in hospital admission and parenteral antimicrobial therapy due to the young age of the patients [39].

There is conflicting information regarding the impact of methicillin resistance on outcome of community-associated *S. aureus* skin infections. One prospective single-center study reported similar outcomes following hospital discharge for patients with MRSA and MSSA skin infections [41]. Lack of incision and drainage was associated with nonresponse at day 30 in the group overall [41]. Another prospective study of patients with community-associated *S. aureus* infections presenting to four Midwestern medical centers found methicillin resistance to be associated with clinical failure, controlling for infection type, underlying illness, and receipt of antimicrobial therapy active against the infecting isolate [42]. A study of cutaneous *S. aureus* infections in pediatric patients in Baltimore found that patients with MRSA SSTIs were significantly more likely to require a drainage procedure [37]. Recurrent *S. aureus* SSTIs in both individuals and households have been described previously with MSSA [43,44], but may be more common with strains of MRSA currently circulating in the community [41,42,45,46]. Similar infections within 30 days after hospital discharge occurred in persons having close contact with 13% of patients with CA-MRSA and 4% of patients with CA-MSSA SSTIs in one prospective study, although this difference was not statistically significant [41]. In another prospective study, relapse (within 2 weeks of completing treatment) or recurrence (2 weeks or more after completing treatment) occurred in 18% of patients with CA-MRSA and 6% of those with CA-MSSA infection ($P < 0.015$) [42]. In a retrospective study of *S. aureus* SSTIs among patients attending a Boston clinic serving a large population of men who have sex with men, 23% of patients with an initial culture-confirmed MRSA SSTI had at least one additional culture-confirmed MRSA SSTI during the study period (1998–2005), while only 4% of MSSA SSTIs identified during the study period were recurrent [46]. An even higher rate of recurrence (71%) following a first episode of culture-proven MRSA SSTI was documented among 62 patients attending an HIV primary care clinic [47]. It is not clear what role persistent colonization versus recurrent exposure from an exogenous source plays in these recurrences.

Although the majority of community-associated *S. aureus* infections are SSTIs, deep-seated and invasive infections also occur. Similar to SSTIs, the proportion of these infections caused by MRSA is increasing. For some syndromes, the emergence of MRSA in the community has been associated with an increase in the overall incidence and/or severity of invasive community-associated *S. aureus* infections. For example, at a children's medical center in Memphis, the overall incidence of acute hematogenous osteoarticular infections (osteomyelitis and septic arthritis) increased from 2.6 to 6.0 per 1000 admissions between 2000 and 2004, and the proportion caused by MRSA increased from 4 to 40% while the proportion caused by MSSA remained stable at 10–13% [48]. The osteoarticular infections caused by MRSA reported in this series were more severe than those caused by MSSA, with an increased prevalence of subperiosteal abscesses, more frequent requirement for surgical intervention, more prolonged duration of fever, and longer hospital stay, which could not be accounted for by delays in institution of appropriate therapy [48]. Other complications, including septic thrombophlebitis, septic pulmonary emboli, and large muscle abscesses, were also more common in the patients with MRSA infection, although the differences were not statistically significant [48]. A pediatric center in Dallas reported significantly increased inflammatory markers on admission, length of hospital stay and antibiotic therapy, and overall rate of complications in children with MRSA as compared with non-MRSA osteomyelitis [49]. Another pediatric center in Houston reported similar findings of increased number of febrile days and hospital days in children with musculoskeletal infections caused by MRSA as compared with MSSA, although there were no significant differences in the final outcome [50]. The same center reported an increase in venous thrombosis associated with staphylococcal osteomyelitis in children, which coincided with the emergence of MRSA as a cause of these infections in the community [51]. Metastatic pulmonary disease due to septic pulmonary emboli was also described as a complication of *S. aureus* musculoskeletal infection at this center [52]. Cases of pyomyositis, typically caused by *S. aureus* but unusual in temperate climates, and acute bacterial myositis, most commonly caused by *Streptococcus pyogenes*, also increased in otherwise healthy children presenting to the pediatric center in Houston from 2000 through 2005 [53]. *Staphylococcus aureus* accounted for 26 (58%) of these cases, with 62% of the *S. aureus* isolates resistant to methicillin. Those patients infected with MRSA required more drainage procedures than the patients with MSSA infections.

Staphylococcus aureus accounts for only about 3% of cases of community-acquired pneumonia (CAP) in which a pathogen is identified [54], but is a recognized cause of influenza-associated CAP [55–57]. A severe necrotizing form of *S. aureus* CAP has been described primarily in adolescents and young adults with preceding or concurrent influenza infection [58–60]. Severe *S. aureus* CAP may occur in the absence of confirmed or suspected influenza infection; however, there is evidence to suggest that influenza and *S. aureus* infection may potentiate one another by facilitating bacterial respiratory tract adhesion and decreasing phagocytic killing, or enhancing viral replication, respectively [61–65]. The case-fatality rate in *S. aureus* CAP case series ranges from 29 to 60%, and patients typically progress from onset of symptoms to death in a matter of days [57–60]. Strains of MRSA associated with SSTIs in the community have also emerged as a cause of severe influenza-associated CAP in the USA [58,60,66,67], although it is not clear whether this has resulted in an increase in the overall incidence of these infections. The proportion of all reported pediatric influenza deaths in which there was an *S. aureus* coinfection increased substantially, from 2 to 30%, in the first 3 years after these deaths were made nationally notifiable in 2004 [68]. Children with *S. aureus* coinfection were significantly older and more likely to have pneumonia and acute respiratory distress syndrome than those who were not coinfected; 60% of the *S. aureus* coinfected children were infected with MRSA.

Reports from several pediatric centers suggest that *S. aureus*, and in particular MRSA, may be replacing *Streptococcus pneumoniae* as the primary cause of pleural empyemas in young children following introduction of the pneumococcal conjugate vaccine in 2000 [69–71]. The proportion of empyema cases caused by *S. aureus* at the previously mentioned pediatric center in Houston increased significantly during 2001–2002 compared with 1999–2000, and the proportion of cases caused by MRSA increased significantly during the period 1993–2002 [71]. The total number of these infections caused by *S. aureus* and MRSA at this center also increased substantially, although the increases were not statistically significant. The empyema cases caused by *S. aureus* occurred primarily in children younger than 1 year old. Patients with MRSA empyema had significantly longer length of hospital stay than patients with MSSA infection; however, no deaths occurred in either group. In a subsequent study from the Houston center, MRSA accounted for over 90% of cases of primary *S. aureus* pneumonia or empyema between August 1, 2001 and June 30, 2004 [52].

Staphylococcus aureus bacteremia can occur in association with virtually any *S. aureus* infection or without obvious preceding focal infection. In a review of data on adult bacteremia from three hospitals, *S. aureus* was the most common cause of clinically significant bacteremia, with about half of these cases being community-onset [72]. Infective endocarditis has been estimated to occur in 5–20% of patients with *S. aureus* bacteremia [73]. *Staphylococcus aureus* differs from many other pathogens in that it can cause infectious endocarditis on a normal native heart valve. Several reports suggest that the proportion of infective endocarditis cases due to *S. aureus* is increasing [74,75]. Endocarditis caused by *S. aureus* is a well-established complication of intravenous drug use. MRSA, including new strains of MRSA that have emerged and become epidemic in the community, has also been described as a cause of community-associated endocarditis in this population [7,76–78]. While infective endocarditis has not frequently been described as a manifestation of CA-MRSA infection in individuals without a history of intravenous drug use, a report from Baltimore, Maryland describes five cases of definite or possible infective endocarditis following MRSA furunculosis in adults without established MRSA risk factors, HIV infection, or history of intravenous drug use [79].

Concomitant with the emergence of MRSA as a community pathogen, MRSA has been described in association with some syndromes infrequently described as manifestations of *S. aureus* infection in the past. For example, 14 previously healthy adolescents presented to a pediatric center in Houston with severe *S. aureus* sepsis and coagulopathy over an 18-month period during 2002 through 2004, compared with only three such cases during the previous 3 years [80]. Of these 14 cases, 12 were caused by MRSA. The primary infection in the majority of these cases was osteomyelitis. Three cases of Waterhouse–Friderichsen syndrome, generally associated with fulminant meningococcemia and characterized by petechial rash, coagulopathy, cardiovascular collapse and bilateral adrenal hemorrhage, were described in association with MRSA (2 cases) and MSSA (1 case) in children in Chicago [81]. Finally, MRSA has been described as an emerging etiology of necrotizing fasciitis, a syndrome most commonly associated with *Streptococcus pyogenes* [82]. MRSA was identified as the etiology in 14 cases of community-onset necrotizing fasciitis and/or necrotizing myositis in adult patients presenting to a medical center in Los Angeles, California during 15 months in 2003 and 2004 [82]. While the majority of the patients had underlying chronic medical problems or injecting drug use, four patients (29%) had no serious coexisting conditions or risk factors. During the study period, 29% of necrotizing fasciitis cases identified at this center were caused by MRSA.

Several staphylococcal diseases, including scalded skin syndrome, food poisoning, and TSS, are mediated by toxins. Staphylococcal food poisoning occurs as a result of ingesting one of several staphylococcal enterotoxins, most commonly enterotoxin A [3,83]. Since it is usually a self-limited disease that rarely leads to systemic infection, and because reporting to state health departments is passive and incomplete, the true incidence of staphylococcal food poisoning is unknown; however, it is considered one of the most common foodborne illnesses [3]. Although TSS is a nationally notifiable disease, reporting is similarly passive and incomplete. Active multistate surveillance for staphylococcal TSS was last conducted in 1986, and confirmed a significant decrease in incidence of menstrual TSS following peak incidence in 1980 [84]. The decrease in incidence followed removal from the market of a brand of highly absorbent tampons that were epidemiologically linked to the disease. A review of passive TSS surveillance in the USA from 1979 through 1996 indicated that the number of TSS cases reported nationwide continued to decline through 1996, as did the proportion of these cases associated with menstruation [85]. Menstrual TSS by definition affects young women. Nonmenstrual TSS also tends to affect young, previously healthy persons and has been more commonly reported among women [85,86]. The case-fatality rate was significantly higher for nonmenstrual TSS compared with menstrual TSS in several published reports [85–87].

Antimicrobial resistance and molecular epidemiology

Since the 1990s, MRSA has accounted for an increasing proportion of community-associated *S. aureus* infections in the USA and elsewhere [15,37,40,88–90]. In a 2004 study of adult patients with purulent SSTIs presenting to emergency departments in 11 US cities, MRSA accounted for 78% of *S. aureus* SSTIs and 59% of SSTIs overall [89]. The proportion of SSTIs from which MRSA was isolated ranged from 15 to 74% by center, but MRSA was the most commonly identified organism in all but one of the centers [89]. MRSA was identified in 86% of 14 severe *S. aureus* sepsis cases identified in adolescents at one center in Houston from August 2002 through January 2004 [80], in 63% of 24 *S. aureus* pyomyositis and myositis cases in children at the same center from 2000 through 2005 [53], and in 88% of 15 severe *S. aureus* CAP cases reported to the CDC in the 2003–2004 influenza season [60]. The proportion of osteomyelitis and septic arthritis cases caused by MRSA increased from 4 to 40% between 2000 and 2004 at a pediatric center in Memphis, while the proportion of these infections caused by MSSA remained stable at 10–13% [48]. Similarly, the proportion of pediatric head and neck abscesses attributed to MRSA increased from zero in July 1999 through December 2001 to 65% in January 2002 through June 2004 at a center in Chicago [91].

Worldwide, the emergence of MRSA as a community pathogen has primarily been associated with strains of MRSA distinct from those historically associated with

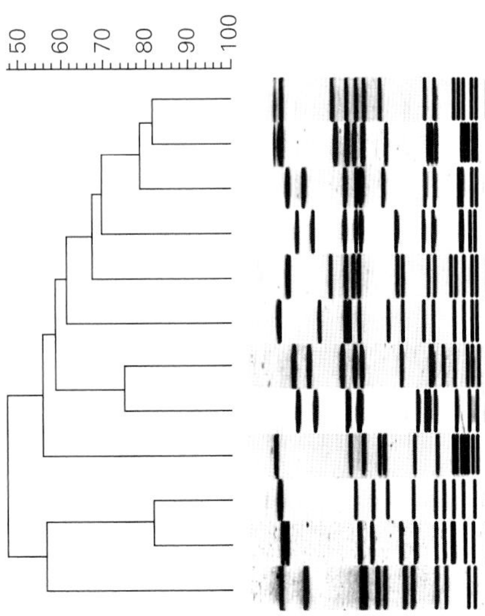

PFT	MLST	SCC*mec*	*pvl*
USA300	8	IV	POS
USA700	72	IV	NEG
USA100	5	II	NEG
USA800	5	IV	NEG
USA400	1	IV	POS
USA500	8	IV, II	NEG
USA1000	59	IV	NEG/POS
USA900	15	MSSA	NEG
USA600	45	II	NEG
USA200	36	II	NEG
USA1100	30	IV	POS
USA1200		MSSA	POS

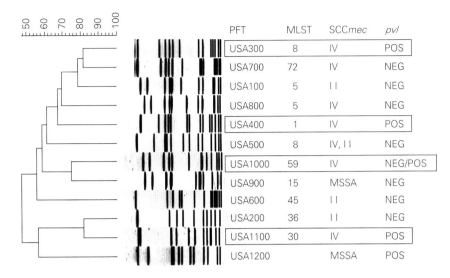

Figure 13.2 Characteristics of pulsed-field types (PFTs) of methicillin-resistant *S. aureus* in the USA. Boxed PFTs on right of diagram indicate historically community-associated strains. MLST, multilocus sequence type; MSSA, methicillin-susceptible *S. aureus*; SCC, staphylococcal cassette chromosome; pvl, Panton–Valentine leukocidin. (From McDougal *et al.* [94] with permission.)

healthcare settings [18,92]. While different strains predominate in different regions of the world, they tend to share some common characteristics, including susceptibility to most classes of antimicrobial agents other than β-lactams, the presence of staphylococcal cassette chromosome (SCC)*mec* type IV or V, the presence of genes encoding Panton–Valentine leukocidin (PVL) and, importantly, a propensity to spread and cause infection among otherwise healthy people in the general community [18,93].

The MRSA pulsed-field gel electrophoresis types (PFTs) associated primarily with community transmission in the USA are USA300, USA400, USA1000, and USA1100, which correspond to multilocus sequence types (ST)8, ST1, ST59, and ST30, respectively [94–96] (Figure 13.2). These are distinct from the predominant MRSA strain associated with the first published report of community MRSA transmission among Detroit intravenous drug users in the early 1980s, which was later described as ST74 [97]. In the late 1990s, when MRSA was first recognized as a significant pathogen in general community settings, predominant MRSA PFTs responsible for community-associated disease varied geographically within the USA. USA400 predominated in the Midwest and Northeast, and was the PFT associated with the deaths of four Midwestern children described in an early report [10], as well as with numerous nonfatal infections including SSTIs [26,36,81]. Subsequently, MRSA PFT USA300 has emerged as the major community PFT in most areas of the country [88,89,98–101], although ST1 (which includes USA400) remained predominant in a study conducted in rural southwestern Alaska through 2006 [102]. MRSA USA1100 (ST30), an occasional cause of CA-MRSA infections in the USA but a predominant cause of these infections in some other countries [103], is genetically related to phage type 80/81 MSSA, which caused epidemic *S. aureus* disease worldwide in the 1950s [104]. MRSA ST80, which has not been assigned a PFT in the USA, is responsible for the majority of CA-MRSA infections in several European countries [105–107].

One unique strain of PFT USA300, termed USA300-0114, has predominated in outbreaks and prevalence studies throughout the USA, suggesting that this strain possesses virulence or transmissibility factors that confer unusual fitness [89,108,109]. Sequencing of the complete genome of this strain identified a mobile genetic element termed arginine catabolic mobile element (ACME) [110]. The authors hypothesized that the products of this gene cluster, also found commonly in *Staphylococcus epidermidis*, enhance the capacity of USA300 strains to survive at low pH on human skin and within phagocytic cells. In a subsequent study, deletion of the ACME element in a rabbit bacteremia model significantly attenuated the competitive fitness of the USA300 mutant strain compared with wild-type USA300 [111]. Analysis of diverse collection of *S. aureus* isolates in the USA and the UK revealed that the ACME-associated *arc*A gene was primarily associated with a subset of USA300 strains that includes USA300-0114, but was also present in some isolates of healthcare-associated MRSA PFT USA100 in the USA and strains of MRSA ST97 and ST1 in the UK [112,113].

PVL is a cytolytic toxin associated with *S. aureus* furuncles and necrotizing pneumonia [114,115]. PVL genes were detected in 98% of MRSA isolates and 42% of MSSA isolates from community-associated SSTIs in a multisite study in the USA conducted in 2004 [89]. In contrast, PVL genes are rarely found in MRSA PFTs more strongly associated with healthcare transmission [116]. PVL genes have been associated with community MRSA strains in most but not all parts of the world. For example, PVL-negative USA400 isolates have been a primary cause of CA-MRSA infections in Western Australia [117,118]. PVL-positive strains of MRSA USA400 have been detected only recently in eastern Australia, in communities where other PVL-positive PFTs are endemic, suggesting horizontal spread of bacteriophage-associated PVL determinants [117]. In contrast, PVL genes were detected in 45% of MRSA isolates obtained from inpatients and outpatients at a group of Japanese hospitals during 1979–1985 but in none of those obtained during the 1990s [119]. The majority of these PVL-positive strains were ST30, which was prevalent in the earlier but not the later period. ST30 has more recently been associated with community transmission in North and South America, Australia, Europe, and Asia [103,105,120–122] and is a descendant of the PVL-positive MSSA phage type 80/81 that caused epidemic hospital- and community-associated disease in the 1950s [104].

PVL has been hypothesized to play a major role in the increased virulence of MRSA strains prevalent in the community. The presence of PVL genes has been associated with more severe local disease, greater systemic inflammatory response and increased complications in children with *S. aureus* (MRSA and MSSA) osteomyelitis [50,123], with secondary pulmonary disease in children with invasive *S. aureus* infections [52], and with decreased survival in patients with community-acquired *S. aureus* pneumonia [114]. However, recent studies comparing the virulence and lethality of PVL-positive MRSA strains and isogenic PVL-negative strains in mouse models have correlated presence of PVL genes with development of necrotizing pneumonia [124] but not with severity of MRSA SSTIs or bloodstream infections [125]. In a rabbit bacteremia model, PVL was found to contribute to pathogenesis during the acute phase of infection [126]. In another study, the quantity of PVL produced *in vitro* by isolates from a variety of MRSA infections did not correlate with severity of infection for MRSA isolates overall or among isolates from patients with a specific clinical syndrome [127]. It is possible that PVL is a key virulence factor in only certain clinical syndromes or that other cofactors are necessary to produce severe disease.

More recently, increased *in vitro* production of a group of peptides related to phenol-soluble modulin (PSM) peptides in *S. epidermidis* has been described in strains of MRSA associated with community versus healthcare transmission [128]. In a mouse bacteremia model, a wild-type strain of MRSA USA400 caused significantly greater mortality compared with an isogenic strain with the gene loci for these peptides deleted. In a similar study using USA300, the strain with the PSM loci deleted had significantly decreased ability to cause skin lesions in mice. These PSM-like peptides were also demonstrated to recruit, activate, and subsequently lyse human neutrophils *in vitro*, indicating that they contribute to strain virulence by eliminating the main cellular defense against *S. aureus* [128]. Additional factors yet to be described, potentially associated with genetic differences in host immune response [129], likely contribute to the wide variability in disease severity observed even among persons infected with a given MRSA PFT such as USA300 or USA400 [130].

One of the defining characteristics of CA-MRSA has been isolate susceptibility to most classes of antimicrobial agents other than β-lactams and macrolides/azalides (e.g., erythromycin, azithromycin) [19]. However, resistance to other antimicrobial agents, including fluoroquinolones, tetracyclines, and clindamycin, also occurs, with prevalence of resistance to these other agents varying geographically [19,89,102,131]. An increasing prevalence of clindamycin resistance among MRSA USA300 isolated from pediatric patients in Houston, particularly those with healthcare risk factors, has been described [20,132]. In contrast, lower rates of clindamycin susceptibility were observed among USA300 MRSA isolates from community-onset versus hospital-onset infections in a San Francisco study [131]. Clindamycin resistance was identified in nearly 50% of MRSA SSTI isolates from outpatients attending a clinic in Boston serving a large population of men who have sex with men during 1998–2005, despite a low prevalence of prior clindamycin use in these patients, indicating that antibiotic exposure is not necessary for acquisition of these resistant strains [46]. MRSA USA300 isolates with multiple resistance to erythromycin, clindamycin, tetracycline, levofloxacin, and mupirocin have been described in adult patients attending outpatient clinics in Boston and San Francisco [133,134]. Resistance determinants to erythromycin, clindamycin, and mupirocin in these isolates was located on a conjugative plasmid from the pSK41 family, which has the capacity to accept additional resistance elements and act as a mechanism of transfer of these elements between *S. aureus* strains [110,135]. Analysis of 825 USA300 MRSA isolates from invasive infections submitted to CDC between 2005 and 2008 revealed resistance to tetracycline in 9% (including three isolates with resistance to both tetracycline and doxycycline conferred by the *tet*M gene), clindamycin in 7%, mupirocin in 3%, trimethoprim–sulfamethoxazole in 1%, and gentamicin in 0.8% [136]. Resistance to one or more of these agents was detected in 9.5% of the isolates, and presence of the pSK41 conjugative plasmid was detected in 3%. Recent case reports have described intermediate susceptibility to vancomycin in USA300 MRSA isolates from patients with recent vancomycin exposure [137,138]. Resistance to at least four classes of non-β-lactam antimicrobials has been described in over 60% of USA1000 (ST59) CA-MRSA SSTI and colonization isolates from children in Taiwan [139].

The *mec*A gene, which confers resistance to methicillin and all β-lactam antimicrobial agents currently available in the USA, is carried on a gene complex known as SCC*mec* [140]. MRSA strains associated with community transmission typically carry SCC*mec* types IV or V, which are smaller and theoretically more easily transferable between organisms than the SCC*mec* types (I–III) characteristic of MRSA strains that predominate in healthcare settings [93]. While SCC*mec* type IV is typical of CA-MRSA isolates, it is also found in some MRSA PFTs associated with healthcare transmission [94].

Strains of MSSA that possess PVL genes and pulsed-field patterns closely related to patterns of MRSA USA300 and USA400 strains have been isolated from patients with community-associated *S. aureus* SSTIs and invasive infections [80,81,89,141]. These strains may represent ancestors of the MRSA strains or MRSA strains that have lost *mec*A. Case reports indicate that these strains and the corresponding MRSA strains have similar virulence potential [80,81]. USA300 strains accounted for an increasing proportion (14–35%) of all invasive MSSA isolates among children treated at a Houston pediatric hospital between 2001 and 2006 [142].

Burden and distribution of disease

The incidence of community-associated *S. aureus* infections is difficult to determine with precision because cultures are often not obtained, particularly from less severe infections. Furthermore, most states do not require reporting of all forms of *S. aureus* infection. However, administrative coding data captured in nationally representative ambulatory care surveys demonstrate significant increases in ambulatory care visits for SSTIs typical of *S. aureus* during the past decade [31,143,144]. Overall rates of visits for SSTIs increased from 32.1 to 48.1 visits per 1000 population between 1997 and 2005, with visits assigned the diagnosis code for abscess/cellulitis accounting for more than 95% of this increase [143]. This corresponded to a total of 14.2 million ambulatory care SSTI visits in 2005 [143]. The largest relative increases in visit rates for these infections occurred in emergency departments (especially in high safety-net-status emergency departments and in the South), among black patients, and among patients younger than 18 years [143]. Similarly, SSTI visits to the Baltimore Veterans Affairs Medical Center Emergency Care service increased from 20 to 61 per 1000 visits during 2001–2005, and the proportion of SSTI cultures at that center which yielded MRSA increased from 4 to 42% ($P < 0.01$), while the proportion that yielded MSSA remained stable (10–13%) [88]. A seasonality has been reported in incidence of *S. aureus* skin infections among children, with an increase in infections occurring during the summer months [38].

Nationally representative hospital discharge surveys have been used to ascertain rates of hospitalizations in which a discharge diagnosis indicating *S. aureus* infection was assigned [145–147]. However, it is generally not possible to determine from administrative coding data whether an infection was community or healthcare associated. In an analysis of national hospital discharge data, hospitalizations with an *S. aureus* diagnosis code other than septicemia or pneumonia in addition to a diagnosis code of cellulitis or abscess increased more than 25% per year from 22 451 in 1999 to 87 500 in 2005, which corresponded to a nearly fourfold increase over the entire time period [145]. Because these types of infections are typically community associated and because increases in hospitalizations for *S. aureus*-related septicemia, pneumonia, and device-associated infections that are typically nosocomial were much less dramatic, the authors attributed their results to a substantial increase in community-associated *S. aureus* infections (including CA-MRSA infections).

In a retrospective study based on review of hospital microbiology records in four metropolitan Connecticut areas in 1998, the population-based incidence of laboratory-confirmed community-onset bacteremic *S. aureus* infections was 17 cases per 100 000 population, making these infections nearly as common as community-onset bacteremic infections due to *Streptococcus pneumoniae* [148]. Males, older adults, blacks, and persons living in urban areas were at greatest risk. The majority (62%) of the community-onset *S. aureus* infections were considered to be healthcare associated. Of the remaining 38%, 85% had at least one underlying medical condition such as diabetes mellitus, cardiovascular disease, injection drug use, or HIV/AIDS. MRSA accounted for 16% of the community-onset cases that were healthcare associated or occurred in patients with underlying medical conditions, but for none of the cases in persons with no underlying conditions [148]. However, as this study preceded the widespread emergence of MRSA as a community pathogen, it is possible that the proportion of these infections caused by MRSA may have subsequently increased.

The population-based incidence of culture-confirmed CA-MRSA infections was determined in surveillance areas of two states (Georgia and Maryland) in 2001–2002, and ranged from 18.0 to 25.7 cases per 100 000 [19] (Figure 13.3). Combined with data from sentinel hospital-laboratory-based surveillance conducted in Minnesota during the same time period, the proportion of all MRSA infections that were CA-MRSA ranged from 8 to 20%. SSTIs accounted for the largest proportion (77%) of all culture-confirmed CA-MRSA infections. Among other types of CA-MRSA infections reported, 10% were wound infections, 6% were invasive (defined as an isolate obtained from a normally sterile site, including bacteremia, septic arthritis, and osteomyelitis), and 2% were pneumonia. In a retrospective population-based study of culture-confirmed MRSA infections among San Francisco residents in 2004–2005, the incidence of community-onset MRSA infection was 316 cases per 100 000; excluding persons who were hospitalized in the year preceding their infection, the incidence was 243 cases per 100 000 [131].

The population-based incidence of culture-confirmed invasive MRSA infections was determined in surveillance areas of nine states in 2005 [21]. Community-associated infections accounted for 14% of these infections, while community-onset infections in persons with healthcare

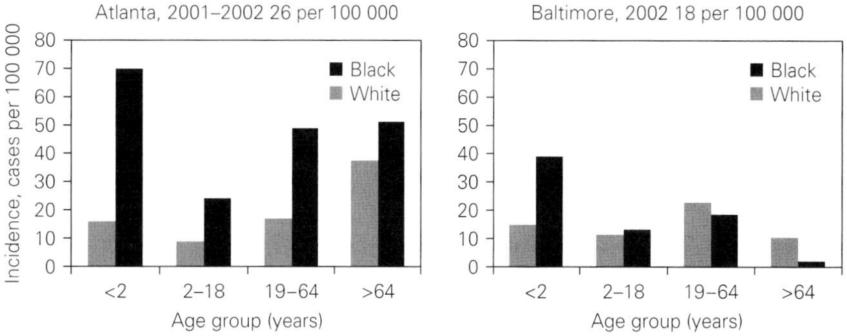

Figure 13.3 Incidence of community-associated methicillin-resistant *S. aureus* infection by age and race in Atlanta and Baltimore. Active Bacterial Core Surveillance System, 2001–2002. (From Fridkin *et al.* [19] with permission.)

risk factors accounted for 58% and hospital-onset infections for 27%. Based on these data, the incidence of invasive CA-MRSA infections was estimated to be 4.6 cases per 100 000 in the USA in 2005, and the incidence of death prior to hospital discharge with these infections was 0.5 per 100 000. Bacteremia was reported as a clinical syndrome for 65% of the patients with invasive CA-MRSA infections. Other clinical syndromes reported included cellulitis (23%), pneumonia (14%), endocarditis (13%), osteomyelitis (8%), and septic shock (4%).

Little information is currently available on trends in population-based incidence of CA-MRSA. In the state of Connecticut, the incidence of invasive CA-MRSA infections increased significantly from 1.1 to 2.8 cases per 100 000 between 2001 and 2006, while the incidence of community-onset MRSA infections in persons with healthcare risk factors remained stable at 15.4 per 100 000 and the incidence of hospital-onset MRSA infections decreased from 10.0 to 7.6 per 100 000 [149]. In addition, there have been reports from individual healthcare facilities documenting increasing numbers of CA-MRSA infections treated at the facility, increasing proportions of all MRSA infections that are community associated, and increasing proportions of all community-associated *S. aureus* infections that are methicillin-resistant [88,99,150,151]. For example, at Texas Children's Hospital in Houston, the number of CA-MRSA infections diagnosed increased 62% between 2001–2002 and 2002–2003, while the annual number of hospital admissions remained stable [99].

To date, reported CA-MRSA infections have disproportionately affected children, young adults, and people from racial or ethnic minorities and low socioeconomic groups [19,116,131,152]. Incidence of these infections has also been higher among males compared with females in some studies [131]. In 2001–2002, the incidence of all culture-confirmed CA-MRSA infections (predominantly SSTIs) in Atlanta and Baltimore was highest among persons less than 2 years of age [19] (Figure 13.3). Among MRSA cases identified at 12 Minnesota laboratories in 2000, the median age of patients with any culture-confirmed CA-MRSA infection was 23 years, compared with 68 years for patients with HA-MRSA infection [116]. In contrast, the incidence

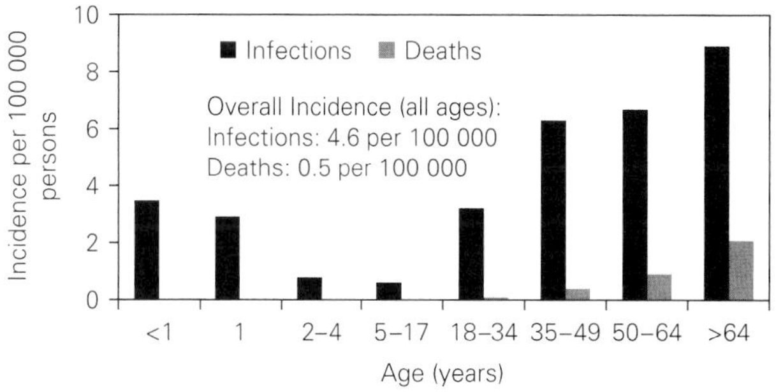

Figure 13.4 Incidence of invasive community-associated methicillin-resistant *S. aureus* infections and deaths by age. Active Bacterial Core Surveillance System, 2005. (Adapted from Klevens *et al.* [21] with permission.)

of invasive CA-MRSA infections in areas of nine states in 2005 was highest in persons aged 65 years or older (8.9 cases per 100 000) and lowest in children aged 5–17 years (0.6 cases per 100 000) (Figure 13.3) [21]. Among children, rates of invasive CA-MRSA infection were highest among infants under 12 months old (3.5 cases per 100 000) and decreased with increasing age [21] (Figure 13.3). Deaths with invasive CA-MRSA infection were also highest among persons aged 65 years or older and were rare in children [21] (Figure 13.4).

Non-white race has been associated with risk of CA-MRSA infection overall [19,31] (Figure 13.3) and with risk of invasive CA-MRSA infection [21]. At a pediatric and women's center in Hawaii, Pacific Islanders represented only 35% of patients served overall in 2002 but accounted for 76% of patients meeting case criteria for CA-MRSA infection [152]. An elevated incidence of CA-MRSA disease has also been reported among Native Americans in a rural Midwest community [153], Alaskan Natives in a remote area of southwestern Alaska [32], and medically underserved patients attending an inner-city soft tissue infection clinic in San Francisco [154]. In Minnesota, the median household income for patients with CA-MRSA infection was lower than that for patients with HA-MRSA infection and considerably lower than the median household income for state residents overall [116]. In San Francisco, the incidence of community-onset MRSA infection was highest in zip codes that included families with the lowest median household incomes [131].

Several published reports have described healthcare-associated MRSA infections caused by PFTs USA300 and USA400 [22,24–27]. For example, USA300 accounted for 20% of MRSA isolates from nosocomial bloodstream infections at an urban public hospital in Atlanta in 2004 [27]. Some of these infections likely represent endogenous infection following acquisition of colonization in the community [131], but outbreaks of infections associated with probable hospital transmission have also been reported [22,26,28]. It remains to be determined whether establishment of these strains in healthcare settings will result in an increase in MRSA-associated morbidity and mortality among hospitalized patients.

Risk factors for transmission

Clusters or outbreaks of *S. aureus* infection or colonization have occurred among inmates in correctional facilities [155], competitive sports participants [108,156–158], military recruits [159], childcare center attendees [160,161], men who have sex with men [162], residents of evacuation shelters [163], full-term infants in newborn nurseries [22,164], and tattoo recipients [165]. However, the majority of infections occur in people who are not members of any of these groups [89].

Factors common across outbreak settings that facilitate the spread of *S.aureus* include crowding; frequent skin-to-skin contact between people; participation in activities that result in abraded or compromised skin surfaces; sharing of potentially contaminated personal items such as towels, sporting equipment, and razors; challenges in maintaining personal cleanliness and hygiene; and limited access to healthcare [108,158,162,166–170]. For example, in a 2002–2003 outbreak of MRSA in a Missouri prison, MRSA infection was significantly associated with a low composite hygiene score based on frequency of hand-washing and showering and number of personal items shared with other inmates [171]. Environmental surfaces with which people have bare skin contact, such as sauna benches, have also been implicated as a possible route of *S. aureus* transmission [168,172,173].

An increase in MRSA USA300 infections not specifically linked to a nursery outbreak has been described among previously healthy term and near-term newborn infants [40]. A maternal history of *S. aureus* infection or SSTI was reported in over 20% of these infants, suggesting that family members are sometimes a source of neonatal MRSA acquisition during or after delivery.

Several patient characteristics and exposures, including age, race, prior antibiotic exposure, homelessness, lack of chronic medical conditions, close contact with someone with a similar infection, and HIV infection, have been associated with methicillin resistance in community-associated *S. aureus* infections [35,37,42,46,89,174–176]. However, these factors have not been consistent across patient populations. For example, white race has been a risk factor for CA-MRSA infection in some populations [35], while black race has been associated with these infections in other populations [89,131,176]. Furthermore, these factors appear to have poor predictive value for discriminating CA-MRSA infection from CA-MSSA infection in individual patients [174].

Frequent exposure to antimicrobial agents may facilitate acquisition of MRSA. For example, in a case–control study conducted during a large community outbreak of MRSA SSTIs in southwestern Alaska, case-patients received significantly more courses of antimicrobial agents for nonskin infections during the 12 months before the outbreak than age-matched controls without SSTIs [172]. In an outbreak of MRSA SSTIs among professional football players, the risk of infection was almost eight times higher among players who received antimicrobial agents in the year preceding the outbreak than among those who did not. Furthermore, the number of antimicrobial prescriptions received in the year before the outbreak was ten times higher among members of the outbreak team than among people of the same age and sex in the general community [108]. In a UK study, risk of CA-MRSA infection in adults increased with number of antimicrobial drug prescriptions received 30–365 days before the index MRSA culture was obtained, and was highest in patients who received quinolones or macrolides during this period [177]. While trimethoprim–sulfamethoxazole exposure has been negatively associated with MRSA colonization or infection in some HIV-infected patients [162,178], trimethoprim–sulfamethoxazole and clindamycin exposure in the previous 12 months were both associated with infection with a multidrug resistant isolate among HIV clinic patients with MRSA USA300 infections in San Francisco [133].

Prevalence and implications of colonization

In 2001–2002, *S. aureus* and MRSA nasal colonization prevalence estimates among noninstitutionalized people in the USA were 32.4% and 0.8%, respectively, corresponding to an estimated 89.4 million and 2.3 million colonized people [179] (Figure 13.5). The prevalence of *S. aureus* colonization was highest in persons aged 6–11 years, whereas MRSA colonization was associated with age 60 years or more and female sex [179]. The prevalence of *S. aureus* colonization decreased to 28.6% in 2003–2004, while the prevalence of MRSA colonization increased to 1.5%; 19.7% of those colonized with MRSA in 2003–2004 carried a PFT associated with community transmission [180,181]. Some studies in specific populations have shown higher MRSA colonization prevalence or greater increases in MRSA colonization prevalence over time. For example, among pediatric patients attending health maintenance visits at

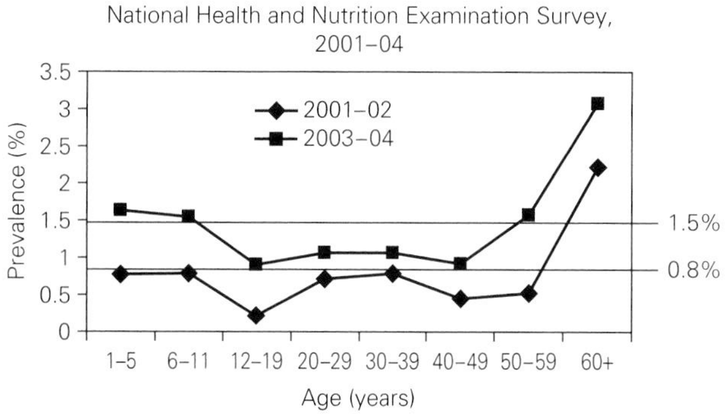

Figure 13.5 Prevalence of methicillin-resistant *S. aureus* colonization by age and survey cycle (N = 18 626). National Health and Nutrition Examination Survey, 2001–2004. (From Gorwitz *et al.* [180] with permission.)

two clinics in Tennessee, MRSA nasal colonization increased from 0.8% in 2001 to 9.2% in 2004 [182]. In addition, 22% of children admitted to a children's hospital in Corpus Christi (or South Texas) during 1 month in 2005 had nasal colonization with MRSA on admission [183], as did 7.3% of adolescent and adult patients admitted to a public urban hospital in Atlanta during a 1-month period in 2003 [184], and 10% of patients of a Dallas HIV clinic during a 2-month period in 2005 [178]. Nasal colonization with *S. aureus* has been identified as a risk factor for subsequent infection [185]. However, few data are available on the association between MRSA colonization and infection in the community. In one study of 812 US Army soldiers presenting for Health Care Specialist training in 2003, nasal colonization with MRSA, as compared with MSSA, was associated with a significantly increased risk of subsequent *S. aureus* SSTI (38% vs. 3%; $P < 0.001$) [186].

Nasal colonization surveys performed in outbreak or highly endemic settings have often failed to identify a substantial pool of MRSA-colonized people [108,168]. Furthermore, nasal MRSA colonization is not always present even in people with active MRSA infections. Among 61 subjects with MRSA SSTIs presenting to a California emergency department, nasal colonization was identified in 21 (34%) [35]. It is possible that some of these people are colonized only at nonnasal sites. The anterior nares have been considered the primary site of MRSA colonization; however, colonization at other sites, such as the pharynx, perineum, rectum, vagina, and axilla, can also occur [161,187]. A study of 67 patients with acute CA-MRSA infections identified MRSA colonization at any of four body sites (nares, axilla, inguinal region, rectum) in 40% of the patients, with nasal and inguinal colonization being most common (identified in 27% and 20% of patients, respectively) [188]. In contrast, in a study of 490 St Louis emergency department patients with skin abscesses (70% confirmed *S. aureus*), 60% of adults and 69% of children were colonized with *S. aureus* in the nares, axilla, and/or groin; the most common site of colonization in adults was the nares (82% of those colonized at any site), while children were equally likely to be colonized in the nares and groin (69% and 70% of those colonized, respectively) [189]. Although colonization screening is not 100% sensitive, failure to identify MRSA colonization at any body site in a substantial proportion of persons with acute CA-MRSA infections suggests that infections may sometimes result from direct inoculation of the infected body site from an exogenous source as opposed to endogenous inoculation from a colonized body site [190].

MRSA isolates with characteristics of USA300 have been detected in vaginal–rectal cultures of pregnant women undergoing prenatal screening for group B streptococcal colonization [191,192]; however, there is currently no evidence to suggest increasing incidence of vertically transmitted, invasive, early-onset neonatal infections due to MRSA. A retrospective study of 5732 pregnant women identified rectovaginal MRSA colonization in 3.5% of the women in late pregnancy, but no cases of early-onset invasive MRSA infection in their newborns [192]. In a prospective study that followed 200 mother–infant pairs until 2 months after delivery, rectovaginal MRSA colonization was detected in 4% of the mothers in late pregnancy and was associated with neonatal MRSA colonization at birth; however, none of the infants colonized with MRSA at birth developed MRSA infections during the first 2 months of life [193]. The implications of maternal MRSA colonization in the vagina and other body sites for the fetus and newborn and appropriate intervention strategies for MRSA-colonized pregnant women require further evaluation.

Prevention and control strategies

No *S. aureus* vaccine is currently available, although such products are under development [194]. Whether an *S. aureus* vaccine, once developed, will prove useful as a prevention strategy in the general population remains to be seen. In the absence of a vaccine, preventing *S. aureus* infections in the community requires an emphasis on general hygiene and wound care. In outbreak settings, strategies focusing on increased awareness, prompt identification and appropriate management of new infections, education about wound care and containment, enhanced hygiene, restricting shared use of potentially contaminated items such as clothing and towels, regular cleaning of frequently touched environmental surfaces, and restricting infected individuals from certain activities if wound drainage cannot be contained appear to have been successful at interrupting transmission [108,156,158,159,168,195].

Regimens to eliminate *S. aureus* colonization have been used in healthcare settings to prevent autoinfection among colonized patients and to control MRSA outbreaks [196]. Decolonization regimens have also been employed in *S. aureus* outbreaks in community settings [197,198]. These regimens have included various combinations of topical and systemic antimicrobial agents and antiseptic body washes and have typically been used as part of multifaceted infection control interventions, which makes it difficult to evaluate the specific contribution of any one component. Data from healthcare settings indicate that intranasal mupirocin can be effective at eliminating *S. aureus* colonization in the short term; however, recolonization is common [199,200].

Data are limited on the effectiveness of decolonization regimens in eliminating *S. aureus* colonization, reducing recurrent infections, or preventing secondary transmission in households or larger aggregate community settings. Two small trials evaluated the use of a monthly 5-day course of nasal mupirocin or a 3-month course of low-dose oral clindamycin to prevent recurrent staphylococcal colonization and infection in nonhospitalized patients with documented recurrent MSSA skin infections [201,202]. Both trials identified significantly fewer SSTI recurrences in the treatment groups. Successful termination of an outbreak of MSSA furunculosis in a German village was reported following decolonization of colonized or infected persons and their family members with a 5-day regimen including intranasal mupirocin; alcohol-based hand sanitizer; bathing, washing hair, and gargling with antiseptic solutions; daily disinfection of personal items; daily washing of clothing and linens; and limited interaction with other village inhabitants [198]. In contrast, a cluster randomized, double-blind, placebo-controlled trial conducted among soldiers attending a 16-week training session found that intranasal mupirocin treatment of soldiers with MRSA nasal colonization upon entry to the training program had no impact on development of MRSA infection among the colonized soldiers or their classmates and also did not prevent new colonization [203]. In another cluster randomized, double-blind, placebo-controlled trial conducted among military trainees, use of chlorhexidine-impregnated cloths for bathing three times a week was not effective in preventing SSTIs. In this study, incident *S. aureus* colonization rates (nasal and axillary) were lower in the intervention group; however, colonization was not a clear risk factor for SSTI [204]. Furthermore, compliance with decolonization regimens may be poor in community settings and widespread or prolonged use of these agents is undesirable due to the promotion of resistance [197,200].

Summary

Staphylococcus aureus has long been a predominant cause of localized and invasive infections in the community. More recently, MRSA has emerged as a cause of community-associated *S. aureus* infections. Strains of MRSA associated with CA-MRSA and HA-MRSA infections initially differed phenotypically and genotypically, but these distinctions are beginning to blur. A small number of MRSA strains have become predominant in the community, and may possess virulence or transmissibility factors conferring increased fitness. While SSTIs are the most common manifestations of both MRSA and MSSA infection in the community, emergence of new MRSA strains in the community may be contributing to an increased overall burden and severity of community-associated *S. aureus* infections. Invasive infections account for a minority of community-associated *S. aureus* infections, and the factors predisposing persons to these invasive manifestations are not well understood. Strategies focusing on increased awareness, prompt recognition and appropriate management of new infections, enhanced hygiene, and maintenance of a clean environment have been successful at limiting transmission of *S. aureus* in the community. Further research is needed to identify the most useful interventions and to develop more effective strategies for prevention and control.

Disclaimer

The findings and conclusions in this report are those of the authors, and do not necessarily represent the views of the Centers for Disease Control and Prevention.

References

1 Lowy FD. *Staphylococcus aureus* infections. N Engl J Med 1998;339:520–32.
2 Travers JB and Mousdicas N. Gram-Positive Infections Associated with Toxin Production. In: Wolff K, Goldsmith LA, Katz SI, Gilchrest BA, Paller AS, and Leffell DJ eds. *Dermatology in General Medicine*, 7th edition. New York, McGraw-Hill, 2008, pp. 1710–1719.
3 Le Loir Y, Baron F, Gautier M. *Staphylococcus aureus* and food poisoning. Genet Mol Res 2003;2:63–76.
4 Waldvogel FA, Papageorgiou PS. Osteomyelitis: the past decade. N Engl J Med 1980;303:360–70.
5 Boyce JM. Methicillin-resistant *Staphylococcus aureus*. Detection, epidemiology, and control measures. Infect Dis Clin North Am 1989;3:901–13.
6 Centers for Disease Control and Prevention. Community-acquired methicillin-resistant *Staphylococcus aureus* infections: Michigan. MMWR 1981;30:185–7.
7 Saravolatz LD, Markowitz N, Arking L, Pohlod D, Fisher E. Methicillin-resistant *Staphylococcus aureus*. Epidemiologic observations during a community-acquired outbreak. Ann Intern Med 1982;96:11–16.
8 Hamoudi AC, Palmer RN, King TL. Nafcillin resistant *Staphylococcus aureus*: a possible community origin. Infect Control 1983;4:153–7.
9 Rathore MH, Kline MW. Community-acquired methicillin-resistant *Staphylococcus aureus* infections in children. Pediatr Infect Dis J 1989;8:645–7.

10 Centers for Disease Control and Prevention. Four pediatric deaths from community-acquired methicillin-resistant *Staphylococcus aureus*: Minnesota and North Dakota, 1997–1999. MMWR 1999;48:707–10.

11 Gorak EJ, Yamada SM, Brown JD. Community-acquired methicillin-resistant *Staphylococcus aureus* in hospitalized adults and children without known risk factors. Clin Infect Dis 1999;29:797–800.

12 Herold BC, Immergluck LC, Maranan MC *et al.* Community-acquired methicillin-resistant *Staphylococcus aureus* in children with no identified predisposing risk. JAMA 1998;279:593–8.

13 Embil J, Ramotar K, Romance L *et al.* Methicillin-resistant *Staphylococcus aureus* in tertiary care institutions on the Canadian prairies 1990–1992. Infect Control Hosp Epidemiol 1994;15:646–51.

14 Maguire GP, Arthur AD, Boustead PJ, Dwyer B, Currie BJ. Emerging epidemic of community-acquired methicillin-resistant *Staphylococcus aureus* infection in the Northern Territory. Med J Aust 1996;164:721–3.

15 Fang YH, Hsueh PR, Hu JJ *et al.* Community-acquired methicillin-resistant *Staphylococcus aureus* in children in northern Taiwan. J Microbiol Immunol Infect 2004;37:29–34.

16 Krishna BV, Patil AB, Chandrasekhar MR. Community-acquired methicillin-resistant *Staphylococcus aureus* infections in a south Indian city. Southeast Asian J Trop Med Public Health 2004;35:371–4.

17 Ribeiro A, Dias C, Silva-Carvalho MC *et al.* First report of infection with community-acquired methicillin-resistant *Staphylococcus aureus* in South America. J Clin Microbiol 2005;43: 1985–8.

18 Vandenesch F, Naimi T, Enright MC *et al.* Community-acquired methicillin-resistant *Staphylococcus aureus* carrying Panton–Valentine leukocidin genes: worldwide emergence. Emerg Infect Dis 2003;9:978–84.

19 Fridkin SK, Hageman JC, Morrison M *et al.* Methicillin-resistant *Staphylococcus aureus* disease in three communities. N Engl J Med 2005;352:1436–44.

20 Kaplan SL, Hulten KG, Gonzalez BE *et al.* Three-year surveillance of community-acquired *Staphylococcus aureus* infections in children. Clin Infect Dis 2005;40:1785–91.

21 Klevens RM, Morrison MA, Nadle J *et al.* Invasive methicillin-resistant *Staphylococcus aureus* infections in the United States. JAMA 2007;298:1763–71.

22 Bratu S, Eramo A, Kopec R *et al.* Community-associated methicillin-resistant *Staphylococcus aureus* in hospital nursery and maternity units. Emerg Infect Dis 2005;11:808–13.

23 Charlebois ED, Perdreau-Remington F, Kreiswirth B *et al.* Origins of community strains of methicillin-resistant *Staphylococcus aureus*. Clin Infect Dis 2004;39:47–54.

24 Healy CM, Hulten KG, Palazzi DL, Campbell JR, Baker CJ. Emergence of new strains of methicillin-resistant *Staphylococcus aureus* in a neonatal intensive care unit. Clin Infect Dis 2004;39:1460–6.

25 Kourbatova EV, Halvosa JS, King MD, Ray SM, White N, Blumberg HM. Emergence of community-associated methicillin-resistant *Staphylococcus aureus* USA 300 clone as a cause of health care-associated infections among patients with prosthetic joint infections. Am J Infect Control 2005;33:385–91.

26 Saiman L, O'Keefe M, Graham PL III *et al.* Hospital transmission of community-acquired methicillin-resistant *Staphylococcus aureus* among postpartum women. Clin Infect Dis 2003;37: 1313–19.

27 Seybold U, Kourbatova EV, Johnson JG *et al.* Emergence of community-associated methicillin-resistant *Staphylococcus aureus* USA300 genotype as a major cause of health care-associated blood stream infections. Clin Infect Dis 2006;42:647–56.

28 James L, Gorwitz RJ, Jones RC *et al.* Methicillin-resistant *Staphylococcus aureus* infections among healthy full-term newborns. Arch Dis Child 2008;93:F40–F44.

29 Darmstadt GL, Lane AT. Impetigo: an overview. Pediatr Dermatol 1994;11:293–303.

30 Demidovich CW, Wittler RR, Ruff ME, Bass JW, Browning WC. Impetigo. Current etiology and comparison of penicillin, erythromycin, and cephalexin therapies. Am J Dis Child 1990; 144:1313–15.

31 McCaig LF, McDonald LC, Mandal S, Jernigan DB. *Staphylococcus aureus*-associated skin and soft tissue infections in ambulatory care. Emerg Infect Dis 2006;12:1715–23.

32 Baggett HC, Hennessy TW, Leman R *et al.* An outbreak of community-onset methicillin-resistant *Staphylococcus aureus* skin infections in southwestern Alaska. Infect Control Hosp Epidemiol 2003;24:397–402.

33 Swanson DL, Vetter RS. Bites of brown recluse spiders and suspected necrotic arachnidism. N Engl J Med 2005;352:700–7.

34 Daum RS. Clinical practice. Skin and soft-tissue infections caused by methicillin-resistant *Staphylococcus aureus*. N Engl J Med 2007;357:380–90.

35 Frazee BW, Lynn J, Charlebois ED, Lambert L, Lowery D, Perdreau-Remington F. High prevalence of methicillin-resistant *Staphylococcus aureus* in emergency department skin and soft tissue infections. Ann Emerg Med 2005;45:311–20.

36 Naimi TS, LeDell KH, Boxrud DJ *et al.* Epidemiology and clonality of community-acquired methicillin-resistant *Staphylococcus aureus* in Minnesota, 1996–1998. Clin Infect Dis 2001;33:990–6.

37 Chen AE, Goldstein M, Carroll K, Song X, Perl TM, Siberry GK. Evolving epidemiology of pediatric *Staphylococcus aureus* cutaneous infections in a Baltimore hospital. Pediatr Emerg Care 2006;22:717–23.

38 Szczesiul JM, Shermock KM, Murtaza UI, Siberry GK. No decrease in clindamycin susceptibility despite increased use of clindamycin for pediatric community-associated methicillin-resistant *Staphylococcus aureus* skin infections. Pediatr Infect Dis J 2007;26:852–4.

39 Centers for Disease Control and Prevention. Community-associated methicillin-resistant *Staphylococcus aureus* infection among healthy newborns: Chicago and Los Angeles County, 2004. MMWR 2006;55:329–32.

40 Fortunov RM, Hulten KG, Hammerman WA, Mason EO Jr, Kaplan SL. Community-acquired *Staphylococcus aureus* infections in term and near-term previously healthy neonates. Pediatrics 2006;118:874–81.

41 Miller LG, Quan C, Shay A *et al.* A prospective investigation of outcomes after hospital discharge for endemic, community-acquired methicillin-resistant and -susceptible *Staphylococcus aureus* skin infection. Clin Infect Dis 2007;44:483–92.

42 Davis SL, Perri MB, Donabedian SM *et al.* Epidemiology and outcomes of community-associated methicillin-resistant *Staphylococcus aureus* infection. J Clin Microbiol 2007;45:1705–11.

43 Hedstrom SA. Treatment and prevention of recurrent staphylococcal furunculosis: clinical and bacteriological follow-up. Scand J Infect Dis 1985;17:55–8.
44 Nahmias AJ, Lepper MH, Hurst V, Mudd S. Epidemiology and treatment of chronic staphylococcal infections in the household. Am J Public Health Nations Health 1962;52:1828–43.
45 David MZ, Mennella C, Mansour M, Boyle-Vavra S, Daum RS. Predominance of methicillin-resistant *Staphylococcus aureus* among pathogens causing skin and soft tissue infections in a large urban jail: risk factors and recurrence rates. J Clin Microbiol 2008;46:3222–7.
46 Szumowski JD, Cohen DE, Kanaya F, Mayer KH. Treatment and outcomes of infections by methicillin-resistant *Staphylococcus aureus* at an ambulatory clinic. Antimicrob Agents Chemother 2007;51:423–8.
47 Graber CJ, Jacobson MA, Perdreau-Remington F, Chambers HF, Diep BA. Recurrence of skin and soft tissue infection caused by methicillin-resistant *Staphylococcus aureus* in a HIV primary care clinic. J Acquir Immune Defic Syndr 2008;49:231–3.
48 Arnold SR, Elias D, Buckingham SC *et al*. Changing patterns of acute hematogenous osteomyelitis and septic arthritis: emergence of community-associated methicillin-resistant *Staphylococcus aureus*. J Pediatr Orthop 2006;26:703–8.
49 Saavedra-Lozano J, Mejias A, Ahmad N *et al*. Changing trends in acute osteomyelitis in children: impact of methicillin-resistant *Staphylococcus aureus* infections. J Pediatr Orthop 2008;28:569–75.
50 Martinez-Aguilar G, Avalos-Mishaan A, Hulten K, Hammerman W, Mason EO Jr, Kaplan SL. Community-acquired, methicillin-resistant and methicillin-susceptible *Staphylococcus aureus* musculoskeletal infections in children. Pediatr Infect Dis J 2004;23:701–6.
51 Gonzalez BE, Teruya J, Mahoney DH Jr *et al*. Venous thrombosis associated with staphylococcal osteomyelitis in children. Pediatrics 2006;117:1673–9.
52 Gonzalez BE, Hulten KG, Dishop MK *et al*. Pulmonary manifestations in children with invasive community-acquired *Staphylococcus aureus* infection. Clin Infect Dis 2005;41:583–90.
53 Pannaraj PS, Hulten KG, Gonzalez BE, Mason EO Jr, Kaplan SL. Infective pyomyositis and myositis in children in the era of community-acquired, methicillin-resistant *Staphylococcus aureus* infection. Clin Infect Dis 2006;43:953–60.
54 Marston BJ, Plouffe JF, File TM Jr *et al*. Incidence of community-acquired pneumonia requiring hospitalization. Results of a population-based active surveillance study in Ohio. The Community-Based Pneumonia Incidence Study Group. Arch Intern Med 1997;157:1709–18.
55 Chickering H, Park J. *Staphylococcus aureus* pneumonia. JAMA 1919;72:617–26.
56 Martin CM, Kunin CM, Gottlieb LS, Finland M. Asian influenza A in Boston, 1957–1958. II. Severe staphylococcal pneumonia complicating influenza. AMA Arch Intern Med 1959;103:532–42.
57 Schwarzmann SW, Adler JL, Sullivan RJ Jr, Marine WM. Bacterial pneumonia during the Hong Kong influenza epidemic of 1968–1969. Arch Intern Med 1971;127:1037–41.
58 Centers for Disease Control and Prevention. Severe methicillin-resistant *Staphylococcus aureus* community-acquired pneumonia associated with influenza: Louisiana and Georgia, December 2006 to January 2007. MMWR 2007;56:325–9.
59 Gillet Y, Vanhems P, Lina G *et al*. Factors predicting mortality in necrotizing community-acquired pneumonia caused by *Staphylococcus aureus* containing Panton–Valentine leukocidin. Clin Infect Dis 2007;45:315–21.
60 Hageman JC, Uyeki TM, Francis JS *et al*. Severe community-acquired pneumonia due to *Staphylococcus aureus*, 2003–04 influenza season. Emerg Infect Dis 2006;12:894–9.
61 Abramson JS, Lewis JC, Lyles DS, Heller KA, Mills EL, Bass DA. Inhibition of neutrophil lysosome–phagosome fusion associated with influenza virus infection in vitro. Role in depressed bactericidal activity. J Clin Invest 1982;69:1393–7.
62 Davison VE, Sanford BA. Adherence of *Staphylococcus aureus* to influenza A virus-infected Madin-Darby canine kidney cell cultures. Infect Immun 1981;32:118–26.
63 Nickerson CL, Jakab GJ. Pulmonary antibacterial defenses during mild and severe influenza virus infection. Infect Immun 1990;58:2809–14.
64 Sanford BA, Ramsay MA. Bacterial adherence to the upper respiratory tract of ferrets infected with influenza A virus. Proc Soc Exp Biol Med 1987;185:120–8.
65 Tashiro M, Ciborowski P, Reinacher M, Pulverer G, Klenk HD, Rott R. Synergistic role of staphylococcal proteases in the induction of influenza virus pathogenicity. Virology 1987; 157:421–30.
66 Francis JS, Doherty MC, Lopatin U *et al*. Severe community-onset pneumonia in healthy adults caused by methicillin-resistant *Staphylococcus aureus* carrying the Panton–Valentine leukocidin genes. Clin Infect Dis 2005;40:100–7.
67 Kallen AJ, Brunkard J, Moore Z *et al*. *Staphylococcus aureus* community-acquired pneumonia during the 2006 to 2007 influenza season. Ann Emerg Med 2009;53:358–65.
68 Finelli L, Fiore A, Dhara R *et al*. Influenza-associated pediatric mortality in the United States: increase of *Staphylococcus aureus* coinfection. Pediatrics 2008;122:805–11.
69 Alfaro C, Fergie J, Purcell K. Emergence of community-acquired methicillin-resistant *Staphylococcus aureus* in complicated parapneumonic effusions. Pediatr Infect Dis J 2005;24:274–6.
70 Buckingham SC, King MD, Miller ML. Incidence and etiologies of complicated parapneumonic effusions in children, 1996 to 2001. Pediatr Infect Dis J 2003;22:499–504.
71 Schultz KD, Fan LL, Pinsky J *et al*. The changing face of pleural empyemas in children: epidemiology and management. Pediatrics 2004;113:1735–40.
72 Weinstein MP, Towns ML, Quartey SM *et al*. The clinical significance of positive blood cultures in the 1990s: a prospective comprehensive evaluation of the microbiology, epidemiology, and outcome of bacteremia and fungemia in adults. Clin Infect Dis 1997;24:584–602.
73 Mylotte JM, McDermott C, Spooner JA. Prospective study of 114 consecutive episodes of *Staphylococcus aureus* bacteremia. Rev Infect Dis 1987;9:891–907.
74 Sanabria TJ, Alpert JS, Goldberg R, Pape LA, Cheeseman SH. Increasing frequency of staphylococcal infective endocarditis. Experience at a university hospital, 1981 through 1988. Arch Intern Med 1990;150:1305–9.
75 Watanakunakorn C, Burkert T. Infective endocarditis at a large community teaching hospital, 1980–1990. A review of 210 episodes. Medicine (Baltimore) 1993;72:90–102.
76 Crane LR, Levine DP, Zervos MJ, Cummings G. Bacteremia in narcotic addicts at the Detroit Medical Center. I. Microbiology,

epidemiology, risk factors, and empiric therapy. Rev Infect Dis 1986;8:364–73.

77 Haque NZ, Davis SL, Manierski CL *et al.* Infective endocarditis caused by USA300 methicillin-resistant *Staphylococcus aureus* (MRSA). Int J Antimicrob Agents 2007;30:72–7.

78 Fleisch F, Zbinden R, Vanoli C, Ruef C. Epidemic spread of a single clone of methicillin-resistant *Staphylococcus aureus* among injection drug users in Zurich, Switzerland. Clin Infect Dis 2001;32:581–6.

79 Bahrain M, Vasiliades M, Wolff M, Younus F. Five cases of bacterial endocarditis after furunculosis and the ongoing saga of community-acquired methicillin-resistant *Staphylococcus aureus* infections. Scand J Infect Dis 2006;38:702–7.

80 Gonzalez BE, Martinez-Aguilar G, Hulten KG *et al.* Severe staphylococcal sepsis in adolescents in the era of community-acquired methicillin-resistant *Staphylococcus aureus*. Pediatrics 2005;115:642–8.

81 Adem PV, Montgomery CP, Husain AN *et al. Staphylococcus aureus* sepsis and the Waterhouse–Friderichsen syndrome in children. N Engl J Med 2005;353:1245–51.

82 Miller LG, Perdreau-Remington F, Rieg G *et al.* Necrotizing fasciitis caused by community-associated methicillin-resistant *Staphylococcus aureus* in Los Angeles. N Engl J Med 2005;352:1445–53.

83 Holmberg SD, Blake PA. Staphylococcal food poisoning in the United States. New facts and old misconceptions. JAMA 1984;251:487–9.

84 Gaventa S, Reingold AL, Hightower AW *et al.* Active surveillance for toxic shock syndrome in the United States, 1986. Rev Infect Dis 1989;11(suppl 1):S28–S34.

85 Hajjeh RA, Reingold A, Weil A, Shutt K, Schuchat A, Perkins BA. Toxic shock syndrome in the United States: surveillance update, 1979–1996. Emerg Infect Dis 1999;5:807–10.

86 Descloux E, Perpoint T, Ferry T *et al.* One in five mortality in non-menstrual toxic shock syndrome versus no mortality in menstrual cases in a balanced French series of 55 cases. Eur J Clin Microbiol Infect Dis 2008;27:37–43.

87 Kain KC, Schulzer M, Chow AW. Clinical spectrum of non-menstrual toxic shock syndrome (TSS): comparison with menstrual TSS by multivariate discriminant analyses. Clin Infect Dis 1993;16:100–6.

88 Johnson JK, Khoie T, Shurland S, Kreisel K, Stine OC, Roghman MC. Skin and soft tissue infections caused by methicillin-resistant *Staphylococcus aureus* USA300 clone. Emerg Infect Dis 2007;13:1195–200.

89 Moran GJ, Krishnadasan A, Gorwitz RJ *et al.* Methicillin-resistant *S. aureus* infections among patients in the emergency department. N Engl J Med 2006;355:666–74.

90 Moran GJ, Amii RN, Abrahamian FM, Talan DA. Methicillin-resistant *Staphylococcus aureus* in community-acquired skin infections. Emerg Infect Dis 2005;11:928–30.

91 Ossowski K, Chun RH, Suskind D, Baroody FM. Increased isolation of methicillin-resistant *Staphylococcus aureus* in pediatric head and neck abscesses. Arch Otolaryngol Head Neck Surg 2006;132:1176–81.

92 Okuma K, Iwakawa K, Turnidge JD *et al.* Dissemination of new methicillin-resistant *Staphylococcus aureus* clones in the community. J Clin Microbiol 2002;40:4289–94.

93 Boyle-Vavra S, Daum RS. Community-acquired methicillin-resistant *Staphylococcus aureus*: the role of Panton–Valentine leukocidin. Lab Invest 2007;87:3–9.

94 McDougal LK, Steward CD, Killgore GE, Chaitram JM, McAllister SK, Tenover FC. Pulsed-field gel electrophoresis typing of oxacillin-resistant *Staphylococcus aureus* isolates from the United States: establishing a national database. J Clin Microbiol 2003;41:5113–20.

95 McDougal LK, Wenming Z, Patel JB, Tenover FC. Characterization of two new community-associated oxacillin-resistant *Staphylococcus aureus* pulsed-field types consisting of U.S. isolates that carry SCC*mec*IV and the Panton–Valentine leukocidin gene [Abstract]. Presented at the 104th General Meeting of the American Society for Microbiology, New Orleans, LA, 2004.

96 Carleton HA, Diep BA, Charlebois ED, Sensabaugh GF, Perdreau-Remington F. Community-adapted methicillin-resistant *Staphylococcus aureus* (MRSA): population dynamics of an expanding community reservoir of MRSA. J Infect Dis 2004;190:1730–8.

97 Johnson LB, Saeed S, Pawlak J, Manzor O, Saravolatz LD. Clinical and laboratory features of community-associated methicillin-resistant *Staphylococcus aureus*: is it really new? Infect Control Hosp Epidemiol 2006;27:133–8.

98 Chavez-Bueno S, Bozdogan B, Katz K *et al.* Inducible clindamycin resistance and molecular epidemiologic trends of pediatric community-acquired methicillin-resistant *Staphylococcus aureus* in Dallas, Texas. Antimicrob Agents Chemother 2005;49:2283–8.

99 Mishaan AM, Mason EO Jr, Martinez-Aguilar G *et al.* Emergence of a predominant clone of community-acquired *Staphylococcus aureus* among children in Houston, Texas. Pediatr Infect Dis J 2005;24:201–6.

100 King MD, Humphrey BJ, Wang YF, Kourbatova EV, Ray SM, Blumberg HM. Emergence of community-acquired methicillin-resistant *Staphylococcus aureus* USA 300 clone as the predominant cause of skin and soft-tissue infections. Ann Intern Med 2006;144:309–17.

101 Bhattacharya D, Carleton H, Tsai CJ, Baron EJ, Perdreau-Remington F. Differences in clinical and molecular characteristics of skin and soft tissue methicillin-resistant *Staphylococcus aureus* isolates between two hospitals in Northern California. J Clin Microbiol 2007;45:1798–803.

102 David MZ, Rudolph KM, Hennessy TW, Boyle-Vavra S, Daum RS. Molecular epidemiology of methicillin-resistant *Staphylococcus aureus*, rural southwestern Alaska. Emerg Infect Dis 2008;14:1693–9.

103 Ma XX, Galiana A, Pedreira W *et al.* Community-acquired methicillin-resistant *Staphylococcus aureus*, Uruguay. Emerg Infect Dis 2005;11:973–6.

104 Robinson DA, Kearns AM, Holmes A *et al.* Re-emergence of early pandemic *Staphylococcus aureus* as a community-acquired meticillin-resistant clone. Lancet 2005;365:1256–8.

105 Holmes A, Ganner M, McGuane S, Pitt TL, Cookson BD, Kearns AM. *Staphylococcus aureus* isolates carrying Panton–Valentine leucocidin genes in England and Wales: frequency, characterization, and association with clinical disease. J Clin Microbiol 2005;43:2384–90.

106 Wannet WJ, Spalburg E, Heck ME *et al.* Emergence of virulent methicillin-resistant *Staphylococcus aureus* strains carrying Panton–Valentine leucocidin genes in The Netherlands. J Clin Microbiol 2005;43:3341–5.

107 Witte W, Braulke C, Cuny C *et al.* Emergence of methicillin-resistant *Staphylococcus aureus* with Panton–Valentine leukocidin

genes in central Europe. Eur J Clin Microbiol Infect Dis 2005;24:1–5.
108 Kazakova SV, Hageman JC, Matava M *et al*. A clone of methicillin-resistant *Staphylococcus aureus* among professional football players. N Engl J Med 2005;352:468–75.
109 Tenover FC, McDougal LK, Goering RV *et al*. Characterization of a strain of community-associated methicillin-resistant *Staphylococcus aureus* widely disseminated in the United States. J Clin Microbiol 2006;44:108–18.
110 Diep BA, Gill SR, Chang RF *et al*. Complete genome sequence of USA300, an epidemic clone of community-acquired meticillin-resistant *Staphylococcus aureus*. Lancet 2006;367:731–9.
111 Diep BA, Stone GG, Basuino L *et al*. The arginine catabolic mobile element and staphylococcal chromosomal cassette *mec* linkage: convergence of virulence and resistance in the USA300 clone of methicillin-resistant *Staphylococcus aureus*. J Infect Dis 2008;197:1523–30.
112 Ellington MJ, Yearwood L, Ganner M, East C, Kearns AM. Distribution of the ACME-arcA gene among methicillin-resistant *Staphylococcus aureus* from England and Wales. J Antimicrob Chemother 2008;61:73–7.
113 Goering RV, McDougal LK, Fosheim GE, Bonnstetter KK, Wolter DJ, Tenover FC. Epidemiologic distribution of the arginine catabolic mobile element among selected methicillin-resistant and methicillin-susceptible *Staphylococcus aureus* isolates. J Clin Microbiol 2007;45:1981–4.
114 Gillet Y, Issartel B, Vanhems P *et al*. Association between *Staphylococcus aureus* strains carrying gene for Panton–Valentine leukocidin and highly lethal necrotising pneumonia in young immunocompetent patients. Lancet 2002;359:753–9.
115 Lina G, Piemont Y, Godail-Gamot F *et al*. Involvement of Panton–Valentine leukocidin-producing *Staphylococcus aureus* in primary skin infections and pneumonia. Clin Infect Dis 1999;29:1128–32.
116 Naimi TS, LeDell KH, Como-Sabetti K *et al*. Comparison of community- and health care-associated methicillin-resistant *Staphylococcus aureus* infection. JAMA 2003;290:2976–84.
117 Coombs GW, Pearson JC, O'Brien FG, Murray RJ, Grubb WB, Christiansen KJ. Methicillin-resistant *Staphylococcus aureus* clones, Western Australia. Emerg Infect Dis 2006;12:241–7.
118 O'Brien FG, Lim TT, Chong FN *et al*. Diversity among community isolates of methicillin-resistant *Staphylococcus aureus* in Australia. J Clin Microbiol 2004;42:3185–90.
119 Ma XX, Ito T, Chongtrakool P, Hiramatsu K. Predominance of clones carrying Panton–Valentine leukocidin genes among methicillin-resistant *Staphylococcus aureus* strains isolated in Japanese hospitals from 1979 to 1985. J Clin Microbiol 2006; 44:4515–27.
120 Coombs GW, Nimmo GR, Bell JM *et al*. Genetic diversity among community methicillin-resistant *Staphylococcus aureus* strains causing outpatient infections in Australia. J Clin Microbiol 2004;42:4735–43.
121 Hsu LY, Tristan A, Koh TH *et al*. Community associated methicillin-resistant *Staphylococcus aureus*, Singapore. Emerg Infect Dis 2005;11:341–2.
122 Pan ES, Diep BA, Carleton HA *et al*. Increasing prevalence of methicillin-resistant *Staphylococcus aureus* infection in California jails. Clin Infect Dis 2003;37:1384–8.
123 Bocchini CE, Hulten KG, Mason EO Jr, Gonzalez BE, Hammerman WA, Kaplan SL. Panton–Valentine leukocidin genes are associated with enhanced inflammatory response and local disease in acute hematogenous *Staphylococcus aureus* osteomyelitis in children. Pediatrics 2006;117:433–40.
124 Labandeira-Rey M, Couzon F, Boisset S *et al*. *Staphylococcus aureus* Panton–Valentine leukocidin causes necrotizing pneumonia. Science 2007;315:1130–3.
125 Voyich JM, Otto M, Mathema B *et al*. Is Panton–Valentine leukocidin the major virulence determinant in community-associated methicillin-resistant *Staphylococcus aureus* disease? J Infect Dis 2006;194:1761–70.
126 Diep BA, Palazzolo-Ballance AM, Tattevin P *et al*. Contribution of Panton–Valentine leukocidin in community-associated methicillin-resistant *Staphylococcus aureus* pathogenesis. PLoS ONE 2008;3:e3198.
127 Hamilton SM, Bryant AE, Carroll KC *et al*. In vitro production of Panton–Valentine leukocidin among strains of methicillin-resistant *Staphylococcus aureus* causing diverse infections. Clin Infect Dis 2007;45:1550–8.
128 Wang R, Braughton KR, Kretschmer D *et al*. Identification of novel cytolytic peptides as key virulence determinants for community-associated MRSA. Nat Med 2007;13:1510–14.
129 Emonts M, Uitterlinden AG, Nouwen JL *et al*. Host polymorphisms in interleukin 4, complement factor H, and C-reactive protein associated with nasal carriage of *Staphylococcus aureus* and occurrence of boils. J Infect Dis 2008;197:1244–53.
130 Nygaard TK, DeLeo FR, Voyich JM. Community-associated methicillin-resistant *Staphylococcus aureus* skin infections: advances toward identifying the key virulence factors. Curr Opin Infect Dis 2008;21:147–52.
131 Liu C, Graber CJ, Karr M *et al*. A population-based study of the incidence and molecular epidemiology of methicillin-resistant *Staphylococcus aureus* disease in San Francisco, 2004–2005. Clin Infect Dis 2008;46:1637–46.
132 Hulten KG, Kaplan SL, Gonzalez BE *et al*. Three-year surveillance of community onset health care-associated *Staphylococcus aureus* infections in children. Pediatr Infect Dis J 2006; 25:349–53.
133 Diep BA, Chambers HF, Graber CJ *et al*. Emergence of multidrug-resistant, community-associated, methicillin-resistant *Staphylococcus aureus* clone USA300 in men who have sex with men. Ann Intern Med 2008;148:249–57.
134 Han LL, McDougal LK, Gorwitz RJ *et al*. High frequencies of clindamycin and tetracycline resistance in methicillin-resistant *Staphylococcus aureus* pulsed-field type USA300 isolates collected at a Boston ambulatory health center. J Clin Microbiol 2007;45:1350–2.
135 Berg T, Firth N, Apisiridej S, Hettiaratchi A, Leelaporn A, Skurray RA. Complete nucleotide sequence of pSK41: evolution of staphylococcal conjugative multiresistance plasmids. J Bacteriol 1998;180:4350–9.
136 McDougal LK, Fosheim GE, Patel JB, Team A. Emergence of resistance among USA300 MRSA isolates causing invasive disease in the U.S. [Abstract]. Presented at the 48th Annual Interscience Conference on Antimicrobial Agents and Chemotherapy (ICAAC) and the Infectious Diseases Society of America (IDSA) 46th Annual Meeting, Washington, DC, 2008.
137 Graber CJ, Wong MK, Carleton HA, Perdreau-Remington F, Haller BL, Chambers HF. Intermediate vancomycin susceptibility in a community-associated MRSA clone. Emerg Infect Dis 2007;13:491–3.

138 Hageman JC, Patel J, Franklin P *et al*. Occurrence of a USA300 vancomycin-intermediate *Staphylococcus aureus*. Diagn Microbiol Infect Dis 2008;62:440–2.
139 Boyle-Vavra S, Ereshefsky B, Wang CC, Daum RS. Successful multiresistant community-associated methicillin-resistant *Staphylococcus aureus* lineage from Taipei, Taiwan, that carries either the novel staphylococcal chromosome cassette *mec* (SCC*mec*) type VT or SCC*mec* type IV. J Clin Microbiol 2005;43:4719–30.
140 Katayama Y, Ito T, Hiramatsu K. A new class of genetic element, staphylococcus cassette chromosome *mec*, encodes methicillin resistance in *Staphylococcus aureus*. Antimicrob Agents Chemother 2000;44:1549–55.
141 Mongkolrattanothai K, Boyle S, Kahana MD, Daum RS. Severe *Staphylococcus aureus* infections caused by clonally related community-acquired methicillin-susceptible and methicillin-resistant isolates. Clin Infect Dis 2003;37:1050–8.
142 McCaskill ML, Mason EO Jr, Kaplan SL, Hammerman W, Lamberth LB, Hulten KG. Increase of the USA300 clone among community-acquired methicillin-susceptible *Staphylococcus aureus* causing invasive infections. Pediatr Infect Dis J 2007;26:1122–7.
143 Hersh AL, Chambers HF, Maselli JH, Gonzales R. National trends in ambulatory visits and antibiotic prescribing for skin and soft-tissue infections. Arch Intern Med 2008;168:1585–91.
144 Pallin DJ, Egan DJ, Pelletier AJ, Espinola JA, Hooper DC, Camargo CA Jr. Increased US emergency department visits for skin and soft tissue infections, and changes in antibiotic choices, during the emergence of community-associated methicillin-resistant *Staphylococcus aureus*. Ann Emerg Med 2008;51:291–8.
145 Klein E, Smith DL, Laxminarayan R. Hospitalizations and deaths caused by methicillin-resistant *Staphylococcus aureus*, United States, 1999–2005. Emerg Infect Dis 2007;13:1840–6.
146 Kuehnert MJ, Hill HA, Kupronis BA, Tokars JI, Solomon SL, Jernigan DB. Methicillin-resistant-*Staphylococcus aureus* hospitalizations, United States. Emerg Infect Dis 2005;11:868–72.
147 Noskin GA, Rubin RJ, Schentag JJ *et al*. The burden of *Staphylococcus aureus* infections on hospitals in the United States: an analysis of the 2000 and 2001 Nationwide Inpatient Sample Database. Arch Intern Med 2005;165:1756–61.
148 Morin CA, Hadler JL. Population-based incidence and characteristics of community-onset *Staphylococcus aureus* infections with bacteremia in 4 metropolitan Connecticut areas, 1998. J Infect Dis 2001;184:1029–34.
149 Petit S, Fraser Z, Mandour M, Hadler JL. Trends in invasive infection with methicillin-resistant *Staphylococcus aureus* (MRSA) in Connecticut, 2001–2006 [Abstract]. Presented at the International Conference on Emerging Infectious Diseases, Atlanta, GA, 2008.
150 Buckingham SC, McDougal LK, Cathey LD *et al*. Emergence of community-associated methicillin-resistant *Staphylococcus aureus* at a Memphis, Tennessee Children's Hospital. Pediatr Infect Dis J 2004;23:619–24.
151 Ochoa TJ, Mohr J, Wanger A, Murphy JR, Heresi GP. Community-associated methicillin-resistant *Staphylococcus aureus* in pediatric patients. Emerg Infect Dis 2005;11:966–8.
152 Estivariz CF, Park SY, Hageman JC *et al*. Emergence of community-associated methicillin resistant *Staphylococcus aureus* in Hawaii, 2001–2003. J Infect 2007;54:349–57.
153 Groom AV, Wolsey DH, Naimi TS *et al*. Community-acquired methicillin-resistant *Staphylococcus aureus* in a rural American Indian community. JAMA 2001;286:1201–5.
154 Young DM, Harris HW, Charlebois ED *et al*. An epidemic of methicillin-resistant *Staphylococcus aureus* soft tissue infections among medically underserved patients. Arch Surg 2004; 139:947–51; discussion 951–3.
155 Centers for Disease Control and Prevention. Methicillin-resistant *Staphylococcus aureus* infections in correctional facilities: Georgia, California, and Texas, 2001–2003. MMWR 2003;52:992–6.
156 Lindenmayer JM, Schoenfeld S, O'Grady R, Carney JK. Methicillin-resistant *Staphylococcus aureus* in a high school wrestling team and the surrounding community. Arch Intern Med 1998;158:895–9.
157 Centers for Disease Control and Prevention. Methicillin-resistant *Staphylococcus aureus* infections among competitive sports participants: Colorado, Indiana, Pennsylvania, and Los Angeles County, 2000–2003. MMWR 2003;52:793–95.
158 Sosin DM, Gunn RA, Ford WL, Skaggs JW. An outbreak of furunculosis among high school athletes. Am J Sports Med 1989;17:828–32.
159 Zinderman CE, Conner B, Malakooti MA, LaMar JE, Armstrong A, Bohnker BK. Community-acquired methicillin-resistant *Staphylococcus aureus* among military recruits. Emerg Infect Dis 2004;10:941–4.
160 Adcock PM, Pastor P, Medley F, Patterson JE, Murphy TV. Methicillin-resistant *Staphylococcus aureus* in two child care centers. J Infect Dis 1998;178:577–80.
161 Shahin R, Johnson IL, Jamieson F, McGeer A, Tolkin J, Ford-Jones EL. Methicillin-resistant *Staphylococcus aureus* carriage in a child care center following a case of disease. Toronto Child Care Center Study Group. Arch Pediatr Adolesc Med 1999; 153:864–8.
162 Lee NE, Taylor MM, Bancroft E *et al*. Risk factors for community-associated methicillin-resistant *Staphylococcus aureus* skin infections among HIV-positive men who have sex with men. Clin Infect Dis 2005;40:1529–34.
163 Centers for Disease Control and Prevention. Infectious disease and dermatologic conditions in evacuees and rescue workers after Hurricane Katrina: multiple states, August–September, 2005. MMWR 2005;54:961–4.
164 Centers for Disease Control and Prevention. Outbreaks of community-associated methicillin-resistant *Staphylococcus aureus* skin infections among healthy newborns: Chicago and Los Angeles County, 2004. MMWR 2006;55:329–32.
165 Centers for Disease Control and Prevention. Methicillin-resistant *Staphylococcus aureus* skin infections among tattoo recipients: Ohio, Kentucky, and Vermont, 2004–2005. MMWR 2006;55:677–9.
166 Bartlett PC, Martin RJ, Cahill BR. Furunculosis in a high school football team. Am J Sports Med 1982;10:371–4.
167 Begier EM, Frenette K, Barrett NL *et al*. A high-morbidity outbreak of methicillin-resistant *Staphylococcus aureus* among players on a college football team, facilitated by cosmetic body shaving and turf burns. Clin Infect Dis 2004;39:1446–53.
168 Coronado F, Nicholas JA, Wallace BJ *et al*. Community-associated methicillin-resistant *Staphylococcus aureus* skin infections in a religious community. Epidemiol Infect 2007;135: 492–501.

169 Decker MD, Lybarger JA, Vaughn WK, Hutcheson RH Jr, Schaffner W. An outbreak of staphylococcal skin infections among river rafting guides. Am J Epidemiol 1986;124:969–76.
170 Nguyen DM, Mascola L, Brancoft E. Recurring methicillin-resistant *Staphylococcus aureus* infections in a football team. Emerg Infect Dis 2005;11:526–32.
171 Turabelidze G, Lin M, Wolkoff B, Dodson D, Gladbach S, Zhu BP. Personal hygiene and methicillin-resistant *Staphylococcus aureus* infection. Emerg Infect Dis 2006;12:422–7.
172 Baggett HC, Hennessy TW, Rudolph K *et al*. Community-onset methicillin-resistant *Staphylococcus aureus* associated with antibiotic use and the cytotoxin Panton–Valentine leukocidin during a furunculosis outbreak in rural Alaska. J Infect Dis 2004;189:1565–73.
173 Landen MG, McCumber BJ, Asam ED, Egeland GM. Outbreak of boils in an Alaskan village: a case-control study. West J Med 2000;172:235–9.
174 Miller LG, Perdreau-Remington F, Bayer AS *et al*. Clinical and epidemiologic characteristics cannot distinguish community-associated methicillin-resistant *Staphylococcus aureus* infection from methicillin-susceptible *S. aureus* infection: a prospective investigation. Clin Infect Dis 2007;44:471–82.
175 Sattler CA, Mason EO Jr, Kaplan SL. Prospective comparison of risk factors and demographic and clinical characteristics of community-acquired, methicillin-resistant versus methicillin-susceptible *Staphylococcus aureus* infection in children. Pediatr Infect Dis J 2002;21:910–17.
176 Skiest DJ, Brown K, Cooper TW, Hoffman-Roberts H, Mussa HR, Elliott AC. Prospective comparison of methicillin-susceptible and methicillin-resistant community-associated *Staphylococcus aureus* infections in hospitalized patients. J Infect 2007;54:427–34.
177 Schneider-Lindner V, Delaney JA, Dial S, Dascal A, Suissa S. Antimicrobial drugs and community-acquired methicillin-resistant *Staphylococcus aureus*, United Kingdom. Emerg Infect Dis 2007;13:994–1000.
178 Cenizal MJ, Hardy RD, Anderson M, Katz K, Skiest DJ. Prevalence of and risk factors for methicillin-resistant *Staphylococcus aureus* (MRSA) nasal colonization in HIV-infected ambulatory patients. J Acquir Immune Defic Syndr 2008; 48:567–71.
179 Kuehnert MJ, Kruszon-Moran D, Hill HA *et al*. Prevalence of *Staphylococcus aureus* nasal colonization in the United States, 2001–2002. J Infect Dis 2006;193:172–9.
180 Gorwitz RJ, Kruszon-Moran D, McAllister SK *et al*. Changes in the prevalence of nasal colonization with *Staphylococcus aureus* in the United States, 2001–2004. J Infect Dis 2008;197:1226–34.
181 Tenover FC, McAllister S, Fosheim G *et al*. Characterization of *Staphylococcus aureus* isolates from nasal cultures collected from individuals in the United States in 2001 to 2004. J Clin Microbiol 2008;46:2837–41.
182 Creech CB II, Kernodle DS, Alsentzer A, Wilson C, Edwards KM. Increasing rates of nasal carriage of methicillin-resistant *Staphylococcus aureus* in healthy children. Pediatr Infect Dis J 2005;24:617–21.
183 Alfaro C, Mascher-Denen M, Fergie J, Purcell K. Prevalence of methicillin-resistant *Staphylococcus aureus* nasal carriage in patients admitted to Driscoll Children's Hospital. Pediatr Infect Dis J 2006;25:459–61.
184 Hidron AI, Kourbatova EV, Halvosa JS *et al*. Risk factors for colonization with methicillin-resistant *Staphylococcus aureus* (MRSA) in patients admitted to an urban hospital: emergence of community-associated MRSA nasal carriage. Clin Infect Dis 2005;41:159–66.
185 Kluytmans J, van Belkum A, Verbrugh H. Nasal carriage of *Staphylococcus aureus*: epidemiology, underlying mechanisms, and associated risks. Clin Microbiol Rev 1997;10:505–20.
186 Ellis MW, Hospenthal DR, Dooley DP, Gray PJ, Murray CK. Natural history of community-acquired methicillin-resistant *Staphylococcus aureus* colonization and infection in soldiers. Clin Infect Dis 2004;39:971–9.
187 Eveillard M, de Lassence A, Lancien E, Barnaud G, Ricard JD, Joly-Guillou ML. Evaluation of a strategy of screening multiple anatomical sites for methicillin-resistant *Staphylococcus aureus* at admission to a teaching hospital. Infect Control Hosp Epidemiol 2006;27:181–4.
188 Yang ES, Tan J, Rieg G, Miller LG. Body site colonization prevalence in patients with community-associated methicillin-resistant *Staphylococcus aureus* infections [Abstract]. In: Program and Abstracts of the 45th Annual Meeting of the Infectious Diseases Society of America. San Diego, CA: Infectious Diseases Society of America, 2007: Abstract 285.
189 Fritz SA, Fritz JM, Mitchell K *et al*. Sites of community-acquired *Staphylococcus aureus* colonization in patients presenting with skin and soft tissue infections [Abstract]. Presented at the 48th Annual Interscience Conference on Antimicrobial Agents and Chemotherapy (ICAAC) and the Infectious Diseases Society of America (IDSA) 46th Annual Meeting, Washington, DC, 2008.
190 Miller LG, Diep BA. Clinical practice: colonization, fomites, and virulence: rethinking the pathogenesis of community-associated methicillin-resistant *Staphylococcus aureus* infection. Clin Infect Dis 2008;46:752–60.
191 Chen KT, Huard RC, Della-Latta P, Saiman L. Prevalence of methicillin-sensitive and methicillin-resistant *Staphylococcus aureus* in pregnant women. Obstet Gynecol 2006;108:482–7.
192 Andrews WW, Schelonka R, Waites K, Stamm A, Cliver SP, Moser S. Genital tract methicillin-resistant *Staphylococcus aureus*: risk of vertical transmission in pregnant women. Obstet Gynecol 2008;111:113–18.
193 Tedeschi S, Sims T, McKenna B, Arnold S, Creech CB. Methicillin-resistant *Staphylococcus aureus* (MRSA) colonization in mothers and newborns [Abstract]. Presented at the 48th Annual Interscience Conference on Antimicrobial Agents and Chemotherapy (ICAAC) and the Infectious Diseases Society of America (IDSA) 46th Annual Meeting, Washington, DC, 2008.
194 Shinefield HR, Black S. Prevention of *Staphylococcus aureus* infections: advances in vaccine development. Expert Rev Vaccines 2005;4:669–76.
195 Wootton SH, Arnold K, Hill HA *et al*. Intervention to reduce the incidence of methicillin-resistant *Staphylococcus aureus* skin infections in a correctional facility in Georgia. Infect Control Hosp Epidemiol 2004;25:402–7.
196 Boyce JM. Preventing staphylococcal infections by eradicating nasal carriage of *Staphylococcus aureus*: proceeding with caution. Infect Control Hosp Epidemiol 1996;17:775–9.
197 Rihn JA, Posfay-Barbe K, Harner CD *et al*. Community-acquired methicillin-resistant *Staphylococcus aureus* outbreak in a local high school football team: unsuccessful interventions. Pediatr Infect Dis J 2005;24:841–3.
198 Wiese-Posselt M, Heuck D, Draeger A *et al*. Successful termination of a furunculosis outbreak due to lukS-lukF-positive,

methicillin-susceptible *Staphylococcus aureus* in a German village by stringent decolonization, 2002–2005. Clin Infect Dis 2007;44:e88–95.

199 Laupland KB, Conly JM. Treatment of *Staphylococcus aureus* colonization and prophylaxis for infection with topical intranasal mupirocin: an evidence-based review. Clin Infect Dis 2003;37:933–8.

200 Loeb M, Main C, Walker-Dilks C, Eady A. Antimicrobial drugs for treating methicillin-resistant *Staphylococcus aureus* colonization. Cochrane Database Syst Rev 2003;4:CD003340.

201 Raz R, Miron D, Colodner R, Staler Z, Samara Z, Keness Y. A 1-year trial of nasal mupirocin in the prevention of recurrent staphylococcal nasal colonization and skin infection. Arch Intern Med 1996;156:1109–12.

202 Klempner MS, Styrt B. Prevention of recurrent staphylococcal skin infections with low-dose oral clindamycin therapy. JAMA 1988;260:2682–5.

203 Ellis MW, Griffith ME, Dooley DP *et al*. Targeted intranasal mupirocin to prevent colonization and infection by community-associated methicillin-resistant *Staphylococcus aureus* strains in soldiers: a cluster randomized controlled trial. Antimicrob Agents Chemother 2007;51:3591–8.

204 Whitman TJ, Wierzba RK, Schlett CD *et al*. Chlorhexidine impregnated cloths to prevent skin and soft tissue infections in marine officer candidates: a cluster randomized, double-blind, controlled trial [Abstract]. Presented at the 48th Annual Interscience Conference on Antimicrobial Agents and Chemotherapy (ICAAC) and the Infectious Disease Society of America (IDSA) 46th Annual Meeting, Washington, DC, 2008.

Chapter 14
Epidemiology of Healthcare-associated *Staphylococcus aureus* Infections

Andrew E. Simor[1] *and Mark Loeb*[2]

[1] Department of Microbiology and Division of Infectious Diseases, University of Toronto, Toronto, Ontario, Canada
[2] Departments of Pathology and Molecular Medicine, Clinical Epidemiology and Biostatistics, McMaster University, Hamilton, Ontario, Canada

Introduction

Staphylococcus aureus is one of the most successful human pathogens, with a global distribution and the potential to cause serious, potentially fatal disease. The organism is well-armed with potent virulence factors, survival fitness, and antimicrobial resistance determinants [1]. *Staphylococcus aureus* may cause infection at any body site, and is among the most common bacterial causes of both community-acquired and healthcare-associated infections. Nosocomial outbreaks of infection caused by *S. aureus* have been recognized for decades. The emergence of a virulent clone, phage type 80/81, was responsible for hospital outbreaks in many parts of the world in the 1950s [2]. Although the frequency of infections caused by phage type 80/81 waned in subsequent decades, methicillin-resistant strains of *S. aureus* (MRSA) became prevalent and spread globally in the late 1970s and 1980s [3]. The introduction and transmission of MRSA in hospital settings appears to be associated with an increase in the overall incidence of nosocomial *S. aureus* infections, rather than just substituting for infections caused by susceptible staphylococcal strains [4–6]. In the past 10 years significant developments in the evolution of *S. aureus* have included the continued worldwide increase in nosocomial MRSA rates [3,7], the development of glycopeptide resistance in staphylococci [8–10], the emergence of community-associated MRSA (CA-MRSA), and their subsequent spread into hospital settings [11,12].

Burden of disease associated with nosocomial *S. aureus* infections

Staphylococcus aureus is a predominant cause of endemic nosocomial infections, and is also responsible for large numbers of healthcare-associated outbreaks of infection. Infection with *S. aureus* occurs in almost 1% of all hospital inpatients, corresponding to approximately 390 000 inpatient infections and at least 2.7 million days of excess hospital stay each year in the USA [13,14]. It has been estimated that approximately half of all *S. aureus* infections in hospitalized patients are nosocomial, and at least 58% are healthcare associated, making the organism one of the most common causes of healthcare-associated infections [14–16]. Using hospital discharge data and infection surveillance data from the National Nosocomial Infections Surveillance (NNIS) system, it was determined that there were an estimated 206 504 *S. aureus* infections (0.58% of hospital admissions) acquired in a healthcare setting in the USA during 1999–2000 [17]. The estimated incidence of nosocomial *S. aureus* infections was 9.13 per 1000 hospital discharges; as 43% of the *S. aureus* isolates were methicillin resistant, the nosocomial MRSA infection rate was 3.95 per 1000 discharges. Approximately 29% of all nosocomial *S. aureus* infections are respiratory, 18% are associated with intravascular catheters, 18% arise from skin or soft tissue, and 13% represent bacteremia without an identified source [15].

In surveillance conducted by the NNIS system in the USA, *S. aureus* was the most common cause of nosocomial infections overall [18]. Many reports have confirmed it to be the leading cause of nosocomial pneumonia and surgical-site infection, and the second most common cause, after coagulase-negative staphylococci, of healthcare-associated bloodstream infections [18–21]. Nosocomial *S. aureus* bacteremia rates have ranged from 0.62 to 1.03 per 1000 admissions, accounting for approximately one-fifth of all nosocomial blood culture isolates [20,22]. These bloodstream infections are most often related to the use of a central venous catheter or some other intravascular device [23,24]. The mean interval between hospital admission and the onset of *S. aureus* bacteremia was found to be 16 days [20].

Typically, *S. aureus* is the most frequently isolated pathogen in adult intensive care unit (ICU) patients [25],

Staphylococci in Human Disease, 2nd edition. Edited by Kent B. Crossley, Kimberly K. Jefferson, Gordon Archer, Vance G. Fowler, Jr.

Table 14.1 Percentage distribution of the most common pathogens associated with hospital-acquired infections in intensive care unit patients in US hospitals participating in the National Nosocomial Infections Surveillance (NNIS) program, 2000–2004. (Data provided by M. Klevens, Centers for Disease Control and Prevention.)

Pathogen	Bloodstream infections	Pneumonia	Surgical-site infections
Staphylococcus aureus	14	26	19
Coagulase-negative staphylococci	35	< 1	13
Enterococcus spp.	16	9	16
Escherichia coli	–	4	6
Klebsiella pneumoniae	–	6	1
Enterobacter spp.	–	–	7
Pseudomonas aeruginosa	–	16	9

and the second most common nosocomial pathogen identified in level-3 high-risk neonatal ICUs [26]. The organism ranks in the top three in frequency as a cause of ICU-acquired primary bacteremia, pneumonia, or surgical-site infection (Table 14.1) [21,24,27,28]. In a point-prevalence survey conducted in 1417 ICUs in 17 European countries, *S. aureus* accounted for 30% of the infections [25]. ICU patients are usually also the major reservoir for MRSA in hospitals [25,29,30].

Healthcare-associated outbreaks of both methicillin-susceptible *S. aureus* (MSSA) and MRSA occur commonly, although in the past 25 years most have been due to MRSA. Outbreaks may occur in adult ICUs [31–33], burn units [34–37], other inpatient hospital units [38–41], neonatal ICUs and nurseries [42–45], and in nursing homes and other long-term care facilities [46–48]. Certain strains of *S. aureus* appear to be associated with an enhanced ability to cause widespread outbreaks of severe infection [2,49,50]. Examples include phage type 80/81 strains of methicillin-susceptible *S. aureus* that were prevalent in the 1950s and 1960s [2], and some of the more recently identified clones of CA-MRSA possessing the Panton–Valentine leukocidin (PVL) gene [51,52].

Healthcare-associated MRSA

In the past decade, rates of infection caused by methicillin-resistant strains of *S. aureus* have continued to increase in most countries around the world, and currently MRSA is the most commonly identified antibiotic-resistant pathogen in hospitalized patients [3,7,29,53]. Most of these infections are healthcare associated, although CA-MRSA have also recently emerged [12]. There is considerable variation in MRSA rates from country to country, and even from hospital to hospital within a country (Figure 14.1) [3,7,54,55]. The explanations for this variability remain unclear, but may be related to differences in diagnostic procedures, antimicrobial utilization patterns, or infection prevention and control practices. MRSA bacteremia (invasive infection) rates appear to correlate well with the overall prevalence and number of new MRSA-infected patients, and therefore may serve as a useful marker in surveillance of the MRSA reservoir and burden of disease [56,57].

In North America, MRSA rates have increased in both US and Canadian hospitals, but are much higher in the USA [29,58]. In US hospitals, the proportion of *S. aureus* resistant to methicillin in ICUs participating in the NNIS system increased from 35.9% in 1992 to 64.4% in 2003, representing an increase of approximately 3% per year (Figure 14.2) [29,59]. The overall prevalence of MRSA in US healthcare facilities in 2006 was found to be 46 per 1000 inpatients; the prevalence of MRSA infections was 34 per 1000 inpatients [60]. The incidence of invasive MRSA infection in the USA was estimated to be 0.2–0.4 per 1000 population overall [11]. In contrast, rates in Canadian hospitals averaged 13% in 2005, and most of these cases represented patients colonized with MRSA who were identified by hospital-based MRSA screening or surveillance [58] (Canadian Nosocomial Infection Surveillance Program, unpublished data). Approximately one-third of hospitalized patients from whom MRSA was recovered had an MRSA infection, giving an infection rate of 2.9 per 1000 admissions; 13% of the infections were associated with bacteremia. A continued increase in MRSA rates in most European countries has also been reported, but with a wide range, from less than 3% of invasive *S. aureus* isolates in the Netherlands and Scandinavian countries to greater than 40% in many countries in southern Europe [7,61,62]. In the UK, approximately one-fifth of all hospital-acquired infections were attributed to MRSA [63].

The prevalence of MRSA colonization on admission to hospital has been reported to range from 1 to 7% in various parts of the world, but appears to be increasing over time [64–69]. Nosocomial acquisition rates of MRSA have been found to vary from 1.7 to 5.4% [70–72], although these findings depend on duration and extent of follow-up. In one study in the USA, the nosocomial MRSA acquisition rate was 5.4 per 100 admissions compared with an acquisition rate of 4.8 per 100 admissions for susceptible strains of *S. aureus* [70].

MRSA is also an important pathogen in long-term care facility residents. The organism may be endemic in nursing homes, especially if neighboring or referring hospitals

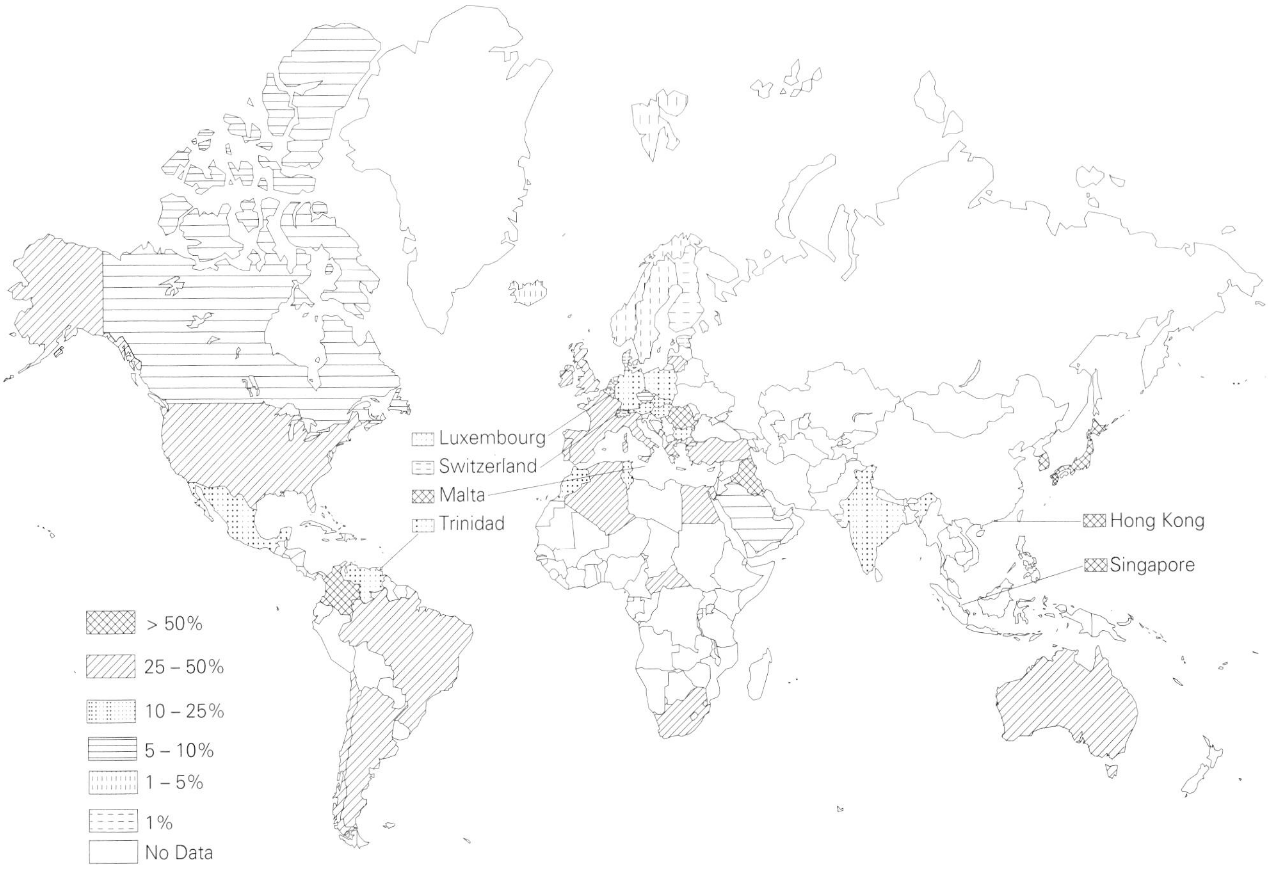

Figure 14.1 Worldwide prevalence of MRSA displayed by country, based on estimates from peer-reviewed studies undertaken since 1998. Reprinted with permission from Elsevier (*The Lancet* 2006;368:874–885).

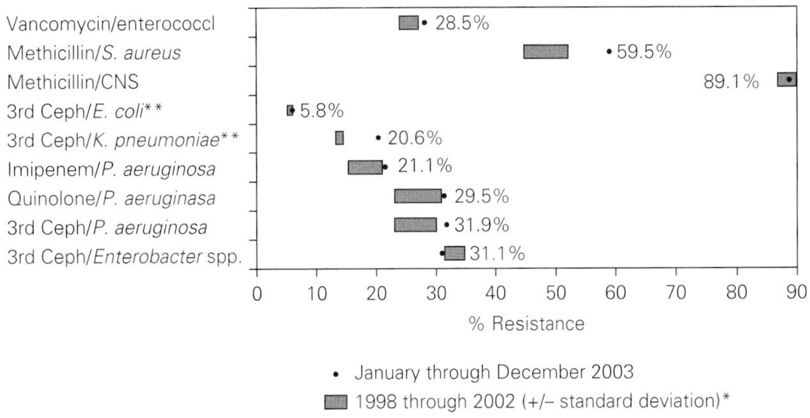

Jan–Dec 2003 No. of Isolates	% increase in resistance (2003 vs 98–02*)
2048	12%
4100	11%
3336	1%
1355	0%
1068	47%
1392	15%
1825	9%
2119	20%
1411	-6%

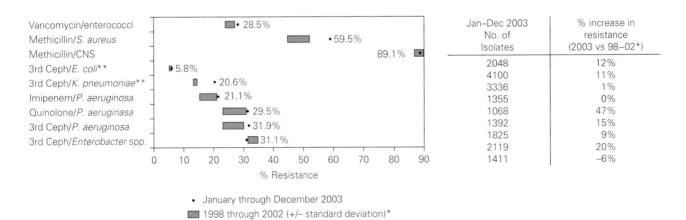

Figure 14.2 Selected antimicrobial-resistant pathogens associated with nosocomial infections in intensive-care unit patients: comparison of resistance rates from January through December 2003 with those from 1998 through 2002. CNS, coagulase-negative staphylococci; 3rd Ceph, resistance to third-generation cephalosporins (ceftriaxone, cefotaxime, or ceftazidime); Quinolone, resistance to either ciprofloxacin or ofloxacin. Percentages indicate increase in resistance rate of current year (January–December 2003) compared with mean rate of resistance over previous 5 years (1998–2002), i.e., [(2003 rate – previous 5-year mean rate)/previous 5-year mean rate] × 100. ** "Resistance" for *E.coli* or *K. pneumoniae* is the rate of nonsusceptibility of these organisms to either third-generation cephalosporins or aztreonam. (From National Nosocomial Infections Surveillance System [29] with permission.)

have high rates of MRSA [73–75]. Transmission of MRSA may occur within long-term care facilities, and may be associated with outbreaks [46–48,76]. It is often assumed that residents of long-term care facilities may serve as a reservoir for MRSA that may spread into hospitals [46,77,78]. Indeed, hospital outbreaks and nosocomial transmission of MRSA have been linked to the admission to hospital of elderly nursing home residents [77]. However, as recent hospitalization is a significant risk factor for MRSA carriage among long-term care facility residents, it is more likely that many, if not most, residents acquire the organism in hospital [75,79–81].

Community-associated MRSA

In the past decade, CA-MRSA have rapidly spread in the USA and in many other parts of the world [11,12,68,82,83]. A relatively small number of unique clones of MRSA, distinct from the classical hospital-acquired strains, have been associated with community-acquired disease. Certain CA-MRSA clones are thought to be genetic descendants of phage type 80/81 *S. aureus* (methicillin susceptible) that have acquired the *mecA* gene with SCC*mec* type IV [84].

Not surprisingly, these CA-MRSA strains have been introduced into healthcare settings, and have proven to be quite capable of being transmitted nosocomially. Transmission among postpartum women and their newborn infants has been described in maternity units, hospital nurseries, and neonatal ICUs [85–88]. Hospital- and healthcare-associated bacteremia, prosthetic joint infections, and other infections have been reported due to CA-MRSA [51,82, 89,90]. In a surveillance study involving dialysis units in the USA, CA-MRSA represented approximately 14% of the MRSA strains responsible for hemodialysis-associated bloodstream infections [91], and the USA300 CA-MRSA clone was the cause of 28% of healthcare-associated bacteremias in a large hospital in Atlanta, Georgia [51].

Glycopeptide resistance in *S. aureus*

Reduced susceptibility to vancomycin in *S. aureus* was first reported from Japan in 1996, and shortly thereafter cases were also reported in the USA and from other countries in Asia, Europe, and South America [10,92]. At present, infections caused by glycopeptide-resistant *S. aureus* remain uncommon in the USA. As of 2007, only 16 infections due to vancomycin-intermediate *S. aureus* (VISA), with vancomycin minimum inhibitory concentrations (MICs) of 4–8 μg/mL, and six epidemiologically unrelated cases caused by vancomycin-resistant *S. aureus* (VRSA), with vancomycin MICs of 16 μg/mL or more, had been reported to the Centers for Disease Control and Prevention. Glycopeptide resistance in *S. aureus* has only been identified in methicillin-resistant strains, and has been associated with prior exposure to vancomycin [8]. Infections caused by VISA or VRSA have not responded adequately to treatment with glycopeptide agents.

Strains of MRSA that exhibit heteroresistance to vancomycin (hetero-VISA) have also been described. The vancomycin MIC for these strains is generally 2 μg/mL, but the isolates contain subpopulations of organisms with reduced killing on exposure to vancomycin *in vitro* [93]. The clinical significance of hetero-VISA strains remains uncertain, although bloodstream infections due to hetero-VISA have been associated with reduced response to glycopeptide therapy and more prolonged bacteremia [94,95].

Risk factors

The relationship between staphylococcal colonization and the development of infection is complex and not well understood, although it is likely related to both host and microbial factors. Nasal carriage of *S. aureus* appears to be a major risk factor for subsequent staphylococcal infection, especially during hospitalization [67,96–99]. Nasal *S. aureus* carriers are more likely than noncarriers to develop nosocomial *S. aureus* bacteremia [relative risk (RR) 3.0, 95% confidence interval (CI) 2.0–4.7], and in most cases the bloodstream isolate is identical (same genotype) to the nasal strain [97,100,101]. In hemodialysis patients, nasal carriage is associated with an increased risk of *S. aureus* bacteremia, and colonization is associated with an increased risk of peritoneal catheter exit-site infections in patients on chronic ambulatory peritoneal dialysis [102,103]. Similarly, colonized patients are at increased risk for developing postoperative surgical-site infections due to *S. aureus*, generally with the same strain as that in the nose [104–109]. Colonization with MRSA appears to pose an even greater risk of subsequent infection. Nasal carriers of MRSA were 3.9 times more likely to develop nosocomial staphylococcal bacteremia than were nasal carriers of susceptible strains of *S. aureus* [96]. Other risk factors that have been reported to be responsible for the development of nosocomial *S. aureus* infection include hemodialysis, diabetes mellitus, cancer, and the presence of an intravascular catheter [13,22,110].

Risk factors for MRSA colonization in hospitalized patients include older age, prolonged hospitalization, use of a feeding tube, presence of skin lesions, wounds or ulcers, and receipt of antibiotics [64,66,69,111,112]. Admission to a hospital room previously occupied by a patient with MRSA was also associated with an increased risk of MRSA acquisition [adjusted odds ratio (OR) 1.4; $P = 0.04$], but this excess risk accounted for less than 5% of all incident MRSA cases [113]. Variables associated with nosocomial MRSA infection have included a history of MRSA colonization, previous hospitalization or surgery, prolonged hospitalization, ICU admission, and prior antimicrobial therapy [110,112,114–116].

Several classes of antimicrobial agents, including β-lactam antibiotics, macrolides, and fluoroquinolones, have been associated with nosocomial acquisition of MRSA [114,117–119]. Treatment with a fluoroquinolone appears to be a risk factor for MRSA acquisition and infection, but not for infection with susceptible strains of *S. aureus* [69,118–120]. *In vitro*, exposure to ciprofloxacin induces upregulation of fibronectin-binding proteins in resistant strains of *S. aureus*, and may thereby promote enhanced staphylococcal adhesion and colonization [121]. At an institutional level, increased antimicrobial utilization of multiple classes of antimicrobial agents correlates with higher MRSA rates [55,120,122,123].

Reservoirs of *S. aureus*

In cross-sectional studies, 20–50% of healthy adults have been found to be colonized with *S. aureus*, and up to 40% are colonized on admission to hospital [105,124–126]. In a recent large population-based survey in the USA, 29% of subjects had nasal colonization with *S. aureus* and 1.5% were colonized with MRSA [127]. Longitudinal studies of staphylococcal colonization have identified three patterns of carriage: (i) persistent or long-term carriage (approximately 20%); (ii) intermittent carriage (approximately 30%); and (iii) noncarriers (approximately 50%) [125,126]. Colonized and infected patients serve as the major reservoir of *S. aureus* in hospitals [31,105,125,128]. Colonizing strains may serve as an endogenous source of infection (the infecting strain arises from the patient's own flora), or the organism may be transmitted to other patients. Patients with unrecognized colonization are most likely to be a source of transmission [129].

The major site of staphylococcal colonization in humans is the anterior nares [124–126], although throat, perineal or gastrointestinal colonization also occur relatively commonly [130–134]. Other body sites that may become colonized with *S. aureus* include the axillae, surgical wounds, decubitus ulcers and other skin lesions, and medical device exit sites [124,125].

Colonized healthcare workers may also be an important source of transmission of *S. aureus* to hospitalized patients [40,135–139]. Nasal colonization with *S. aureus* is a risk factor for hand carriage of the organism among hospital staff [140]. Hand carriage may arise from the healthcare worker's own flora, or may come from contact with another colonized or infected individual, or with the hospital environment [141]. When isolates have been typed by pulsed-field gel electrophoresis (PFGE), it has been found that the *S. aureus* isolates on the hands of healthcare workers have been acquired from an exogenous source approximately half the time, and from apparent self-inoculation from the nose about half the time [140]. Although hand carriage of *S. aureus* is often transient, the organism may remain viable on hands for at least several hours [136–138]. In studies done before the widespread use of gloves in hospitals, more than 20% of random hand cultures of nurses yielded *S. aureus*, with median colony counts ranging from several hundred to 40 000 cfu [142,143].

Several studies have documented that the hospital environment of patients with *S. aureus* colonization or infection is commonly contaminated, and both MSSA and MRSA strains may survive for months on dry surfaces [39,144,145]. Up to 54% of surface cultures in the rooms of patients with MRSA (including mattresses, pillows, furniture, and medical equipment) have yielded the organism, and the environmental isolates have often been the same strain as those recovered from the patient [141,146–148]. Even higher rates of environmental contamination have been reported in burn units, especially in hydrotherapy rooms and equipment [34–36,149]. Room surfaces of patients with MRSA colonization experiencing diarrhea have a high rate of environmental contamination [150]. *Staphylococcus aureus* has been recovered from stethoscopes [151], blood pressure cuffs [152,153], phlebotomy tourniquets [154,155], hospital computer keyboards [156], and hospital pens [157]. In addition, hospital air sample cultures taken from patient rooms may also yield *S. aureus* [148]. Despite the ease with which *S. aureus* and MRSA are recovered from the hospital environment, the role of the environment in the transmission of staphylococci remains uncertain [141,145,158,159].

Transmission of *S. aureus*

Transmission of *S. aureus* in hospitals and other healthcare facilities is usually mediated by direct contact with a colonized healthcare worker, although airborne transmission and transmission following contact with the contaminated environment may also occur. Hand carriage of *S. aureus* by hospital personnel may be transient [136–138] but has been implicated as the major mode of staphylococcal transmission in various healthcare settings [31,34,135,138,139,160, 161]. Personnel may contaminate their hands (or gloves) by touching colonized or infected wounds or wound dressings [136], or by touching dry and intact skin colonized with *S. aureus* [31,160]. Clothing or gowns worn by healthcare workers may also become contaminated with *S. aureus* and thereby become a source of subsequent hand colonization and transmission [141,162]. The hands (or gloves) of personnel may also become colonized with staphylococci after contact with the contaminated hospital environment [36,141].

Airborne transmission of *S. aureus* appears to be less important than transmission by direct contact. However, airborne transmission has occasionally been described in newborn nurseries [163,164] and in burn units [35,36]. Airborne transmission in burn units has been linked to the extensive shedding of colonized skin cells, leading to an increased load of organisms in burn unit air samples [36]. Similarly, there may be potential for airborne spread when changing wound dressings of patients with large draining wounds, or in the presence of areas of dermatitis that are colonized or infected with *S. aureus* [164]. Contamination of hospital ventilation grilles with MRSA leading to airborne spread was thought to have occurred in outbreaks in an ICU and on an orthopedic surgery unit [165,166].

Airborne dispersal of *S. aureus* from the nose as a source of infection appears to be relatively uncommon, and is probably related to the load of organisms colonizing the anterior nares [167]. However, individuals with a heavy growth of *S. aureus* in the nose and a concomitant upper respiratory tract infection may be at increased risk of shedding the organism into the air and environment. Experimental rhinovirus infection of adults with nasal *S. aureus* colonization increased dispersal of the organism into the air, particularly with sneezing, which caused a fourfold to fivefold increase in airborne dispersal of *S. aureus* [168,169]. Increased staphylococcal shedding from the nose has also occurred with natural viral respiratory infections, and this has been associated with outbreaks of *S. aureus* infection [33,41,170]. The terms "cloud baby" and "cloud adult" have been used to describe this phenomenon [33,170].

There have been relatively few examples of *S. aureus* transmission clearly linked to an environmental source. *Staphylococcus aureus* may be transferred from colonized patients to ultrasound equipment, probes, and gel [171], and an outbreak of staphylococcal pyoderma in a neonatal clinic was attributed to exposure to contaminated ultrasound gel [172]. Contamination of surfaces and equipment in a dental procedure room appeared to contribute to spread of MRSA to dental patients [173]. An outbreak of mupirocin-resistant MRSA involving patients on a dermatology ward was thought to have been related to contamination of a blood pressure cuff and a communal shower [152]. Contaminated ultrasonic nebulizers were identified as the likely source of a hospital outbreak in the Netherlands [174]. Other rarely reported modes of nosocomial *S. aureus* transmission have included transmission of MRSA through food contaminated by a dietary worker [175], and transfer of MRSA from donor to recipients during implantation of harvested organs for transplantation [176].

Rates of nosocomial transmission of *S. aureus* have been determined infrequently. In one study, the MRSA transmission rate was calculated to be 0.17 transmissions per colonized patient-week during a hospital outbreak, and most transmissions originated from unisolated patients [129]. The rate of transmission of MRSA from patients on contact isolation was 0.009 transmissions per day as compared with a rate of 0.14 transmissions per day from unisolated patients. In a hospital with a low endemic rate of MRSA infections, and not experiencing an outbreak, the MRSA transmission rate was determined to be 0.048 transmissions per day [65]. In a recent study, approximately 13% of hospital inpatients with MRSA sharing the same room acquired the organism within 10 days after exposure was recognized [177].

Variables that may affect the likelihood of nosocomial transmission of *S. aureus* include microbial, host, and environmental factors. Certain strains of *S. aureus* appear to be more virulent and to have an enhanced capacity to be spread within healthcare facilities [2,49]. The microbial characteristics responsible for the rapid dissemination of these strains remain uncertain. Various host factors have been determined to increase the risk of *S. aureus* acquisition in hospitals, including hospitalization in high-risk units such as burn units, ICUs, or neonatal nurseries [24,25,31,35], surgical procedures, and the presence of intravascular catheters [22–24,110]. Prior antimicrobial therapy may increase the risk of acquiring an antibiotic-resistant strain of *S. aureus* [69,118,120,136].

Several studies have identified overcrowding and understaffing in hospital units as major contributors to nosocomial *S. aureus* transmission, especially in adult and neonatal ICUs, and in burn units [34,42,45,178,179]. Colonization pressure (defined as the number of MRSA-carrier patient-days/total number of patient-days) has been determined to be a significant risk factor for nosocomial MRSA transmission and acquisition in several studies [30,180–182]. During prospective surveillance in an ICU, nosocomial acquisition of MRSA was associated with severity of illness, the number of new imported cases of MRSA, nursing workload, and weekly colonization pressure; in a multivariate analysis, the weekly colonization pressure was the only independent predictive factor for MRSA acquisition [180]. In this study, if the weekly colonization pressure was greater than 30%, the risk of MRSA acquisition was nearly fivefold higher (RR 4.9, 95% CI 1.2–19.9; $P < 0.0001$).

Epidemiological typing of *S. aureus*

Several phenotypic and genotypic methods have been used for epidemiological typing of *S. aureus* in order to track transmission. DNA fingerprinting by pulse field gel electrophoresis (PFGE) has been standardized and has become very useful for investigating nosocomial staphylococcal outbreaks [183–185]. All staphylococcal strains are typeable, and the method is reproducible and able to distinguish different clones (Figure 14.3). PFGE typing has also been used to characterize national and international clones of MRSA [185,186]. However, sequence-based typing methods such as multilocus sequence typing, based on the sequence polymorphism of fragments of seven

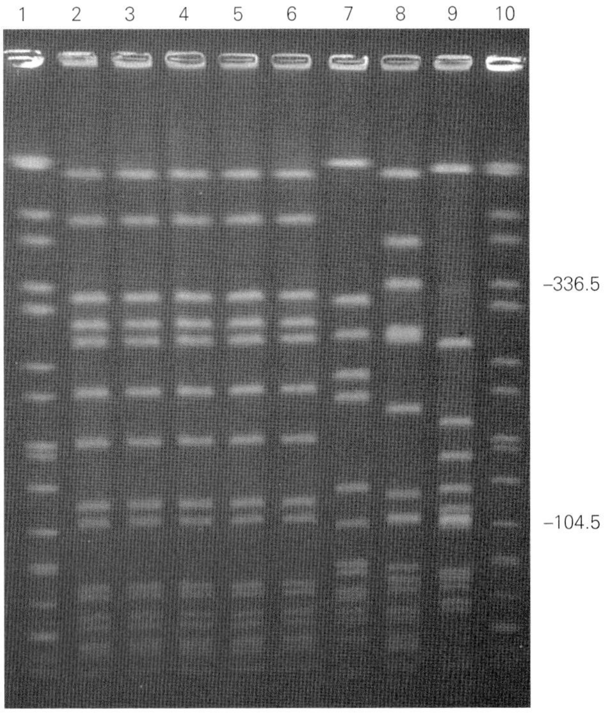

Figure 14.3 Pulsed-field gel electrophoresis profiles of *Sma*I-digested genomic DNA of methicillin-resistant *Staphylococcus aureus* (MRSA). Lanes 1 and 10, *Salmonella* serotype Braenderup H9812 (molecular size marker); lanes 2–6, identical strains of MRSA recovered from five patients on a surgical unit during an outbreak; lanes 7–9, sporadic and epidemiologically unrelated strains of MRSA.

housekeeping genes, and sequencing the polymorphic X region (Fc-binding region) of the staphylococcal protein A gene (*spa*-typing) have become more important methods for designating *S. aureus* lineages in long-term national or international surveillance [185,187,188].

Impact and outcome

Invasive *S. aureus* infections, whether community acquired or nosocomial and whether due to antibiotic-susceptible or -resistant strains, are associated with increased morbidity and mortality. In-hospital death rates have been found to be twofold to fivefold higher for those with *S. aureus* infection as compared with those without staphylococcal infection, even if low-risk hospital patients are excluded from the analysis [13,14]. Case-fatality rates for invasive *S. aureus* infections have been reported to range from 10 to 34% [13–15,22,189–191]. In a British study, *S. aureus* bacteremia was associated with increased in-hospital mortality, with an adjusted OR for dying with infection due to a susceptible strain of *S. aureus* of 7.0 (95% CI 5.1–9.8; 27% mortality) and an OR for dying with MRSA bacteremia of 13.8 (95% CI 10.2–18.6; 34% mortality) [6]. Nosocomial pneumonia due to *S. aureus* also appears to be independently associated with increased mortality (OR 1.58, 95% CI 1.32–1.89; $P < 0.0001$) [21]. Predictors of mortality in patients with *S. aureus* infection have included older age, diabetes mellitus, acute renal failure, pulmonary source of infection, and the presence of shock [15,189,190,192].

In addition to its impact on mortality, *S. aureus* infection increases the length of hospital stay by a median of as many as 12 days [19,193]. The median length of hospital stay has been reported to be 4–7 days longer for patients with nosocomial bacteremia caused by susceptible strains of *S. aureus* as compared with uninfected controls, and MRSA bacteremia has been associated with a median excess length of stay of 9–12 days [16,194]. Ventilator-associated pneumonia and surgical-site infections caused by *S. aureus* have also been associated with increased attributable length of hospitalization [195,196].

As hospital lengths of stay increase with nosocomial staphylococcal infections, associated costs also rise. Incremental hospital charges attributed to *S. aureus* infections were estimated to be approximately $14.5 billion in the USA in 2003 [13]. In New York City hospitals in 1995, the direct attributable medical cost per patient with MSSA was determined to be $31 500, and the mean cost for an MRSA infection was found to be $34 000 [14]. The increased costs associated with MRSA were attributed to the longer hospital stay, the higher costs of antimicrobial treatment, and the costs of isolation procedures. In Canada, the mean attributable costs associated with an MRSA infection were CAN$14 360, with a mean cost of CAN$1363 for each colonized patient [197]. Median hospital costs attributed to nosocomial MRSA bacteremia have ranged from $6916 to $27 083, compared with a median cost of $9661 for bacteremia with MSSA [16,194,198]. Median hospital costs associated with surgical-site infections caused by susceptible *S. aureus* were found to be $52 791, as compared with a median of $92 363 for MRSA surgical-site infections ($P < 0.001$) [195].

Is methicillin resistance in *S. aureus* associated with a worse outcome?

The risk of adverse outcomes in hospitalized patients with MRSA infection has often been found to be higher than that in patients with infections due to MSSA [16,191, 195,198]. Although some studies did not find that the outcome associated with MRSA bacteremia was different from that associated with infection due to susceptible *S. aureus* [6,189,199–201], most studies, including two meta-analyses, have found that methicillin resistance is a significant and independent risk factor for mortality in patients with bacteremic *S. aureus* infections even when logistic regression analysis was done to adjust for potential confounders such as age, presence of comorbidities, source of infection, and severity of illness [191,192,198,202–206]. The observed differences in *S. aureus*-related mortality may be explained by differences in patient characteristics and underlying comorbidities, enhanced virulence of MRSA strains, delays in starting effective antimicrobial treatment, or diminished effectiveness of available therapy (such as vancomycin).

In studies examining outcome in patients with nosocomial or ventilator-associated staphylococcal pneumonia, increased mortality in patients with infection due to MRSA was identified in a small number of investigations [61,207]. However, in these studies, the MRSA patients tended to be older and to have other risk factors for mortality. In studies where potential confounders were controlled, there was no apparent difference in mortality in patients with pneumonia due to MRSA as compared with infection with *S. aureus* susceptible to methicillin [208–211]. In some studies of surgical-site infections, patients with MRSA had significantly increased mortality compared with patients with infection due to susceptible strains, although this finding has not been confirmed in other investigations [195,212,213].

Strategies to reduce the risk of healthcare-associated *S. aureus* infections

Various strategies for reducing the risk of acquisition and transmission of *S. aureus* infections within healthcare settings have been attempted, including elimination of staphylococcal colonization, surveillance, enhanced hand hygiene, and use of isolation, cohorting and barrier precautions. The approach is frequently multifaceted where one or more of these and other interventions are implemented. Although such a strategy may increase the likelihood of success, it makes it difficult to determine which factor(s) is important. As a result, data regarding the effectiveness of infection control interventions for reducing the risk of *S. aureus* or MRSA infections are sparse. A recent review of studies that evaluated the effectiveness of a range of interventions to prevent and control the transmission of MRSA in hospital settings assessed the role of screening, use of surveillance data, isolation and cohorting, decolonization, and environmental cleaning [214]. The reviewers assessed evidence from four systematic reviews, 24 nonexperimental studies, five economic evaluations, and one international guideline. With the exception of decolonization, where randomized controlled trial evidence exits, the grade of evidence for the other categories was Grade III, referring to "evidence from non-experimental descriptive studies."

Reduction of *S. aureus* colonization or infection

A common approach for reducing the risk of staphylococcal infection in those colonized with the organism is decolonization (elimination of staphylococcal carriage) using topical or systemic antimicrobials [215]. Most published experience with staphylococcal decolonization has involved the use of intranasal application of mupirocin calcium ointment. A number of studies have found that topical therapy with mupirocin is able to eradicate nasal *S. aureus* colonization in healthcare workers, and this effect persists for at least 4 weeks [216–218]. Mupirocin has also been effective in eradicating *S. aureus* nasal carriage in HIV-infected patients and in those undergoing long-term hemodialysis [219,220]. Treatment with oral rifampin has been found to be effective for the eradication of *S. aureus* carriage, although development of antimicrobial resistance during and after treatment occurs in a considerable proportion of patients [221]. These studies provide evidence that elimination of staphylococcal carriage may be feasible in various patient populations, but do not address the question of whether such an approach reduces the risk of infection.

A study to determine the efficacy of perioperative nasopharyngeal and oropharyngeal decontamination with 0.12% chlorhexidine gluconate was performed in patients undergoing cardiac surgery [222]. A significant reduction in *S. aureus* nasal carriage was found in the chlorhexidine gluconate group as compared with those in the placebo group (57.5% vs. 18.1%; $P < 0.001$). The incidence of nosocomial infection in the chlorhexidine gluconate group and placebo group was 19.8% and 26.2%, respectively [absolute risk reduction (ARR) 6.4%, 95% CI 1.1–11.7; $P = 0.002$]. In particular, lower respiratory tract infections and deep surgical-site infections were less common in the chlorhexidine gluconate group (ARR 6.5%, 95% CI 2.3–10.7; $P = 0.002$) than in the placebo group (ARR 3.2%, 95% CI 0.9–5.5; $P = 0.002$).

There is little evidence that preoperative treatment with mupirocin reduces the risk of surgical-site infections. In a large, double-blind, randomized controlled trial, 4030 surgical patients were allocated to either intranasal administration of mupirocin (twice daily for up to 5 days) or to placebo [107]. There was no difference in overall surgical-site infection rates or in the rate of surgical-site infections due to *S. aureus*. However, in a secondary analysis of 891 nasal *S. aureus* carriers, there were significantly fewer mupirocin-treated patients who developed nosocomial *S. aureus* infection (4%) compared with placebo recipients (7.7%). Smaller randomized controlled trials in gastrointestinal, orthopedic, and cardiac surgery patients also failed to detect a protective effect of preoperative treatment with intranasal mupirocin [109,223,224].

Two studies have evaluated the efficacy of mupirocin for the prevention of nosocomial *S. aureus* infections in nonsurgical patients. One study involved patients in four hospitals in the Netherlands who were randomized to receive treatment with either intranasal mupirocin ointment or placebo for 5 days [100]. In subsequent follow-up, there were no statistically significant differences in the rates of nosocomial *S. aureus* infections (mupirocin 2.6%; placebo 2.8%), mortality (mupirocin 3.0%; placebo 2.8%), or duration of hospitalization (median for both, 8 days). The second investigation was a placebo-controlled randomized study done in two long-term care facilities [225]. In this study, there was a trend toward a reduction in staphylococcal infections in those who had received a 14-day course of mupirocin compared with those who had received a placebo, but this was not statistically significant. These results would suggest that mupirocin is ineffective in reducing risks of healthcare-associated *S. aureus* infections in nonsurgical patients.

A systematic review has addressed the issue of whether mupirocin therapy can reduce the rate of *S. aureus* infection among patients undergoing long-term hemodialysis or peritoneal dialysis [226]. Ten randomized trials and cohort studies were reviewed, including a total of 2445 patients. Use of mupirocin reduced the rate of *S. aureus* infections by 68% (95% CI 57–76) among all patients undergoing dialysis; risk reductions were 80% (95% CI 65–89) among patients undergoing hemodialysis and 63% (95% CI 50–73) among patients undergoing peritoneal dialysis. When the data were stratified by type of infection, *S. aureus* bacteremia was found to be reduced by 78% among patients undergoing hemodialysis, and peritonitis and exit-site infections were found to be reduced by 66% and 62%, respectively, among patients undergoing peritoneal dialysis. These results indicate that mupirocin prophylaxis reduces the rate of *S. aureus* infection in the dialysis population. However, in one study, long-term follow-up of these patients identified a substantial risk of the emergence of mupirocin resistance over time [227].

Reduction of MRSA colonization or infection

Eradication of MRSA carriage, if effective, could be used to prevent the development of subsequent infection in colonized patients, or as part of infection control strategies to limit transmission of the organism in healthcare settings. In a systematic review [228], six randomized controlled trials of topical or systemic agents used for MRSA decolonization in hospitalized or long-term care facility patients were identified (Table 14.2) [229–234]. Three of the trials included a placebo or no-treatment group, and eradication of MRSA on day 14 after treatment was the most frequently reported outcome. No statistically significant difference in MRSA eradication was identified in any of the studies, although most were small and not adequately powered. Only one study in this review reported data regarding MRSA infection: Harbarth *et al.* [233] randomized 102 patients in a Swiss university hospital to 5 days of treatment with mupirocin ointment or to placebo. Although mupirocin was no more effective than placebo in eliminating MRSA colonization, there were fewer MRSA infections (7%) in the mupirocin-treated group compared with the placebo group (14% infection rate) (RR 0.47, 95% CI 0.13–1.70).

Table 14.2 Summary of characteristics and results of randomized clinical trials of antimicrobial agents used for eradication of methicillin-resistant *Staphylococcus aureus* (MRSA) colonization.

Study	*N*	Interventions	Follow-up (days)	Results
Peterson *et al.*, 1990 [229]	21	Ciprofloxacin + rifampin ×14 days vs. TMP–SMX + rifampin ×14 days	180	30% eradication with ciprofloxacin vs. 40% with TMP–SMX (RR 0.6, 95% CI 0.2–1.9)
Walsh *et al.*, 1993 [230]	80	Novobiocin + rifampin ×7 days vs. TMP–SMX + rifampin ×7 days	14	67% eradication with novobiocin vs. 53% with TMP–SMX (RR 1.3, 95% CI 0.9–1.6)
Muder *et al.*, 1994 [231]	35	Rifampin ×5 days vs. minocycline ×5 days vs. rifampin + minocycline ×5 days vs. no treatment	90	70% eradication with rifampin vs. 14% with no treatment (RR 4.9, 95% CI 0.8–31.5) 38% eradication with minocycline vs. 14% with no treatment (RR 2.6, 95% CI 0.35–19.9) 50% eradication with rifampin + minocycline vs. 14% with no treatment (RR 3.5, 95% CI 0.5–23.8)
Parras *et al.*, 1995 [232]	72	Mupirocin ointment ×5 days vs. fusidic acid ointment + TMP–SMX ×5 days	90	74% eradication with mupirocin vs. 71% fusidic acid + TMP–SMX (RR 1.1, 95% CI 0.6–1.9)
Harbarth *et al.*, 1999 [233]	102	Mupirocin ointment vs. placebo ×5 days	26	25% eradication with mupirocin vs. 18% with placebo (RR 1.4, 95% CI 0.6–3.0)
Chang *et al.*, 2000 [234]	16	Fusidic acid orally ×7 days vs. no treatment	14–77	33% eradication with fusidic acid vs. 50% with no treatment (RR 0.7, 95% CI 0.2–2.4)
Simor *et al.*, 2007 [235]	112	2% chlorhexidine gluconate washes, 2% mupirocin ointment intranasally, and oral rifampin and doxycycline ×7 days vs. no treatment	90	32% eradication with treatment vs. 74% with no treatment (RR 2.29, 95% CI 1.28–4.13)

RR, relative risk of MRSA eradication; TMP–SMX, trimethoprim–sulfamethoxazole.

In a recently published study, inpatients colonized with MRSA were randomized to a regimen consisting of both topical and systemic antimicrobials (2% chlorhexidine gluconate washes and 2% mupirocin ointment applied intranasally, with oral rifampin and doxycycline for 7 days) or to no treatment [235]. Follow-up samples for MRSA culture were obtained from the nares, perineum, skin lesions, and catheter exit sites monthly for up to 8 months. At 3 months of follow-up, 64 (74%) of those treated had culture results negative for MRSA compared with 8 (32%) of those not treated ($P = 0.0001$) (Table 14.2). This difference remained significant at 8 months of follow-up, at which time 54% of those treated had culture results negative for MRSA. Mupirocin resistance emerged in 5% of follow-up isolates. This study is the first trial to show efficacy of the combination of topical and systemic antimicrobials for long-term eradication of MRSA carriage, but it did not address the issue of infection prevention.

Variables that have been associated with persistence or recolonization with MRSA following attempts to decolonize have included MRSA present at more than one anatomical site, prior exposure to fluoroquinolones, and the presence of mupirocin resistance [235,236]. Mupirocin resistance rates in staphylococci have increased in many parts of the world [237], and the development of resistance is often associated with extensive mupirocin use [227,238,239].

Effect of infection control interventions

Several reports describe control of large MRSA outbreaks or a substantial reduction in MRSA rates in endemic settings over prolonged periods of time [56,129,240–245]. Most of these studies have involved implementation of multiple concomitant or sequential interventions including the use of single rooms or isolation wards, staff cohorting, contact screening, handwashing education, use of barrier precautions, use of chlorhexidine soap, or MRSA decolonization therapy. Therefore, it is not possible to determine which interventions have been most important. Moreover, there have been other reports suggesting failure of similar control measures in preventing MRSA spread or reducing endemic rates after long-term follow-up [246,247]. Unfortunately, most of the studies assessing the effectiveness of isolation procedures or infection control measures in reducing MRSA transmission have had significant methodological weaknesses, and plausible alternate explanations for observed reductions in MRSA rates could not always be excluded [214,248]. However, the evidence available does provide support for a range of interventions that are likely to contribute to the prevention and control of MRSA within healthcare facilities.

In a multifaceted intervention that included high-risk patient screening, contact isolation, a computerized alert system, and a hand hygiene campaign based on the use of alcohol hand rub, a decrease in nosocomial MRSA rates from 0.6 cases per 100 admissions in 1993 to 0.24 cases per 100 admissions in 1997 ($P < 0.001$) was observed [56]. A decrease in MRSA infection and bacteremia rates was also observed. This study is generally considered the best evidence for the role of hand hygiene in reducing the spread of MRSA.

In another study, the effectiveness of isolation rooms for reducing the spread of MRSA was questioned [63]. The study was conducted in ICUs over 1 year, and in the middle 6 months patients colonized with MRSA were not moved to a single room or cohort-nursed unless they were colonized with other multiresistant pathogens. Patient care included the use of gloves and gowns during patient contact. There was no evidence of increased MRSA transmission during this phase of the study, suggesting that there was no need for use of isolation rooms in ICUs where MRSA is endemic. However, this interpretation of the study results was criticized in an accompanying editorial because of inadequate MRSA screening on admission to the units, and poor compliance with hand hygiene during the study [249]. In another study, a statistical model was used to determine that, on a surgical unit, dedicated cohort facilities would help limit the spread of MRSA [181]. This model predicted that the risk of MRSA acquisition would increase by 160% per year in the absence of cohort facilities.

Contact isolation (including hand hygiene and use of gloves, gown and mask) appeared to be effective in controlling an MRSA outbreak in a neonatal ICU [129]. The rate of transmission of MRSA from patients on contact precautions was approximately 16-fold lower than that from patients not on contact precautions (0.0009 transmissions per day on isolation compared with 0.14 transmissions per day unisolated; $P < 0.0001$). Other interventions that were implemented in order to control this outbreak included weekly surveillance cultures to detect MRSA, hand hygiene campaigns, and decolonization therapy for selected patients. Several other studies have also confirmed the effectiveness of contact precautions in combination with other measures in limiting the spread of MRSA in healthcare facilities [30,56,245].

There have been few comparative evaluations of the role of gowns in preventing nosocomial transmission of MRSA. In one study that attempted to address this issue, MRSA transmission on units where gloves and gowns were used as part of a standard isolation protocol was compared with that on units where gowns were not used [250]. Over 2 years, the units with use of gloves and gown had 0.1 fewer new MRSA transmissions per ward per month compared with the glove-use only units, but this difference was not statistically significant.

Data regarding the utility of masks in preventing transmission of MRSA are also limited. In an experimental setting, wearing a surgical facemask did not reduce the airborne dispersal of *S. aureus* from nasal carriers [251]. However, wearing a mask may offer healthcare providers some protection from becoming colonized. In one study, healthcare workers wearing masks in addition to gloves and gowns when in contact with MRSA patients had reduced nasal, pharyngeal, and hand carriage of MRSA [252]. Although this study did not determine the effect of wearing masks on rates of MRSA acquisition in hospital, the results do suggest that wearing a mask may prevent transient MRSA carriage by hospital staff, thereby decreasing the risk of nosocomial MRSA transmission.

A great deal of attention has been paid to the role of active surveillance to identify individuals asymptomatically colonized with MRSA in order to reduce transmission. It is recognized that clinical cultures are an insensitive method for detecting MRSA, and miss the significant reservoir of asymptomatically colonized patients admitted to healthcare facilities [253,254]. Consequently, even though there are no definitive studies (i.e., randomized controlled trials) that establish the efficacy of MRSA screening or surveillance in reducing nosocomial transmission of the organism, numerous recommendations for this as an infection control strategy have been made [255–259]. These recommendations and guidelines are based on the results of many studies supporting the effectiveness and cost-effectiveness of screening high-risk hospitalized patients for MRSA carriage in association with subsequently decreased MRSA infection rates [65,245,255,260–263]. However, to be effective, MRSA screening must be linked to hand hygiene policies and implementation of contact precautions [129,263,264]. Two recent studies employed universal MRSA admission screening using rapid molecular assays (multiplex polymerase chain reaction), along with implementation of contact isolation and decolonization of MRSA carriers [263,265]. In one study, using historic controls, there was a substantial and sustained decrease in nosocomial MRSA infections [263]. However, in the other investigation, using a crossover study design, there was no reduction in MRSA acquisition or infection rates [265]. The results of a recently conducted randomized controlled trial evaluating the effectiveness of MRSA active surveillance in ICUs are likely to be published in the near future.

Patients who should be considered for MRSA screening on admission to hospital include those thought to be at "high-risk" for being colonized (e.g., known to have been infected or colonized with MRSA in the past, direct transfer from another healthcare facility, recent hospitalization, or residence in a long-term care facility) [65,255,256,259,261]. Other risk groups may include injecting drug users, patients infected with HIV, and those who are homeless or incarcerated. Another approach may be to screen all patients admitted to high-risk units such as ICUs [245,259,260]. There is no evidence that routine screening of staff working in healthcare facilities is warranted, although such screening should be considered in the setting of an outbreak with ongoing transmission despite implementation of control measures [259]. Recommended sites for MRSA screening include the anterior nares, the perineum or groin, skin lesions and wounds, and medical device and catheter exit sites. The application of newer molecular assays has the potential to increase sensitivity and reduce turn-around times for the detection of MRSA directly from screening specimens [266–268]. Several such commercial tests are currently being evaluated, and their cost-effectiveness is also being assessed.

Adapting an approach that differs from laboratory-based surveillance, Curran *et al.* [269] used statistical process control charts to monitor MRSA acquisition over nearly 4 years. Monthly feedback to ward and medical staff of individual rates of MRSA acquisition was provided, and was associated with a 50% reduction in nosocomial MRSA rates. An important limitation of this study was the absence of a concurrent control group; the data obtained in this study were compared with historical data. However, the study does suggest that regular feedback of surveillance data to healthcare staff may influence behavior that would have an impact on the transmission of nosocomial pathogens. Other investigators have also shown that it may be possible to reduce MRSA infection rates without performing active surveillance cultures [270]. In this study, conducted in an ICU, implementation of evidence-based infection prevention and control interventions was associated with decreasing MRSA infection rates, attributed to a decrease in overall rates of device-related healthcare-associated infections.

The role of the inanimate hospital environment in *S. aureus* or MRSA transmission remains uncertain. Studies have demonstrated that it is possible to reduce hospital environmental contamination with MRSA using cleaning and disinfection protocols [271,272]. In one study, the critical infection control measure that appeared to be responsible for termination of an MRSA outbreak was continuous, thorough attention to environmental cleaning and dust removal [272].

In summary, a review of existing data suggests that successful MRSA infection control measures in healthcare facilities include screening or surveillance of high-risk patients, compliance with good hand hygiene practices, use of contact precautions, and attention to adequate environmental cleaning. Future studies should be designed to better define the effectiveness of these and other infection prevention and control strategies.

References

1 Lowy FD. *Staphylococcus aureus* infections. N Engl J Med 1998; 339:520–32.

2 Williams REO. Epidemic staphylococci. Lancet 1959;i:190–5.
3 Grundmann H, Aires de Sousa M, Boyce J, Tiemersma E. Emergence and resurgence of meticillin-resistant *Staphylococcus aureus* as a public-health threat. Lancet 2006;368:874–85.
4 Boyce JM, White RL, Spruill EY. Impact of methicillin-resistant *Staphylococcus aureus* on the incidence of nosocomial staphylococcal infections. J Infect Dis 1983;148:763.
5 Stamm AM, Long MN, Belcher B. Higher overall nosocomial infection rate because of increased attack rate of methicillin-resistant *Staphylococcus aureus*. Am J Infect Control 1993;21: 70–4.
6 Wyllie DH, Crook DW, Peto TEA. Mortality after *Staphylococcus aureus* bacteraemia in two hospitals in Oxfordshire, 1997–2003: cohort study. BMJ 2006;333:281–7.
7 Tiemersma EW, Bronzwaer SLAM, Lyytikäinen O *et al.* Methicillin-resistant *Staphylococcus aureus* in Europe, 1999–2002. Emerg Infect Dis 2004;10:1627–34.
8 Fridkin SK, Hageman J, McDougal LK *et al.* Epidemiological and microbiological characterization of infections caused by *Staphylococcus aureus* with reduced susceptibility to vancomycin, United States, 1997–2001. Clin Infect Dis 2003;36:429–39.
9 Chang S, Sievert DM, Hageman JC *et al.* Infection with vancomycin-resistant *Staphylococcus aureus* containing the *vanA* resistance gene. N Engl J Med 2003;348:1342–7.
10 Appelbaum PC. The emergence of vancomycin-intermediate and vancomycin-resistant *Staphylococcus aureus*. Clin Microbiol Infect 2006;12(suppl 1):16–23.
11 Fridkin SK, Hageman JC, Morrison M *et al.* Methicillin-resistant *Staphylococcus aureus* disease in three communities. N Engl J Med 2005;352:1436–44.
12 Deresinski S. Methicillin-resistant *Staphylococcus aureus*: an evolutionary, epidemiologic, and therapeutic odyssey. Clin Infect Dis 2005;40:562–73.
13 Noskin GA, Rubin RJ, Schentag JJ *et al.* National trends in *Staphylococcus aureus* infection rates: impact on economic burden and mortality over a 6-year period (1998–2003). Clin Infect Dis 2007;45:1132–40.
14 Rubin RJ, Harrington CA, Poon A, Dietrich K, Greene JA, Moiduddin A. The economic impact of *Staphylococcus aureus* infection in New York city hospitals. Emerg Infect Dis 1999; 5:9–17.
15 Laupland KB, Church DL, Mucenski M, Sutherland LR, Davies HD. Population-based study of the epidemiology of and the risk factors for invasive *Staphylococcus aureus* infections. J Infect Dis 2003;187:1452–9.
16 Cosgrove SE, Qi Y, Kaye KS, Harbarth S, Karchmer AW, Carmeli Y. The impact of methicillin resistance in *Staphylococcus aureus* bacteremia on patient outcomes: mortality, length of stay, and hospital charges. Infect Control Hosp Epidemiol 2005;26:166–74.
17 Kuehnert MJ, Hill HA, Kupronis BA, Tokars JI, Solomon SL, Jernigan DB. Methicillin-resistant *Staphylococcus aureus* hospitalizations, United States. Emerg Infect Dis 2005;11:868–72.
18 Hospital Infections Program, National Center for Infectious Diseases, Centers for Disease Control and Prevention, Public Health Service, US Department of Health and Human Services. National Nosocomial Infections Surveillance (NNIS) system report: data summary from January 1990–May 1999, issued June 1999. Am J Infect Control 1999;26:520–32.
19 Pittet D, Wenzel RP. Nosocomial bloodstream infections: secular trends in rates, mortality, and contribution to total hospital deaths. Arch Intern Med 1995;155:1177–84.
20 Wisplinghoff H, Bischoff T, Tallent SM, Seifert H, Wenzel RP, Edmond MB. Nosocomial bloodstream infections in US hospitals: analysis of 24,179 cases from a prospective nationwide surveillance study. Clin Infect Dis 2004;39:309–17.
21 Kollef MH, Shorr A, Tabak YP, Gupta V, Liu LZ, Johannes RS. Epidemiology and outcomes of health-care-associated pneumonia. Results from a large US database of culture-positive pneumonia. Chest 2005;128:3854–62.
22 Jensen AG, Wachmann CH, Poulsen KB *et al.* Risk factors for hospital-acquired *Staphylococcus aureus* bacteremia. Arch Intern Med 1999;159:1437–44.
23 Steinberg JP, Clark CC, Hackman BO. Nosocomial and community-acquired *Staphylococcus aureus* bacteremias from 1980 to 1993: impact of intravascular devices and methicillin resistance. Clin Infect Dis 1996;23:255–9.
24 Richards MJ, Edwards JR, Culver DH, Gaynes RP, and the National Nosocomial Infections Surveillance System. Nosocomial infections in combined medical–surgical intensive care units in the United States. Infect Control Hosp Epidemiol 2000; 21:510–15.
25 Vincent J-L, Bihari DJ, Suter PM *et al.* The prevalence of nosocomial infection in intensive care units in Europe. Results of the European Prevalence of Infection in Intensive Care (EPIC) Study. JAMA 1995;274:639–44.
26 Gaynes RP, Edwards JR, Jarvis WR, Culver DH, Tolson JS, Martone WJ. Nosocomial infections among neonates in high-risk nurseries in the United States. National Nosocomial Infections Surveillance System. Pediatrics 1996;98:357–61.
27 Ibrahim EH, Ward S, Sherman G, Kollef MH. A comparative analysis of patients with early-onset vs late-onset nosocomial pneumonia in the ICU setting. Chest 2000;117:1434–42.
28 Richards MJ, Edwards JR, Culver DH, Gaynes RP, and the National Nosocomial Infections Surveillance System. Nosocomial infections in medical intensive care units in the United States. Crit Care Med 1999;27:887–92.
29 National Nosocomial Infections Surveillance (NNIS) System. National Nosocomial Infections Surveillance (NNIS) System report, data summary from January 1992 through June 2004, issued October 2004. Am J Infect Control 2004;32:470–85.
30 Lucet J-C, Paoletti X, Lolom L *et al.* Successful long-term program for controlling methicillin-resistant *Staphylococcus aureus* in intensive care units. Intensive Care Med 2005;31:1051–7.
31 Thompson RL, Cabezudo I, Wenzel RP. Epidemiology of nosocomial infections caused by methicillin-resistant *Staphylococcus aureus*. Ann Intern Med 1982;97:309–17.
32 Hartstein AI, Denny MA, Morthland VH, LeMonte AM, Pfaller MA. Control of methicillin-resistant *Staphylococcus aureus* in a hospital and an intensive care unit. Infect Control Hosp Epidemiol 1995;16:405–11.
33 Sherertz RJ, Reagan DR, Hampton KD *et al.* A cloud adult: the *Staphylococcus aureus*–virus interaction revisited. Ann Intern Med 1996;124:539–47.
34 Arnow PM, Allyn PA, Nichols EM, Hill DL, Pezzlo MA, Bartlett RH. Control of methicillin-resistant *Staphylococcus aureus* in a burn unit: role of nurse staffing. J Trauma 1982;22:954–9.
35 Boyce JM, White RL, Causey WA, Lockwood WR. Burn units as a source of methicillin-resistant *Staphylococcus aureus* infections. JAMA 1983;249:2803–7.

36 Rutala WA, Katz EBS, Sherertz RJ, Sarubbi FA Jr. Environmental study of a methicillin-resistant *Staphylococcus aureus* epidemic in a burn unit. J Clin Microbiol 1983;18:683–8.

37 Meier PA, Carter CD, Wallace SE, Hollis RJ, Pfaller MA, Herwaldt LA. A prolonged outbreak of methicillin-resistant *Staphylococcus aureus* in the burn unit of a tertiary medical center. Infect Control Hosp Epidemiol 1996;17:798–802.

38 Locksley RM, Cohen ML, Quinn TC *et al.* Multiply antibiotic-resistant *Staphylococcus aureus*: introduction, transmission, and evolution of nosocomial infection. Ann Intern Med 1982;97: 317–24.

39 Bartzokas CA, Paton JH, Gibson MF, Graham R, McLoughlin GA, Croton RS. Control and eradication of methicillin-resistant *Staphylococcus aureus* on a surgical unit. N Engl J Med 1984;311: 1422–5.

40 Reboli AC, John JF Jr, Platt CG, Cantey JR. Methicillin-resistant *Staphylococcus aureus* outbreak at a Veterans Affairs Medical Center: importance of carriage of the organism by hospital personnel. Infect Control Hosp Epidemiol 1990;11:291–6.

41 Boyce JM, Opal SM, Potter-Bynoe G, Medeiros AA. Spread of methicillin-resistant *Staphylococcus aureus* in a hospital after exposure to a health care worker with chronic sinusitis. Clin Infect Dis 1993;17:495–504.

42 Haley RW, Bregman DA. The role of understaffing and overcrowding in recurrent outbreaks of staphylococcal infection in a neonatal special-care unit. J Infect Dis 1982;145:875–85.

43 Coovadia YM, Bhana RH, Johnson AP, Haffejee I, Marples RR. A laboratory-confirmed outbreak of rifampicin-methicillin resistant *Staphylococcus aureus* (MRSA) in a newborn nursery. J Hosp Infect 1989;14:303–12.

44 Haley RW, Cushion NB, Tenover FC *et al.* Eradication of endemic methicillin-resistant *Staphylococcus aureus* infections from a neonatal intensive care unit. J Infect Dis 1995;171:614–24.

45 Andersen BM, Lindemann R, Bergh K *et al.* Spread of methicillin-resistant *Staphylococcus aureus* in a neonatal intensive unit associated with understaffing, overcrowding and mixing of patients. J Hosp Infect 2002;50:18–24.

46 Thomas JC, Bridge J, Waterman S, Vogt J, Kilman L, Hancock G. Transmission and control of methicillin-resistant *Staphylococcus aureus* in a skilled nursing facility. Infect Control Hosp Epidemiol 1989;10:106–10.

47 Cox RA, Bowie PES. Methicillin-resistant *Staphylococcus aureus* colonization in nursing home residents: a prevalence study in Northamptonshire. J Hosp Infect 1999;43:115–22.

48 Drinka P, Faulks JT, Gauerke C, Goodman B, Stemper M, Reed K. Adverse events associated with methicillin-resistant *Staphylococcus aureus* in a nursing home. Arch Intern Med 2001;161:2371–7.

49 Cox RA, Conquest C, Mallaghan C, Marples RR. A major outbreak of methicillin-resistant *Staphylococcus aureus* caused by a new phage-type (EMRSA-16). J Hosp Infect 1995;29:87–106.

50 Aires de Sousa M, Sanches IS, Ferro ML *et al.* Intercontinental spread of a multidrug-resistant methicillin-resistant *Staphylococcus aureus* clone. J Clin Microbiol 1998;36:2590–6.

51 Seybold U, Kourbatova EV, Johnson JG *et al.* Emergence of community-associated methicillin-resistant *Staphylococcus aureus* USA300 genotype as a major cause of health care-associated blood stream infections. Clin Infect Dis 2006;42:647–56.

52 King MD, Humphrey BJ, Wang YF, Kourbatova EV, Ray SM, Blumberg HM. Emergence of community-acquired methicillin-resistant *Staphylococcus aureus* USA 300 clone as the predominant cause of skin and soft-tissue infections. Ann Intern Med 2006;144:309–17.

53 Diekema DJ, Pfaller MA, Schmitz FJ *et al.* Survey of infections due to *Staphylococcus* species: frequency of occurrence and antimicrobial susceptibility of isolates collected in the United States, Canada, Latin America, Europe, and the Western Pacific region for the SENTRY Antimicrobial Surveillance Program, 1997–1999. Clin Infect Dis 2001;32(suppl 2):S114–S132.

54 Voss A, Milatovic D, Wallrauch-Schwarz C, Rosdahl VT, Braveny I. Methicillin-resistant *Staphylococcus aureus* in Europe. Eur J Clin Microbiol Infect Dis 1994;13:50–5.

55 Meyer E, Schwab F, Gastmeier P, Jonas D, Rueden H, Daschner FD. Methicillin-resistant *Staphylococcus aureus* in German intensive care units during 2000–2003: data from Project SARI (Surveillance of Antimicrobial Use and Antimicrobial Resistance in Intensive Care Units). Infect Control Hosp Epidemiol 2006; 27:146–54.

56 Harbarth S, Martin Y, Rohner P, Henry N, Auckenthaler R, Pittet D. Effect of delayed infection control measures on a hospital outbreak of methicillin-resistant *Staphylococcus aureus*. J Hosp Infect 2000;46:43–9.

57 Speller DCE, Johnson AP, James D, Marples RR, Charlett A, George RC. Resistance to methicillin and other antibiotics in isolates of *Staphylococcus aureus* from blood and cerebrospinal fluid, England and Wales, 1989–95. Lancet 1997;350:323–5.

58 Simor AE, Ofner-Agostini M, Gravel D *et al.* Surveillance for methicillin-resistant *Staphylococcus aureus* in Canadian hospitals: a report update from the Canadian Nosocomial Infection Surveillance Program. Canada Communicable Dis Rep 2005; 31:33–40.

59 Klevens RM, Edwards JR, Tenover FC *et al.* Changes in the epidemiology of methicillin-resistant *Staphylococcus aureus* in intensive care units in US hospitals, 1992–2003. Clin Infect Dis 2006;42:389–91.

60 Jarvis WR, Schlosser J, Chinn RY, Tweeten S, Jackson M. National prevalence of methicillin-resistant *Staphylococcus aureus* in inpatients at US health care facilities, 2006. Am J Infect Control 2007;35:631–7.

61 Gastmeier P, Sohr D, Geffers C, Behnke M, Daschner F, Rüden H. Mortality risk factors with nosocomial *Staphylococcus aureus* infections in intensive care units: results from the German Nosocomial Infection Surveillance System (KISS). Infection 2005;33:50–5.

62 European Antimicrobial Resistance Surveillance System (EARSS). Annual Report 2005. Available at www.earss.rivm.nl.

63 Cepeda JA, Whitehouse T, Cooper B *et al.* Isolation of patients in single rooms or cohorts to reduce spread of MRSA in intensive-care units: prospective two-centre study. Lancet 2005;365:295–304.

64 Troillet N, Carmeli Y, Samore MH *et al.* Carriage of methicillin-resistant *Staphylococcus aureus* at hospital admission. Infect Control Hosp Epidemiol 1998;19:181–5.

65 Papia G, Louie M, Tralla A, Johnson C, Collins V, Simor AE. Screening high-risk patients for methicillin-resistant *Staphylococcus aureus* on admission to the hospital: is it cost-effective? Infect Control Hosp Epidemiol 1999;20:473–7.

66 Jernigan JA, Pullen AL, Flowers L, Bell M, Jarvis WR. Prevalence of and risk factors for colonization with methicillin-resistant *Staphylococcus aureus* at the time of hospital admission. Infect Control Hosp Epidemiol 2003;24:409–14.

67 Davis KA, Stewart JJ, Crouch HK, Florez CE, Hospenthal DR. Methicillin-resistant *Staphylococcus aureus* (MRSA) nares colonization at hospital admission and its effect on subsequent MRSA infection. Clin Infect Dis 2004;39:776–82.
68 Hidron AI, Kourbatova EV, Halvosa JS *et al*. Risk factors for colonization with methicillin-resistant *Staphylococcus aureus* (MRSA) in patients admitted to an urban hospital: emergence of community-associated MRSA nasal carriage. Clin Infect Dis 2005;41:159–66.
69 Harbarth S, Sax H, Frankhauser-Rodriguez C, Schrenzel J, Agostinho A, Pittet D. Evaluating the probability of previously unknown carriage of MRSA at hospital admission. Am J Med 2006;119:275.e15–275.e23.
70 Jernigan JA, Clemence MA, Stott GA *et al*. Control of methicillin-resistant *Staphylococcus aureus* at a university hospital: one decade later. Infect Control Hosp Epidemiol 1995;16:686–96.
71 Fishbain JT, Lee JC, Nguyen HD *et al*. Nosocomial transmission of methicillin-resistant *Staphylococcus aureus*: a blinded study to establish baseline acquisition rates. Infect Control Hosp Epidemiol 2003;24:415–21.
72 Rioux C, Armand-Lefevre L, Guerinot W, Andremont A, Lucet J-C. Acquisition of methicillin-resistant *Staphylococcus aureus* in the acute care setting: incidence and risk factors. Infect Control Hosp Epidemiol 2007;28:733–6.
73 Muder RR, Brennen C, Wagener MM *et al*. Methicillin-resistant staphylococcal colonization and infection in a long-term care facility. Ann Intern Med 1991;114:107–12.
74 Bradley SF, Terpenning MS, Ramsey MA *et al*. Methicillin-resistant *Staphylococcus aureus*: colonization and infection in a long-term care facility. Ann Intern Med 1991;115:417–22.
75 Bradley SF. *Staphylococcus aureus* infections and antibiotic resistance in older adults. Clin Infect Dis 2002;34:211–16.
76 Kotilainen P, Routumaa M, Peltonen R *et al*. Eradication of methicillin-resistant *Staphylococcus aureus* from a health center ward and associated nursing home. Arch Intern Med 2001;161: 859–63.
77 Hsu CCS, Macaluso CP, Special L, Hubble RH. High rate of methicillin resistance of *Staphylococcus aureus* isolated from hospitalized nursing home patients. Arch Intern Med 1988; 148:569–70.
78 Goodall B, Tompkins DS. Methicillin-resistant staphylococcal infections: nursing homes act as a reservoir. BMJ 1994; 308:58.
79 Murphy S, Denman S, Bennett RG, Greenough WB III, Lindsay J, Zelesnick LB. Methicillin-resistant *Staphylococcus aureus* colonization in a long-term-care facility. J Am Geriatr Soc 1992;40: 213–17.
80 von Baum H, Schmidt C, Svoboda D, Bock-Hensley O, Wendt C. Risk factors for methicillin-resistant *Staphylococcus aureus* carriage in residents of German nursing homes. Infect Control Hosp Epidemiol 2002;23:511–15.
81 Simor AE, Ofner-Agostini M, Paton S *et al*. Clinical and epidemiologic features of methicillin-resistant *Staphylococcus aureus* in elderly hospitalized patients. Infect Control Hosp Epidemiol 2005;26:838–41.
82 Linde H, Wagenlehner F, Strommenger B *et al*. Healthcare-associated outbreaks and community-acquired infections due to MRSA carrying the Panton–Valentine leucocidin gene in southeastern Germany. Eur J Clin Microbiol Infect Dis 2005; 24:419–22.
83 Hota B, Ellenbogen C, Hayden MK, Aroutcheva A, Rice TW, Weinstein RA. Community-associated methicillin-resistant *Staphylococcus aureus* skin and soft tissue infections at a public hospital. Do public housing and incarceration amplify transmission? Arch Intern Med 2007;167:1026–33.
84 Robinson DA, Kearns AM, Holmes A *et al*. Re-emergence of early pandemic *Staphylococcus aureus* as a community-acquired meticillin-resistant clone. Lancet 2005;365:1256–8.
85 Saiman L, O'Keefe M, Graham PL III *et al*. Hospital transmission of community-acquired methicillin-resistant *Staphylococcus aureus* among postpartum women. Clin Infect Dis 2003;37:1313–19.
86 Healy CM, Hulten KG, Palazzi DL, Campbell JR, Baker CJ. Emergence of new strains of methicillin-resistant *Staphylococcus aureus* in a neonatal intensive care unit. Clin Infect Dis 2004;39:1460–6.
87 Bratu S, Eramo A, Kopec R *et al*. Community-associated methicillin-resistant *Staphylococcus aureus* in hospital nursery and maternity units. Emerg Infect Dis 2005;11:808–13.
88 Regev-Yochay G, Rubinstein E, Barzilai A *et al*. Methicillin-resistant *Staphylococcus aureus* in neonatal intensive care unit. Eur J Clin Microbiol Infect Dis 2005;11:453–6.
89 Kourbatova EV, Halvosa JS, King MD, Ray SM, White N, Blumberg HM. Emergence of community-associated methicillin-resistant *Staphylococcus aureus* USA 300 clone as a cause of health care-associated infections among patients with prosthetic joint infections. Am J Infect Control 2005;33:385–91.
90 Gonzalez BE, Rueda AM, Shelburne SA, Musher DM, Hamill RJ, Hultén KG. Community-associated strains of methicillin-resistant *Staphylococcus aureus* as the cause of healthcare-associated infection. Infect Control Hosp Epidemiol 2006;27: 1051–6.
91 Collins A, Forrest B, Klevens RM *et al*. Invasive methicillin-resistant *Staphylococcus aureus* infections among dialysis patients: United States, 2005. MMWR 2007;56:197–9.
92 Smith TL, Pearson ML, Wilcox KR *et al*. Emergence of vancomycin resistance in *Staphylococcus aureus*. N Engl J Med 1999; 340:493–501.
93 Charles PGP, Ward PB, Johnson PDR, Howden BP, Grayson ML. Clinical features associated with bacteremia due to heterogeneous vancomycin-intermediate *Staphylococcus aureus*. Clin Infect Dis 2004;38:448–51.
94 Ariza J, Pujol M, Cabo J *et al*. Vancomycin in surgical infections due to meticillin-resistant *Staphylococcus aureus* with heterogeneous resistance to vancomycin. Lancet 1999;353:1587–8.
95 Khosrovaneh A, Riederer K, Saeed S *et al*. Frequency of reduced vancomycin susceptibility and heterogeneous subpopulation in persistent or recurrent methicillin-resistant *Staphylococcus aureus* bacteremia. Clin Infect Dis 2004;38:1328–30.
96 Pujol M, Peña C, Pallares R *et al*. Nosocomial *Staphylococcus aureus* bacteremia among nasal carriers of methicillin-resistant and methicillin-susceptible strains. Am J Med 1996;100:509–16.
97 von Eiff C, Becker K, Machka K, Stammer H, Peters G. Nasal carriage as a source of *Staphylococcus aureus* bacteremia. N Engl J Med 2001;344:11–16.
98 Huang SS, Platt R. Risk of methicillin-resistant *Staphylococcus aureus* infection after previous infection or colonization. Clin Infect Dis 2003;36:281–5.
99 Wertheim HFL, Melles DC, Vos MC *et al*. The role of nasal carriage in *Staphylococcus aureus* infections. Lancet Infect Dis 2005;5:751–62.

100 Wertheim HFL, Vos MC, Ott A *et al.* Mupirocin prophylaxis for nosocomial *Staphylococcus aureus* infections in non-surgical patients. Ann Intern Med 2004;140:419–25.
101 Wertheim HFL, Vos MC, Ott A *et al.* Risk and outcome of nosocomial *Staphylococcus aureus* bacteraemia in nasal carriers versus non-carriers. Lancet 2004;364:703–5.
102 Luzar MA, Coles GA, Faller B *et al. Staphylococcus aureus* nasal carriage and infection in patients on continuous ambulatory peritoneal dialysis. N Engl J Med 1990;322:505–9.
103 Kluytmans JAJW, Manders M-J, van Bommel E, Verbrugh H. Elimination of nasal carriage of *Staphylococcus aureus* in hemodialysis patients. Infect Control Hosp Epidemiol 1996;17:793–7.
104 Kluytmans JAJW, Mouton JW, VandenBergh MFQ *et al.* Reduction of surgical-site infections in cardiothoracic surgery by elimination of nasal carriage of *Staphylococcus aureus*. Infect Control Hosp Epidemiol 1996;17:780–5.
105 Wenzel RP, Perl TM. The significance of nasal carriage of *Staphylococcus aureus* and the incidence of postoperative wound infection. J Hosp Infect 1995;31:13–24.
106 Kluytmans JAJW, Mouton JW, Ijzerman EPF *et al.* Nasal carriage of *Staphylococcus aureus* as a major risk factor for wound infections after cardiac surgery. J Infect Dis 1995;171:216–19.
107 Perl TM, Cullen JJ, Wenzel RP *et al.* Intranasal mupirocin to prevent postoperative *Staphylococcus aureus* infections. N Engl J Med 2002;346:1871–7.
108 Kalmeijer MD, van Nieuwland-Bollen E, Bogaers-Hofman D, de Baere GAJ, Kluytmans JAJW. Nasal carriage of *Staphylococcus aureus* is a major risk factor for surgical-site infections in orthopedic surgery. Infect Control Hosp Epidemiol 2000; 21:319–23.
109 Kalmeijer MD, Coertjens H, van Nieuwland-Bollen PM *et al.* Surgical site infections in orthopedic surgery: the effect of mupirocin nasal ointment in a double-blind, randomized, placebo-controlled study. Clin Infect Dis 2002;35:353–8.
110 Pujol M, Peña C, Pallares R, Ayats J, Ariza J, Gudiol F. Risk factors for nosocomial bacteremia due to methicillin-resistant *Staphylococcus aureus*. Eur J Clin Microbiol Infect Dis 1994;13: 96–102.
111 Lucet J-C, Chevret S, Durand-Zaleski I, Chastang C, Régnier B. Prevalence and risk factors for carriage of methicillin-resistant *Staphylococcus aureus* at admission to the intensive care unit. Results of a multicenter study. Arch Intern Med 2003;163:181–8.
112 Asensio A, Guerrero A, Quereda C, Lizán M, Martinez-Ferrer M. Colonization and infection with methicillin-resistant *Staphylococcus aureus*: associated factors and eradication. Infect Control Hosp Epidemiol 1996;17:20–8.
113 Huang SS, Datta R, Platt R. Risk of acquiring antibiotic-resistant bacteria from prior room occupants. Arch Intern Med 2006;166:1945–51.
114 Graffunder EM, Venezia RA. Risk factors associated with nosocomial methicillin-resistant *Staphylococcus aureus* (MRSA) infection including previous use of antimicrobials. J Antimicrob Chemother 2002;49:999–1005.
115 Lodise TP Jr, McKinnon PS, Rybak M. Prediction model to identify patients with *Staphylococcus aureus* bacteremia at risk for methicillin resistance. Infect Control Hosp Epidemiol 2003;24:655–61.
116 Oztoprak N, Cevik MA, Akinci E *et al.* Risk factors for ICU-acquired methicillin-resistant *Staphylococcus aureus* infections. Am J Infect Control 2006;34:1–5.
117 Monnet DL, Archibald LK, Phillips L, Tenover FC, McGowan JE Jr, Gaynes RP. Antimicrobial use and resistance in eight US hospitals: complexities of analysis and modeling. Infect Control Hosp Epidemiol 1998;19:388–94.
118 Weber SG, Gold HS, Hooper DC, Karchmer AW, Carmeli Y. Fluoroquinolones and the risk for methicillin-resistant *Staphylococcus aureus* in hospitalized patients. Emerg Infect Dis 2003;9:1415–22.
119 LeBlanc L, Pépin J, Toulouse K *et al.* Fluoroquinolones and risk for methicillin-resistant *Staphylococcus aureus*, Canada. Emerg Infect Dis 2006;12:1398–405.
120 Muller A, Mauny F, Talon D, Donnan PT, Harbarth S, Bertrand X. Effect of individual- and group-level antibiotic exposure on MRSA isolation: a multilevel analysis. J Antimicrob Chemother 2006;58:578–81.
121 Li D, Renzoni A, Estoppey T *et al.* Induction of fibronectin adhesions in quinolone-resistant *Staphylococcus aureus* by subinhibitory levels of ciprofloxacin or by sigma B transcription factor activity is mediated by two separate pathways. Antimicrob Agents Chemother 2005;49:916–24.
122 Monnet DL. Methicillin-resistant *Staphylococcus aureus* and its relationship to antimicrobial use: possible implications for control. Infect Control Hosp Epidemiol 1998;19:552–9.
123 Crowcroft NS, Ronveaux O, Monnet DL, Mertens R. Methicillin-resistant *Staphylococcus aureus* and antimicrobial use in Belgian hospitals. Infect Control Hosp Epidemiol 1999;20:31–6.
124 Williams REO. Healthy carriage of *Staphylococcus aureus*: its prevalence and importance. Bacteriol Rev 1963;27:56–71.
125 Kluytmans J, van Belkum A, Verbrugh H. Nasal carriage of *Staphylococcus aureus*: epidemiology, underlying mechanisms, and associated risks. Clin Microbiol Rev 1997;10:505–20.
126 Kluytmans JAJW, Wertheim HFL. Nasal carriage of *Staphylococcus aureus* and prevention of nosocomial infections. Infection 2005;33:3–8.
127 Gorwitz RJ, Kruszon-Moran D, McAllister SK *et al.* Changes in the prevalence of nasal colonization with *Staphylococcus aureus* in the United States, 2001–2004. J Infect Dis 2008;197:1226–34.
128 Blok HEM, Troelstra A, Kamp-Hopmans TEM *et al.* Role of healthcare workers in outbreaks of methicillin-resistant *Staphylococcus aureus*: a 10-year evaluation from a Dutch university hospital. Infect Control Hosp Epidemiol 2003;24:679–85.
129 Jernigan JA, Titus MG, Gröschel DHM, Getchell-White SL, Farr BM. Effectiveness of contact isolation during a hospital outbreak of methicillin-resistant *Staphylococcus aureus*. Am J Epidemiol 1996;143:496–504.
130 Boe J, Solberg CO, Vogelsang TM, Wormnes A. Perineal carriers of staphylococci. BMJ 1964;2:280–1.
131 Rimland D, Roberson B. Gastrointestinal carriage of methicillin-resistant *Staphylococcus aureus*. J Clin Microbiol 1986;24: 137–8.
132 Boyce JM, Havill NL, Maria B. Frequency and possible infection control implications of gastrointestinal colonization with methicillin-resistant *Staphylococcus aureus*. J Clin Microbiol 2005;43:5992–5.
133 Nilsson P, Ripa T. *Staphylococcus aureus* throat colonization is more frequent than colonization in the anterior nares. J Clin Microbiol 2006;44:3334–9.
134 Mertz D, Frei R, Jaussi B *et al.* Throat swabs are necessary to reliably detect carriers of *Staphylococcus aureus*. Clin Infect Dis 2007;45:475–7.

135 Rammelkamp CH Jr, Mortimer EA Jr, Wolinky E. Transmission of streptococcal and staphylococcal infections. Ann Intern Med 1964;60:753–8.

136 Crossley K, Landesman B, Zaske D. An outbreak of infections caused by strains of *Staphylococcus aureus* resistant to methicillin and aminoglycosides. II. Epidemiologic studies. J Infect Dis 1979;139:280–7.

137 Cookson B, Peters B, Webster M, Phillips I, Rahman M, Noble W. Staff carriage of epidemic methicillin-resistant *Staphylococcus aureus*. J Clin Microbiol 1989;27:1471–6.

138 Boyce JM. Methicillin-resistant *Staphylococcus aureus* in hospitals and long-term care facilities: microbiology, epidemiology, and preventive measures. Infect Control Hosp Epidemiol 1992; 13:725–37.

139 Vonberg R-P, Stamm-Balderjahn S, Hansen S *et al.* How often do asymptomatic healthcare workers cause methicillin-resistant *Staphylococcus aureus* outbreaks? A systematic evaluation. Infect Control Hosp Epidemiol 2006;27:1123–7.

140 Tammelin A, Klötz F, Hambraeus A, Stahle E, Ransjö U. Nasal and hand carriage of *Staphylococcus aureus* in staff at a department for thoracic and cardiovascular surgery: endogenous or exogenous source? Infect Control Hosp Epidemiol 2003;24: 686–9.

141 Boyce JM, Potter-Bynoe G, Chenevert C, King T. Environmental contamination due to methicillin-resistant *Staphylococcus aureus*: possible infection control implications. Infect Control Hosp Epidemiol 1997;18:622–7.

142 Ojajärvi J. Effectiveness of hand washing and disinfection methods in removing transient bacteria after patient nursing. J Hyg (Camb) 1980;85:193–203.

143 Ayliffe GAJ, Babb JR, Davies JG, Lilly HA. Hand disinfection: a comparison of various agents in laboratory and ward studies. J Hosp Infect 1988;11:226–43.

144 Beard-Pegler MA, Stubbs E, Vickery AM. Observations on the resistance to drying of staphylococcal strains. J Med Microbiol 1988;26:251–5.

145 Hardy KJ, Oppenheim BA, Gossain S, Gao F, Hawkey PM. A study of the relationship between environmental contamination with methicillin-resistant *Staphylococcus aureus* (MRSA) and patients' acquisition of MRSA. Infect Control Hosp Epidemiol 2006;27:127–32.

146 Blythe D, Keenlyside D, Dawson SJ, Galloway A. Environmental contamination due to methicillin-resistant *Staphylococcus aureus* (MRSA). J Hosp Infect 1998;38:67–70.

147 Ndawula EM, Brown L. Mattresses as reservoirs of epidemic methicillin-resistant *Staphylococcus aureus*. Lancet 1991;337:488.

148 Sexton T, Clarke P, O'Neill E, Dillane T, Humphreys H. Environmental reservoirs of methicillin-resistant *Staphylococcus aureus* in isolation rooms: correlation with patient isolates and implications for hospital hygiene. J Hosp Infect 2006;62: 187–94.

149 Embil JM, McLeod JA, Al-Barrak AM *et al.* An outbreak of methicillin-resistant *Staphylococcus aureus* on a burn unit: potential role of contaminated hydrotherapy equipment. Burns 2001;27:681–8.

150 Boyce JM, Havill NL, Otter JA, Adams NMT. Widespread environmental contamination associated with patients with diarrhea and methicillin-resistant *Staphylococcus aureus* colonization of the gastrointestinal tract. Infect Control Hosp Epidemiol 2007;28:1142–7.

151 Marinella MA, Pierson C, Chenoweth C. The stethoscope. A potential source of nosocomial infection? Arch Intern Med 1997;157:786–90.

152 Layton MC, Perez M, Heald P, Patterson JE. An outbreak of mupirocin-resistant *Staphylococcus aureus* on a dermatology ward associated with an environmental reservoir. Infect Control Hosp Epidemiol 1993;14:369–75.

153 Walker N, Gupta R, Cheesbrough J. Blood pressure cuffs: friend or foe? J Hosp Infect 2006;63:167–9.

154 Berman DS, Schaeffler S, Simberkoff MS, Rahal JJ. Tourniquets and nosocomial methicillin-resistant *Staphylococcus aureus* infections. N Engl J Med 1986;315:514–15.

155 Leitch A, McCormick I, Gunn I, Gillispie T. Reducing the potential for phlebotomy tourniquets to act as a reservoir for meticillin-resistant *Staphylococcus aureus*. J Hosp Infect 2006;63: 428–31.

156 Devine J. Cooke RPD, Wright EP. Is methicillin-resistant *Staphylococcus aureus* (MRSA) contamination of ward-based computer terminals a surrogate marker for nosocomial MRSA transmission and handwashing compliance? J Hosp Infect 2001;48:72–5.

157 French G, Rayner D, Branson M, Walsh M. Contamination of doctors' and nurses' pens with nosocomial pathogens. Lancet 1998;351:213.

158 Hota B. Contamination, disinfection, and cross-colonization: Are hospital surfaces reservoirs for nosocomial infection? Clin Infect Dis 2004;39:1182–9.

159 Wilson AP, Hayman S, Whitehouse T *et al.* Importance of the environment for patient acquisition of methicillin-resistant *Staphylococcus aureus* in the intensive care unit: a baseline study. Crit Care Med 2007;35:2275–9.

160 Mortimer EA, Lipsitz PJ, Wolinsky E, Gonzaga AJ, Rammelkamp CH. Transmission of staphylococci between newborns: importance of the hands of personnel. Am J Dis Child 1962;104:289–95.

161 Klimek JJ, Marsik FJ, Bartlett RC, Weir B, Shea P, Quintiliani R. Clinical, epidemiologic and bacteriologic observations of an outbreak of methicillin-resistant *Staphylococcus aureus* at a large community hospital. Am J Med 1976;61:340–5.

162 Hare R, Ridley M. Further studies on the transmission of *Staph. aureus*. BMJ 1958;1:69–73.

163 Wolinsky E, Lipsitz PJ, Mortimer EA Jr, Rammelkamp CH Jr. Acquisition of staphylococci by newborns. Direct versus indirect transmission. Lancet 1960;ii:620–2.

164 Mortimer EA, Wolinsky E, Gonzaga AJ, Rammelkamp CH. Role of airborne transmission in staphylococcal infections. BMJ 1966;1:319–22.

165 Wagenvoort JHT, Davies BI, Westermann EJA, Werink TJ, Toenbreker HMJ. MRSA from air-exhaust channels. Lancet 1993;341:840–1.

166 Kumari DNP, Haji TC, Keer V, Hawkey PM, Duncanson V, Flower E. Ventilation grilles as a potential source of methicillin-resistant *Staphylococcus aureus* causing an outbreak on an orthopaedic ward at a district general hospital. J Hosp Infect 1998;39:127–33.

167 White A. Relation between quantitative nasal cultures and dissemination of staphylococci. J Lab Clin Med 1961;58:273–7.

168 Bassetti S, Bischoff WE, Walter M *et al.* Dispersal of *Staphylococcus aureus* into the air associated with a rhinovirus infection. Infect Control Hosp Epidemiol 2005;26:196–203.

169 Bischoff WE, Wallis ML, Tucker BK *et al.* "Gesundheit!" sneezing, common colds, allergies, and *Staphylococcus aureus* dispersion. J Infect Dis 2006;194:1119–26.
170 Eichenwald H, Kotsevalov O, Fasso LA. The "cloud baby": an example of bacterial–viral interaction. Am J Dis Child 1960; 100:161–73.
171 Ohara T, Hoh Y, Itoh K. Ultrasound instruments as possible vectors of staphylococcal infection. J Hosp Infect 1998;40:73–7.
172 Weist K, Wendt C, Petersen LR, Versmold H, Ruden H. An outbreak of pyodermas among neonates caused by ultrasound gel contaminated with methicillin-susceptible *Staphylococcus aureus*. Infect Control Hosp Epidemiol 2000;21:761–4.
173 Kurita H, Kurashina K, Honda T. Nosocomial transmission of methicillin-resisant *Staphylococcus aureus* via the surfaces of the dental operatory. Br Dent J 2006;201:297–300.
174 Schultsz C, Meester HHM, Kranenburg AMH *et al.* Ultrasonic nebulizers as a potential source of methicillin-resistant *Staphylococcus aureus* causing an outbreak in a university tertiary care hospital. J Hosp Infect 2003;55:269–75.
175 Kluytmans J, van Leeuwen W, Goessens W *et al.* Food-initiated outbreak of methicillin-resistant *Staphylococcus aureus* analyzed by pheno- and genotyping. J Clin Microbiol 1995;33:1121–8.
176 Johnston L, Chui L, Chang N *et al.* Cross-Canada spread of methicillin-resistant *Staphylococcus aureus* via transplant organs. Clin Infect Dis 1999;29:819–23.
177 Moore C, Dhaliwal J, Tong A *et al.* Risk factors for methicillin-resistant *Staphylococcus aureus* (MRSA) acquisition in roommate contacts of patients colonized or infected with MRSA in an acute-care hospital. Infect Control Hosp Epidemiol 2008;29: 600–6.
178 Vicca AF. Nursing staff workload as a determinant of methicillin-resistant *Staphylococcus aureus* spread in an adult intensive therapy unit. J Hosp Infect 1999;43:109–13.
179 Borg MA, Suda D, Scicluna E. Time-series analysis of the impact of bed occupancy rates on the incidence of methicillin-resistant *Staphylococcus aureus* infection in overcrowded general wards. Infect Control Hosp Epidemiol 2008;29:496–502.
180 Merrer J, Santoli F, Appéré De Vecchi C, Tran B, De Jonghe B, Outin H. "Colonization pressure" and risk of acquisition of methicillin-resistant *Staphylococcus aureus* in a medical intensive care unit. Infect Control Hosp Epidemiol 2000;21:718–23.
181 Talon DT, Vichard P, Muller A, Bertin M, Jeunet L, Bertrand X. Modelling the usefulness of a dedicated cohort facility to prevent the dissemination of MRSA. J Hosp Infect 2003;54:57–62.
182 Eveillard M, Lancien E, Hidri N *et al.* Estimation of methicillin-resistant *Staphylococcus aureus* transmission by considering colonization pressure at the time of hospital admission. J Hosp infect 2005;60:27–31.
183 Bannerman TL, Hancock GA, Tenover FC, Miller JM. Pulsed-field gel electrophoresis as a replacement for bacteriophage typing of *Staphylococcus aureus*. J Clin Microbiol 1995;33:551–5.
184 Mulvey MR, Chui L, Ismail J *et al.* Development of a Canadian standardized protocol for subtyping methicillin-resistant *Staphylococcus aureus* using pulsed-field gel electrophoresis. J Clin Microbiol 2001;39:3481–5.
185 Hallin M, Deplano A, Denis O, DeMendoça R, DeRyck R, Struelens MJ. Validation of pulsed-field gel electrophoresis and *spa* typing for long-term, nationwide epidemiological surveillance studies of *Staphylococcus aureus* infections. J Clin Microbiol 2007;45:127–33.
186 McDougal LK, Steward CD, Killgore GE, Chaitram JM, McAllister SK, Tenover FC. Pulsed-field gel electrophoresis typing of oxacillin-resistant *Staphylococcus aureus* isolates from the United States: establishing a national database. J Clin Microbiol 2003;41:5113–20.
187 Enright MC, Day NPJ, Davies CE, Peacock SJ, Spratt BG. Multilocus sequence typing for characterization of methicillin-resistant and methicillin-susceptible clones of *Staphylococcus aureus*. J Clin Microbiol 2000;38:1008–15.
188 Christianson S, Golding GR, Campbell J; Canadian Nosocomial Infection Surveillance Program, Mulvey MR. Comparative genomics of Canadian epidemic lineages of methicillin-resistant *Staphylococcus aureus*. J Clin Microbiol 2007;45:1904–11.
189 Mylotte JM, Tayara A. *Staphylococcus aureus* bacteremia: predictors of 30-day mortality in a large cohort. Clin Infect Dis 2000;31:1170–4.
190 Jensen AG, Wachmann CH, Espersen F, Scheibel J, Skinhøj P, Frimodt-Møller N. Treatment and outcome of *Staphylococcus aureus* bacteremia. A prospective study of 278 cases. Arch Intern Med 2002;162:25–32.
191 Cosgrove SE, Sakoulas G, Perencevich EN, Schwaber MJ, Karchmer AW, Carmeli Y. Comparison of mortality associated with methicillin-resistant and methicillin-susceptible *Staphylococcus aureus* bacteremia: a meta-analysis. Clin Infect Dis 2003; 36:53–9.
192 Conterno LO, Wey SB, Castelo A. Risk factors for mortality in *Staphylococcus aureus* bacteremia. Infect Control Hosp Epidemiol 1998;19:32–7.
193 Wakefield DS, Pfaller MA, Hammons GT, Massanari RM. Use of the Appropriateness Evaluation Protocol for estimating the incremental costs associated with nosocomial infections. Med Care 1987;25:481–8.
194 Abramson MA, Sexton DJ. Nosocomial methicillin-resistant and methicillin-susceptible *Staphylococcus aureus* primary bacteremia: at what costs? Infect Control Hosp Epidemiol 1999; 20:408–11.
195 Engemann JJ, Carmeli Y, Cosgrove SE *et al.* Adverse clinical and economic outcomes attributable to methicillin resistance among patients with *Staphylococcus aureus* surgical site infection. Clin Infect Dis 2003;36:592–8.
196 Shorr AF, Tabak YP, Gupta V, Johannes RS, Liu LZ, Kollef MH. Morbidity and cost burden of methicillin-resistant *Staphylococcus aureus* in early ventilator-associated pneumonia. Crit Care 2006;10:R97.
197 Kim T, Oh PI, Simor AE. The economic impact of methicillin-resistant *Staphylococcus aureus* in Canadian hospitals. Infect Control Hosp Epidemiol 2001;22:99–104.
198 Reed SD, Friedman JY, Engemann JJ *et al.* Costs and outcomes among hemodialysis-dependent patients with methicillin-resistant or methicillin-susceptible *Staphylococcus aureus* bacteremia. Infect Control Hosp Epidemiol 2005;26:175–83.
199 Harbarth S, Rutschmann O, Sudre P, Pittet D. Impact of methicillin resistance on the outcome of patients with bacteremia caused by *Staphylococcus aureus*. Arch Intern Med 1998;158: 182–9.
200 Soriano A, Martínez JA, Mensa J *et al.* Pathogenic significance of methicillin resistance for patients with *Staphylococcus aureus* bacteremia. Clin Infect Dis 2000;30:368–73.
201 Guilarde AO, Turchi MD, Martelli CMT, Primo MGB. *Staphylococcus aureus* bacteraemia: incidence, risk factors and

predictors for death in a Brazilian teaching hospital. J Hosp Infect 2006;63:330–6.

202 Whitby M, McLaws M-L, Berry G. Risk of death from methicillin-resistant *Staphylococcus aureus* bacteraemia: a meta-analysis. Med J Aust 2001;175:264–7.

203 Romero-Vivas J, Rubio M, Fernandez C, Picazo JJ. Mortality associated with nosocomial bacteremia due to methicillin-resistant *Staphylococcus aureus*. Clin Infect Dis 1995;21:1417–23.

204 Blot SI, Vandewoude KH, Hoste EA, Colardyn FA. Outcome and attributable mortality in critically ill patients with bacteremia involving methicillin-susceptible and methicillin-resistant *Staphylococcus aureus*. Arch Intern Med 2002;162: 2229–35.

205 Melzer M, Eykyn SJ, Gransden WR, Chinn S. Is methicillin-resistant *Staphylococcus aureus* more virulent than methicillin-susceptible *S. aureus*? A comparative cohort study of British patients with nosocomial infection and bacteremia. Clin Infect Dis 2003;37:1453–60.

206 Shurland S, Zhan M, Bradham DD, Roghmann M-C. Comparison of mortality risk associated with bacteremia due to methicillin-resistant and methicillin-susceptible *Staphylococcus aureus*. Infect Control Hosp Epidemiol 2007;28:273–9.

207 Rello J, Torres A, Ricart M *et al.* Ventilator-associated pneumonia by *Staphylococcus aureus*. Comparison of methicillin-resistant and methicillin-sensitive episodes. Am J Respir Crit Care Med 1994;150:1545–9.

208 González C, Rubio M, Romero-Vivas J, González M, Picazo JJ. Bacteremic pneumonia due to *Staphylococcus aureus*: a comparison of disease caused by methicillin-resistant and methicillin-susceptible organisms. Clin Infect Dis 1999;29:1171–7.

209 Combes A, Luyt C-E, Fagon J-Y *et al.* Impact of methicillin resistance on outcome of *Staphylococcus aureus* ventilator-associated pneumonia. Am J Respir Crit Care Med 2004;170:786–92.

210 DeRyke CA, Lodise TP Jr, Rybak MJ, McKinnon PS. Epidemiology, treatment, and outcomes of nosocomial bacteremic *Staphylococcus aureus* pneumonia. Chest 2005;128:1414–22.

211 Zahar J-R, Clec'h C, Tafflet M *et al.* Is methicillin resistance associated with a worse prognosis in *Staphylococcus aureus* ventilator-associated pneumonia? Clin Infect Dis 2005;41: 1224–31.

212 Mekontso-Dessap A, Kirsch M, Brun-Buisson C, Loisance D. Poststernotomy mediastinitis due to *Staphylococcus aureus*: comparison of methicillin-resistant and methicillin-susceptible cases. Clin Infect Dis 2001;32:877–83.

213 Combes A, Trouillet J-L, Joly-Guillou M-L, Chastre J, Gibert C. The impact of methicillin resistance on the outcome of poststernotomy mediastinitis due to *Staphylococcus aureus*. Clin Infect Dis 2004;38:822–9.

214 Loveday HP, Pellowe CM, Jones SRLJ, Pratt RJ. A systematic review of the evidence for interventions for the prevention and control of meticillin-resistant *Staphylococcus aureus* (1996–2004): report to the Joint MRSA Working Part (Subgroup A). J Hosp Infect 2006;63(suppl 1):S45– S70.

215 Laupland KB, Conly JM. Treatment of *Staphylococcus aureus* colonization and prophylaxis for infection with topical intranasal mupirocin: an evidence-based review. Clin Infect Dis 2003;37: 933–8.

216 Doebbeling BN, Breneman DL, Neu HC *et al.* Elimination of *Staphylococcus aureus* nasal carriage in health care workers: analysis of six clinical trials with calcium mupirocin ointment. Clin Infect Dis 1993;17:466–74.

217 Fernandez C, Gaspar C, Torrellas A *et al.* A double-blind, randomized, placebo-controlled clinical trial to evaluate the safety and efficacy of mupirocin calcium ointment for eliminating nasal carriage of *Staphylococcus aureus* among hospital personnel. J Antimicrob Chemother 1995;35:399–408.

218 Soto NE, Vaghjimal A, Stahl-Avicolli A, Protic JR, Lutwick LI, Chapnick EK. Bacitracin versus mupirocin for *Staphylococcus aureus* nasal colonization. Infect Control Hosp Epidemiol 1999;20:351–3.

219 Martin JN, Perdreau-Remington F, Kartalija M *et al.* A randomized clinical trial of mupirocin in the eradication of *Staphylococcus aureus* nasal carriage in human immunodeficiency virus disease. J Infect Dis 1999;180:896–9.

220 Watanakunakorn C, Brandt J, Durkin P, Santore S, Bota B, Stahl CJ. The efficacy of mupirocin ointment and chlorhexidine body scrubs in the eradication of nasal carriage of *Staphylococcus aureus* among patients undergoing long-term hemodialysis. Am J Infect Control 1992;20:138–41.

221 Falagas ME, Bliziotis IA, Fragoulis KN. Oral rifampin for eradication of *Staphylococcus aureus* carriage from healthy and sick populations: a systematic review of the evidence from comparative trials. Am J Infect Control 2007;35:106–14.

222 Segers P, Speekenbrink RGH, Ubbink DT, van Ogtrop ML, de Mol BA. Prevention of nosocomial infection in cardiac surgery by decontamination of the nasopharynx and oropharynx with chlorhexidine gluconate: a randomized controlled trial. JAMA 2006;296:2460–6.

223 Suzuki Y, Kamigaki T, Fujino Y, Tominaga M, Ku Y, Kuroda Y. Randomized clinical trial of preoperative intranasal mupirocin to reduce surgical-site infection after digestive surgery. Br J Surg 2003;90:1072–5.

224 Konvalinka A, Errett L, Fong IW. Impact of treating *Staphylococcus aureus* nasal carriers on wound infections in cardiac surgery. J Hosp Infect 2006;64:162–8.

225 Mody L, Kauffman CA, McNeil SA, Galecki AT, Bradley SF. Mupirocin-based decolonization of *Staphylococcus aureus* carriers in residents of two long-term care facilities: a randomized, double-blind, placebo-controlled trial. Clin Infect Dis 2003;37: 1467–74.

226 Tacconelli E, Carmeli Y, Aizer A, Ferreira G, Foreman MG, D'Agata EMC. Mupirocin prophylaxis to prevent *Staphylococcus aureus* infection in patients undergoing dialysis: a meta-analysis. Clin Infect Dis 2003;37:1629–38.

227 Pérez-Fontán M, Rosales M, Rodríguez-Carmona A, García Falcón T, Valdés F. Mupirocin resistance after long-term use for *Staphylococcus aureus* colonization in patients undergoing chronic peritoneal dialysis. Am J Kidney Dis 2002;39:337–41.

228 Loeb M, Main C, Walker-Dilks C, Eady A. Antimicrobial agents for treating methicillin resistant *Staphylococcus aureus*. Cochrane Database Syst Rev 2003;CD003340.

229 Peterson LR, Quick JN, Jensen B *et al.* Emergence of ciprofloxacin resistance in nosocomial methicillin-resistant *Staphylococcus aureus* isolates. Resistance during ciprofloxacin plus rifampin therapy for methicillin-resistant *S. aureus* colonization. Arch Intern Med 1990;150:2151–5.

230 Walsh TJ, Standiford HC, Reboli AC *et al.* Randomized double-blinded trial of rifampin with either novobiocin or trimethoprim-sulfamethoxazole against methicillin-resistant

Staphylococcus aureus colonization: prevention of antimicrobial resistance and effect of host factors on outcome. Antimicrob Agents Chemother 1993;37:1134–42.
231 Muder RR, Boldin M, Brennen C *et al.* A controlled trial of rifampicin, minocycline, and rifampicin plus minocycline for eradication of methicillin-resistant *Staphylococcus aureus* in long-term care patients. J Antimicrob Chemother 1994;34: 189–90.
232 Parras F, del Carmen Guerrero M, Bouza E *et al.* Comparative study of mupirocin and oral co-trimoxazole plus topical fusidic acid in eradication of nasal carriage of methicillin-resistant *Staphylococcus aureus*. Antimicrob Agents Chemother 1995;39: 175–9.
233 Harbarth S, Dharan S, Liassine N, Herrault P, Auckenthaler R, Pittet D. Randomized, placebo-controlled, double-blind trial to evaluate the efficacy of mupirocin for eradicating carriage of methicillin-resistant *Staphylococcus aureus*. Antimicrob Agents Chemother 1999;43:1412–16.
234 Chang S-C, Hsieh S-M, Chen M-L, Sheng W-H, Chen Y-C. Oral fusidic acid fails to eradicate methicillin-resistant *Staphylococcus aureus* colonization and results in emergence of fusidic acidresistant strains. Diagn Microbiol Infect Dis 2000;36:131–6.
235 Simor AE, Phillips E, McGeer A *et al.* Randomized controlled trial of chlorhexidine gluconate for washing, intranasal mupirocin, and rifampin and doxycycline versus no treatment for the eradication of methicillin-resistant *Staphylococcus aureus* colonization. Clin Infect Dis 2007;44:178–85.
236 Harbarth S, Liassine N, Dharan S, Herrault P, Auckenthaler R, Pittet D. Risk factors for persistent carriage of methicillin-resistant *Staphylococcus aureus*. Clin Infect Dis 2000;31:1380–5.
237 Cookson BD. The emergence of mupirocin resistance: a challenge to infection control and antibiotic prescribing practice. J Antimicrob Chemother 1998;41:11–18.
238 Miller MA, Dascal A, Portnoy J, Mendelson J. Development of mupirocin resistance among methicillin-resistant *Staphylococcus aureus* after widespread use of nasal mupirocin ointment. Infect Control Hosp Epidemiol 1996;17:811–13.
239 Vasquez JE, Walker ES, Franzus BW, Overbay BK, Reagan DR, Sarubbi FA. The epidemiology of mupirocin resistance among methicillin-resistant *Staphylococcus aureus* at a Veterans Affairs hospital. Infect Control Hosp Epidemiol 2000;21:459–64.
240 Murray-Leisure KA, Geib S, Graceley D *et al.* Control of epidemic methicillin-resistant *Staphylococcus aureus*. Infect Control Hosp Epidemiol 1990;11:343–50.
241 Coello R, Jiménez J, García M *et al.* Prospective study of infection, colonization and carriage of methicillin-resistant *Staphylococcus aureus* in an outbreak affecting 990 patients. Eur J Clin Microbiol Infect Dis 1994;13:74–81.
242 Duckworth GJ, Lothian JLE, Williams JD. Methicillin-resistant *Staphylococcus aureus*: report of an outbreak in a London teaching hospital. J Hosp Infect 1988;11:1–15.
243 Pittet D, Hugonnet S, Harbarth S *et al.* Effectiveness of a hospital-wide programme to improve compliance with hand hygiene. Lancet 2000;356:1307–12.
244 Tomic V, Sorli PS, Trinkaus D, Sorli J, Widmer AF, Trampuz A. Comprehensive strategy to prevent nosocomial spread of methicillin-resistant *Staphylococcus aureus* in a highly endemic setting. Arch Intern Med 2004;164:2038–43.
245 Huang SS, Yokoe DS, Hinrichsen VL *et al.* Impact of routine intensive care unit surveillance cultures and resultant barrier precautions on hospital-wide methicillin-resistant *Staphylococcus aureus* bacteremia. Clin Infect Dis 2006;43:971–8.
246 Faoagali JL, Thong ML, Grant D. Ten years' experience with methicillin-resistant *Staphylococcus aureus* in a large Australian hospital. J Hosp Infect 1992;20:113–19.
247 Farrington M, Redpath C, Trundle C, Coomber S, Brown NM. Winning the battle but losing the war: methicillin-resistant *Staphylococcus aureus* (MRSA) at a teaching hospital. Q J Med 1998;91:539–48.
248 Cooper BS, Stone SP, Kibbler CC *et al.* Isolation measures in the hospital management of methicillin resistant *Staphylococcus aureus* (MRSA): systematic review of the literature. BMJ 2004;329:533.
249 Huskins WC, Goldmann DA. Controlling methicillin-resistant *Staphylococcus aureus*, aka "Superbug". Lancet 2005;365:273–5.
250 Grant J, Ramman-Haddad L, Dendukuri N, Libman MD. The role of gowns in preventing nosocomial transmission of methicillin-resistant *Staphylococcus aureus* (MRSA): gown use in MRSA control. Infect Control Hosp Epidemiol 2006;27:191–4.
251 Bischoff WE, Tucker BK, Wallis ML *et al.* Preventing the airborne spread of *Staphylococcus aureus* by persons with the common cold: effect of surgical scrubs, gowns, and masks. Infect Control Hosp Epidemiol 2007;28:1148–54.
252 Lacey S, Flaxman D, Scales J, Wilson A. The usefulness of masks in preventing transient carriage of epidemic methicillin-resistant *Staphylococcus aureus* by healthcare workers. J Hosp Infect 2001;48:308–11.
253 Salgado CD, Farr BM. What proportion of hospital patients colonized with methicillin-resistant *Staphylococcus aureus* are identified by clinical microbiological cultures? Infect Control Hosp Epidemiol 2006;27:116–21.
254 Furuno JP, Harris AD, Wright M-O *et al.* Value of performing active surveillance cultures on intensive care unit discharge for detection of methicillin-resistant *Staphylococcus aureus*. Infect Control Hosp Epidemiol 2007;28:666–70.
255 Rubinovitch B, Pittet D. Screening for methicillin-resistant *Staphylococcus aureus* in the endemic hospital: what have we learned? J Hosp Infect 2001;47:9–18.
256 Arnold MS, Dempsey JM, Fishman M, McAuley PJ, Tibert C, Vallande NC. The best hospital practices for controlling methicillin-resistant *Staphylococcus aureus*: on the cutting edge. Infect Control Hosp Epidemiol 2002;23:69–76.
257 Farr BM, Jarvis WR. Would active surveillance cultures help control healthcare-related methicillin-resistant *Staphylococcus aureus* infections? Infect Control Hosp Epidemiol 2002;23:65–8.
258 Muto CA, Jernigan JA, Ostrowsky BE *et al.* SHEA guidelines for preventing nosocomial transmission of multidrug-resistant strains of *Staphylococcus aureus* and *Enterococcus*. Infect Control Hosp Epidemiol 2003;24:362–86.
259 Coia JE, Duckworth GJ, Edwards DI *et al.* Guidelines for the control and prevention of meticillin-resistant *Staphylococcus aureus* (MRSA) in healthcare facilities by the Joint BSAC/HIS/ICNA Working Party on MRSA. J Hosp Infect 2006;63(suppl 1): S1–S44.
260 Chaix C, Durand-Zaleski I, Alberti C, Brun-Buisson C. Control of endemic methicillin-resistant *Staphylococcus aureus*. A cost–benefit analysis in an intensive care unit. JAMA 1999;282: 1745–51.
261 Karchmer TB, Durbin LJ, Simonton BM, Farr BM. Cost-effectiveness of active surveillance cultures and contact/droplet

precautions for control of methicillin-resistant *Staphylococcus aureus*. J Hosp Infect 2002;51:126–32.

262 Farr BM. Prevention and control of methicillin-resistant *Staphylococcus aureus* infections. Curr Opin Infect Dis 2004;17: 317–22.

263 Robicsek A, Beaumont JL, Paule SM *et al.* Universal surveillance for methicillin-resistant *Staphylococcus aureus* in 3 affiliated hospitals. Ann Intern Med 2008;148:409–18.

264 Diekema DJ, Edmond MB. Look before you leap: active surveillance for multidrug-resistant organisms. Clin Infect Dis 2007;44:1101–7.

265 Harbarth S, Fankhauser C, Schrenzel J *et al.* Universal screening for methicillin-resistant *Staphylococcus aureus* at hospital admission and nosocomial infection in surgical patients. JAMA 2008;299:1149–57.

266 Francois P, Pittet D, Bento M *et al.* Rapid detection of methicillin-resistant *Staphylococcus aureus* directly from sterile or nonsterile clinical samples by a new molecular assay. J Clin Microbiol 2003;41:254–60.

267 Huletsky A, Giroux R, Rossbach V *et al.* New real-time PCR assay for rapid detection of methicillin-resistant *Staphylococcus aureus* directly from specimens containing a mixture of staphylococci. J Clin Microbiol 2004;42:1875–84.

268 de San N, Denis O, Gasasira M-F, De MendonHa, Nonhoff C, Struelens MJ. Controlled evaluation of the IDI-MRSA assay for detection of colonization by methicillin-resistant *Staphylococcus aureus* in diverse mucocutaneous specimens. J Clin Microbiol 2007;45:1098–1101.

269 Curran ET, Benneyan JC, Hood J. Controlling methicillin-resistant *Staphylococcus aureus*: a feedback approach using annotated statistical process control charts. Infect Control Hosp Epidemiol 2002;23:13–18.

270 Edmond MB, Ober JF, Bearman G. Active surveillance cultures are not required to control MRSA infections in the critical care setting. Am J Infect Control 2008;36:461–3.

271 Fitzpatrick F, Murphy OM, Brady A, Prout S, Fenelon LE. A purpose built MRSA cohort unit. J Hosp Infect 2000;46:271–9.

272 Rampling A, Wiseman S, Davis L *et al.* Evidence that hospital hygiene is important in the control of methicillin-resistant *Staphylococcus aureus*. J Hosp Infect 2001;49:109–16.

Chapter 15
Epidemiology of Coagulase-negative Staphylococci and Infections Caused by these Organisms

Kathie L. Rogers[1], *Paul D. Fey*[1,2] *and Mark E. Rupp*[2]
[1] Department of Pathology and Microbiology and [2] Department of Internal Medicine, University of Nebraska Medical Center, Omaha, Nebraska, USA

Introduction

Coagulase-negative staphylococci (CoNS) are the most abundant microbes inhabiting normal human skin and mucous membranes [1–7]. Owing to their ubiquitous nature, they are frequently encountered as contaminants of clinical cultures. Although CoNS are normally harmless commensal flora, because of relatively recent changes in the practice of medicine they have emerged as formidable pathogens [8–10]. *Staphylococcus epidermidis* is the most common cause of primary bacteremia and is a frequent cause of surgical-site infections and infections of indwelling medical devices [11]. It owes its pathogenic success to two major features: its natural niche on human skin and its ability to adhere to biomaterials and form a biofilm [12]. Infections due to *S. epidermidis* are often indolent and may be clinically difficult to diagnose. Differentiation of culture contamination from true infection can at times be challenging. Treatment of CoNS is complicated by increasing rates of antibiotic resistance, by the effect of biofilms on host defense and antimicrobial susceptibility, and by the frequent need to remove infected prosthetic devices in order to exact cure. An increased understanding of the epidemiology and pathogenesis of CoNS should ultimately lead to improved techniques in differentiating CoNS contaminants from pathogens, better treatment modalities, and more effective preventive techniques.

This chapter covers the epidemiology of CoNS and in particular *S. epidermidis*. In addition, a brief description of pathogenesis and antimicrobial resistance is included. Short sections on major clinical entities caused by CoNS are provided and, where appropriate, the reader is referred to other areas of the book for additional, more detailed information.

Staphylococci in Human Disease, 2nd edition. Edited by Kent B. Crossley, Kimberly K. Jefferson, Gordon Archer, Vance G. Fowler, Jr.

History

Staphylococcus epidermidis, a member of the coagulase-negative *Staphylococcus* group, was first described in 1880 by Pasteur and Ogston [13]. In 1884, Rosenbach separated white colonies of staphylococci from yellow *Staphylococcus aureus* colonies and named them *Staphylococcus albus* [14]. In 1961, *Staphylococcus*, *Micrococcus*, and *Planococcus* were categorized under the family Micrococcaceae due to their Gram-positive catalase-positive phenotypes.

Currently, the *Staphylococcus* genus is included in the Staphylococcaceae family in the order Bacillales. The genus includes more than 40 species, of which most are unable to produce free coagulase, the major distinguishing factor used to divide the staphylococci for diagnostic purposes. Of this noncoagulase-producing subset, 14 species are isolated from human sources [9], some of these only rarely (Table 15.1). Seven species have been positively identified as having pathogenic potential in humans [15]. This chapter primarily covers the four species most commonly isolated from human infections or disease [9], with greater emphasis placed on *S. epidermidis*, the most commonly isolated CoNS species in human infections [16]. *Staphylococcus epidermidis*, *Staphylococcus haemolyticus*, *Staphylococcus lugdunensis*, and *Staphylococcus saprophyticus* all have individual niches and virulence factors that allow them to exist primarily as normal commensal flora on human skin and mucous membranes; in unique circumstances, however, they have the ability to cause infections.

Historically, CoNS were generally considered to be skin contaminants when isolated from microbiological cultures [17,18]. Beginning in the 1950s, a handful of reports documented cases of native valve endocarditis and septicemia caused by CoNS [19–21]. For example, Smith *et al.* [18] determined that 1.5% of cases of septicemia diagnosed at the University of Iowa between 1936 and 1955 were authentically caused by CoNS. In the 1960s, there were increasing numbers of reports of nosocomial infections

Table 15.1 *Staphylococcus* species.

Staphylococcus arlettae
Staphylococcus aureus[1]
Staphylococcus auricularis[1]
Staphylococcus capitis[1]
Staphylococcus caprae[1]
Staphylococcus carnosus[1]
Staphylococcus caseolyticus
Staphylococcus chromogenes
Staphylococcus cohnii[1]
Staphylococcus condimenti
Staphylococcus delphini
Staphylococcus epidermidis[1]
Staphylococcus equorum
Staphylococcus felis
Staphylococcus fleuretti
Staphylococcus gallinarum
Staphylococcus haemolyticus[1]
Staphylococcus hominis[1]
Staphylococcus hyicus
Staphylococcus intermedius
Staphylococcus kloosii
Staphylococcus lentus
Staphylococcus lugdunensis[1]
Staphylococcus lutrae
Staphylococcus muscae
Staphylococcus nepalensis
Staphylococcus pasteuri[1]
Staphylococcus pettenkoferi[1]
Staphylococcus piscifermentans
Staphylococcus pseudintermedius
Staphylococcus pulvereri
Staphylococcus saccharolyticus[1]
Staphylococcus saprophyticus[1]
Staphylococcus schleiferi[1]
Staphylococcus sciuri
Staphylococcus simiae
Staphylococcus simulans[1]
Staphylococcus succinus
Staphylococcus vitulinus
Staphylococcus warneri[1]
Staphylococcus xylosus[1]

[1] Isolated from human specimens.

due to CoNS in patients who had prosthetic medical devices, including prosthetic joints, artificial heart valves, and cerebrospinal fluid (CSF) shunts [22]. Concurrent with these reports, Wilson and Stuart [23] noted that 4.4% of 1200 infected wound cultures yielded a pure culture of CoNS, and the clinical significance of *S. saprophyticus* as a cause of urinary tract infections in young women was first recognized [24]. In the 1970s the clinical significance of CoNS became increasingly obvious as numerous reports of well-defined infection due to CoNS were published [25–28]. For example, Pulverer [29] noted that of 2276 peritoneal or ventriculoatrial shunt placement surgeries, 8% became infected and 58% of these infections were due to CoNS.

Prior to the 1980s, simply identifying CoNS to the species level was difficult as no standardized laboratory methods or guidelines existed. In addition, molecular tools were lacking to prove whether isolates obtained over time from the same culture sources were indistinguishable. Notably, many of the different species of CoNS had yet to be identified and characterized [2,30–32].

Almost all infections due to CoNS are nosocomial in origin [33]. This can be directly attributable to the prodigious increase in the number of implanted devices used in healthcare as well as the increased number of immunocompromised patients [34]. Beginning in the 1970s the National Nosocomial Infections Surveillance (NNIS) system was developed to monitor the incidence of healthcare-associated infections and their associated risk factors [35]. In the 1970s, NNIS reported that fewer than 4% of hospital-acquired infections were due to *S. epidermidis*, thus ranking them as the eighth most common cause of nosocomial infection [36]. However, by the 1990s, NNIS reported that CoNS ranked as the number one cause of nosocomial primary bloodstream infection and were second only to *S. aureus* as a cause of surgical-site infections [34]. In the late 1990s, CoNS were implicated in 45% of primary bloodstream infections in medical/surgical intensive care patients [37,38]. CoNS are now recognized as causing a myriad of infections, including bacteremia, CSF shunt infections, continuous ambulatory peritoneal dialysis (CAPD)-related peritonitis, endophthalmitis, genitourinary prostheses infections, infections of breast implants, intravascular device infections, native valve endocarditis, prosthetic joint infections, prosthetic valve endocarditis, surgical-site infections, urinary tract infections, vascular graft infections, and infections in high-risk populations such as neonates and organ transplant recipients [9].

Of the CoNS group, *S. epidermidis* is the species most often isolated from human specimens [1–7,39]. Healthy human skin supports CoNS populations of ten to 10^6 cfu/cm^2. Aptly named, *S. epidermidis* is the most prevalent species found on human skin and mucous membranes, with the average person consistently carrying 10–24 different strains [3,40]. Typically, in healthy immunocompetent individuals, the organism resides harmlessly on the skin and is even beneficial in the maintenance of healthy epidermis [41]. Due to the varying characteristics of human skin, including moisture content, nutrient substances, pH range, and temperature, *S. epidermidis* has had to adapt to a variety of environmental conditions.

The presence of an implanted medical device is the single most important risk factor for infection due to CoNS [15,42,43]. *Staphylococcus epidermidis* can cause infection in all types of prosthetic medical devices [9]. The factors that allow *S. epidermidis* to create such varied infections are multiple, but a prime factor is simply its location and abundance on human skin and mucous membranes [3,44]. This allows for easy access to any transcutaneous device and ready contamination of surgically implanted devices.

Pathogenesis

The ability to produce biofilm is a significant factor in the pathogenesis of infections due to *S. epidermidis*. Studies have shown that biofilm maturation occurs in two stages [45]. First, the organism must adhere to the biomaterial and then it must proliferate and produce a biofilm. Existence in a biofilm rather than as planktonic cells may also describe the state of the organism in its natural skin environment. It is this ability of *S. epidermidis* to form a biofilm which allows it to be unsurpassingly successful as a pathogen of prosthetic devices. In the first step of biofilm formation, adherence, the organism binds to the biomaterial surface via nonspecific factors such as van der Waals forces, surface charge, and hydrophobic interactions. This initial binding is temporary and reversible.

In the second phase of adherence, specific attachment occurs via adhesins that bind to host extracellular matrix molecules. This specific type of linkage is possible because the surface of an implanted device rapidly becomes coated after insertion with a conditioning film consisting of human plasma proteins and cellular elements. Specific attachment is irreversible and paves the way for biofilm maturation consisting of proliferation of bacterial cells and accumulation of an extracellular polysaccharide.

There are currently 10 putative adhesins found in *S. epidermidis* [46] (summarized in Table 15.2). At least six of these have been more fully characterized. Aae (autolysin/adhesin from *S. epidermidis*) [47] binds fibrinogen, vitronectin, and fibronectin. Similar to Aae is GehD (glycerol ester hydrolase D), which functions as a lipase but also binds collagen [48]. Fbe (fibrinogen-binding protein of *S. epidermidis*), also identified as SdrG (serine-aspartate repeat protein G), binds fibrinogen [49] and shows significant homology to clumping factor (Clf)A and ClfB in *S. aureus*. Similar to SdrG is SdrF, which binds to collagen [50]. Another autolysin, AtlE, functions as a vitronectin-binding protein [51]. Embp (extracellular matrix-binding

Table 15.2 Virulence and adaptive factors found in *Staphylococcus epidermidis*.

Attachment to host and/or polystyrene	
Aae	Binds fibrinogen, vitronectin, and fibronectin
AtlE	Binds vitronectin
Bhp	Binds polystyrene
δ-Toxin	Inhibits binding of polystyrene
EbpS	Binds elastin
EmbP	Binds fibronectin
Fbe (SdrG)	Binds fibrinogen
GehD	Binds collagen
ScaA (Aae)	Binds fibrinogen, vitronectin, and fibronectin
ScaB	Unknown ligand
SdrF	Binds collagen
SdrG (Fbe)	Binds fibrinogen
Ssp1	Binds polystyrene
Ssp2	Binds polystyrene
Teichoic acid	Binds fibronectin
Biofilm maturation	
Polysaccharide intercellular adhesin	Accumulation, cell–cell adhesion, and hemagglutination
Aap	Accumulation
Bhp	Cell–cell adhesion
Phenol-soluble modulins	Biofilm dispersion
Virulence factors	
Peptidoglycan/teichoic acid	Induce IL-6, IL-1, and TNF-α; enhance fibronectin binding
Poly-γ-glutamic acid	Immune system modulation
Phenol-soluble modulins	Immune system modulation
Other virulence factors	
Fatty acid-modifying enzyme	Allows persistence on skin
Lipases	Allows persistence on skin; aids survival in abscesses
Proteases	Allows persistence on skin; immune system modulation
δ-Toxin	Immune modulation

IL, interleukin; TNF, tumor necrosis factor.

protein) binds to fibronectin [52]. ScaA and ScaB (staphylococcal conserved antigens A and B) have both been shown to be ligand-binding proteins [53]. EbpS (elastin-binding protein S) is another adhesin which, as its name implies, binds elastin [54]. Nearly one-third (30%) of the cell wall of *S. epidermidis* consists of a glycerol teichoic acid. Teichoic acid enhances binding to fibronectin [55] and along with peptidoglycan induces the production of interleukin (IL)-1, IL-6 and tumor necrosis factor (TNF)-α [56,57]. Finally, *S. epidermidis* also manifests two surface proteins, Ssp1 and Ssp2, which assist in the binding to polystyrene surfaces [58].

Once bound to either the conditioning film on an indwelling medical device or on compromised valvular tissue (infective endocarditis), the bacteria next establishes a sustained biofilm community (Figure 15.1). The matrix of *S. epidermidis* biofilm consists primarily of polysaccharide intercellular adhesin (PIA). PIA is necessary for biofilm formation [59], mediates hemagglutination and bacterial aggregation, and is necessary for virulence in animal models [60]. PIA is produced by enzymes encoded by the *ica* (intercellular adhesin) operon consisting of the *icaA*, *icaD*, *icaB*, *icaC*, and *icaR* genes. *ica*ADBC transcription, and thus PIA production, is regulated by a variety of factors including SarA, σ^B, and IcaR, a *tet*R family transcriptional regulator transcribed divergently from *ica*ADBC. *ica*ADBC transcription, and thus PIA production, is also regulated by a wide variety of environmental signals including the presence of ethanol, anaerobiosis, and those regulated by the tricarboxylic acid cycle [61–64]. PIA allows cells in the biofilm to be tolerant of antimicrobials [65] as well as to avoid immune system extirpation [66]. Although not all strains of *S. epidermidis* contain the *ica* locus [67], studies have shown that those strains that are *ica*-positive are more often isolated as a cause of nosocomial infections than those which are *ica*-negative [68–70]. In addition to the polysaccharide PIA, a protein known as accumulation-associated protein (Aap) is involved in agglomeration of cells. Aap is secreted into the biofilm as well as being cell-wall bound [71]. Another protein called Bhp (Bap homolog protein) is involved in the formation of a biofilm by some strains of *S. epidermidis* [72].

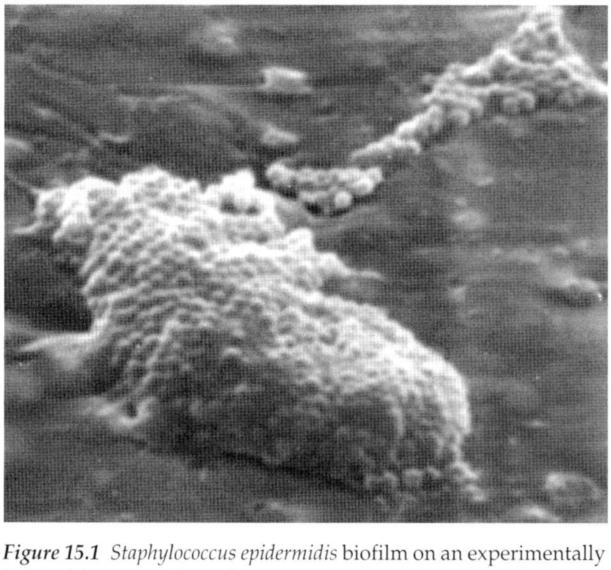

Figure 15.1 *Staphylococcus epidermidis* biofilm on an experimentally infected intravascular catheter.

Once the biofilm has matured, the bacteria exist in a variety of metabolic states in which some are actively replicating while others are relatively quiescent [73]. The final stage of the biofilm maturation process consists of biofilm maintenance and dispersion. In this phase, some cells are actively or passively dispelled from the biofilm community to presumably metastasize to distant sites, thus beginning the entire biofilm formation process anew. Some of the proteins known to be involved in the dispersion activity include a small group of peptides known as phenol-soluble modulins (PSMs) [74]. *Staphylococcus epidermidis* encodes for three of these peptides, designated PSMα, PSMβ, and PSMγ, and they have been shown to have a role in both immune system modulation [75] and biofilm dispersion [74,76].

Although biofilm is recognized as the primary virulence factor in *S. epidermidis*, at least two other virulence traits have been identified. These include the previously mentioned PSMs, which modulate an immune response in the host [74,75], and the production of poly-γ-glutamic acid (PGA). PGA is an anionic extracellular polymer, which in *Bacillus anthracis* produces a capsule that functions to mediate immune system evasion. In *S. epidermidis*, all strains studied so far contain the *cap* operon responsible for the formation of PGA [77]. The molecule appears to play a role in both the commensal lifestyle by allowing survival in a high-salt environment (i.e., human skin) and is also necessary for full production of a biofilm on indwelling devices [74]. PGA appears to help the organism resist antibacterial peptides produced by host immune cells as well as evade phagocytosis [77]. Lastly, *S. epidermidis* produces δ-toxin with significant amino acid similarity to the δ-toxin of *S. aureus* [78], a molecule which may form pores in the membranes of host red blood cells [76].

Epidemiology and specific clinical conditions

In the 1990s, CoNS caused 11% of all nosocomial infections [33,79,80]. It is estimated that just over 2 million nosocomial infections occur annually in the USA and therefore over 200 000 are due to CoNS [80]. This is exceeded only by infections caused by *Escherichia coli* and *S. aureus* [10]. Much of this increase is due to rising rates of CoNS bloodstream and surgical-site infections. Generally, CoNS bloodstream infections predominate when large numbers of intravenous catheters are used in high-risk patient populations, such as neonates or neutropenic oncology patients [81]. Surgical-site infections due to CoNS are more common at surgical centers that perform implantation of prosthetic medical devices [82–84].

Community-acquired strains of CoNS are more likely to cause an infection in patients with a short hospital stay and are usually methicillin susceptible [85]. Patients with a longer hospital stay are likely to become colonized by CoNS strains carried by the hospital staff or found on hospital environmental surfaces, and nosocomial infections occurring in this patient population reflect this colonization [86–90]. These CoNS strains are usually multiply antibiotic resistant and produce biofilm [70,89,91,92]. Airborne transmission of these organisms has also been occasionally documented [25,93].

Because these infections are often difficult to eradicate, prevention of the infection is a primary goal of healthcare practitioners. Prevention of CoNS infections begins with classical infection control measures, especially hand hygiene of healthcare personnel [94]. Other means for reduction include the education of healthcare workers involved in the insertion and care of intravenous catheters, with emphasis on the necessity of maintaining maximal sterility during insertion and strict adherence to aseptic technique whenever the catheter is manipulated [94–96]. Measures to prevent surgical-site infections due to CoNS include patient skin preparation with preoperative antiseptic showering and appropriate application of antiseptics in the operating room, preoperative hand and forearm antisepsis of the surgical team, use of antimicrobial prophylaxis when indicated, proper environmental controls in the surgical suite, and proper care of the surgical wound [97].

Bacteremia and intravascular catheter-associated infection

CoNS are now recognized as the most common cause of nosocomial bloodstream infections and are responsible for 30% of these infections [10,37]. The vast majority of the CoNS bloodstream infections are associated with vascular catheters, usually central venous catheters (CVCs) and less frequently peripheral venous catheters. However, because peripheral venous catheters are more frequently utilized, they are responsible for a large number of infections annually [96,98–100]. CoNS bloodstream infections not associated with intravenous devices are generally found in profoundly neutropenic patients as a consequence of a breakdown in normal mucosal barriers [101–103].

Staphylococcal vascular catheter infections are discussed more thoroughly in Chapter 18. Briefly, infection of short-term nontunneled CVCs occurs most commonly due to migration of skin commensal organisms via the cutaneous catheter tract. Conversely, the longer a short-term catheter stays in place, and also for tunneled CVCs, hub colonization and migration of organisms via the luminal surface becomes an increasingly important route of infection [96,98]. The staphylococcal isolates causing these infections often come from the skin of the patient, but may also be acquired from hospital personnel or the hospital environment [104–106]. Occasionally, catheters may become hematogenously seeded from another focus of infection or via infusate contamination [96].

Diagnosing CoNS bacteremia has historically been difficult and many investigators have attempted to create means to delineate contaminants from true pathogens [107–111]. Because CoNS comprise such a large subset of the human skin commensal flora (as high as 10^3–10^6 cfucm^2 of skin surface [3]) they are often found as contaminants in blood cultures. Typical blood culture contamination rates for most hospitals range from 1 to 3%, and 25–75% of the contaminants are CoNS [112–115]. It has been suggested that determination of true bacteremia can be made in several ways. The Centers for Disease Control and Prevention (CDC) differentiates laboratory-confirmed bloodstream infection (most often due to infected intravascular catheters) from secondary bacteremia (due to infection at another site) by defining primary bacteremia in patients greater than 1 year of age in the following manner:

1 recognized pathogen in the blood from one or more blood cultures and the pathogen is not related to an infection at another site; or

2 fever, chills, or hypotension (not related to infection at another site) and a common skin contaminant is isolated from at least two blood cultures drawn on separate occasions, and the organism is not related to infection at another site [116].

When diagnosing a bloodstream infection due to CoNS, it is imperative that at least two separate blood cultures be obtained, and if the patient has an indwelling CVC, that one of the blood cultures be collected through the catheter [117,118]. Means to differentiate true bacteremia from contamination include consideration of the microbe recovered from the blood, clinical presentation, number of positive cultures, and incubation time to positivity. An incubation time to positivity of less than 25 hours has been considered consistent with true bacteremia [119–121]. In addition, the "differential time to positivity" test can be used to determine whether a vascular catheter is the source of bacteremia [119–123]. This test is predicated on the principle that a blood culture bottle with a higher bacterial inoculum will reveal bacterial growth (i.e., turn positive) more quickly than a bottle with a lower inoculum. Therefore, in the case of a catheter-associated bacteremia, the blood drawn from the catheter should have a higher inoculum, and turn positive more quickly, than blood obtained from the peripheral bloodstream. A number of investigators have shown that a 2-hour cutoff time is a reasonably sensitive and specific means to define catheter-associated bacteremia [119,120,124]. In addition to a supportive differential time to positivity test result, the two CoNS isolates should have the same pulsed-field gel electrophoresis (PFGE) pattern and the same antibiogram [125]. When only a single blood culture is drawn and reveals growth, the best determinants of true bacteremia are the time to positivity (again less than 25 hours) and "slime" production (i.e., PIA) [125]. Generally, clinical signs of CoNS bloodstream infection include classic signs of sepsis using the criteria of Bates [126,127] and the presence of fever (> 38°C), leukocytosis, anemia, and hypotension. If the catheter is removed and sent for culture, the semi-quantitative culture method described by Maki *et al.* [128] may help determine the diagnosis of catheter infection. Other techniques used to culture the catheter include sonication or flushing of the catheter segment [122,129,130].

Often, these infections are difficult to eradicate due to the presence of a biofilm rendering the cells tolerant to antimicrobials and resistant to host immune responses [131,132]. Frequently, the catheter must be removed for successful treatment. Mortality as high as 28% (range 3–28% depending on the study cited) has been noted [81,98,99,133–135]. Novel approaches that have been proposed for prevention or treatment of CVC-associated CoNS infection include coating catheters with various antibiotics or antiseptics, flushing or locking the catheter with a variety of antimicrobial solutions, administration of lysostaphin to help eradicate staphylococcal biofilms, or applying a low-voltage charge across the catheter to electrostatically inhibit microbial adherence [136–141]. Undoubtedly, as our population ages, increasing numbers of patients will require intravenous catheters, making CoNS bacteremia a continuing threat [142] (see Chapter 18 for additional information).

Endocarditis

Native valve endocarditis due to CoNS is a rare phenomenon that occurs in approximately 5–8% of endocarditis cases [143–145]. This infection is due to hematogenous seeding of previously damaged or malformed heart valves and endocardium [146]. The diagnosis of endocarditis is based on demonstration of high-grade bacteremia; observation of supporting clinical findings such as splinter hemorrhages, petechiae, and a cardiac murmur; documentation of consistent laboratory findings such as elevated inflammatory markers and microscopic hematuria; and echocardiographic observation of valvular vegetations or a perivalvular abscess [147]. Patients with native valve CoNS endocarditis often have a very complicated clinical course due to embolic events, rhythm conduction abnormalities, and congestive heart failure [148,149]. Mortality may be as high as 36% [148–151]. More than half of these cases require valve replacement [151].

Unlike native valve endocarditis, in which CoNS are a relatively unlikely etiology, 17% of prosthetic valve endocarditis cases occurring within 2 months of valvular surgery and 20% of cases occurring after 2 months are due to CoNS, usually *S. epidermidis*, with rare cases caused by *S. haemolyticus*, *S. cohnii*, or *S. lugdunensis* [26,149,152–156]. Prosthetic valve endocarditis due to CoNS may occur within days of surgery or may develop after 1 year or more, with the greatest number of cases occurring at about 6 weeks after surgery [155,157–159]. The organisms isolated within 1 year of surgery are generally methicillin resistant (87%) and are probably inoculated at the time of surgery [147]. Those isolates obtained 1 year or more after surgery are often methicillin susceptible [89] and are probably the result of transient bacteremia from the patient's endogenous skin flora. Patients who develop endocarditis within the first few months following surgery generally have involvement of the sewing ring and adjacent myocardium [147]. Signs and symptoms include fever, a new regurgitant murmur, and prosthetic valve dysfunction or failure [149]. Cases of late-onset endocarditis due to CoNS present with valve dysfunction with splenomegaly, progressive congestive heart failure, dehiscence of the prosthetic valve, cardiac conduction abnormalities, and worsening regurgitant murmur [147,149,160]. Diagnosis is made by recovery of CoNS from two or more blood cultures, serial electrocardiography, transesophogeal echocardiography, and histopathological evidence of endocarditis at the time of surgery [160–164]. Because mortality rates as high as 43–74% are observed in patients with CoNS prosthetic valve endocarditis, an aggressive combined medical and surgical therapeutic approach should be initiated [147,165,166]. Typically, antibiotic therapy consists of vancomycin with the addition of gentamicin and/or rifampin [147,167–170]. Often surgery to remove the infected valve is necessary [147].

The use of antibiotics as prophylaxis in valve replacement surgery is enigmatic. Prophylaxis has been documented to cause an alteration in skin flora and increase the number of hospital strains resistant to antibiotics [170–172]. In addition, cephalosporin prophylaxis (the most commonly used agent) does not offer coverage against the most frequent causative organisms, namely methicillin-resistant strains of *S. epidermidis* [173]. If an institution has a substantial number of patients with methicillin-resistant CoNS sternal wound infections or prosthetic valve endocarditis, vancomycin prophylaxis is suggested [174]. A recent study provides evidence to support this position [170] (Chapter 16 also addresses infective endocarditis due to staphylococci).

Vascular graft infection

Intraabdominal vascular graft infections are most frequently due to CoNS (32%) or to *S. aureus* (28%) [175,176]. Generally, *S. aureus* infections occur within days of the graft surgery while CoNS infections are much more indolent and on average manifest 41 months after surgery [176–179]. The organisms causing these infections are believed to have been inoculated at the time of surgery due to their multiply antibiotic-resistant profile and the perioperative isolation of *S. epidermidis* from implanted grafts [177,180,181]. Infections are most likely to occur in either aortofemoral or femoropopliteal grafts with a groin incision, while fewer infections are found in aortoiliac grafts [182]. The major risk factor for development of these infections is the use of a groin incision, with minor risk factors reported to include diabetes mellitus, emergency aortic aneurysm repair, inguinal surgical-site infection, hematoma, lymphocele, or an infected lower extremity wound at the time of surgery [183–185].

Symptoms of CoNS infections that occur within 30 days of surgery usually include fever, cellulitis, increased white blood cell count, abscess formation, and purulent drainage from the incision site [176,177,182]. Later-onset infections due to CoNS may manifest as a false aneurysm, fistula formation, hemorrhage at the anastomosis site, inguinal sinus tract, or gastrointestinal bleeding [176,182,183,186]. Diagnosis is confirmed by physical examination, which often reveals erythema or purulent drainage at the incisional site, the formation of a false aneurysm, or development of a sinus tract at the site of the vascular anastomosis [178,186]. If graft material is removed, then it is necessary to incubate the material in broth in order to maximize the recovery of the small numbers of *S. epidermidis* cells found within the biofilm [177,187,188].

The infected graft must always be replaced and local abscesses drained [176]. These infections are associated with high morbidity and mortality [189]. Lower extremity amputation is ultimately required in 15–30% of patients with CoNS infections of aortofemoral grafts and in 36–53% of those with infections of femoropoliteal grafts [190,191]. Mortality rates vary from 10 to 50% with infections of aortic grafts and from 10 to 25% with infections of femoropopliteal grafts [183,185,186,189].

Central nervous system infection

CSF shunt infections were first described by Schimke *et al.* in 1961 [192]. Currently the infection rate for ventriculoatrial and ventriculoperitoneal shunt procedures ranges between 2 and 30%, with 40–60% of these infections due to CoNS, and *S. epidermidis* comprising 90% of this subset [28,193–195]. About 80% of shunt infections manifest clinically within 4 months of shunt placement [28,196]. Risk factors include age less than 6 months at time of shunt placement, replacement of an infected shunt with new apparatus, dermatitis on the scalp at time of shunt insertion, wound dehiscence postoperatively, scalp necrosis, length of the surgical procedure, experience and proficiency of the surgeon placing the shunt, and intraoperative use of a neuroendoscope [193,194,197].

Signs of an infected shunt include fever, erythema at the incision site, nausea, vomiting, increased intracranial pressure, and shunt malfunction [28,198,199]. About one-third of patients will exhibit clinical signs of meningitis [28]. In cases of prolonged infection, glomerulonephritis may occur due to deposition of immune complexes in the kidney [200]. Diagnosis can be made by culturing CSF from the cerebral ventricles or the shunt, from culturing the shunt itself or, if signs of meningitis are present, from culturing CSF obtained via lumbar puncture [196,201]. Positive blood cultures are observed in cases of ventriculoatrial shunt infection [196]. For epidural catheters, which may be in place for up to 2 weeks, neither positive skin cultures obtained near the catheter insertion site nor quantitative culture of the catheter itself is diagnostic of deep-seated infection, as positive cultures for CoNS generally indicate colonization or a superficial site infection and not an epidural abscess [202]. The literature indicates that prophylaxis prior to shunt placement as well as the use of antibiotic-coated catheters may decrease the likelihood of CSF shunt infection [203–205]. Central nervous system infections due to staphylococci are more completely addressed in Chapter 20.

Endophthalmitis

CoNS account for 40–60% of cases of endophthalmitis following ocular surgery or trauma and *S. epidermidis* is the most common causative organism [206–208]. Symptoms of endophthalmitis, which usually begin within days to weeks following surgery, often include pain and decreased vision and may also include photophobia, headache, and purulent discharge. Generally there is no fever and the presence of leukocytosis is variable [208–210]. Diagnosis is made by physical examination and evaluation of ocular structures using echography or ultrasound as well as microbiological evaluation of specimens of aqueous and vitreous fluids [208–212]. Physical examination often reveals conjunctival injection, hypopyon, corneal edema, and diminished or absent red reflex. Careful interpretation of cultures that grow CoNS is necessary as these organisms often colonize conjunctival surfaces and eyelids, and subsequently contaminate specimens received for culture [212,213]. Typically, infections due to *S. epidermidis* and other CoNS respond more favorably to antibiotic therapy than do those caused by Gram-negative rods or other Gram-positive cocci [207,212,214,215]. The treatment success rate for CoNS endophthalmitis using intravenous and intravitreal antibiotic administration is greater than 70% with complete visual perspicuity [212]. Diseases of the eye due to staphylococci are addressed in more detail in Chapter 21.

Urinary tract infection

Urinary tract infections due to CoNS fall into two major groups. The first is due to *S. saprophyticus*, primarily affecting young females [216]. The second group, those urinary tract infections caused by non-*S. saprophyticus* CoNS, are uncommon and occur almost exclusively in hospitalized patients with underlying urinary tract abnormalities [217,218]. The majority of these patients have a urinary catheter in place and have recently undergone urinary tract surgery or kidney transplantation, experienced kidney stone disease, or have a neurogenic bladder or obstructive uropathy. CoNS cause less than 5% of nosocomial urinary tract infections, with *S. epidermidis* isolated in 90% of the diagnosed cases in this subset [218]. Risk factors, besides the aforementioned urinary tract complications, include advanced age (> 50 years) and extended length of hospital stay [219]. These organisms are usually methicillin resistant and treatment consists of appropriate antibiotic therapy based on the susceptibility profile of the organism [218]. Urinary tract infections due to staphylococci are also addressed in Chapter 24.

Infection of penile prostheses and synthetic urinary sphincters

Staphylococcus epidermidis is responsible for 40–50% of infections of synthetic urinary sphincters and penile prostheses, in which an overall infection rate of 2–8% is observed [220–224]. CoNS infections of penile prostheses are often indolent and may take many weeks, or up to a year, to clinically manifest from the date of implantation [223,225]. Those with infected prostheses exhibit local pain, swelling, induration, and erythema of the penis; occasionally fistula formation is observed, and malfunction or impairment of the device is frequent [220–222]. Rarely do systemic signs of infection occur. Diagnosis is made clinically and by culture of any drainage or irrigation fluid, or by culture of the device itself [222]. In mild cases, treatment may consist of antibiotic therapy alone, although device removal is often required [222,226]. Currently, the emphasis is on prevention of these infections by use of fastidious surgical technique, intraoperative antibiotic prophylaxis, and use of antibiotic-coated prostheses [222,227,228].

Peritoneal dialysis catheter infection and peritonitis

As many as 40% of patients undergoing CAPD are diagnosed with peritonitis within the first year [229,230]. Improvements in catheter connections and the introduction of dialysate in plastic bags rather than glass bottles have helped lower the incidence, but the overall rate of peritonitis remains 0.5–6.3 episodes per patient-year [229–232]. CoNS account for 25–50% of these infections, with *S. epidermidis* comprising 80% of this group [233–235]. Other CoNS isolated include *S. haemolyticus*, *S. capitis*, *S. warneri*, and *S. simulans* [235]. Symptoms of infection include abdominal pain, fever, nausea, and diarrhea [236,237]. Diagnosis is made by the presence of cloudy dialysate fluid with a white blood cell count of more than $100/mm^3$, the majority of these cells consisting of polymorphonuclear cells, and a positive bacterial culture [231]. It is necessary to culture large volumes of fluid (> 100 mL), or to use a filter technique or broth enrichment, to detect small numbers of organisms when culturing the dialysate. However, care must be taken as it may be difficult to differentiate contaminants from causative pathogens [238,239]. Antibiotic therapy is usually successful in the treatment of CoNS peritonitis and catheter removal is generally not necessary [231,240]. Although historically most of these infections were caused by methicillin-susceptible strains, the antimicrobial susceptibility pattern has recently shifted. In 1992, an 18.9% methicillin-resistance rate was observed in CoNS strains causing CAPD peritonitis compared with a rate of 73.9% in 1998 [230,240–242].

Infection of breast implants

Infections of implants used for augmentation mammoplasty are infrequent, but are generally caused by *S. aureus* with *S. epidermidis* a close second [243,244]. *Staphylococcus epidermidis* inhabits the glandular tissue ducts of the breast and from there gains access to the space surrounding the implant [244,245]. This may cause an acute infection that generally occurs within weeks of surgery, with symptoms of drainage, erythema, pain, and swelling [243,246]. Diagnosis is made via culture of the drainage or fluid surrounding the implant or of the implant itself [247]. Treatment consists of antibiotic therapy and removal, with or without replacement, of the implants [248,249]. Indolent infections due to CoNS have been described resulting in capsule formation and contracture of the implant [250,251].

Prosthetic joint infection

The frequency of prosthetic joint infection ranges from less than 2% in new joint placements up to 5% in repeat arthroplasty procedures [252]. In the 1960s, when hip replacement surgery first became available, *S. aureus* was the most common etiology of arthroplasty infection, but in the last half of the 1970s CoNS became the preeminent cause and are now responsible for 30–43% of infections [253,254]. Risk factors include remote infection at the time of surgery, prolonged duration of the surgical procedure, rheumatoid arthritis, previous surgery involving the joint, or an underlying malignancy [253,255,256]. There are three recognized time-points in infection manifestation: stage 1 infections occur within 3 months of surgery and generally consist of infected hematomas caused by *S. aureus*; stage 2 infections are diagnosed between 3 months and 2 years after surgery and are usually caused by CoNS; and stage 3 infections generally occur more than 2 years following surgery and are due to the hematogenous spread of bacteria introduced from dental, intraabdominal, or urinary tract sources; these are rarely due to CoNS [255]. Signs and symptoms of stage 2 infections due to CoNS include pain at the joint, fever, swelling, joint dislocation, and drainage [255]. Diagnosis is based on Gram stain and culture of infected material and may be aided by finding an increased erythrocyte sedimentation rate and by radionuclide scan results [257–259]. The recovery of organisms can be optimized by sonication of the prosthesis at the time of removal [259,260]. Surgery is almost always necessary for treatment, with removal of the infected device and débridement of the surrounding bone, as osteomyelitis is consistently present [252]. Emphasis is placed on prevention of infections as the treatment is so onerous [261–263]. Prevention strategies include the use of laminar flow operating suites, antimicrobial prophylaxis, and antibiotic-impregnated bone cement [263–265]. Chapter 22 discusses these infections in more detail.

Surgical-site infections

There are three classes of surgical-site infection: class 1, superficial incisional infections; class 2, deep incisional infections; and class 3, organ/space infections. Class 1 and 2 surgical-site infections are the most common, accounting for 60–70% of all such reported infections. Class 3 surgical-site infections make up the other 30% of reported cases [116,266,267]. *Staphylococus aureus* is the most common cause of surgical-site infection, with CoNS being the second most frequent agents isolated [116,268]. Of this CoNS group of isolates, *S. epidermidis* is the species most commonly noted, with *S. lugdunensis*, *S. schleiferi*, and *S. caprae* less frequently isolated [269–271]. CoNS are most frequently recovered from class 1 surgical-site infections but less often from class 2 surgical-site infections [266,272]. Risk factors for these infections include severity of underlying disease, obesity, very young (neonate) or advanced age, nutritional status, length of surgical procedure, trauma and condition of the skin at the site of surgery, experience of surgical staff, and number of procedures performed at the healthcare institution [79,273–276].

Signs of a surgical-site infection include swelling, warmth and erythema at the incisional site, wound drainage, an increased peripheral white blood cell count, and fever [277]. Class 1 infections generally occur 3–7 days after surgery. Diagnosis of surgical-site infections should follow the CDC guidelines [278] and include culture of the causative bacteria from the site. These cultures need careful interpretation as CoNS are common contaminants in surgical incisional cultures if the specimens are not properly collected [267,278]. Generally, CoNS are interpreted to be the etiological agent of the surgical-site infection if they are the predominant or only isolate from an abscess or purulent drainage and/or are repeatedly cultured from the same source [79,278]. Morbidity due to CoNS surgical-site infections varies broadly and is dependent on the classification of the infection and the overall health status of the patient [279]. Treatment can range from topical wound care and antimicrobial therapy to surgical débridement and systemic antibiotic treatment [280,281]. As in other types of nosocomial infections, the emphasis is on prevention of these infections [282] and the CDC offers detailed guidelines for this purpose [268]. Surgical-site infections and surgical prophylaxis are further addressed in Chapter 17.

Other types of infection

In addition to the infections listed above, there are many other potential sites of CoNS infection. These infections have been documented with virtually all synthetic implantable devices and as the list of such items in use in today's healthcare environment grows, it can be expected that infections due to CoNS will also continue to increase in number.

Special host populations

Transplant patients

Transplant patients are susceptible to CoNS infections due to their state of immunosuppression and lengthy periods of intravascular catheterization [86,102,103]. These infections are most often manifest as an *S. epidermidis* bloodstream infection due to an infected intravenous catheter or, more rarely, because of a breakdown of mucosal integrity [283]. IL-2 therapy has also been associated with *S. epidermidis* bacteremia [284]. Other nosocomial infections due to CoNS that may occur less frequently in this patient population include endocarditis, mediastinitis, and infections of any synthetic materials used to abet the transplantation process [9,285,286]. Infections in immunocompromised patients are addressed more thoroughly in Chapter 28.

Neonates

Much of the recent increase in overall total numbers of CoNS bacteremia is due to infections in the neonatal intensive care unit (NICU) [287–289]. Studies have reported CoNS bacteremia rates as high as 22% in low-birthweight babies and these organisms account for 73% of all NICU bacteremias as well as 31% of all nosocomial infections in these units [287]. Babies become colonized with CoNS on their skin, nares, umbilicus, and pharynx within days of their admission to the NICU [290,291]. The organisms isolated in these cases do not originate from the mother and are not acquired at the time of birth [292]. Instead, these CoNS strains stem from the hospital environment and healthcare workers. *Staphylococus epidermidis* is the most common species causing these infections, along with lesser numbers of infections due to *S. haemolyticus*, *S. capitis*, and *S. warneri* [293–295]. Risk factors for developing CoNS bacteremia in these circumstances include low birthweight (< 1500 g), the presence and duration of use of CVCs, mechanical ventilation, and total parenteral nutrition (especially with intravenous lipid emulsions) [296–298]. Signs of CoNS bacteremia may include abdominal distension, apnea, bradycardia, inability to maintain body temperature, feeding difficulties, lethargy, neutropenia, thrombocytopenia, hyperglycemia, metabolic acidosis, as well as local signs of infection at the insertion site of the catheter [299–302]. Although most bloodstream infections occur in infants with indwelling catheters, some cases are also found when no intravenous catheters are present [302,303]. These may be the result of skin lesions, or repiratory or gastrointestinal colonization by these organisms. Besides bacteremia, CoNS can also cause skin infections, pneumonia, urinary tract infections, enterocolitis, and even meningitis in the newborn [290,304–307]. CoNS infections infrequently result in mortality in these infants but are often associated with morbidity requiring many additional days of care in the hospital on antimicrobial therapy [301,304].

Diagnosis of neonatal CoNS infections is arduous for several reasons, including difficulty in obtaining blood from low-birthweight neonates, the small volume of the sample obtained (generally 0.1–1.0 mL), and the fact that oftentimes only a single blood culture is obtained [107,109,302]. It is usually necessary to correlate other laboratory findings (e.g., increased C-reactive protein or increased number of immature neutrophils) along with the clinical presentation and the blood culture results to make the diagnosis [299,301,302]. Other CoNS infections in this patient population are diagnosed by the careful interpretation of culture results obtained from the site of the suspected infection, correlated with the clinical presentation of the neonate [303]. Studies have shown that multiply antibioticresistant, *ica*-positive clones of *S. epidermidis* are successful at becoming endemic opportunists and may exist for as long as a decade in the NICU environment [291].

Species and molecular typing methods

The CoNS were originally divided on the basis of colony morphology and biochemical tests by Baird-Parker in the 1960s [308]. Originally consisting of only *S. epidermidis* subgroups II–VI, they were then subdivided by Baird-Parker into two species, *epidermidis* and *saprophyticus* with several subgroups in both of these categories [309]. Eventually, it became clear that there were more species of CoNS and that further differentiation tests and divisions were necessary. In the 1970s, Kloos and Musselwhite [3], developed a method for identifying CoNS to the species level involving an array of morphological descriptions, biochemical testing, physiological testing, susceptibility testing results, and cell wall characterization. Using this schema, several new species were defined. Soon after, a simplified method for identifying relevant (human and animal) species of CoNS in the clinical laboratory was proposed by the same group [310]. This identification scheme involved 10 biochemical tests, novobiocin susceptibility, hemolysis, coagulase production, and reduction of nitrate. These have been adapted and utilized in rapid identification kits as well as the automated systems currently used in most clinical laboratories.

As CoNS are often found as culture contaminants, it is recognized that, as an aid in diagnosis and therapy, accurate determination of species/strain is often imperative. In addition to biochemical tests, other typing analyses have historically included the use of the antibiogram, phage typing, multilocus enzyme electrophoresis, and plasmid profiling [311–314]. More recently, DNA-based techniques have been used to characterize CoNS. These techniques include ribotyping, restriction fragment length polymorphism (RFLP) analysis, polymerase chain reaction (PCR)-based locus-specific RFLP analysis, random amplified polymorphic DNA assays, repetitive extragenic palindromic elements (REP)-PCR, amplified fragment length polymorphism testing, PFGE, PCR amplification of ribosomal DNA spacer regions and tRNA intergenic regions, and finally genomic DNA sequencing [315–317]. A survey of the literature supports the notion that, of these methods, PFGE has been used most often and remains the most discriminatory method used in epidemiological typing. Although PFGE is an excellent technique for exploring local epidemiological questions, it is not an appropriate tool to address questions of population structure.

To address questions of population biology, multilocus sequence typing (MLST) has been recently developed for use in *S. epidermidis*. MLST typically involves the partial sequencing and subsequent comparison of seven conserved housekeeping genes. Three MLST schemes have been proposed for *S. epidermidis*, with the most recent scheme proposed by Miragaia *et al.* [318] providing the highest level of discrimination. Using MLST, several conclusions about the population structure of *S. epidermidis* can be inferred. First, there are at least nine major clonal lineages of *S. epidermidis*; however, a single clonal lineage, CC2 or ST2 [319], is predominant worldwide. Second, SCC*mec* (encoding *mecA*, which confers resistance to oxacillin) has been introduced into multiple *S. epidermidis* backgrounds at multiple times. Lastly, those isolates that do not encode the *icaADBC* operon have the same sequence type as those isolates that do encode *icaADBC* [320]. These data suggest that *icaADBC*-negative isolates do not comprise a separate population and that *icaADBC*-negative isolates have arisen from *icaADBC*-positive isolates, possibly through the deletion of *icaADBC*. Finally, Monk and Archer [320] have recently demonstrated that PCR and DNA sequence analysis of the repeat regions of both *sdrG* (fibrinogen-binding protein Fbe) and *aap* (accumulation-associated protein) in conjunction with MLST further enhances the discriminatory power of these methodologies.

Antimicrobial resistance

β-Lactam agents

A constant theme in both the history and immediate story of *S. epidermidis* is the organism's resistance to antimicrobials [321]. Studies posit that an individual with an infection caused by a more resistant staphylococcal strain will have a worse clinical outcome than the same infection caused by a more susceptible strain [322]. When reviewing antimicrobial resistance in CoNS, it is necessary to distinguish hospital-acquired strains from community strains. Typically, those isolates causing disease in the community have lower rates of resistance than isolates acquired in the hospital environment [323,324]. Most notably, nosocomial isolates of CoNS possess the *mec*A gene, which confers resistance to methicillin and all the β-lactam antibiotics. As a consequence, susceptibility testing of CoNS is usually dichotomized into methicillin-resistant and -susceptible categories. Resistance to antimicrobials is generally classified by the mechanism of resistance into three different classes: (i) specific or general efflux pumps that remove the antibiotic from the cell, preventing accumulation (and action) of the drug [325]; (ii) modification of the bacterial target of the drug (e.g., the ribosome); or (iii) inactivation of the antimicrobial agent. Acquisition of resistance can occur by either mutation of a bacterial gene or genes or by the accretion of a resistance gene or genes via genetic transfer (transduction, conjugation, or transformation) [326]. The staphylococci contain a number of plasmids and transposons, both important mechanisms for the horizontal transfer of antimicrobial resistance genes [327].

Penicillin was the first antibiotic used successfully for the treatment of staphylococci [328] and is a cell-wall biosynthesis inhibitor. Shortly after its introduction in the 1940s, β-lactamase-producing penicillin-resistant strains of *S. epidermidis* were described and currently greater than 90% of strains isolated from infections are resistant to penicillin [329]. Methicillin was marketed in 1960 to help nullify this increasing resistance. Methicillin-resistant strains of *S. epidermidis* were quickly reported. By 1980, about 20% of *S. epidermidis* strains isolated from hospital patients were methicillin resistant and by 1989, 60% of these isolates were resistant. During the 1990s, resistance rates for CoNS ranged globally from 75 to 90% [329]. In addition to resistance to all β-lactam agents, methicillin-resistant CoNS are oftentimes resistant to multiple classes of other antibiotic agents.

Non-β-lactam agents

The glycopeptide vancomycin (so named because of its use in "vanquishing" penicillin-resistant staphylococci) [330,331] was developed in the 1950s and until the 1990s *S. epidermidis* remained susceptible to this drug. Since then, there have been increasing reports of both vancomycin-intermediate as well as vancomycin-resistant strains, and overall minimum inhibitory concentration "creep" [331]. Glycopeptides with greater potency against staphylococci that are in various stages of development include telavancin, dalbovancin, and oritavancin [332].

The aminoglycosides, first isolated in the 1940s and 1950s, are protein synthesis inhibitors and are also able to disrupt the bacterial membrane and advance their own uptake into bacterial cells. This property may explain why they are able to act synergistically with the β-lactams. Gentamicin is sometimes used for the treatment of severe *S. epidermidis* infections along with vancomycin and rifampin especially if bacteremia is also present. Unfortunately, 62% of methicillin-resistant CoNS are also resistant to gentamicin [329].

The tetracyclines were first identified in 1948 and work by inhibiting protein synthesis. Worldwide, in the 1990s, methicillin-resistant CoNS averaged about 22% resistance to tetracyclines. The macrolide–lincosamide–streptogramin B (MLS_B) group of antibiotics are structurally related protein synthesis inhibitors. The macrolides include erythromycin (introduced in 1952), and two related compounds, clarithromycin (1991) and azithromycin (1991). Resistance to erythromycin for methicillin-resistant CoNS is generally 75%. The only lincosamide available in the USA is clindamycin, which was introduced in 1966. Resistance to this drug is currently around 50% for methicillin-resistant CoNS and 10% for methicillin-sensitive CoNS. The streptogramins were first isolated in 1953 and currently the only drug of this class available in the USA is quinipristin/dalfopristin, introduced in 1999. Resistance to quinupristin/dalfopristin for both methicillin-resistant CoNS and methicillin-sensitive CoNS is generally less than 2% [326]. Chloramphenicol (introduced in 1949) inhibits protein synthesis. Resistance rates for methicillin-resistant CoNS, although generally low, vary by geographic region, from 6.7% in the USA to 44.8% in Latin American nations. However, due to the small risk of irreversible aplastic anemia associated with chloramphenicol, it is rarely used in the USA. The sulfonamides and trimethoprim are usually given as combination therapy, and interfere with the biosynthesis of tetrahydrofolic acid [333,334]. Methicillin-resistant CoNS average 60% resistance rates to this antimicrobial, while methicillin-sensitive CoNS exhibit about a 17% resistance rate. The oxazolidinone linezolid, introduced in 2001, is the first drug in a completely synthetic class of protein synthesis inhibitors. Currently, resistance in CoNS is very rare (1%). Rifampin, a member of the rifamycin class of antibiotics introduced in 1971, prevents transcription of bacterial mRNA [335,336]. Mutations conferring resistance to this drug readily occur, and therefore if rifampin is used it should be combined with another antimicrobial [326]. Currently, resistance rates average about 2% for methicillin-sensitive CoNS and 13% for methicillin-resistant CoNS. The fluoroquinolones are a synthetic class serendipitously discovered during the synthesis of the antimalarial agent chloroquine. In staphylococci, topoisomerase IV is the primary target of action for this antibiotic. There are several quinolones currently used in the USA and resistance rates for ciprofloxacin average about 8% for methicillin-sensitive CoNS and greater than 50% for methicillin-resistant CoNS. Daptomycin, a lipopeptide, received approval from the Food and Drug Administration in 2003. It acts by binding to the cell membrane, causing rapid depolarization of the membrane without lysis of the organism and cell death [337]. Thus far, for CoNS, resistance rates are very low (< 1%). Antibiotic resistance is covered in more detail in Chapters 8, 9, and 10).

Coagulase-negative staphylococci other than *S. epidermidis*

Staphylococcus haemolyticus

Staphylococcus haemolyticus is most often a nosocomial pathogen that has historically been multiply antibiotic resistant [338]. Its natural niche on humans (it is also found on primates and some domestic animals) includes the axillae, inguinal region, and the perineum [3,339]. It has been implicated in a variety of human infections including urinary tract infections, bacteremia, native valve endocarditis, and orthopedic infections [115]. Of the CoNS, it is second only to *S. epidermidis* in frequency of isolation from blood cultures [9]. It has been implicated in outbreaks, most often in NICUs [340]. *Staphylococcus haemolyticus* contains several putative virulence genes including lipases, proteases, and lyases [340]. As previously noted, it is often multiply antibiotic resistant and historically acquired methicillin and glycopeptide resistance earlier than most other staphylococcal species [341]. It is believed this is due to a copious number of insertion sequences (IS elements), many of them highly homologous [341,342]. The glycopeptide-resistant strains possess highly cross-linked peptidoglycan with additional serine instead of glycine in their cross-bridges [341,342].

Staphylococcus lugdunensis

Staphylococcus lugdunensis, first described in 1988 in Lyon, France, has been reported to cause up to 44% of cases of CoNS native valve endocarditis. It has also been implicated as a cause of skin and soft tissue infections and post-operative wound infections, especially those occurring below the navel [343]. Other infections due to *S. lugdunensis* include indwelling catheter and prosthetic device infections, osteomyelitis, peritonitis, and septic arthritis, all most often with corresponding bacteremia. Unlike the often indolent chronic infections due to *S. epidermidis*, *S. lugdunensis* typically results in an acute infection more similar to that caused by *S. aureus* [344].

Normally found on human skin as a commensal, in particular in the inguinal area, the organism is of greater virulence than many other species of CoNS due to several factors. These include the production of clumping factor as well as a thermostable DNase (both of these sometimes responsible for its misidentification in the clinical laboratory as *S. aureus*). In addition, *S. lugdunensis* produces an extracellular glycocalyx that allows it to infect foreign bodies as well as interfere with prostaglandin E_2 production, which inhibits T-cell expansion and modulates TNF-α and nitric oxide, thus impeding macrophage function [344–347]. The microorganism also produces lipase, esterase, a fatty acid-modifying enzyme (FAME), as well as a synergistic hemolysin (SLUSH) which interacts with the previously mentioned factors allowing them to act synergistically to facilitate tissue invasion [348]. The microbe binds to collagen, fibronectin, fibrinogen, human IgG, laminin, plasminogen, thrombospondin, and vitronectin [346,347]. The organism also expresses a von Willebrand factor-binding protein that possibly plays a primary role in bacterial attachment to minute vascular lesions, the inceptive step in bacterial endocarditis [349]. When subjected to PFGE or plasmid profiling restriction endonuclease analysis, *S. lugdunensis* exhibits high genotypic uniformity [350]. This may partially explain its fortuitously susceptible antibiotic profile. Typically, only 25% of strains are positive for β-lactamase and methicillin resistance is rare [351].

Staphylococcus saprophyticus

Staphylococcus saprophyticus is second only to *E. coli* as a causative agent of uncomplicated urinary tract infections in young (18–35 years old) women [352–359]. This organism chiefly causes acute urinary tract infections, including cystitis, pyelonephritis (occasionally associated with renal calculus), and urethritis. These urinary tract infections have a seasonal predilection (late summer to early autumn), often follow sexual intercourse, may occur concomitant with vaginal candidiasis, or shortly after a menstrual period [354,356,357]. Rare exceptional cases of native valve endocarditis, endophthalmitis after cataract surgery, and septicemia have also been cited in the literature [359]. *Staphylococcus saprophyticus* is normally found colonizing the rectum or urogenital tracts of approximately 10% of young females [358]. It is also occasionally found on other mammals and in contaminated food of animal origin.

Recent whole-genome sequencing of the organism demonstrated that none of the virulence genes associated with *S. aureus* nor any of the extracellular matrix-binding proteins found in *S. aureus* or *S. epidermidis* are found in its genome [360]. However, the presence of several unique genes in the chromosome allow *S. saprophyticus* to be uniquely equipped to cause urinary tract infections. *Staphylococcus saprophyticus* exhibits hemagglutination mediated by the cell wall-anchored protein UafA [361,362], which correlates with adherence to human ureteral epithelial cells [362]. The organism also has many transporter proteins and systems that allow rapid adaptation to the human urine environment with its constantly fluctuating urea concentration, pH, osmolarity, and inorganic ions. This species also contains two plasmids each encoding a putative water channel aquaporin Z gene (*aqpZ*) that may also assist with osmotic balance. Although *S. saprophyticus* encodes for the urease operon *ureABCEFGD*, also found in *S. epidermidis* and *S. aureus*, it produces urease in much greater amounts, thus allowing it to utilize the urea found in urine as a source of nitrogen [363].

Staphylococcus saprophyticus is often identified in the clinical laboratory via its resistance to novobiocin [364]. Although resistant to nalidixic acid, *S. saprophyticus* is generally susceptible to aminoglycosides, fluoroquinolones, glycopeptides, lincosamides, and methicillin. It varies in its susceptibility to erythromycin, penicillin, and tetracycline [365]. It is most often treated with urinary tract antimicrobials but occasional therapeutic failures have been reported with nitrofurantoin and the sulfonamides [355,359].

Conclusions

In *S. epidermidis*, we have witnessed the emergence of a microbe as a nosocomial pathogen. As the number of patients in hospital with invasive vascular catheters and prosthetic devices continues to increase, we will most likely witness a concomitant rise in CoNS nosocomial infections. In addition, the large expansion in the number of immunocompromised patients, the continued escalation of antimicrobial use, and the inadequate application of infection control practices contribute to the problem. Because treatment of CoNS prosthetic device infections is quite onerous and generally requires removal of the device, increased emphasis must be placed on prevention of these infections. At present this may be accomplished by consistent application of good infection control practices, adherence to antimicrobial stewardship recommendations, and introduction of medical devices coated with various antiseptics or antibiotics. In the future, with improved understanding of the pathogenesis of these infections, it is hoped that new and innovative devices may be developed that are less infection prone or that means to prevent bacterial adherence and biofilm production may be discovered.

References

1 Ayliffe GA. The effect of antibacterial agents on the flora of the skin. J Hosp Infect 1980;1:111–24.

2 Kloos WE. Natural populations of the genus *Staphylococcus*. Annu Rev Microbiol 1980;34:559–92.

3 Kloos WE, Musselwhite MS. Distribution and persistence of *Staphylococcus* and *Micrococcus* species and other aerobic bacteria on human skin. Appl Microbiol 1975;30:381–5.

4 Leeming JP, Holland KT, Cunliffe WJ. The microbial ecology of pilosebaceous units isolated from human skin. J Gen Microbiol 1984;130:803–7.

5 Marples MJ. The normal microbial flora of the skin. Soc Appl Bacteriol Symp Ser 1974;3:7–12.

6 McBride ME, Duncan WC, Knox JM. The environment and the microbial ecology of human skin. Appl Environ Microbiol 1977;33:603–8.

7 Noble WC, Somerville DA. Microbiology of Human Skin. Philadelphia: WB Saunders, 1974.

8 Weinstein RA. Nosocomial infection update. Emerg Infect Dis 1998;4:416–20.

9 Boyce JM. Coagulase-negative staphylococci. In: Mayhall CG, ed. Hospital Epidemiology and Infection Control, 3rd edn. Philadelphia: Lippincott, Williams and Wilkins, 2004:495–516.

10 National Nosocomial Infections Surveillance System, Division of Healthcare Quality Promotion, National Center for Infectious Diseases. National Nosocomial Infections Surveillance (NNIS) System Report, Data Summary from January 1992 to June 2001. Am J Infect Control 2001;29:404–21.

11 National Nosocomial Infections Surveillance System. Data summary from October 1986 to April 1996. Am J Infect Control 1996;24:380–8.

12 O'Gara JP, Humphreys H. *Staphylococcus epidermidis* biofilms: importance and implications. J Med Microbiol 2001;50:582–7.

13 Ogston A. Report upon micro-organisms in surgical diseases. BMJ 1881;1:369–75.

14 Rosenbach FJ. Mikro-Organismen bei den Wund-Infections. Bergman JF, ed. Wiesbaden, 1884.

15 Heilmann C, Peters G. Biology and pathogenicity of *Staphylococcus epidermidis*. In: Fischetti VA, Novick RP, Ferretti JJ, Portnoy DA, Rood JI, eds. Gram-positive Pathogens, 2nd edn. Washington, DC: ASM Press, 2006:560–71.

16 Refsahl K, Andersen BM. Clinically significant coagulase-negative staphylococci: identification and resistance patterns. J Hosp Infect 1992;22:19–31.

17 Forse RA, Dixon C, Bernard K, Martinez L, McLean AP, Meakins JL. *Staphylococcus epidermidis*: an important pathogen. Surgery 1979;86:507–14.

18 Smith IM, Beals PD, Kingsbury KR, Hasenclever HF. Observations on *Staphylococcus albus* septicemia in mice and men. AMA Arch Intern Med 1958;102:375–88.

19 Denton C, Pappas EG, Uricchio JF, Goldberg H, Likoff W. Bacterial endocarditis following cardiac surgery. Circulation 1957;15:525–31.

20 Koiwai EK, Nahas HC. Subacute bacterial endocarditis following cardiac surgery. AMA Arch Surg 1956;73:272–8.

21 Pulverer G, Halswick R. [Coagulase-negative staphylococci (*Staphylococcus albus*) as pathogens.] Dtsch Med Wochenschr 1967;92:1141–5.

22 Callaghan RP, Cohen SJ, Stewart GT. Septicaemia due to colonization of Spitz-Holter valves by staphylococci. Five cases treated with methicillin. BMJ 1961;1:860–3.

23 Wilson TS, Stuart RD. *Staphylococcus albus* in wound infection and in septicemia. Can Med Assoc J 1965;93:8–16.

24 Pereira AT. Antigenic structure of staphylococci. Ann Ist Super Sanita 1965;1:487–99.

25 Blakemore WS, McGarrity GJ, Thurer RJ, Wallace HW, MacVaugh H III, Coriell LL. Infection by air-borne bacteria with cardiopulmonary bypass. Surgery 1971;70:830–8.

26 Dismukes WE, Karchmer AW, Buckley MJ, Austen WG, Swartz MN. Prosthetic valve endocarditis. Analysis of 38 cases. Circulation 1973;48:365–77.
27 Holt RJ. The colonization of ventriculoatrial shunts by coagulase-negative staphylococci. In: Finland WM, Bartmann K, eds. Bacterial Infections: Changes in their Causative Agents, Trends and Possible Basis. Stuttgart: Springer-Verlag, 1971:81–7.
28 Schoenbaum SC, Gardner P, Shillito J. Infections of cerebrospinal fluid shunts: epidemiology, clinical manifestations, and therapy. J Infect Dis 1975;131:543–52.
29 Pulverer G. On the pathogenicity of coagulase-negative staphylococci. In: Jelijszewics J, ed. The Staphylococci: Proceedings of V International Symposium on Staphylococci and Staphylococcal Infections. Stuttgart: Gustav Fischer Verlag, 1985:1–9.
30 Kloos WE. Systematics and the natural history of staphylococci 1. Soc Appl Bacteriol Symp Ser 1990;19:25S–37S.
31 Schleifer KH, Kloos WE. Isolation and characterization of staphylococci from human skin. I. Amended description of *Staphylococcus epidermidis* and *Staphylococcus saprophyticus* and descriptions of three new species: *Staphylococcus cohnii, Staphylococcus haemolyticus*, and *Staphylococcus xylosus*. Int J Syst Bacteriol 1975;25:50–61.
32 Schleifer KH, Kloos WE. A simple test system for the separation of staphylococci from micrococci. J Clin Microbiol 1975;1:337–8.
33 Schaberg DR, Culver DH, Gaynes RP. Major trends in the microbial etiology of nosocomial infection. Am J Med 1991;91(3B):72S–75S.
34 Richards MJ, Edwards JR, Culver DH, Gaynes RP. Nosocomial infections in combined medical–surgical intensive care units in the United States. Infect Control Hosp Epidemiol 2000;21:510–15.
35 Richards C, Emori TG, Edwards J, Fridkin S, Tolson J, Gaynes R. Characteristics of hospitals and infection control professionals participating in the National Nosocomial Infections Surveillance System 1999. Am J Infect Control 2001;29:400–3.
36 National Nosocomial Infections Surveillance System. National Nosocomial Infections Surveillance (NNIS) System Report, Annual Summary 1979. Atlanta, GA: Centers for Disease Control and Prevention, 1979.
37 Richards MJ, Edwards JR, Culver DH, Gaynes RP. Nosocomial infections in medical intensive care units in the United States. National Nosocomial Infections Surveillance System. Crit Care Med 1999;27:887–92.
38 Rupp ME. Nosocomial bloodstream infections. In: Mayhall CG, ed. Hospital Epidemiology and Infection Control, 3rd edn. Philadelphia: Lippincott, Williams and Wilkins, 2004:253–66.
39 Jenny D. [Bacterial flora of the skin and its resistance status.] Dermatologica 1967;134:293–300.
40 Brown E, Wenzel RP, Hendley JO. Exploration of the microbial anatomy of normal human skin by using plasmid profiles of coagulase-negative staphylococci: search for the reservoir of resident skin flora. J Infect Dis 1989;160:644–50.
41 Chiller K, Selkin BA, Murakawa GJ. Skin microflora and bacterial infections of the skin. J Invest Dermatol Symp Proc 2001;6:170–4.
42 Gandelman G, Frishman WH, Wiese C *et al.* Intravascular device infections: epidemiology, diagnosis, and management. Cardiol Rev 2007;15:13–23.
43 Lew DP, Pittet D, Waldvogel FA. Infections that complicate the insertion of prosthetic devices. In: Mayhall CG, ed. Hospital Epidemiology and Infection Control, 3rd edn. Philadelphia: Lippincott, Williams and Wilkins, 2004:1181–206.
44 Otto M. Virulence factors of the coagulase-negative staphylococci. Front Biosci 2004;9:841–63.
45 von Eiff C, Peters G, Heilmann C. Pathogenesis of infections due to coagulase-negative staphylococci. Lancet Infect Dis 2002;2:677–85.
46 Yao Y, Sturdevant DE, Villaruz A, Xu L, Gao Q, Otto M. Factors characterizing *Staphylococcus epidermidis* invasiveness determined by comparative genomics. Infect Immun 2005;73:1856–60.
47 Heilmann C, Thumm G, Chhatwal GS, Hartleib J, Uekotter A, Peters G. Identification and characterization of a novel autolysin (Aae) with adhesive properties from *Staphylococcus epidermidis*. Microbiology 2003;149:2769–78.
48 Longshaw CM, Farrell AM, Wright JD, Holland KT. Identification of a second lipase gene, *gehD*, in *Staphylococcus epidermidis*: comparison of sequence with those of other staphylococcal lipases. Microbiology 2000;146:1419–27.
49 Davis SL, Gurusiddappa S, McCrea KW, Perkins S, Hook M. SdrG, a fibrinogen-binding bacterial adhesin of the microbial surface components recognizing adhesive matrix molecules subfamily from *Staphylococcus epidermidis*, targets the thrombin cleavage site in the Bbeta chain. J Biol Chem 2001;276:27799–805.
50 Arrecubieta C, Lee MH, Macey A, Foster TJ, Lowy FD. SdrF, a *Staphylococcus epidermidis* surface protein, binds type I collagen. J Biol Chem 2007;282:18767–76.
51 Heilmann C, Hussain M, Peters G, Gotz F. Evidence for autolysin-mediated primary attachment of *Staphylococcus epidermidis* to a polystyrene surface. Mol Microbiol 1997;24:1013–24.
52 Williams RJ, Henderson B, Sharp LJ, Nair SP. Identification of a fibronectin-binding protein from *Staphylococcus epidermidis*. Infect Immun 2002;70:6805–10.
53 Pourmand MR, Clarke SR, Schuman RF, Mond JJ, Foster SJ. Identification of antigenic components of *Staphylococcus epidermidis* expressed during human infection. Infect Immun 2006;74:4644–54.
54 Downer R, Roche F, Park PW, Mecham RP, Foster TJ. The elastin-binding protein of *Staphylococcus aureus* (EbpS) is expressed at the cell surface as an integral membrane protein and not as a cell wall-associated protein. J Biol Chem 2002;277:243–50.
55 Hussain M, Heilmann C, Peters G, Herrmann M. Teichoic acid enhances adhesion of *Staphylococcus epidermidis* to immobilized fibronectin. Microb Pathog 2001;31:261–70.
56 Jones KJ, Perris AD, Vernallis AB, Worthington T, Lambert PA, Elliott TS. Induction of inflammatory cytokines and nitric oxide in J774.2 cells and murine macrophages by lipoteichoic acid and related cell wall antigens from *Staphylococcus epidermidis*. J Med Microbiol 2005;54:315–21.
57 Mattsson E, Van Dijk H, Verhoef J, Norrby R, Rollof J. Supernatants from *Staphylococcus epidermidis* grown in the presence of different antibiotics induce differential release of tumor necrosis factor alpha from human monocytes. Infect Immun 1996;64:4351–5.
58 Veenstra GJ, Cremers FF, van Dijk H, Fleer A. Ultrastructural organization and regulation of a biomaterial adhesin of *Staphylococcus epidermidi*s. J Bacteriol 1996;178:537–41.
59 Fey PD, Ulphani JS, Gotz F, Heilmann C, Mack D, Rupp ME. Characterization of the relationship between polysaccharide

intercellular adhesin and hemagglutination in *Staphylococcus epidermidis*. J Infect Dis 1999;179:1561–4.
60 Rupp ME, Fey PD. In vivo models to evaluate adhesion and biofilm formation by *Staphylococcus epidermidis*. Methods Enzymol 2001;336:206–15.
61 Conlon KM, Humphreys H, O'Gara JP. Regulation of *icaR* gene expression in *Staphylococcus epidermidis*. FEMS Microbiol Lett 2002;216:171–7.
62 Conlon KM, Humphreys H, O'Gara JP. *icaR* encodes a transcriptional repressor involved in environmental regulation of *ica* operon expression and biofilm formation in *Staphylococcus epidermidis*. J Bacteriol 2002;184:4400–8.
63 Handke LD, Slater SR, Conlon KM *et al.* SigmaB and SarA independently regulate polysaccharide intercellular adhesin production in *Staphylococcus epidermidis*. Can J Microbiol 2007; 53:82–91.
64 Tormo MA, Marti M, Valle J *et al.* SarA is an essential positive regulator of *Staphylococcus epidermidis* biofilm development. J Bacteriol 2005;187:2348–56.
65 Arciola CR, Campoccia D, Gamberini S *et al.* Antibiotic resistance in exopolysaccharide-forming *Staphylococcus epidermidis* clinical isolates from orthopaedic implant infections. Biomaterials 2005;26:6530–5.
66 Vuong C, Voyich JM, Fischer ER *et al.* Polysaccharide intercellular adhesin (PIA) protects *Staphylococcus epidermidis* against major components of the human innate immune system. Cell Microbiol 2004;6:269–75.
67 Cafiso V, Bertuccio T, Santagati M *et al.* Presence of the *ica* operon in clinical isolates of *Staphylococcus epidermidis* and its role in biofilm production. Clin Microbiol Infect 2004;10: 1081–8.
68 Arciola CR, Baldassarri L, Montanaro L. In catheter infections by *Staphylococcus epidermidis* the intercellular adhesion (*ica*) locus is a molecular marker of the virulent slime-producing strains. J Biomed Mater Res 2002;59:557–62.
69 Galdbart JO, Allignet J, Tung HS, Ryden C, El Solh N. Screening for *Staphylococcus epidermidis* markers discriminating between skin-flora strains and those responsible for infections of joint prostheses. J Infect Dis 2000;182:351–5.
70 Arciola CR, Baldassarri L, Montanaro L. Presence of *icaA* and *icaD* genes and slime production in a collection of staphylococcal strains from catheter-associated infections. J Clin Microbiol 2001;39:2151–6.
71 Hussain M, Herrmann M, von Eiff C, Perdreau-Remington F, Peters G. A 140-kilodalton extracellular protein is essential for the accumulation of *Staphylococcus epidermidis* strains on surfaces. Infect Immun 1997;65:519–24.
72 Tormo MA, Knecht E, Gotz F, Lasa I, Penades JR. Bap-dependent biofilm formation by pathogenic species of *Staphylococcus*: evidence of horizontal gene transfer? Microbiology 2005;151: 2465–75.
73 Rani SA, Pitts B, Beyenal H *et al.* Spatial patterns of DNA replication, protein synthesis, and oxygen concentration within bacterial biofilms reveal diverse physiological states. J Bacteriol 2007;189:4223–33.
74 Yao Y, Sturdevant DE, Otto M. Genomewide analysis of gene expression in *Staphylococcus epidermidis* biofilms: insights into the pathophysiology of *S. epidermidis* biofilms and the role of phenol-soluble modulins in formation of biofilms. J Infect Dis 2005;191:289–98.
75 Liles WC, Thomsen AR, O'Mahony DS, Klebanoff SJ. Stimulation of human neutrophils and monocytes by staphylococcal phenol-soluble modulin. J Leukoc Biol 2001;70:96–102.
76 Vuong C, Durr M, Carmody AB, Peschel A, Klebanoff SJ, Otto M. Regulated expression of pathogen-associated molecular pattern molecules in *Staphylococcus epidermidis*: quorum-sensing determines pro-inflammatory capacity and production of phenol-soluble modulins. Cell Microbiol 2004;6:753–9.
77 Kocianova S, Vuong C, Yao Y *et al.* Key role of poly-gamma-DL-glutamic acid in immune evasion and virulence of *Staphylococcus epidermidis*. J Clin Invest 2005;115:688–94.
78 McKevitt AI, Bjornson GL, Mauracher CA, Scheifele DW. Amino acid sequence of a deltalike toxin from *Staphylococcus epidermidis*. Infect Immun 1990;58:1473–5.
79 Emori TG, Gaynes RP. An overview of nosocomial infections, including the role of the microbiology laboratory. Clin Microbiol Rev 1993;6:428–42.
80 National Nosocomial Infections Surveillance System, Division of Healthcare Quality Promotion, National Center for Infectious Diseases. National Nosocomial Infections Surveillance (NNIS) System Report. Am J Infect Control 2003;31:481–98.
81 Banerjee SN, Emori TG, Culver DH *et al.* Secular trends in nosocomial primary bloodstream infections in the United States, 1980–1989. National Nosocomial Infections Surveillance System. Am J Med 1991;91(3B):86S–89S.
82 Gaynes RP, Martone WJ, Culver DH *et al.* Comparison of rates of nosocomial infections in neonatal intensive care units in the United States. National Nosocomial Infections Surveillance System. Am J Med 1991;91(3B):192S–196S.
83 Marples RR, Hone R, Notley CM, Richardson JF, Crees-Morris JA. Ivestigation of coagulase-negative staphylococci from infections in surgical patients. Zentralbl Bakteriol [Orig A] 1978;241:140–56.
84 Ajemian E, Andrews L, Hryb K, Klimek JJ. Hospital-acquired infections after arthroscopic knee surgery: a probable environmental source. Am J Infect Control 1987;15:159–62.
85 Cove JH, Eady EA, Cunliffe WJ. Skin carriage of antibiotic-resistant coagulase-negative staphylococci in untreated subjects. J Antimicrob Chemother 1990;25:459–69.
86 Bender JW, Hughes WT. Fatal *Staphylococcus epidermidis* sepsis following bone marrow transplantation. Johns Hopkins Med J 1980;146:13–15.
87 Boyce JM. Environmental contamination makes an important contribution to hospital infection. J Hosp Infect 2007;65(suppl 2): 50–4.
88 Pittet D, Allegranzi B, Sax H *et al.* Evidence-based model for hand transmission during patient care and the role of improved practices. Lancet Infect Dis 2006;6:641–52.
89 Archer GL. Alteration of cutaneous staphylococcal flora as a consequence of antimicrobial prophylaxis. Rev Infect Dis 1991;13(suppl 10):S805–S809.
90 Varaldo PE, Cipriani P, Foca A *et al.* Identification, clinical distribution, and susceptibility to methicillin and 18 additional antibiotics of clinical *Staphylococcus* isolates: nationwide investigation in Italy. J Clin Microbiol 1984;19:838–43.
91 Dryden MS, Talsania H, McCann M, Cookson BD, Phillips I. The epidemiology of ciprofloxacin resistance in coagulase-negative staphylococci in CAPD patients. Epidemiol Infect 1992;109:97–112.

92 Frebourg NB, Lefebvre S, Baert S, Lemeland JF. PCR-based assay for discrimination between invasive and contaminating *Staphylococcus epidermidis* strains. J Clin Microbiol 2000;38: 877–80.

93 Aglietti P, Salvati EA, Wilson PD Jr, Kutner LJ. Effect of a surgical horizontal unidirectional filtered air flow unit on wound bacterial contamination and wound healing. Clin Orthop Relat Res 1974;101:99–104.

94 Voss A, Meis JF. Hand hygiene and health-care-associated infections. Lancet Infect Dis 2007;7:304–5; author reply 305–306.

95 Lavery I, Ingram P. Prevention of infection in peripheral intravenous devices. Nurs Stand 2006;20:49–56.

96 O'Grady NP, Alexander M, Dellinger EP *et al.* Guidelines for the prevention of intravascular catheter-related infections. MMWR 2002;51(RR-10):1–29.

97 Dellinger EP, Hausmann SM, Bratzler DW *et al.* Hospitals collaborate to decrease surgical site infections. Am J Surg 2005; 190:9–15.

98 Eggimann P, Sax H, Pittet D. Catheter-related infections. Microbes Infect 2004;6:1033–42.

99 Martin MA, Pfaller MA, Wenzel RP. Coagulase-negative staphylococcal bacteremia. Mortality and hospital stay. Ann Intern Med 1989;110:9–16.

100 Pfaller MA, Herwaldt LA. Laboratory, clinical, and epidemiological aspects of coagulase-negative staphylococci. Clin Microbiol Rev 1988;1:281–99.

101 Herwaldt LA, Hollis RJ, Boyken LD, Pfaller MA. Molecular epidemiology of coagulase-negative staphylococci isolated from immunocompromised patients. Infect Control Hosp Epidemiol 1992;13:86–92.

102 Wade JC, Schimpff SC, Newman KA, Wiernik PH. *Staphylococcus epidermidis*: an increasing cause of infection in patients with granulocytopenia. Ann Intern Med 1982;97:503–8.

103 Winston DJ, Dudnick DV, Chapin M, Ho WG, Gale RP, Martin WJ. Coagulase-negative staphylococcal bacteremia in patients receiving immunosuppressive therapy. Arch Intern Med 1983;143:32–6.

104 Mermel LA. Prevention of central venous catheter-related infections: what works other than impregnated or coated catheters? J Hosp Infect 2007;65(suppl 2):30–3.

105 Mermel LA, McCormick RD, Springman SR, Maki DG. The pathogenesis and epidemiology of catheter-related infection with pulmonary artery Swan–Ganz catheters: a prospective study utilizing molecular subtyping. Am J Med 1991;91(3B):197S–205S.

106 Parisi JT. Epidemiologic markers in *Staphylococcus epidermidis* infections. In: Leive L, (ed). Microbiology – 1986. Washington, DC: American Society for Microbiology, 1986, pp. 139–144.

107 Beekmann SE, Diekema DJ, Doern GV. Determining the clinical significance of coagulase-negative staphylococci isolated from blood cultures. Infect Control Hosp Epidemiol 2005;26: 559–66.

108 Haimi-Cohen Y, Shafinoori S, Tucci V, Rubin LG. Use of incubation time to detection in BACTEC 9240 to distinguish coagulase-negative staphylococcal contamination from infection in pediatric blood cultures. Pediatr Infect Dis J 2003; 22:968–74.

109 Huang YC, Wang YH, Chou YH, Lien RI. Significance of coagulase-negative staphylococci isolated from a single blood culture from neonates in intensive care. Ann Trop Paediatr 2006;26:311–18.

110 Muller-Premru M, Cernelc P. Molecular epidemiology of catheter-related bloodstream infections caused by coagulase-negative staphylococci in haematological patients with neutropenia. Epidemiol Infect 2004;132:921–5.

111 Tokars JI. Predictive value of blood cultures positive for coagulase-negative staphylococci: implications for patient care and health care quality assurance. Clin Infect Dis 2004;39:333–41.

112 Herwaldt LA, Geiss M, Kao C, Pfaller MA. The positive predictive value of isolating coagulase-negative staphylococci from blood cultures. Clin Infect Dis 1996;22:14–20.

113 Souvenir D, Anderson DE Jr, Palpant S *et al.* Blood cultures positive for coagulase-negative staphylococci: antisepsis, pseudobacteremia, and therapy of patients. J Clin Microbiol 1998; 36:1923–6.

114 Weinstein MP, Towns ML, Quartey SM *et al.* The clinical significance of positive blood cultures in the 1990s: a prospective comprehensive evaluation of the microbiology, epidemiology, and outcome of bacteremia and fungemia in adults. Clin Infect Dis 1997;24:584–602.

115 Archer GL, Climo MW. *Staphylococcus epidermidis* and other coagulase-negative staphylococci. In: Mandell GL, Bennett JE, Dolin R, eds. Principles and Practice of Infectious Diseases. Philadelphia: Elsevier Churchill Livingstone, 2005:2352–60.

116 National Healthcare Safety Network, Division of Healthcare Quality Improvement, National Center for Infectious Diseases. The National Healthcare Safety Network Manual. Patient Safety Component Protocol. Atlanta, GA: Centers for Disease Control and Prevention, 2008.

117 Capdevila JA, Planes AM, Palomar M *et al.* Value of differential quantitative blood cultures in the diagnosis of catheter-related sepsis. Eur J Clin Microbiol Infect Dis 1992;11:403–7.

118 Richter SS, Beekmann SE, Croco JL *et al.* Minimizing the workup of blood culture contaminants: implementation and evaluation of a laboratory-based algorithm. J Clin Microbiol 2002;40:2437–44.

119 Martinez JA, Pozo L, Almela M *et al.* Microbial and clinical determinants of time-to-positivity in patients with bacteraemia. Clin Microbiol Infect 2007;13:709–16.

120 Yebenes JC, Serra-Prat M, Miro G, Sauca G, Capdevila JA. Differences in time to positivity can affect the negative predictive value of blood cultures drawn through a central venous catheter. Intensive Care Med 2006;32:1442– 3.

121 Raad I, Hanna HA, Alakech B, Chatzinikolaou I, Johnson MM, Tarrand J. Differential time to positivity: a useful method for diagnosing catheter-related bloodstream infections. Ann Intern Med 2004;140:18 –25.

122 Sherertz RJ. Update on vascular catheter infections. Curr Opin Infect Dis 2004;17:303–7.

123 Catton JA, Dobbins BM, Kite P *et al.* In situ diagnosis of intravascular catheter-related bloodstream infection: a comparison of quantitative culture, differential time to positivity, and endoluminal brushing. Crit Care Med 2005;33:787–91.

124 Chatzinikolaou I, Hanna H, Hachem R, Alakech B, Tarrand J, Raad I. Differential quantitative blood cultures for the diagnosis of catheter-related bloodstream infections associated with short- and long-term catheters: a prospective study. Diagn Microbiol Infect Dis 2004;50:167–72.

125 Garcia P, Benitez R, Lam M *et al.* Coagulase-negative staphylococci: clinical, microbiological and molecular features to predict true bacteraemia. J Med Microbiol 2004;53:67–72.

126 Bates DW, Lee TH. Rapid classification of positive blood cultures. Prospective validation of a multivariate algorithm. JAMA 1992;267:1962–6.

127 Bates DW, Cook EF, Goldman L, Lee TH. Predicting bacteremia in hospitalized patients. A prospectively validated model. Ann Intern Med 1990;113:495–500.

128 Maki DG, Weise CE, Sarafin HW. A semiquantitative culture method for identifying intravenous-catheter-related infection. N Engl J Med 1977;296:1305–9.

129 Bouza E, Alvarado N, Alcala L *et al*. A prospective, randomized, and comparative study of 3 different methods for the diagnosis of intravascular catheter colonization. Clin Infect Dis 2005;40:1096–100.

130 Safdar N, Fine JP, Maki DG. Meta-analysis: methods for diagnosing intravascular device-related bloodstream infection. *Ann Intern* 2005;142:451–466.

131 Donlan RM. Role of biofilms in antimicrobial resistance. ASAIO J 2000;46:S47–S52.

132 Mack D, Horstkotte MA, Rohde H, Knobloch JKM. Coagulase-negative staphylococci. In: Pace JL, Rupp ME, Finch RG eds. Biofilms, Infection, and Antimicrobial Therapy. CRC Press, Taylor & Francis, Boca Raton 2006:109–153.

133 Blot SI, Depuydt P, Annemans L *et al*. Clinical and economic outcomes in critically ill patients with nosocomial catheter-related bloodstream infections. Clin Infect Dis 2005;41:1591–8.

134 Digiovine B, Chenoweth C, Watts C, Higgins M. The attributable mortality and costs of primary nosocomial bloodstream infections in the intensive care unit. Am J Respir Crit Care Med 1999;160:976–81.

135 Fidalgo S, Vazquez F, Mendoza MC, Perez F, Mendez FJ. Bacteremia due to *Staphylococcus epidermidis*: microbiologic, epidemiologic, clinical, and prognostic features. Rev Infect Dis 1990;12:520–8.

136 Sheng WH, Ko WJ, Wang JT, Chang SC, Hsueh PR, Luh KT. Evaluation of antiseptic-impregnated central venous catheters for prevention of catheter-related infection in intensive care unit patients. Diagn Microbiol Infect Dis 2000;38:1–5.

137 Rupp ME, Lisco SJ, Lipsett PA *et al*. Effect of a second-generation venous catheter impregnated with chlorhexidine and silver sulfadiazine on central catheter-related infections: a randomized, controlled trial. Ann Intern Med 2005;143:570–80.

138 Brun-Buisson C, Doyon F, Sollet JP, Cochard JF, Cohen Y, Nitenberg G. Prevention of intravascular catheter-related infection with newer chlorhexidine–silver sulfadiazine-coated catheters: a randomized controlled trial. Intensive Care Med 2004;30:837–43.

139 Shah A, Mond J, Walsh S. Lysostaphin-coated catheters eradicate *Staphylococccus aureus* challenge and block surface colonization. Antimicrob Agents Chemother 2004;48:2704–7.

140 Wu JA, Kusuma C, Mond JJ, Kokai-Kun JF. Lysostaphin disrupts *Staphylococcus aureus* and *Staphylococcus epidermidis* biofilms on artificial surfaces. Antimicrob Agents Chemother 2003; 47:3407–14.

141 Elliott TS. Line-associated bacteraemias. Commun Dis Rep CDR Rev 1993;3:R91–R96.

142 Liang SY, Mackowiak PA. Infections in the elderly. Clin Geriatr Med 2007;23:441–56, viii.

143 Demitrovicova A, Hricak V, Karvay M, Krcmery V. Endocarditis due to coagulase-negative staphylococci: data from a 22-years national survey. Scand J Infect Dis 2007;39:655–6.

144 Hricak V, Kovacik J, Marks P, West D, Kromery V Jr. Aetiology and outcome in 53 cases of native valve staphylococcal endocarditis. Postgrad Med J 1999;75:540–3.

145 Hricak V, Matejicka F, Sedlak T *et al*. Native valve staphylococcal endocarditis: etiology, risk factors and outcome in 53 cases. J Chemother 1998;10:360–8.

146 Paneth M. Native and prosthetic valve endocarditis. Thorac Cardiovasc Surg 1982;30:362–4.

147 Karchmer AW, Archer GL, Dismukes WE. *Staphylococcus epidermidis* causing prosthetic valve endocarditis: microbiologic and clinical observations as guides to therapy. Ann Intern Med 1983;98:447–55.

148 Caputo GM, Archer GL, Calderwood SB, DiNubile MJ, Karchmer AW. Native valve endocarditis due to coagulase-negative staphylococci. Clinical and microbiologic features. Am J Med 1987;83:619–25.

149 Whitener C, Caputo GM, Weitekamp MR, Karchmer AW. Endocarditis due to coagulase-negative staphylococci. Microbiologic, epidemiologic, and clinical considerations. Infect Dis Clin North Am 1993;7:81–96.

150 Chu VH, Cabell CH, Abrutyn E *et al*. Native valve endocarditis due to coagulase-negative staphylococci: report of 99 episodes from the International Collaboration on Endocarditis Merged Database. Clin Infect Dis 2004;39:1527–30.

151 Etienne J, Eykyn SJ. Increase in native valve endocarditis caused by coagulase negative staphylococci: an Anglo-French clinical and microbiological study. Br Heart J 1990;64:381–4.

152 Wang A, Athan E, Pappas PA *et al*. Contemporary clinical profile and outcome of prosthetic valve endocarditis. JAMA 2007; 297:1354–61.

153 Calderwood SB, Swinski LA, Karchmer AW, Waternaux CM, Buckley MJ. Prosthetic valve endocarditis. Analysis of factors affecting outcome of therapy. J Thorac Cardiovasc Surg 1986; 92:776–83.

154 Calderwood SB, Swinski LA, Waternaux CM, Karchmer AW, Buckley MJ. Risk factors for the development of prosthetic valve endocarditis. Circulation 1985;72:31–7.

155 Ivert TS, Dismukes WE, Cobbs CG, Blackstone EH, Kirklin JW, Bergdahl LA. Prosthetic valve endocarditis. Circulation 1984; 69:223–32.

156 Karchmer AW, Dismukes WE, Buckley MJ, Austen WG. Late prosthetic valve endocarditis: clinical features influencing therapy. Am J Med 1978;64:199–206.

157 Boyce JM, Potter-Bynoe G, Opal SM, Dziobek L, Medeiros AA. A common-source outbreak of *Staphylococcus epidermidis* infections among patients undergoing cardiac surgery. J Infect Dis 1990;161:493–9.

158 Petheram IS, Boyce JM. Prosthetic valve endocarditis: a review of 24 cases. Thorax 1977;32:478–85.

159 van den Broek PJ, Lampe AS, Berbee GA, Thompson J, Mouton RP. Epidemic of prosthetic valve endocarditis caused by *Staphylococcus epidermidis*. BMJ 1985;291:949–50.

160 Hammond GW, Stiver HG. Combination antibiotic therapy in an outbreak of prosthetic endocarditis caused by *Staphylococcus epidermidis*. Can Med Assoc J 1978;118:524–30.

161 Abrutyn E, Cabell CH, Fowler VG *et al*. Medical treatment of endocarditis. Curr Infect Dis Rep 2007;9:271–82.

162 Chu VH, Bayer AS. Use of echocardiography in the diagnosis and management of infective endocarditis. Curr Infect Dis Rep 2007;9:283–90.

163 Lester SJ, Wilansky S. Endocarditis and associated complications. Crit Care Med 2007;35(8 suppl):S384–S391.
164 Paterick TE, Paterick TJ, Nishimura RA, Steckelberg JM. Complexity and subtlety of infective endocarditis. Mayo Clin Proc 2007;82:615–21.
165 Brown PD. Surgery for infective endocarditis. Curr Infect Dis Rep 2007;9:291–6.
166 Kobasa WD, Kaye KL, Shapiro T, Kaye D. Therapy for experimental endocarditis due to *Staphylococcus epidermidis*. Rev Infect Dis 1983;5(suppl 3):S533–S537.
167 Karchmer AW. Staphylococcal endocarditis. Laboratory and clinical basis for antibiotic therapy. Am J Med 1985;78(6B): 116–27.
168 Massanari RM, Donta ST. The efficacy of rifampin as adjunctive therapy in selected cases of staphylococcal endocarditis. Chest 1978;73:371–5.
169 Patel SM, Saravolatz LD. Monotherapy versus combination therapy. Med Clin North Am 2006;90:1183–95.
170 Winston LG, Bolger AF. Modern epidemiology, prophylaxis, and diagnosis and therapy for infective endocarditis. Curr Cardiol Rep 2006;8:102–8.
171 Archer GL, Armstrong BC. Alteration of staphylococcal flora in cardiac surgery patients receiving antibiotic prophylaxis. J Infect Dis 1983;147:642–9.
172 Wilson W, Taubert KA, Gewitz M *et al*. Prevention of Infective endocarditis: guidelines from the American Heart Association. A guideline from the American Heart Association Rheumatic Fever, Endocarditis, and Kawasaki Disease Committee, Council on Cardiovascular Disease in the Young, and the Council on Clinical Cardiology, Council on Cardiovascular Surgery and Anesthesia, and the Quality of Care and Outcomes Research Interdisciplinary Working Group. Circulation 2007;116:1736–54.
173 Archer GL, Vazquez GJ, Johnston JL. Antibiotic prophylaxis of experimental endocarditis due to methicillin-resistant *Staphylococcus epidermidis*. J Infect Dis 1980;142:725–31.
174 Bratzler DW, Houck PM. Antimicrobial prophylaxis for surgery: an advisory statement from the National Surgical Infection Prevention Project. Clin Infect Dis 2004;38:1706–15.
175 Henke PK, Bergamini TM, Rose SM, Richardson JD. Current options in prosthetic vascular graft infection. Am Surg 1998; 64:39–45; discussion 46.
176 O'Brien T, Collin J. Prosthetic vascular graft infection. Br J Surg 1992;79:1262–7.
177 Bandyk DF, Berni GA, Thiele BL, Towne JB. Aortofemoral graft infection due to *Staphylococcus epidermidis*. Arch Surg 1984;119: 102–8.
178 Bandyk DF, Esses GE. Prosthetic graft infection. Surg Clin North Am 1994;74:571–90.
179 Kaebnick HW, Bandyk DF, Bergamini TW, Towne JB. The microbiology of explanted vascular prostheses. Surgery 1987; 102:756–62.
180 Bunt TJ. Sources of *Staphylococcus epidermidis* at the inguinal incision during peripheral revascularization. Am Surg 1986; 52:472–3.
181 Wooster DL, Louch RE, Krajden S. Intraoperative bacterial contamination of vascular grafts: a prospective study. Can J Surg 1985;28:407–9.
182 Bunt TJ. Vascular graft infections: an update. Cardiovasc Surg 2001;9:225–33.
183 Lorentzen JE. Graft infection. Introduction. Acta Chir Scand Suppl 1987;538:70–1.
184 Lorentzen JE, Nielsen OM, Arendrup H *et al*. Vascular graft infection: an analysis of sixty-two graft infections in 2411 consecutively implanted synthetic vascular grafts. Surgery 1985;98:81–6.
185 Richet HM, Chidiac C, Prat A *et al*. Analysis of risk factors for surgical wound infections following vascular surgery. Am J Med 1991;91(3B):170S–172S.
186 Golan JF. Vascular graft infection. Infect Dis Clin North Am 1989;3:247–58.
187 Bergamini TM, Bandyk DF, Govostis D, Vetsch R, Towne JB. Identification of *Staphylococcus epidermidis* vascular graft infections: a comparison of culture techniques. J Vasc Surg 1989; 9:665–70.
188 Tollefson DF, Bandyk DF, Kaebnick HW, Seabrook GR, Towne JB. Surface biofilm disruption. Enhanced recovery of microorganisms from vascular prostheses. Arch Surg 1987;122:38–43.
189 Liekweg WG Jr, Greenfield LJ. Vascular prosthetic infections: collected experience and results of treatment. Surgery 1977;81: 335–42.
190 Chang JK, Calligaro KD, Ryan S, Runyan D, Dougherty MJ, Stern JJ. Risk factors associated with infection of lower extremity revascularization: analysis of 365 procedures performed at a teaching hospital. Ann Vasc Surg 2003;17:91–6.
191 Goeau-Brissonniere OA, Coggia M. Arterial prosthetic infections. In: Waldvogel FA, Bisno AL eds. *Infections Associated with Indwelling Medical Devices*, 3rd ed. ASM Press, Washington DC. 2000:127–144.
192 Schimke RT, Black PH, Mark VH, Swartz MN. Indolent *Staphylococcus albus* or *aureus* bacteremia after ventriculoatriostomy. Role of foreign body in its initiation and perpetuation. N Engl J Med 1961;264:264–70.
193 Blomstedt GC. Infections in neurosurgery: a retrospective study of 1143 patients and 1517 operations. Acta Neurochir (Wien) 1985;78:81–90.
194 Renier D, Lacombe J, Pierre-Kahn A, Sainte-Rose C, Hirsch JF. Factors causing acute shunt infection. Computer analysis of 1174 operations. J Neurosurg 1984;61:1072–8.
195 Stromblad LG, Schalen C, Steen A, Sundbarg G, Kamme C. Bacterial contamination in cerebrospinal fluid shunt surgery. Scand J Infect Dis 1987;19:211–14.
196 Venes JL. Infections of CSF shunt and intracranial pressure monitoring devices. Infect Dis Clin North Am 1989;3:289–99.
197 McGirt MJ, Zaas A, Fuchs HE, George TM, Kaye K, Sexton DJ. Risk factors for pediatric ventriculoperitoneal shunt infection and predictors of infectious pathogens. Clin Infect Dis 2003; 36:858–62.
198 Sarguna P, Lakshmi V. Ventriculoperitoneal shunt infections. Indian J Med Microbiol 2006;24:52–4.
199 Wang KW, Chang WN, Shih TY *et al*. Infection of cerebrospinal fluid shunts: causative pathogens, clinical features, and outcomes. Jpn J Infect Dis 2004;57:44–8.
200 Dobrin RS, Day NK, Quie PG *et al*. The role of complement, immunoglobulin and bacterial antigen in coagulase-negative staphylococcal shunt nephritis. Am J Med 1975;59:660–73.
201 Thomson RB Jr, Bertram H. Laboratory diagnosis of central nervous system infections. Infect Dis Clin North Am 2001; 15:1047–71.
202 Sanchez-Mora D, Mermel L, Parenteau S *et al*., eds. Epidural Catheter Infection: Epidemiology and Pathogenesis. Proceedings

of the 33rd Interscience Conference on Antimicrobial Agents and Chemotherapy, New Orleans, LA, 1993.
203 Langley JM, LeBlanc JC, Drake J, Milner R. Efficacy of antimicrobial prophylaxis in placement of cerebrospinal fluid shunts: meta-analysis. Clin Infect Dis 1993;17:98–103.
204 Ratilal B, Costa J, Sampaio C. Antibiotic prophylaxis for surgical introduction of intracranial ventricular shunts. Cochrane Database Syst Rev 2006;3:CD005365.
205 Sciubba DM, Stuart RM, McGirt MJ *et al.* Effect of antibiotic-impregnated shunt catheters in decreasing the incidence of shunt infection in the treatment of hydrocephalus. J Neurosurg 2005;103(2 suppl):131–6.
206 Davis JL, Koidou-Tsiligianni A, Pflugfelder SC, Miller D, Flynn HW Jr, Forster RK. Coagulase-negative staphylococcal endophthalmitis. Increase in antimicrobial resistance. Ophthalmology 1988;95:1404–10.
207 Driebe WT Jr, Mandelbaum S, Forster RK, Schwartz LK, Culbertson WW. Pseudophakic endophthalmitis. Diagnosis and management. Ophthalmology 1986;93:442–8.
208 Weber DJ, Hoffman KL, Thoft RA, Baker AS. Endophthalmitis following intraocular lens implantation: report of 30 cases and review of the literature. Rev Infect Dis 1986;8:12–20.
209 Carlson A, Tetz MR, Apple DJ. Infectious complications of modern cataract surgery and intraocular lens implantation. Infect Dis Clin North Am 1998;3:339–55.
210 Lemley CA, Han DP. Endophthalmitis: a review of current evaluation and management. Retina 2007;27:662–80.
211 Chiquet C, Lina G, Benito Y *et al.* Polymerase chain reaction identification in aqueous humor of patients with postoperative endophthalmitis. J Cataract Refract Surg 2007;33:635–41.
212 Diamond JG. Intraocular management of endophthalmitis. A systematic approach. Arch Ophthalmol 1981;99:96–9.
213 Callegan MC, Gilmore MS, Gregory M *et al.* Bacterial endophthalmitis: therapeutic challenges and host–pathogen interactions. Prog Retin Eye Res 2007;26:189–203.
214 Al-Omran AM, Abboud EB, Abu El-Asrar AM. Microbiologic spectrum and visual outcome of posttraumatic endophthalmitis. Retina 2007;27:236–42.
215 Gregory M, Callegan MC, Gilmore MS. Role of bacterial and host factors in infectious endophthalmitis. Chem Immunol Allergy 2007;92:266–75.
216 Hovelius B, Mardh PA. *Staphylococcus saprophyticus* as a common cause of urinary tract infections. Rev Infect Dis 1984;6:328–37.
217 Lewis JF, Brake SR, Anderson DJ, Vredeveld GN. Urinary tract infection due to coagulase-negative staphylococcus. Am J Clin Pathol 1982;77:736–9.
218 Nicolle LE, Hoban SA, Harding GK. Characterization of coagulase-negative staphylococci from urinary tract specimens. J Clin Microbiol 1983;17:267–71.
219 Maskell R. Importance of coagulase-negative staphylococci as pathogens in the urinary tract. Lancet 1974;i:1155–8.
220 Blum MD. Infections of genitourinary prostheses. Infect Dis Clin North Am 1989;3:259–74.
221 Carson CC. Infections in genitourinary prostheses. Urol Clin North Am 1989;16:139–47.
222 Carson CC. Diagnosis, treatment and prevention of penile prosthesis infection. Int J Impot Res 2003;15(suppl 5):S139–S146.
223 Montague DK. Periprosthetic infections. J Urol 1987;138:68–9.
224 Thomalla JV, Thompson ST, Rowland RG, Mulcahy JJ. Infectious complications of penile prosthetic implants. J Urol 1987;138:65–7.
225 Kabalin JN, Kessler R. Infectious complications of penile prosthesis surgery. J Urol 1988;139:953–5.
226 Sadeghi-Nejad H. Penile prosthesis surgery: a review of prosthetic devices and associated complications. J Sex Med 2007;4:296–309.
227 Abouassaly R, Montague DK. Penile prosthesis coating and the reduction of postoperative infection. Curr Urol Rep 2004;5:460–6.
228 Droggin D, Shabsigh R, Anastasiadis AG. Antibiotic coating reduces penile prosthesis infection. J Sex Med 2005;2:565–8.
229 Gokal R. Peritonitis in continuous ambulatory peritoneal dialysis. J Antimicrob Chemother 1982;9:417–20.
230 Zelenitsky S, Barns L, Findlay I *et al.* Analysis of microbiological trends in peritoneal dialysis-related peritonitis from 1991 to 1998. Am J Kidney Dis 2000;36:1009–13.
231 Rubin J, Rogers WA, Taylor HM *et al.* Peritonitis during continuous ambulatory peritoneal dialysis. Ann Intern Med 1980;92:7–13.
232 Rubin JE, Marquardt E, Pierre M, Maxey RW. Improved training techniques and UltraBag system resulted in lowered peritonitis rate in an inner-city population. Adv Perit Dial 1995;11:208–9.
233 Beard-Pegler MA, Gabelish CL, Stubbs E *et al.* Prevalence of peritonitis-associated coagulase-negative staphylococci on the skin of continuous ambulatory peritoneal dialysis patients. Epidemiol Infect 1989;102:365–78.
234 Eisenberg ES, Ambalu M, Szylagi G, Aning V, Soeiro R. Colonization of skin and development of peritonitis due to coagulase-negative staphylococci in patients undergoing peritoneal dialysis. J Infect Dis 1987;156:478–82.
235 Gruer LD, Bartlett R, Ayliffe GA. Species identification and antibiotic sensitivity of coagulase-negative staphylococci from CAPD peritonitis. J Antimicrob Chemother 1984;13:577–83.
236 Vas S, Oreopoulos DG. Infections in patients undergoing peritoneal dialysis. Infect Dis Clin North Am 2001;15:743–74.
237 Vas SI. Infections of continuous ambulatory peritoneal dialysis catheters. Infect Dis Clin North Am 1989;3:301–28.
238 Knight KR, Polak A, Crump J, Maskell R. Laboratory diagnosis and oral treatment of CAPD peritonitis. Lancet 1982;ii:1301–4.
239 Vas SI, Law L. Microbiological diagnosis of peritonitis in patients on continuous ambulatory peritoneal dialysis. J Clin Microbiol 1985;21:522–3.
240 Vas SI, Keane WF. Treatment of peritonitis: update or new course. Perit Dial Int 2000;20:384–5.
241 Troidle LK, Kliger AS, Finkelstein FO. Challenges of managing chronic peritoneal dialysis-associated peritonitis. Perit Dial Int 1999;19:315–18.
242 Vas SI. Etiology and treatment of peritonitis. Trans Am Soc Artif Intern Organs 1984;30:682–4.
243 Brand KG. Infection of mammary prostheses: a survey and the question of prevention. Ann Plast Surg 1993;30:289–95.
244 Freedman AM, Jackson IT. Infections in breast implants. Infect Dis Clin North Am 1989;3:275–87.
245 Dobke MK, Svahn JK, Vastine VL, Landon BN, Stein PC, Parsons CL. Characterization of microbial presence at the surface of silicone mammary implants. Ann Plast Surg 1995;34:563–9; disscusion 570–1.

246 Virden CP, Dobke MK, Stein P, Parsons CL, Frank DH. Subclinical infection of the silicone breast implant surface as a possible cause of capsular contracture. Aesthetic Plast Surg 1992;16:173–9.
247 Vinh DC, Embil JM. Infection in breast implants. Lancet Infect Dis 2005;5:462–3; author reply 463.
248 Chun JK, Schulman MR. The infected breast prosthesis after mastectomy reconstruction: successful salvage of nine implants in eight consecutive patients. Plast Reconstr Surg 2007;120: 581–9.
249 Spear SL, Howard MA, Boehmler JH, Ducic I, Low M, Abbruzzesse MR. The infected or exposed breast implant: management and treatment strategies. Plast Reconstr Surg 2004;113:1634–44.
250 Siggelkow W, Klosterhalfen B, Klinge U, Rath W, Faridi A. Analysis of local complications following explantation of silicone breast implants. Breast 2004;13:122–8.
251 Spear SL, Low M, Ducic I. Revision augmentation mastopexy: indications, operations, and outcomes. Ann Plast Surg 2003;51: 540–6.
252 Lentino JR. Prosthetic joint infections: bane of orthopedists, challenge for infectious disease specialists. Clin Infect Dis 2003;36:1157–61.
253 Fitzgerald RH. Infections of hip prostheses and artificial joints. Infect Dis Clin North Am 1989;3:329–38.
254 Sampedro MF, Patel R. Infections associated with long-term prosthetic devices. Infect Dis Clin North Am 2007;21:785–819.
255 Gillespie WJ. Infection in total joint replacement. Infect Dis Clin North Am 1990;4:465–84.
256 Kettlekamp DB. Infected total joint replacement. Arch Surg 1977;112:552–3.
257 Anguita-Alonso P, Hanssen AD, Patel R. Prosthetic joint infection. Expert Rev Anti Infect Ther 2005;3:797–804.
258 Rand JA, Brown ML. The value of indium 111 leukocyte scanning in the evaluation of painful or infected total knee arthroplasties. Clin Orthop Relat Res 1990;259:179–82.
259 Trampuz A, Zimmerli W. Prosthetic joint infections: update in diagnosis and treatment. Swiss Med Wkly 2005;135:243–51.
260 Trampuz A, Piper KE, Jacobson MJ *et al.* Sonication of removed hip and knee prostheses for diagnosis of infection. N Engl J Med 2007;357:654–63.
261 Lidwell OM, Elson RA, Lowbury EJ *et al.* Ultraclean air and antibiotics for prevention of postoperative infection. A multicenter study of 8,052 joint replacement operations. Acta Orthop Scand 1987;58:4–13.
262 Norden CW. A critical review of antibiotic prophylaxis in orthopedic surgery. Rev Infect Dis 1983;5:928–32.
263 Norden CW. Prevention of bone and joint infections. Am J Med 1985;78(6B):229–32.
264 Laurent F, Bignon A, Goldnadel J *et al.* A new concept of gentamicin loaded HAP/TCP bone substitute for prophylactic action: in vitro release validation. J Mater Sci Mater Med 2008;19:947–51.
265 Lidgren L. Joint prosthetic infections: a success story. Acta Orthop Scand 2001;72:553–6.
266 Gaynes RP, Culver DH, Horan TC, Edwards JR, Richards C, Tolson JS. Surgical site infection (SSI) rates in the United States, 1992–1998: the National Nosocomial Infections Surveillance System basic SSI risk index. Clin Infect Dis 2001;33(suppl 2): S69–S77.
267 Society for Hospital Epidemiology of America, Association for Practitioners in Infection Control, Centers for Disease Control Surgical Infection Society. Consensus paper on the surveillance of surgical wound infections. Infect Control Hosp Epidemiol 1992;13:599–605.
268 Mangram AJ, Horan TC, Pearson ML, Silver LC, Jarvis WR. Guideline for prevention of surgical site infection, 1999. Hospital Infection Control Practices Advisory Committee. Infect Control Hosp Epidemiol 1999;20:250–78.
269 Hernandez JL, Calvo J, Sota R, Aguero J, Garcia-Palomo JD, Farinas MC. Clinical and microbiologic characteristics of 28 patients with *Staphylococcus schleiferi* infection. *Eur J Clin Microbiol Infect Dis* 2001;20:153–8.
270 Kawamura Y, Hou XG, Sultana F *et al.* Distribution of *Staphylococcus* species among human clinical specimens and emended description of *Staphylococcus caprae*. J Clin Microbiol 1998;36:2038–42.
271 Kluytmans J, Berg H, Steegh P, Vandenesch F, Etienne J, van Belkum A. Outbreak of *Staphylococcus schleiferi* wound infections: strain characterization by randomly amplified polymorphic DNA analysis, PCR ribotyping, conventional ribotyping, and pulsed-field gel electrophoresis. J Clin Microbiol 1998;36: 2214–19.
272 Culver DH, Horan TC, Gaynes RP *et al.* Surgical wound infection rates by wound class, operative procedure, and patient risk index. National Nosocomial Infections Surveillance System. Am J Med 1991;91(3B):152S–157S.
273 Kaya E, Yetim I, Dervisoglu A, Sunbul M, Bek Y. Risk factors for and effect of a one-year surveillance program on surgical site infection at a university hospital in Turkey. Surg Infect (Larchmt) 2006;7:519–26.
274 Leong G, Wilson J, Charlett A. Duration of operation as a risk factor for surgical site infection: comparison of English and US data. J Hosp Infect 2006;63:255–62.
275 Muilwijk J, van den Hof S, Wille JC. Associations between surgical site infection risk and hospital operation volume and surgeon operation volume among hospitals in the Dutch nosocomial infection surveillance network. Infect Control Hosp Epidemiol 2007;28:557–63.
276 Wilson JA, Clark JJ. Obesity: impediment to postsurgical wound healing. Adv Skin Wound Care 2004;17:426–35.
277 Van Natta TL. Surgical infections. In: Bongard FS, Sue DY, Vintch JRE, eds. Current Diagnosis and Treatment Critical Care, 3rd edn. New York: McGraw Hill Medical, 2008:397–408.
278 Horan TC, Gaynes RP, Martone WJ, Jarvis WR, Emori TG. CDC definitions of nosocomial surgical site infections, 1992: a modification of CDC definitions of surgical wound infections. Infect Control Hosp Epidemiol 1992;13:606–8.
279 Huebner J, Goldmann DA. Coagulase-negative staphylococci: role as pathogens. Annu Rev Med 1999;50:223–36.
280 Homer-Vanniasinkam S. Surgical site and vascular infections: treatment and prophylaxis. Int J Infect Dis 2007;11(suppl 1): S17–S22.
281 Nichols RL. Postoperative infections in the age of drug-resistant gram-positive bacteria. Am J Med 1998;104(5A):11S–16S.
282 Nichols RL. Preventing surgical site infections. Clin Med Res 2004;2:115–18.
283 Costa SF, Barone AA, Miceli MH *et al.* Colonization and molecular epidemiology of coagulase-negative staphylococcal

bacteremia in cancer patients: a pilot study. Am J Infect Control 2006;34:36–40.
284 Richards JM, Gilewski TA, Vogelzang NJ. Association of interleukin-2 therapy with staphylococcal bacteremia. Cancer 1991;67:1570–5.
285 Eykyn SJ. Staphylococcal sepsis. The changing pattern of disease and therapy. Lancet 1988;i:100–4.
286 Singh N. Nosocomial infections in solid organ transplant recipients. In: Mayhall CG, ed. Hospital Epidemiology and Infection Control, 3rd edn. Philadelphia: Lippincott, Williams and Wilkins, 2004:985–1010.
287 Anday EK, Talbot GH. Coagulase-negative *Staphylococcus* bacteremia: a rising threat in the newborn infant. Ann Clin Lab Sci 1985;15:246–51.
288 Goldmann DA, Durbin WA Jr, Freeman J. Nosocomial infections in a neonatal intensive care unit. J Infect Dis 1981;144:449–59.
289 Kumar SP, Delivoria-Papadopoulos M. Infections in newborn infants in a special care unit. A changing pattern of infection. Ann Clin Lab Sci 1985;15:351–6.
290 Hubner J, Kropec A. Cross infections due to coagulase-negative staphylococci in high-risk patients. Zentralbl Bakteriol 1995; 283:169–74.
291 Huebner J, Pier GB, Maslow JN *et al.* Endemic nosocomial transmission of *Staphylococcus epidermidis* bacteremia isolates in a neonatal intensive care unit over 10 years. J Infect Dis 1994; 169:526–31.
292 Finelli L, Livengood JR, Saiman L. Surveillance of pharyngeal colonization: detection and control of serious bacterial illness in low birth weight infants. Pediatr Infect Dis J 1994;13:854–9.
293 Low DE, Schmidt BK, Kirpalani HM *et al.* An endemic strain of *Staphylococcus haemolyticus* colonizing and causing bacteremia in neonatal intensive care unit patients. Pediatrics 1992;89: 696–700.
294 Raimundo O, Heussler H, Bruhn JB *et al.* Molecular epidemiology of coagulase-negative staphylococcal bacteraemia in a newborn intensive care unit. J Hosp Infect 2002;51:33–42.
295 Van Der Zwet WC, Debets-Ossenkopp YJ, Reinders E *et al.* Nosocomial spread of a *Staphylococcus capitis* strain with heteroresistance to vancomycin in a neonatal intensive care unit. J Clin Microbiol 2002;40:2520–5.
296 Avila-Figueroa C, Goldmann DA, Richardson DK, Gray JE, Ferrari A, Freeman J. Intravenous lipid emulsions are the major determinant of coagulase-negative staphylococcal bacteremia in very low birth weight newborns. Pediatr Infect Dis J 1998; 17:10–17.
297 Brodie SB, Sands KE, Gray JE *et al.* Occurrence of nosocomial bloodstream infections in six neonatal intensive care units. Pediatr Infect Dis J 2000;19:56–65.
298 Freeman J, Goldmann DA, Smith NE, Sidebottom DG, Epstein MF, Platt R. Association of intravenous lipid emulsion and coagulase-negative staphylococcal bacteremia in neonatal intensive care units. N Engl J Med 1990;323:301–8.
299 Healy CM, Palazzi DL, Edwards MS, Campbell JR, Baker CJ. Features of invasive staphylococcal disease in neonates. Pediatrics 2004;114:953–61.
300 Kudawla M, Dutta S, Narang A. Validation of a clinical score for the diagnosis of late onset neonatal septicemia in babies weighing 1000–2500 g. J Trop Pediatr 2008;54:66–9.
301 Munson DP, Thompson TR, Johnson DE, Rhame FS, VanDrunen N, Ferrieri P. Coagulase-negative staphylococcal septicemia: experience in a newborn intensive care unit. J Pediatr 1982;101:602–5.
302 Schmidt BK, Kirpalani HM, Corey M, Low DE, Philip AG, Ford-Jones EL. Coagulase-negative staphylococci as true pathogens in newborn infants: a cohort study. Pediatr Infect Dis J 1987;6:1026–31.
303 Noel GJ, Edelson PJ. *Staphylococcus epidermidis* bacteremia in neonates: further observations and the occurrence of focal infection. Pediatrics 1984;74:832–7.
304 Hall SL. Coagulase-negative staphylococcal infections in neonates. Pediatr Infect Dis J 1991;10:57–67.
305 Venkatesh MP, Placencia F, Weisman LE. Coagulase-negative staphylococcal infections in the neonate and child: an update. Semin Pediatr Infect Dis 2006;17:120–7.
306 von Eiff C, Proctor RA, Peters G. Coagulase-negative staphylococci. Pathogens have major role in nosocomial infections. Postgrad Med 2001;110:63–4, 69–70, 73–6.
307 Weisman LE. Coagulase-negative staphylococcal disease: emerging therapies for the neonatal and pediatric patient. Curr Opin Infect Dis 2004;17:237–41.
308 Baird-Parker AC. A classification of micrococci and staphylococci based on physiological and biochemical tests. J Gen Microbiol 1963;30:409–27.
309 Baird-Parker AC. Staphylococci and their classification. Ann NY Acad Sci 1965;128:4–25.
310 Kloos WE, Schleifer KH. Simplified scheme for routine identification of human *Staphylococcus* species. J Clin Microbiol 1975;1:82–8.
311 Casey AL, Worthington T, Lambert PA, Elliott TS. Evaluation of routine microbiological techniques for establishing the diagnosis of catheter-related bloodstream infection caused by coagulase-negative staphylococci. J Med Microbiol 2007;56: 172–6.
312 Combe M, Lemeland J, Pestel-Caron M, Pons J. Multilocus enzyme analysis in aerobic and anaerobic bacteria using gel electrophoresis-nitrocellulose blotting. FEMS Microbiol Lett 2000;185:169–74.
313 Parisi JT, Lampson BC, Hoover DL, Khan JA. Comparison of epidemiologic markers for *Staphylococcus epidermidis*. J Clin Microbiol 1986;24:56–60.
314 Schlichting C, Branger C, Fournier JM *et al.* Typing of *Staphylococcus aureus* by pulsed-field gel electrophoresis, zymotyping, capsular typing, and phage typing: resolution of clonal relationships. J Clin Microbiol 1993;31:227–32.
315 Thomas JC, Vargas MR, Miragaia M, Peacock SJ, Archer GL, Enright MC. Improved multilocus sequence typing scheme for *Staphylococcus epidermidis*. J Clin Microbiol 2007;45:616–19.
316 Turner KM, Feil EJ. The secret life of the multilocus sequence type. Int J Antimicrob Agents 2007;29:129–35.
317 Wang XM, Noble L, Kreiswirth BN *et al.* Evaluation of a multilocus sequence typing system for *Staphylococcus epidermidis*. J Med Microbiol 2003;52:989–98.
318 Miragaia M, Thomas JC, Couto I, Enright MC, de Lencastre H. Inferring a population structure for *Staphylococcus epidermidis* from multilocus sequence typing data. J Bacteriol 2007;189: 2540–52.
319 Kozitskaya S, Olson ME, Fey PD, Witte W, Ohlsen K, Ziebuhr W. Clonal analysis of *Staphylococcus epidermidis* isolates carrying or lacking biofilm-mediating genes by multilocus sequence typing. J Clin Microbiol 2005;43:4751–7.

320 Monk AB, Archer GL. Use of outer surface protein repeat regions for improved genotyping of *Staphylococcus epidermidis*. J Clin Microbiol 2007;45:730–5.

321 Hamilton-Miller JM, Iliffe A. Antimicrobial resistance in coagulase-negative staphylococci. J Med Microbiol 1985;19:217–26.

322 Hamilton-Miller JM. Antibiotic resistance from two perspectives: man and microbe. Int J Antimicrob Agents 2004;23:209–12.

323 O'Kane GM, Gottlieb T, Bradbury R. Staphylococcal bacteraemia: the hospital or the home? A review of *Staphylococcus aureus* bacteraemia at Concord Hospital in 1993. Aust NZ J Med 1998;28:23–7.

324 Rao GG. Risk factors for the spread of antibiotic-resistant bacteria. Drugs 1998;55:323–30.

325 Nikaido H. Prevention of drug access to bacterial targets: permeability barriers and active efflux. Science 1994;264:382–8.

326 Mascaretti OA. Bacteria versus Antibacterial Agents, An Integrated Approach. Washington, DC: ASM Press, 2003.

327 Udo EE, Love H, Grubb WB. Intra- and inter-species mobilisation of non-conjugative plasmids in staphylococci. J Med Microbiol 1992;37:180–6.

328 Fleming A. In vitro tests of penicillin potency. Lancet 1942;i:732.

329 Diekema DJ, Pfaller MA, Schmitz FJ *et al*. Survey of infections due to *Staphylococcus* species: frequency of occurrence and antimicrobial susceptibility of isolates collected in the United States, Canada, Latin America, Europe, and the Western Pacific region for the SENTRY Antimicrobial Surveillance Program, 1997–1999. Clin Infect Dis 2001;32(suppl 2):S114–S132.

330 Jones RN. Microbiological features of vancomycin in the 21st century: minimum inhibitory concentration creep, bactericidal/static activity, and applied breakpoints to predict clinical outcomes or detect resistant strains. Clin Infect Dis 2006; 42(suppl 1):S13–S24.

331 Kollef MH. Limitations of vancomycin in the management of resistant staphylococcal infections. Clin Infect Dis 2007; 45(suppl 3):S191–S195.

332 Lentino JR, Narita M, Yu VL. New antimicrobial agents as therapy for resistant gram-positive cocci. Eur J Clin Microbiol Infect Dis 2008;27:3–15.

333 Hitchings GH. Mechanism of action of trimethoprim–sulfamethoxazole. J Infect Dis 1973;128(suppl):433–6.

334 Angehrn P, Then R. Investigations on the mode of action of the combination sulfamethoxazole–trimethoprim. Chemotherapy 1973;19:1–10.

335 Furesz S. Chemical and biological properties of rifampicin. Antibiot Chemother 1970;16:316–51.

336 Frank LA. Clinical pharmacology of rifampin. J Am Vet Med Assoc 1990;197:114–17.

337 Steenbergen JN, Alder J, Thorne GM, Tally FP. Daptomycin: a lipopeptide antibiotic for the treatment of serious Gram-positive infections. J Antimicrob Chemother 2005;55:283–8.

338 Tristan A, Lina G, Etienne J, Vandenesch F. Biology and pathogenicity of staphylococci other than *Staphylococcus aureus* and *Staphylococcus epidermidis*. In: Fischetti VA, Novick RP, Ferretti JJ, Portnoy DA, Rood JI, eds. Gram-positive Pathogens, 2nd edn. Washington, DC: ASM Press, 2006:572–86.

339 Bannerman TL. *Staphylococcus* and *Micrococcus* and other catalase-positive cocci that grow aerobically. In: Murray PR, Baron EJ, Jorgenson JH, Pfaller MA, Yolken RH, eds. Manual of Clinical Microbiology, 8th edn. Washington, DC: ASM Press, 2003:384–404.

340 Takeuchi F, Watanabe S, Baba T *et al*. Whole-genome sequencing of *Staphylococcus haemolyticus* uncovers the extreme plasticity of its genome and the evolution of human-colonizing staphylococcal species. J Bacteriol 2005;187:7292–308.

341 Nunes AP, Teixeira LM, Iorio NL *et al*. Heterogeneous resistance to vancomycin in *Staphylococcus epidermidis*, *Staphylococcus haemolyticus* and *Staphylococcus warneri* clinical strains: characterisation of glycopeptide susceptibility profiles and cell wall thickening. Int J Antimicrob Agents 2006;27:307–15.

342 Giovanetti E, Biavasco F, Pugnaloni A, Lupidi R, Biagini G, Varaldo PE. An electron microscopic study of clinical and laboratory-derived strains of teicoplanin-resistant *Staphylococcus haemolyticus*. Microb Drug Resist 1996;2:239–43.

343 van der Mee-Marquet N, Achard A, Mereghetti L, Danton A, Minier M, Quentin R. *Staphylococcus lugdunensis* infections: high frequency of inguinal area carriage. J Clin Microbiol 2003; 41:1404–9.

344 Hebert GA. Hemolysins and other characteristics that help differentiate and biotype *Staphylococcus lugdunensis* and *Staphylococcus schleiferi*. J Clin Microbiol 1990;28:2425–31.

345 Lambe DW Jr, Ferguson KP, Keplinger JL, Gemmell CG, Kalbfleisch JH. Pathogenicity of *Staphylococcus lugdunensis*, *Staphylococcus schleiferi*, and three other coagulase-negative staphylococci in a mouse model and possible virulence factors. Can J Microbiol 1990;36:455–63.

346 Mitchell J, Tristan A, Foster TJ. Characterization of the fibrinogen-binding surface protein Fbl of *Staphylococcus lugdunensis*. Microbiology 2004;150:3831–41.

347 Paulsson M, Petersson AC, Ljungh A. Serum and tissue protein binding and cell surface properties of *Staphylococcus lugdunensis*. J Med Microbiol 1993;38:96–102.

348 Donvito B, Etienne J, Denoroy L, Greenland T, Benito Y, Vandenesch F. Synergistic hemolytic activity of *Staphylococcus lugdunensis* is mediated by three peptides encoded by a non-agr genetic locus. Infect Immun 1997;65:95–100.

349 Nilsson M, Bjerketorp J, Wiebensjo A, Ljungh A, Frykberg L, Guss B. A von Willebrand factor-binding protein from *Staphylococcus lugdunensis*. FEMS Microbiol Lett 2004;234:155–61.

350 Mateo M, Maestre JR, Aguilar L *et al*. Genotypic versus phenotypic characterization, with respect to susceptibility and identification, of 17 clinical isolates of *Staphylococcus lugdunensis*. J Antimicrob Chemother 2005;56:287–91.

351 Hellbacher C, Tornqvist E, Soderquist B. *Staphylococcus lugdunensis*: clinical spectrum, antibiotic susceptibility, and phenotypic and genotypic patterns of 39 isolates. Clin Microbiol Infect 2006;12:43–9.

352 Gillespie WA, Sellin MA, Gill P, Stephens M, Tuckwell LA, Hilton AL. Urinary tract infection in young women, with special reference to *Staphylococcus saprophyticus*. J Clin Pathol 1978;31:348–50.

353 Wallmark G, Arremark I, Telander B. *Staphylococcus saprophyticus*: a frequent cause of acute urinary tract infection among female outpatients. J Infect Dis 1978;138:791–7.

354 Jordan PA, Iravani A, Richard GA, Baer H. Urinary tract infection caused by *Staphylococcus saprophyticus*. J Infect Dis 1980;142: 510–15.

355 Gerber MA, Baldovi V. *Staphylococcus saprophyticus* urinary tract infection. Clin Pediatr 1982;21:378–9.

356 Marrie TJ, Kwan C, Noble MA, West A, Duffield L. *Staphylococcus saprophyticus* as a cause of urinary tract infections. J Clin Microbiol 1982;16:427–31.
357 Pead L, Maskell R, Morris J. *Staphylococcus saprophyticus* as a urinary pathogen: a six year prospective survey. BMJ 1985;291: 1157–9.
358 Rupp ME, Soper DE, Archer GL. Colonization of the female genital tract with *Staphylococcus saprophyticus*. J Clin Microbiol 1992;30:2975–9.
359 Mardh PA, Hovelius B. *Staphylococcus saprophyticus* infections. Lancet 1977;ii:875.
360 Kuroda M, Yamashita A, Hirakawa H *et al.* Whole genome sequence of *Staphylococcus saprophyticus* reveals the pathogenesis of uncomplicated urinary tract infection. Proc Natl Acad Sci USA 2005;102:13272–7.
361 Beuth J, Ko HL, Schumacher-Perdreau F, Peters G, Heczko P, Pulverer G. Hemagglutination by *Staphylococcus saprophyticus* and other coagulase-negative staphylococci. Microb Pathog 1988;4:379–83.
362 Meyer HG, Wengler-Becker U, Gatermann SG. The hemagglutinin of *Staphylococcus saprophyticus* is a major adhesin for uroepithelial cells. Infect Immun 1996;64:3893–6.
363 Gatermann S, John J, Marre R. *Staphylococcus saprophyticus* urease: characterization and contribution to uropathogenicity in unobstructed urinary tract infection of rats. Infect Immun 1989;57:110–16.
364 Nicolle LE, Harding GK. Susceptibility of clinical isolates of *Staphylococcus saprophyticus* to fifteen commonly used antimicrobial agents. Antimicrob Agents Chemother 1982;22:895–6.
365 Richardson JF. Frequency of resistance to trimethoprim among isolates of *Staphylococcus epidermidis* and *Staphylococcus saprophyticus*. J Antimicrob Chemother 1983;11:163–7.

Section III
Diseases Caused by Staphylococci

Chapter 16
Staphylococcus aureus Bacteremia and Endocarditis

Zeina A. Kanafani[1], *Sara E. Cosgrove*[2] *and Vance G. Fowler Jr*[3]
[1] Division of Infectious Diseases, American University of Beirut Medical Center, Beirut, Lebanon
[2] Division of Infectious Diseases, Johns Hopkins University School of Medicine, Baltimore, Maryland, USA
[3] Division of Infectious Diseases, Duke University Medical Center, Durham, North Carolina, USA

Bacteremia and endocarditis

Staphylococcus aureus is a major cause of bloodstream infections, in both the hospital and community settings. Recent evidence has shown that the incidence of *S. aureus* bacteremia (SAB) has increased significantly [1–3]. The impact of this increasing frequency has been amplified by the concomitant rise in the rates of antibiotic resistance among *S. aureus* isolates [4–6]. While the majority of superficial skin infections caused by *S. aureus* are easily treated, invasive *S. aureus* infections such as bacteremia and infective endocarditis often lead to serious sequelae and high mortality rates [7,8]. According to recent estimates, the burden of SAB is significant. In one study, the mean infection-related costs in patients with prosthetic devices and SAB amounted to $67 439 for hospital-acquired infections and $37 868 for community-acquired infections [9]. Prompt diagnosis and initiation of appropriate therapy remain a challenge but are essential goals in the approach to patients with SAB and *S. aureus* infective endocarditis (SAIE).

Epidemiology

SAB has been traditionally categorized according to the presumed place of acquisition of the infection. In addition to the traditional designations of hospital-acquired (nosocomial) and community-acquired infections, nonnosocomial healthcare-associated infection has recently emerged in importance. This shift likely reflects the increased emphasis on delivery of healthcare outside the hospital [10]. In many places, methicillin-resistant *S. aureus* (MRSA) now account for the majority of nosocomial and nonnosocomial healthcare-associated infections [11].

Staphylococci in Human Disease, 2nd edition. Edited by Kent B. Crossley, Kimberly K. Jefferson, Gordon Archer, Vance G. Fowler, Jr.
 ISBN 978-14051-6332-3.

Nosocomial SAB

Staphylococcus aureus is the second most common organism isolated from blood cultures in hospitalized patients [12,13]. The incidence of SAB is increasingly steadily, an observation that has been ascribed to the use of invasive procedures and implantable devices in a growing population of patients [3]. From 1980 to 1989, the National Nosocomial Infections Surveillance (NNIS) System of the Centers for Disease Control and Prevention (CDC) reported increases in the rates of SAB ranging from 176% in large teaching hospitals to 283% in nonteaching hospitals [1]. A similar trend has been observed in European hospitals. For example, between 1995 and 2001, there was a 55% increase in the incidence of SAB in Finland [14]. Significant increases in rates of SAB have also been reported in Denmark [15] and the UK [16].

Community-acquired SAB

Traditionally, injection drug users (IDUs) constituted the bulk of patients presenting with community-acquired SAB [17,18]. Unhygienic handling of needles places IDUs at risk for SAB and right-sided SAIE. Over the past several years, there has been emergence of community-acquired MRSA (CA-MRSA) infections, mainly skin infections and pneumonia, in patients who have not had any prior healthcare contact [19,20] (see Chapter 13). Although bacteremia is a rare occurrence in the setting of superficial skin infections, deep abscesses can be complicated by SAB [21,22]. In addition, CA-MRSA pneumonia can manifest as a fulminant disease with extensive pulmonary necrosis and frequently bacteremia [23–25]. For example, a recent report in *Morbidity and Mortality Weekly Report* described 10 cases of CA-MRSA necrotizing pneumonia between December 2006 and January 2007 in Georgia and Louisiana. All episodes followed an influenza virus infection or an influenza-like illness in case patients. The average duration of symptoms was 3.5 days, and mortality was 60% [26].

Healthcare-associated SAB

Healthcare-associated infections occur in patients who receive healthcare outside the hospital setting. Examples include hemodialysis recipients, individuals residing in long-term care facilities, those receiving home healthcare, those receiving intravascular therapy at home or in an outpatient facility, and those who have been hospitalized within 90 days. SAB has been increasingly encountered in this population of patients, primarily because of the expanding use of intravascular catheters [3,10]. In a large prospective cohort study, 37% of patients admitted with bloodstream infections had healthcare-associated bacteremia [10]. Recent evidence suggests that a significant portion of healthcare-associated MRSA bloodstream infections are caused by strains associated with episodes of community-acquired infection [27,28].

Staphylococcus aureus endocarditis

Infective endocarditis complicates the course of SAB in around 12% of cases [29–31]. Probably because of the increasing rates of SAB, the frequency of SAIE has also increased [32–35]. *Staphylococcus aureus* is now the leading cause of both native [8,36] and prosthetic [37] valve endocarditis in many parts of the world. The increasing frequency of infective endocarditis caused by *S. aureus* is due in large part to the emergence of healthcare-associated SAIE [8,33,35,38]. A growing number of patients are at risk of *S. aureus* bloodstream infections because of the use of interventional procedures, intravascular catheters, and implantable devices. In contrast to IDU-associated and community-acquired infections, healthcare-associated SAIE exhibits distinct characteristics. For example, healthcare-associated SAIE is more clinically occult, more frequently caused by MRSA, and is associated with a higher mortality than other forms of SAIE [8]. The increased availability and use of echocardiography in the evaluation of patients with SAB has also likely contributed to the increased recognition of underlying endocarditis [39].

Risk factors for development of SAB

The risk factors for hospital-acquired and healthcare-associated SAB include healthcare-related factors (e.g., surgical wounds, intravascular catheters, invasive devices) [40] and comorbid patient conditions (e.g., advanced age [41], diabetes mellitus, end-stage renal disease, immunosuppression). In a prospective case–control study of hospitalized Danish patients, the presence of a central venous catheter was the single greatest risk factor for the development of SAB [42]. On the other hand, community-acquired SAB traditionally affects IDUs and otherwise healthy patients with infections at various sites [43]. While true community-acquired SAB is relatively uncommon, its presence is strongly associated with underlying infectious complications [31,43,44].

Risk factors for complicated SAB

The single most important aspect in the management of SAB is to identify the extent of infection. Distinguishing patients with complicated SAB guides pivotal medical and surgical management decisions, yet is often difficult. For this reason, the possibility of complications, including infective endocarditis, should be considered in every patient with SAB. Approximately one-third of patients with SAB develop one or more complications [17,31,45–47]. Although the majority of these complications are present at the time of initial evaluation, some may only become clinically apparent several weeks later. Almost any site of the body may be involved. In one large retrospective study, common sites of metastatic disease were kidneys (29%), central nervous system (28%), skin (16%), intervertebral disk (15%), lungs (15%), liver/spleen (13%), bone (11%), joints (10%), and heart valves (8%). Importantly, more than one metastatic site of infection was present in half of the cases [17].

Conditions that predispose patients with SAB to develop distant foci of infection include (i) old age [48], IDU [44,49], and comorbid conditions such as hemodialysis [50] and HIV infection [51]; (ii) underlying cardiac disease, such as native valvular abnormalities, congenital heart disease, and prior infective endocarditis [52,53]; and (iii) prosthetic implants, such as orthopedic implants [54], prosthetic valves [55], and intracardiac devices [56]. In fact, the risk of infective endocarditis in patients with prosthetic cardiac valves and cardiac devices (permanent pacemakers or cardioverters-defibrillators) who develop SAB is exceedingly high (~ 50%) [56–58]. However, the absence of the aforementioned risk factors does not exclude the presence of metastatic disease. Additional factors that were found to predict disseminated infection in patients with SAB include the following:

- community-onset SAB [31,43,44], due in part to the typically prolonged disease course and duration of bacteremia prior to detection;
- persistent fever (> 38.0°C) more than 72 hours following the initial positive blood culture [31];
- positive blood culture 2–4 days after the initial diagnosis of SAB [31];
- absence of a primary source of infection [44].

It is important to emphasize that SAIE frequently arises as a consequence of dissemination from a primary identifiable source of infection [38]. Thus, the presence of an identifiable source of infection does not exclude the presence of complicated bacteremia in a patient with SAB.

As prompt recognition of complications of SAB is essential to the optimal management of patients, simple clinical identifiers were evaluated for their ability to predict the presence of complications in over 700 patients with SAB [31]. A positive follow-up blood culture at 48–96 hours was the strongest predictor of complicated SAB. A 5-point scoring system, based on positive follow-up blood culture

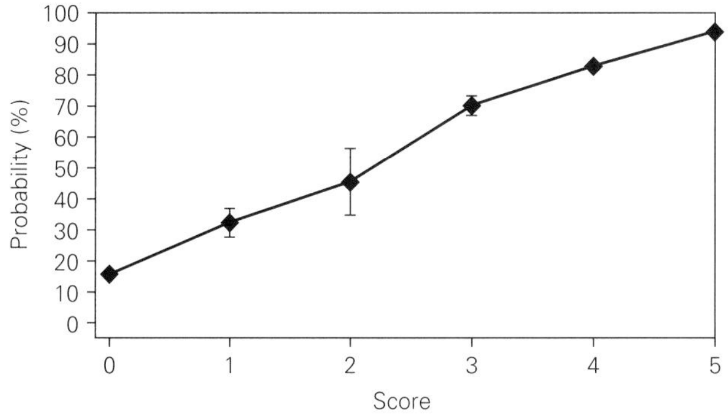

Figure 16.1 Association between *Staphylococcus aureus* bacteremia (SAB) score and probability of complicated SAB. *Staphylococcus aureus* bacteremia score derived from sum of individual risk factors: 1 point for community-acquired SAB, skin examination findings suggesting the presence of acute systemic infection, and persistent fever at 72 hours; 2 points for positive follow-up blood culture result at 48–96 hours. The bars indicate range of predicted probabilities of complicated SAB for each corresponding risk score (only one way to achieve a score of 0, 4, or 5). (From Fowler *et al.* [31] with permission.)

(2 points), community-acquired infection, persistent fever at 72 hours, and skin examination showing evidence of acute systemic infection (1 point each), accurately identified complicated SAB (Figure 16.1).

Clinical manifestations of SAB and SAIE

The clinical features of SAB are nonspecific. When present, symptoms range from fever and chills to septic shock. Symptoms in elderly or immunosuppressed patients with SAB can be limited to confusion or tachycardia. Any patient complaining of focal pain indicates the possibility of underlying complications of SAB and should be aggressively pursued if no firm alternate explanation can be identified. Back pain is a nonspecific but uniform complaint of paraspinous complications of SAB, including vertebral osteomyelitis [59,60] (Figure 16.2), psoas or epidural abscess [61] (Figure 16.3), and occasionally infective endocarditis [62]. Joint pain in a patient with SAB, especially if accompanied by erythema or effusion, should raise concern for septic arthritis and should be evaluated accordingly. This concern is particularly true among patients with prosthetic joints who develop SAB, for whom the risk of arthroplasty involvement is at least 25% [54]. The abrupt onset of abdominal pain in a patient with SAB or endocarditis can herald splenic or mesenteric infarction.

A careful physical examination is a critical aspect in the management of every patient with SAB. Findings such as an inflamed insertion site, a tender thrombotic "cord" adjacent to an intravenous catheter, cutaneous infarcts or peripheral emboli, a new or changing cardiac flow murmur, joint swelling, and spinal tenderness may be indicative of the presence of metastatic complications and

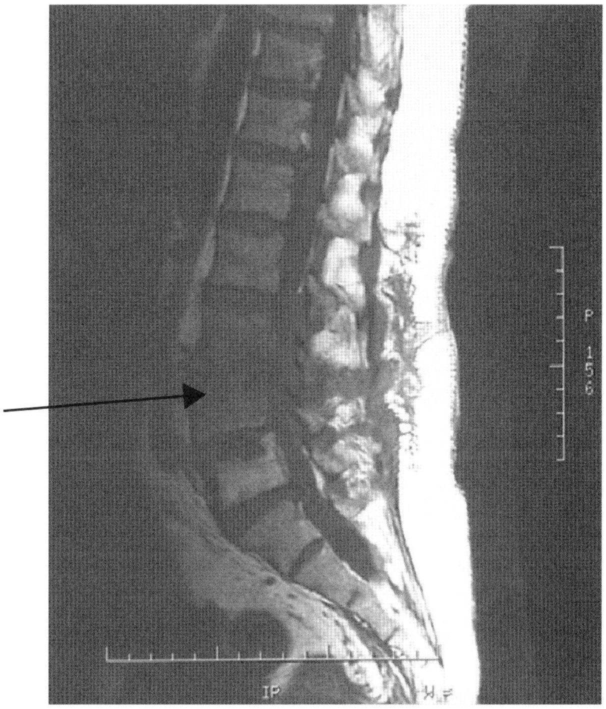

Figure 16.2 Vertebral osteomyelitis (arrow) in a patient with complicated *S. aureus* bacteremia.

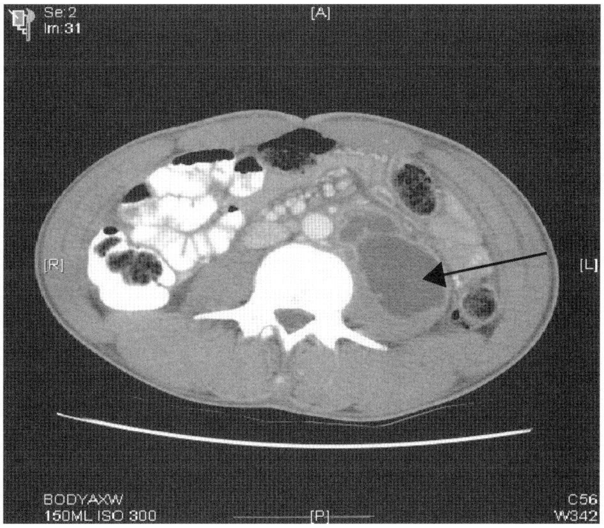

Figure 16.3 Psoas abscess (arrow) in a patient with complicated *S. aureus* bacteremia.

should be pursued. Echocardiography and radiographic imaging guided by the patient's signs and symptoms are valuable tools for the detection of distant foci of infection, a crucial step in the management of patients with SAB.

In cases of complicated infective endocarditis, specific clinical manifestations may be apparent, such as congestive heart failure, evidence of severe valvular dysfunction, heart block, neurological manifestations (with cerebral emboli or mycotic aneurysms), or pleural effusion.

Diagnosis of SAB

The diagnosis of SAB is straightforward, and relies on the isolation of the bacterium in blood cultures. Because *S. aureus* is almost never a contaminant [63] and because the mortality of untreated SAB is over 80% [64], the identification of *S. aureus* from even a single blood culture in a patient with signs and symptoms of infection is probably clinically significant and should be treated. During outbreaks, molecular typing is useful for recognizing the epidemic strain [65,66]. Patient antibodies to a variety of *S. aureus* antigens, including peptidoglycan, teichoic acid, *S. aureus* ultrasonicate, whole *S. aureus* cells, α-toxin, lipase, and capsular polysaccharide, have been evaluated but lack clinical utility [67,68].

Diagnosis of SAIE

While the presence of physical examination findings such as new cardiac murmur, conjunctival hemorrhage, Osler nodes, Janeway lesions, or peripheral cutaneous infarcts (see Plate 16.1) are critical clues in the diagnosis of infective endocarditis, most patients with SAIE in the current era do not have these telltale physical findings that historically were used to diagnose this condition [8,38,52,69]. Consequently, physical examination alone is insufficient to exclude the diagnosis of SAIE [52,69].

Echocardiography has been advocated in patients with SAB in order to optimize the timely detection of endocarditis. Transthoracic echocardiography (TTE) is a widely available noninvasive screening modality in the setting of SAB; however, it has limited sensitivity in detecting vegetations (64%) [70]. On the other hand, transesophageal echocardiography (TEE) offers significant advantages over TTE in evaluating patients with SAB, including higher sensitivity in detecting infective endocarditis (90%) [71–74], improved identification of the complications of infective endocarditis [75–77], and an enhanced ability to exclude infective endocarditis in patients with native valves (negative predictive value 100%) [78,79]. Whether TTE or TEE should be employed in the initial screening of the patient presenting with SAB remains a controversial issue. TEE is likely to be helpful in guiding the duration of therapy in patients with catheter-associated SAB or for patients at higher risk of infective endocarditis or associated complications by either providing evidence to support abbreviating a course of parenteral therapy to 2 weeks (e.g., in selected patients with intravascular catheter-associated SAB) or by demonstrating the need for more intensive therapy (e.g., prolonged duration of antibiotic therapy or cardiac surgery).

Treatment

Successful management of SAB depends primarily on determining the extent of infection and then on making appropriate decisions about choice and length of therapy. A routine infectious disease service consultation is recommended as this will result in better detection of complications and ensures adherence to standards of care [80].

Removal of the source of infection

Failure to remove infected intravascular catheters and implantable prostheses has been strongly correlated with recurrence of SAB. Among 244 hospitalized patients with SAB, 56% of the 23 patients whose infected foreign bodies were not removed experienced relapse of infection or death, compared with 16% of the 221 patients whose devices were removed or who did not have a device ($P < 0.01$) [45]. In another study in patients with permanent pacemakers or implantable cardiac defibrillators and SAB, failure to remove the device was associated with increased risk of recurrent bacteremia or death (52.4% vs. 25%) [56]. In the event of a nonremovable focus of infection, such as an abscess or musculoskeletal infection, surgical drainage and débridement becomes essential whenever possible.

Traditional indications for surgical intervention for infective endocarditis have included congestive heart failure, myocardial invasion, high risk for embolic complications, and failure to respond to antimicrobial therapy [81]. A series of studies suggests that patients with SAIE are likely to benefit from early surgical intervention [82–87]. In one study, early surgery significantly improved survival rates in patients with native or prosthetic valve SAIE, but did not improve survival in patients with other pathogens [83]. The exact role, indications, and timing of early surgery in SAIE have yet to be determined; however, it is likely that early surgical intervention will be beneficial to many patients.

Duration of therapy

The duration of antimicrobial therapy depends on the extent of infection. A summary of generally accepted treatment durations is provided in Table 16.1. Patients with SAB complicated by metastatic infection should be treated for at least 4 weeks with intravenous antibiotics. Patients with uncomplicated catheter-related SAB were traditionally treated with 4 weeks of intravenous antibiotics [88]. However, in the 1980s, clinicians increasingly began to abbreviate the duration of therapy for intravascular catheter-associated SAB to 10–14 days, combined with catheter removal. In 1993, a metaanalysis by Jernigan and Farr concluded that until a means existed to identify patients who may safely receive short-course therapy, patients with uncomplicated catheter-associated SAB should be treated with antibiotics for more than 2 weeks. In 1998, an algorithm developed by Fowler *et al.* [45] proposed the use of clinical and TEE criteria to identify candidates for 2-week (short-course) therapy. The algorithm included the following criteria: (i) catheter-associated SAB, with prompt removal of the intravenous catheter; (ii) infective endocarditis excluded by TEE; (iii) no implanted prostheses (e.g., prosthetic valves, cardiac devices, or prosthetic

Table 16.1 Proposed antimicrobial regimens for patients with *Staphylococcus aureus* bacteremia and endocarditis.[1]

Categories of infection	Patients with MSSA infection	Patients with MRSA infection or penicillin allergy	Duration of treatment
Simple bacteremia[2]	Nafcillin/oxacillin 2 g i.v. every 4 hours[3]	Vancomycin[4] 30 mg/kg daily in two doses *or* daptomycin 6 mg/kg once daily	1 week if all criteria below[2] are met *and* no valvular abnormalities
Uncomplicated bacteremia[2]	Nafcillin/oxacillin 2 g i.v. every 4 hours[3]	Vancomycin[4] 30 mg/kg daily in two doses *or* daptomycin 6 mg/kg once daily	2 weeks if all criteria below[2] are met; otherwise > 2 weeks
Complicated bacteremia	Nafcillin/oxacillin 2 g i.v. every 4 hours[3]	Vancomycin[4] 30 mg/kg daily in two doses *or* daptomycin 6 mg/kg once daily	4–8 weeks[5]
Uncomplicated right-sided native valve endocarditis	Nafcillin/oxacillin 2 g i.v. every 4 hours[3] + gentamicin 3 mg/kg daily in three doses for 3–5 days	Vancomycin[4] 30 mg/kg daily in two doses *or* daptomycin 6 mg/kg once daily	2–4 weeks
Complicated right-sided native valve endocarditis	Nafcillin/oxacillin 2 g i.v. every 4 hours[3] ± gentamicin 3 mg/kg daily in three doses for 3–5 days	Vancomycin[4] 30 mg/kg daily in two doses *or* daptomycin 6 mg/kg once daily	4–6 weeks
Left-sided native valve endocarditis	Nafcillin/oxacillin 2 g i.v. every 4 hours[3] ± gentamicin 3 mg/kg daily in three doses for 3–5 days	Vancomycin[4] 30 mg/kg daily in two doses	4–6 weeks
Prosthetic valve endocardiis	Nafcillin/oxacillin 2 g i.v. every 4 hours[3] + rifampin 300 mg i.v./p.o. every 8 hours + gentamicin 3 mg/kg daily in three doses for 2 weeks	Vancomycin[4] 30 mg/kg daily in two doses + gentamicin 3 mg/kg daily in three doses for 2 weeks	≥ 6 weeks

[1] Suggestions are intended to be generalized recommendations rather than hard and fast rules, and should never replace clinical judgment.
[2] Defined as a patient with catheter-associated *S. aureus* bacteremia in which the implicated catheter is removed and all the following criteria are met: (i) endocarditis should be excluded with TEE; (ii) the patient should have no implanted prostheses (e.g., prosthetic valves, cardiac devices, or arthroplasties); (iii) follow-up blood cultures drawn 2–4 days after initial set of blood cultures must be negative for *S. aureus*; (iv) the patient should defervesce within 72 hours of initiating effective antistaphylococcal therapy; and (v) the patient should have no localizing signs or symptoms of metastatic staphylococcal infection.
[3] Cefazolin 2 g i.v. every 8 hours is an alternative to semisynthetic penicillins in patients with MSSA infection.
[4] Dose adjusted to maintain a target serum trough level of 15–20 μg/mL.
[5] Depending on type of complication and individual patient circumstances.
MSSA, methicillin-susceptible *S. aureus*; MRSA, methicillin-resistant *S. aureus*.

joints); (iv) negative repeat blood cultures 2–4 days after the initial set of blood cultures; (v) defervescence within 72 hours of initiating effective antistaphylococcal therapy; and (vi) no clinical evidence of metastatic staphylococcal infection. Although this treatment strategy was shown to be cost-effective [89], it has not yet been validated in an appropriately designed clinical trial.

Antimicrobial therapy of SAB and SAIE

β-Lactams

Although antistaphylococcal penicillins remain the treatment of choice for SAB caused by methicillin-sensitive *S. aureus* (MSSA), their use has been greatly handicapped by the increasing prevalence of MRSA strains. Patients with MSSA bacteremia experienced shorter durations of bacteremia and were less likely to relapse than similar patients who received vancomycin [30].

Cefazolin is a familiar and trusted alternative to the antistaphylococcal penicillins. Although there have been reports of increased hydrolysis of cefazolin by *S. aureus* [90], the clinical significance of these findings is unknown. Moreover, in a recent prospective study in hemodialysis-dependent patients with MSSA bacteremia, patients treated with cefazolin were at a lower risk of experiencing treatment failure than those receiving vancomycin [91]. Given this observation, the use of vancomycin to treat MSSA infections should be restricted to patients who have a history of allergy to β-lactams.

Vancomycin

Vancomycin has long been the mainstay of therapy for MRSA bacteremia and endocarditis. Although it still maintains *in vitro* activity against the majority of MRSA isolates, clinical cure rates in serious infections have been disappointing. Vancomycin has been associated with prolonged duration of bacteremia in the treatment of MRSA bacteremia and endocarditis [92,93]. Treatment failure rates exceeding 40% have been quoted for SAB [94] and *S. aureus* pneumonia [95]. In general, infections due to MRSA isolates with vancomycin minimum inhibitory concentrations (MICs) of 2 μg/mL are associated with worse clinical outcomes [94,96,97] and higher mortality [98]. Prior exposure to vancomycin and ICU stay at the time of infection are independent predictors of high MIC values [99]. Although current guidelines recommend achieving serum vancomycin troughs of 10–20 μg/mL [81], the ideal vancomycin trough level continues to be an area of active investigation [96,100].

The addition of rifampin to the treatment regimen has not shown benefit in MRSA bacteremia or native valve endocarditis [92]. In addition, the use of rifampin in native valve endocarditis is associated with significant hepatotoxicity and drug–drug interactions. However, if rifampin is used, this should be done after the clearance of bacteremia to minimize the risk developing resistance [101]. Similarly, the initial use of synergistic gentamicin has not been shown to improve outcome in patients with MRSA bacteremia and native valve endocarditis, although it appears to reduce the duration of bacteremia by about a day in patients with MSSA native valve endocarditis [102,103]. Consequently, the administration of gentamicin in these patients is now considered optional and should be weighed against the potential for nephrotoxicity [81].

Daptomycin

Daptomycin is a concentration-dependent bactericidal cyclic lipopeptide that was approved by the Food and Drug Administration in 2006 for the treatment of SAB and right-sided SAIE. In a prospective randomized trial of 235 patients with SAB or SAIE, daptomycin 6 mg/kg once daily was found to be as effective as standard therapy, consisting of initial low-dose short-course gentamicin plus either vancomycin or an antistaphylococcal penicillin [104]. It should be noted, however, that isolates from six of the 19 daptomycin-treated patients who failed therapy demonstrated the emergence of resistance to daptomycin while on therapy. All these patients required, but did not receive, adjunctive surgical therapy for their infection (e.g., drainage of abscess, surgical débridement). Several other investigators have reported a potential association between resistance to vancomycin and resistance to daptomycin in *S. aureus* [105–108]. This finding suggests that susceptibility testing to daptomycin should be repeated in patients with persistently positive cultures who do not respond rapidly to daptomycin therapy. Of note, daptomycin should not be used in patients with pneumonia since it is inactivated by pulmonary surfactant [109].

Other agents

Linezolid is a bacteriostatic oxazolidinone with activity against MRSA. Its use in MRSA bacteremia and endocarditis has had conflicting results. Although anecdotal case reports describe successful outcomes [110], there have been several cases of clinical failure with linezolid [111–113] and a recent FDA advisory letter detailed a higher rate of Gram-negative sepsis in a clinical trial evaluating linezolid in the treatment of catheter-related bloodstream infections [114]. Therefore, linezolid is not recommended for the treatment of SAB and SAIE.

Quinupristin–dalfopristin, a streptogramin antibiotic, has been used as salvage therapy in patients with MRSA infections who are failing or are intolerant of traditional therapy. Overall clinical success rates were 70% with bacteremia and 54% with endocarditis [115]. The cost, the requirement for administration by central catheter, and the side-effect profile have all limited the use of quinupristin–dalfopristin [116].

Trimethoprim–sulfamethoxazole (TMP–SMX) was compared with vancomycin in a randomized controlled trial in 101 IDUs with *S. aureus* infections [117]. In this study, over half of patients had an intravascular infection including tricuspid valve endocarditis, thrombophlebitis, pseudoaneurysm, or bacteremia. Cure rates were 86% for patients treated with TMP–SMX compared with 98% for those who received vancomycin, although all 47 patients with MRSA infection in both arms were cured. These results, and those from a recent study demonstrating that TMP–SMX is rapidly bactericidal against MRSA isolates *in vitro*, make this drug a potential agent for a salvage regimen for MRSA bacteremia and endocarditis [118].

Investigational agents

The lipoglycopeptides dalbavancin, telavancin and oritavancin and the broad-spectrum cephalosporins ceftobiprole and ceftaroline are currently under investigation for the treatment of various MRSA infections including bacteremia and endocarditis. However, no clinical data are currently available.

Infections of cardiac devices

Included under this heading are prosthetic cardiac valves, implantable pacemakers and defibrillators, and ventricular assist devices. While these devices are essential in the management of a growing population of patients, infection is a feared complication as it carries significant morbidity and mortality. *Staphylococcus aureus* is now the most common cause of prosthetic valve endocarditis [37], and is also a major cause of infections involving pacemakers [56], implantable defibrillators [58], and pocket and driveline infections with ventricular assist devices [119].

The clinical manifestations of prosthetic valve endocarditis resemble those of native valve endocarditis and might be subtle. However, prosthetic valve dysfunction or embolic phenomena can sometimes dominate the picture [120–122]. With other devices, infections can present as bloodstream infections or as device pocket infections. In the latter, local signs of inflammation are often present, such as erythema, local tenderness, and wound drainage.

In advanced cases, a sinus tract may form or the device might erode through the overlying skin.

The management of cardiac device infections is complicated by the difficulty of eradicating *S. aureus* from the surface of prosthetic material due to the adherence and biofilm-formation properties of the organism. Surgical intervention to remove the infected device is therefore standard of care in the successful treatment of patients with such infections [123,124]. The optimal timing of device reimplantation has been highly debated. Most infectious disease clinicians recommend deferring reimplantation of the permanent device, if possible, until blood cultures have been negative and the patient has received parenteral antibiotics for at least 7 days.

Metastatic sites of infection

In adults, *S. aureus* is the most common cause of hematogenous vertebral osteomyelitis. In a retrospective analysis of 40 patients with *S. aureus* hematogenous vertebral osteomyelitis, 55% of cases occurred following invasive procedures [125]. Neurological abnormalities were found in 48% of cases, and 60% of patients had an epidural, paraspinous, or psoas abscess detected by neuroimaging. The infection was cured in 83% (24/29) of evaluable patients, but 50% of cured patients were left with infection-related sequelae. Intravenous antibiotic therapy for at least 8 weeks was the only clinical factor associated with cure.

Septic arthritis develops in 4–10% of patients with SAB [17,31,126]. Patients who suffer from rheumatoid arthritis are especially predisposed to develop polyarticular *S. aureus* septic arthritis [127]. Although the knee is the most frequently involved, any joint can occasionally be infected [128].

Septic thrombophlebitis occurs in patients with infected vascular catheters or in IDUs [129]. In one prospective observational cohort study that evaluated consecutive patients with central venous catheter-associated SAB with venous ultrasound, over 70% of patients had evidence of thrombosis by diagnostic imaging [130]. Importantly, most of these patients had no evidence of obstructive venous thrombosis by physical examination. Patients with septic thrombophlebitis commonly present with persistent bacteremia. In patients with superficial thrombophlebitis, surgical excision of the infected vein is often necessary. For infections involving central veins, surgical options are limited. Treatment of central vein septic thrombophlebitis generally involves extended courses of parenteral antibiotics and frequently long-term anticoagulation.

References

1 Banerjee SN, Emori TG, Culver DH *et al.* Secular trends in nosocomial primary bloodstream infections in the United States, 1980–1989. National Nosocomial Infections Surveillance System. Am J Med 1991;91(3B):86S–89S.

2 Edmond MB, Wallace SE, McClish DK, Pfaller MA, Jones RN, Wenzel RP. Nosocomial bloodstream infections in United States hospitals: a three-year analysis. Clin Infect Dis 1999;29:239–44.

3 Steinberg JP, Clark CC, Hackman BO. Nosocomial and community-acquired *Staphylococcus aureus* bacteremias from 1980 to 1993: impact of intravascular devices and methicillin resistance. Clin Infect Dis 1996;23:255–9.

4 Calfee DP, Durbin LJ, Germanson TP, Toney DM, Smith EB, Farr BM. Spread of methicillin-resistant *Staphylococcus aureus* (MRSA) among household contacts of individuals with nosocomially acquired MRSA. Infect Control Hosp Epidemiol 2003; 24:422–6.

5 Enright MC, Robinson DA, Randle G, Feil EJ, Grundmann H, Spratt BG. The evolutionary history of methicillin-resistant *Staphylococcus aureus* (MRSA). Proc Natl Acad Sci USA 2002;99: 7687–92.

6 Herold BC, Immergluck LC, Maranan MC *et al.* Community-acquired methicillin-resistant *Staphylococcus aureus* in children with no identified predisposing risk. JAMA 1998;279:593–8.

7 Fowler VG Jr, Justice A, Moore C *et al.* Risk factors for hematogenous complications of intravascular catheter-associated *Staphylococcus aureus* bacteremia. Clin Infect Dis 2005;40:695–703.

8 Fowler VG Jr, Miro JM, Hoen B *et al. Staphylococcus aureus* endocarditis: a consequence of medical progress. JAMA 2005;293: 3012–21.

9 Chu VH, Crosslin DR, Friedman JY *et al. Staphylococcus aureus* bacteremia in patients with prosthetic devices: costs and outcomes. Am J Med 2005;118:1416.

10 Friedman ND, Kaye KS, Stout JE *et al.* Health care-associated bloodstream infections in adults: a reason to change the accepted definition of community-acquired infections. Ann Intern Med 2002;137:791–7.

11 Klevens RM, Morrison MA, Nadle J *et al.* Invasive methicillin-resistant *Staphylococcus aureus* infections in the United States. JAMA 2007;298:1763–71.

12 Martone WJ, Jarvis WR, Culver DH. Hospital infections. In: Bennett JV, Brachman PS, eds. Incidence and Nature of Endemic and Epidemic Nosocomial Infections. Boston: Little Brown, 1992:577–96.

13 Wisplinghoff H, Bischoff T, Tallent SM, Seifert H, Wenzel RP, Edmond MB. Nosocomial bloodstream infections in US hospitals: analysis of 24,179 cases from a prospective nationwide surveillance study. Clin Infect Dis 2004;39:309–17.

14 Lyytikainen O, Ruotsalainen E, Jarvinen A, Valtonen V, Ruutu P. Trends and outcome of nosocomial and community-acquired bloodstream infections due to *Staphylococcus aureus* in Finland, 1995–2001. Eur J Clin Microbiol Infect Dis. 2005;24:399–404.

15 Benfield T, Espersen F, Frimodt-Moller N *et al.* Increasing incidence but decreasing in-hospital mortality of adult *Staphylococcus aureus* bacteraemia between 1981 and 2000. Clin Microbiol Infect 2007;13:257–63.

16 Wyllie DH, Crook DW, Peto TE. Mortality after *Staphylococcus aureus* bacteraemia in two hospitals in Oxfordshire, 1997–2003: cohort study. BMJ 2006;333:281.

17 Lautenschlager S, Herzog C, Zimmerli W. Course and outcome of bacteremia due to *Staphylococcus aureus*: evaluation of different clinical case definitions. Clin Infect Dis 1993;16:567–73.

18 Mylotte JM, McDermott C, Spooner JA. Prospective study of 114 consecutive episodes of *Staphylococcus aureus* bacteremia. Rev Infect Dis 1987;9:891–907.
19 Pan ES, Diep BA, Carleton HA *et al*. Increasing prevalence of methicillin-resistant *Staphylococcus aureus* infection in California jails. Clin Infect Dis 2003;37:1384–8.
20 Purcell K, Fergie JE. Exponential increase in community-acquired methicillin-resistant *Staphylococcus aureus* infections in South Texas children. Pediatr Infect Dis J 2002;21:988–9.
21 Baggett HC, Hennessy TW, Leman R *et al*. An outbreak of community-onset methicillin-resistant *Staphylococcus aureus* skin infections in southwestern Alaska. Infect Control Hosp Epidemiol 2003;24:397–402.
22 Lindenmayer JM, Schoenfeld S, O'Grady R, Carney JK. Methicillin-resistant *Staphylococcus aureus* in a high school wrestling team and the surrounding community. Arch Intern Med 1998;158:895–9.
23 Gillet Y, Issartel B, Vanhems P *et al*. Association between *Staphylococcus aureus* strains carrying gene for Panton–Valentine leukocidin and highly lethal necrotising pneumonia in young immunocompetent patients. Lancet 2002;359:753–9.
24 Gonzalez BE, Martinez-Aguilar G, Hulten KG *et al*. Severe staphylococcal sepsis in adolescents in the era of community-acquired methicillin-resistant *Staphylococcus aureus*. Pediatrics 2005;115:642–8.
25 Mongkolrattanothai K, Boyle S, Kahana MD, Daum RS. Severe *Staphylococcus aureus* infections caused by clonally related community-acquired methicillin-susceptible and methicillin-resistant isolates. Clin Infect Dis 2003;37:1050–8.
26 Centers for Disease Control and Prevention. Severe methicillin-resistant *Staphylococcus aureus* community-acquired pneumonia associated with influenza: Louisiana and Georgia, December 2006–January 2007. MMWR 2007;56:325–9.
27 Maree CL, Daum RS, Boyle-Vavra S, Matayoshi K, Miller LG. Community-associated methicillin-resistant *Staphylococcus aureus* isolates causing healthcare-associated infections. Emerg Infect Dis 2007;13:236–42.
28 Seybold U, Kourbatova EV, Johnson JG *et al*. Emergence of community-associated methicillin-resistant *Staphylococcus aureus* USA300 genotype as a major cause of health care-associated blood stream infections. Clin Infect Dis 2006;42:647–56.
29 Chang FY, MacDonald BB, Peacock JE Jr *et al*. A prospective multicenter study of *Staphylococcus aureus* bacteremia: incidence of endocarditis, risk factors for mortality, and clinical impact of methicillin resistance. Medicine (Baltimore) 2003;82:322–32.
30 Chang FY, Peacock JE Jr, Musher DM *et al*. *Staphylococcus aureus* bacteremia: recurrence and the impact of antibiotic treatment in a prospective multicenter study. Medicine (Baltimore) 2003; 82:333–9.
31 Fowler VG Jr, Olsen MK, Corey GR *et al*. Clinical identifiers of complicated *Staphylococcus aureus* bacteremia. Arch Intern Med 2003;163:2066–72.
32 Cabell CH, Jollis JG, Peterson GE *et al*. Changing patient characteristics and the effect on mortality in endocarditis. Arch Intern Med 2002;162:90–4.
33 Fernandez-Guerrero ML, Verdejo C, Azofra J, de Gorgolas M. Hospital-acquired infectious endocarditis not associated with cardiac surgery: an emerging problem. Clin Infect Dis 1995; 20:16–23.
34 Sanabria TJ, Alpert JS, Goldberg R, Pape LA, Cheeseman SH. Increasing frequency of staphylococcal infective endocarditis. Experience at a university hospital, 1981 through 1988. Arch Intern Med 1990;150:1305–9.
35 Watanakunakorn C, Burkert T. Infective endocarditis at a large community teaching hospital, 1980–1990. A review of 210 episodes. Medicine (Baltimore) 1993;72:90–102.
36 Miro JM, Anguera I, Cabell CH *et al*. *Staphylococcus aureus* native valve infective endocarditis: report of 566 episodes from the International Collaboration on Endocarditis Merged Database. Clin Infect Dis 2005;41:507–14.
37 Wang A, Athan E, Pappas PA *et al*. Contemporary clinical profile and outcome of prosthetic valve endocarditis. JAMA 2007;297:1354–61.
38 Fowler VG Jr, Sanders LL, Kong LK *et al*. Infective endocarditis due to *Staphylococcus aureus*: 59 prospectively identified cases with follow-up. Clin Infect Dis 1999;28:106–14.
39 Petti CA, Fowler VG Jr. *Staphylococcus aureus* bacteremia and endocarditis. Cardiol Clin 2003;21:219–33, vii.
40 Musher DM, Lamm N, Darouiche RO, Young EJ, Hamill RJ, Landon GC. The current spectrum of *Staphylococcus aureus* infection in a tertiary care hospital. Medicine (Baltimore) 1994; 73:186–208.
41 McClelland RS, Fowler VG Jr, Sanders LL *et al*. *Staphylococcus aureus* bacteremia among elderly vs younger adult patients: comparison of clinical features and mortality. Arch Intern Med 1999;159:1244–7.
42 Jensen AG, Wachmann CH, Poulsen KB *et al*. Risk factors for hospital-acquired *Staphylococcus aureus* bacteremia. Arch Intern Med 1999;159:1437–44.
43 Willcox PA, Rayner BL, Whitelaw DA. Community-acquired *Staphylococcus aureus* bacteraemia in patients who do not abuse intravenous drugs. Q J Med 1998;91:41–7.
44 Nolan CM, Beaty HN. *Staphylococcus aureus* bacteremia. Current clinical patterns. Am J Med 1976;60:495–500.
45 Fowler VG Jr, Sanders LL, Sexton DJ *et al*. Outcome of *Staphylococcus aureus* bacteremia according to compliance with recommendations of infectious diseases specialists: experience with 244 patients. Clin Infect Dis 1998;27:478–86.
46 Libman H, Arbeit RD. Complications associated with *Staphylococcus aureus* bacteremia. Arch Intern Med 1984;144:541–5.
47 Ringberg H, Thoren A, Lilja B. Metastatic complications of *Staphylococcus aureus* septicemia. To seek is to find. Infection 2000;28:132–6.
48 Werner GS, Schulz R, Fuchs JB *et al*. Infective endocarditis in the elderly in the era of transesophageal echocardiography: clinical features and prognosis compared with younger patients. Am J Med 1996;100:90–7.
49 Miro JM, del Rio A, Mestres CA. Infective endocarditis in intravenous drug abusers and HIV-1 infected patients. Infect Dis Clin North Am 2002;16:273–95, vii–viii.
50 Marr KA, Kong L, Fowler VG *et al*. Incidence and outcome of *Staphylococcus aureus* bacteremia in hemodialysis patients. Kidney Int 1998;54:1684–9.
51 Jacobson MA, Gellermann H, Chambers H. *Staphylococcus aureus* bacteremia and recurrent staphylococcal infection in patients with acquired immunodeficiency syndrome and AIDS-related complex. Am J Med 1988;85:172–6.
52 Espersen F, Frimodt-Moller N. *Staphylococcus aureus* endocarditis. A review of 119 cases. Arch Intern Med 1986;146:1118–21.

53 Lamas CC, Eykyn SJ. Bicuspid aortic valve. A silent danger: analysis of 50 cases of infective endocarditis. Clin Infect Dis 2000;30:336–41.
54 Murdoch DR, Roberts SA, Fowler VG Jr *et al.* Infection of orthopedic prostheses after *Staphylococcus aureus* bacteremia. Clin Infect Dis 2001;32:647–9.
55 Fang G, Keys TF, Gentry LO *et al.* Prosthetic valve endocarditis resulting from nosocomial bacteremia. A prospective, multicenter study. Ann Intern Med 1993;119:560–7.
56 Chamis AL, Peterson GE, Cabell CH *et al. Staphylococcus aureus* bacteremia in patients with permanent pacemakers or implantable cardioverter-defibrillators. Circulation 2001;104:1029–33.
57 El-Ahdab F, Benjamin DK Jr, Wang A *et al.* Risk of endocarditis among patients with prosthetic valves and *Staphylococcus aureus* bacteremia. Am J Med 2005;118:225–9.
58 Uslan DZ, Sohail MR, St Sauver JL *et al.* Permanent pacemaker and implantable cardioverter defibrillator infection: a population-based study. Arch Intern Med 2007;167:669–75.
59 Jensen AG, Espersen F, Skinhoj P, Frimodt-Moller N. Bacteremic *Staphylococcus aureus* spondylitis. Arch Intern Med 1998;158: 509–17.
60 McHenry MC, Easley KA, Locker GA. Vertebral osteomyelitis: long-term outcome for 253 patients from 7 Cleveland-area hospitals. Clin Infect Dis 2002;34:1342–50.
61 Darouiche RO. Spinal epidural abscess. N Engl J Med 2006; 355:2012–20.
62 Watanakunakorn C. *Staphylococcus aureus* endocarditis at a community teaching hospital, 1980 to 1991. An analysis of 106 cases. Arch Intern Med 1994;154:2330–5.
63 Weinstein MP, Towns ML, Quartey SM *et al.* The clinical significance of positive blood cultures in the 1990s: a prospective comprehensive evaluation of the microbiology, epidemiology, and outcome of bacteremia and fungemia in adults. Clin Infect Dis 1997;24:584–602.
64 Skinner D, Keefer CS. Significance of bacteremia caused by *Staphylococcus aureus*. Arch Intern Med 1941;68:851–75.
65 Branchini ML, Morthland VH, Tresoldi AT, Von Nowakonsky A, Dias MB, Pfaller MA. Application of genomic DNA subtyping by pulsed field gel electrophoresis and restriction enzyme analysis of plasmid DNA to characterize methicillin-resistant *Staphylococcus aureus* from two nosocomial outbreaks. Diagn Microbiol Infect Dis 1993;17:275–81.
66 van Belkum A, Bax R, Peerbooms P, Goessens WH, van Leeuwen N, Quint WG. Comparison of phage typing and DNA fingerprinting by polymerase chain reaction for discrimination of methicillin-resistant *Staphylococcus aureus* strains. J Clin Microbiol 1993;31:798–803.
67 Ryding U, Espersen F, Soderquist B, Christensson B. Evaluation of seven different enzyme-linked immunosorbent assays for serodiagnosis of *Staphylococcus aureus* bacteremia. Diagn Microbiol Infect Dis 2002;42:9–15.
68 Wise KA, Tosolini FA. Detection of teichoic acid antibodies in *Staphylococcus aureus* infections. Pathology 1992;24:102–8.
69 Roder BL, Wandall DA, Frimodt-Moller N, Espersen F, Skinhoj P, Rosdahl VT. Clinical features of *Staphylococcus aureus* endocarditis: a 10-year experience in Denmark. Arch Intern Med 1999;159:462–9.
70 Mugge A. Echocardiographic detection of cardiac valve vegetations and prognostic implications. Infect Dis Clin North Am 1993;7:877–98.
71 Abraham J, Mansour C, Veledar E, Khan B, Lerakis S. *Staphylococcus aureus* bacteremia and endocarditis: the Grady Memorial Hospital experience with methicillin-sensitive *S. aureus* and methicillin-resistant *S. aureus* bacteremia. Am Heart J 2004; 147:536–9.
72 Chamis AL, Gesty-Palmer D, Fowler VG, Corey GR. Echocardiography for the diagnosis of *Staphylococcus aureus* infective endocarditis. Curr Infect Dis Rep 1999;1:129–35.
73 Fowler VG Jr, Li J, Corey GR *et al.* Role of echocardiography in evaluation of patients with *Staphylococcus aureus* bacteremia: experience in 103 patients. J Am Coll Cardiol 1997;30:1072–8.
74 Sullenberger AL, Avedissian LS, Kent SM. Importance of transesophageal echocardiography in the evaluation of *Staphylococcus aureus* bacteremia. J Heart Valve Dis 2005;14:23–8.
75 Daniel WG, Mugge A, Martin RP *et al.* Improvement in the diagnosis of abscesses associated with endocarditis by transesophageal echocardiography. N Engl J Med 1991;324:795–800.
76 De Castro S, d'Amati G, Cartoni D *et al.* Valvular perforation in left-sided infective endocarditis: a prospective echocardiographic evaluation and clinical outcome. Am Heart J 1997;134: 656–64.
77 Habib G, Guidon C, Tricoire E, Djiane V, Monties JR, Luccioni R. Papillary muscle rupture caused by bacterial endocarditis: role of transesophageal echocardiography. J Am Soc Echocardiogr 1994;7:79–81.
78 Lowry RW, Zoghbi WA, Baker WB, Wray RA, Quinones MA. Clinical impact of transesophageal echocardiography in the diagnosis and management of infective endocarditis. Am J Cardiol 1994;73:1089–91.
79 Sochowski RA, Chan KL. Implication of negative results on a monoplane transesophageal echocardiographic study in patients with suspected infective endocarditis. J Am Coll Cardiol 1993; 21:216–21.
80 Jenkins TC, Price CS, Sabel AL, Mehler PS, Burman WJ. Impact of routine infectious diseases service consultation on the evaluation, management, and outcomes of *Staphylococcus aureus* bacteremia. Clin Infect Dis 2008;46:1000–8.
81 Baddour LM, Wilson WR, Bayer AS *et al.* Infective endocarditis: diagnosis, antimicrobial therapy, and management of complications. A statement for healthcare professionals from the Committee on Rheumatic Fever, Endocarditis, and Kawasaki Disease, Council on Cardiovascular Disease in the Young, and the Councils on Clinical Cardiology, Stroke, and Cardiovascular Surgery and Anesthesia, American Heart Association: endorsed by the Infectious Diseases Society of America. Circulation 2005;111:e394–e434.
82 Aksoy O, Sexton DJ, Wang A *et al.* Early surgery in patients with infective endocarditis: a propensity score analysis. Clin Infect Dis 2007;44:364–72.
83 Bishara J, Leibovici L, Gartman-Israel D *et al.* Long-term outcome of infective endocarditis: the impact of early surgical intervention. Clin Infect Dis 2001;33:1636–43.
84 Chu VH, Cabell CH, Benjamin DK Jr *et al.* Early predictors of in-hospital death in infective endocarditis. Circulation 2004; 109:1745–9.
85 D'Agostino RS, Miller DC, Stinson EB *et al.* Valve replacement in patients with native valve endocarditis: what really determines operative outcome? Ann Thorac Surg 1985;40:429–38.
86 John MD, Hibberd PL, Karchmer AW, Sleeper LA, Calderwood SB. *Staphylococcus aureus* prosthetic valve endocarditis: optimal

management and risk factors for death. Clin Infect Dis 1998; 26:1302–9.

87 Mullany CJ, McIsaacs AI, Rowe MH, Hale GS. The surgical treatment of infective endocarditis. World J Surg 1989;13:132–6; discussion 136.

88 Wilson R, Hamburger M. Fifteen years' experience with staphylococcus septicemia in a large city hospital: analysis of fifty-five cases in the Cincinnati General Hospital 1940 to 1954. Am J Med 1957;22:437–57.

89 Rosen AB, Fowler VG Jr, Corey GR *et al.* Cost-effectiveness of transesophageal echocardiography to determine the duration of therapy for intravascular catheter-associated *Staphylococcus aureus* bacteremia. Ann Intern Med 1999;130:810–20.

90 Nannini EC, Singh KV, Murray BE. Relapse of type A beta-lactamase-producing *Staphylococcus aureus* native valve endocarditis during cefazolin therapy: revisiting the issue. Clin Infect Dis 2003;37:1194–8.

91 Stryjewski ME, Szczech LA, Benjamin DK Jr *et al.* Use of vancomycin or first-generation cephalosporins for the treatment of hemodialysis-dependent patients with methicillin-susceptible *Staphylococcus aureus* bacteremia. Clin Infect Dis 2007;44:190–6.

92 Levine DP, Fromm BS, Reddy BR. Slow response to vancomycin or vancomycin plus rifampin in methicillin-resistant *Staphylococcus aureus* endocarditis. Ann Intern Med 1991;115:674–80.

93 Siegman-Igra Y, Reich P, Orni-Wasserlauf R, Schwartz D, Giladi M. The role of vancomycin in the persistence or recurrence of *Staphylococcus aureus* bacteraemia. Scand J Infect Dis 2005;37:572–8.

94 Sakoulas G, Moise-Broder PA, Schentag J, Forrest A, Moellering RC Jr, Eliopoulos GM. Relationship of MIC and bactericidal activity to efficacy of vancomycin for treatment of methicillin-resistant *Staphylococcus aureus* bacteremia. J Clin Microbiol 2004;42:2398–402.

95 Moise PA, Schentag JJ. Vancomycin treatment failures in *Staphylococcus aureus* lower respiratory tract infections. Int J Antimicrob Agents 2000;16(suppl 1):S31–S34.

96 Hidayat LK, Hsu DI, Quist R, Shriner KA, Wong-Beringer A. High-dose vancomycin therapy for methicillin-resistant *Staphylococcus aureus* infections: efficacy and toxicity. Arch Intern Med 2006;166:2138–44.

97 Maclayton DO, Suda KJ, Coval KA, York CB, Garey KW. Case-control study of the relationship between MRSA bacteremia with a vancomycin MIC of 2 microg/mL and risk factors, costs, and outcomes in inpatients undergoing hemodialysis. Clin Ther 2006;28:1208–16.

98 Soriano A, Marco F, Martinez JA *et al.* Influence of vancomycin minimum inhibitory concentration on the treatment of methicillin-resistant *Staphylococcus aureus* bacteremia. Clin Infect Dis 2008;46:193–200.

99 Lodise TP, Miller CD, Graves J *et al.* Predictors of high vancomycin MIC values among patients with methicillin-resistant *Staphylococcus aureus* bacteraemia. J Antimicrob Chemother 2008;62:1138–41.

100 Jeffres MN, Isakow W, Doherty JA *et al.* Predictors of mortality for methicillin-resistant *Staphylococcus aureus* health-care-associated pneumonia: specific evaluation of vancomycin pharmacokinetic indices. Chest 2006;130:947–55.

101 Simon GL, Smith RH, Sande MA. Emergence of rifampin-resistant strains of *Staphylococcus aureus* during combination therapy with vancomycin and rifampin: a report of two cases. Rev Infect Dis 1983;5(suppl 3):S507–S508.

102 Abrams B, Sklaver A, Hoffman T, Greenman R. Single or combination therapy of staphylococcal endocarditis in intravenous drug abusers. Ann Intern Med 1979;90:789–91.

103 Korzeniowski O, Sande MA. Combination antimicrobial therapy for *Staphylococcus aureus* endocarditis in patients addicted to parenteral drugs and in nonaddicts: a prospective study. Ann Intern Med 1982;97:496–503.

104 Fowler VG Jr, Boucher HW, Corey GR *et al.* Daptomycin versus standard therapy for bacteremia and endocarditis caused by *Staphylococcus aureus*. N Engl J Med 2006;355:653–65.

105 Cui L, Tominaga E, Neoh HM, Hiramatsu K. Correlation between reduced daptomycin susceptibility and vancomycin resistance in vancomycin-intermediate *Staphylococcus aureus*. Antimicrob Agents Chemother 2006;50:1079–82.

106 Mwangi MM, Wu SW, Zhou Y *et al.* Tracking the in vivo evolution of multidrug resistance in *Staphylococcus aureus* by whole-genome sequencing. Proc Natl Acad Sci USA 2007;104:9451–6.

107 Patel JB, Jevitt LA, Hageman J, McDonald LC, Tenover FC. An association between reduced susceptibility to daptomycin and reduced susceptibility to vancomycin in *Staphylococcus aureus*. Clin Infect Dis 2006;42:1652–3.

108 Sakoulas G, Alder J, Thauvin-Eliopoulos C, Moellering RC Jr, Eliopoulos GM. Induction of daptomycin heterogeneous susceptibility in *Staphylococcus aureus* by exposure to vancomycin. Antimicrob Agents Chemother 2006;50:1581–5.

109 Silverman JA, Mortin LI, Vanpraagh AD, Li T, Alder J. Inhibition of daptomycin by pulmonary surfactant: in vitro modeling and clinical impact. J Infect Dis 2005;191:2149–52.

110 Woods CW, Cheng AC, Fowler VG Jr *et al.* Endocarditis caused by *Staphylococcus aureus* with reduced susceptibility to vancomycin. Clin Infect Dis 2004;38:1188–91.

111 Ben Mansour EH, Jacob E, Monchi M *et al.* Occurrence of MRSA endocarditis during linezolid treatment. Eur J Clin Microbiol Infect Dis 2003;22:372–3.

112 Corne P, Marchandin H, Macia JC, Jonquet O. Treatment failure of methicillin-resistant *Staphylococcus aureus* endocarditis with linezolid. Scand J Infect Dis 2005;37:946–9.

113 Ruiz ME, Guerrero IC, Tuazon CU. Endocarditis caused by methicillin-resistant *Staphylococcus aureus*: treatment failure with linezolid. Clin Infect Dis 2002;35:1018–20.

114 Food and Drug Administration. Safety alerts for drugs, biologics, medical devices, and dietary supplements. 2007. http://www.fda.gov/medwatch/safety/2007/safety07.htm#Zyvox. Last accessed May 23, 2009.

115 Drew RH, Perfect JR, Srinath L, Kurkimilis E, Dowzicky M, Talbot GH. Treatment of methicillin-resistant *Staphylococcus aureus* infections with quinupristin–dalfopristin in patients intolerant of or failing prior therapy. For the Synercid Emergency-Use Study Group. J Antimicrob Chemother 2000;46:775–84.

116 Eliopoulos GM, Wennersten CB. Antimicrobial activity of quinupristin–dalfopristin combined with other antibiotics against vancomycin-resistant enterococci. Antimicrob Agents Chemother 2002;46:1319–24.

117 Markowitz N, Quinn EL, Saravolatz LD. Trimethoprim–sulfamethoxazole compared with vancomycin for the treatment of *Staphylococcus aureus* infection. Ann Intern Med 1992; 117:390–8.

118 Kaka AS, Rueda AM, Shelburne SA III, Hulten K, Hamill RJ, Musher DM. Bactericidal activity of orally available agents against methicillin-resistant *Staphylococcus aureus*. J Antimicrob Chemother 2006;58:680–3.

119 Deng MC, Loebe M, El-Banayosy A *et al*. Mechanical circulatory support for advanced heart failure: effect of patient selection on outcome. Circulation 2001;103:231–7.

120 Keyser DL, Biller J, Coffman TT, Adams HP Jr. Neurologic complications of late prosthetic valve endocarditis. Stroke 1990;21:472–5.

121 Masur H, Johnson WD Jr. Prosthetic valve endocarditis. J Thorac Cardiovasc Surg 1980;80:31–7.

122 Tornos P, Sanz E, Permanyer-Miralda G, Almirante B, Planes AM, Soler-Soler J. Late prosthetic valve endocarditis. Immediate and long-term prognosis. Chest 1992;101:37–41.

123 Baddour LM, Bettmann MA, Bolger AF *et al*. Nonvalvular cardiovascular device-related infections. Circulation 2003;108: 2015–31.

124 Chua JD, Wilkoff BL, Lee I, Juratli N, Longworth DL, Gordon SM. Diagnosis and management of infections involving implantable electrophysiologic cardiac devices. Ann Intern Med 2000;133: 604–8.

125 Priest DH, Peacock JE Jr. Hematogenous vertebral osteomyelitis due to *Staphylococcus aureus* in the adult: clinical features and therapeutic outcomes. South Med J 2005;98:854–62.

126 Lamas C, Boia M, Eykyn SJ. Osteoarticular infections complicating infective endocarditis: a study of 30 cases between 1969 and 2002 in a tertiary referral centre. Scand J Infect Dis 2006;38: 433–40.

127 Dubost JJ, Soubrier M, Sauvezie B. Pyogenic arthritis in adults. Joint Bone Spine 2000;67:11–21.

128 Ross JJ, Hu LT. Septic arthritis of the pubic symphysis: review of 100 cases. Medicine (Baltimore) 2003;82:340–5.

129 Levine DP, Crane LR, Zervos MJ. Bacteremia in narcotic addicts at the Detroit Medical Center. II. Infectious endocarditis: a prospective comparative study. Rev Infect Dis 1986;8:374–96.

130 Crowley AL, Peterson GE, Benjamin DK Jr *et al*. Venous thrombosis in patients with short- and long-term central venous catheter-associated *Staphylococcus aureus* bacteremia. Crit Care Med 2008;36:385–90.

131 Jernigan JA, Farr BM. Short-course therapy of catheter-related *Staphylococcus aureus* bacteremia: a meta-analysis. *Ann Intern Med* 1993;119:304–11.

Chapter 17
Surgical-site Infections and Surgical Prophylaxis

Deverick J. Anderson and Keith S. Kaye
Duke University Medical Center, Durham, North Carolina, USA

Introduction

Significant advances have been made in the field of surgery and infection control over the past 150–200 years. Improved knowledge regarding the pathophysiology of postsurgical infection has led to numerous improvements in infection prevention. As medicine has advanced, however, new infection risks have been introduced. Over the past 50 years, the frequency of surgical procedures has increased, procedures have become more invasive, a greater proportion of operative procedures include insertion of foreign objects, and procedures are performed on an increasingly morbid patient population. As a result, surgical-site infections (SSIs), particularly those caused by *Staphylococcus aureus*, remain a leading cause of morbidity and mortality in modern healthcare. Recently, improvements in surgical care have been reached through the implementation of performance processes and measures. Several nationwide quality improvement initiatives have introduced evidence-based performance measures specifically targeting infection prevention in patients undergoing surgical procedures.

Epidemiology and pathogenesis

Epidemiology

SSIs are a devastating and common complication of hospitalization, occurring in 2–5% of patients undergoing surgery in the USA [1]. Given the high number of surgical procedures performed in the USA, this translates into 300 000–500 000 SSIs each year [2]. SSI is the second most common type of healthcare-associated infection [3].

Staphylococcus aureus is the most common cause of SSI. It is the primary pathogen in 20% of SSIs among hospitals that report to the Centers for Disease Control and Prevention (CDC) (Table 17.1) [4] and causes as many as 37% of SSIs that occur in community hospitals [5]. The prevalence of SSIs due to *S. aureus* has increased over the past few decades. From 1992 to 2002, the proportion of SSIs caused by *S. aureus* increased from 16.6 to 30.9% among patients undergoing coronary artery bypass grafting, cholecystectomy, colectomy, and total hip replacement at hospitals reporting SSI data to the CDC [6]. The proportion of *S. aureus* SSIs caused by methicillin-resistant *S. aureus* (MRSA) increased from 9 to 49% during 1992–2002 [6]. MRSA has also emerged as the single most commonly isolated organism from surgical wounds in community hospitals [5].

Table 17.1 The 10 most common pathogens in surgical-site infections among hospitals that report to the CDC [4,9].

Pathogen	Infections (%)
Staphylococcus aureus	20
Coagulase-negative staphylococci	14
Enterococci	12
Pseudomonas aeruginosa	8
Escherichia coli	8
Enterobacter species	7
Proteus mirabilis	3
Streptococci	3
Klebsiella pneumoniae	3
Candida albicans	2

Pathogenesis

The likelihood that an SSI will occur is a complex relationship between microbial characteristics, patient characteristics, and surgical characteristics (e.g., introduction of foreign material, amount of damage to tissues).

Microbial characteristics

Even with expert technique and technology, microbial contamination of surgical sites is universal. The period of greatest risk for infection is from the time of incision to the time of wound closure [7]. Pathogens that lead to SSI typically arise from the patient's endogenous flora and less commonly are acquired exogenously from the operating room environment.

Staphylococci in Human Disease, 2nd edition. Edited by Kent B. Crossley, Kimberly K. Jefferson, Gordon Archer, Vance G. Fowler, Jr.
 ISBN 978-14051-6332-3.

Endogenous contamination

Gram-positive cocci from a patient's endogenous flora at or near the site of surgery remain the leading cause of SSI [8]. More specifically, *S. aureus*, coagulase-negative staphylococci, and enterococci are the three organisms most commonly isolated from SSI and account for close to 50% of all isolates [9]. Gram-negative bacilli, including *Escherichia coli*, *Pseudomonas aeruginosa*, *Enterobacter* species, *Proteus mirabilis*, and *Klebsiella pneumoniae*, account for 30% of isolates. When surgery involves the respiratory, gastrointestinal, or genitourinary tracts, infections may be polymicrobial and may include both aerobic and anaerobic organisms. Of the bacterial skin flora, 20% reside in skin appendages such as sebaceous glands, hair follicles, and sweat glands [10]. Thus, modern methods of preoperative and perioperative antisepsis can reduce but not eliminate contamination of the surgical site by endogenous skin flora of the surgical patient.

Inoculation of the surgical site by endogenous flora from remote sites on the patient has also been proven to occur. Ingenious experiments using human albumin microspheres as tracer particles have revealed that all surgical wounds are contaminated with particles (skin squames) from endogenous sites that are remote and distant in location relative to the wound [11]. Finally, postsurgical inoculation of the surgical site secondary to a remote focus of infection (such as *S. aureus* pneumonia) is an infrequent cause of SSI [12].

Exogenous contamination

Exogenous sources of contamination, including colonized or infected surgical personnel, the operating room environment, and surgical instruments, are occasionally implicated in the pathogenesis of SSI. Infections due to exogenous sources most commonly occur sporadically, but several exogenous point-source outbreaks have been reported. For example, surgical personnel carriage of group A β-hemolytic streptococci has been implicated in outbreaks of SSI [13–17]. Additionally, unusual environmental pathogens are occasionally implicated in SSI.

Surgical personnel colonized with *S. aureus* are occasionally blamed for SSIs due to *S. aureus*. The association of colonized surgical personnel and outbreaks of SSI due to *S. aureus* was first described in 1939. Devenish *et al.* [18] described two surgeons with *S. aureus* colonization in the nares. One of the two surgeons had much higher rates of SSI and was subsequently found to have *S. aureus* colonization on his hands and frequent punctures in his gloves. Another outbreak of SSI due to *S. aureus* was described in children undergoing cardiothoracic surgery. Three of four infection strains were identical by pulsed-field gel electropheresis. None of the children were colonized with the epidemic strain, but approximately 25% of operating room personnel were colonized [19]. Finally, another outbreak of SSI due to *S. aureus* in patients admitted to a surgical intensive care unit described a "cloud person" as an exogenous disseminator of *S. aureus* [20]. One resident who had a persistent upper respiratory tract infection during the epidemic was ultimately found to be colonized with the epidemic strain. Further experimentation revealed that rhinoviral infection led to a large increase in the number of colony-forming units of *S. aureus* released into the air by the individual [20]. Although exogenous *S. aureus* sources can cause SSI, this occurs rarely as endogenous sources of *S. aureus* are much more common.

Burden of inoculation

While many other factors contribute to the risk of surgical site infection, the burden of pathogens inoculated into a surgical wound remains one of the most well-understood and accepted risk factors. The greater the degree of surgical wound contamination, the higher the risk for infection. Even in the setting of appropriate antimicrobial prophylaxis, the risk of SSI increases as total bacterial burden in the surgical wound increases [21]. Generally, wound contamination with greater than 10^5 microorganisms is required to cause SSI [22].

When foreign bodies are present, the bacterial inoculum required to cause SSI is much lower [23]. For example, human volunteer studies involving foreign bodies have demonstrated that the presence of surgical sutures decreases the required inoculum from 10^6 to 10^2 organisms [24]. Other models have demonstrated that as few as 10 cfu of *S. aureus* in the presence of polytetrafluoroethylene vascular grafts [25] or 1 cfu of *S. aureus* in the proximity of dextran beads can cause SSI [26].

Virulence factors of S. aureus

Staphylococcus aureus has intrinsic virulence factors that greatly enhance its ability to cause infection. For example, *S. aureus* possesses MSCRAMMs (microbial surface components recognizing adhesive matrix molecules) that allow improved adhesion to collagen, fibrin, fibronectin, and other extracellular matrix proteins [26,27]. Also *S. aureus* has the ability to produce a glycocalyx-rich biofilm that shields the organism from the immune system and most antimicrobial agents [28]. Once firmly entrenched in the wound, *S. aureus* produces exotoxins that lead to host tissue damage [29], interfere with leukocyte phagocytosis [30], and alter cellular metabolism [31].

Antimicrobial resistance sometimes plays an important role in SSI pathogenesis. Some strains of *S. aureus* harbor the type A variant of staphylococcal β-lactamase, which degrades less stable cephalosporins such as cefazolin, an agent commonly used for perioperative antimicrobial prophylaxis [32]. Animal models have demonstrated that the number of colony-forming units required to cause SSI is significantly smaller in strains that harbor the type A β-lactamase compared with non-β-lactamase-producing strains of *S. aureus* [33].

Local and systemic host defense mechanisms

Neutrophils and neutrophil-mediated killing by reactive oxygen intermediates are believed to be the most important component of host defense against SSI [34]. Unfortunately, the process of surgery itself impairs neutrophil function, decreases levels of circulating HLA-DR antigens [35], and decreases T-cell proliferation and response [36]. For example, the microbicidal activity of neutrophils harvested after surgery is 25% less than neutrophils harvested prior to surgery, and this activity remains reduced for 9 days after surgery [37]. Neutrophils also exhibit reduced chemotaxis and diminished superoxide production in the setting of perioperative hypothermia [38]. Thus, the process of surgery itself acts as an immunosuppressant that leads to a higher risk of infection due to *S. aureus* and other pathogens.

Damaged tissue

Damaged and devitalized tissue may also promote SSI by providing an environment for potential pathogens to elude host defense mechanisms [34]. *In vitro* models suggest that thermally damaged tissue leads to activation and fixation of complement and subsequent inhibition of neutrophil activity [39].

Risk factors

Most risk factors for SSI pertain to all pathogens and are not specific for *S. aureus*. Risk factors for SSI are typically separated into patient-related (preoperative), procedure-related (perioperative), and postoperative categories (Table 17.2).

Table 17.2 Risk factors for, and current recommendations to decrease, the risk of surgical-site infection.

Risk factor	Recommendation
Intrinsic, patient-related (preoperative)	
Unmodifiable	
Age	No formal recommendation: relationship to increased risk of SSI may be secondary to comorbidities or immunosenescence [42,44,48]
Modifiable	
Glucose control, diabetes	Control serum blood glucose levels [188]
Obesity	Increase dosing of perioperative antimicrobial agent for morbidly obese patients [144]
Smoking cessation	Encourage smoking cessation within 30 days of procedure [188]
Immunosuppressive medications	No formal recommendation [188]; in general, avoid immunosuppressive medications in perioperative period if possible
Nutrition	Do not delay surgery to enhance nutritional support [188]
Remote sites of infection	Identify and treat all remote infections prior to elective procedures [188]
Preoperative hospitalization	Keep preoperative stay as short as possible [188]
Extrinsic, procedure-related (perioperative)	
Preparation of patient	
Hair removal	Do not remove unless presence of hair will interfere with the operation [188]; if hair removal is necessary, remove by clipping and do not shave
Skin preparation	Wash and clean skin around incision site [188]
Preoperative shower	Bathe with antiseptic agent the night before the procedure [188]
Chlorhexidine nasal and oropharyngeal rinse	No formal recommendation in most recent guidelines [189]; recent randomized controlled trial of cardiac surgeries showed decreased incidence of postoperative nosocomial infections [132]
Surgical scrub (surgeon hands and forearms)	Use appropriate antiseptic agent to perform 2–5 min preoperative surgical scrub [188]
Incision site	Use appropriate antiseptic agent [188]
Antimicrobial prophylaxis	Administer only when indicated [188]
Timing	Administer within 1 hour of incision to maximize tissue concentration [188]
Choice	Select appropriate agents based on surgical procedure, most common pathogens causing SSI for a specific procedure, and published recommendations [188]
Duration of therapy	Stop agent within 24 hours after the procedure [188]
Surgeon skill/technique	Handle tissue carefully and eradicate dead space [188]
Incision time	No formal recommendation in most recent guidelines [188]; minimize as much as possible [80]
Maintain oxygenation with supplemental O_2	No formal recommendation in most recent guidelines [188]: randomized controlled trials have reported conflicting results in colorectal procedures [105,106,189]
Maintain normothermia	Avoid hypothermia in surgical patients whenever possible by actively warming the patient to > 36°C, particularly in colorectal surgery [102]
Operating room characteristics	
Ventilation	Follow American Institute of Architects' recommendations [188]
Traffic	Minimize traffic [188]
Environmental surfaces	Use an EPA-approved hospital disinfectant to clean visibly soiled or contaminated surfaces and equipment [188]

Preoperative risk factors

Intrinsic patient-related risk factors

Investigators have reported contradictory results about the relationship between increasing age and risk of SSI. Several investigators have concluded that increasing age is associated with a greater risk of all types of postoperative infections; in some of these studies, increasing age was associated with an increased risk of development of SSI [40–44]. In other studies, however, advanced age was associated with a decreased risk of SSI [45–47]. In a recent cohort study of over 144 000 patients, increasing age independently predicted an increased risk of SSI until age 65 years, but above 65 years increasing age independently predicted a decreased risk of SSI [48]. The authors hypothesized that decreased risk of SSI in patients older than 65 years of age might represent surgical patient selection bias or a "hardy survivor" effect.

Lack of independence is a strong predictor of SSI specifically due to MRSA. A recent study of 150 patients with SSI caused by MRSA demonstrated that patients who required assistance with activities of daily living were at twofold to fourfold higher risk of developing SSI caused by MRSA than were either uninfected patients or patients with SSI caused by methicillin-sensitive *S. aureus* (MSSA) [49]. Of note, this association was independent of age.

Modifiable patient-related risk factors

Diabetes mellitus

Diabetes and hyperglycemia are important risk factors for SSI [50–55]. Elevated serum glucose in both the preoperative and postoperative periods has been associated with increased risk of SSI [54,55].

Obesity

Obesity is another well-established risk factor for SSI. Several investigators have shown that obesity leads to a twofold to sixfold increased rate of SSI compared with that in nonobese patients [53,56–58]. Possible explanations for increased rates of SSI among obese patients include decreased tissue oxygenation [59], poor wound closure, and/or inadequate dosing of perioperative antimicrobial prophylaxis.

Smoking/tobacco use

Cigarette smoking and tobacco use prior to a surgical procedure increase the risk of SSI by twofold to 16-fold compared with nonsmokers [58,60,61]. Smoking causes peripheral tissue hypoxia [62,63], decreased collagen synthesis [64], and interferes with the oxidative killing mechanisms of host neutrophils [65,66].

Nutrition

Malnutrition, defined in different studies as either weight loss prior to surgery or low serum albumin, has been associated with an increased risk of SSI in some [41,67–70] but not all [71] procedures. Additionally, studies concerning the utility of preoperative, perioperative, or postoperative total parenteral nutrition or total enteral nutrition have provided inconsistent and generally unfavorable results [72–74].

Disinfection of the patient

Preoperative showering with agents such as chlorhexidine has been shown to reduce bacterial colonization of the skin, but this has not consistently translated into decreased rates of SSI [75,76]. Colonization with *S. aureus* is strongly associated with increased risk of SSI [77,78], but studies examining the utility of *S. aureus* nasal decolonization with antimicrobial agents (e.g., mupirocin) have been inconsistent (see sections on prevention and treatment below).

Extrinsic procedure-related perioperative risk factors

Wound class

The National Research Council created a classification that is commonly used to predict the risk of SSI based on the level of perioperative contamination [79]. Surgical wounds are classified as clean, clean-contaminated, contaminated, or dirty and infected (Table 17.3). Wound class primarily reflects the degree of endogenous bacterial contamination (skin or viscera) but, in practice, remains only a moderate predictor of risk of infection [80]. When appropriate preoperative antibiotics are administered, the risk of infection is 0.8% for clean wounds, 1.3% for clean-contaminated wounds, and 10.2% for contaminated wounds [81].

Table 17.3 Surgical-site classification scheme as developed by the National Research Council. (Adapted from Berard & Gandon [79] with permission.)

Clean surgical sites
No inflammation is encountered
Respiratory, alimentary, and genitourinary tracts are not entered
If drainage is necessary, closed drainage is used
Clean-contaminated surgical sites
Respiratory, alimentary, or genitourinary tract is entered under controlled conditions without unusual contamination
Contaminated surgical sites
Open, fresh accidental wounds or operations with major breaks in usual sterile technique or gross spillage from the gastrointestinal tract
Entry into the genitourinary tract with infected urine or biliary tract with infected bile
Acute nonpurulent inflammation is encountered
Dirty and infected surgical sites
Old traumatic wounds with retained devitalized tissue, foreign bodies, or fecal contamination
Perforated viscus or pus is encountered

Length of surgery

Increased operative duration is a risk factor for SSI [42,79,82–84]. According to the SENIC study, the risk of SSI increases dramatically after 2 hours of operative time [80]. In general, risk of SSI doubles with each additional hour of operative time. For example, in a recent multicenter prospective cohort study of SSI following abdominal surgery in 4700 patients, rates of postoperative infection were 6.3% for procedures lasting 1 hour, 12.2% for procedures lasting 1–2 hours, and 27.7% for procedures lasting longer than 2 hours [42]. The National Nosocomial Infection Surveillance (NNIS) System publishes operation-specific cut-points from data obtained from hospitals that report to the CDC. Procedures that last longer than the 75th percentile of the duration of the specific procedure are at higher risk for SSI [85]. In fact, surgical procedures lasting longer than the 75th percentile are specifically at higher risk for SSI due to MRSA [86].

Surgical technique

Despite the lack of controlled data, there is consensus among authorities that the single most important factor for prevention of SSI is good surgical technique [7,34,87]. When discussing SSI prevention, experts often describe the importance of maintaining hemostasis while preserving blood flow and tissue oxygenation, preventing hypothermia, carefully handling tissues, removing necrotic or damaged tissue, and eradicating dead space.

Hair removal

Compared with depilatory techniques or no hair removal, preoperative shaving leads to increased rates of SSI by causing microscopic abrasions of the skin that become foci for bacterial growth [82,88,89]. In fact, some studies suggest that any form of hair removal (shaving, depilatory, or clipping) leads to increased rates of SSI and should thus be avoided when possible [88,90,91]. Thus current recommendations state that hair should not be removed from the surgical site unless the hair will interfere with the procedure [9]. If hair removal is necessary, the hair should be removed with electric clippers immediately prior to surgery.

Perioperative and postoperative hyperglycemia

Hyperglycemia leads to decreased host immune responses by impairing the function of neutrophils and mononuclear phagocytes. Diabetes mellitus and postoperative hyperglycemia are both clearly associated with increased risk of SSI [54,92]. In a retrospective study of 8910 patients undergoing cardiac surgery, rates of SSI decreased substantially after implementing an intensive intravenous insulin regimen to maintain postoperative glucose below 200 mg/dL for the first 48 hours after surgery [54].

Hypothermia

Surgical patients may become hypothermic, defined as a core body temperature below 36°C, as a result of exposure to cold ambient temperatures in the operating room, anesthesia, changes in body heat distribution, or intentionally induced hypothermia such as during some cardiac surgeries [93–95]. Hypothermia increases the risk of SSI through thermoregulatory vasoconstriction and impaired immunity. Vasoconstriction is universal in patients with hypothermia [96] and leads to decreased partial pressure of oxygen in tissues [97], decreased microbial killing [98], impaired chemotaxis and phagocytosis by granulocytes, and decreased motility of macrophages [99,100]. Randomized controlled trials of patients undergoing elective hernia repair, varicose vein surgery, breast surgery, or colon surgery have demonstrated that patients who received aggressive warming therapy (either a warming blanket prior to surgery or 30 min of preoperative local warming to the surgical site) had lower rates of SSI than controls [101,102].

Hypoxia

In vitro studies, animal studies, and observational human studies support the value of increased tissue oxygen tension as an important factor in decreasing the risk of SSI [63,65,98,103,104]. Thus far, three randomized clinical trials have compared $F\text{IO}_2$ of 80% to $F\text{IO}_2$ of 30–35% during the intraoperative and postoperative periods; two of these studies showed a significant decrease in the rate of SSI [105,106], while the third actually showed a significant increase in the rate of SSI. Of note, both studies in favor of supplemental oxygen included patients who underwent colorectal surgery, while the study reporting adverse effects of supplemental oxygen included all types of patients. When the results of the three studies are pooled, the rate of SSI decreases from 15.2% in patients who received 30–35% $F\text{IO}_2$ to 11.5% in patients who received 80% $F\text{IO}_2$ during surgery (3.7% absolute risk reduction; $P = 0.10$) [107].

Operating room characteristics

The degree of microbial contamination of the operating room air is directly proportional to the number of people in the room [108]. Although hands and arms are scrubbed and covered during surgery, other body parts, hair, and skin remain exposed. In fact, tracer particle experiments have demonstrated that aerosolized droplets from the hair, skin, and oropharynx of operating room personnel, including ancillary staff, are universally transported to the surgical field [11,109,110]. Traffic in and out of the operating room should be limited, and operating room doors should be kept closed throughout procedures except as needed for passage of equipment, necessary personnel, and the patient [9].

Postoperative risk factors

Several risk factors that occur during the perioperative period (e.g., glucose control, oxygenation, hypothermia) remain important during the immediate postoperative period. Two additional variables that are present exclusively in the postoperative period are wound care and blood transfusions.

Postoperative wound care is determined by the technique used for closure of the surgical site. The majority of wounds are closed primarily (i.e., skin edges are approximated with sutures or staples) and these wounds should be kept clean by covering with a sterile dressing for 24–48 hours after surgery [111]. If a wound is left open to heal by secondary intent, the wound should be packed with sterile gauze. In general, the exact impact of postoperative wound care on the risk of SSI is unknown. Further studies are needed to determine appropriate duration of wound care and type of materials. However, a recent study with a quasi-experimental design concluded that antimicrobial-impregnated dressings decreased the risk of SSI and particularly SSI due to MRSA [112].

A metaanalysis of 20 studies of the associated risk of SSI following receipt of blood products demonstrated that patients who received even a single unit of blood in the immediate postoperative period were at increased risk for SSI [odds ratio (OR) 3.45] [113]. Furthermore, the risk of SSI increases as the total volume of transfusion increases [114].

Prevention

An important component of improving outcomes of surgical patients is addressing all modifiable risk factors for SSI during the perioperative period. However, few interventions are supported by data from randomized controlled trials and even less data are available regarding risk factor modifications that specifically prevent SSI due to *S. aureus*. Table 17.2 summarizes important risk factors and current guidelines for addressing each risk factor in an effort to decrease the risk of SSI.

Antiseptic agents to decrease microbial burden: preparation of the patient and the surgical team

Showering or bathing with an antiseptic agent such as chlorhexidine, povidone-iodine, or triclorcarban-medicated soap decreases the number of endogenous microbial flora on the skin by as much as twofold [115,116]. However, despite the proven reduction in preoperative microbial burden, this intervention has not yet been clearly demonstrated to lower rates of SSI in clinical trials [76,117,118].

Antiseptic agents commonly used to prepare the patient's skin in the operating room include alcohol-containing solutions, chlorhexidine gluconate, and povidone-iodine, all of which have activity against *S. aureus*. Advantages of alcohol-containing solutions include availability, overall level of experience and track record with use of these agents for patient preparation, low cost, and effectiveness [119]. However, two major disadvantages include the flammability of alcohol agents and the potential ineffectiveness of alcohol in eliminating bacterial and fungal spores [119,120].

Both chlorhexidine gluconate and povidone-iodine are effective antiseptics with broad spectra of antimicrobial activity and are good alternatives to alcohol-containing solutions. Chlorhexidine gluconate reduces endogenous flora to a greater extent and has greater residual activity after one application than povidone-iodine [119,121–123]. The relative efficacy of these agents specifically against *S. aureus* has not been formally studied.

Several agents are available for antiseptic surgical hand scrubbing. In many European countries, alcohol-containing solutions are the gold standard, while in the USA povidone-iodine and chlorhexidine gluconate are the agents of choice [124–126]. No clinical trials have evaluated the impact of antiseptic agent choice on the risk of SSI. The optimum duration of presurgical scrubbing is not known, but studies suggest that 2–5 min is as effective as 10 min [127–129]. Typically, the first scrub of the day should include a thorough cleansing underneath fingernails. Fingernails should be kept short and artificial fingernails should not be worn by any healthcare personnel [130,131].

Decolonization of *S. aureus* carriage

Colonization with *S. aureus* is strongly associated with increased risk of SSI due to *S. aureus* [77,78]. Studies examining the utility of preoperative *S. aureus* nasal decolonization with antimicrobial agents have produced inconsistent results. A recent randomized controlled trial examined the utility of oral and nasal rinses with chlorhexidine gluconate (0.12%) prior to cardiothoracic surgery for the prevention of postoperative nosocomial infections [132]. The frequency of postoperative pneumonias and number of postoperative bacteremias were both decreased in the chlorhexidine-treated group. While the overall number of SSIs was not different in the two groups, the number of deep SSIs was significantly decreased in the chlorhexidine-treated group (1.9% vs. 5.2%; $P = 0.002$). Given the proven benefit, low toxicity, and lack of emerging resistance in long-term clinical studies [133], preoperative treatment with chlorhexidine represents a promising intervention for the prevention of SSIs, particularly among cardiothoracic surgery patients.

Studies examining the efficacy of decolonization of *S. aureus* with mupirocin, a topical antibiotic, have generally shown that it is effective at decolonization, but the impact on SSI remains unclear. One study reported that, regardless of *S. aureus* carrier status, the preoperative application of mupirocin to the nares of operative patients led to a 67% decrease in rate of SSI compared with historical controls following cardiothoracic surgery (from 7.3% to 2.8%) [134]. More recently, an analysis of 854 consecutive cardiothoracic patients who received intranasal mupirocin compared with 992 consecutive cardiothoracic patients who did not receive intranasal mupirocin showed that the overall rate of SSI was lower in the mupirocin-treated group (0.9% vs. 2.7%; $P = 0.005$) [133]. However, these findings were not fully corroborated in a recent double-blind randomized controlled trial in which 1933 surgical patients randomized to receive preoperative mupirocin were compared with 1931 randomized to placebo [135]. Treatment with mupirocin led to lower rates of *S. aureus* colonization and lower rates of overall postoperative nosocomial infections due to *S. aureus* (3.8% vs. 7.6%; $P = 0.02$) but did not lead to a significant decrease in the rate of SSI due to *S. aureus* (3.6% vs. 5.8%; OR 2.9, 95% CI 0.8–3.4) [135].

Unfortunately, *S. aureus* resistance to mupirocin has rapidly emerged in some institutions [136,137]. The emergence of mupirocin resistance is concerning and can negate the efficacy of preoperative decolonization. The efficacy and practical use of mupirocin for prevention of SSI due to *S. aureus* remains controversial and unresolved.

Perioperative antimicrobial prophylaxis

The goal of surgical antimicrobial prophylaxis is to reduce the concentration of potential pathogens at or in close proximity to the surgical incision. The appropriate use of perioperative antimicrobial prophylaxis is a well-proven intervention to reduce the risk of SSI in elective procedures [9,21,138]. Four principles override the use of prophylactic antimicrobial use.

1 Use antimicrobial prophylaxis for all elective operations that require entry into a hollow viscus (i.e., clean-contaminated and contaminated procedures), operations that involve insertion of an intravascular prosthetic device or prosthetic joint, or operations in which an SSI would pose catastrophic risk (e.g., clean surgery where bone is incised such as a craniotomy) [34,139–141].

2 Use antimicrobial agents that are safe, cost-effective, and bactericidal against expected pathogens for specific surgical procedures [9].

3 Time the infusion so that a bactericidal concentration of the agent is present in tissue and serum at the time of incision [138].

4 Maintain therapeutic levels of the agent in tissue and serum throughout the entire operation [139,142,143].

Table 17.4 summarizes surgical procedures for which antimicrobial prophylaxis is indicated, typical pathogens that cause SSI, and recommended doses of antimicrobial agents. Of note, larger doses of antimicrobial agents are required to achieve effective drug levels in obese patients [144]. Agents recommended for antimicrobial prophylaxis typically have time-dependent bactericidal activity.

Administering antimicrobial prophylaxis shortly before incision reduces the rate of SSI [138]. The optimal administration time for maximizing drug concentration at incision typically occurs within 1–2 hours before surgery. For some agents such as cefazolin (1–2 g i.v.), the optimal administration time is within 30 min before incision [145]. The importance of appropriate timing of perioperative antimicrobial prophylaxis has been demonstrated in both animal and human studies. Guinea-pig model studies have demonstrated that antibiotics given shortly before or at the time of *S. aureus* intradermal inoculation led to a decrease in subsequent wound induration compared with antibiotics given 1, 2, and 4 hours after inoculation [146,147]. This finding was corroborated in a retrospective study of approximately 3000 patients undergoing inpatient elective clean or clean-contaminated procedures. The lowest rates of infection occurred in the group of patients who received antimicrobial prophylaxis within 1 hour before incision [138]. Rates of SSI increased linearly with increasing time prior to or after incision. If a procedure is expected to last several hours, additional agents should be infused intraoperatively [9]. For example, cefazolin should be re-infused if a procedure lasts longer than 3–4 hours.

Single-dose antimicrobial prophylaxis is equivalent to multiple perioperative doses for the prevention of SSI. A metaanalysis of over 40 studies comparing single doses of parenteral antimicrobials to placebo or multiple doses in hysterectomies, cesarean sections, colorectal procedures, gastric, biliary and transurethral operations and cardiothoracic procedures demonstrated that administration of multiple doses of antibiotics provided no benefit over a single dose [148]. A more recent systematic review of 28 prospective randomized studies comparing single versus multiple doses of perioperative antimicrobials also concluded that there was no additional benefit of more than a single prophylactic dose [142].

The routine use of vancomycin for antimicrobial prophylaxis is not currently recommended [149]. A recent metaanalysis of seven studies comparing glycopeptides to β-lactam antimicrobial prophylaxis prior to cardiothoracic surgery showed that there was no difference in rates of SSI between the two classes of antibiotics, supporting the view that β-lactam antibiotics should remain the agents of choice [150]. In particular, some experts are concerned that the widespread use of vancomycin for surgical prophylaxis may exacerbate the increasing rates of vancomycin-resistant enterococci [149]. Instead, the use of vancomycin should be reserved for specific clinical circumstances, such as during a proven outbreak of SSI due to MRSA, if there is a "high" prevalence of MRSA in the hospital (note that there is no specific incidence of MRSA defined as "high"), or for patients identified to be at increased risk for SSI due to MRSA (e.g., prior history of MRSA infection or colonization) [151]. When vancomycin is used, careful planning is necessary to allow for the longer infusion time required with this drug (typically 1–2 hours).

Quality improvement programs, process measures, and bundles to decrease the risk of SSI

Increased emphasis has been placed on measuring, implementing, and improving specific processes proven to

Table 17.4 Elective procedures for which antimicrobial prophylaxis is indicated, typical infecting organisms, and recommended antimicrobial agent. (Adapted from Mangram *et al.* [9] and Anon. [190].)

Procedure	Pathogen	Agent and dose[1]
Cardiac		
Prosthetic valve, coronary bypass graft, pacemaker placement, other	*S. aureus*, coagulase-negative staphylococci	Cefazolin 1–2 g i.v. or cefuroxime 1–2 g i.v. or vancomycin 1 g i.v.
Gastrointestinal		
High-risk[2] esophageal, gastric, duodenal	Enteric Gram-negative bacilli, streptococci, anaerobes	Cefazolin 1–2 g i.v.
High-risk[3] biliary	Enteric Gram-negative bacilli, anaerobes	Cefazolin 1–2 g i.v.
Colorectal, nonperforated appendectomy	Enteric Gram-negative bacilli, enterococci, anaerobes	Cefoxitin 1–2 g i.v. or cefotetan 1–2 g i.v. or cefazolin 1–2 g i.v. + metronidazole 0.5 g i.v.
Orthopedic		
Prosthetic joint replacement, internal fixation with hardware, trauma	*S. aureus*, coagulase-negative staphylococci, Gram-negative bacilli	Cefazolin 1–2 g i.v. or vancomycin 1 g i.v.
Thoracic (noncardiac)		
Lobectomy, pneumonectomy, other	*S. aureus*, coagulase-negative staphylococci, *Streptococcus pneumoniae*, Gram-negative bacilli	Cefazolin 1–2 g i.v. or cefuroxime 1–2 g i.v. or vancomycin 1 g i.v.
Vascular		
Arterial surgery involving prosthetic material, abdominal aorta or a groin incision, lower extremity amputation for ischemia	*S. aureus*, coagulase-negative staphylococci, Gram-negative bacilli, clostridia	Cefazolin 1–2 g i.v. or vancomycin 1 g i.v.
Obstetric and gynecological		
Hysterectomy, high-risk[4] cesarean section	Enteric Gram-negative bacilli, anaerobes, group B streptococci, enterococci	Cefazolin 1–2 g i.v. or cefoxitin 1–2 g i.v. or cefotetan 1–2 g i.v.
Genitourinary		
High-risk[5] procedures	Enteric Gram-negative bacilli, enterococci	Ciprofloxacin 400 mg i.v. or 500 mg p.o.
Neurosurgery		
Craniotomy	*S. aureus*, coagulase-negative staphylococci	Cefazolin 1–2 g i.v. or vancomycin 1 g i.v.
Head and neck		
Major procedures with incision through oropharyngeal mucosa	*S. aureus*, oropharyngeal anaerobes, streptococci	Clindamycin 600–900 mg i.v. + gentamicin 1.5 mg/kg i.v. or cefazolin 1–2 g i.v.
Ophthalmic		
Anterior segment resection, vitrectomy, other	*S. aureus*, coagulase-negative staphylococci, streptococci, Gram-negative bacilli	Multiple topical drops over 2–24 hours of gentamicin, tobramycin, ciprofloxacin, ofloxacin or cefazolin 100 mg subconjunctivally

[1] Note that although vancomycin is included as a recommended agent for some procedures, it should only be used for patients with proven β-lactam allergy or in hospitals with high endemic rates of methicillin-resistant *S. aureus*.
[2] High risk defined as obesity, esophageal obstruction, or decreased gastric motility.
[3] High risk defined as age > 70 years, obstructive jaundice, common duct stone, or acute cholecystitis.
[4] High risk defined as active labor or premature rupture of membranes.
[5] High risk defined as urine culture positive or unavailable, transrectal prostate biopsy, presence of urinary catheter prior to procedure.

prevent SSI. The Surgical Infection Prevention Project (SIP) [152–154], Surgical Care Improvement Project (SCIP) [152], and the Institute for Healthcare Improvement's 100K Lives and 5 Million Lives campaigns [155] have employed complementary effective strategies and "bundles" for SSI prevention.

Clinical manifestations

The diagnosis of SSI can be difficult. Discrimination between infectious and noninfectious postoperative inflammation poses a diagnostic challenge, as symptoms such as fever and erythema might be present in both scenarios. SSI

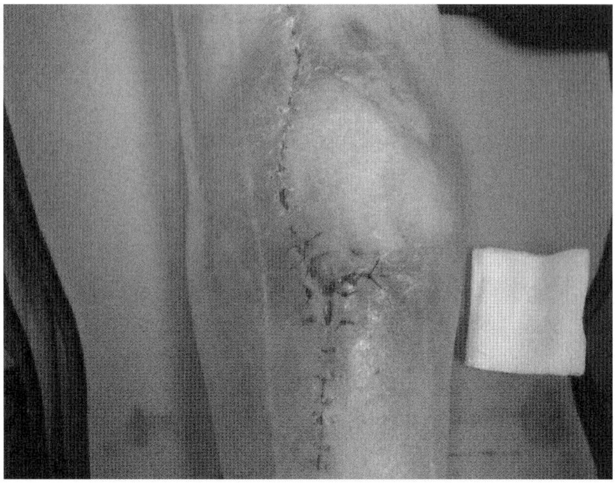

Figure 17.1 Superficial incisional *S. aureus* surgical-site infection with poor wound healing following a complicated total knee replacement. (Photograph courtesy of Milford Marchant MD.)

rarely occurs during the first 48 hours after surgery [156]. Instead, patients with an SSI initially manifest symptoms within a week of surgery. Most infections present with pain and clinical signs ranging from local induration to warmth, erythema, and swelling in the area of the surgical wound. The presence of pus and a wound culture obtained under sterile conditions that grows *S. aureus* are clear indications of infection. Infection may occur at the surgical site at any depth from the skin to the deepest cavity exposed during the course of the surgical procedure. Occasionally, infections may only involve the organ upon which surgery was performed. In this situation, superficial signs of infection might be absent and presenting symptoms might include organ dysfunction and signs and symptoms of a deep abscess.

Cellulitis is infection-related erythema of skin. In cases of superficial incisional SSI, cellulitis occurs adjacent to the surgical wound, often without drainage or fluctuance (Figure 17.1). Abscess refers to a localized collection of purulent material within tissue. A stitch-abscess is a boil that occurs at the site of a surgical suture that does not extend into the surgical wound. In contrast, wound abscesses extend into and sometimes through surgical planes. Necrotizing soft-tissue infections invade tissue widely and rapidly, causing widespread tissue necrosis. When a necrotizing infection involves fascia, the infection is referred to as necrotizing fasciitis. Postoperative necrotizing fasciitis is currently quite rare. Myonecrosis refers to involvement of underlying muscle. Patients with SSI and, in particular, SSI due to *S. aureus* are at risk for sepsis and septic shock. In some instances, sepsis may be the first sign of an SSI.

Diagnosis

The CDC has developed standardized surveillance criteria for defining SSI that are widely used [157] (Table 17.5).

Table 17.5 Criteria for defining a surgical-site infection (SSI)[1]. (Adapted from Horan *et al.* [157] with permission.)

Incisional SSI

Superficial

Infection involves skin or subcutaneous tissue of the incision *and* at least one of the following:

- Purulent drainage, with or without laboratory confirmation, from the superficial incision
- Organisms isolated from an aseptically obtained culture from the superficial incision
- At least one of the following signs or symptoms: pain, localized swelling, erythema, or heat and superficial incision is deliberately opened by surgeon, unless incision is culture-negative
- Diagnosis of superficial incisional SSI by surgeon

Deep

Infection involves deep soft tissues (e.g., fascial and muscle layers) of the incision *and* at least one of the following:

- Purulent drainage from the deep incision, excluding organ/space[2]
- A deep incision that spontaneously dehisces or is deliberately opened by the surgeon when a patient has one or more of the following signs/symptoms: fever (> 38°C), localized pain, unless site is culture-negative
- An abscess or other evidence of infection is found on direct examination, during repeat surgery, or by histopathological or radiological examination[3]
- Diagnosis of deep incisional SSI by surgeon

Organ/space SSI

Infection involves any part of the anatomy (e.g., organs or organ spaces) that was opened or manipulated during an operation *and* at least one of the following:

- Purulent drainage from a drain placed through the stab wound into the organ/space
- Organisms isolated from an aseptically obtained culture from the organ/space
- An abscess or other evidence of infection involving organ/space that is found on examination (physical, histopathological, or radiological) or during repeat surgery
- Diagnosis of organ/space SSI by surgeon

[1] For all classifications, infection is defined as occurring within 30 days after the operation if no implant is placed or within 1 year if an implant is in place and the infection is related to the incision.

[2] Report infection that involves both superficial and deep incision sites as a deep incisional SSI.

[3] Report an organ/space SSI that drains through the incision as a deep incisional SSI.

SSIs are classified as either incisional or organ/space (Figure 17.2). Incisional SSIs are further classified into superficial (involving only skin or subcutaneous tissue of the incision; see Figure 17.1) or deep (involving fascia and/or muscular layers). Organ/space SSIs include infections in any other anatomical site that was opened or manipulated during surgery.

Serum laboratory tests can be suggestive but not confirmatory for SSI. For example, basic hematological abnormalities such as increasing white blood cell count and neutrophil concentration are suggestive of infection. Leukocytosis of more than 15 000/mm^3 in the setting of hyponatremia (sodium < 135 mEq/L) is predictive of

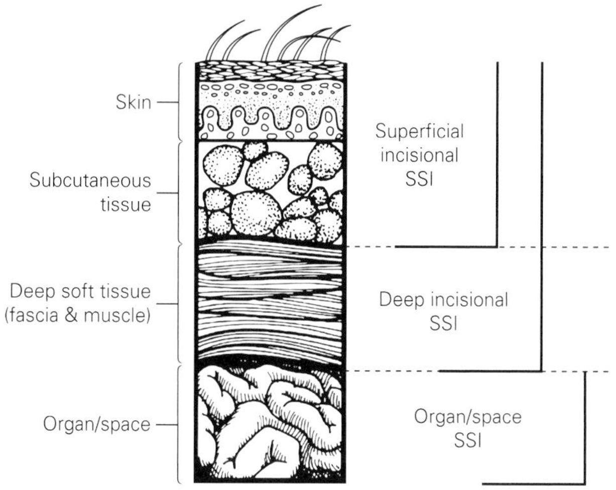

Figure 17.2 CDC classification of surgical-site infection. (From Horan *et al.* [157] with permission.)

necrotizing soft-tissue infection [158]. Cultures are not mandatory for the management of superficial incisional SSIs, especially if incision and drainage is curative and antibiotics are not needed. Cultures, ideally obtained in the operative setting, should be sent on all suspected cases of deep and organ/space infections in order to guide therapy and determine the susceptibility of the infecting organism. A wound culture growing *S. aureus* should never be considered to be a contaminant. Radiographic studies may be adjunctive for the diagnosis of SSI. Computed tomography is more reliable than plain radiographs for the detection of free air in soft tissue.

Surveillance for SSI

Successful infection control programs use epidemiologically sound definitions of infection and effective surveillance methods, stratify SSI rates according to risk factors for infection, and provide routine data feedback to surgeons and hospital leadership [159]. Infection control programs serve several purposes, including (i) providing comparative risk-adjusted data that can document success and detect deficiencies, (ii) providing a benchmark for SSI rates to help measure improvement efforts and effects of changes in technique or clinical care, and (iii) documenting data pertaining to the quality of care for internal and external reviewers. The majority of SSIs are diagnosable within 21 days of surgery [160,161].

Treatment

Surgical opening of the incision with removal of necrotic tissue is the primary and most important aspect of therapy for many types of SSI [156]. Incision and drainage of superficial incisional SSIs may be all that is necessary for cure in many cases, particularly if the area of induration is less than 5 cm [156,162]. Deep and organ/space infections almost universally require drainage of accumulated pus, most often by surgical débridement. Type of débridement and duration of antimicrobial therapy depend on the type of procedure and type of SSI.

According to expert opinion, postoperative patients with a temperature above 38.5°C or a heart rate above 110 bpm generally require antibiotics as well as opening of the suture line [156]. However, no data exist to guide the use of specific agents or duration of therapy for SSI due to *S. aureus*. The antimicrobial agent and length of therapy for SSI due to *S. aureus* are typically determined by the location of the infection (e.g., mediastinum, abdominal cavity, joint), the completeness of surgical débridement, the depth of infection, the presence of prosthetic material placed during surgery, and whether the *S. aureus* pathogen is methicillin resistant. As a rule of thumb, systemic antimicrobial therapy should be started as soon as a deep or organ/space SSI is suspected [163]. First-generation cephalosporins and antistaphylococcal penicillins are frequently used for antimicrobial treatment of SSI due to MSSA [164]. Rifampin, a bactericidal agent with excellent biofilm penetration, can be added as adjunctive antimicrobial therapy but should never be used as a single agent [165]. Patients with SSI due to MRSA are typically treated with vancomycin, the treatment of choice for infections caused by MRSA [156]. Of note, however, as many as 25% of patients with SSI due to MRSA do not receive appropriate antimicrobial therapy even after culture results are available [166].

Other agents with activity against MRSA, including linezolid, daptomycin, and tigecycline, have received Food and Drug Administration (FDA) indications for treatment of complicated skin and skin structure infections and thus represent alternatives to vancomycin for the treatment of SSI due to MRSA. Data comparing these agents with vancomycin for the treatment of SSI due to MRSA have been limited to subset analyses of larger trials. A recent subset analysis of a prospective randomized controlled trial comparing linezolid with vancomycin for the treatment of skin and soft tissue infections focused exclusively on patients with SSI [167]. Linezolid and vancomycin were equivalent with respect to clinical resolution of symptoms of SSI, but linezolid led to higher rates of microbial cure 7 days after therapy than vancomycin (84% vs. 58%; $P = 0.007$), particularly in patients with SSI due to MRSA (87% vs. 48%; $P = 0.002$) [167]. If linezolid therapy is administered for more than 2 weeks, hematological monitoring, including platelet counts, must be performed at least weekly given the increased risk of bone marrow suppression associated with the use of linezolid [168]. Both daptomycin and tigecycline have FDA indications for skin and soft tissue infections, but data on SSIs are lacking [169,170].

Prosthetic joint infection due to *S. aureus* is a unique problem. Surgical treatment for prosthetic joint infection includes the following strategies: débridement with retention of the prosthesis, one- or two-stage exchange with reimplantation, resection arthroplasty, and amputation [171]. In all strategies, débridement is a key component, as removal of foreign materials such as wires, bone wax, and devitalized tissues improves the likelihood of cure [172]. One-stage exchange involves débridement, removal of the prosthetic joint, and immediate reimplantation of a new prosthesis. Two-stage exchange involves débridement and removal of the infected prosthesis followed by a delay (often up to 6–8 weeks) prior to reimplantation with a new prosthesis. Antimicrobial therapy is typically administered for the duration of the delay between removal of infected prosthesis and reimplantation. The choice between modalities for surgical treatment is a matter of clinical judgment that may be influenced by the operative findings, type of pathogen, and/or the skill or experience of individual surgeons. If *S. aureus* infection is identified quickly, early surgical débridement can lead to successful maintenance of the prosthesis [173]. Débridement with retention of the implant can be effective if the following conditions are met: signs and symptoms of prosthetic joint infection with *S. aureus* are detected within 3 weeks of implantation, the implant remains stable, the surrounding soft tissue remains in good condition, and the patient can receive both intravenous and oral antibiotics [171]. Intravenous antimicrobial therapy for 2–4 weeks is then followed by 3 months of oral antimicrobial therapy for hip prostheses and by 6 months of such therapy for knee prostheses [174]. If signs and symptoms occur more than 3 weeks after the implantation of the prosthesis, then the infected prosthesis should be removed. Patients with prosthetic joint infection due to MSSA and intact surrounding soft tissues can often be treated with a one-stage exchange [175]. Patients with either compromised soft tissue or infection due to MRSA should undergo a two-stage exchange. Patients with prosthetic joint infection due to MRSA should undergo 6–8 weeks of intravenous antimicrobial therapy after explantation of the infected prosthesis prior to reimplantation [171].

Adjunctive therapy with antibiotic-impregnated devices and wound-closure devices are frequently provided for the treatment of prosthetic joint infection due to *S. aureus*. Vancomycin-impregnated cement beads and PROSTOLAC (prosthesis of antibiotic-loaded acrylic cement) may be used during revision arthroplasties for infected joints [176]. Animal models suggest that surgically implanted absorbable gentamicin-impregnated sponges may assist in the cure of MRSA joint infection [177]. Animal models also show that vacuum-assisted closure devices may assist with healing of infected surgical wounds by optimizing blood flow, decreasing tissue edema, and removing fluid and dead space from the wound [178]. Clinical trials have been limited to small case series and cohort studies [179, 180]. No randomized controlled trials in humans have yet proven the benefits or cost-effectiveness of antibiotic-impregnated beads or vacuum-assisted closure devices.

Outcomes

Despite improvements in surgical technique, advances in infection control practices, improved understanding of the pathogenesis of wound infection, and the widespread use of prophylactic perioperative antibiotics, SSIs remain a leading cause of morbidity and mortality. SSIs due to *S. aureus* are associated with particularly severe patient outcomes. Patients with any type of postoperative *S. aureus* infection are at risk for adverse outcomes including 2 weeks of additional hospitalization, more than $49 000 of attributable extra costs, and a 5% increase in the mortality rate [181]. In one case–control study comparing elderly patients with SSI due to *S. aureus* with uninfected elderly surgical patients, patients with SSI due to *S. aureus* were at fivefold increased risk of death, had a 2.5-fold increased duration of hospitalization, and had an excess of $41 000 of attributable charges per SSI [182]. In an another matched outcomes study comparing 121 patients with SSI due to MRSA with 193 uninfected postoperative control patients, patients with SSI due to MRSA had more than an 11-fold increase in mortality, $29 000 of additional attributable costs, and approximately 2 extra weeks of hospitalization [183].

Patients with infections due to MRSA have worse outcomes and accumulate more hospital costs than patients with infections due to MSSA [184,185] and this trend is no different in SSI. A matched outcomes study comparing 127 patients with SSI due to MRSA with 173 patients with SSI due to MSSA demonstrated that patients with SSI due to MRSA had 3.4-fold higher mortality rates and $13 900 per SSI higher costs than patients with SSI due to MSSA [183]. A cohort study of 441 SSIs due to Gram-positive bacteria reported that patients with SSI due to MRSA had almost 50 days of additional hospitalization than patients with SSI due to MSSA (71.9 days vs. 26.6 days; $P < 0.05$) [186]. In addition, one study examined the attributable impact of methicillin resistance in patients undergoing cardiothoracic surgery. Patients with mediastinitis due to MRSA had approximately fivefold higher rates of mortality at 1 year compared to patients with mediastinitis due to MSSA (74% vs. 16%; $P = 0.04$) [187].

Conclusion

SSI due to *S. aureus* is a major concern in the modern healthcare system. Given its current trajectory, SSIs due to *S. aureus* will likely account for an increasingly greater proportion of healthcare resources, patient suffering, and death. As SSI continues to gain public attention and becomes a target for patient safety initiatives, improved compliance with proven preventive measures and development of novel approaches to SSI prevention will hopefully help to improve the prevention and management of SSI due to *S. aureus*.

References

1 Anderson DJ, Kaye KS, Classen D *et al*. Infect Control Hosp Epidemiol 2008;29:S51–S61.

2 Cruse P. Wound infection surveillance. Rev Infect Dis 1981;3: 734–7.

3 Wenzel RP. Health care-associated infections: major issues in the early years of the 21st century. Clin Infect Dis 2007;45 (suppl 1):S85–S88.

4 National Nosocomial Infections Surveillance (NNIS) System. Data summary from October 1986 to April 1996, issued May 1996. A report from the National Nosocomial Infections Surveillance (NNIS) System. Am J Infect Control 1996;24:380–8.

5 Anderson DJ, Sexton DJ, Kanafani ZA, Auten G, Kaye KS. Severe surgical site infection in community hospitals: epidemiology, key procedures, and the changing prevalence of methicillin-resistant *Staphylococcus aureus*. Infect Control Hosp Epidemiol 2007;28:1043–57.

6 Jernigan JA. Is the burden of *Staphylococcus aureus* among patients with surgical-site infections growing? Infect Control Hosp Epidemiol 2004;25:457–60.

7 Wong ES. Surgical site infections. In: Mayhall CG, ed. Hospital Epidemiology and Infection Control, 3rd edn. Baltimore: Lippincott, Williams and Wilkins, 2004;287–306.

8 Altemeier WA, Culbertson WR, Hummel RP. Surgical considerations of endogenous infections: sources, types, and methods of control. Surg Clin North Am 1968;48:227–40.

9 Mangram AJ, Horan TC, Pearson ML, Silver LC, Jarvis WR. Guideline for prevention of surgical site infection, 1999. Hospital Infection Control Practices Advisory Committee. Infect Control Hosp Epidemiol 1999;20:250–78; quiz 279–80.

10 Tuazon CU. Skin and skin structure infections in the patient at risk: carrier state of *Staphylococcus aureus*. Am J Med 1984; 76(5A):166–71.

11 Wiley AM, Ha'eri GB. Routes of infection. A study of using "tracer particles" in the orthopedic operating room. Clin Orthop Relat Res 1979;139:150–5.

12 Edwards LD. The epidemiology of 2056 remote site infections and 1966 surgical wound infections occurring in 1865 patients: a four year study of 40,923 operations at Rush-Presbyterian-St. Luke's Hospital, Chicago. Ann Surg 1976;184:758–66.

13 Berkelman RL, Martin D, Graham DR *et al*. Streptococcal wound infections caused by a vaginal carrier. JAMA 1982;247: 2680–2.

14 McIntyre DM. An epidemic of *Streptococcus pyogenes* puerperal and postoperative sepsis with an unusual carrier site: the anus. Am J Obstet Gynecol 1968;101:308–14.

15 Stamm WE, Feeley JC, Facklam RR. Wound infections due to group A streptococcus traced to a vaginal carrier. J Infect Dis 1978;138:287–92.

16 Schaffner W, Lefkowitz LB Jr, Goodman JS, Koenig MG. Hospital outbreak of infections with group A streptococci traced to an asymptomatic anal carrier. N Engl J Med 1969;280:1224–5.

17 Gyrska P. Postoperative streptococcal wound infection. The anatomy of an epidemic. JAMA 1970;213:1189–91.

18 Devenish EA, Lond MS, Miles AA. Control of *Staphylococcus aureus* in an operating theatre. Lancet 1939;233:1088–94.

19 Weber S, Herwaldt LA, McNutt LA *et al*. An outbreak of *Staphylococcus aureus* in a pediatric cardiothoracic surgery unit. Infect Control Hosp Epidemiol 2002;23:77–81.

20 Sheretz RJ, Reagan DR, Hampton KD *et al*. A cloud adult: the *Staphylococcus aureus*–virus interaction revisited. Ann Intern Med 1996;124:539–47.

21 Houang ET, Ahmet Z. Intraoperative wound contamination during abdominal hysterectomy. J Hosp Infect 1991;19:181–9.

22 Krizek TJ, Robson MC. Evolution of quantitative bacteriology in wound management. Am J Surg 1975;130:579–84.

23 James RC, Macleod CJ. Induction of staphylococcal infections in mice with small inocula introduced on sutures. Br J Exp Pathol 1961;42:266–77.

24 Elek SD, Conen PE. The virulence of *Staphylococcus pyogenes* for man: a study of the problems of wound infection. Br J Exp Pathol 1957;38:573–86.

25 Arbeit RD, Dunn RM. Expression of capsular polysaccharide during experimental focal infection with *Staphylococcus aureus*. J Infect Dis 1987;156:947–52.

26 Froman G, Switalski LM, Speziale P, Hook M. Isolation and characterization of a fibronectin receptor from *Staphylococcus aureus*. J Biol Chem 1987;262:6564–71.

27 Switalski LM, Patti JM, Butcher W, Gristina AG, Speziale P, Hook M. A collagen receptor on *Staphylococcus aureus* strains isolated from patients with septic arthritis mediates adhesion to cartilage. Mol Microbiol 1993;7:99–107.

28 Mayberry-Carson KJ, Tober-Meyer B, Smith JK, Lambe DW Jr, Costerton JW. Bacterial adherence and glycocalyx formation in osteomyelitis experimentally induced with *Staphylococcus aureus*. Infect Immun 1984;43:825–33.

29 Rogolsky M. Nonenteric toxins of *Staphylococcus aureus*. Microbiol Rev 1979;43:320–60.

30 Dossett JH, Kronvall G, Williams RC Jr, Quie PG. Antiphagocytic effects of staphylococcal protein A. J Immunol 1969;103:1405–10.

31 Dellinger EP. Surgical infections and choice of antibiotics. In: Sabiston DC, ed. Textbook of Surgery, 15th edn. Philadelphia: WB Saunders, 1997:264–280.

32 Kernodle DS, Classen DC, Burke JP, Kaiser AB. Failure of cephalosporins to prevent *Staphylococcus aureus* surgical wound infections. JAMA 1990;263:961–6.

33 Kernodle DS, Voladri RK, Kaiser AB. Beta-lactamase production diminishes the prophylactic efficacy of ampicillin and cefazolin in a guinea pig model of *Staphylococcus aureus* wound infection. J Infect Dis 1998;177:701–6.

34 Kernodle DS, Kaiser AB. Surgical and trauma related infections. In: Mandell GL, Bennett JE, Dolin R, eds. Principles and Practice of Infectious Diseases, 5th edn, vol 2. New York: Churchill Livingstone, 2000.

35 Cheadle WG, Hershman MJ, Wellhausen SR, Polk HC Jr. HLA-DR antigen expression on peripheral blood monocytes correlates with surgical infection. Am J Surg 1991;161:639–45.

36 Hensler T, Hecker H, Heeg K *et al*. Distinct mechanisms of immunosuppression as a consequence of major surgery. Infect Immun 1997;65:2283–91.

37 El-Maallem H, Fletcher J. Effects of surgery on neutrophil granulocyte function. Infect Immun 1981;32:38–41.

38 Clardy CW, Edwards KM, Gay JC. Increased susceptibility to infection in hypothermic children: possible role of acquired neutrophil dysfunction. Pediatr Infect Dis 1985;4:379–82.

39 Yamada Y, Hefter K, Burke JF, Gelfand JA. An in vitro model of the wound microenvironment: local phagocytic cell abnormalities associated with in situ complement activation. J Infect Dis 1987;155:998–1004.

40 de Boer AS, Mintjes-de Groot AJ, Severijnen AJ, van den Berg JM, van Pelt W. Risk assessment for surgical-site infections in orthopedic patients. Infect Control Hosp Epidemiol 1999;20: 402–7.
41 Scott JD, Forrest A, Feuerstein S, Fitzpatrick P, Schentag JJ. Factors associated with postoperative infection. Infect Control Hosp Epidemiol 2001;22:347–51.
42 Pessaux P, Msika S, Atalla D, Hay JM, Flamant Y. Risk factors for postoperative infectious complications in noncolorectal abdominal surgery: a multivariate analysis based on a prospective multicenter study of 4718 patients. Arch Surg 2003; 138:314–24.
43 Polly SM, Sanders WE Jr. Surgical infections in the elderly: prevention, diagnosis, and treatment. Geriatrics 1977;32:88–90, 95–7.
44 Raymond DP, Pelletier SJ, Crabtree TD, Schulman AM, Pruett TL, Sawyer RG. Surgical infection and the aging population. Am Surg 2001;67:827–32; discussion 832–3.
45 Byrne DJ, Lynch W, Napier A, Davey P, Malek M, Cuschieri A. Wound infection rates: the importance of definition and post-discharge wound surveillance. J Hosp Infect 1994;26: 37–43.
46 Delgado-Rodriguez M, Gomez-Ortega A, Sillero-Arenas M, Llorca J. Epidemiology of surgical-site infections diagnosed after hospital discharge: a prospective cohort study. Infect Control Hosp Epidemiol 2001;22:24–30.
47 Haley RW, Hooton TM, Culver DH *et al.* Nosocomial infections in U.S. hospitals, 1975–1976: estimated frequency by selected characteristics of patients. Am J Med 1981;70:947–59.
48 Kaye KS, Schmit K, Pieper C *et al.* The effect of increasing age on the risk of surgical site infection. J Infect Dis 2005;191: 1056–62.
49 Anderson DJ, Chen LF, Schmader KE *et al.* Poor functional status as a risk factor for surgical site infection due to methicillin-resistant *Staphylococcus aureus*. Infect Control Hosp Epidemiol 2008;29:832–9.
50 Gadaleta D, Risucci DA, Nelson RL *et al.* Effects of morbid obesity and diabetes mellitus on risk of coronary artery bypass grafting. Am J Cardiol 1992;70:1613–14.
51 Grossi EA, Esposito R, Harris LJ *et al.* Sternal wound infections and use of internal mammary artery grafts. J Thorac Cardiovasc Surg 1991;102:342–6; discussion 346–7.
52 Hoogwerf BJ, Sheeler LR, Licata AA. Endocrine management of the open heart surgical patient. Semin Thorac Cardiovasc Surg 1991;3:75–80.
53 Lilienfeld DE, Vlahov D, Tenney JH, McLaughlin JS. Obesity and diabetes as risk factors for postoperative wound infections after cardiac surgery. Am J Infect Control 1988;16:3–6.
54 Zerr KJ, Furnary AP, Grunkemeier GL, Bookin S, Kanhere V, Starr A. Glucose control lowers the risk of wound infection in diabetics after open heart operations. Ann Thorac Surg 1997; 63:356–61.
55 Wilson SJ, Sexton DJ. Elevated preoperative fasting serum glucose levels increase the risk of postoperative mediastinitis in patients undergoing open heart surgery. Infect Control Hosp Epidemiol 2003;24:776–8.
56 Choban PS, Heckler R, Burge JC, Flancbaum L. Increased incidence of nosocomial infections in obese surgical patients. Am Surg 1995;61:1001–5.
57 Nystrom PO, Jonstam A, Hojer H, Ling L. Incisional infection after colorectal surgery in obese patients. Acta Chir Scand 1987;153:225–7.
58 Nagachinta T, Stephens M, Reitz B, Polk BF. Risk factors for surgical-wound infection following cardiac surgery. J Infect Dis 1987;156:967–73.
59 Kabon B, Nagele A, Reddy D *et al.* Obesity decreases perioperative tissue oxygenation. Anesthesiology 2004;100:274–80.
60 Sorensen LT, Hemmingsen U, Kallehave F *et al.* Risk factors for tissue and wound complications in gastrointestinal surgery. Ann Surg 2005;241:654–8.
61 Sorensen LT, Horby J, Friis E, Pilsgaard B, Jorgensen T. Smoking as a risk factor for wound healing and infection in breast cancer surgery. Eur J Surg Oncol 2002;28:815–20.
62 Jensen JA, Goodson WH, Hopf HW, Hunt TK. Cigarette smoking decreases tissue oxygen. Arch Surg 1991;126:1131–4.
63 Hopf HW, Hunt TK, West JM *et al.* Wound tissue oxygen tension predicts the risk of wound infection in surgical patients. Arch Surg 1997;132:997–1004; discussion 1005.
64 Jorgensen LN, Kallehave F, Christensen E, Siana JE, Gottrup F. Less collagen production in smokers. Surgery 1998;123:450–5.
65 Allen DB, Maguire JJ, Mahdavian M *et al.* Wound hypoxia and acidosis limit neutrophil bacterial killing mechanisms. Arch Surg 1997;132:991–6.
66 Sorensen LT, Nielsen HB, Kharazmi A, Gottrup F. Effect of smoking and abstention on oxidative burst and reactivity of neutrophils and monocytes. Surgery 2004;136:1047–53.
67 Klein JD, Hey LA, Yu CS *et al.* Perioperative nutrition and postoperative complications in patients undergoing spinal surgery. Spine 1996;21:2676–82.
68 Malone DL, Genuit T, Tracy JK, Gannon C, Napolitano LM. Surgical site infections: reanalysis of risk factors. J Surg Res 2002;103:89–95.
69 Windsor JA, Hill GL. Protein depletion and surgical risk. Aust NZ J Surg 1988;58:711–15.
70 Windsor JA, Hill GL. Weight loss with physiologic impairment. A basic indicator of surgical risk. Ann Surg 1988;207:290–6.
71 Ulicny KS Jr, Hiratzka LF, Williams RB *et al.* Sternotomy infection: poor prediction by acute phase response and delayed hypersensitivity. Ann Thorac Surg 1990;50:949–58.
72 Brennan MF, Pisters PW, Posner M, Quesada O, Shike M. A prospective randomized trial of total parenteral nutrition after major pancreatic resection for malignancy. Ann Surg 1994;220: 436–41; discussion 441–4.
73 Veterans Affairs Total Parenteral Nutrition Cooperative Study Group. Perioperative total parenteral nutrition in surgical patients. N Engl J Med 1991;325:525–32.
74 Muller JM, Brenner U, Dienst C, Pichlmaier H. Preoperative parenteral feeding in patients with gastrointestinal carcinoma. Lancet 1982;i:68–71.
75 Kaul AF, Jewett JF. Agents and techniques for disinfection of the skin. Surg Gynecol Obstet 1981;152:677–85.
76 Rotter ML, Larsen SO, Cooke EM *et al.* A comparison of the effects of preoperative whole-body bathing with detergent alone and with detergent containing chlorhexidine gluconate on the frequency of wound infections after clean surgery. The European Working Party on Control of Hospital Infections. J Hosp Infect 1988;11:310–20.

77 Perl TM, Golub JE. New approaches to reduce *Staphylococcus aureus* nosocomial infection rates: treating *S. aureus* nasal carriage. Ann Pharmacother 1998;32:S7–S16.
78 Kluytmans JA, Mouton JW, Ijzerman EP *et al.* Nasal carriage of *Staphylococcus aureus* as a major risk factor for wound infections after cardiac surgery. J Infect Dis 1995;171:216–19.
79 Berard F, Gandon J. Postoperative wound infections: the influence of ultraviolet irradiation of the operating room and of various other factors. Ann Surg 1964;160(suppl 1):1–192.
80 Haley RW, Culver DH, Morgan WM, White JW, Emori TG, Hooton TM. Identifying patients at high risk of surgical wound infection. A simple multivariate index of patient susceptibility and wound contamination. Am J Epidemiol 1985;121:206–15.
81 Olson M, O'Connor M, Schwartz ML. Surgical wound infections. A 5-year prospective study of 20,193 wounds at the Minneapolis VA Medical Center. Ann Surg 1984;199:253–9.
82 Cruse PJ, Foord R. The epidemiology of wound infection. A 10-year prospective study of 62,939 wounds. Surg Clin North Am 1980;60:27–40.
83 Ridgeway S, Wilson J, Charlet A, Kafatos G, Pearson A, Coello R. Infection of the surgical site after arthroplasty of the hip. J Bone Joint Surg Br 2005;87:844–50.
84 Simchen E, Stein H, Sacks TG, Shapiro M, Michel J. Multivariate analysis of determinants of postoperative wound infection in orthopaedic patients. J Hosp Infect 1984;5:137–46.
85 Culver DH, Horan TC, Gaynes RP *et al.* Surgical wound infection rates by wound class, operative procedure, and patient risk index. National Nosocomial Infections Surveillance System. Am J Med 1991;91(3B):152S–157S.
86 Harbarth S, Huttner B, Gervaz P *et al.* Risk factors for methicillin-resistant *Staphylococcus aureus* surgical site infection. Infect Control Hosp Epidemiol 2008;29:890–3.
87 American College of Surgeons Committee on Control of Surgical Infections. Manual on Control of Infection in Surgical Patients. Philadelphia: JB Lippincott, 1984.
88 Mishriki SF, Law DJ, Jeffery PJ. Factors affecting the incidence of postoperative wound infection. J Hosp Infect 1990;16:223–30.
89 Seropian R, Reynolds BM. Wound infections after preoperative depilatory versus razor preparation. Am J Surg 1971;121: 251–4.
90 Moro ML, Carrieri MP, Tozzi AE, Lana S, Greco D. Risk factors for surgical wound infections in clean surgery: a multicenter study. Italian PRINOS Study Group. Ann Ital Chir 1996;67: 13–19.
91 Winston KR. Hair and neurosurgery. Neurosurgery 1992;31: 320–9.
92 Latham R, Lancaster AD, Covington JF, Pirolo JS, Thomas CS. The association of diabetes and glucose control with surgical-site infections among cardiothoracic surgery patients. Infect Control Hosp Epidemiol 2001;22:607–12.
93 Sessler DI. Mild perioperative hypothermia. N Engl J Med 1997;336:1730–7.
94 Sessler DI, McGuire J, Hynson J, Moayeri A, Heier T. Thermoregulatory vasoconstriction during isoflurane anesthesia minimally decreases cutaneous heat loss. Anesthesiology 1992; 76:670–5.
95 Matsukawa T, Sessler DI, Sessler AM *et al.* Heat flow and distribution during induction of general anesthesia. Anesthesiology 1995;82:662–73.
96 Sessler DI, Rubinstein EH, Moayeri A. Physiologic responses to mild perianesthetic hypothermia in humans. Anesthesiology 1991;75:594–610.
97 Chang N, Mathes SJ. Comparison of the effect of bacterial inoculation in musculocutaneous and random-pattern flaps. Plast Reconstr Surg 1982;70:1–10.
98 Hohn DC, MacKay RD, Halliday B, Hunt TK. Effect of O_2 tension on microbicidal function of leukocytes in wounds and in vitro. Surg Forum 1976;27:18–20.
99 Leijh PC, van den Barselaar MT, van Zwet TL, Dubbeldeman-Rempt I, van Furth R. Kinetics of phagocytosis of *Staphylococcus aureus* and *Escherichia coli* by human granulocytes. Immunology 1979;37:453–65.
100 van Oss CJ, Absolom DR, Moore LL, Park BH, Humbert JR. Effect of temperature on the chemotaxis, phagocytic engulfment, digestion and O_2 consumption of human polymorphonuclear leukocytes. J Reticuloendothel Soc 1980;27:561–5.
101 Melling AC, Ali B, Scott EM, Leaper DJ. Effects of preoperative warming on the incidence of wound infection after clean surgery: a randomised controlled trial. Lancet 2001;358:876–80.
102 Kurz A, Sessler DI, Lenhardt R. Perioperative normothermia to reduce the incidence of surgical-wound infection and shorten hospitalization. Study of Wound Infection and Temperature Group. N Engl J Med 1996;334:1209–15.
103 Hunt TK, Linsey M, Grislis H, Sonne M, Jawetz E. The effect of differing ambient oxygen tensions on wound infection. Ann Surg 1975;181:35–9.
104 Knighton DR, Fiegel VD, Halverson T, Schneider S, Brown T, Wells CL. Oxygen as an antibiotic. The effect of inspired oxygen on bacterial clearance. Arch Surg 1990;125:97–100.
105 Belda FJ, Aguilera L, Garcia de la Asuncion J *et al.* Supplemental perioperative oxygen and the risk of surgical wound infection: a randomized controlled trial. JAMA 2005;294:2035–42.
106 Greif R, Akca O, Horn EP, Kurz A, Sessler DI. Supplemental perioperative oxygen to reduce the incidence of surgical-wound infection. N Engl J Med 2000;342:161–7.
107 Dellinger EP. Increasing inspired oxygen to decrease surgical site infection: time to shift the quality improvement research paradigm. JAMA 2005;294:2091–2.
108 Ayliffe GA. Role of the environment of the operating suite in surgical wound infection. Rev Infect Dis 1991;13(suppl 10): S800–S804.
109 Ha'eri GB, Wiley AM. The efficacy of standard surgical face masks: an investigation using "tracer particles". Clin Orthop Relat Res 1980;148:160–2.
110 Letts RM, Doermer E. Conversation in the operating theater as a cause of airborne bacterial contamination. J Bone Joint Surg Am 1983;65:357–62.
111 Morain WD, Colen LB. Wound healing in diabetes mellitus. Clin Plast Surg 1990;17:493–501.
112 Mueller SW, Krebsbach LE. Impact of an antimicrobial-impregnated gauze dressing on surgical site infections including methicillin-resistant *Staphylococcus aureus* infections. Am J Infect Control 2008;36:651–5.
113 Hill GE, Frawley WH, Griffith KE, Forestner JE, Minei JP. Allogeneic blood transfusion increases the risk of postoperative bacterial infection: a meta-analysis. J Trauma 2003;54: 908–14.

114 Claridge JA, Sawyer RG, Schulman AM, McLemore EC, Young JS. Blood transfusions correlate with infections in trauma patients in a dose-dependent manner. Am Surg 2002;68:566–72.
115 Garibaldi RA. Prevention of intraoperative wound contamination with chlorhexidine shower and scrub. J Hosp Infect 1988;11(suppl B):5–9.
116 Hayek LJ, Emerson JM, Gardner AM. A placebo-controlled trial of the effect of two preoperative baths or showers with chlorhexidine detergent on postoperative wound infection rates. J Hosp Infect 1987;10:165–72.
117 Leigh DA, Stronge JL, Marriner J, Sedgwick J. Total body bathing with "Hibiscrub" (chlorhexidine) in surgical patients: a controlled trial. J Hosp Infect 1983;4:229–35.
118 Lynch W, Davey PG, Malek M, Byrne DJ, Napier A. Cost-effectiveness analysis of the use of chlorhexidine detergent in preoperative whole-body disinfection in wound infection prophylaxis. J Hosp Infect 1992;21:179–91.
119 Larson E. Guideline for use of topical antimicrobial agents. Am J Infect Control 1988;16:253–66.
120 Ritter MA, French ML, Eitzen HE, Gioe TJ. The antimicrobial effectiveness of operative-site preparative agents: a microbiological and clinical study. J Bone Joint Surg Am 1980;62:826–8.
121 Brown TR, Ehrlich CE, Stehman FB, Golichowski AM, Madura JA, Eitzen HE. A clinical evaluation of chlorhexidine gluconate spray as compared with iodophor scrub for preoperative skin preparation. Surg Gynecol Obstet 1984;158:363–6.
122 Lowbury EJ, Lilly HA. Use of 4 per cent chlorhexidine detergent solution (Hibiscrub) and other methods of skin disinfection. BMJ 1973;1:510–15.
123 Aly R, Maibach HI. Comparative antibacterial efficacy of a 2-minute surgical scrub with chlorhexidine gluconate, povidoneiodine, and chloroxylenol sponge-brushes. Am J Infect Control 1988;16:173–7.
124 Hardin WD Jr. Handwashing and patient skin preparation. In: Malangoni MA, ed. Critical Issues in Operating Room Management. Philadelphia: Lippincott-Raven, 1997;133–49.
125 Lowbury EJ, Lilly HA, Ayliffe GA. Preoperative disinfection of surgeons' hands: use of alcoholic solutions and effects of gloves on skin flora. BMJ 1974;4:369–72.
126 Rotter ML. Hygienic hand disinfection. Infect Control 1984;5: 18–22.
127 Galle PC, Homesley HD, Rhyne AL. Reassessment of the surgical scrub. Surg Gynecol Obstet 1978;147:215–18.
128 O'Shaughnessy M, O'Malley VP, Corbett G, Given HF. Optimum duration of surgical scrub-time. Br J Surg 1991;78:685–6.
129 Wheelock SM, Lookinland S. Effect of surgical hand scrub time on subsequent bacterial growth. AORN J 1997;65:1087–92, 1094–8.
130 Pottinger J, Burns S, Manske C. Bacterial carriage by artificial versus natural nails. Am J Infect Control 1989;17:340–4.
131 Association of Operating Room Nurses. Standards, Recommended Practices, Guidelines. Denver: AORN, 1999.
132 Segers P, Speekenbrink RG, Ubbink DT, van Ogtrop ML, de Mol BA. Prevention of nosocomial infection in cardiac surgery by decontamination of the nasopharynx and oropharynx with chlorhexidine gluconate: a randomized controlled trial. JAMA 2006;296:2460–6.
133 Cimochowski GE, Harostock MD, Brown R, Bernardi M, Alonzo N, Coyle K. Intranasal mupirocin reduces sternal wound infection after open heart surgery in diabetics and nondiabetics. Ann Thorac Surg 2001;71:1572–8; discussion 1578–9.
134 Kluytmans JA, Mouton JW, VandenBergh MF *et al*. Reduction of surgical-site infections in cardiothoracic surgery by elimination of nasal carriage of *Staphylococcus aureus*. Infect Control Hosp Epidemiol 1996;17:780–5.
135 Perl TM, Cullen JJ, Wenzel RP *et al*. Intranasal mupirocin to prevent postoperative *Staphylococcus aureus* infections. N Engl J Med 2002;346:1871–7.
136 Perl TM. Prevention of *Staphylococcus aureus* infections among surgical patients: beyond traditional perioperative prophylaxis. Surgery 2003;134(5 suppl):S10–S17.
137 Miller MA, Dascal A, Portnoy J, Mendelson J. Development of mupirocin resistance among methicillin-resistant *Staphylococcus aureus* after widespread use of nasal mupirocin ointment. Infect Control Hosp Epidemiol 1996;17:811–13.
138 Classen DC, Evans RS, Pestotnik SL, Horn SD, Menlove RL, Burke JP. The timing of prophylactic administration of antibiotics and the risk of surgical-wound infection. N Engl J Med 1992;326:281–6.
139 Anon. Antimicrobial prophylaxis in surgery. Med Lett Drugs Ther 1997;39:97–101.
140 Ehrenkranz NJ. Antimicrobial prophylaxis in surgery: mechanisms, misconceptions, and mischief. Infect Control Hosp Epidemiol 1993;14:99–106.
141 Nichols RL. Surgical antibiotic prophylaxis. Med Clin North Am 1995;79:509–22.
142 McDonald M, Grabsch E, Marshall C, Forbes A. Single- versus multiple-dose antimicrobial prophylaxis for major surgery: a systematic review. Aust NZ J Surg 1998;68:388–96.
143 Nichols RL. Antibiotic prophylaxis in surgery. J Chemother 1989;1:170–8.
144 Forse RA, Karam B, MacLean LD, Christou NV. Antibiotic prophylaxis for surgery in morbidly obese patients. Surgery 1989;106:750–6; discussion 756–7.
145 Page CP, Bohnen JM, Fletcher JR, McManus AT, Solomkin JS, Wittmann DH. Antimicrobial prophylaxis for surgical wounds. Guidelines for clinical care. Arch Surg 1993;128:79–88.
146 Burke JF. The effective period of preventive antibiotic action in experimental incisions and dermal lesions. Surgery 1961;50: 161–8.
147 Miles AA, Miles EM, Burke J. The value and duration of defence reactions of the skin to the primary lodgement of bacteria. Br J Exp Pathol 1957;38:79–96.
148 DiPiro JT, Cheung RP, Bowden TA Jr, Mansberger JA. Single dose systemic antibiotic prophylaxis of surgical wound infections. Am J Surg 1986;152:552–9.
149 Recommendations of the Hospital Infection Control Practices Advisory Committee (HICPAC). Recommendations for preventing the spread of vancomycin resistance. MMWR 1995; 44(RR-12):1–13.
150 Bolon MK, Morlote M, Weber SG, Koplan B, Carmeli Y, Wright SB. Glycopeptides are no more effective than beta-lactam agents for prevention of surgical site infection after cardiac surgery: a meta-analysis. Clin Infect Dis 2004;38:1357–63.
151 Dodds Ashley ES, Carroll DN, Engemann JJ *et al*. Risk factors for postoperative mediastinitis due to methicillin-resistant *Staphylococcus aureus*. Clin Infect Dis 2004;38:1555–60.
152 Bratzler DW, Hunt DR. The surgical infection prevention and surgical care improvement projects: national initiatives to

improve outcomes for patients having surgery. Clin Infect Dis 2006;43:322–30.

153 Bratzler DW, Houck PM. Antimicrobial prophylaxis for surgery: an advisory statement from the National Surgical Infection Prevention Project. Clin Infect Dis 2004;38:1706–15.

154 Dellinger EP, Hausmann SM, Bratzler DW *et al.* Hospitals collaborate to decrease surgical site infections. Am J Surg 2005; 190:9–15.

155 Institute of Healthcare Improvement. A resource from the Institute of Healthcare Improvement. 2007. http://www.ihi.org, accessed September 2008.

156 Stevens DL, Bisno AL, Chambers HF *et al.* Practice guidelines for the diagnosis and management of skin and soft-tissue infections. Clin Infect Dis 2005;41:1373–406.

157 Horan TC, Gaynes RP, Martone WJ, Jarvis WR, Emori TG. CDC definitions of nosocomial surgical site infections, 1992: a modification of CDC definitions of surgical wound infections. Infect Control Hosp Epidemiol 1992;13:606–8.

158 Wall DB, Klein SR, Black S, de Virgilio C. A simple model to help distinguish necrotizing fasciitis from nonnecrotizing soft tissue infection. J Am Coll Surg 2000;191:227–31.

159 Society for Hospital Epidemiology of America, Association for Practitioners in Infection Control, Centers for Disease Control and Surgical Infection Society. Consensus paper on the surveillance of surgical wound infections. Infect Control Hosp Epidemiol 1992;13:599–605.

160 Weigelt JA, Dryer D, Haley RW. The necessity and efficiency of wound surveillance after discharge. Arch Surg 1992;127:77–81; discussion 81–2.

161 Sands K, Vineyard G, Platt R. Surgical site infections occurring after hospital discharge. J Infect Dis 1996;173:963–70.

162 Lee MC, Rios AM, Aten MF *et al.* Management and outcome of children with skin and soft tissue abscesses caused by community-acquired methicillin-resistant *Staphylococcus aureus*. Pediatr Infect Dis J 2004;23:123–7.

163 Karra R, McDermott L, Connelly S, Smith P, Sexton DJ, Kaye KS. Risk factors for 1-year mortality after postoperative mediastinitis. J Thorac Cardiovasc Surg 2006;132:537–43.

164 Lewis RT. Soft tissue infections. World J Surg 1998;22:146–51.

165 Widmer AF, Gaechter A, Ochsner PE, Zimmerli W. Antimicrobial treatment of orthopedic implant-related infections with rifampin combinations. Clin Infect Dis 1992;14:1251–3.

166 Kaye KS, Anderson DJ, Choi Y, Link K, Thacker P, Sexton DJ. The deadly toll of invasive methicillin-resistant *Staphylococcus aureus* infection in community hospitals. Clin Infect Dis 2008; 46:1568–77.

167 Weigelt J, Kaafarani HM, Itani KM, Swanson RN. Linezolid eradicates MRSA better than vancomycin from surgical-site infections. Am J Surg 2004;188:760–6.

168 Gerson SL, Kaplan SL, Bruss JB *et al.* Hematologic effects of linezolid: summary of clinical experience. Antimicrob Agents Chemother 2002;46:2723–6.

169 Arbeit RD, Maki D, Tally FP, Campanaro E, Eisenstein BI. The safety and efficacy of daptomycin for the treatment of complicated skin and skin-structure infections. Clin Infect Dis 2004;38:1673–81.

170 Ellis-Grosse EJ, Babinchak T, Dartois N, Rose G, Loh E. The efficacy and safety of tigecycline in the treatment of skin and skin-structure infections: results of 2 double-blind phase 3 comparison studies with vancomycin-aztreonam. Clin Infect Dis 2005;41(suppl 5):S341–S353.

171 Zimmerli W, Trampuz A, Ochsner PE. Prosthetic-joint infections. N Engl J Med 2004;351:1645–54.

172 El Oakley RM, Wright JE. Postoperative mediastinitis: classification and management. Ann Thorac Surg 1996;61:1030–6.

173 Brandt CM, Sistrunk WW, Duffy MC *et al. Staphylococcus aureus* prosthetic joint infection treated with debridement and prosthesis retention. Clin Infect Dis 1997;24:914–19.

174 Zimmerli W, Widmer AF, Blatter M, Frei R, Ochsner PE. Role of rifampin for treatment of orthopedic implant-related staphylococcal infections: a randomized controlled trial. Foreign-Body Infection (FBI) Study Group. JAMA 1998;279:1537–41.

175 Callaghan JJ, Katz RP, Johnston RC. One-stage revision surgery of the infected hip. A minimum 10-year followup study. Clin Orthop Relat Res 1999;369:139–43.

176 Youngman JR, Ridgway GL, Haddad FS. Antibiotic-loaded cement in revision joint replacement. Hosp Med 2003;64:613–16.

177 Owen MR, Moores AP, Coe RJ. Management of MRSA septic arthritis in a dog using a gentamicin-impregnated collagen sponge. J Small Anim Pract 2004;45:609–12.

178 Morykwas MJ, Argenta LC, Shelton-Brown EI, McGuirt W. Vacuum-assisted closure: a new method for wound control and treatment: animal studies and basic foundation. Ann Plast Surg 1997;38:553–62.

179 Heller L, Levin SL, Butler CE. Management of abdominal wound dehiscence using vacuum assisted closure in patients with compromised healing. Am J Surg 2006;191:165–72.

180 Schaffzin DM, Douglas JM, Stahl TJ, Smith LE. Vacuum-assisted closure of complex perineal wounds. Dis Colon Rectum 2004; 47:1745–8.

181 Noskin GA, Rubin RJ, Schentag JJ *et al.* The burden of *Staphylococcus aureus* infections on hospitals in the United States: an analysis of the 2000 and 2001 Nationwide Inpatient Sample Database. Arch Intern Med 2005;165:1756–61.

182 McGarry SA, Engemann JJ, Schmader K, Sexton DJ, Kaye KS. Surgical-site infection due to *Staphylococcus aureus* among elderly patients: mortality, duration of hospitalization, and cost. Infect Control Hosp Epidemiol 2004;25:461–7.

183 Engemann JJ, Carmeli Y, Cosgrove SE *et al.* Adverse clinical and economic outcomes attributable to methicillin resistance among patients with *Staphylococcus aureus* surgical site infection. Clin Infect Dis 2003;36:592–8.

184 Cosgrove SE, Qi Y, Kaye KS, Harbarth S, Karchmer AW, Carmeli Y. The impact of methicillin resistance in *Staphylococcus aureus* bacteremia on patient outcomes: mortality, length of stay, and hospital charges. Infect Control Hosp Epidemiol 2005;26: 166–74.

185 Cosgrove SE, Sakoulas G, Perencevich EN, Schwaber MJ, Karchmer AW, Carmeli Y. Comparison of mortality associated with methicillin-resistant and methicillin-susceptible *Staphylococcus aureus* bacteremia: a meta-analysis. Clin Infect Dis 2003;36:53–9.

186 Gleason TG, Crabtree TD, Pelletier SJ *et al.* Prediction of poorer prognosis by infection with antibiotic-resistant Gram-positive cocci than by infection with antibiotic-sensitive strains. Arch Surg 1999;134:1033–40.

187 Mekontso-Dessap A, Kirsch M, Brun-Buisson C, Loisance D. Poststernotomy mediastinitis due to *Staphylococcus aureus*:

comparison of methicillin-resistant and methicillin-susceptible cases. Clin Infect Dis 2001;32:877–83.

188 Mangram AJ, Horan TC, Pearson ML, Silver LC, Jarvis WR. Guideline for Prevention of Surgical Site Infection, 1999. Centers for Disease Control and Prevention (CDC) Hospital Infection Control Practices Advisory Committee. Am J Infect Control 1999;27:97–132; quiz 133–4; discussion 96.

189 Pryor KO, Fahey TJ III, Lien CA, Goldstein PA. Surgical site infection and the routine use of perioperative hyperoxia in a general surgical population: a randomized controlled trial. JAMA 2004;291:79–87.

190 Anon. Antimicrobial prophylaxis in surgery. Med Lett Drugs Ther 2001;43:92–7.

Chapter 18
Infections of Intravascular Catheters and Vascular Devices

Hidetaka Yanagi[1] *and Robert J. Sherertz*[2]
[1] Tokai University School of Medicine, Division of General Internal Medicine, Isehara, Kanagawa, Japan
[2] Wake Forest University School of Medicine, Section on Infectious Diseases, Winston-Salem, North Carolina, USA

Introduction

Infections involving intravascular devices are a leading cause of morbidity and mortality in hospitalized patients. Since such infections are the most common reason for device failure, an improved understanding of these infections can decrease morbidity, mortality, and healthcare costs. Various kinds of intravascular devices are currently in clinical use, and the use of each has been complicated by infection. The rates of infections vary significantly among the different devices [1–3] (Table 18.1). Recent data have shown that the incidence of catheter-related bloodstream infection (BSI) has been decreasing [4]. Increased use of evidence-based procedures and better understanding of the pathogenesis might have contributed to this improvement [5–7]. We discuss vascular catheters as the prototype of such devices since much more is known about them and some of the findings related to these devices are applicable to other intravascular devices.

Table 18.1 Device-related infections associated with devices other than central venous catheters.[1]

Type of device	Incidence of infection (%)
Peripheral venous catheter	0.08–1.9
Vena cava filters	Rare
Pacemakers	0.13–19.9
Defibrillators	0–3.2
Left ventricular assist device	25–70
Ventriculoatrial shunt	2.4–9.4
Atrial septal defect closure devices	Rare
Vascular graft including hemodialysis	1–6
Coronary artery stents	Rare
Intraaortic balloon pumps	5–26
Peripheral vascular stents	Rare
Pulmonary artery catheter	0–5.3
Peripheral arterial catheter	0–5.6

[1] Data from references 1–4.

Staphylococci in Human Disease, 2nd edition. Edited by Kent B. Crossley, Kimberly K. Jefferson, Gordon Archer, Vance G. Fowler, Jr.
 ISBN 978-14051-6332-3.

Central venous catheter-related infection

The most common cause of primary BSI is intravascular device-related infection [8]. In the USA it is estimated that 200 000–400 000 nosocomial BSIs occur each year [9] and that these infections may be responsible for at least 5000 deaths annually. The attributable cost of each catheter-associated BSI is reported to be approximately $11 971 [95% confidence interval (CI) $6732–$18 352], with a yearly impact in the USA estimated to be $1.8 billion [10]. Most central venous catheter (CVC)-related BSIs occur in patients in intensive care units (ICUs), followed by patients with long-term catheters placed for cancer and hemodialysis.

Staphylococci are the most common cause of CVC-related infection. *Staphylococcus aureus* CVC-related infections are felt to be more severe due to the frequency of hematogenous complications in patients with this infection. In contrast, coagulase-negative staphylococci (CoNS) are the most common cause of CVC-related infection but these infections are generally milder.

Epidemiology

Infections related to the use of intravascular devices account for 10–20% of all nosocomial infections. In one study, these infections increased ICU length of stay by 2.41 days (95% CI 0.08–3.09 days) and hospital length of stay by 7.54 days (95% CI 3.99–11.09 days) after adjusting for underlying severity of illness [11]. The crude mortality rates of patients with CVC-related BSIs range from 12 to 35% [12–14]; however, attributable mortality has been said to range from 0 to 10% [14].

Since 1970, the National Nosocomial Infection Surveillance System (NNIS) of the Centers for Disease Control and Prevention (CDC) has been gathering data on the incidence and etiologies of hospital-acquired BSIs. During 1992–2004, NNIS hospitals reported ICU rates of

Table 18.2 Pooled means of the distribution of central venous catheter-related bloodstream infection rates in hospitals reporting to the National Nosocomial Infection Surveillance System, January 2002 through June 2004.

Type of intensive care unit	Pooled mean per 1000 catheter-days
Coronary	3.5
Cardiothoracic	2.7
Medical	5.1
Major teaching hospitals	3.9
All others	3.3
Neurosurgical	4.6
Pediatric	6.6
Surgical	4.6
Trauma	7.4
Burn	7.0
Respiratory	4.8
Neonatal	
Weight ≤ 1000 g	9.1
Weight 1001–1500 g	5.4
Weight 1501–2500 g	4.1
Weight > 2500 g	3.5

CVC-associated BSI ranging from 2.7 (in a cardiothoracic ICU) to 9.1 (in a neonatal nursery for infants weighing < 1000 g) BSIs per 1000 CVC-days (Table 18.2) [4]. Infection rates are influenced by patient-related parameters (e.g., severity of illness, comorbid conditions), catheter-related parameters (e.g., catheter placement conditions, catheter type), and healthcare-related factors (e.g., hospital size, procedure volume, and skill of personnel in catheter insertion and maintenance) [15].

The types of organisms most frequently isolated in hospital-acquired BSIs vary over time. During 1986–1989, CoNS followed by *S. aureus* were the most frequently reported causes of BSIs, representing 27% and 16% of BSIs respectively [16]. Pooled data from 1992–1999 demonstrate that CoNS followed by enterococci were the most frequently isolated in hospital-acquired BSIs, accounting for 37.3% and 13.5% respectively. *Staphylococcus aureus* represented 12.6% of reported hospital-acquired BSIs during this period [17]. A recent prospective study from a cardiothoracic ICU found that CoNS followed by Gram-negative rods, *S. aureus*, and yeasts were the most frequently isolated causes of hospital-acquired BSIs, accounting for 37.9%, 24.1%, and 20.7%, respectively [18] (Table 18.3).

Table 18.3 Most common pathogens isolated from hospital-acquired bloodstream infections. (From Centers for Disease Control and Prevention [157] with permission.)

Pathogen (%)	1986–1989 (%)	1992–1999 (%)
Coagulase-negative staphylococci	27	37
Staphylococcus aureus	16	13
Enterococcus	8	13
Gram-negative rods	19	14
Escherichia coli	6	2
Enterobacter	5	5
Pseudomonas aeruginosa	4	4
Klebsiella pneumoniae	4	3
Candida spp.	8	8

Pathogenesis

In catheters placed for a short period (≤ 8 days), catheter colonization is most likely to result from skin microorganisms (75–90%), followed by the catheter hub/lumen (10–50%), hematogenous seeding (3–10%, but up to 50% in ICU patients), and infusate (2–3%) [19,20] (Figure 18.1). For long-term catheters (> 8 days), the source of colonization is most commonly the hub/lumen (66%) followed by the skin (26%). Several studies have demonstrated that

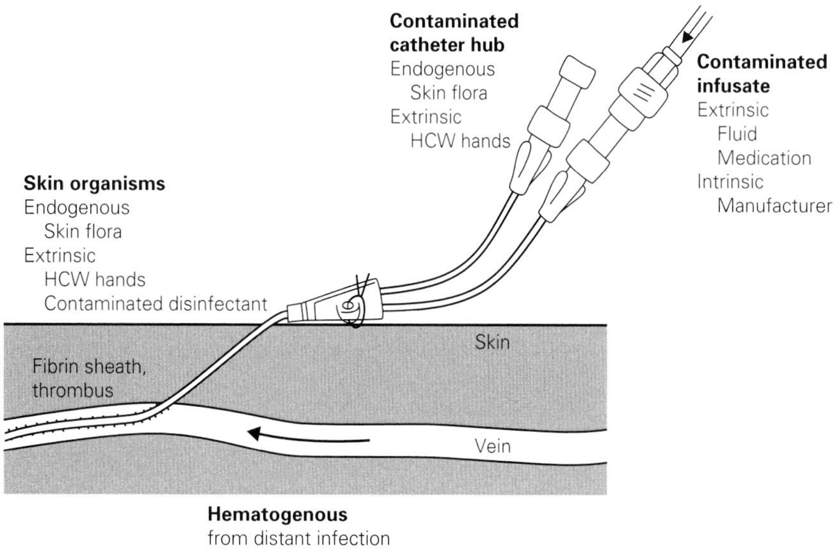

Figure 18.1 Sources of vascular catheter infection. HCW, healthcare worker. (From Crnich & Maki [155] with permission.)

Table 18.4 Risk factors for intravascular catheter-related infection.

Host factors	
	Extremes of age
	Immunosuppression
	Loss of skin integrity (burn, psoriasis, etc.)
	Staphylococcal colonization of the nose
	Severity of underlying diseases
	Distant infection
Catheter factors	
	Duration of catheterization
	Catheter composition and antimicrobial coating
	Catheter manipulation
	Site of insertion
	Type of dressing
	Insertion condition (sterile barriers, skin disinfection)
	Catheter care personnel
	Antithrombotics
Microbial factors	
	S. aureus MSCRAMMs
	S. epidermidis polysaccharide intercellular adhesins
	Small-colony variants

MSCRAMMs, microbial surface components recognizing adhesive matrix molecules.

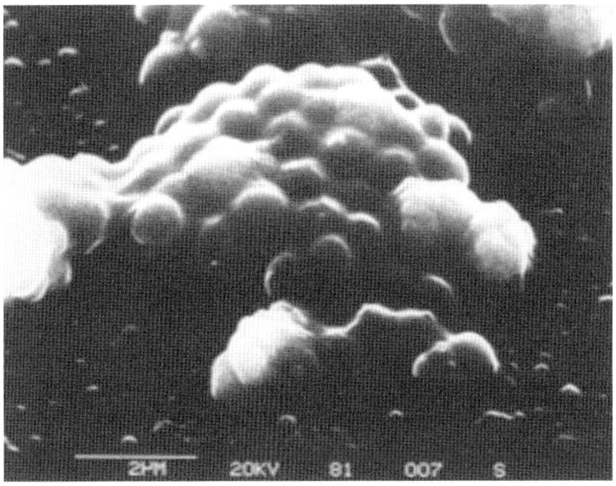

Figure 18.2 Vascular catheter biofilm showing staphylococci in association with proteins and glycocalyx. (From von Eiff *et al.* [156] with permission.)

clinical findings correlate well with quantitative catheter cultures, and that the more microorganisms isolated from the surface of the catheter, the greater the likelihood of insertion site erythema and/or catheter-related BSIs [21–24].

Factors affecting catheter colonization and infection include those that relate to the host, the catheter, and the causative microorganism [25] (Table 18.4). Although most host factors cannot generally be altered, intravascular catheter infection has been associated with modifiable factors including catheter- and operator-associated factors. Silicone catheters have a greater risk of infection than catheters made of other materials. This is thought to be related to excessive complement activation [19]. Unfortunately, there is no good alternative material to silicone for long-term catheters. In addition, certain catheter materials, such as silicone, are more prone to thrombosis than others, which might predispose to catheter colonization and catheter-related infection [20]. A number of studies have demonstrated that heparin-bonded catheters reduce catheter-related thrombosis and catheter-related infection [26]. However, in these studies heparin is attached to the catheter via benzalkonium chloride, which has antibacterial activity and may be responsible for the reduction in infection rates [20]. Other modifiable factors include infection control interventions such as use of maximum sterile barriers, chlorhexidine skin preparation, antiinfective catheter coatings, and antiinfective flush solutions [19]. These are discussed in the section on prevention.

Microbial adherence to a biomaterial is an early essential event in the pathogenesis of a prosthetic device infection [27]. The process of adherence can be divided into four stages: attachment, adhesion, aggregation, and dispersion. The stages of adhesion and aggregation are mediated by specific adhesin–receptor interactions. Both *S. aureus* and *Staphylococus epidermidis* possess unique factors that predispose to intravascular device-related infections. *Staphylococcus aureus* can adhere to host proteins (e.g., fibronectin, fibrinogen, fibrin, collagen, bone sialoprotein, laminin, elastin, and extracellular matrix protein) commonly present on intravascular catheters [28]. In contrast, *S. epidermidis* adheres to polymer surfaces more readily than do other pathogens [29]. Most strains of both *S. aureus* and *S. epidermidis* produce an extracellular polysaccharide often referred to as biofilm (Figure 18.2). Initial attachment appears to occur via a protein autolysin. Subsequent adherence and biofilm formation are mediated by polysaccharide intercellular adhesin (PIA) [30]. In a rat model, *S. epidermidis* isolates lacking protein autolysin or PIA are significantly less likely to cause catheter infection, bacteremia, and metastatic infection [31]. Interestingly, the *ica* operon encoding PIA in *S. epidermidis* can also be found in *S. aureus* isolates from patients with catheter-related infection [32]. The *ica* locus appears to be regulated by the *agr* quorum-sensing system. Isolates of *S. aureus* that are *agr*-positive are much less likely to form biofilms than *agr*-negative strains (78% vs. 6%) [33,34].

A variant subpopulation of *S. aureus* has been reported to be defective in electron transport [35]. These bacteria grow slowly and are referred to as small-colony variants. These have been associated with persistent infections and are more resistant to many antibiotics. When an infection is unusually resistant to therapy, persistent for a long time, or fails apparently adequate antimicrobial therapy, clinicians should consider these strains [36–38].

Clinical manifestation and diagnosis

Clinical findings are not sufficient for establishing the diagnosis of intravascular device-related infection because of their poor specificity and sensitivity [39,40]. The most common and sensitive clinical findings, such as fever with or without chills, have poor specificity, whereas erythema, fluctuance, or purulence around the catheter insertion site have better specificity but poor sensitivity. The presence of inflammation may be helpful for diagnosis of peripheral catheter-related infections but is rare in CVC-related infections. Maki *et al.* [41] reported that local signs of inflammation were present in only 64% of catheters that were positive on semiquantitative culture, and in as many as 18% of culture-negative ones. If there is no laboratory confirmation, cure of sepsis syndrome or decrease in fever after removal of the catheter in question from a patient with BSI may suggest catheter-related infection [42]. Blood cultures positive for *S. aureus*, CoNS, or *Candida* in any catheterized patient should increase suspicion of catheter-related BSIs [39,43,44]. Patients with catheter-tip cultures positive for *S. aureus* have a high risk of developing bacteremia, whereas those catheters positive for CoNS do not [45].

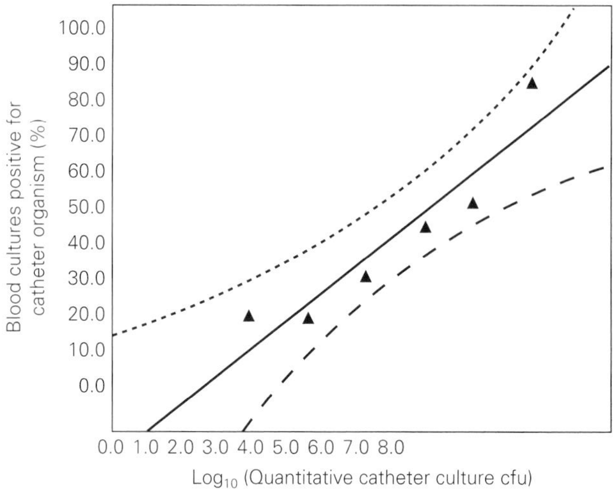

Figure 18.3 Quantitative relationship between the number of organisms removed from catheters by sonication and the frequency of positive blood cultures for the same organisms. The solid line is the linear regression line; the dashed lines are 95% confidence limits. (From Sherertz *et al.* [21] with permission.)

Intravenous catheter cultures

Conventionally, a definite diagnosis of catheter-related infection requires removal of the catheter or a guidewire exchange for culture of the catheter tip. Qualitative broth culture of the catheter tip was the only method available until 1977. Broth cultures are highly sensitive, and have high negative predictive value when they are sterile in the absence of antibiotic therapy. Unfortunately, they have a high frequency of false-positive diagnoses of catheter-related infection [41]. Therefore, this method is not recommended [39].

Semiquantitative (roll plate) or quantitative (vortex or sonication) catheter culture techniques are the most reliable diagnostic methodologies. They have greater specificity in the identification of catheter-related infection compared with qualitative cultures [46]. A study looking at 780 catheter-tip cultures in critically ill patients demonstrated that the sensitivity and specificity were 92% and 83%, respectively, with a negative predictive value of 99.8% when 5 cfu or more was used to define a positive result [47]. Using a threshold of 15 and 50 cfu, Rello *et al.* [48] reported that sensitivity and specificity were satisfactory, but the positive predictive value remained less than 50% irrespective of the thresholds. Quantitative catheter-tip culture methods using vortexing in sterile water with a threshold of 10^3 cfu/mL was reported to be 97.5% sensitive and 88% specific for the diagnosis of catheter-related infections [23]. Sherertz *et al.* [21] reported that another technique utilizing sonication to dislodge microorganisms from the catheter had similar excellent sensitivity and specificity (Figure 18.3). As the use of antimicrobial-coated catheters becomes more common, the current definitions of catheter colonization and catheter-related infection may need to be modified, since these coatings could result in false-negative cultures [49].

Guidewire exchange of CVCs suspicious for catheter-related infection with subsequent culture has been proposed as a compromise solution. If the first catheter is found to be significantly colonized, the second catheter can be removed and a new line inserted at a new site. Guidewire exchange can avoid mechanical complications associated with puncture of a new site [42], and has been shown not to increase patient risk in at least one randomized clinical trial [50].

Quantitative blood cultures of peripheral and CVC blood samples

Quantitative blood culture techniques (without removal of catheters) have been developed as an alternative for diagnosis of catheter-related infection, especially in patients with limited vascular access. This technique utilizes quantitative culture of paired blood samples, one obtained via the catheter hub and the other through a peripheral venipuncture site. Several studies using this method have demonstrated that a significant differential colony count of 2–10 : 1 for the CVC versus the peripheral vein culture is indicative of catheter-related infection, with a specificityof 90–100% and a sensitivity of approximately 80% [51–54]. Moreover, Capdevila *et al.* [52] showed that among tunneled catheters, a quantitative blood culture from the CVC with at least 100 cfu/mL may be diagnostic without a simultaneously taken peripheral blood culture. This technique is currently rarely used in clinical practice, primarily because it is relatively labor-intensive and expensive.

Differential time to positivity for CVC versus peripheral blood cultures

This new method has a good correlation with quantitative blood cultures when the blood obtained for culture through a catheter becomes positive 2 hours or more before the peripheral blood culture. Blot *et al.* [55] showed that there is a linear relationship between the initial concentration of various microorganisms and the time to positivity of cultures, and the differential time to positivity (DTP) has 100% specificity and 96.4% sensitivity when a cutoff limit of 120 min was chosen. This method resulted in comparative accuracy to quantitative blood cultures and had greater cost-effectiveness when investigated in both tunneled and nontunneled catheters in cancer patients. DTP had a sensitivity of 81% and a specificity of 92% for short-term catheters and a sensitivity of 93% and a specificity of 75% for long-term catheters. The specificity was reduced in patients being treated with antibiotics at the time of the cultures [56,57]. The DTP approach offers a significant advantage over catheter culture methods [58], and has good sensitivity and specificity [59].

Management of catheter-related infections

Systemic antibiotics

The initial antibiotic choice should be based on the severity of illness, the risk factors for infection, the anticipated pathogen, and local microbiological susceptibility data. Vancomycin is usually recommended because of the frequency of CoNS and *S. aureus* as causes of catheter-associated infection. Further empirical coverage for enteric Gram-negative rods and *Pseudomonas aeruginosa* is often required.

There are no compelling data to support specific recommendations in terms of the duration of therapy for catheter-related infections except for *S. aureus* infections. These issues are discussed in detail in the consensus catheter infection management paper by Mermel *et al.* [39]. If there is an immediate response to initial empiric therapy, most immunocompetent patients without underlying valvular heart disease or an intravascular prosthetic device can be treated for 10–14 days of antimicrobial treatment after removal of the catheter(s) for pathogens other than CoNS and *S. aureus*. Since CoNS are usually intrinsically resistant to multiple antibiotics, empiric therapy with vancomycin should be started and may be changed to semisynthetic penicillin depending on the susceptibility pattern [39,60]. If the CVC is removed, the duration of systemic antibiotic therapy for CoNS is generally 5–7 days.

For *S. aureus* catheter-related BSIs, β-lactam antibiotics should be used if possible [61,62]. If a patient is allergic to penicillin without anaphylaxis or angioedema, a first-generation cephalosporin can be used. Those with anaphylactic reactions to β-lactam antibiotics can be treated with vancomycin, linezolid, quinupristin–dalfopristin, or daptomycin. Daptomycin is approved by the Food and Drug Administration for the treatment of bacteremia and right-sided endocarditis due to methicillin-sensitive *S. aureus* or methicillin-resistant *S. aureus* (MRSA) [63].

While the optimal duration of treatment for *S. aureus* catheter-related BSIs is unknown, Rosen *et al.* [64] suggested in a cost-effectiveness study on the duration of treatment for intravascular catheter-associated *S. aureus* bacteremia that treating selected patients for 2 weeks instead of 4–6 weeks was safe if the patient had negative transesophageal echocardiography. However, definitive guidelines await an adequately designed randomized clinical trial.

Removal of the catheter

Catheter removal should be considered in most patients with catheter-related BSIs. However, nontunneled CVCs in patients with fever and mild to moderate disease do not necessarily need to be removed. Rijnders *et al.* [50] studied 80 ICU patients with suspected catheter-related infections in a randomized trial and reported that there was no significant difference in outcomes between the group receiving standard of care and that receiving watchful waiting, and there was a 60% reduction in the number of catheters removed in the watchful waiting group. However, if blood culture results are positive or if the catheter has been exchanged over a guidewire and the tip culture is positive by quantitative or semiquantitative cultures, then the catheter should be removed and a new one inserted at a different site [65].

Benjamin *et al.* [66] studied pediatric patients with catheter-related BSIs and found that infants who had four blood cultures positive for CoNS were at significantly increased risk for end-organ damage and death, compared with those who had three or fewer positive blood cultures for CoNS (odds ratio 29.58). These authors recommended that the catheter be removed once a neonate has three or more positive blood cultures for CoNS.

Surgically implantable vascular devices, such as Hickman, Broviac or Groshong catheters or a Portacath, are usually hard to remove. It is therefore important to be convinced that the patient has a true catheter-related BSI rather than colonization or infection at another site. One should not remove the tunneled catheter only because the patient is febrile and one of the blood cultures is positive for CoNS. In this case, one should repeat blood cultures to ensure that it is a true catheter-related BSI [23,67]. Findings consistent with BSI caused by CoNS include multiple positive blood cultures, quantitative blood cultures drawn from a catheter with 100 cfu/mL or more, isolation of the same microorganisms from catheter-tip and percutaneous blood cultures, and a DTP of more than 2 hours [56,68]. In patients with catheter-related BSI secondary to CoNS without evidence of persistent bacteremia or local metastatic complications, the catheter can be retained with an approximate 80% success rate [69].

For patients with *S. aureus* catheter-related BSIs, removal of vascular catheters has been associated with a more rapid response to therapy and a higher cure rate in observational studies [70–72]. The exception might be a patient with a long-term tunneled catheter infected with *S. aureus*, negative transesophageal echocardiography, and prompt clearing of blood cultures after initiation of antibiotic therapy. In this case, intravenous antibiotics in combination with antibiotic lock therapy could potentially result in clinical cure and catheter salvage [73].

Patients with complicated device infections, such as tunnel infection or port abscess, need removal of the catheter and an adequate course of antibiotic therapy. Patients with septic thrombosis or infective endocarditis require removal of the catheter and 4–6 weeks of antibiotic treatment. Patients with osteomyelitis require removal of the catheter and 6–8 weeks of antibiotic therapy [74].

AIDS has been reported to be an adverse prognostic factor in patients with *S. aureus* bacteremia, and a longer course of therapy has been recommended for such patients [75,76].

Antibiotic lock therapy

Eradication of microorganisms from the surface of the catheter is often impossible. Bacteria on the catheter surface aggregate in a hydrated polymeric matrix of their own synthesis to form biofilm, and are then resistant to the host immune response and the activity of antimicrobials [77,78].

Antibiotic lock therapy provides a new approach to treatment without removing the catheter: parenteral antibiotics are infused through the catheter and then "locked" into the catheter in a supratherapeutic concentration over a 12-hour period. Several open trials of antibiotic lock therapy of tunneled catheter-related bacteremia, with or without concomitant parenteral therapy, have reported a response and catheter salvage without recurrence in 138 (82.6%) of 167 episodes. In comparison with administration of parenteral antibiotics alone, treatment including antibiotic lock therapy was significantly associated with catheter salvage (relative risk 1.24, 95% CI 1.13–1.36; $P = 0.0001$) [39]. Usually, antibiotic solutions containing the appropriate antimicrobial agents in a concentration of 1–5 mg/L are locked in the catheter lumen during periods when the catheter is not in use [79–82]. Vancomycin has been used at a concentration of 1–5 mg/mL. The usual duration of antibiotic lock therapy has been 2 weeks.

In an *in vitro* study, Raad *et al.* [83] reported that minocycline, daptomycin, and tigecycline were more efficacious in inhibiting MRSA in biofilm than linezolid, vancomycin, and the negative control ($P < 0.001$) after the first day of exposure to lock therapy with these antibiotics. When rifampin was used alone, it was the least effective in eradicating MRSA in biofilm, as it was associated with the emergence of resistance. However, when rifampin was used in combination with other antibiotics, the combinations were significantly more effective in rapidly eliminating MRSA in biofilim than each of the antibiotics alone.

In addition, combination lock therapy with antibiotics and ethanol may be useful. Sherertz *et al.* [84] examined the relative efficacies of vancomycin, ciprofloxacin, minocycline, minocycline–rifampin, ciprofloxacin–rifampin, vancomycin–rifampin, ethanol, ethylenediaminetetraacetic acid (EDTA), minocycline–EDTA, and taurolidine (2%)–polyvinylpyrrolidone (5%) at killing *S. aureus*, *S. epidermidis*, *P. aeruginosa*, and *Candida albicans* growing in biofilms. Minocycline–EDTA, taurolidine (2%)–polyvinylpyrrolidone (5%), and ethanol were significantly more active than traditional lock solutions of minocycline, rifampin, ciprofloxacin, and vancomycin. In another *in vitro* study, Raad *et al.* [85] studied the activity of minocycline, EDTA, and 25% ethanol, alone or in combination, against MRSA and *Candida parapsilosis* catheter-related BSI strains in an established model of biofilm colonization. They found that minocycline–EDTA in 25% ethanol was highly effective at rapidly eradicating *S. aureus* and *C. parapsilosis* embedded in biofilm adhering to catheter segments.

The first randomized controlled trial examining the efficacy of antibiotic lock therapy by Rijnders *et al.* [86] demonstrated that failure to cure the catheter-related BSI occurred in 33% (7 of 22) in the antibiotic lock therapy arm and in 57% (13 of 23) in the placebo arm (hazard ratio 0.55; $P = 0.10$). A relapse with the same strain occurred in 3 of 21 in the treatment arm and 9 of 23 in the placebo group ($P = 0.06$). Fortun *et al.* [87] retrospectively studied 48 episodes of catheter-related bacteremia in patients with Hickman catheters or totally implantable reservoirs using vancomycin for Gram-positive infections and ciprofloxacin or gentamicin for Gram-negative bacilli. They reported that successful treatment was achieved in 84% in the antibiotic lock treatment group and in 65% in the control group ($P = 0.27$). However, antibiotic lock therapy was successful in 93% of episodes caused by CoNS, whereas failure was observed in two-thirds of *S. aureus* catheter-related bacteremia.

Dannenberg *et al.* [88] used systemic antibiotics in combination with ethanol to treat 24 episodes of catheter-related infections and compared this therapy with 15 episodes treated with systemic antibiotics alone. The ethanol-lock technique consists of filling and closing the catheter lumen with 74% ethanol solution for 20–24 hours. They reported that 67% of the ethanol group had no relapse after 4 weeks compared with 47% of the control group. No severe clinical side effects associated with ethanol-lock therapy were observed even in children. In another retrospective study of pediatric patients with persistent bacteremia associated with long-term intravascular devices, Onland *et al.* [89] demonstrated that of 51 ethanol-lock treatments in 40 children, no catheters were removed because of persistent infection, 88% (45 of 51) of the treated

Table 18.5 Summary of the efficacy of approaches to prevent catheter-related bloodstream infections: incidence per 1000 catheter-days.

Intervention	Control	Treatment	*P*	Reference
Education	3.3	2.4	< 0.001	Sherertz *et al.* [6]
Evidence-based interventions	2.7	0	< 0.002	Pronovost *et al.* [5]
Education based on CDC guidelines	45.9	9.9	< 0.001	Rosenthal *et al.* [92]
Self-study module	4.9	2.1	0.03	Warren *et al.* [90]
Vancomycin/heparin lock solution	17.8	2.3	0.005	Garland *et al.* [120]
Second-generation CSS catheter	24.1	13.3	< 0.01	Rupp *et al.* [128]
Minocycline–rifampin catheter	3.1	0.7	0.02	Hanna *et al.* [131]

CSS, chlorhexidine–silver sulfadiazine.

episodes cleared without recurrence, and 12 of 16 (75%) polymicrobial infections and 33 of 35 (94%) monomicrobial ones were successfully treated. There were no adverse reactions reported. Based on these studies, a prospective randomized study should be designed to establish the efficacy of the ethanol-lock technique in the treatment of device-related BSIs.

Prevention

For effective prevention, a basic understanding of the underlying mechanisms is essential. These include the pathogenesis and epidemiology as well as risk factors and have been discussed previously in this chapter. Other important ways to reduce the frequency of these infections include the following (Table 18.5).

Quality assurance and continuing education

Continuing education of healthcare workers involved in catheterization has been demonstrated to be beneficial in preventing catheter-related infection [5,6,90–92]. Sherertz *et al.* [6] reported that a 1-day course educating physicians in training about infection control practices and procedures of vascular access insertion resulted in a reduction of the infection rate from 3.3 to 2.4 per 1000 CVC-days. Eggimann *et al.* [91] demonstrated that implementation of a comprehensive educational strategy directed at reduction of catheter-related infections in ICU patients led to a reduction in incidence density of BSIs from 11.3 to 3.8 episodes per 1000 patients-days (relative risk 0.33, 95% CI 0.20–0.56). In a recent prospective study investigating the use of five evidence-based procedures (hand-washing, using full barrier precautions during insertion of CVCs, cleaning the skin with chlorhexidine, avoiding the femoral site if possible, and removing unnecessary catheters), Pronovost *et al.* [5] demonstrated that the intervention resulted in a large and sustained reduction in the median rates of catheter-related BSI from 2.7 infections per 1000 catheter-days at baseline to zero at 3 months after implementation of the study intervention ($P \leq 0.002$).

On the other hand, insertion and maintenance of intravascular catheters by inexperienced staff can increase the risk for catheter colonization and catheter-related BSIs, although the efficacy of dedicated teams for intravenous catheter insertion and maintenance has not been established [93,94]. It has been demonstrated that infection risk might increase with nursing staff reduction below a critical level [95]. Giving treatment advice semiautomatically via an email increased compliance with the Infectious Disease Society of America's catheter-related infection guideline. Rijnders *et al.* [96] used email to distribute treatment advice for catheter-related infection, which increased compliance from 66% to 85% ($P < 0.01$).

The situation with peripheral arterial lines appears to be different from that with CVCs. Rijnders *et al.* [97] reported that full sterile barriers did not reduce the risk of infection in a randomized trial studying the use of full sterile barriers in 373 patients requiring arterial lines inserted in the radial or dorsalis pedis arteries. This might suggest that contamination of arterial catheters does not commonly occur at the time of insertion with minimal sterile technique unlike with CVCs.

Site of catheter insertion

The internal jugular vein has been associated with a lower risk of mechanical complication but a higher risk for infection, whereas the opposite holds for the subclavian vein, although no randomized trial has satisfactorily compared these catheter sites [98,99]. Femoral catheters have been associated with a higher risk for deep venous thrombosis than internal jugular or subclavian catheters [100–102]. Nahum *et al.* [103] evaluated the efficacy of a subcutaneous tunnel for femoral catheters in a randomized trial in 98 children in a cardiac care unit. The authors found that subcutaneous tunneling of CVCs in the femoral site is a safe procedure and significantly decreases the rate of CVC colonization, although there was no difference in catheter-related infection rates. Timsit *et al.* [104] found similar results in adult patients, and reported a significant reduction in colonization as well as catheter-related bacteremia ($P < 0.05$). Two studies of heparin-bonded femoral catheters found a significant reduction in catheter colonization, catheter-related bacteremia, and catheter-associated thrombosis [26,105]. Further study will be needed to determine which approach would be better.

Cutaneous antisepsis

The use of 2% chlorhexidine-based preparations is recommended as a result of several studies showing a greater efficacy of chlorhexidine over povidone-iodine [106–108].

Catheter site dressings

A large controlled trial studying peripheral catheters demonstrated that the rate of colonization among catheters covered with transparent dressings (5.7%) is comparable to that of those dressed with gauze (4.6%) [109]. A metaanalysis also showed that there is no difference in the risk for catheter-related BSIs between transparent and gauze dressings [110].

Antimicrobial prophylaxis

Systemic antimicrobial prophylaxis during catheter insertion is still debatable. Two studies examined vancomycin prophylaxis, both of which demonstrated a reduction in morbidity but not in mortality [111,112]. A recent metaanalysis also showed that vancomycin or teicoplanin decreased the risk for Gram-positive infections [113]. However, because the prophylactic use of vancomycin is an important risk factor for selection of vancomycin-resistant enterococci, routine use of systemic antibiotics cannot be recommended [15].

Antibiotic/antiseptic ointments

In a randomized trial, the use of topical povidone-iodine ointment at the catheter insertion site in 129 patients on hemodialysis resulted in reduction in the incidence of catheter-related BSIs [114]. In a recent study, Johnson *et al.* [115] demonstrated in 50 hemodialysis patients with tunneled cuffed catheters that mupirocin ointment applied to the catheter site three times a week was associated with a significantly lower rate of catheter-related bacteremia (7% vs. 35%; $P < 0.01$), even in patients without prior nasal colonization with *S. aureus*. Moreover, significant mupirocin resistance was not seen. Use of polyantibiotic ointment (consisting of polymyxin, neomycin, and bacitracin) led to indeterminate results, although its use was associated with an increased frequency of *Candida* colonization [15,116].

Anticoagulants/thrombolytics

A metaanalysis evaluating the benefit of heparin prophylaxis in patients with short-term catheters reported a decrease in the incidence of catheter-associated thrombosis but not catheter-related infection [117]. In patients with long-term CVCs, low-dose warfarin has been shown to reduce the incidence of catheter thrombosis but not the incidence of catheter-related BSIs [118]. Urokinase catheter flushes do not reduce the risk of infection [119].

Antibiotic lock prophylaxis

Although there have been studies showing the efficacy of vancomycin lock prophylaxis in high-risk cancer patients and ICU patients, it is not routinely recommended because of increased risk for selection of vancomycin-resistant enterococci [120–122]. Minocycline–EDTA used as a flush solution reduced the risk of catheter-related bacteremia. In a randomized controlled trial, Bleyer *et al.* found that in 60 patients undergoing hemodialysis through catheters, those who was randomized to minocycline and EDTA did better than those to heparin as a flush solution in terms of significant catheter colonization (1 of 11 vs. 9 of 14, respectively; $P = 0.005$).

In a randomized controlled trial investigating the efficacy of a citrate/taurolidine-containing lock solution in hemodialysis patients, Betjes and van Agteren [123] found that although there was no difference in the incidence of catheter colonization, four cases with sepsis occurred in the control group as opposed to no sepsis episodes in the citrate/taurolidine-treated group. In another recent study, Allon [124] reported that use of a taurolidine/citrate lock solution was associated with an increase in the bacteremia-free survival of catheters at 90 days in hemodialysis patients.

A recent review and metaanalysis reported a significant reduction in the frequency of BSI where antimicrobial lock solutions were used. Development of resistance was documented in 1 of 924 patients. Trials with nonantimicrobial solutions (e.g., citrate) were more difficult to assess because of the use of other preventive measures (e.g., mupirocin nasal decolonization) [125].

Antimicrobial/antiseptic-impregnated catheters

The two best-studied catheters in clinical use are the catheter impregnated with chlorhexidine and silver sulfadiazine and the catheter coated with minocycline and rifampin.

Chlorhexidine–silver sulfadiazine catheters

A first-generation catheter is coated with chlorhexidine and silver sulfadiazine only on the external luminal surface. A metaanalysis showed that these catheters reduced the risk of catheter-related bacteremia with a summary odds ratio of 0.56 (95% CI 0.37–0.84; $P = 0.005$) [126]. A second-generation catheter is coated with chlorhexidine and silver sulfadiazine on both the internal and external luminal surfaces. The external surface coating of chlorhexidine is combined with silver sulfadiazine, while the internal surface is coated with chlorhexidine alone. A cost-effectiveness analysis suggested that the use of chlorhexidine–silver sulfadiazine catheters should lead to cost savings of $68–391 per catheter [127]. In a recent multicenter, randomized, controlled trial examining 780 patients in ICUs, Rupp *et al.* [128] found that use of second-generation chlorhexidine–silver sulfadiazine catheters was associated with a reduced incidence of catheter colonization (24.1 vs. 13.3 colonized catheters per 1000 catheter-days;

$P < 0.01$). However, there was no difference in the incidence of catheter-related BSI.

Minocycline–rifampin catheters

In a multicenter randomized trial, Darouiche *et al.* [129] found that catheters impregnated with minocycline and rifampin were associated with lower rates of catheter-related bacteremia. These catheters were one-third as likely to be colonized as catheters impregnated with chlorhexidine and silver sulfadiazine only on the external surface [28 of 356 (7.9%) vs. 87 of 382 (22.8%); $P < 0.001$], and catheter-related BSI was only one-twelfth as likely in catheters impregnated with minocycline and rifampin compared with those impregnated with chlorhexidine and silver sulfadiazine [1 of 356 (0.3%) vs. 13 of 382 (3.4%); $P < 0.002$]. A prospective surveillance study investigating patients in ICUs demonstrated that use of catheters impregnated with minocycline and rifampin was associated with a significant decrease in nosocomial BSIs. The rate of nosocomial BSI decreased from 8.3 to 3.5 per 1000 patient-days ($P < 0.01$) in the medical ICU [130]. The same group conducted a prospective randomized trial examining the efficacy of long-term catheters impregnated with minocycline and rifampin in cancer patients and found that use of these catheters resulted in a catheter-related BSI rate of 0.25 per 1000 catheter-days compared with 1.28 per 1000 catheter-days in the control group ($P = 0.003$) [131]. Although resistance to minocycline or rifampin was not observed in clinical trials, this remains a concern since an *in vitro* study suggested this possibility [132].

Infections associated with hemodialysis

Infections are the second leading cause of mortality among this population. Many of these infections are due to sepsis, primarily arising from the vascular access site. Bacteremia alone represents almost 11% of mortality in hemodialysis patients [133]. The type of vascular access used in this setting includes native arteriovenous fistulas, arteriovenous grafts, permanent or temporary catheters, and implanted port devices [134].

Epidemiology

The incidence of hemodialysis access-associated bacteremia has recently ranged from 0.31 to 1.2 infections per 1000 patient-days [135,136]. Older age, uninsured, having Medicaid insurance, a history of hospitalization, HIV infection, and previous history of bacteremia were associated with a higher risk of bacteremia [137,138]. The primary risk factor for access-associated infection is access type. Risk is highest for catheters, intermediate for grafts, and lowest for native arteriovenous fistulas [137]. Placement of a fistula or grafts should be pursued whenever possible instead of CVCs for permanent vascular access in dialysis patients. However, catheter use increased from 13% in 1995 to 26% in 2002, despite the effort to reduce the number of patients dialyzed through catheters [139].

The majority of bacteremias associated with hemodialysis catheters are due to *S. aureus* (32%) or CoNS (32%), followed by Gram-negative bacilli (18%) and nonstaphylococcal Gram-positive cocci including enterococci (12%) [135]. The increasing prevalence of antimicrobial resistance has been an issue in hemodialysis patients. In the USA, the majority of the patients with vancomycin-intermediate *S. aureus* had received dialysis, and the first patient reported to be infected with vancomycin-resistant *S. aureus* was a hemodialysis patient [140,141].

Clinical manifestations and diagnosis

Clinical manifestations include erythema, edema, exudate, induration, purulence, fever, chills, and hypotension. Drainage from the exit site should be sent for culture. Two sets of blood culture should be obtained, one through the catheter and the other through a peripheral vein before antimicrobial therapy is started. However, avoidance of peripheral venipuncture in hemodialysis patients may be considered because it might preclude placement of a new arteriovenous fistula at the venipuncture site [142].

Management

Initial empiric antimicrobial therapy should be directed against both Gram-positive and Gram-negative microorganisms, given the immunocompromised status of hemodialysis patients. Vancomycin is usually necessary because of the high prevalence of MRSA in most dialysis units. Subsequent directed therapy should be based on blood culture results. If the blood culture is positive for a β-lactam-susceptible microorganism, vancomycin should be discontinued, and nafcillin, oxacillin or cefazolin should be used unless contraindicated because vancomycin has been associated with a higher rate of treatment failure and recurrence [62]. Management of bacteremia associated with indwelling cuffed hemodialysis catheters has been controversial. Attempts to salvage catheters in such patients with systemic antimicrobial therapy alone are rarely successful [143]. If the causative organism is *S. aureus*, tunneled hemodialysis catheters should be removed, and duration of antimicrobial therapy should be determined as discussed previously. CoNS can be treated without removal of the catheter if the patient is not critically ill, subsequent blood cultures became negative quickly, and there is no evidence of infectious complications.

Prevention

The most basic strategy for prevention of catheter-related BSI is to minimize the use of catheters. General preventive measures, such as keeping maximal sterile barriers when inserting the catheter, hold for hemodialysis patients as well. Other selected recommendations for prevention of hemodialysis catheter-related BSI include the following.

- Use the catheter exclusively for hemodialysis, unless there is no alternative.
- Ensure optimal adequacy of hemodialysis.
- Prevent or treat malnutrition.
- Maintain optimum hemoglobin concentration.
- Avoid iron overload.
- Use a dialysis membrane that causes the lowest degree of complement and leukocyte activation.
- Administer nasal mupirocin in documented *S. aureus* carriers who have had an *S. aureus* catheter-related bacteremia and continue to need the hemodialysis catheter.
- Apply povidone-iodine or mupirocin ointment at the catheter site unless incompatible with the catheter material.
- An antibiotic lock solution may be used when there is a history of multiple catheter-related BSIs [134,144].

Vascular graft infection

The development of a synthetic arterial prosthesis was a great advance in vascular surgery, with which complex revascularization can be performed with good long-term clinical outcome. However, arterial graft infection continues to be a challenging issue [145]. The pathogenesis of infections of vascular grafts is similar to that of other intravascular device-related infections. Staphylococci are inoculated into the wound during the surgery, adhere to the prosthesis, proliferate in the local environment of the foreign body, and cause a clinical infection. It has been shown that contamination of the graft and native arterial wall with staphylococci is common during surgery [146]. Both contiguous spread and hematogenous seeding can occur [2].

Epidemiology

The incidence of prosthetic vascular graft infection is variable depending on the anatomic location of the device. For aortic grafts limited to the abdomen, graft-related infections occur in 1% or less of recipients. The incidence of infection is higher (1.5–2%) for aortic grafts extending to the femoral location. Infrainguinal vascular grafts originating in the groin are at highest risk for infection (6%). The most common pathogens isolated from infected grafts are *S. aureus* (43–64%) and *S. epidermidis* (up to 14%) [147,148]. Especially in late-onset infections, less virulent organisms that are part of the normal skin flora such as *Corynebacterium* spp. and *Propionibacterium acnes* can be the causative pathogens.

Clinical manifestations and diagnosis

The clinical presentation of vascular graft infection is variable. In early graft infections, local inflammatory findings indicating surgical-site infection are present. Even when these findings appear to be limited to superficial soft tissue structures overlaying the graft, graft infection should be included in the differential diagnosis. Abscess formation, sinus tract formation, hemorrhage, graft occlusion, pseudoaneurysm, graft exposure, and poor tissue incorporation can develop. Septic emboli and distal tissue ischemia may also be seen. Systemic signs of sepsis can accompany the local findings, particularly when more aggressive pathogens, including *S. aureus*, are present. On the other hand, late graft infection is characterized less often by systemic toxicity. Significant and sometimes fatal delays in diagnosis are not uncommon in these cases [149]. Cutaneous sinus tracts, lack of graft incorporation by surrounding tissue, anastomotic aneurysm, and graft-enteric erosions or fistula may occur. Hemorrhage can develop and be life-threatening. For one-third of patients, the clinical presentation of anastomotic pseudoaneurysm is an emergency in terms of threat to life or limb.

Computed tomography (CT) is the diagnostic test of choice for infected grafts [150]. However, magnetic resonance imaging (MRI) has also been proposed as a technique for determining the presence of graft infection. Due to its ability to distinguish between fluid and surrounding tissue and to provide information about inflammation, it may become the preferred method for diagnosing graft infection. In a study comparing the usefulness of MRI and CT, MRI was demonstrated to be superior to CT for detecting the presence and the extension of prosthetic graft infection [151].

Management

For patients with vascular graft infection, the initial treatment should be directed at sepsis control and reestablishment of flow to the distal tissue [152]. Complete graft excision along with surrounding tissue débridement is the most effective treatment strategy in eliminating the source of infection. Treatment strategies of revascularization following graft excision have been controversial and included extraanatomic bypass grafting, *in situ* prosthetic graft replacement, *in situ* allograft replacement, and *in situ* autologous graft replacement. Advantages of *in situ* allografts and autologous vein grafts include the reduced likelihood of new graft infection, reduced rates of lower extremity amputation, elimination of need for a second operation for a staged extraanatomic bypass, avoidance of creating an aortic stump, and lack of anatomic limitations to placement. Rifampin-bonded prosthetic grafts are beneficial for patients who are poor surgical candidates. The long-term patency of the autologous vein graft is a major advantage of this type of *in situ* graft, whereas the prolonged operative time required for venectomy is the disadvantage.

Specimens for culture should be sent at the time of graft excision. Prenteral broad-spectrum antibiotics should be initiated before graft excision, followed by long-term culture-directed antimicrobial therapy and subsequent oral suppressive therapy sometimes for life [145].

Prevention

Whenever possible, reestablishing satisfactory immune defenses and an acceptable nutritional status should be achieved. The importance of strict adherence to the principles of surgical asepsis should be emphasized. In some debilitated patients, prosthetic grafting should be avoided except for limb salvage [145]. Prophylactic antibiotics should be used; the use of cefazolin has been shown to decrease infection significantly in a controlled trial [153]. A recent metaanalysis using a fixed-effect model revealed that systemic antibiotics decreased the graft infection rate (relative risk 0.31, 95% CI 0.11–0.85; $P < 0.02$), but using a random-effects model caused loss of statistical significance ($P = 0.06$). There was no evidence of a significantly greater reduction in wound infection with comparable regimens of first- or second-generation cephalosporins, penicillin/β-lactamse inhibitors, aminoglycosides, or the glycopeptides vancomycin or teicoplanin [154], although theoretically antibiotics with activity against MRSA will be increasingly effective given the increasing frequency of MRSA and methicillin-resistant *S. epidermidis* infections. Rifampin graft bonding, suction wound drainage, or a preoperative bathing or shower regimen with antiseptic agents did not confer any benefit in reducing wound infection [154].

References

1 Mayhall CG. Peripheral vascular catheters. In: Seifert H, Jansen B, Farr BM, eds. Catheter-related Infections, 2nd edn. New York: Marcel Dekker, 2005:327–77.

2 Baddour LM, Wilson WR. Infections of prosthetic valves and other cardiovascular devices. In: Mandell G, Bennett J, Dolin R, eds. Principles and Practice of Infectious Diseases, 6th edn. Philadelphia: Churchill Livingstone, 2005:1024–32.

3 Mermel LA, Maki DG. Infectious complications of pulmonary artery catheters, Cordis introducers, and peripheral arterial catheters. In: Seifert H, Jansen B, Farr BM, eds. Catheter-related Infections, 2nd edn. New York: Marcel Dekker, 2005:379–423.

4 National Nosocomial Infections Surveillance (NNIS) System Report. Data summary from January 1992 through June 2004, issued October 2004. Am J Infect Control 2004;32:470–85.

5 Pronovost P, Needham D, Berenholtz S *et al.* An intervention to decrease catheter-related bloodstream infections in the ICU. N Engl J Med 2006;355:2725–32.

6 Sherertz RJ, Ely EW, Westbrook DM *et al.* Education of physicians-in-training can decrease the risk for vascular catheter infection. Ann Intern Med 2000;132:641–8.

7 Raad II, Hohn DC, Gilbreath BJ *et al.* Prevention of central venous catheter-related infections by using maximal sterile barrier precautions during insertion. Infect Control Hosp Epidemiol 1994; 15:231–8.

8 Maki DG. Nosocomial bacteremia. An epidemiologic overview. Am J Med 1981;70:719–32.

9 Mermel LA. Prevention of intravascular catheter-related infections. Ann Intern Med 2000;132:391–402.

10 Mayor S. Hospital acquired infections kill 5000 patients a year in England. BMJ 2000;321:1370.

11 Warren DK, Quadir WW, Hollenbeak CS, Elward AM, Cox MJ, Fraser VJ. Attributable cost of catheter-associated bloodstream infections among intensive care patients in a nonteaching hospital. Crit Care Med 2006;34:2084–9.

12 Pittet D, Tarara D, Wenzel RP. Nosocomial bloodstream infection in critically ill patients. Excess length of stay, extra costs, and attributable mortality. JAMA 1994;271:1598–601.

13 Dimick JB, Pelz RK, Consunji R, Swoboda SM, Hendrix CW, Lipsett PA. Increased resource use associated with catheter-related bloodstream infection in the surgical intensive care unit. Arch Surg 2001;136:229–34.

14 Rello J, Ochagavia A, Sabanes E *et al.* Evaluation of outcome of intravenous catheter-related infections in critically ill patients. Am J Respir Crit Care Med 2000;162:1027–30.

15 O'Grady NP, Alexander M, Dellinger EP *et al.* Guidelines for the prevention of intravascular catheter-related infections. Infect Control Hosp Epidemiol 2002;23:759–69.

16 Schaberg DR, Culver DH, Gaynes RP. Major trends in the microbial etiology of nosocomial infection. Am J Med 1991; 91(3B):72S–75S.

17 National Nosocomial Infections Surveillance (NNIS) System Report. Data summary from January 1990 to May 1999, issued June 1999. Am J Infect Control 1999;27:520–32.

18 Bouza E, Alvarado N, Alcala L, Perez MJ, Rincon C, Munoz P. A randomized and prospective study of 3 procedures for the diagnosis of catheter-related bloodstream infection without catheter withdrawal. Clin Infect Dis 2007;44:820–6.

19 Sherertz R. Pathogenesis of vascular catheter infections. In: Seifert H, Jansen B, Farr BM, eds. Catheter-related Infections, 2nd edn. New York: Marcel Dekker, 2005:23–36.

20 Sherertz RJ. Pathogenesis of vascular catheter infection. In: Waldvogel FA, Bisno AL, eds. Infections Associated with Indwelling Medical Devices, 3rd edn. Washington: ASM Press, 2000:111–25.

21 Sherertz RJ, Raad II, Belani A *et al.* Three-year experience with sonicated vascular catheter cultures in a clinical microbiology laboratory. J Clin Microbiol 1990;28:76–82.

22 Cleri DJ, Corrado ML, Seligman SJ. Quantitative culture of intravenous catheters and other intravascular inserts. J Infect Dis 1980;141:781–6.

23 Brun-Buisson C, Abrouk F, Legrand P, Huet Y, Larabi S, Rapin M. Diagnosis of central venous catheter-related sepsis. Critical level of quantitative tip cultures. Arch Intern Med 1987;147: 873–7.

24 Siegman-Igra Y, Anglim AM, Shapiro DE, Adal KA, Strain BA, Farr BM. Diagnosis of vascular catheter-related bloodstream infection: a meta-analysis. J Clin Microbiol 1997;35:928–36.

25 Rupp ME. Infections of intravascular catheters and vascular devices. In: Crossley KB, Archer GL, eds. The Staphylococci in Human Disease. Philadelphia: Churchill Livingstone, 1997: 379–412.

26 Pierce CM, Wade A, Mok Q. Heparin-bonded central venous lines reduce thrombotic and infective complications in critically ill children. Intensive Care Med 2000;26:967–72.

27 Gristina AG. Biomaterial-centered infection: microbial adhesion versus tissue integration. Science 1987;237:1588–95.

28 Herrmann M, Vaudaux PE, Pittet D *et al.* Fibronectin, fibrinogen, and laminin act as mediators of adherence of clinical

staphylococcal isolates to foreign material. J Infect Dis 1988; 158:693–701.
29 Gray ED, Peters G, Verstegen M, Regelmann WE. Effect of extracellular slime substance from *Staphylococcus epidermidis* on the human cellular immune response. Lancet 1984;i:365–7.
30 Mack D, Haeder M, Siemssen N, Laufs R. Association of biofilm production of coagulase-negative staphylococci with expression of a specific polysaccharide intercellular adhesin. J Infect Dis 1996;174:881–4.
31 Rupp ME, Fey PD, Heilmann C, Gotz F. Characterization of the importance of *Staphylococcus epidermidis* autolysin and polysaccharide intercellular adhesin in the pathogenesis of intravascular catheter-associated infection in a rat model. J Infect Dis 2001;183:1038–42.
32 Arciola CR, Baldassarri L, Montanaro L. Presence of icaA and icaD genes and slime production in a collection of staphylococcal strains from catheter-associated infections. J Clin Microbiol 2001;39:2151–6.
33 Vuong C, Saenz HL, Gotz F, Otto M. Impact of the agr quorum-sensing system on adherence to polystyrene in *Staphylococcus aureus*. J Infect Dis 2000;182:1688–93.
34 Vuong C, Kocianova S, Yao Y, Carmody AB, Otto M. Increased colonization of indwelling medical devices by quorum-sensing mutants of *Staphylococcus epidermidis* in vivo. J Infect Dis 2004;190:1498–505.
35 Proctor RA, Kahl B, von Eiff C, Vaudaux PE, Lew DP, Peters G. Staphylococcal small colony variants have novel mechanisms for antibiotic resistance. Clin Infect Dis 1998;27(suppl 1):S68–S74.
36 von Eiff C, Vaudaux P, Kahl BC *et al.* Bloodstream infections caused by small-colony variants of coagulase-negative staphylococci following pacemaker implantation. Clin Infect Dis 1999;29:932–4.
37 Kahl B, Herrmann M, Everding AS *et al.* Persistent infection with small colony variant strains of *Staphylococcus aureus* in patients with cystic fibrosis. J Infect Dis 1998;177:1023–9.
38 Proctor RA. Microbial pathogenic factors: small-colony variants. In: Waldvogel FA, Bisno AL, eds. Infections Associated with Indwelling Medical Devices, 3rd edn. Washington: ASM Press, 2000:41–54.
39 Mermel LA, Farr BM, Sherertz RJ *et al.* Guidelines for the management of intravascular catheter-related infections. Clin Infect Dis 2001;32:1249–72.
40 Raad II, Sabbagh MF, Rand KH, Sherertz RJ. Quantitative tip culture methods and the diagnosis of central venous catheter-related infections. Diagn Microbiol Infect Dis 1992;15:13–20.
41 Maki DG, Weise CE, Sarafin HW. A semiquantitative culture method for identifying intravenous-catheter-related infection. N Engl J Med 1977;296:1305–9.
42 Blot F. Diagnosis of catheter-related infections. In: Seifert H, Jansen B, Farr BM, eds. Catheter-related Infections, 2nd edn. New York: Marcel Dekker, 2005:37–76.
43 Kiehn TE, Armstrong D. Changes in the spectrum of organisms causing bacteremia and fungemia in immunocompromised patients due to venous access devices. Eur J Clin Microbiol Infect Dis 1990;9:869–72.
44 Raad II, Bodey GP. Infectious complications of indwelling vascular catheters. Clin Infect Dis 1992;15:197–208.
45 Peacock SJ, Eddleston M, Emptage A, King A, Crook DW. Positive intravenous line tip cultures as predictors of bacteraemia. J Hosp Infect 1998;40:35–8.
46 Raad I, Costerton W, Sabharwal U, Sacilowski M, Anaissie E, Bodey GP. Ultrastructural analysis of indwelling vascular catheters: a quantitative relationship between luminal colonization and duration of placement. J Infect Dis 1993;168:400–7.
47 Moyer MA, Edwards LD, Farley L. Comparative culture methods on 101 intravenous catheters. Routine, semiquantitative, and blood cultures. Arch Intern Med 1983;143:66–9.
48 Rello J, Coll P, Prats G. Evaluation of culture techniques for diagnosis of catheter-related sepsis in critically ill patients. Eur J Clin Microbiol Infect Dis 1992;11:1192–3.
49 Schmitt SK, Knapp C, Hall GS, Longworth DL, McMahon JT, Washington JA. Impact of chlorhexidine–silver sulfadiazine-impregnated central venous catheters on in vitro quantitation of catheter-associated bacteria. J Clin Microbiol 1996;34:508–11.
50 Rijnders BJ, Peetermans WE, Verwaest C, Wilmer A, Van Wijngaerden E. Watchful waiting versus immediate catheter removal in ICU patients with suspected catheter-related infection: a randomized trial. Intensive Care Med 2004;30:1073–80.
51 Raucher HS, Hyatt AC, Barzilai A *et al.* Quantitative blood cultures in the evaluation of septicemia in children with Broviac catheters. J Pediatr 1984;104:29–33.
52 Capdevila JA, Planes AM, Palomar M *et al.* Value of differential quantitative blood cultures in the diagnosis of catheter-related sepsis. Eur J Clin Microbiol Infect Dis 1992;11:403–7.
53 Flynn PM, Shenep JL, Barrett FF. Differential quantitation with a commercial blood culture tube for diagnosis of catheter-related infection. J Clin Microbiol 1988;26:1045–6.
54 Fan ST, Teoh-Chan CH, Lau KF. Evaluation of central venous catheter sepsis by differential quantitative blood culture. Eur J Clin Microbiol Infect Dis 1989;8:142–4.
55 Blot F, Schmidt E, Nitenberg G *et al.* Earlier positivity of central-venous- versus peripheral-blood cultures is highly predictive of catheter-related sepsis. J Clin Microbiol 1998;36:105–9.
56 Raad I, Hanna HA, Alakech B, Chatzinikolaou I, Johnson MM, Tarrand J. Differential time to positivity: a useful method for diagnosing catheter-related bloodstream infections. Ann Intern Med 2004;140:18–25.
57 Blot F, Nitenberg G, Chachaty E *et al.* Diagnosis of catheter-related bacteraemia: a prospective comparison of the time to positivity of hub-blood versus peripheral-blood cultures. Lancet 1999;354:1071–7.
58 Sherertz RJ. Update on vascular catheter infections. Curr Opin Infect Dis 2004;17:303–7.
59 Seifert H, Cornely O, Seggewiss K *et al.* Bloodstream infection in neutropenic cancer patients related to short-term nontunnelled catheters determined by quantitative blood cultures, differential time to positivity, and molecular epidemiological typing with pulsed-field gel electrophoresis. J Clin Microbiol 2003;41:118–23.
60 Archer GL, Climo MW. *Staphylococcus epidermidis* and other coagulase-negative staphylococci. In: Mandell G, Bennett J, Dolin R, eds. Principles and Practice of Infectious Diseases, 6th edn. Philadelphia: Churchill Livingstone, 2005:2352–60.
61 Chang FY, Peacock JE Jr, Musher DM *et al. Staphylococcus aureus* bacteremia: recurrence and the impact of antibiotic treatment in a prospective multicenter study. Medicine (Baltimore) 2003; 82:333–9.
62 Stryjewski ME, Szczech LA, Benjamin DK Jr *et al.* Use of vancomycin or first-generation cephalosporins for the treatment of hemodialysis-dependent patients with methicillin-susceptible

Staphylococcus aureus bacteremia. Clin Infect Dis 2007;44: 190–6.

63 Fowler VG Jr, Boucher HW, Corey GR *et al.* Daptomycin versus standard therapy for bacteremia and endocarditis caused by *Staphylococcus aureus*. N Engl J Med 2006;355:653–65.

64 Rosen AB, Fowler VG Jr, Corey GR *et al.* Cost-effectiveness of transesophageal echocardiography to determine the duration of therapy for intravascular catheter-associated *Staphylococcus aureus* bacteremia. Ann Intern Med 1999;130:810–20.

65 Pettigrew RA, Lang SD, Haydock DA, Parry BR, Bremner DA, Hill GL. Catheter-related sepsis in patients on intravenous nutrition: a prospective study of quantitative catheter cultures and guidewire changes for suspected sepsis. Br J Surg 1985;72:52–5.

66 Benjamin DK Jr, Miller W, Garges H *et al.* Bacteremia, central catheters, and neonates: when to pull the line. Pediatrics 2001; 107:1272–6.

67 Widmer AF, Nettleman M, Flint K, Wenzel RP. The clinical impact of culturing central venous catheters. A prospective study. Arch Intern Med 1992;152:1299–302.

68 Herwaldt LA, Geiss M, Kao C, Pfaller MA. The positive predictive value of isolating coagulase-negative staphylococci from blood cultures. Clin Infect Dis 1996;22:14–20.

69 Raad I, Davis S, Khan A, Tarrand J, Elting L, Bodey GP. Impact of central venous catheter removal on the recurrence of catheter-related coagulase-negative staphylococcal bacteremia. Infect Control Hosp Epidemiol 1992;13:215–21.

70 Fowler VG Jr, Sanders LL, Sexton DJ *et al.* Outcome of *Staphylococcus aureus* bacteremia according to compliance with recommendations of infectious diseases specialists: experience with 244 patients. Clin Infect Dis 1998;27:478–86.

71 Dugdale DC, Ramsey PG. *Staphylococcus aureus* bacteremia in patients with Hickman catheters. Am J Med 1990;89:137–41.

72 Malanoski GJ, Samore MH, Pefanis A, Karchmer AW. *Staphylococcus aureus* catheter-associated bacteremia. Minimal effective therapy and unusual infectious complications associated with arterial sheath catheters. Arch Intern Med 1995;155:1161–6.

73 Capdevila JA, Segarra A, Planes AM *et al.* Successful treatment of haemodialysis catheter-related sepsis without catheter removal. Nephrol Dial Transplant 1993;8:231–4.

74 Mayhall CG. Diagnosis and management of infections of implantable devices used for prolonged venous access. Curr Clin Top Infect Dis 1992;12:83–110.

75 Jacobson MA, Gellermann H, Chambers H. *Staphylococcus aureus* bacteremia and recurrent staphylococcal infection in patients with acquired immunodeficiency syndrome and AIDS-related complex. Am J Med 1988;85:172–6.

76 Mortara LA, Bayer AS. *Staphylococcus aureus* bacteremia and endocarditis. New diagnostic and therapeutic concepts. Infect Dis Clin North Am 1993;7:53–68.

77 Costerton JW, Stewart PS, Greenberg EP. Bacterial biofilms: a common cause of persistent infections. Science 1999;284:1318–22.

78 Zimmerli W, Frei R, Widmer AF, Rajacic Z. Microbiological tests to predict treatment outcome in experimental device-related infections due to *Staphylococcus aureus*. J Antimicrob Chemother 1994;33:959–67.

79 Gaillard JL, Merlino R, Pajot N *et al.* Conventional and non-conventional modes of vancomycin administration to decontaminate the internal surface of catheters colonized with coagulase-negative staphylococci. JPEN J Parenter Enteral Nutr 1990;14:593–7.

80 Arnow PM, Kushner R. *Malassezia furfur* catheter infection cured with antibiotic lock therapy. Am J Med 1991;90:128–30.

81 Messing B, Peitra-Cohen S, Debure A, Beliah M, Bernier JJ. Antibiotic-lock technique: a new approach to optimal therapy for catheter-related sepsis in home-parenteral nutrition patients. JPEN J Parenter Enteral Nutr 1988;12:185–9.

82 Cowan CE. Antibiotic lock technique. J Intraven Nurs 1992; 15:283–7.

83 Raad I, Hanna H, Jiang Y *et al.* Comparative activities of daptomycin, linezolid, and tigecycline against catheter-related methicillin-resistant *Staphylococcus* bacteremic isolates embedded in biofilm. Antimicrob Agents Chemother 2007;51:1656–60.

84 Sherertz RJ, Boger MS, Collins CA, Mason L, Raad II. Comparative in vitro efficacies of various catheter lock solutions. Antimicrob Agents Chemother 2006;50:1865–8.

85 Raad I, Hanna H, Dvorak T, Chaiban G, Hachem R. Optimal antimicrobial catheter lock solution, using different combinations of minocycline, EDTA, and 25-percent ethanol, rapidly eradicates organisms embedded in biofilm. Antimicrob Agents Chemother 2007;51:78–83.

86 Rijnders BJ, Van Wijngaerden E, Vandecasteele SJ, Stas M, Peetermans WE. Treatment of long-term intravascular catheter-related bacteraemia with antibiotic lock: randomized, placebo-controlled trial. J Antimicrob Chemother 2005;55:90–4.

87 Fortun J, Grill F, Martin-Davila P *et al.* Treatment of long-term intravascular catheter-related bacteraemia with antibiotic-lock therapy. J Antimicrob Chemother 2006;58:816–21.

88 Dannenberg C, Bierbach U, Rothe A, Beer J, Korholz D. Ethanol-lock technique in the treatment of bloodstream infections in pediatric oncology patients with broviac catheter. J Pediatr Hematol Oncol 2003;25:616–21.

89 Onland W, Shin CE, Fustar S, Rushing T, Wong WY. Ethanol-lock technique for persistent bacteremia of long-term intravascular devices in pediatric patients. Arch Pediatr Adolesc Med 2006;160:1049–53.

90 Warren DK, Zack JE, Cox MJ, Cohen MM, Fraser VJ. An educational intervention to prevent catheter-associated bloodstream infections in a nonteaching, community medical center. Crit Care Med 2003;31:1959–63.

91 Eggimann P, Harbarth S, Constantin MN, Touveneau S, Chevrolet JC, Pittet D. Impact of a prevention strategy targeted at vascular-access care on incidence of infections acquired in intensive care. Lancet 2000;355:1864–8.

92 Rosenthal VD, Guzman S, Pezzotto SM, Crnich CJ. Effect of an infection control program using education and performance feedback on rates of intravascular device-associated bloodstream infections in intensive care units in Argentina. Am J Infect Control 2003;31:405–9.

93 Soifer NE, Borzak S, Edlin BR, Weinstein RA. Prevention of peripheral venous catheter complications with an intravenous therapy team: a randomized controlled trial. Arch Intern Med 1998;158:473–7.

94 Tomford JW, Hershey CO, McLaren CE, Porter DK, Cohen DI. Intravenous therapy team and peripheral venous catheter-associated complications. A prospective controlled study. Arch Intern Med 1984;144:1191–4.

95 Fridkin SK, Pear SM, Williamson TH, Galgiani JN, Jarvis WR. The role of understaffing in central venous catheter-associated bloodstream infections. Infect Control Hosp Epidemiol 1996; 17:150–8.

96 Rijnders BJ, Vandecasteele SJ, Van Wijngaerden E, De Munter P, Peetermans WE. Use of semiautomatic treatment advice to improve compliance with Infectious Diseases Society of America guidelines for treatment of intravascular catheter-related infection: a before-after study. Clin Infect Dis 2003;37: 980–3.

97 Rijnders BJ, Van Wijngaerden E, Wilmer A, Peetermans WE. Use of full sterile barrier precautions during insertion of arterial catheters: a randomized trial. Clin Infect Dis 2003;36:743–8.

98 Richet H, Hubert B, Nitemberg G *et al.* Prospective multicenter study of vascular-catheter-related complications and risk factors for positive central-catheter cultures in intensive care unit patients. J Clin Microbiol 1990;28:2520–5.

99 Horowitz HW, Dworkin BM, Savino JA, Byrne DW, Pecora NA. Central catheter-related infections: comparison of pulmonary artery catheters and triple lumen catheters for the delivery of hyperalimentation in a critical care setting. JPEN J Parenter Enteral Nutr 1990;14:588–92.

100 Merrer J, De Jonghe B, Golliot F *et al.* Complications of femoral and subclavian venous catheterization in critically ill patients: a randomized controlled trial. JAMA 2001;286:700–7.

101 Durbec O, Viviand X, Potie F, Vialet R, Albanese J, Martin C. A prospective evaluation of the use of femoral venous catheters in critically ill adults. Crit Care Med 1997;25:1986–9.

102 Joynt GM, Kew J, Gomersall CD, Leung VY, Liu EK. Deep venous thrombosis caused by femoral venous catheters in critically ill adult patients. Chest 2000;117:178–83.

103 Nahum E, Levy I, Katz J *et al.* Efficacy of subcutaneous tunneling for prevention of bacterial colonization of femoral central venous catheters in critically ill children. Pediatr Infect Dis J 2002;21:1000–4.

104 Timsit JF, Bruneel F, Cheval C *et al.* Use of tunneled femoral catheters to prevent catheter-related infection. A randomized, controlled trial. Ann Intern Med 1999;130:729–35.

105 Krafte-Jacobs B, Sivit CJ, Mejia R, Pollack MM. Catheter-related thrombosis in critically ill children: comparison of catheters with and without heparin bonding. J Pediatr 1995;126:50–4.

106 Mimoz O, Karim A, Mercat A *et al.* Chlorhexidine compared with povidone-iodine as skin preparation before blood culture. A randomized, controlled trial. Ann Intern Med 1999;131: 834–7.

107 Mimoz O, Pieroni L, Lawrence C *et al.* Prospective, randomized trial of two antiseptic solutions for prevention of central venous or arterial catheter colonization and infection in intensive care unit patients. Crit Care Med 1996;24:1818–23.

108 Humar A, Ostromecki A, Direnfeld J *et al.* Prospective randomized trial of 10% povidone-iodine versus 0.5% tincture of chlorhexidine as cutaneous antisepsis for prevention of central venous catheter infection. Clin Infect Dis 2000;31:1001–7.

109 Maki DG, Ringer M. Evaluation of dressing regimens for prevention of infection with peripheral intravenous catheters. Gauze, a transparent polyurethane dressing, and an iodophor-transparent dressing. JAMA 1987;258:2396–403.

110 Hoffmann KK, Weber DJ, Samsa GP, Rutala WA. Transparent polyurethane film as an intravenous catheter dressing. A meta-analysis of the infection risks. JAMA 1992;267:2072–6.

111 Kacica MA, Horgan MJ, Ochoa L, Sandler R, Lepow ML, Venezia RA. Prevention of Gram-positive sepsis in neonates weighing less than 1500 grams. J Pediatr 1994;125:253–8.

112 Spafford PS, Sinkin RA, Cox C, Reubens L, Powell KR. Prevention of central venous catheter-related coagulase-negative staphylococcal sepsis in neonates. J Pediatr 1994;125:259–63.

113 van de Wetering MD, van Woensel JB. Prophylactic antibiotics for preventing early central venous catheter Gram-positive infections in oncology patients. Cochrane Database Syst Rev 2003;2:CD003295.

114 Levin A, Mason AJ, Jindal KK, Fong IW, Goldstein MB. Prevention of hemodialysis subclavian vein catheter infections by topical povidone-iodine. Kidney Int 1991;40:934–8.

115 Johnson DW, van Eps C, Mudge DW *et al.* Randomized, controlled trial of topical exit-site application of honey (Medihoney) versus mupirocin for the prevention of catheter-associated infections in hemodialysis patients. J Am Soc Nephrol 2005;16:1456–62.

116 Jansen B, Kohnen W. Prevention and control of catheter-related infections. In: Seifert H, Jansen B, Farr BM, eds. Catheter-related Infections, 2nd edn. New York: Marcel Dekker, 2005: 89–139.

117 Randolph AG, Cook DJ, Gonzales CA, Andrew M. Benefit of heparin in central venous and pulmonary artery catheters: a meta-analysis of randomized controlled trials. Chest 1998;113: 165–71.

118 Bern MM, Lokich JJ, Wallach SR *et al.* Very low doses of warfarin can prevent thrombosis in central venous catheters. A randomized prospective trial. Ann Intern Med 1990;112:423–8.

119 Aquino VM, Sandler ES, Mustafa MM, Steele JW, Buchanan GR. A prospective double-blind randomized trial of urokinase flushes to prevent bacteremia resulting from luminal colonization of subcutaneous central venous catheters. J Pediatr Hematol Oncol 2002;24:710–13.

120 Garland JS, Alex CP, Henrickson KJ, McAuliffe TL, Maki DG. A vancomycin-heparin lock solution for prevention of nosocomial bloodstream infection in critically ill neonates with peripherally inserted central venous catheters: a prospective, randomized trial. Pediatrics 2005;116:e198–e205.

121 Henrickson KJ, Axtell RA, Hoover SM *et al.* Prevention of central venous catheter-related infections and thrombotic events in immunocompromised children by the use of vancomycin/ciprofloxacin/heparin flush solution: a randomized, multicenter, double-blind trial. J Clin Oncol 2000;18:1269–78.

122 Carratala J, Niubo J, Fernandez-Sevilla A *et al.* Randomized, double-blind trial of an antibiotic-lock technique for prevention of Gram-positive central venous catheter-related infection in neutropenic patients with cancer. Antimicrob Agents Chemother 1999;43:2200–4.

123 Betjes MG, van Agteren M. Prevention of dialysis catheter-related sepsis with a citrate-taurolidine-containing lock solution. Nephrol Dial Transplant 2004;19:1546–51.

124 Allon M. Prophylaxis against dialysis catheter-related bacteremia with a novel antimicrobial lock solution. Clin Infect Dis 2003;36:1539–44.

125 Yahav D, Rozen-Zvi B, Gafter-Gvili A *et al.* Antimicrobial lock solutions for the prevention of infections associated with intravascular catheters in patients undergoing hemodialysis: systematic review and meta-analysis of randomized, controlled trials. Clin Infect Dis 2008;47:83–93.

126 Veenstra DL, Saint S, Saha S, Lumley T, Sullivan SD. Efficacy of antiseptic-impregnated central venous catheters in preventing

catheter-related bloodstream infection: a meta-analysis. JAMA 1999;281:261–7.
127 Veenstra DL, Saint S, Sullivan SD. Cost-effectiveness of antiseptic-impregnated central venous catheters for the prevention of catheter-related bloodstream infection. JAMA 1999;282: 554–60.
128 Rupp ME, Lisco SJ, Lipsett PA *et al.* Effect of a second-generation venous catheter impregnated with chlorhexidine and silver sulfadiazine on central catheter-related infections: a randomized, controlled trial. Ann Intern Med 2005;143:570–80.
129 Darouiche RO, Raad II, Heard SO *et al.* A comparison of two antimicrobial-impregnated central venous catheters. Catheter Study Group. N Engl J Med 1999;340:1–8.
130 Hanna HA, Raad II, Hackett B *et al.* Antibiotic-impregnated catheters associated with significant decrease in nosocomial and multidrug-resistant bacteremias in critically ill patients. Chest 2003;124:1030–8.
131 Hanna H, Benjamin R, Chatzinikolaou I *et al.* Long-term silicone central venous catheters impregnated with minocycline and rifampin decrease rates of catheter-related bloodstream infection in cancer patients: a prospective randomized clinical trial. J Clin Oncol 2004;22:3163–71.
132 Tambe SM, Sampath L, Modak SM. In vitro evaluation of the risk of developing bacterial resistance to antiseptics and antibiotics used in medical devices. J Antimicrob Chemother 2001;47:589–98.
133 Arduino MJ, Tokars JI. Why is an infection control program needed in the hemodialysis setting? Nephrol News Issues 2005;19:44, 46–49.
134 Tokars JI, Klevens RM. Infections associated with hemodialysis vascular access and with catheters used for hemodialysis. In: Seifert H, Jansen B, Farr BM, eds. Catheter-related Infections, 2nd edn. New York: Marcel Dekker, 2005:499–514.
135 Tokars JI, Miller ER, Stein G. New national surveillance system for hemodialysis-associated infections: initial results. Am J Infect Control 2002;30:288–95.
136 Hoen B, Paul-Dauphin A, Hestin D, Kessler M. EPIBACDIAL: a multicenter prospective study of risk factors for bacteremia in chronic hemodialysis patients. J Am Soc Nephrol 1998;9: 869–76.
137 Powe NR, Jaar B, Furth SL, Hermann J, Briggs W. Septicemia in dialysis patients: incidence, risk factors, and prognosis. Kidney Int 1999;55:1081–90.
138 Tokars JI, Light P, Anderson J *et al.* A prospective study of vascular access infections at seven outpatient hemodialysis centers. Am J Kidney Dis 2001;37:1232–40.
139 Finelli L, Miller JT, Tokars JI, Alter MJ, Arduino MJ. National surveillance of dialysis-associated diseases in the United States, 2002. Semin Dial 2005;18:52–61.
140 Fridkin SK. Vancomycin-intermediate and -resistant *Staphylococcus aureus*: what the infectious disease specialist needs to know. Clin Infect Dis 2001;32:108–15.
141 Anon. *Staphylococcus aureus* resistant to vancomycin: United States, 2002. MMWR 2002;51:565–7.
142 Berns JS, Tokars JI. Preventing bacterial infections and antimicrobial resistance in dialysis patients. Am J Kidney Dis 2002;40:886–98.
143 Marr KA, Sexton DJ, Conlon PJ, Corey GR, Schwab SJ, Kirkland KB. Catheter-related bacteremia and outcome of attempted catheter salvage in patients undergoing hemodialysis. Ann Intern Med 1997;127:275–80.
144 Taal MW, Fluck RJ, McIntyre CW. Preventing catheter related infections in haemodialysis patients. Curr Opin Nephrol Hypertens 2006;15:599–602.
145 Goëau-Brissonnière OA, Coggia M. Arterial prosthetic infections. In: Waldvogel FA, Bisno AL, eds. Infections Associated with Indwelling Medical Devices, 3rd edn. Washington: ASM Press, 2000:127–44.
146 Wooster DL, Louch RE, Krajden S. Intraoperative bacterial contamination of vascular grafts: a prospective study. Can J Surg 1985;28:407–9.
147 Scobie K, McPhail N, Barber G, Elder R. Bacteriologic monitoring in abdominal aortic surgery. Can J Surg 1979;22:368–71.
148 Speziale F, Rizzo L, Sbarigia E *et al.* Bacterial and clinical criteria relating to the outcome of patients undergoing *in situ* replacement of infected abdominal aortic grafts. Eur J Vasc Endovasc Surg 1997;13:127–33.
149 Yeager RA, McConnell DB, Sasaki TM, Vetto RM. Aortic and peripheral prosthetic graft infection: differential management and causes of mortality. Am J Surg 1985;150:36–43.
150 Wilson SE. New alternatives in management of the infected vascular prosthesis. Surg Infect (Larchmt) 2001;2:171–5.
151 Olofsson PA, Auffermann W, Higgins CB, Rabahie GN, Tavares N, Stoney RJ. Diagnosis of prosthetic aortic graft infection by magnetic resonance imaging. J Vasc Surg 1988;8: 99–105.
152 Mussa FF, Hedayati N, Zhou W *et al.* Prevention and treatment of aortic graft infection. Expert Rev Anti Infect Ther 2007; 5:305–15.
153 Kaiser AB, Clayson KR, Mulherin JL Jr *et al.* Antibiotic prophylaxis in vascular surgery. Ann Surg 1978;188:283–9.
154 Stewart AH, Eyers PS, Earnshaw JJ. Prevention of infection in peripheral arterial reconstruction: a systematic review and meta-analysis. J Vasc Surg 2007;46:148–55.
155 Crnich CJ, Maki DG. The promise of novel technology for the prevention of intravascular device-related bloodstream infection. I. Pathogenesis and short-term devices. Clin Infect Dis 2002;34:1232–42.
156 von Eiff C, Peters G, Heilmann C. Pathogenesis of infections due to coagulase negative staphylococci. Lancet Infect Dis 2002;2:677–85.
157 Centers for Disease Control and Prevention. Guidelines for the prevention of intravascular catheter-related infections. MMWR 2002;51(RR-10):4.
158 Bleyer AJ *et al.* A randomized, controlled trial of a vascular catheter flush solution (minocylcine-EDTA) in temporary hemodialysis access. *Infection Control and Hospital Epidemiology* 2005;26:520–4.

Chapter 19
Skin and Soft Tissue Infections

Martin E. Stryjewski[1,2], *Esteban C. Nannini*[3,4] *and G. Ralph Corey*[2]

[1] Department of Medicine and Division of Infectious Diseases, Centro de Educación Médica e Investigaciones Clínicas "Norberto Quirno," CEMIC, Buenos Aires, Argentina
[2] Division of Infectious Diseases, Duke Clinical Research Institute, Durham, North Carolina, USA
[3] Division of Infectious Diseases, Sanatorio Parque and [4]Facultad de Ciencias Médicas, Rosario, Argentina

Introduction and epidemiology

Staphylococcus aureus is the most common pathogen responsible for skin and soft tissue infections (SSTIs) worldwide. The spectrum of SSTIs associated with this microorganism ranges from mild superficial to invasive life-threatening diseases encompassing a variety of entities (Table 19.1). Most of these infections are cared for in the outpatient setting and are among the most frequent causes of medical visits. Based on a survey of physician offices, hospital outpatient, and emergency departments in the USA between 2001 and 2003, the National Ambulatory Medical Care Surveys (NAMCS) and the National Hospital Ambulatory Medical Care Surveys (NHAMCS) estimate the number of ambulatory care visits for SSTIs to be 11.6 million, with a visit rate of 410.7 per 10 000 person-years [1]. Cellulitis and abscesses represent more than 50% of these visits [1]. Compared with a similar report from 1992–1994, several important differences are noted: increases of 59% and 31% in hospital outpatient and emergency department visits, a 32% decrease in impetigo, and a 26% rise in cellulitis and abscesses [1]. These changes are related to a dramatic increase in cutaneous infections caused by community-associated methicillin-resistant *S. aureus* (CA-MRSA) strains. Indeed, strains of CA-MRSA carrying the staphylococcal cassette chromosome (SCC)*mec* type IV (usually clone USA300) and Panton–Valentine leukocidin have now been reported as the most prevalent cause of staphylococcal community-onset SSTI, particularly abscesses and cellulitis [2–7]. Infections caused by CA-MRSA are discussed in detail in Chapter 29.

Though most patients with SSTI can be treated in the outpatient setting, 4% do require hospitalization [1]. As expected the hospitalization rate is higher among patients with SSTI seeking care in emergency departments; 13.6% of patients presenting to emergency departments are

Table 19.1 Skin and skin-structure infections associated with *S. aureus*.

Primary pyodermas
Impetigo: affects children; *S. aureus* is the most common cause
Folliculitis
Furuncles and carbuncles
Paronychia
Erysipelas: very rarely caused by *S. aureus*
Infectious cellulitis
Botryomycosis (cutaneous form): very rare; several cases described in patients with HIV infection
Secondary to preexisting skin lesions
Hidradenitis suppurativa
Blistering skin diseases
Bullous impetigo: affects children; *S. aureus* phage group II
Scalded skin syndrome (Ritter's disease): diffuse form of bullous impetigo
Subcutaneous tissue infections
Abscesses: *S. aureus* is the most frequent cause; most frequent form of infection caused by CA-MRSA; PVL-positive strains tend to cause abscesses; drainage is the most important treatment modality
Necrotizing fasciitis: polymicrobial (more common) or monomicrobial; frequent underlying diabetes; early suspicion is crucial in management
Systemic syndromes mediated by toxins and affecting the skin
Staphylococcal toxic shock syndrome (see Chapter 25)
Purpura fulminans: very rare, with severe presentation and high mortality; described for both MRSA and MSSA; usually strains carrying superantigen toxins (SEB, SEC, TSST-1)
Henoch–Schönlein purpura: very rare; believed to be associated with superantigen activity
Waterhouse–Friderichsen syndrome: very rare; described in association with respiratory infections
Scarlet fever: very rarely caused by *S. aureus*; strains carrying enterotoxins (e.g., SEB)

CA-MRSA, community-acquired methicillin-resistant *S. aureus*; MRSA, methicillin-resistant *S. aureus*; MSSA, methicillin-susceptible *S. aureus*; PVL, Panton–Valentine leukocidin; TSST, toxic shock syndrome toxin.

Staphylococci in Human Disease, 2nd edition. Edited by Kent B. Crossley, Kimberly K. Jefferson, Gordon Archer, Vance G. Fowler, Jr.
 ISBN 978-14051-6332-3.

hospitalized [1]. Many of these patients require surgical interventions, which are often associated with significant morbidity and expense. For example, in 2004 there were 368 000 surgical procedures associated with SSTIs (débridement of wound, infection, or burn) in the USA [8].

Described risk factors associated with SSTIs potentially caused by *S. aureus* in the USA include emergency department care, male sex, payment by Medicaid, younger age, and being a resident from the southern and western areas of the country [1]. Other risk factors specifically related to CA-MRSA infection are more fully elucidated in Chapter 29.

Impetigo

The incidence of impetigo is estimated to be 20.6 per 1000 person-years (age < 18 years), with higher rates during the summer months and in rural areas [9]. Until the early 1980s, *Streptococcus pyogenes* was the predominant agent causing this disease but in the last 20 years it has been supplanted by *S. aureus* [10–13]. However, mixed infection with both pathogens still occurs in 15–20% of cases [10,11].

Nasal colonization by the infecting *S. aureus* strain usually precedes the appearance of the skin lesions [13]. Impetigo often develops at sites of prior injury or damage such as insect bites, abrasions, varicella lesions, and burns (Table 19.2). The presence of the exfoliative toxin ETB in *S. aureus* strains causing nonbullous impetigo is associated with an increased number and size of skin lesions [14].

Lesions of impetigo usually begin as vesicles, which become pustules and then rupture leaving an erythematous base. When the purulent discharge dries, it forms the honey-crusted exudates that characterize the infection. Lesions are usually painless but the associated pruritus can lead to scratching which can spread the disease [15]. Impetigo is a superficial infection that does not cause dermis infiltration or ulcer formation and therefore heals without scarring. Regional lymphadenopathy is common and half of the subjects have leukocytosis, although constitutional symptoms are usually absent. Cultures from skin lesions often reveal the offending agent, most commonly *S. aureus*.

Even though impetigo is a self-limited disease of about 2 weeks' duration, the administration of antimicrobials reduces the length of illness, the contagious period, the risk of local outbreaks, and the likelihood of the nowadays very rare poststreptococcal glomerulonephritis [16,17]. Localized disease can be effectively treated with topical antibiotics such as mupirocin or fusidic acid (not available in the USA) cream with fewer side effects than oral agents [17–19]. However, increasing rates of mupirocin resistance in *S. aureus* strains in some areas is worrisome [20]. Topical

Table 19.2 Risk factors for development of skin and skin-structure related infections caused by *S. aureus*.

SSTI	Risk factor	Comment
Impetigo	Any type of injury to skin site (e.g., insect bites, abrasions, varicella lesions, burns)	
Recurrent furunculosis	Nasal carriage of *S. aureus*[1]	Outbreaks of staphylococcal skin disease might occur in closed environment
	Close contact with someone with furunculosis	
	Diabetes	
	Obesity	
	Use of corticosteroids or cytotoxic agents	
	Immunosuppression	
	Lower serum mannose-binding lectin levels	Hereditary predisposition
Infective cellulitis	Disruption of skin integrity (ulcers, wounds)	
	Prior episode of cellulitis	
	Injection drug users	At site of injection (also a common risk factor for abscesses)
	Venous or lymphatic leg edema	Lower-extremity cellulitis
	Presence of *S. aureus* in toe webs	Lower-extremity cellulitis
Pyomyositis (temperate climate)	HIV infection	
	Diabetes mellitus	
	Injection drug users	
Necrotizing fasciitis	Diabetes, immunosuppression	
Puerperal infectious mastitis	Cracking of nipples	
	Obstruction to lactiferous ducts	
	Prior episode of mastitis	

[1] Nasal carriage of *S. aureus* predisposes to superficial and invasive staphylococcal infections. Risk factors for this condition overlap with overall risk factors for *S. aureus* infection: diabetes mellitus, chronic skin diseases, patients undergoing haemodialysis or continuous peritoneal dialysis, infection with HIV, obesity, and a history of cerebrovascular accident.

retapamulin, a novel pleuromutilin antimicrobial agent, has recently been shown to be an effective alternative [21]. For more extensive or systemic disease, oral antimicrobials are preferred. Since *S. aureus* is the most frequent pathogen, penicillinase-resistant penicillins, amoxicillin–clavulanate, and first-generation cephalosporins are recommended [11,22,23]. While erythromycin has been extensively used in the past, it is now a less desirable therapeutic option [17] because of emergence of resistance in *S. aureus* [12] and a higher rate of side effects than topical treatment [24]. MRSA strains, including CA-MRSA, have also been implicated in cases of impetigo and will require alternative antibiotics.

Blistering skin diseases

Bullous impetigo and staphylococcal scalded-skin syndrome (SSSS) are considered different expressions of the same disease, the former being the localized and the latter the systemic form of the disease. Both entities are produced by strains of *S. aureus* that produce exfoliative toxins and are classified within phage group 2. There are three types of exfoliative toxin, ETA, ETB, and ETD, but only the first two have been clearly associated with human disease and are encoded by the *eta* and *etb* genes, located in the chromosome and on a plasmid, respectively [25]. Prevalence of *S. aureus* strains harboring the *eta* and/or *etb* genes ranges from 1.2 to 6.2% of the isolates in different parts of the world [25–27]. These exfoliative toxins, acting as serine proteases, cleave human desmoglein 1 (Dsg1) at a crucial site, inhibiting its function [28–30]. This cleavage causes loss of adhesion of keratinocytes under the stratum corneum, with resulting blister formation in the epidermis. Dsg1 is a transmembrane structural skin protein that mediates keratinocyte adhesion in the granular layer and is present throughout the epithelium. Interestingly, this protein is also inactivated by anti-Dsg1 antibodies in immune-mediated diseases such as pemphigus foliaceus.

SSSS, known as Ritter's disease or pemphigus neonatorum, is characterized by widespread blister formation and exfoliation. This syndrome is most common in newborns, infants, and children. The increased prevalence in children may be related to low titers of anti-exfoliative toxin antibodies in this population. The exfoliative toxin-producing *S. aureus* isolate can usually be recovered from distant sites such as throat, nose, eyes, and ears [31]. SSSS commonly presents with abrupt onset of fever and progressive erythroderma or scarlatiniform rash followed by generalized blister formation [32]. New bullae continue to appear during the first 2 or 3 days of illness followed by spontaneous exfoliation. The Nikolsky sign (detachment of epidermis with application of light lateral pressure over perilesional normal-appearing skin) is frequently positive. "Dry" underlying skin represents a subcorneal blistering process such as seen in SSSS; obtaining a "wet" response implies an intraepidermal blistering process as seen in pemphigus vulgaris, toxic epidermal necrolysis (TEN), or Steven–Johnson syndrome (SJS) [33]. The bullae seen in SSSS are extremely tender and flaccid and more commonly affect the flexures; occasionally, large areas of the skin may be involved [32]. The bulla progressively enlarges and ruptures, draining clear fluid; the denuded skin is brightly erythematous giving the scalded appearance. The lack of mucous membrane involvement differentiates SSSS from the more severe TEN (Lyell syndrome) which, together with SJS, are severe forms of drug reactions having different pathological findings on skin biopsy (i.e., keratinocyte apoptosis and dermoepidermal splitting) [34,35]. With supportive care and appropriate antibiotics the skin heals in about 2 weeks, giving a mortality rate in children of less than 5% [30,32,36,37]. The identification of the primary site of staphylococcal infection is crucial in the management of SSSS [19]. Infection control measures should be implemented since the spread of these exfoliative toxin-producing strains has been associated with local outbreaks of SSSS, especially among neonates [38].

Bullous impetigo accounts for 10–30% of cases of impetigo [11] and affects primarily newborns and young children. This disease begins with the formation of fluid-filled vesicles, followed by single or several flaccid bullae arising over intact skin with a positive Nikolsky sign ("wet"). The liquid from the bullae is yellowish and, if cultured, the exfoliative toxin-producing *S. aureus* strain can be isolated [32]. Patients suffering from bullous impetigo can be treated with topical antibiotics such as mupirocin or fusidic acid cream similar to patients with nonbullous impetigo [18,19]. As in other SSTIs, MRSA strains are becoming more prevalent [39,40] and will require empiric treatment with an agent active against MRSA, especially in severe cases.

Folliculitis, furuncles, and carbuncles

Folliculitis is a localized infection deep within the hair follicle [15]. The lesions consist of small (< 5 mm), tender, pruritic papules with an erythematous and sometimes indurated base surrounding the hair follicle [41] (see Plate 19.1). Generalized symptoms are absent. A distinctive chronic form of folliculitis affecting the bearded areas of the face is called sycosis barbae.

A furuncle (or boil) is an extension of preceding folliculitis into the subcutaneous tissue resulting in a painful, indurated, and reddish nodule of 1–2 cm in diameter. This lesion affects hairy areas of the body subject to friction and perspiration such as the face, neck, axillae, buttocks, and extremities [15,41]. Following nodule formation a small abscess develops in the dermis [41]. Next, the furuncle becomes fluctuant with a yellowish top, subsiding after the spontaneous drainage of purulent material. Gradual resolution without treatment generally ensues. Furuncles are often multiple and have a tendency to recur. The infecting strain can spread to other subjects, leading to local outbreaks of disease [42–44].

Carbuncles are characterized by the coalescence of multiple furuncles, producing a painful inflammatory mass with purulent material draining from multiple involved hair follicles (see Plate 19.2). Located most frequently at the base of the neck, buttocks, or thighs, these abscesses tend to affect diabetic subjects. Carbuncles often extend into the subcutaneous tissue and are frequently associated with fever and malaise. In addition they may be a source of bacteremia.

If subjects with large-sized furuncles or carbuncles have signs and symptoms of systemic involvement, Gram stain and cultures of purulent secretions and peripheral blood cultures should be obtained [45]; a surgical consultation should also be considered. Severe *S. aureus* disease such as bacteremia, pneumonia, fasciitis, or arthritis should be suspected in young patients with furuncles presenting with symptoms of sepsis [46]. Of note, cases of native valve endocarditis following furunculosis caused by CA-MRSA have been reported [47].

Treatment of folliculitis usually requires only topical antiseptics, although occasionally lesions might recur. Furuncles commonly respond to moist heat, thought to accelerate drainage; larger lesions and carbuncles require either incision and drainage or more extensive surgical débridement. Antibiotics are usually reserved for those subjects with systemic symptoms or associated cellulitis. Early surgical intervention is essential in many of these patients [15,45]. Staphylococcal skin infections arising around the nose or upper lip can rarely result in life-threatening septic thrombosis of the cavernous sinus [48] and therefore should be treated more aggressively with antibiotics and drainage.

Abscesses

Staphylococus aureus is among the most common causes of skin and skin structure-related abscesses [1,4,49,50]. As mentioned earlier, CA-MRSA has become the predominant cause of abscesses, often affecting young and healthy people, in the USA [3,4,6]. Certain groups of patients such as injection drug users (IDUs) (e.g., "skin poppers") are at risk of suffering recurrent skin abscesses [51,52], particularly caused by MRSA [53]. Abscesses produced by staphylococci occur more often on the extremities and in the pelvic area [49], although in IDUs the infected area is dictated by the site of injection. Abscesses are usually suspected by the presence of painful red nodules surrounded by an erythematous swollen area (see Plates 19.3 and 19.4); a pustule on the top of the lesion is common [45]. Leukocytosis is frequent. In medically underserved populations (homeless and IDUs), abscesses produced by *S. aureus*, particularly MRSA, are often accompanied by surrounding cellulitis [53]. Surprisingly, fever is uncommon (< 10%) [54], although the amount of pus drained per lesion (an average of 15 mL) is significant [53]. Importantly, epidermal inclusion cysts are frequently infected by *S. aureus* and streptococci and can mimic abscesses [55]. Interestingly, the bacteriology of inflamed and noninflamed epidermal inclusion cysts is undistinguishable [56]. As a result, the majority of physicians prescribe antibiotics for inflamed epidermal cysts [57].

Diagnosis of abscesses relies on clinical findings and can be confirmed and/or assessed by soft tissue ultrasound. Clinical examination has a sensitivity of 86% and a specificity of 70% in the diagnosis of abscesses, while soft tissue ultrasound has a sensitivity of 98% and a specificity of 88% [58]. When ultrasound findings disagree with clinical examination, ultrasound findings are correct more than 90% of the time [58]. In the era of CA-MRSA, the practice of requesting cultures should be emphasized [59,60].

Incision and drainage is the main treatment for patients with skin abscesses [4,45,54,61–65]. Several studies have shown that antibiotic therapy provides only marginal [5,61] benefit in patients with abscesses undergoing surgical drainage [4–6,54,61–63]. Therefore, all patients with abscesses should undergo incision and open drainage (preferred) or needle aspiration [45]. In a prospective observational study, children with abscesses larger than 5 cm in diameter were more likely to fail incision and drainage without antibiotic therapy [63]. A recent survey indicated that the majority of physicians prescribe antimicrobials (often inadequate ones) for patients with skin abscesses [66]. Antibiotics should be used in patients with large, dangerous, or difficult to drain collections, as well as in patients with surrounding cellulitis, cutaneous gangrene, and systemic signs of infection as well as in patients who are immunocompromised [45].

Cellulitis

Cellulitis refers to an acute pyogenic inflammation of the dermis and subcutaneous tissues [67]. A conservative estimate of the frequency of cellulitis puts the incidence rate at 24.6 per 1000 person-years [68]. Cellulitis is most frequently caused by streptococci and staphylococci [69]. *S. aureus*, particularly CA-MRSA, is becoming, in certain regions of the USA, the most common cause of SSTIs in both adults and children [3,4,6]. Other than studies on

CA-MRSA and recent clinical trials, most of the research done on cellulitis has not specifically focused on *S. aureus*.

Several factors have been independently associated with cellulitis of the lower extremities among hospitalized patients. Obesity, history of cellulitis or saphenous vein stripping especially when associated with chronic lower extremity edema, chronic cutaneous lesions such as ulcers especially in patients with diabetes mellitus, and tinea pedis [70–74] are all predisposing conditions for cellulitis (see Table 19.2). In addition, the presence of *S. aureus* in toe webs has also been associated with cellulitis [71], although clones isolated from the webs were not always responsible for the infections [75] (Table 19.2). Although cellulitis in the lower extremities is most common, other factors such as injection drug use, lymph node dissection after mastectomy, radiation, oral hygiene, facial acne, and both intentional and unintentional wounds predispose to cellulitis of the rest of the body [51,52]. Indeed, local risk factors seem to be the most important determinants for the occurrence of cellulitis [71,76,77].

Innate immunity seems to play a role in limiting the infection to a single anatomic location. Patients with infective cellulitis have overexpression of the mRNA for two important endogenous antimicrobial peptides, cathelicidin and human β-defensin 2, in both infected and distal normally appearing skin [78].

The physical examination of patients with cellulitis reveals a spreading area of edema, erythema, tenderness, and warmth (see Plate 19.5). In some instances an entry site can be identified (see Plate 19.6). In contrast to erysipelas, cellulitis does not have a sharply demarcated border between involved and uninvolved skin and is not elevated above the level of surrounding skin [45], although this distinction is often difficult in clinical practice. Indeed, in certain parts of Europe the terms "cellulitis" and "erysipelas" refer to the same disease [71]. *S. aureus* is an uncommon cause of erysipelas, which is usually caused by streptococci [15,79].

Vesicles or bullae filled with clear fluid are common in patients with cellulitis; localized petechiae or ecchymosis can be seen in the affected area. Lymphangitis and regional lymphadenopathy may occur during the course of the infection. Although any site of the skin can be involved (see Plates 19.6 and 19.7), cellulitis occurs more frequently in the lower extremities (> 70% of the cases) [45,80]. Orbital infections and periorbital cellulitis are also commonly associated with *S. aureus*, including CA-MRSA [81–83]. Aside from mastitis, *S. aureus* is an unusual cause of cellulitis of the breast following axillary lymph node dissection [84,85]. Systemic signs (e.g., fever, tachycardia) are frequently mild although in some instances the infection can be severe. Concomitant bacteremia is relatively uncommon in cellulitis [80,86]. Shock is present in less than 5% of cases and is associated with increased mortality [69].

Outcomes at 30 days are similar in patients hospitalized with SSTIs produced by CA-MRSA or methicillin-susceptible *S. aureus* (MSSA) [7]. Patients with multiple comorbid conditions, cutaneous necrosis, hypoalbuminemia, and renal insufficiency are more likely to have local or systemic complications [69]. Recurrence is common in cellulitis; in fact, 20–50% of patients with cellulitis have suffered a previous episode in the past [69,70,77]. Certain clinical characteristics, such as involvement of the tibial area, ipsilateral dermatitis, and cancer, are predictors of recurrence [87].

The isolation of a bacterial pathogen in subjects with cellulitis is difficult. Cultures are reportedly positive in 20–28% of biopsies and 10–15% of needle aspirations (in the leading edge of the erythema), although in our hands this rate is significantly lower. Gram stains are rarely helpful [88]. Overall, blood cultures are positive in 4% or less of cases and they are not considered cost-effective in either adults or children [86,89], although they should be obtained in elderly patients (especially those with systemic symptoms), in those with severe/extensive infection, and in immunocompromised patients [86,89,90].

A large proportion of patients with cellulitis produced by *S. aureus* can be treated with oral therapy for 5–10 days. In fact, 5 days of therapy is as effective as 10 days in patients with uncomplicated disease [91]. Parenteral therapy, usually for 7–14 days, is indicated in patients with systemic signs of infection (e.g., fever, tachycardia, or hypotension), immunosuppression, dangerous locations (e.g., periorbital), or extensive involvement at presentation. There is a wide variety of agents that can be used to treat SSTIs produced by *S. aureus* including MRSA (see Table 19.3). In patients with erysipelas, time of healing is shortened by 1 day with prednisolone [92]. In order to avoid recurrences, correction of predisposing factors such as dermatitis, leg edema, and toe-web colonization should be addressed [45]. Prophylactic antibiotics have been suggested as beneficial, particularly in patients without risk factors and in those with recurrent streptococcal infections [93,94].

Necrotizing fasciitis

Necrotizing fasciitis is an uncommon life-threatening infection characterized by widespread necrosis of subcutaneous tissues and fascia [95,96]. The disease is often polymicrobial [95,97,98]. When necrotizing fasciitis is monomicrobial, *S. pyogenes* is the most common pathogen isolated [95,97]. *S. aureus* is frequently involved in polymicrobial and, less commonly, monomicrobial forms of the disease [96–101].

Necrotizing fasciitis due to *S. aureus* affects patients of all ages [99,100,102] and can occur in any area of the body [103], although the extremities are most frequently involved

[98]. Patients with necrotizing fasciitis due to *S. aureus* often have diabetes mellitus [98,99,104–106], although other types of immunosuppression can be present [107,108].

While necrotizing fasciitis is usually a rapidly progressive infection [99,105,109], *S. aureus* can also produce a subacute form of the disease [104,110]. Subacute necrotizing fasciitis has been described for both MRSA, including CA-MRSA [104], and MSSA [110] and appears to have a low mortality although morbidity remains high [104]. *S. aureus*, including CA-MRSA [111], can also produce Fournier gangrene, a particular type of necrotizing infection affecting the perineum [112,113]. Necrotizing fasciitis due to *S. aureus* can be associated with bacteremia [104–106,109], septic shock [106], or staphylococcal toxic shock syndrome [107].

The clinical diagnosis of necrotizing fasciitis can be quite difficult. A clinical score (Laboratory Risk Indicator for Necrotizing Fasciitis or LRINEC) has been proposed to distinguish necrotizing fasciitis from other SSTIs [114]. Similarly, magnetic resonance imaging (MRI) has been used with significant success in the differentiation of necrotizing fasciitis from cellulitis. Nevertheless, when this life-threatening infection is suspected, surgical exploration is mandatory. Frozen biopsies during surgical exploration can contribute to earlier recognition of the disease and improve clinical outcomes [115].

Regardless of the etiological agent, the main treatment of necrotizing fasciitis is surgery [45,116]. A prompt surgical exploration with extensive débridement of necrotic tissue is crucial. Aggressive surgical management [117], particularly early débridement [97], is associated with decreased mortality. Multiple surgeries are often required; in some cases amputations cannot be avoided [105].

Antibiotic therapy is important in helping to control the infection and prevent relapses. Concomitant antibiotic therapy should be intravenous, usually for 2–4 weeks, until the infection is totally under control and no further surgical interventions are needed. Then therapy can be continued with a short course of oral antibiotics. Several different antibiotics, often in combination, have been used in patients with necrotizing fasciitis due to *S. aureus*. Oxacillin [101,109,110], clindamycin, and vancomycin [7, 102] have been used for MSSA. Vancomycin [100,101,104], teicoplanin [101], ciprofloxacin [101], and clindamycin [104] have been used to treat necrotizing infections produced by MRSA. Clindamycin and linezolid have the theoretical advantage of inhibiting production of several exotoxins in both MSSA or MRSA although no comparative clinical data exist [118].

Limb loss in patients with nonclostridial necrotizing infections occurs in 20% [119]. Overall mortality in patients with necrotizing fasciitis is 34% [97]. Mortality in patients with necrotizing fasciitis in which *S. aureus* is involved was 14% (8 of 59), which is certainly lower than that associated with clostridial infection [119].

Pyomyositis

Pyomyositis is a primary suppurative infection of skeletal muscle, commonly associated with abscess formation [120,121]. *S. aureus* is the most common cause of pyomyositis [122,123]. The infection has been classically described in the tropics as affecting all age groups (although more common in children and young people) [123,124]. In temperate climates, pyomyositis is a rare disease that often affects individuals with some degree of immunosuppression (e.g., HIV infection, diabetes mellitus, IDUs) [52,120,121,125–127] (see Table 19.2). However, the distinction between tropical and temperate pyomyositis is somewhat arbitrary. Healthy people can have pyomyositis in temperate climates and HIV may underlie the tropical form of the disease [120,121,127]. Pyomyositis is thought to be produced by hematogenous seeding [120,121]. A history of muscle trauma is frequently found, suggesting that a muscle lesion or bleeding may predispose tissue to being seeded during an intermittent bacteremia [123]. Although the disease has usually been caused by MSSA, recent reports suggest that CA-MRSA is now a growing cause of pyomyositis in the USA [128,129].

Muscles of the thighs (quadriceps) and pelvis (psoas and gluteus) are the most commonly affected [121]. Most patients have involvement of a single muscle or muscle group [121,122]. Different from necrotizing fasciitis and myonecrosis, pyomyositis often has a subacute course [121]. Localized pain and fever are very common [122]. Involved muscles are tender and indurated at early stages while an abscess forms. Swelling and edema of overlying tissues along with systemic signs of infection are frequent during late stages of the disease [121]. Involvement of anterior tibial muscles can result in compartment syndrome [130]. Leukocytosis is frequent but serum creatine kinase is usually within normal limits [122,128]. Rarely, pyomyositis is associated with toxic shock syndrome [131]. In temperate climates concomitant bacteremia is present in 17–37% of patients [122]. Except in patients with HIV, recurrence is uncommon [122].

Imaging methods are essential to confirm the diagnosis of pyomyositis. Plain radiography can be helpful for excluding gross bone infections and ultrasound for ruling out deep venous thrombosis. Computed tomography and particularly magnetic radionuclide imaging are excellent imaging methods for confirming and assessing the extent of pyomyositis [121,132–134]. Gallium scans are very sensitive in the detection of pyomyositis but specificity and localization are often inadequate [135]. Imaging studies are also helpful during the follow-up period.

The mainstay treatment of pyomyositis is surgical drainage of collections accompanied by antibiotic therapy. The vast majority of patients recover without sequelae [121]. Parenteral antibiotics are frequently needed for 10–14 days or until collections are drained and systemic signs of infection have resolved. Then, a switch to oral therapy can be made and maintained for another 2–3 weeks [122].

Mastitis

Mastitis refers to an inflammatory process in the breast, usually secondary to bacterial infection. The infection involves the interlobular connective tissue and/or obstructed ducts. Epidemic outbreaks of nosocomial mastitis caused by *S. aureus* used to be frequent when mothers and neonates had longer hospital stays [136]. Nowadays, most cases of infectious mastitis are acute and sporadic (non-epidemic). Mastitis is uncommon in children; it affects predominantly neonates and female adolescents, periods in which breast enlargement takes place [137]. The majority of cases of mastitis occurs in mothers during the first 8 weeks after birth [138]. The exact incidence of acute infectious puerperal mastitis is difficult to estimate because individual definitions were established in each study; reported incidence rates range from 2.9% [139] to 17.3% [140] of lactating mothers.

The development of infectious mastitis requires the presence of milk stasis or engorgement plus a potential route for microorganisms. Therefore, cracking of nipples, obstructions to lactiferous ducts, and prior history of mastitis [140,141] are all risk factors for puerperal mastitis [142]. Longer duration of breast-feeding does not increase the risk of puerperal mastitis [140,142].

S. aureus has been isolated in patients with puerperal mastitis in 30–50% of cases [143]. Coagulase-negative staphylococci (CoNS), streptococci (including *Streptococcus agalactiae*), Gram-negative bacilli such as *Escherichia coli*, and anaerobes such as *Propionibacterium acne* are more rarely associated with mastitis [138,143]. The microorganisms involved represent mothers' skin flora and infants' oral or nasal flora. Nursing mothers with sore cracked nipples have higher chances of being colonized by *S. aureus* [144]. These same breast-feeding mothers have a 12–35% chance of having an episode of infectious mastitis [145]. Also, a significant association between the infant's (and not the mother's) nasal carriage of *S. aureus* and mastitis has been described [146]. The pathogenic role of *S. aureus* in women with mastitis is highlighted by its association with poorer outcomes compared with mastitis caused by other microorganisms [147].

A prospective study found that, at presentation, 80% and 20% of puerperal mothers with breast infection had mastitis and abscess, respectively [148]. In addition, in 10–20% of cases, puerperal mastitis is complicated by breast abscesses [138,143]. No differences in demographics and overall risk factors were found between women with infectious mastitis and those with breast abscesses [148]. About 10% of women with puerperal mastitis have recurrence of disease [148]. Based on clinical symptoms and the number of leukocytes and bacterial cells in the milk, different stages of breast inflammation can be established in puerperal women. Patients with benign milk stasis and noninfectious inflammation usually respond to conservative treatment measures. These women present with low-grade fever, a swollen breast, and high leukocyte count ($> 10^6$/mL) but with insignificant bacterial counts in the milk. If stasis and breast inflammation persist, the clinical picture may progress to infectious mastitis; in this case, the patient may present with a swollen, red and hot breast as well as high-grade fever and a significant number of bacterial cells in the expressed milk ($> 10^3$ cfu/mL) [149,150].

However, the diagnosis of infectious mastitis is usually made on clinical grounds. The most frequent symptoms are pain in the breast and axillae, chills, fever, and myalgias. Breast examination reveals unilateral edema, erythema, and tenderness in a wedge-shaped area representing a lactiferous area. If a breast abscess is present, a localized breast mass with fluctuance is frequently observed. Also a fissure, crack or fungal infection of the nipple may be found on examination. High fever and leukocytosis are frequent [151]. Obtaining a milk sample for culture is not part of the standard practice and in fact milk culture is positive in more than 80% of healthy mothers [152]. However, milk culture may be useful in selected circumstances (e.g., abscess formation or persistent fever) [147]. Breast ultrasound is recommended if the presence of an abscess is suspected on physical examination [153].

Clinical presentation and physical findings of nonpuerperal mastitis in children does not differ from that observed in adults and *S. aureus* has also been implicated in the majority of the cases reported in children and neonates [137,154,155]. If the inflammatory process in the breast does not respond to a trial of effective antistaphylococcal antibiotics, inflammatory breast cancer should be suspected, especially in women above 40 years old [156].

Conservative measures are critical in the management of puerperal mastitis. Continued lactation, which allows proper drainage of the breast, is important [151]; if breast-feeding of the affected side is not possible (the baby may reject the salty taste of infected milk), a breast pump can be used. Warm moist heat should be applied to the inflamed breast. In addition, increased fluid intake, bed-rest, analgesics, and antipyretics are important. If a breast abscess is diagnosed, it can be effectively treated by percutaneous drainage [153,157] or by incision and drainage, depending on the experience and availability of these procedures. Antibiotics are indicated in the nursing mother with mastitis if systemic symptoms are present, although selected cases resolve with conservative measures only. Most of the studies evaluating the treatment of infectious mastitis were done more than 20 years ago and have not focused on the type of antibiotic prescribed. Agents with activity against MSSA and streptococci, such as the penicillinase-resistant penicillins or cephalosporins, are usually administered. Other agents with activity against MRSA might be required since the emergence of CA-MRSA in postpartum mastitis [158] and breast abscess [159].

Hidradenitis suppurativa

Hidradenitis suppurativa, also known as Verneuil's disease or acne inverse, is a chronic relapsing inflammatory skin disease originating in the hair follicle and characterized by recurrent draining sinuses and abscesses affecting skin folds that carry apocrine glands, especially in the axillae and the anogenital region [160]. Hidradenitis suppurativa affects more women than men and frequently occurs between puberty and menopause, suggesting a hormonal component in the pathogenesis. A genetic factor is also present with autosomal dominant inheritance and a possible association with other disorders such as acne conglobata and dissecting cellulitis of the scalp (the follicular occlusion triad). This recurrent disease could lead to periods of inflammation, secondary bacterial infections, and disfiguring lesions. It has been suggested that microorganisms inside the inflamed apocrine glands play a pathogenic role [161]. The predominant aerobic microorganisms are *S. aureus*, CoNS, *S. pyogenes* and anaerobes such as *Peptostreptococcus* spp., *Prevotella* spp., microaerophilic streptococci, *Fusobacterium* spp., and *Bacteroides* spp. [160–162]. Antibiotics should target cultured microorganisms during flare-ups; in extended disease, extensive surgical treatment is necessary [162].

Botryomycosis

Botryomycosis is a very rare, chronic granulomatous disease produced by nonbranching bacteria and characterized by the presence of granules within suppurative foci [163,164]. The name of the disease comes from the Greek *botrys* meaning "bunch of grapes" and *mykes* because originally it was thought to be the result of a fungal infection. *S. aureus* is the most common cause of botryomycosis [164]. The pathophysiology of the disease is still poorly understood. Immunological deficiencies in the host [165–167] as well as weakly virulent bacterial strains have been postulated to be involved in this chronic infection.

Botryomycosis is usually described in patients with diabetes, poor hygiene, alcoholism, or HIV [164,167]. Adults and children are both affected [163,164,168]. The disease most commonly involves skin and subcutaneous tissues although visceral lesions (e.g., lung) have been described [164]. Skin lesions are chronic and can adopt various forms such as nodules, sinuses, fistulas, ulcers, and verrucous lesions [167,169]. Hands and feet are more commonly affected. Differential diagnoses include mycetoma, actinomycosis, sporotrichosis, cutaneous leishmaniasis, tuberculosis, and cancer. MRI can be helpful to determine the extent of the lesions [170].

Definitive diagnosis of botryomycosis relies on the identification of nonfilamentous bacteria in granules from pus of draining lesions or biopsies [164]. An eosinophilic matrix, probably representing antigen–antibody precipitation, can surround the offending microorganisms (Splendore–Hoeppli phenomenon) [171]. Treatment requires several weeks of antibiotics combined occasionally with surgical resection.

Skin and soft tissue infections caused by coagulase-negative staphylococci

It is often difficult to distinguish between colonization and infection when a CoNS strain is isolated from an infected skin site. However, several reports have well-documented infections caused by several species of CoNS, including *Staphylococcus epidermidis*, *Staphylococcus haemolyticus*, *Staphylococcus saprophyticus*, and *Staphylococcus lugdunensis* [172]. Very rarely, *Staphylococcus sciuri* can cause SSTI in humans [173]. CoNS have also been implicated in exacerbations of hidradenitis suppurativa. [161]. *S. lugdunensis* appears to be more virulent than other CoNS species and has been associated with superficial skin abscesses, particularly gluteal abscess, and sebaceous gland infection [174,175]. Other CoNS species such as *S. epidermidis* and *S. warneri* can also be isolated although they are less frequently considered clinically significant [175]. If the SSTI is associated with foreign material (e.g., pacemaker pocket infection), CoNS are more often a true pathogen [176]. Overall, CoNS display higher resistance rates to multiple antibiotics. As a consequence non-β-lactam antibiotics are required.

Colonization, outbreaks, and recurrent infection

The anterior nares are considered the colonization niche of *S. aureus*. Hands have been described as the typical vector used by the colonizing *S. aureus* strain to reach the subject's anterior nares [177], where they multiply and are then transferred to altered skin sites on the carrier or their contacts [178]. *S. aureus* survives in the vestibulum nasi within the nostril, evading several host immune responses such as immunoglobulins, lysozyme, lactoferrin, and antimicrobial peptides (defensins and cathelicidins) [179]. The *S. aureus* clumping factor B, surface protein G, and teichoic acid are the necessary factors needed for bacterial binding to nasal epithelial cells; the adhesive matrix molecules called MSCRAMMs (microbial surface components recognizing adhesive matrix molecules) may well have a role in attaching to the mucosal lining when a breach is present [179]. Strains of *S. aureus* can survive for days and even months on dry surfaces [180,181] explaining, at least in part, the tendency of this microorganism to cause recurrent disease. Innate immunity can play a role in predisposing certain patients to recurrent skin infections produced by *S. aureus*. As an example, patients with atopic dermatitis have a deficit in expression of endogenous antimicrobial peptides such as human β-defensin 2 and cathelicidin [182] resulting in more frequent *S. aureus* colonization of involved skin. (See Chapter 12 for a detailed discusion of nasal colonization.)

The prevalence of nasal *S. aureus* colonization in the general population of the USA was 32.4% in a national survey in 2001–2002 [183]. Among men, higher rates were observed in non-Hispanic whites and Mexican Americans, with no race/ethnicity differences noted in women [183]. Carriage of *S. aureus* is classified as intermittent (60%), persistent (20%), or absent/never colonized (20%) [178,184,185]. Host factors are clearly implicated in determining the subject's nasal carrier state [186]; for example, persistent *S. aureus* nasal carriage is significantly associated with particular polymorphisms in the glucocorticoid receptor gene [187]. Overall, a higher rate of nasal carriage has been reported among subjects with diabetes mellitus (both insulin and noninsulin dependent), chronic skin diseases (e.g., eczema), end-stage renal disease undergoing dialysis, HIV infection, obesity, and a history of cerebrovascular accident [178,179]. *S. aureus* can also be isolated from extranasal sites: skin, pharynx, perineum, chronic ulcers, open wounds, and other areas with disrupted skin integrity such as the site of a tracheostomy or gastrotomy.

Subjects with staphylococcal skin infections who are carriers of *S. aureus* have a high risk of developing recurrent episodes of skin infection [188]. In fact, 80% of subjects with recurrent staphylococcal skin infection carry the same *S. aureus* strain in their nares [179,189].

Close contacts of subjects with furunculosis produced by *S. aureus* are at risk of becoming colonized and/or of developing staphylococcal skin disease with the same strains [190]. Factors such as the extent of colonization (i.e., the number of positive skin sites), the patient's hygiene practices, and certain host determinants will affect the contact's overall risk of SSTI. For example, family members suffering from furunculosis had lower serum mannose-binding lectin levels than those without skin disease [191].

Transmission of *S. aureus* from person to person and its ability to survive on inanimate materials [180] explain, at least in part, the development of local outbreaks of staphylococcal skin disease in closed communities and the tendency of this microorganism to cause recurrent disease. Outbreaks affecting family members [42,192], sports teammates [44,193–195], prisoners in correctional facilities [196], firefighters [42], and steam bath users [43] have been described for both MRSA [43,190,193] and MSSA [42,197]. Recurrence of staphylococcal skin disease in patients with abscesses, cellulitis, and furuncles was 15%, up to 3 months after the initial episode [7].

Even though there has not been sufficient evidence to recommend universal nasal decolonization of *S. aureus* [198,199], subjects with recurrent staphylococcal skin disease may well benefit from this approach. Decolonization can be achieved with antiseptics and/or antibiotics. Bathing with an antiseptic solution such as chlorhexidine gluconate when combined with nasal decolonization, adequate personal hygiene and thorough cleaning of personal items will help decrease recurrence rates of skin infections [42]. Decolonization with topical mupirocin (2% ointment twice daily for 5 days each month for 1 year) in subjects with recurrent furunculosis was associated with significantly less skin infection episodes than in a placebo group ($P < 0.002$) [188], although many subjects in the mupirocin arm during follow-up were culture-positive [188]. Failures of *S. aureus* eradication could be explained, at least in part, by development of mupirocin resistance [200].

Prophylactic oral antibiotics may have a role in preventing recurrent disease. Low-dose clindamycin (150 mg/day) for 3 months in patients with recurrent staphylococcal skin infections produced a significant reduction in the recurrence rate when compared with placebo and in about 50% of the subjects the effect lasted for more than 9 months [201]. Other topical and systemic antibiotics (or combinations) have been tested in clinical trials of decolonization that were not specifically designed for patients with recurrent skin disease. These include novobiocin or trimethoprim–sulfamethoxazole (TMP–SMX) plus rifampin [202], TMP–SMX with topical fusidic acid [203], and intranasal mupirocin with oral rifampin plus doxycycline [200]. Rifampin-containing regimens appear to be associated with higher success rates [204], although this drug should not be used as monotherapy since development of resistance occurs rapidly.

Antibacterial therapy

Skin and soft tissue infections due to MSSA

A large list of approved agents is available to treat patients with SSTI due to MSSA (Table 19.3). Antistaphylococcal penicillins (e.g., nafcillin) and first-generation cephalosporins (e.g., cefazolin, cephalexin) are preferred. In patients with immediate-type hypersensitivity to β-lactams, treatment options include clindamycin, TMP–SMX, long-acting tetracyclines, vancomycin, daptomycin, linezolid, and tigecycline. Recent evidence suggests that vancomycin is an inferior agent for the treatment of *S. aureus* infections. However, such evidence is derived from patients with invasive infections (i.e., bacteremia, endocarditis) [205–208] and not from patients with SSTIs due to MSSA. Topical

Table 19.3 FDA-approved and off-label agents for the treatment of skin and soft tissue infection caused by *S. aureus*.[1]

Only approved for MSSA

Antistaphylococcal penicillins (e.g., nafcillin): used commonly for treatment of SSTI
First-generation cephalosporins (e.g., cephalexin, cefazolin, cefadroxil): used commonly for treatment of SSTI
Second-generation cephalosporins (e.g., cefaclor, cefuroxime): use cefaclor for uncomplicated SSTI only
Third-generation cephalosporins (e.g., ceftriaxone, cefditoren): use cefditoren for uncomplicated SSTI only
Fourth-generation cephalosporins (cefepime): use cefepime for uncomplicated SSTI only
Ampicillin–sulbactam: used commonly for treatment of diabetic foot infection
Amoxicillin–clavulanate: used commonly for treatment of diabetic foot infection
Piperacillin–tazobactam: used commonly for treatment of diabetic foot infection
Ticarcillin–clavulanate: used commonly for treatment of diabetic foot infection
Carbapenems (imipenem, meropenem, ertapenem): used commonly for treatment of diabetic foot infection
Macrolides (erythromycin, azithromycin, clarithromycin): only approved for uncomplicated SSTI
Quinupristin–dalfopristin: rarely used
Tetracyclines (e.g., minocycline, doxycycline): limited data but probably effective
Quinolones (e.g., ciprofloxacin, moxifloxacin, levofloxacin (use with caution because of resistance may arise during treatment))
Clindamycin: increasing resistance
Retapamulin (topical): only approved for impetigo

Approved for both MSSA and MRSA

Vancomycin: most common intravenous therapy for SSTI due to MRSA
Linezolid: superior to vancomycin (in patients with MRSA) in open-label study [209]
Daptomycin: not inferior to vancomycin; < 50 microbiologically evaluable patients with MRSA treated with the agent in registrational studies[2] [210]
Tigecycline: not inferior to vancomycin; < 50 microbiologically evaluable patients with MRSA treated with the agent in registrational studies[2] [211]
Mupirocin: only approved for topical use (nasal decolonization and impetigo)

Off-label (agents used in clinical practice without adequate evidence from clinical trials)

MSSA or MRSA

Trimethoprim–sulfamethoxazole: not approved for *S. aureus* infections though probably effective; coverage against *Streptococcus pyogenes* is unknown
Rifampin: not approved for *S. aureus* infections; no evidence of effectiveness either as monotherapy or as combined agent; monotherapy associated with rapid emergence of resistance

MRSA

Clindamycin: approved for *S. aureus* infections (not specifically for MRSA); resistance rates rising
Tetracyclines (e.g., minocycline): approved for *S. aureus* infections (not specifically for MRSA); limited evidence of efficacy

[1] Teicoplanin has been approved in Europe and South America but not in the USA.
[2] Information available at http://www.accessdata.fda.gov/scripts/cder/drugsatfda/index.cfm
MRSA, methicillin-resistant *S. aureus*; MSSA, methicillin-susceptible *S. aureus*; SSTI, skin and soft tissue infection.

antibiotics for superficial *S. aureus* infections include mupirocin, retapamulin (only approved for impetigo), and fusidic acid [21]. Fusidic acid is not approved in the USA.

Skin and soft tissue infections due to MRSA

Patients requiring parenteral therapy

When MRSA is being considered (e.g., in areas with a high prevalence of CA-MRSA or in healthcare-related infections) vancomycin is still the drug of choice. Vancomycin has the most supporting evidence of any drug in patients with SSTIs due to MRSA, is safe, and is inexpensive [209–211]. However, vancomycin has been associated with clinical failures in invasive *S. aureus* infection when the minimum inhibitory concentration (MIC) was 1 μg/mL or more [212].

Other approved antibiotics for treating patients with SSTIs due to MRSA include linezolid [209], daptomycin [210], and tigecycline [211] (Table 19.3). Investigational agents with activity against MRSA include telavancin [213,214], dalbavancin [215], oritavancin [216], iclaprim [217], ceftaroline [218], and ceftobiprole [219,220]. All these agents have completed or are undergoing phase III trials in patients with SSTI.

Patients requiring oral or topical therapy

Linezolid is the only drug with an oral formulation approved by the Food and Drug Administration (FDA) for treatment of SSTIs caused by MRSA. The oral formulation has excellent bioavailability and does not need adjustment in patients with renal dysfunction [221].

Although not FDA approved, other antibiotics have activity against MRSA. Clindamycin has been successfully used to treat children with SSTI due to MRSA [222] and it has the potential advantage of enhancing phagocytosis

[223] and inhibiting toxin production [118]. Susceptibility testing should be done when considering use of this drug since resistance to clindamycin is increasing. TMP–SMX has been used in a single clinical trial against *S. aureus*, including subjects with SSTI [224]. Importantly, no failures occurred in patients infected with MRSA. Long-acting tetracyclines (e.g., minocycline, doxycycline) were effective in small series of patients with SSTI produced by MRSA [225]. There are no robust data to support the use of these drugs in serious infections produced by MRSA. For this reason the National Institutes of Health has funded a large ongoing clinical trial to determine their efficacy.

Acknowledgments

We want to thank Dr Fabián Herrera (Centro de Educación Médica e Investigaciones Clínicas, CEMIC, Buenos Aires, Argentina), Dr Carlos Lovesio (Sanatorio Parque, Rosario, Argentina), and Dr Claude S. Burton (Duke University Medical Center, Durham, North Carolina, USA) for providing the excellent clinical pictures.

References

1 McCaig LF, McDonald LC, Mandal S, Jernigan DB. *Staphylococcus aureus*-associated skin and soft tissue infections in ambulatory care. Emerg Infect Dis 2006;12:1715–23.

2 Moellering RC Jr. The growing menace of community-acquired methicillin-resistant *Staphylococcus aureus*. Ann Intern Med 2006;144:368–70.

3 King MD, Humphrey BJ, Wang YF, Kourbatova EV, Ray SM, Blumberg HM. Emergence of community-acquired methicillin-resistant *Staphylococcus aureus* USA 300 clone as the predominant cause of skin and soft-tissue infections. Ann Intern Med 2006;144:309–17.

4 Moran GJ, Krishnadasan A, Gorwitz RJ *et al*. Methicillin-resistant *S. aureus* infections among patients in the emergency department. N Engl J Med 2006;355:666–74.

5 Ruhe JJ, Smith N, Bradsher RW, Menon A. Community-onset methicillin-resistant *Staphylococcus aureus* skin and soft-tissue infections: impact of antimicrobial therapy on outcome. Clin Infect Dis 2007;44:777–84.

6 Fridkin SK, Hageman JC, Morrison M *et al*. Methicillin-resistant *Staphylococcus aureus* disease in three communities. N Engl J Med 2005;352:1436–44.

7 Miller LG, Quan C, Shay A *et al*. A prospective investigation of outcomes after hospital discharge for endemic, community-acquired methicillin-resistant and -susceptible *Staphylococcus aureus* skin infection. Clin Infect Dis 2007;44:483–92.

8 Centers for Disease Control and Prevention, National Center for Health Statistics. Vital and Health Statistics. National Hospital Discharge Survey: 2004 Annual Summary with Detailed Diagnosis and Procedure Data. U.S. Department of Health and Human Services 2006;13[162].

9 Koning S, Mohammedamin RS, van der Wouden JC, van Suijlekom-Smit LW, Schellevis FG, Thomas S. Impetigo: incidence and treatment in Dutch general practice in 1987 and 2001. Results from two national surveys. Br J Dermatol 2006;154:239–43.

10 Schachner LA. Treatment of uncomplicated skin and skin infections in the pediatric and adolescent patient populations. J Drugs Dermatol 2005;4(6 suppl):s30–s33.

11 Demidovich CW, Wittler RR, Ruff ME, Bass JW, Browning WC. Impetigo. Current etiology and comparison of penicillin, erythromycin, and cephalexin therapies. Am J Dis Child 1990;144:1313–15.

12 Dagan R, Bar-David Y. Double-blind study comparing erythromycin and mupirocin for treatment of impetigo in children: implications of a high prevalence of erythromycin-resistant *Staphylococcus aureus* strains. Antimicrob Agents Chemother 1992;36:287–90.

13 Dajani AS, Ferrieri P, Wannamaker LW. Natural history of impetigo. II. Etiologic agents and bacterial interactions. J Clin Invest 1972;51:2863–71.

14 Koning S, van Belkum A, Snijders S *et al*. Severity of nonbullous *Staphylococcus aureus* impetigo in children is associated with strains harboring genetic markers for exfoliative toxin B, Panton–Valentine leukocidin, and the multidrug resistance plasmid pSK41. J Clin Microbiol 2003;41:3017–21.

15 Lopez FA, Lartchenko S. Skin and soft tissue infections. Infect Dis Clin North Am 2006;20:759–72, v–vi.

16 Koning S, van Suijlekom-Smit LW, Nouwen JL *et al*. Fusidic acid cream in the treatment of impetigo in general practice: double blind randomised placebo controlled trial. BMJ 2002;324:203–6.

17 Koning S, Verhagen AP, van Suijlekom-Smit LW, Morris A, Butler CC, van der Wouden JC. Interventions for impetigo. Cochrane Database Syst Rev 2004;2:CD003261.

18 Mertz PM, Marshall DA, Eaglstein WH, Piovanetti Y, Montalvo J. Topical mupirocin treatment of impetigo is equal to oral erythromycin therapy. Arch Dermatol 1989;125:1069–73.

19 Johnston GA. Treatment of bullous impetigo and the staphylococcal scalded skin syndrome in infants. Expert Rev Anti Infect Ther 2004;2:439–46.

20 Yun HJ, Lee SW, Yoon GM *et al*. Prevalence and mechanisms of low- and high-level mupirocin resistance in staphylococci isolated from a Korean hospital. J Antimicrob Chemother 2003;51:619–23.

21 Oranje AP, Chosidow O, Sacchidanand S *et al*. Topical retapamulin ointment, 1%, versus sodium fusidate ointment, 2%, for impetigo: a randomized, observer-blinded, noninferiority study. Dermatology 2007;215:331–40.

22 Cole C, Gazewood J. Diagnosis and treatment of impetigo. Am Fam Physician 2007;75:859–64.

23 Darmstadt GL, Lane AT. Impetigo: an overview. Pediatr Dermatol 1994;11:293–303.

24 McLinn S. A bacteriologically controlled, randomized study comparing the efficacy of 2% mupirocin ointment (Bactroban) with oral erythromycin in the treatment of patients with impetigo. J Am Acad Dermatol 1990;22:883–5.

25 Becker K, Friedrich AW, Lubritz G, Weilert M, Peters G, von Eiff C. Prevalence of genes encoding pyrogenic toxin superantigens and exfoliative toxins among strains of *Staphylococcus aureus* isolated from blood and nasal specimens. J Clin Microbiol 2003;41:1434–9.

26 Piemont Y, Rasoamananjara D, Fouace JM, Bruce T. Epidemio-

logical investigation of exfoliative toxin-producing *Staphylococcus aureus* strains in hospitalized patients. J Clin Microbiol 1984;19:417–20.

27 Adesiyun AA, Lenz W, Schaal KP. Exfoliative toxin production by *Staphylococcus aureus* strains isolated from animals and human beings in Nigeria. Microbiologica 1991;14:357–62.

28 Amagai M, Matsuyoshi N, Wang ZH, Andl C, Stanley JR. Toxin in bullous impetigo and staphylococcal scalded-skin syndrome targets desmoglein 1. Nat Med 2000;6:1275–7.

29 Hanakawa Y, Schechter NM, Lin C *et al.* Molecular mechanisms of blister formation in bullous impetigo and staphylococcal scalded skin syndrome. J Clin Invest 2002;110:53–60.

30 Ladhani S. Understanding the mechanism of action of the exfoliative toxins of *Staphylococcus aureus*. FEMS Immunol Med Microbiol 2003;39:181–9.

31 Lina G, Gillet Y, Vandenesch F, Jones ME, Floret D, Etienne J. Toxin involvement in staphylococcal scalded skin syndrome. Clin Infect Dis 1997;25:1369–73.

32 Patel GK, Finlay AY. Staphylococcal scalded skin syndrome: diagnosis and management. Am J Clin Dermatol 2003;4:165–75.

33 Salopek TG. Nikolsky's sign: is it "dry" or is it "wet"? Br J Dermatol 1997;136:762–7.

34 Abe R, Shimizu T, Shibaki A, Nakamura H, Watanabe H, Shimizu H. Toxic epidermal necrolysis and Stevens–Johnson syndrome are induced by soluble Fas Ligand. Am J Pathol 2003;162:1515–20.

35 Bastuji-Garin S, Rzany B, Stern RS, Shear NH, Naldi L, Roujeau JC. Clinical classification of cases of toxic epidermal necrolysis, Stevens–Johnson syndrome, and erythema multiforme. Arch Dermatol 1993;129:92–6.

36 Stanley JR, Amagai M. Pemphigus, bullous impetigo, and the staphylococcal scalded-skin syndrome. N Engl J Med 2006;355: 1800–10.

37 Yamasaki O, Yamaguchi T, Sugai M *et al.* Clinical manifestations of staphylococcal scalded-skin syndrome depend on serotypes of exfoliative toxins. J Clin Microbiol 2005;43:1890–3.

38 El Helali N, Carbonne A, Naas T *et al.* Nosocomial outbreak of staphylococcal scalded skin syndrome in neonates: epidemiological investigation and control. J Hosp Infect 2005;61:130–8.

39 Yamaguchi T, Yokota Y, Terajima J *et al.* Clonal association of *Staphylococcus aureus* causing bullous impetigo and the emergence of new methicillin-resistant clonal groups in Kansai district in Japan. J Infect Dis 2002;185:1511–16.

40 Noguchi N, Nakaminami H, Nishijima S, Kurokawa I, So H, Sasatsu M. Antimicrobial agent of susceptibilities and antiseptic resistance gene distribution among methicillin-resistant *Staphylococcus aureus* isolates from patients with impetigo and staphylococcal scalded skin syndrome. J Clin Microbiol 2006; 44:2119–25.

41 Nichols RL, Florman S. Clinical presentations of soft-tissue infections and surgical site infections. Clin Infect Dis 2001; 33(suppl 2):S84–S93.

42 Wiese-Posselt M, Heuck D, Draeger A *et al.* Successful termination of a furunculosis outbreak due to lukS-lukF-positive, methicillin-susceptible *Staphylococcus aureus* in a German village by stringent decolonization, 2002–2005. Clin Infect Dis 2007;44:e88–e95.

43 Landen MG, McCumber BJ, Asam ED, Egeland GM. Outbreak of boils in an Alaskan village: a case–control study. West J Med 2000;172:235–9.

44 Decker MD, Lybarger JA, Vaughn WK, Hutcheson RH Jr, Schaffner W. An outbreak of staphylococcal skin infections among river rafting guides. Am J Epidemiol 1986;124:969–76.

45 Stevens DL, Bisno AL, Chambers HF *et al.* Practice guidelines for the diagnosis and management of skin and soft-tissue infections. Clin Infect Dis 2005;41:1373–406.

46 Moreillon P, Que Y, Glauser MP. *Staphylococcus aureus* (including staphylococcal toxic shock). In: Mandell GL, Bennett JE, Dolin R, eds. Principles and Practice of Infectious Diseases, 6th edn. Philadelphia: Elsevier Churchill Livingstone, 2005:2321–51.

47 Bahrain M, Vasiliades M, Wolff M, Younus F. Five cases of bacterial endocarditis after furunculosis and the ongoing saga of community-acquired methicillin-resistant *Staphylococcus aureus* infections. Scand J Infect Dis 2006;38:702–7.

48 Ebright JR, Pace MT, Niazi AF. Septic thrombosis of the cavernous sinuses. Arch Intern Med 2001;161:2671–6.

49 Talbot TR, Nania JJ, Wright PW, Jones I, Aronsky D. Evaluation of the microbiology of soft-tissue abscesses in the era of community-associated strains of methicillin-resistant *Staphylococcus aureus*: an argument for empirical contact precautions. Infect Control Hosp Epidemiol 2007;28:730–2.

50 Entin MA. Infections of the hand. Surg Clin North Am 1964; 44:981–93.

51 Binswanger IA, Kral AH, Bluthenthal RN, Rybold DJ, Edlin BR. High prevalence of abscesses and cellulitis among community-recruited injection drug users in San Francisco. Clin Infect Dis 2000;30:579–81.

52 Ebright JR, Pieper B. Skin and soft tissue infections in injection drug users. Infect Dis Clin North Am 2002;16:697–712.

53 Young DM, Harris HW, Charlebois ED *et al.* An epidemic of methicillin-resistant *Staphylococcus aureus* soft tissue infections among medically underserved patients. Arch Surg 2004;139: 947–51.

54 Paydar KZ, Hansen SL, Charlebois ED, Harris HW, Young DM. Inappropriate antibiotic use in soft tissue infections. Arch Surg 2006;141:850–4; discussion 855–6.

55 Brook I. Microbiology and management of infected neck cysts. J Oral Maxillofac Surg 2005;63:392–5.

56 Diven DG, Dozier SE, Meyer DJ, Smith EB. Bacteriology of inflamed and uninflamed epidermal inclusion cysts. Arch Dermatol 1998;134:49–51.

57 Poonawalla T, Uchida T, Diven DG. Survey of antibiotic prescription use for inflamed epidermal inclusion cysts. J Cutan Med Surg 2006;10:79–84.

58 Squire BT, Fox JC, Anderson C. ABSCESS: applied bedside sonography for convenient evaluation of superficial soft tissue infections. Acad Emerg Med 2005;12:601–6.

59 Grayson ML. The treatment triangle for staphylococcal infections. N Engl J Med 2006;355:724–7.

60 Heilpern KL. Skin and soft tissue abscesses: the case for culturing abscess fluid. Ann Emerg Med 2007;50:64–6.

61 Macfie J, Harvey J. The treatment of acute superficial abscesses: a prospective clinical trial. Br J Surg 1977;64:264–6.

62 Llera JL, Levy RC. Treatment of cutaneous abscess: a double-blind clinical study. Ann Emerg Med 1985;14:15–19.

63 Lee MC, Rios AM, Aten MF *et al.* Management and outcome of children with skin and soft tissue abscesses caused by community-acquired methicillin-resistant *Staphylococcus aureus*. Pediatr Infect Dis J 2004;23:123–7.

64 Hankin A, Everett WW. Are antibiotics necessary after incision and drainage of a cutaneous abscess? Ann Emerg Med 2007; 50:49–51.

65 Rajendran PM, Young D, Maurer T *et al.* Randomized, double-blind, placebo-controlled trial of cephalexin for treatment of uncomplicated skin abscesses in a population at risk for community-acquired methicillin-resistant *Staphylococcus aureus* infection. Antimicrob Agents Chemother 2007;51:4044–8.

66 Rajendran PM, Young DM, Maurer T, Chambers HF, Jacobson MA, Harris HW. Antibiotic use in the treatment of soft tissue abscesses: a survey of current practice. Surg Infect (Larchmt) 2007;8:237–8.

67 Swartz MN. Clinical practice. Cellulitis. N Engl J Med 2004;350: 904–12.

68 Ellis Simonsen SM, van Orman ER, Hatch BE *et al.* Cellulitis incidence in a defined population. Epidemiol Infect 2006;134:293–9.

69 Carratala J, Roson B, Fernandez-Sabe N *et al.* Factors associated with complications and mortality in adult patients hospitalized for infectious cellulitis. Eur J Clin Microbiol Infect Dis 2003;22:151–7.

70 Bjornsdottir S, Gottfredsson M, Thorisdottir AS *et al.* Risk factors for acute cellulitis of the lower limb: a prospective case–control study. Clin Infect Dis 2005;41:1416–22.

71 Dupuy A, Benchikhi H, Roujeau JC *et al.* Risk factors for erysipelas of the leg (cellulitis): case–control study. BMJ 1999; 318:1591–4.

72 Semel JD, Goldin H. Association of athlete's foot with cellulitis of the lower extremities: diagnostic value of bacterial cultures of ipsilateral interdigital space samples. Clin Infect Dis 1996;23: 1162–4.

73 Baddour LM, Bisno AL. Recurrent cellulitis after saphenous venectomy for coronary bypass surgery. Ann Intern Med 1982; 97:493–6.

74 Baddour LM, Bisno AL. Recurrent cellulitis after coronary bypass surgery. Association with superficial fungal infection in saphenous venectomy limbs. JAMA 1984;251:1049–52.

75 Baddour LM. Cellulitis syndromes: an update. Int J Antimicrob Agents 2000;14:113–16.

76 Woo PC, Lum PN, Wong SS, Cheng VC, Yuen KY. Cellulitis complicating lymphoedema. Eur J Clin Microbiol Infect Dis 2000;19:294–7.

77 Koutkia P, Mylonakis E, Boyce J. Cellulitis: evaluation of possible predisposing factors in hospitalized patients. Diagn Microbiol Infect Dis 1999;34:325–7.

78 Stryjewski ME, Hall RP, Chu VH *et al.* Expression of antimicrobial peptides in the normal and involved skin of patients with infective cellulitis. J Infect Dis 2007;196:1425–30.

79 Bisno AL, Stevens DL. Streptococcal infections of skin and soft tissues. N Engl J Med 1996;334:240–5.

80 Peralta G, Padron E, Roiz MP *et al.* Risk factors for bacteremia in patients with limb cellulitis. Eur J Clin Microbiol Infect Dis 2006;25:619–26.

81 Rodriguez Ferran L, Puigarnau Vallhonrat R, Fasheh Youssef W, Ribo Aristazabal J, Luaces Cubells C, Pou Fernandez J. [Orbital and periorbital cellulitis. Review of 107 cases.] An Esp Pediatr 2000;53:567–72.

82 Blomquist PH. Methicillin-resistant *Staphylococcus aureus* infections of the eye and orbit (an American Ophthalmological Society thesis). Trans Am Ophthalmol Soc 2006;104:322–45.

83 Rutar T, Chambers HF, Crawford JB *et al.* Ophthalmic manifestations of infections caused by the USA300 clone of community-associated methicillin-resistant *Staphylococcus aureus*. Ophthalmology 2006;113:1455–62.

84 Simon MS, Cody RL. Cellulitis after axillary lymph node dissection for carcinoma of the breast. Am J Med 1992;93: 543–8.

85 Mertz KR, Baddour LM, Bell JL, Gwin JL. Breast cellulitis following breast conservation therapy: a novel complication of medical progress. Clin Infect Dis 1998;26:481–6.

86 Perl B, Gottehrer NP, Raveh D, Schlesinger Y, Rudensky B, Yinnon AM. Cost-effectiveness of blood cultures for adult patients with cellulitis. Clin Infect Dis 1999;29:1483–8.

87 McNamara DR, Tleyjeh IM, Berbari EF *et al.* A predictive model of recurrent lower extremity cellulitis in a population-based cohort. Arch Intern Med 2007;167:709–15.

88 Duvanel T, Auckenthaler R, Rohner P, Harms M, Saurat JH. Quantitative cultures of biopsy specimens from cutaneous cellulitis. Arch Intern Med 1989;149:293–6.

89 Sadow KB, Chamberlain JM. Blood cultures in the evaluation of children with cellulitis. Pediatrics 1998;101(3):e4.

90 Eron LJ, Lipsky BA. Use of cultures in cellulitis: when, how, and why? Eur J Clin Microbiol Infect Dis 2006;25:615–17.

91 Hepburn MJ, Dooley DP, Skidmore PJ, Ellis MW, Starnes WF, Hasewinkle WC. Comparison of short-course (5 days) and standard (10 days) treatment for uncomplicated cellulitis. Arch Intern Med 2004;164:1669–74.

92 Bergkvist PI, Sjobeck K. Antibiotic and prednisolone therapy of erysipelas: a randomized, double blind, placebo-controlled study. Scand J Infect Dis 1997;29:377–82.

93 Wang JH, Liu YC, Cheng DL *et al.* Role of benzathine penicillin G in prophylaxis for recurrent streptococcal cellulitis of the lower legs. Clin Infect Dis 1997;25:685–9.

94 Duvanel T, Merot Y, Harms M, Saurat JH. Prophylactic antibiotics in erysipelas. Lancet 1985;i:1401.

95 Green RJ, Dafoe DC, Raffin TA. Necrotizing fasciitis. Chest 1996;110:219–29.

96 Childers BJ, Potyondy LD, Nachreiner R *et al.* Necrotizing fasciitis: a fourteen-year retrospective study of 163 consecutive patients. Am Surg 2002;68:109–16.

97 McHenry CR, Piotrowski JJ, Petrinic D, Malangoni MA. Determinants of mortality for necrotizing soft-tissue infections. Ann Surg 1995;221:558–63; discussion 563–5.

98 Brook I, Frazier EH. Clinical and microbiological features of necrotizing fasciitis. J Clin Microbiol 1995;33:2382–7.

99 Regev A, Weinberger M, Fishman M, Samra Z, Pitlik SD. Necrotizing fasciitis caused by *Staphylococcus aureus*. Eur J Clin Microbiol Infect Dis 1998;17:101–3.

100 Hsieh WS, Yang PH, Chao HC, Lai JY. Neonatal necrotizing fasciitis: a report of three cases and review of the literature. Pediatrics 1999;103(4):e53.

101 Lee YT, Lin JC, Wang NC, Peng MY, Chang FY. Necrotizing fasciitis in a medical center in northern Taiwan: emergence of methicillin-resistant *Staphylococcus aureus* in the community. J Microbiol Immunol Infect 2007;40:335–41.

102 Dehority W, Wang E, Vernon PS, Lee C, Perdreau-Remington F, Bradley J. Community-associated methicillin-resistant *Staphylococcus aureus* necrotizing fasciitis in a neonate. Pediatr Infect Dis J 2006;25:1080–1.

103 Mohammedi I, Ceruse P, Duperret S, Vedrinne J, Bouletreau P. Cervical necrotizing fasciitis: 10 years' experience at a single institution. Intensive Care Med 1999;25:829–34.

104 Miller LG, Perdreau-Remington F, Rieg G *et al.* Necrotizing fasciitis caused by community-associated methicillin-resistant *Staphylococcus aureus* in Los Angeles. N Engl J Med 2005;352: 1445–53.

105 Morgan WR, Caldwell MD, Brady JM, Stemper ME, Reed KD, Shukla SK. Necrotizing fasciitis due to a methicillin-sensitive *Staphylococcus aureus* isolate harboring an enterotoxin gene cluster. J Clin Microbiol 2007;45:668–71.

106 Cheng NC, Chang SC, Kuo YS, Wang JL, Tang YB. Necrotizing fasciitis caused by methicillin-resistant *Staphylococcus aureus* resulting in death. A report of three cases. J Bone Joint Surg Am 2006;88:1107–10.

107 Omland LH, Rasmussen SW, Hvolris J, Friis-Moller A. Necrotizing fasciitis caused by TSST-1 producing penicillin-sensitive *Staphylococcus aureus*: a case report. Acta Orthop 2007; 78:296–7.

108 Jarrett P, Ha T, Oliver F. Necrotizing fasciitis complicating disseminated cutaneous herpes zoster. Clin Exp Dermatol 1998;23:87–8.

109 Lee YT, Chou TD, Peng MY, Chang FY. Rapidly progressive necrotizing fasciitis caused by *Staphylococcus aureus*. J Microbiol Immunol Infect 2005;38:361–4.

110 Saliba WR, Goldstein LH, Raz R, Mader R, Colodner R, Elias MS. Subacute necrotizing fasciitis caused by gas-producing *Staphylococcus aureus*. Eur J Clin Microbiol Infect Dis 2003;22: 612–14.

111 Kalorin CM, Tobin EH. Community associated methicillin resistant *Staphylococcus aureus* causing Fournier's gangrene and genital infections. J Urol 2007;177:967–71.

112 Basoglu M, Gul O, Yildirgan I, Balik AA, Ozbey I, Oren D. Fournier's gangrene: review of fifteen cases. Am Surg 1997;63: 1019–21.

113 Eke N. Fournier's gangrene: a review of 1726 cases. Br J Surg 2000;87:718–28.

114 Wong CH, Khin LW, Heng KS, Tan KC, Low CO. The LRINEC (Laboratory Risk Indicator for Necrotizing Fasciitis) score: a tool for distinguishing necrotizing fasciitis from other soft tissue infections. Crit Care Med 2004;32:1535–41.

115 Stamenkovic I, Lew PD. Early recognition of potentially fatal necrotizing fasciitis. The use of frozen-section biopsy. N Engl J Med 1984;310:1689–93.

116 Anaya DA, Dellinger EP. Necrotizing soft-tissue infection: diagnosis and management. Clin Infect Dis 2007;44:705–10.

117 Bilton BD, Zibari GB, McMillan RW, Aultman DF, Dunn G, McDonald JC. Aggressive surgical management of necrotizing fasciitis serves to decrease mortality: a retrospective study. Am Surg 1998;64:397–400.

118 Stevens DL, Ma Y, Salmi DB, McIndoo E, Wallace RJ, Bryant AE. Impact of antibiotics on expression of virulence-associated exotoxin genes in methicillin-sensitive and methicillin-resistant *Staphylococcus aureus*. J Infect Dis 2007;195:202–11.

119 Anaya DA, McMahon K, Nathens AB, Sullivan SR, Foy H, Bulger E. Predictors of mortality and limb loss in necrotizing soft tissue infections. Arch Surg 2005;140:151–7; discussion 158.

120 Small LN, Ross JJ. Tropical and temperate pyomyositis. Infect Dis Clin North Am 2005;19:981–9, x–xi.

121 Bickels J, Ben-Sira L, Kessler A, Wientroub S. Primary pyomyositis. J Bone Joint Surg Am 2002;84A:2277–86.

122 Crum NF. Bacterial pyomyositis in the United States. Am J Med 2004;117:420–8.

123 Chauhan S, Jain S, Varma S, Chauhan SS. Tropical pyomyositis (myositis tropicans): current perspective. Postgrad Med J 2004; 80:267–70.

124 Scriba J. Beitrang zur Aetiologie der myositis acuta. Deutche Zeit Chir 1885;22:497–502.

125 Levin MJ, Gardner P, Waldvogel FA. An unusual infection due to *Staphylococcus aureus*. N Engl J Med 1971;284:196–8.

126 Hsueh PR, Hsiue TR, Hsieh WC. Pyomyositis in intravenous drug abusers: report of a unique case and review of the literature. Clin Infect Dis 1996;22:858–60.

127 Gibson RK, Rosenthal SJ, Lukert BP. Pyomyositis. Increasing recognition in temperate climates. Am J Med 1984;77:768–72.

128 Pannaraj PS, Hulten KG, Gonzalez BE, Mason EO Jr, Kaplan SL. Infective pyomyositis and myositis in children in the era of community-acquired, methicillin-resistant *Staphylococcus aureus* infection. Clin Infect Dis 2006;43:953–60.

129 Fowler A, Mackay A. Community-acquired methicillin-resistant *Staphylococcus aureus* pyomyositis in an intravenous drug user. J Med Microbiol 2006;55:123–5.

130 Cone LA, Lamb RB, Graff-Radford A *et al.* Pyomyositis of the anterior tibial compartment. Clin Infect Dis 1997;25:146–8.

131 Immerman RP, Greenman RL. Toxic shock syndrome associated with pyomyositis caused by a strain of *Staphylococcus aureus* that does not produce toxic-shock-syndrome toxin-1. J Infect Dis 1987;156:505–7.

132 Tumeh SS, Butler GJ, Maguire JH, Nagel JS. Pyogenic myositis: CT evaluation. J Comput Assist Tomogr 1988;12:1002–5.

133 Karmazyn B, Kleiman MB, Buckwalter K, Loder RT, Siddiqui A, Applegate KE. Acute pyomyositis of the pelvis: the spectrum of clinical presentations and MR findings. Pediatr Radiol 2006;36:338–43.

134 Struk DW, Munk PL, Lee MJ, Ho SG, Worsley DF. Imaging of soft tissue infections. Radiol Clin North Am 2001;39:277–303.

135 Lamki L, Willis RB. Radionuclide findings of pyomyositis. Clin Nucl Med 1982;7:465–7.

136 Gibberd GF. Sporadic and epidemic puerperal breast infections; a contrast in morbid anatomy and clinical signs. Am J Obstet Gynecol 1953;65:1038–41.

137 Faden H. Mastitis in children from birth to 17 years. Pediatr Infect Dis J 2005;24:1113.

138 Michie C, Lockie F, Lynn W. The challenge of mastitis. Arch Dis Child 2003;88:818–21.

139 Kaufmann R, Foxman B. Mastitis among lactating women: occurrence and risk factors. Soc Sci Med 1991;33:701–5.

140 Amir LH, Forster DA, Lumley J, McLachlan H. A descriptive study of mastitis in Australian breastfeeding women: incidence and determinants. BMC Public Health 2007;7:62.

141 Jonsson S, Pulkkinen MO. Mastitis today: incidence, prevention and treatment. Ann Chir Gynaecol Suppl 1994;208:84–7.

142 Foxman B, D'Arcy H, Gillespie B, Bobo JK, Schwartz K. Lactation mastitis: occurrence and medical management among 946 breastfeeding women in the United States. Am J Epidemiol 2002;155:103–14.

143 Hager WD, Barton JR. Treatment of sporadic acute puerperal mastitis. Infect Dis Obstet Gynecol 1996;4:97–101.

144 Livingstone VH, Willis CE, Berkowitz J. *Staphylococcus aureus* and sore nipples. Can Fam Physician 1996;42:654–9.
145 Livingstone V, Stringer LJ. The treatment of *Staphyloccocus aureus* infected sore nipples: a randomized comparative study. J Hum Lact 1999;15:241–6.
146 Amir LH, Garland SM, Lumley J. A case–control study of mastitis: nasal carriage of *Staphylococcus aureus*. BMC Fam Pract 2006;7:57.
147 Osterman KL, Rahm VA. Lactation mastitis: bacterial cultivation of breast milk, symptoms, treatment, and outcome. J Hum Lact 2000;16:297–302.
148 Dener C, Inan A. Breast abscesses in lactating women. World J Surg 2003;27:130–3.
149 Thomsen AC, Espersen T, Maigaard S. Course and treatment of milk stasis, noninfectious inflammation of the breast, and infectious mastitis in nursing women. Am J Obstet Gynecol 1984;149:492–5.
150 Thomsen AC, Hansen KB, Moller BR. Leukocyte counts and microbiologic cultivation in the diagnosis of puerperal mastitis. Am J Obstet Gynecol 1983;146:938–41.
151 Barbosa-Cesnik C, Schwartz K, Foxman B. Lactation mastitis. JAMA 2003;289:1609–12.
152 Eidelman AI, Szilagyi G. Patterns of bacterial colonization of human milk. Obstet Gynecol 1979;53:550–2.
153 O'Hara RJ, Dexter SP, Fox JN. Conservative management of infective mastitis and breast abscesses after ultrasonographic assessment. Br J Surg 1996;83:1413–14.
154 Walsh M, McIntosh K. Neonatal mastitis. Clin Pediatr 1986;25: 395–9.
155 Stricker T, Navratil F, Forster I, Hurlimann R, Sennhauser FH. Nonpuerperal mastitis in adolescents. J Pediatr 2006;148:278–81.
156 Dahlbeck SW, Donnelly JF, Theriault RL. Differentiating inflammatory breast cancer from acute mastitis. Am Fam Physician 1995;52:929–34.
157 Berna-Serna JD, Madrigal M. Percutaneous management of breast abscesses. An experience of 39 cases. Ultrasound Med Biol 2004;30:1–6.
158 Reddy P, Qi C, Zembower T, Noskin GA, Bolon M. Postpartum mastitis and community-acquired methicillin-resistant *Staphylococcus aureus*. Emerg Infect Dis 2007;13:298–301.
159 Moazzez A, Kelso RL, Towfigh S, Sohn H, Berne TV, Mason RJ. Breast abscess bacteriologic features in the era of community-acquired methicillin-resistant *Staphylococcus aureus* epidemics. Arch Surg 2007;142:881–4.
160 Mortimer PS, Lunniss PJ. Hidradenitis suppurativa. J R Soc Med 2000;93:420–2.
161 Lapins J, Jarstrand C, Emtestam L. Coagulase-negative staphylococci are the most common bacteria found in cultures from the deep portions of hidradenitis suppurativa lesions, as obtained by carbon dioxide laser surgery. Br J Dermatol 1999;140:90–5.
162 Shah N. Hidradenitis suppurativa: a treatment challenge. Am Fam Physician 2005;72:1547–52.
163 Winslow DJ. Botryomycosis. Am J Pathol 1959;35:153–67.
164 Neafie RC, Marty AM. Unusual infections in humans. Clin Microbiol Rev 1993;6:34–56.
165 Brunken RC, Lichon-Chao N, van der Broek H. Immunologic abnormalities in botryomycosis. A case report with review of the literature. J Am Acad Dermatol 1983;9:428–34.
166 Shapiro RL, Duquette JG, Nunes I *et al.* Urokinase-type plasminogen activator-deficient mice are predisposed to staphylococcal botryomycosis, pleuritis, and effacement of lymphoid follicles. Am J Pathol 1997;150:359–69.
167 de Vries HJ, van Noesel CJ, Hoekzema R, Hulsebosch HJ. Botryomycosis in an HIV-positive subject. J Eur Acad Dermatol Venereol 2003;17:87–90.
168 Gavin PJ, Das L, Chadwick EG, Yogev R. Botryomycosis in a child with acquired immunodeficiency syndrome. Pediatr Infect Dis J 2000;19:900–1.
169 Yencha MW, Walker CW, Karakla DW, Simko EJ. Cutaneous botryomycosis of the cervicofacial region. Head Neck 2001;23: 594–8.
170 Chu WO, Fruauff A, Rivas R, Donovan V. Cutaneous botryomycosis: MR findings. AJR Am J Roentgenol 1994;163:647–8.
171 Schlossberg D, Pandey M, Reddy R. The Splendore–Hoeppli phenomenon in hepatic botryomycosis. J Clin Pathol 1998;51: 399–400.
172 Herchline TE, Ayers LW. Occurrence of *Staphylococcus lugdunensis* in consecutive clinical cultures and relationship of isolation to infection. J Clin Microbiol 1991;29:419–21.
173 Shittu A, Lin J, Morrison D, Kolawole D. Isolation and molecular characterization of multiresistant *Staphylococcus sciuri* and *Staphylococcus haemolyticus* associated with skin and soft-tissue infections. J Med Microbiol 2004;53:51–5.
174 Sanchez P, Buezas V, Maestre JR. [*Staphylococcus lugdunensis* infection: report of thirteen cases.] Enferm Infecc Microbiol Clin 2001;19:475–8.
175 Tan TY, Ng SY, Ng WX. Clinical significance of coagulase-negative staphylococci recovered from nonsterile sites. J Clin Microbiol 2006;44:3413–14.
176 Da Costa A, Lelievre H, Kirkorian G *et al.* Role of the preaxillary flora in pacemaker infections: a prospective study. Circulation 1998;97:1791–5.
177 Wertheim HF, van Kleef M, Vos MC, Ott A, Verbrugh HA, Fokkens W. Nose picking and nasal carriage of *Staphylococcus aureus*. Infect Control Hosp Epidemiol 2006;27:863–7.
178 Kluytmans J, van Belkum A, Verbrugh H. Nasal carriage of *Staphylococcus aureus*: epidemiology, underlying mechanisms, and associated risks. Clin Microbiol Rev 1997;10:505–20.
179 Wertheim HF, Melles DC, Vos MC *et al.* The role of nasal carriage in *Staphylococcus aureus* infections. Lancet Infect Dis 2005; 5:751–62.
180 Kramer A, Schwebke I, Kampf G. How long do nosocomial pathogens persist on inanimate surfaces? A systematic review. BMC Infect Dis 2006;6:130.
181 Huang R, Mehta S, Weed D, Price CS. Methicillin-resistant *Staphylococcus aureus* survival on hospital fomites. Infect Control Hosp Epidemiol 2006;27:1267–9.
182 Ong PY, Ohtake T, Brandt C *et al.* Endogenous antimicrobial peptides and skin infections in atopic dermatitis. N Engl J Med 2002;347:1151–60.
183 Kuehnert MJ, Kruszon-Moran D, Hill HA *et al.* Prevalence of *Staphylococcus aureus* nasal colonization in the United States, 2001–2002. J Infect Dis 2006;193:172–9.
184 Eriksen NH, Espersen F, Rosdahl VT, Jensen K. Carriage of *Staphylococcus aureus* among 104 healthy persons during a 19-month period. Epidemiol Infect 1995;115:51–60.
185 Nouwen JL, Ott A, Kluytmans-Vandenbergh MF *et al.* Predicting the *Staphylococcus aureus* nasal carrier state: derivation and validation of a "culture rule". Clin Infect Dis 2004;39:806–11.

186 Nouwen J, Boelens H, van Belkum A, Verbrugh H. Human factor in *Staphylococcus aureus* nasal carriage. Infect Immun 2004;72:6685–8.

187 van den Akker EL, Nouwen JL, Melles DC *et al.* *Staphylococcus aureus* nasal carriage is associated with glucocorticoid receptor gene polymorphisms. J Infect Dis 2006;194:814–18.

188 Raz R, Miron D, Colodner R, Staler Z, Samara Z, Keness Y. A 1-year trial of nasal mupirocin in the prevention of recurrent staphylococcal nasal colonization and skin infection. Arch Intern Med 1996;156:1109–12.

189 Toshkova K, Annemuller C, Akineden O, Lammler C. The significance of nasal carriage of *Staphylococcus aureus* as risk factor for human skin infections. FEMS Microbiol Lett 2001;202: 17–24.

190 Baggett HC, Hennessy TW, Rudolph K *et al.* Community-onset methicillin-resistant *Staphylococcus aureus* associated with antibiotic use and the cytotoxin Panton–Valentine leukocidin during a furunculosis outbreak in rural Alaska. J Infect Dis 2004; 189:1565–73.

191 Kars M, van Dijk H, Salimans MM, Bartelink AK, van de Wiel A. Association of furunculosis and familial deficiency of mannose-binding lectin. Eur J Clin Invest 2005;35:531–4.

192 Zimakoff J, Rosdahl VT, Petersen W, Scheibel J. Recurrent staphylococcal furunculosis in families. Scand J Infect Dis 1988;20:403–5.

193 Nguyen DM, Mascola L, Brancoft E. Recurring methicillin-resistant *Staphylococcus aureus* infections in a football team. Emerg Infect Dis 2005;11:526–32.

194 Centers for Disease Control and Prevention. Methicillin-resistant *Staphylococcus aureus* infections among competitive sports participants: Colorado, Indiana, Pennsylvania, and Los Angeles County, 2000–2003. MMWR 2003;52:793–5.

195 Kazakova SV, Hageman JC, Matava M *et al.* A clone of methicillin-resistant *Staphylococcus aureus* among professional football players. N Engl J Med 2005;352:468–75.

196 Centers for Disease Control and Prevention. Methicillin-resistant *Staphylococcus aureus* infections in correctional facilities: Georgia, California, and Texas, 2001–2003. MMWR 2003;52: 992–6.

197 Nolte O, Haag H, Zimmerman A, Geiss HK. *Staphylococcus aureus* positive for Panton–Valentine leukocidin genes but susceptible to methicillin in patients with furuncles. Eur J Clin Microbiol Infect Dis 2005;24:477–9.

198 Loeb M, Main C, Walker-Dilks C, Eady A. Antimicrobial drugs for treating methicillin-resistant *Staphylococcus aureus* colonization. Cochrane Database Syst Rev 2003;4:CD003340.

199 Laupland KB, Conly JM. Treatment of *Staphylococcus aureus* colonization and prophylaxis for infection with topical intranasal mupirocin: an evidence-based review. Clin Infect Dis 2003;37: 933–8.

200 Simor AE, Phillips E, McGeer A *et al.* Randomized controlled trial of chlorhexidine gluconate for washing, intranasal mupirocin, and rifampin and doxycycline versus no treatment for the eradication of methicillin-resistant *Staphylococcus aureus* colonization. Clin Infect Dis 2007;44:178–85.

201 Klempner MS, Styrt B. Prevention of recurrent staphylococcal skin infections with low-dose oral clindamycin therapy. JAMA 1988;260:2682–5.

202 Walsh TJ, Standiford HC, Reboli AC *et al.* Randomized double-blinded trial of rifampin with either novobiocin or trimethoprim–sulfamethoxazole against methicillin-resistant *Staphylococcus aureus* colonization: prevention of antimicrobial resistance and effect of host factors on outcome. Antimicrob Agents Chemother 1993;37:1334–42.

203 Parras F, Guerrero MC, Bouza E *et al.* Comparative study of mupirocin and oral co-trimoxazole plus topical fusidic acid in eradication of nasal carriage of methicillin-resistant *Staphylococcus aureus*. Antimicrob Agents Chemother 1995;39:175–9.

204 Falagas ME, Bliziotis IA, Fragoulis KN. Oral rifampin for eradication of *Staphylococcus aureus* carriage from healthy and sick populations: a systematic review of the evidence from comparative trials. Am J Infect Control 2007;35:106–14.

205 Small PM, Chambers HF. Vancomycin for *Staphylococcus aureus* endocarditis in intravenous drug users. Antimicrob Agents Chemother 1990;34:1227–31.

206 Chang FY, Peacock JE Jr, Musher DM *et al.* *Staphylococcus aureus* bacteremia: recurrence and the impact of antibiotic treatment in a prospective multicenter study. Medicine (Baltimore) 2003; 82:333–9.

207 Fortun J, Navas E, Martinez-Beltran J *et al.* Short-course therapy for right-side endocarditis due to *Staphylococcus aureus* in drug abusers: cloxacillin versus glycopeptides in combination with gentamicin. Clin Infect Dis 2001;33:120–5.

208 Stryjewski ME, Szczech LA, Benjamin DK Jr *et al.* Use of vancomycin or first-generation cephalosporins for the treatment of hemodialysis-dependent patients with methicillin-susceptible *Staphylococcus aureus* bacteremia. Clin Infect Dis 2007;44:190–6.

209 Weigelt J, Itani K, Stevens D, Lau W, Dryden M, Knirsch C. Linezolid versus vancomycin in treatment of complicated skin and soft tissue infections. Antimicrob Agents Chemother 2005; 49:2260–6.

210 Arbeit RD, Maki D, Tally FP, Campanaro E, Eisenstein BI. The safety and efficacy of daptomycin for the treatment of complicated skin and skin-structure infections. Clin Infect Dis 2004; 38:1673–81.

211 Ellis-Grosse EJ, Babinchak T, Dartois N, Rose G, Loh E. The efficacy and safety of tigecycline in the treatment of skin and skin-structure infections: results of 2 double-blind phase 3 comparison studies with vancomycin–aztreonam. Clin Infect Dis 2005;41(suppl 5):S341–S353.

212 Hidayat LK, Hsu DI, Quist R, Shriner KA, Wong-Beringer A. High-dose vancomycin therapy for methicillin-resistant *Staphylococcus aureus* infections: efficacy and toxicity. Arch Intern Med 2006;166:2138–44.

213 Stryjewski ME, O'Riordan WD, Lau WK *et al.* Telavancin versus standard therapy for treatment of complicated skin and soft-tissue infections due to Gram-positive bacteria. Clin Infect Dis 2005;40:1601–7.

214 Stryjewski ME, Chu VH, O'Riordan WD *et al.* Telavancin versus standard therapy for treatment of complicated skin and skin structure infections caused by Gram-positive bacteria: FAST 2 study. Antimicrob Agents Chemother 2006;50: 862–7.

215 Jauregui LE, Babazadeh S, Seltzer E *et al.* Randomized, double-blind comparison of once-weekly dalbavancin versus twice-daily linezolid therapy for the treatment of complicated skin and skin structure infections. Clin Infect Dis 2005;41:1407–15.

216 Ward KE, Mersfelder TL, LaPlante KL. Oritavancin: an investigational glycopeptide antibiotic. Expert Opin Investig Drugs 2006;15:417–29.

217 Kohlhoff SA, Sharma R. Iclaprim. Expert Opin Investig Drugs 2007;16:1441–8.
218 Talbot GH, Thye D, Das A, Ge Y. Phase 2 study of ceftaroline versus standard therapy in treatment of complicated skin and skin structure infections. Antimicrob Agents Chemother 2007; 51:3612–16.
219 Bush K, Heep M, Macielag MJ, Noel GJ. Anti-MRSA beta-lactams in development, with a focus on ceftobiprole: the first anti-MRSA beta-lactam to demonstrate clinical efficacy. Expert Opin Investig Drugs 2007;16:419–29.
220 Noel GJ. Clinical profile of ceftobiprole, a novel beta-lactam antibiotic. Clin Microbiol Infect 2007;13(suppl 2):25–9.
221 Moellering RC. Linezolid: the first oxazolidinone antimicrobial. Ann Intern Med 2003;138:135–42.
222 Purcell K, Fergie J. Epidemic of community-acquired methicillin-resistant *Staphylococcus aureus* infections: a 14-year study at Driscoll Children's Hospital. Arch Pediatr Adolesc Med 2005;159:980–5.
223 Milatovic D, Braveny I, Verhoef J. Clindamycin enhances opsonization of *Staphylococcus aureus*. Antimicrob Agents Chemother 1983;24:413–17.
224 Markowitz N, Quinn EL, Saravolatz LD. Trimethoprim–sulfamethoxazole compared with vancomycin for the treatment of *Staphylococcus aureus* infection. Ann Intern Med 1992;117:390–8.
225 Ruhe JJ, Monson T, Bradsher RW, Menon A. Use of long-acting tetracyclines for methicillin-resistant *Staphylococcus aureus* infections: case series and review of the literature. Clin Infect Dis 2005;40:1429–34.

Chapter 20
Central Nervous System Infections

Karen L. Roos
Indiana University School of Medicine, Indianapolis, Indiana, USA

Introduction

The staphylococci are important causative organisms of cerebrospinal fluid (CSF) shunt infections, acute purulent meningitis, brain abscess associated with trauma, spinal and cranial subdural empyema, and epidural abscess. Coagulase-negative staphylococci (CoNS) and *Staphylococcus aureus* are the etiological organisms in most CSF shunt infections. The staphylococci typically enter the shunt system from a contaminated wound or from the patient's skin surface at operation.

Staphylococci are the causative organisms in cases of meningitis that develop as a complication of a neurosurgical procedure, from a parameningeal focus of infection, as a congenital anomaly, or during the course of endocarditis. *Staphylococcus aureus* is a common causative organism of brain abscess that develops as a result of cranial trauma, either penetrating wounds of the brain or craniotomy. *Staphylococcus aureus* causes most cases of spinal subdural empyema and 15–25% of cases of cranial subdural empyema. CoNS are isolated on rare occasions from cranial subdural empyemas. *Staphylococcus aureus* is the causative organism in 50–60% of spinal epidural abscesses and in most cranial epidural abscesses that occur as a complication of craniotomy or compound skull fracture.

The chapter is divided into sections on each of the important central nervous system (CNS) infections caused by staphylococci: CSF shunt infections, meningitis, brain abscess, subdural empyema, and epidural abscess. Each section is subdivided into a discussion of the pathogenesis, clinical manifestations, diagnostic studies, surgical and antimicrobial therapy, and prognosis.

Cerebrospinal fluid shunt infections

The staphylococci have always been the predominant organisms causing infection in patients with CSF shunts. The ventriculoperitoneal (VP) shunt is the most common device in use today for surgical decompression of hydrocephalus. The VP shunt drains CSF from the ventricle to the peritoneal cavity [1]. The ventriculoatrial (VA) shunt is a similar device that drains CSF from the ventricle through the internal jugular vein into the right atrium; it is used much less frequently than the VP shunt [2]. Most shunts in use today have a flushing device or a differential pressure valve and contain a reservoir that facilitates access to the shunt system [3].

The risks of infection during initial insertion of a CSF shunt and for each subsequent revision procedure are approximately equal, averaging 13.2% [3–5]. The overall infection rate for VP and VA shunts are similar. Approximately 70% of infections of VP and VA shunts develop within 2 months of the surgical procedure and 78% occur within 4 months [6–8].

Pathogenesis

That most shunt infections develop with 2 months of insertion suggests that bacteria most often enter the shunt system during the surgical procedure. The bacteria involved in early shunt infection gain entry into the lumen of the shunt from a contaminated wound or from the patient's skin surface at operation [6,9,10].

CoNS are normally considered organisms of low virulence. Their place as the leading cause of infection in CSF shunts is attributed to several properties, such as the ability to adhere to catheter surfaces, to grow and proliferate on the inner and outer surfaces of catheters in the absence of externally supplied nutrients, and to produce a mucoid substance. The most common species of CoNS that colonizes shunts is *Staphylococcus epidermidis* (Table 20.1). These organisms produce a large amount of a mucoid substance (slime) during growth that confers three advantages: (i) facilitation of bacterial adhesion to the wall of the shunt lumen and to its valves, (ii) protection of the bacterial cell from the action of lysozyme, and (iii) protection against the action of antibiotics [11,12].

In addition to the inherent properties of the staphylococci that potentiate the development of shunt infections, the shunt itself interferes with host defenses, increasing the pathogenicity of bacteria [13]. Although white blood

Staphylococci in Human Disease, 2nd edition. Edited by Kent B. Crossley, Kimberly K. Jefferson, Gordon Archer, Vance G. Fowler, Jr.
 ISBN 978-14051-6332-3.

Reference	Coagulase-negative staphylococci (%)	*S. aureus* (%)	gram-negative bacilli (%)	Streptococci (%)	Other (%)
Schoenbaum *et al.* [8]	60.3	25.0	5.9	8.8	
Ein *et al.* [32]	64.0	12.0	16.0		8.0
Pople *et al.* [4]	67.0				
Walters *et al.* [5]	48.0	26.0	11.0	9.0	6.0
Forward *et al.* [6]	53.8	17.9	17.9	10.3	0.1
Mean	58.6	20.2	12.7	9.4	4.7

Table 20.1 Bacteriology of CSF shunt infections.

cells (WBCs) that adhere to a surface may engulf any bacteria they contact, WBCs adhere poorly to shunt catheters and consequently are less able to phagocytose bacteria. In addition, an important enzyme in the internal microbicidal system of neutrophils, myeloperoxidase (MPO), becomes deficient in this system. WBCs exocytose MPO when contacting various components of the shunt system and, because neutrophils are mature cells, they are unable to synthesize additional MPO. As they become MPO deficient, they lose their ability to kill intracellular bacteria [14]. For these reasons, among others, the host is unable to limit the spread of CNS shunt infection.

The operative shunt infection rate is age dependent. Infants of 1–6 months of age have a significantly higher incidence of shunt infection than do those older than 6 months of age [4]. This increased susceptibility to shunt infections has been attributed to both quantitative and qualitative differences in the skin bacterial flora between younger infants and older children [4,15].

Clinical manifestations

The initial symptoms of shunt infection are nonspecific and include fever, nausea, vomiting, and lethargy. Fever is the most common manifestation of shunt infection but is not invariably present [8]. Fever is often the sole manifestation of infection in patients with VA shunts, while those with infected VP shunts are more likely to present with signs of shunt malfunction or of inflammation around the shunt reservoir or along the course of the tubing [5,6,8]. Signs of shunt malfunction include enlarging cranial circumference, a tense nonpulsatile fontanelle, and papilledema; these are secondary to progressive hydrocephalus [16]. In one series, fever and cough were the initial symptoms in 6 of 19 patients with infected VA shunts, in contrast to 7 of 21 patients with infected VP shunts who presented with complaints of abdominal pain [6]. Severe abdominal pain and prominent signs of peritonitis dominated the clinical picture in seven children with infected VP shunts [17]. Meningeal signs are not a common presentation of shunt infection, occurring in less than one-third of patients [8]. In a recent review of shunt infections in adults, fever was the most common manifestation [18]. Other evidence of infection (e.g., neck stiffness or local signs of infection) was present in only about half of patients.

Diagnosis

CSF obtained from lumbar puncture is often not diagnostic of shunt infection. There is usually only a modest inflammatory reaction in the CSF, with an average WBC count of 75–100/mm^3 [6]. CSF protein concentration is elevated and there is only a mild degree of hypoglycorrhachia [3,6,7]. Because CSF shunt infections are often indolent, the peripheral WBC count may not be elevated. In one series, the WBC count was greater than 20 000/mm^3 in 25% of cases with active disease [8].

The procedure of choice for the definitive diagnosis of a shunt infection is aspiration of the shunt reservoir or valve to obtain CSF for examination and culture. Cultures of CSF obtained by this technique are almost always positive. In contrast, CSF cultures obtained by lumbar puncture are often negative. CSF cultures were positive in 20 of 21 and in 34 of 36 specimens obtained by direct aspiration of the shunt in two representative series [6,8] (Table 20.1).

Patients with infected VA shunts generally have bacteremia and positive blood cultures. For example, in one series, 13 of 17 patients with infected VA shunts had positive blood cultures [6]. In another series, 95% of patients with infected VA shunts from whom blood specimens were obtained had positive cultures. The VP shunt apparatus is not in direct contact with the bloodstream and, as such, patients with VP shunt infections almost never have positive blood cultures [8].

The first manifestation of a CoNS VA shunt infection may be hypocomplementemic glomerulonephritis. Patients typically develop hematuria, proteinuria, anemia, and azotemia; if severe, the nephrotic syndrome or progressive renal insufficiency may develop [19–21]. The renal disease develops between 1 month and 6 years after insertion of a VA shunt and is associated with CoNS or other organisms (e.g., diphtheroids) [20]. Renal disease is the result of an immunological response to the infection. Bacterial antigens form immune complexes with host antibody and complement. The deposition of these immune complexes in the kidney may lead to shunt nephritis [20,22]. The presentation of hematuria, anemia, and proteinuria in patients with VA shunts should suggest shunt infection.

Both serum C-reactive protein (CRP) and polymerase chain reaction (PCR) for bacterial DNA have been suggested for diagnosis of shunt infection. The serum CRP is nonspecific and appears in serum in response to infection and to acute tissue damage or destruction. The value of this test is limited, as CRP is present in the serum after shunt operation alone, presumably as a result of the tissue damage that occurs during shunt insertion. In this setting, its presence does not indicate infection. In addition, the test may be falsely negative in cases of colonization of the shunt [23]. Thus, detection of elevated concentrations of serum CRP is not helpful in the diagnosis of CNS shunt infection.

PCR is increasingly used in the diagnosis of CNS infections. A number of primers are available for detection of Gram-positive or gram-negative bacterial DNA and the conserved 16S ribosomal RNA for *Staphylococcus* species, methicillin-resistant *S. aureus* (MRSA), and *Propionibacterium acnes*. Theoretically, the PCR result can be available in much less time than the culture result and may identify an etiology in patients with negative cultures [24]. The principal limitation of PCR is that the detection of microbial DNA does not necessarily correlate with the existence of living microorganisms [25]. A positive finding may indicate colonization, contamination, or infection.

Treatment

VP or VA shunt infections caused by CoNS or *S. aureus* have been managed by one of several methods. One approach involves removal of the shunt, with administration of systemic and intraventricular antibiotics. An external ventricular drain or intermittent ventricular taps can be used transiently to maintain ventricular decompression in order to control intracranial pressure and for the administration of antibiotics. Alternatively, the peritoneal end of the shunt catheter is externalized and attached to a closed-system sterile drainage apparatus. After a course of systemic and intraventricular antibiotic therapy, a new catheter is inserted and attached to the distal end of the shunt, or the shunt is removed and immediately replaced followed by antibiotic therapy. Another method is to treat the infection with antibiotics without removal or replacement of the shunt. This is less successful with *S. aureus* than with other pathogens but may be appropriate in patients with CoNS infection [26].

Most published series and investigators with extensive clinical experience in the area favor early shunt removal as the definitive procedure for therapy of infected shunts. When the infected shunt is removed, an external ventricular drain is used temporarily, antibiotics are administered by the parenteral or intraventricular route, and when the CSF is sterile the shunt is replaced. Another therapeutic option is removal of the colonized shunt with immediate replacement by a new shunt followed by a course of antibiotics. Contraindications to immediate replacement of the shunt include the presence of organisms in the CSF and an infected wound near the operative site [8]. Immediate replacement of the shunt is technically difficult with a functioning system because the ventricles are small. In addition, removal of a peritoneal catheter may be difficult due to adhesions, and replacement of a VA shunt requires sacrifice of the vein [27]. Immediate replacement of an infected shunt may result in an increase in the subsequent infection rate [28,29]. An external ventricular drain can be used temporarily to treat hydrocephalus and has the added advantage of providing a means for administration of intraventricular antibiotics. The disadvantages of this temporizing technique are the hazards of disconnection of the system and the risks of superinfection in the ventriculostomy [30].

In patients with VP shunts who experience malfunction of the distal intraperitoneal catheter or show evidence of intraperitoneal infection, the distal end of the shunt can be temporarily externalized and attached to a closed-system drainage apparatus while the infection is treated. Patients with VA shunts who develop bacteremia or shunt nephritis should have the shunt revised to a VP shunt whenever possible [7].

Antimicrobial therapy

Methicillin-resistant CoNS are the predominant cause of CSF shunt infections. Vancomycin is bactericidal against MRSA and CoNS, but penetrates the CSF poorly after parenteral administration in the absence of meningeal inflammation [31,32]. Once-daily intraventricular vancomycin administration results in antimicrobial concentrations in the CSF much in excess of the minimum bactericidal concentration (MBC) of most susceptible strains [27]. The current practice for treatment of methicillin-resistant CoNS shunt infections is a combination of intravenous vancomycin (2–4 g daily in two to four divided doses in adults, 40 mg/kg daily in children in divided doses every 6–8 hours) and either intrashunt or intraventricular vancomycin (20 mg once daily in adults, 10 mg once daily in children) and rifampin (20 mg/kg daily in two divided doses to a maximum of 600 mg twice a day) [33]. Because infection around the shunt may not be reached with intraventricular therapy, this route does not replace systemic antibiotic therapy [34].

Rifampin is among the most active antibiotics against CoNS and is also extremely potent against *S. aureus in vitro* [34–36]. Rifampin penetrates the CSF well, achieving concentrations as high as 1000 times the minimum inhibitory concentration (MIC) of CoNS [7,37]. However, resistance develops rapidly to rifampin when it is used alone, and addition of a second agent is necessary to prevent the emergence of rifampin-resistant strains. The combination of oral rifampin (900–1200 mg daily in adults, 20 mg/kg daily in children in divided doses every 8 hours) and intravenous vancomycin (2 g daily in adults, 40 mg/kg daily in children) has been successful in eradicating CSF shunt infections due to CoNS [36,38,39]. However, there are reports in European literature of isolation of rifampin-resistant strains of MRSA during or after therapy for MRSA infections with vancomycin and rifampin [40–42].

For methicillin-susceptible CoNS and methicillin-susceptible *S. aureus* (MSSA) shunt infections, intravenous nafcillin (9–12 g daily or 300 mg/kg daily in divided doses every 4 hours) is the recommended antimicrobial agent. For intraventricular therapy, vancomycin is preferred over nafcillin.

The role of antibiotic prophylaxis in shunt surgery is controversial. Clinical trials have included small numbers of patients, and the antibiotics used in some series have not been active against CoNS. The organisms involved in early shunt infection contaminate the shunt system at operation. Careful surgical technique, including the surgeon changing gloves before handling the shunt and the isolation of wound edges with antiseptic-soaked packs during surgery, and measures to reduce the skin bacterial population at surgery are more accepted practices to prevent shunt infection than is the use of prophylactic antibiotic therapy [4]. Antibiotic-impregnated shunts may reduce the incidence of shunt infections, but to date this has not been clearly demonstrated in clinical trials [43].

Meningitis

The staphylococci rarely cause acute purulent meningitis, accounting for only 1–8% of cases in reported series of bacterial meningitis [44–54] (Table 20.2). Staphylococcal meningitis usually develops from a parameningeal focus of infection, during the course of staphylococcal bacteremia or endocarditis, in association with congenital anomalies, or after a neurosurgical procedure. *Staphylococcus aureus* is the causative organism in the vast majority of cases of staphylococcal meningitis, except when meningitis develops as a complication of an intraventricular shunting device.

The conditions associated with staphylococcal meningitis have changed over time. The records of patients with staphylococcal meningitis during the 10-year period from 1932 to 1942 were compared with the records of patients seen during 1949 to 1959. All the patients seen from 1932 to 1942 had a focus of infection outside the CNS prior to the development of meningitis. Staphylococci gained entry to the meninges by direct spread from facial or paraspinal infections or by hematogenous dissemination from a more distal site. In contrast, meningitis developed after an invasive diagnostic or neurosurgical procedure in the majority of patients seen from 1949 to 1959 [45]. Similarly, in a review of 33 cases of *S. aureus* meningitis seen at the Mayo Clinic from 1948 to 1962, most developed postoperatively after craniotomy for brain tumors, shunt insertions for hydrocephalus, or laminectomies for herniated disks, and that continues to be the case today [50]. In addition, staphylococcal meningitis may develop as a complication of intracranial pressure monitoring devices and external ventricular drains.

Table 20.2 Incidence of *S. aureus* as an etiological agent in cases of bacterial meningitis.

Reference	Total cases	No. due to *S. aureus*
Schlesinger *et al.* [44]	363	21 (5.8%)
Mulcare & Harter [45]	637	13 (2.0%)
Swartz & Dodge [46]	207	13 (6.3%)
Studdert [47]	115	7 (6.1%)
Geiseler *et al.* [48]	1316	11 (0.8%)
Roberts *et al.* [49]	710	21 (3.0%)
Wellman & Senft [50]	294	23 (7.8%)
Carson & Koch [51]	354	6 (1.7%)
Carpenter & Petersdorf [52]	209	8 (3.8%)
Smith [53]	409	6 (1.5%)
Kneebone [54]	237	7 (2.9%)

Parameningeal focus

Several possible parameningeal foci of infection may result in staphylococcal meningitis: (i) underlying infection in the facial sinuses or bones of the skull, (ii) subdural empyema, (iii) cranial or spinal epidural abscess, (iv) rupture of a cerebral abscess into the ventricle or subarachnoid space, and (v) fracture of the cranial bones. Staphylococcal meningitis may thus complicate osteomyelitis of the frontal bone, facial cellulitis, chronic mastoiditis, sinusitis, and epidural spinal abscess [46,47,49]. Sinus infection can readily spread to the meninges because of close proximity to the intracranial compartment. Infection can gain access through the thin mucosal barrier that separates the meninges from the sinus cavity [55].

Fracture of the petrous bone may lead to meningitis. Typically, there is only a brief period of otorrhea, but CSF continually leaks into the eustachian tube, producing rhinorrhea. Organisms may then gain access to the middle ear and meninges by this route [46].

Meningitis may develop after even relatively minor head injuries. During the first few days following a head injury, pneumococci are the most common cause of meningitis but as the interval between the head injury and the development of meningitis lengthens beyond 5 days, other organisms, including *S. aureus*, assume increasing predominance among the causative agents [34]. The head injury may not be severe or produce CSF rhinorrhea, yet meningitis may still occur. A fracture through the cribriform plate may trap a small piece of meninges and its vascular connections, which may then serve as a conduit into the CNS for the ingress of microorganisms from the nasal cavity [46].

Staphylococcal bacteremia

Staphylococci may infect the meninges hematogenously by dissemination from sites outside the CNS. Meningitis may complicate up to 20% of cases of staphylococcal bacteremia [56]. Most frequently, the source of sepsis is either a skin infection or endocarditis. The staphylococci do not readily infect normal skin, but infection may develop in postoperative wounds, burns, and decubitus ulcers. Indwelling intravenous catheters and arteriovenous shunts or fistulas are also sources of *S. aureus* sepsis. The majority of patients with *S. aureus* bacteremia have severe underlying diseases, such as chronic renal failure, diabetes mellitus, malignancies, or alcoholism [57,58].

A recent study from Denmark reported 96 cases of bacteremia-associated meningitis among 12 480 cases of *S. aureus* bacteremia in that country during 1991–2000 [59]. Most of these cases were community acquired (81 of 96). The median age was 67 years. A primary focus was unknown in 61% of cases, while 57 of 61 cases had an additional secondary focus of infection which was most often osteomyelitis. Most patients had fever (85%) or mental status changes (74%). Slightly over half (56%) of patients died.

Acute purulent meningitis is the most common presentation of *S. aureus* endocarditis with nervous system involvement [60,61]. Meningitis develops during the course of staphylococcal endocarditis when infected emboli lodge in meningeal vessels, or by spread of infection from brain infarcted by septic emboli, or as an inflammatory reaction to infarction or hemorrhage elsewhere within the brain. Characteristic of meningeal involvement in this setting are signs and symptoms of meningitis and the finding of a sterile CSF pleocytosis [62]. Encephalitic symptoms are frequent due to the conspicuous presence of multiple cerebral microabscesses.

Congenital dermal sinus and myelomeningocele

Congenital dermal sinuses are midline defects or tracts lined with stratified squamous epithelium [63]. They may be found anywhere in the midline along the craniospinal axis but are most common in the lumbosacral and occipital regions [46]. Dermal sinus tracts are often not recognized until a child develops recurrent or unexplained meningitis. The sinus tract provides a pathway for entry into the subarachnoid space by skin organisms. *Staphylococcus aureus* is a common causative agent of meningitis in this clinical setting. In children with meningitis due to *S. aureus*, careful search of the entire skin surface along the midline should be performed for evidence of a dermal sinus opening. These openings are often inconspicuous and may have the appearance of a dimple or tiny pinhole from which coarse black hairs may emerge [64,65].

Expansion of the sinus into a cyst may occur at any point along a congenital dermal sinus. Such a cyst is termed "epidermoid" when its capsule is lined with stratified squamous epithelium and it contains only epithelial debris; it is termed "dermoid" if its structure contains, in addition to epithelium of the epidermal type, an underlying layer comparable to the dermis. The cyst contents of a dermoid include glandular secretory products, desquamating epithelial cells, and hair [64–66]. Dermoids and epidermoids may occur in the cerebellum or fourth ventricle and may be manifested clinically by focal or obstructive symptoms, but more commonly are recognized because of recurrent meningitis, of which *S. aureus* is a common cause [63,67,68].

In infants with neural tube defects, *S. aureus* and *Escherichia coli* predominate as the causative organisms of meningitis. In one series of 262 cases of spina bifida cystica (meningomyelocele 249, meningocele 13) in neonates and infants, there were 33 cases of bacterial meningitis and *S. aureus* was responsible for the majority of cases. These patients developed either an ascending infection from the meningomyelocele or developed the infection from the investigation or treatment of the associated hydrocephalus [69].

In anatomically normal full-term neonates, staphylococcal meningitis is rare [70]. Sepsis due to *S. aureus* has become an increasing problem in preterm and low-birth-weight infants, especially those requiring neonatal intensive care unit support and monitoring, often with intravascular catheters. In the neonate, *S. aureus* bacteremia results in meningeal invasion in approximately 25% of cases [71].

Neurosurgical procedures

Staphylococcal meningitis may follow any type of invasive neurosurgical procedure, but most frequently it complicates shunting operations for hydrocephalus. Meningitis related to an indwelling CSF shunt usually produces a less intense CSF inflammatory response than meningitis of other etiologies and is a more indolent infection. Patients generally have a favorable outcome.

Staphylococcal meningitis may develop as a complication from the use of subcutaneous and Ommaya reservoirs for the administration of intrathecal chemotherapy in patients with carcinomatous meningitis. Limited data are available regarding the infection rate in this setting, but in one series 4 of 31 patients developed CSF infections with CoNS. These infections were attributed to the natural colonization of the skin surface with CoNS and the necessity to puncture the reservoir twice weekly for 8–12 weeks to administer chemotherapy, with frequent potential for breaches in sterile technique [72].

Clinical manifestations and diagnosis

The presenting signs and symptoms of staphylococcal meningitis are typical of other forms of bacterial meningitis. Patients usually have fever, nuchal rigidity, headache, nausea and vomiting, and photophobia. They may also complain of myalgias and arthralgias and usually have some degree of altered mental status, ranging from lethargy to coma [57]. The CSF examination generally reveals a marked pleocytosis with a preponderance of polymorphonuclear leukocytes, a low glucose concentration, and an elevated protein concentration. Gram-positive cocci in clusters may be demonstrated on Gram's stain of the sediment. The organism is more difficult to demonstrate by Gram's stain and in culture of CSF from patients who develop staphylococcal meningitis following shunting procedures and during the course of staphylococcal bacteremia, as compared with patients with staphylococcal meningitis in association with a parameningeal focus of infection [49].

The peripheral WBC count is often elevated, with a predominance of polymorphonuclear leukocytes and a left shift. The serum sodium concentration may be low [46]. Patients who develop meningitis in the course of staphylococcal sepsis should have positive blood cultures [44]. Computed tomography (CT) and magnetic resonance imaging (MRI) are not helpful in differential diagnosis but may reveal diffuse meningeal enhancement after contrast administration. However, CT or MRI is often obtained in patients with staphylococcal meningitis to evaluate the possibility of a parameningeal focus of infection or of cerebral abscess formation by these organisms.

Therapy

Vancomycin is the first-line treatment for patients with staphylococcal meningitis; however, therapy should be switched to oxacillin or nafcillin if susceptibility tests indicate that these antibiotics would be appropriate [73]. Isolates of *S. aureus* with low-level resistance to vancomycin have been described in infections originating in the skin [74].

Meningitis due to MRSA can be treated with vancomycin or rifampin plus vancomycin. Systemically administered vancomycin penetrates poorly into the CSF in the absence of meningeal inflammation [31]. Vancomycin entry into CSF in the presence of meningeal inflammation has not been well documented *in vivo* in humans; however, it has been successful in therapy for many different kinds of meningitis [34]. The recommended intravenous dose of vancomycin for staphylococcal meningitis is 2–4 g daily for adults (every 6–12 hours) and 40 mg/kg daily for children and neonates. If intravenous vancomycin fails to control the infection, either intrathecal or intraventricular vancomycin (10 mg once daily in children, 20 mg once daily in adults) may be added. Intraventricular instillation is the preferred route, as intralumbar administration of vancomycin may not result in adequate concentrations within the cerebral ventricles. Concentrations of drug in the CSF (i.e., CSF bactericidal titers) should be monitored closely to gauge the response to therapy [75]. A vancomycin concentration of 50–80 mg/L from a CSF sample obtained 15–30 min after drug administration (peak concentration) is desirable [11].

Rifampin is active against CoNS [34,36]. It penetrates the CSF well, although resistance develops rapidly to rifampin when used alone. The addition of a second antibiotic often prevents the emergence of rifampin-resistant strains. The combination of oral rifampin (900–1200 mg daily in adults, 20 mg/kg daily in children in divided doses every 8 hours) and intravenous vancomycin has been successful in eradicating meningitis due to *S. aureus* and CoNS [36,39,44].

Prognosis

Patients with staphylococcal meningitis as a result of bacteremic spread from a site of infection outside the CNS tend to have a more fulminant course and a higher mortality compared with other groups with this form of meningitis. This may be related to the presence of severe and/or several underlying diseases(s) in most of these patients. Meningitis related to a ventricular shunt tends to be more insidious in onset, runs a more benign course, and has a much lower mortality rate [44].

At least one-third of surviving patients with bacterial meningitis have some degree of permanent neurologic sequelae. There are limited data on long-term outcome in patients who have had staphylococcal meningitis. However, as all types of purulent meningitis produce similar pathophysiological changes in the nervous system, the reported neurological sequelae from other types of bacterial meningitis can be expected to occur following staphylococcal meningitis.

Brain abscess

The organisms most commonly isolated from brain abscesses are streptococci, staphylococci, anaerobes (*Peptococcus* sp., *Fusobacterium* sp. and *Bacteroides* sp.), *Candida*, *Nocardia asteroides*, and *Aspergillus* [75–81]. In the pre-antibiotic era, most organisms isolated from brain abscesses were *S. aureus* or aerobic and microaerophilic streptococci. During the pre-penicillin era and in the early years thereafter, *S. aureus* was the causative organism in 25–31% of brain abscesses [82–84]. Since then, increased recognition of parasitic and fungal organisms as a cause of brain abscess in organ transplant and immunosuppressed patients has led to a decrease in the relative incidence of *S. aureus* brain abscess.

Epidemiology and pathogenesis

Bacteria may reach the brain either by direct spread from a contiguous cranial site of infection such as otitis media, odontogenic infection, frontal sinusitis, or mastoiditis, or by retrograde septic thrombophlebitis from these areas of infection. Brain abscesses also develop following cranial trauma, either surgical or accidental, or as a result of hematogenous spread from a remote site of infection, such as bacterial endocarditis, cyanotic congenital heart disease with paradoxic emboli, and acute or chronic pulmonary infections [85–87]. Approximately 30% of brain abscesses are cryptogenic without an identifiable associated condition.

The patient's primary underlying condition is often predictive of the causative organism(s) and of the location of the abscess within the brain [82]. Brain abscess due to *S. aureus* most commonly develops as a result of cranial

(a) (b) (c)

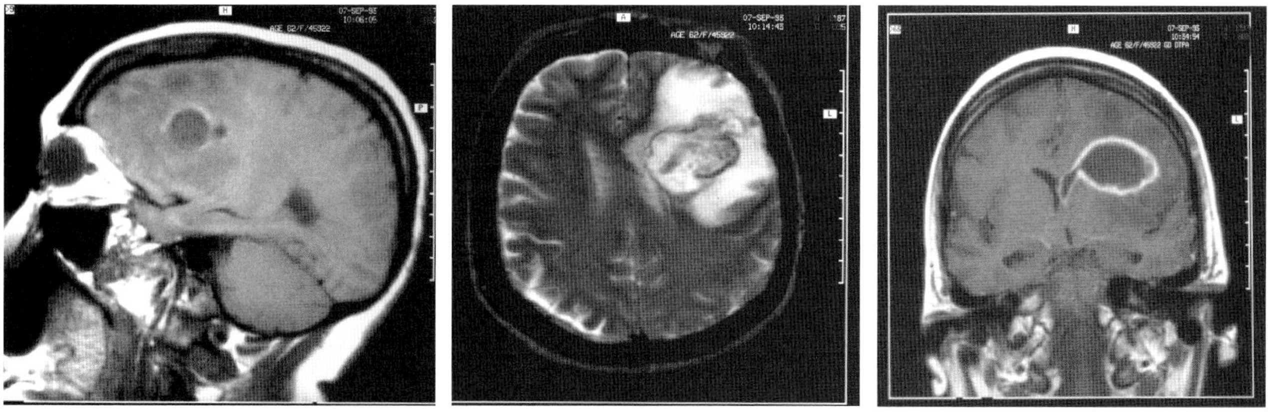

Figure 20.1 Brain abscess caused by *Staphylococcus aureus*. (a) Sagittal noncontrast T1-weighted MRI scan demonstrates a frontal lobe abscess as a spherical zone of low signal intensity outlined by a uniformly thin rim of short T1 value, surrounded by a large area of cerebral edema. A small "daughter" loculation is seen budding from the posterior aspect of the main lesion. (b) Axial T2-weighted scan: the complex abscess morphology demonstrates a thin rim of relatively low signal intensity interposed between the bright signal of the abscess content and the surrounding frontal edema, which extends into the corpus callosum. (c) Coronal postcontrast T1-weighted scan showing intense uniform contrast enhancement throughout the capsule of the abscess. The medial margin of the lesion has reached the lateral ventricle and associated ventriculitis is indicated by enhancement of the ventricular margins and increased signal intensity of the fluid within the left frontal horn as compared with normal CSF. A thin communication between the abscess and the ventricle suggests that the lesion has ruptured into the ventricular cavity. (Images courtesy of Dr Douglas H. Yock Jr, Department of Radiology, Abbott-Northwestern Hospital, Minneapolis, Minnesota, USA.)

trauma, either penetrating wounds of the brain or neurosurgical procedures [85,86,88–92]. Brain abscess caused by this organism may also develop secondary to otogenic infections or endocarditis. Most brain abscesses develop in the temporal and frontal lobes (Figure 20.1) [87,88,92]. Abscesses that develop as a result of direct spread of infection from the frontal, ethmoidal, or sphenoidal sinuses are usually found in the frontal lobes. Abscesses that are the result of direct spread from the middle ear or mastoid usually occur in the temporal lobe or cerebellum. Metastatic abscesses that are the result of infection elsewhere in the body can occur throughout the brain, but tend to form primarily in areas supplied by the middle cerebral artery [82].

Brain abscesses in infants and children are commonly associated with cyanotic congenital heart disease or develop from ear, nose, and throat infections, but can also arise following head trauma or a neurosurgical procedure [87,93–95]. Because a brain abscess is thought to develop only in an area of ischemia or infarction [96], children with cyanotic congenital heart disease are especially susceptible to this complication. The most important predisposing factor is polycythemia, which induces intravascular thrombosis and reduces blood flow in the microcirculation of the brain leading to brain hypoxia or infarct. In addition, the presence of a right-to-left shunt may preclude filtering of virulent bacteria by the lungs. Bacteria reach the brain and are able to establish infection in areas of focal cerebral damage secondary to hypoxemia [86,94,97,98].

Pathology

Results of animal experiments suggest that for bacterial invasion of brain parenchyma to occur, preexisting or concomitant areas of ischemia, necrosis or hypoxia in brain tissue must be present [86]. The intact brain parenchyma is relatively resistant to infection [85]. Once bacteria have established infection, brain abscess formation often evolves through four stages, regardless of the infecting organism: early cerebritis, late cerebritis, early capsule formation, and late capsule formation.

The findings in the experimental *S. aureus* brain abscess model suggest that infection with this organism results in extensive destruction of white matter with relative sparing of gray matter, a quantitative difference in the formation of the capsule between the cortical and ventricular sides of the abscess, early spread of infection to the ventricle, and, most importantly, areas of extension of the inflammatory process beyond the confines of the collagenous capsule. The latter finding, and the early appearance of ependymitis, has not been seen in experimental brain abscess caused by less virulent organisms, including streptococci, gram-negative aerobic bacilli, and anaerobes [99].

Signs and symptoms

In children and adults, the most common symptom of brain abscess is headache, which occurs in at least 75% of patients [85,100]. More than half of patients have vomiting or focal neurological deficit, the most common of which is hemiparesis [85,92]. One-third of patients present with new-onset focal or generalized seizure activity [85,93]. Frontal lobe abscesses are more prone to produce seizures than those in other locations [100]. Brain abscess presents as an expanding intracranial mass lesion, rather than as a systemic infectious process. As such, fever is present in only half of patients and usually is not very striking [85].

The findings on neurological examination are related to both the site of the abscess and the presence of raised intracranial pressure (ICP). In cases of frontal or parietal lobe abscess, hemiparesis is the most common localizing sign. Patients with temporal lobe abscess may have language disturbance or hemianopsia. Cerebellar abscess is manifest by nystagmus and ataxia [89]. Patients with expanding mass lesions and increased ICP often have alterations in consciousness ranging from lethargy to irritability, confusion, or coma [85]. There may be papilledema, and deficits of cranial nerves III and VI, if raised ICP is present. Patients with brain abscess may present with signs of meningitis if the abscess ruptures into the ventricle or if the infection spreads to the subarachnoid space. Infants with brain abscess usually present with seizures, irritability, failure to thrive, or an enlarging head [98].

Diagnosis

Patients with brain abscess may have a leukocytosis or elevated erythrocyte sedimentation rate. However, in a significant proportion of patients, laboratory evidence for infection in the peripheral blood is lacking [85].

When a brain abscess is suspected, examination of the CSF should be avoided because of the danger of herniation of the brainstem and the low likelihood that spinal fluid will demonstrate the organism. In one series, lumbar puncture was performed in 140 patients with brain abscess; 41 patients showed significant deterioration in the level of consciousness during the subsequent 48 hours, and 25 of these patients died [84]. In another series, 4 of 27 patients with brain abscess who underwent lumbar puncture died within 24 hours after the procedure [101]. Although it is thought safe by some to perform lumbar puncture if only a small amount of CSF is removed, the inadvertent creation of a hole in the theca after the needle is withdrawn may allow slow seepage of CSF, resulting in clinical deterioration within several hours after the procedure [102].

Unless there has been extension of the abscess to the meninges or ventricle, bacteria are detected by Gram's stain or culture of CSF obtained by lumbar puncture in less than 10% of patients [101,103]. An elevated cell count in the CSF is directly related to the stage of encapsulation of the abscess and its proximity to the meningeal or ventricular surfaces, and usually ranges from a few to several hundred cells [104]. Polymorphonuclear leukocytes or lymphocytes may predominate. The protein concentration is moderately elevated, up to a few hundred milligrams per deciliter, in patients with unruptured abscesses [85]. The CSF glucose concentration is normal in the vast majority of patients. The finding of hypoglycorrhachia usually indicates that the meninges have been breached by bacteria [104] or suggests an alternative diagnosis.

CT revolutionized the clinical evaluation of patients with suspected or proven brain abscess. MRI has further improved the ability to detect these lesions. On CT an abscess in the early cerebritis stage has the appearance of a focal low-density lesion, with faint contrast enhancement at the lesion edge early in this stage and more prominent contrast enhancement with a complete ring around the lesion by the end of this stage. Delayed scans, obtained 30 min after the infusion of intravenous contrast, show diffusion of contrast into the low-density center [105]. On MRI, the cerebritis stage appears as an area of low signal intensity on T1-weighted scans and increased signal intensity on T2-weighted images [106].

In the capsule stage, on CT the brain abscess has the appearance of a low-density lesion surrounded by a homogeneous ring of contrast enhancement and a surrounding area of low-density edema. On MRI, the capsule is hyperintense on T1-weighted scans and hypointense on T2-weighted images. There is marked contrast enhancement of the abscess capsule following use of the paramagnetic contrast agent gadolinium-diethylenetriaminepentaacetic acid (Gd-DTPA). The surrounding edema is hypointense on T1-weighted and hyperintense on T2-weighted images [107]. A brain abscess is hyperintense on diffusion-weighted MRI.

The Gd-DTPA-enhanced MRI scan is superior to CT in differentiating the three components of a brain abscess: the central core, the surrounding area of ring enhancement, and the area of edema around the abscess. Similarly, MRI is able to detect a decrease in the size of any of the three regions of a brain abscess before these changes are seen on CT and is therefore most useful in the assessment of therapeutic response [108]. Furthermore, MRI is superior to CT in detecting posterior fossa lesions.

Treatment

Systemic antibiotic therapy alone may be successful in eradicating brain abscesses characterized in the cerebritis stage by CT or MRI, as well as lesions less than 3 cm in diameter [109]. The choice of agent(s) to treat a brain abscess should not only be made on the basis of susceptibility of potential organisms but should also include consideration of the antibiotic's ability to penetrate the blood–brain barrier and to penetrate and be effective in brain abscess pus. The ability of some antibiotics to penetrate brain tissue has been studied sparingly *in vivo*. Frame *et al.* [110] examined penetration of nafcillin and methicillin into the brain tissue of patients given single intravenous doses before craniotomy and brain biopsy for diagnostic purposes. Nafcillin and methicillin each penetrated brain tissue after a 2-g infusion, but nafcillin more predictably exceeded the MICs for *S. aureus* isolates than did methicillin [107]. Permeability of antibiotics into brain tissue is enhanced by the local inflammation and the alteration in the blood–brain barrier that occurs in areas of cerebritis [86].

Despite the presence in abscess cavities of potentially therapeutic concentrations of antimicrobial agents, organisms often persist in the purulent core [111]. This persistence of viable organisms in abscess pus in the presence of therapeutic concentrations of antibiotics has been attributed to inactivation of some agents by bacterial or leukocytic enzymes [101]. DeLouvois and colleagues [112,113] examined the antibiotic concentrations in brain abscess pus from 32 patients. Benzylpenicillin (penicillin G) was detectable in samples of pus obtained from patients receiving doses exceeding 4 million units daily; however, when penicillin was added to pus, up to 90% of the drug was inactivated within 1 hour *in vitro* in 4 of 22 specimens. The antibiotic of choice for a brain abscess that is small or in the cerebritis stage, as determined by MRI or CT, and in which methicillin-sensitive staphylococci are suspected or grown is nafcillin 2 g i.v. every 4 hours [114]. Parenteral therapy is often continued for 6–8 weeks, but the optimal duration of treatment is unknown and must be individualized. Vancomycin is recommended for patients who are allergic to penicillin or from whom MRSA has been isolated.

In addition to appropriate antimicrobial therapy, an abscess beyond the cerebritis stage should be managed by aspiration or excision. There are several potential advantages of aspiration. First, it decreases the size of the intracranial mass, and in this way decreases ICP. Second, by removal of purulent material, it may decrease the likelihood of inactivation of antibiotics by bacterial or leukocytic enzymes in the pus. Third, aspiration facilitates the diagnosis. Finally, duration of therapy is potentially shortened. The risks of aspiration are abscess rupture into the ventricle or leakage into the subarachnoid space [92].

Excision is the definitive procedure and should be undertaken when antibiotics and aspiration cannot control the infection and, whenever possible, in lesions that are greater than 4 cm in size on CT [105]. Excision (or aspiration) is relatively contraindicated in the early stages of abscess formation, before a capsule has formed, due to the risk of hemorrhage, or if an abscess is deep in the brain or in vital structures. A major complication of excision is the likelihood of a permanent neurological deficit. With the use of CT and ICP monitoring devices, an increasing number of patients have been successfully managed with systemic antibiotic therapy and aspiration of the abscess alone [85, 115–118]. Because of the risk of a permanent neurological deficit with excision, the surgical method preferred for children and infants is drainage or repeated aspiration [87,93].

The use of steroids in the management of brain abscess is both beneficial and problematic. The effect of the expanding mass leading to increased ICP and herniation of the brainstem is a major threat to the patient's life. Steroids decrease the endothelial permeability of the vessels associated with the inflammatory response around the abscess, and subsequently decrease cerebral edema [86]. However, this effect on the permeability of vessels may also result in decreased diffusion of antimicrobial agents into the site of infection [86,101]. Steroids have a role in the management of increased ICP secondary to brain abscess edema, and should be used in conjunction with other measure to decrease ICP (i.e., mannitol and hyperventilation). A monitoring device may be inserted and used to track elevations in ICP. In the absence of cerebral edema associated with a brain abscess, steroid therapy is probably not beneficial.

Morbidity and mortality

Since 1975, there has been a significant reduction in mortality associated with brain abscess reported in all major series [87,94,98,119]. This reduction in mortality has been attributed to improvement in culture technique with better identification of the infecting organisms, and to the contribution of CT and MRI in the diagnosis and management of this infection [98,120]. Mortality of brain abscess in recent series has ranged from 0 to 24%.

The major morbidity from brain abscess is associated with surgical intervention, and includes permanent neurological deficit and postoperative epilepsy. The incidence of neurological sequelae, ranging from minor to incapacitating deficits, is reported at approximately 30–55% [90,101]. The incidence of postoperative seizure disorder ranges from 30 to 50% in reported series and the onset may be delayed for 6–12 months following surgery [100,121].

Subdural empyema

Subdural empyema is a pyogenic infection of the space between the dura and the arachnoid. Most of these infections are confined to the subdural space over the dorsolateral surface of one cerebral hemisphere; however, the exudate may spread under the falx to the contralateral side, resulting in bilateral collections of pus over both hemispheres or in the parafalcine space [122,123]. Although rare, empyemas also develop in the subdural structures of the posterior fossa and of the spinal cord [124,125]. Subdural empyema represents 13–20% of localized intracranial infections [126–128].

Etiology and pathogenesis

Paranasal sinusitis, especially frontal sinusitis, is the most common predisposing condition leading to the development of a subdural empyema, accounting for 50–80% of cases. In the pre-antibiotic era, otitis media was the prominent predisposing condition; however, the decreased incidence of chronic otitis since the advent of antimicrobial agents has reduced the incidence of middle ear infections as the source of subdural empyema to 10–20% of cases [124,128]. Infection in the sinuses or the middle ear reaches the subdural space either through communicating veins that drain these areas and connect with the dural venous sinuses or by direct spread of infection through bone [129–131]. The highest incidence of subdural empyema is between 10 and 25 years of age [124,128,132]. At this age, the posterior wall of the frontal sinus is developing and, as such, may be an incomplete barrier to intracranial spread of organisms that cause sinusitis [132]. However, the most important pathophysiological antecedent of subdural empyema is septic thrombophlebitis of the mucosal veins of the sinuses, which results in retrograde extension of infection with drainage of bacteria into the regional dural veins, and then into the superior sagittal sinus [128]. Subdural empyemas may also result from direct infection of the subdural space during a neurosurgical procedure, such as drainage of a subdural hematoma, or may result from hematogenous spread of infection from a distant site, such as suppuration in the lung [127,128,133]. Subdural empyema in infants usually represents an infected subdural effusion associated with bacterial meningitis [130,134].

Once infection is established in the subdural space, evolution of an empyema tends to be remarkably rapid. The empyema, aided by gravity, extends chiefly in a posterior direction, but also extends medially over the tentorium and toward the falx [135,136]. Reaction of the mesothelial cells of the dura attempts to limit the spread of infection, but this is rarely effective, and the exudate spreads extensively throughout the subdural space [136]. Septic thrombophlebitis extends in a retrograde fashion from the dural sinuses to the cortical veins. Cortical venous infarction may follow and is largely responsible for the severe symptoms, particularly the focal signs, which develop in the course of this illness [131]. Hemorrhagic necrosis of cortical and subcortical tissue is the result of venous thrombosis and infarction [136]. These areas of cerebral necrosis, in addition to producing neurological deficits, are also particularly suitable for the formation of a brain abscess. A coexistent cerebral abscess has been reported in up to 24% of cases of subdural empyema [122,128].

Although cortical vein thrombosis and brain abscess are frequently associated with subdural empyema, purulent meningitis occurs in only 14% of adults with this infection [126]. An inflammatory reaction is present within the subarachnoid space, but bacteria do not usually cross the arachnoid membrane. In infants and children under 5 years of age, purulent meningitis and subdural empyema are frequently associated; however, the pathophysiological process is different from that which occurs in adults. Subdural fluid collections complicate bacterial meningitis in infants and children by effusion of fluid through irritated or damaged capillary walls in the arachnoid [137]. When this collection of fluid becomes infected, a subdural empyema results. The causative organism is that of the meningitis itself [126,130]. The incidence of this complication of meningitis in infants is approximately 2% but is very rare in adults.

Table 20.3 Bacteriology of subdural empyema in cases with only single bacterial isolates.[1]

Staphylococci
S. aureus 17.4%
Coagulase-negative 2.3%
Streptococci
Aerobic 40.7%
Microaerobic 4.6%
Anaerobic 19.8%
Aerobic gram-negative bacilli 12.8%
Haemophilus influenzae 2.3%

[1] Data from references 122, 130, 135 and 146.

Most subdural empyemas develop over the convexity of the cerebral hemispheres. Posterior fossa and spinal subdural empyemas, although uncommon, do occur. Posterior fossa subdural empyemas develop either by direct extension of an otogenic infection or by spread from supratentorial subdural empyema complicating acute frontal sinusitis [124]. Spinal subdural empyemas are almost always metastatic in origin [128,138,139].

Bacteriology

Most empyemas are associated with sinusitis or otitis and are caused by those organisms typically isolated from chronic, rather than acute, sinusitis or otitis [122–132]. The staphylococci are the causative organisms in 15–25% of cases [128] (Table 20.3). *Staphylococcus aureus* is responsible for most cases; on rare occasions, CoNS are isolated. Aerobic streptococci are the causative organisms in 30–50% of cases of subdural empyema.

Anaerobic organisms are isolated from 15–25% of cases, and aerobic gram-negative bacilli from 5–10% of cases [126–128]. *Staphylococcus aureus* is the causative organism in most cases of spinal subdural empyema [125].

Signs and symptoms

The initial signs and symptoms of subdural empyema are those of infection, focal brain ischemia or infarction, and increased ICP. Most patients complain of headache, often localized initially to the side of the infection. The headache then becomes more severe and generalized and is followed by a change in the patient's level of consciousness, progressing from confusion and somnolence to stupor and coma. The disturbance of consciousness reflects the increase in ICP. Fever, chills, and nuchal rigidity are present in most cases. Focal neurological deficits are present in 80–90% of patients and most often are hemiparesis or hemiplegia, paralysis of horizontal gaze to the contralateral side of the lesion, and focal or generalized seizures. A left-sided empyema will often produce a disturbance of language. Orbital swelling may develop in patients with subdural empyema originating from the frontal sinus [128,129,131].

In addition to symptoms of severe headache and vomiting, patients with posterior fossa subdural empyemas may have cerebellar signs, cranial nerve deficits, and pupillary abnormalities. Most will have marked nuchal rigidity [124]. A typical presentation of spinal subdural empyema consists of backache without vertebral column percussion tenderness, fever, radicular pain, and early symptoms of spinal cord compression or cauda equina involvement [125].

Infants with subdural empyemas usually demonstrate early signs of irritability, poor feeding or increase in head size, followed by hemiparesis, convulsions, stupor, and coma. Examination may reveal increased head size and a bulging fontanelle. Papilledema is unusual and fever may be absent in this age group [126].

Diagnosis

The differential diagnosis of subdural empyema includes bacterial meningitis, superior sagittal sinus thrombosis, epidural abscess, and cerebral abscess. Bacterial meningitis and subdural empyema may present in a similar fashion, with disturbances of consciousness, fever and nuchal rigidity; however, meningitis in adults, unlike subdural empyema, is not generally associated with focal neurological deficits, especially of the severity described above, at least at the time of presentation [122]. The clinical presentation of a superior sagittal sinus thrombosis is characterized by bilateral signs, alternating or ascending hemiparesis, severe headache, and focal or generalized seizures. Patients with epidural abscess are often not as ill as patients with subdural empyema and rarely have nuchal rigidity. The presentation of a cerebral abscess is very similar to that of a subdural empyema, except that the initial stage of a cerebral abscess is milder and more insidious in onset, and nuchal rigidity rarely occurs unless the abscess has ruptured into the ventricle [131]. Fever occurs in only about 50% of patients with a brain abscess and, although more common with subdural empyema, is unreliable in distinguishing the two syndromes.

During the early stages of a subdural empyema, before the development of focal neurological deficits and raised ICP, meningitis can usually be excluded by examination of the CSF. There is a mild to moderate degree of pleocytosis in the spinal fluid, consisting predominantly of polymorphonuclear leukocytes. The protein concentration is mildly elevated, and the glucose concentration is usually normal. In most series, bacteria were not demonstrated by smears or by culture of CSF obtained by lumbar puncture [122,129,131,140,141].

Because of the strong association of subdural empyema with underlying paranasal sinus infection, plain radiography of the skull and sinuses may be very useful in confirming sinus infection or demonstrating osteomyelitis of the skull [127,141]. A subdural empyema can be identified on CT by the appearance of a crescentic or lentiform-shaped area of low density adjacent to the inner border of the skull [142]. The empyema consists of an inflammatory exudate and thus appears denser than CSF. There may also be evidence of inward displacement of the interface between gray matter and white matter resulting from the presence of fluid in the subdural space. After contrast administration, dense enhancement of the medial membrane of the subdural collection is evident by the time the lesion is 3 weeks old [140].

However, CT initially may be normal or show only nonspecific hemisphere swelling [141–143]. Failure to identify a subdural empyema by CT may occur if the scan is performed before the empyema is fully developed [140]. Small interhemispheric subdural empyemas are difficult to demonstrate on CT. A subdural empyema is well visualized by MRI. MRI is very sensitive for the detection of fluid collections in the subdural space, for differentiating noninfected subdural effusions from infected empyemas, and for distinguishing between a subdural empyema and an epidural collection. MRI also visualizes the complications associated with a subdural empyema more readily (i.e., cortical vein thrombosis, cerebritis, brain abscess, and edema) than does CT [144] (Figure 20.2).

In infants, the diagnosis can often be made by subdural taps, if the subdural empyema is overlying the lateral convexity of the cerebral hemisphere and the pus is not loculated or highly viscous. However, interhemispheric subdural empyemas can be missed by this procedure [130].

Therapy

The treatment of subdural empyema consists of antibiotic therapy, immediate surgical drainage of the empyema and infected sinuses, and management of increased ICP, when present [125]. Nafcillin, oxacillin, or vancomycin are the recommended antimicrobial agents if staphylococci are suspected. Although there are reports of successful management of subdural empyemas without surgery [145], these are rare and prompt surgical intervention is recommended. Craniotomy is the preferred treatment [127,133, 146–148], although the placement of multiple burr holes has been recommended by some [135,149]. Antibiotics should be continued for at least 3 weeks after surgical drainage [122]. Increased ICP can be treated with mannitol (1.0 g/kg i.v.), hyperventilation, or dexamethasone (10 mg i.v., followed by 4 mg every 6 hours) [126].

Outcome

From 1950 to 1975, the mortality rate from subdural empyema was 25–40% [122,127,129,135]. The current mortality rate is 15–20% [132,146]. This reduction in mortality has been attributed to improved diagnostic methods and to the use of intensive care facilities [128]. Delay in surgical intervention is the one factor that correlates most with an unfavorable outcome [122–149].

(a) (b) (c)

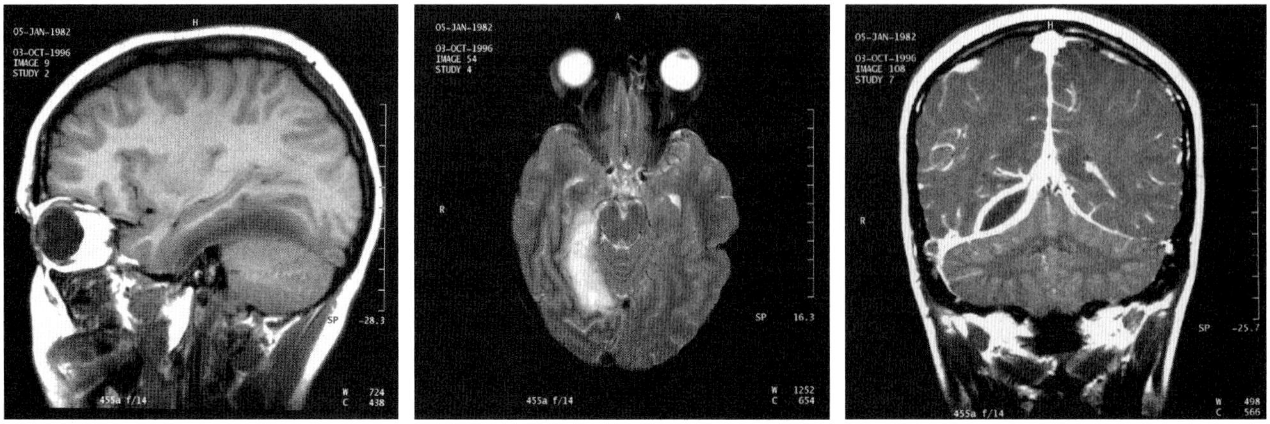

Figure 20.2 Subdural empyema. (a) Sagittal noncontrast T1-weighted MRI scan demonstrates a low-signal fluid collection along the superior surface of the tentorium extending from the petrous bone. (a) and (c) also show a thrombus in the right transverse sinus which is an associated complication of the right-sided mastoiditis. (b) On axial T2-weighted scan, the empyema is seen as a high-signal intensity zone paralleling the surface of the tentorium. (c) Coronal postcontrast T1-weighted scan. The low-signal intensity empyema is outlined by a uniform thin rim of enhancement. (Images courtesy of Dr Douglas H. Yock Jr, Department of Radiology, Abbott-Northwestern Hospital, Minneapolis, Minnesota, USA.)

Spinal subdural empyema

Most infections of the spinal subdural space are the result of hematogenous spread of infection from a distant source, most often a cutaneous infection. *Staphylococus aureus* is a common organism isolated from spinal subdural empyemas. The empyema is usually posterior to the cord, and involves the thoracic and lumbar segments predominantly [126]. The clinical presentation includes fever, back pain without vertebral column percussion tenderness, radicular pain, and early symptoms of spinal cord compression or cauda equina involvement. The diagnosis is made by spinal MRI. Therapy includes laminectomy with exploration and lavage of the subdural space and antibiotics. Because of the frequency with which *S. aureus* is isolated from this infection, agents effective against this organism (e.g., nafcillin or vancomycin) are the best empirical therapy until the results of Gram's stain and culture are known.

Epidural abscess

Staphylococus aureus and gram-negative bacilli are the most common organisms implicated in infections of the spinal epidural space. An epidural abscess can also develop between the dura and the inner table of the skull; when this occurs as a complication of craniotomy or compound skull fracture, *S. aureus* is the most common infecting organism. Spinal and cranial epidural abscess are discussed separately.

Spinal epidural abscess

A spinal epidural abscess is a collection of purulent material outside the dura matter within the spinal canal [150]. The clinical signs of this infection tend to evolve rapidly, over days, from back pain to root pain to paresis followed by paralysis. Immediate recognition and surgical decompression are required to prevent permanent paralysis.

Anatomy

The most common location for an epidural abscess is the posterior thoracic or lower lumbar epidural space [151]. The anterior epidural space is only a potential space, as the dura is virtually adherent to the posterior surface of the vertebral bodies and ligaments along the ventral aspect of the spinal canal [152]. In contrast, the posterior epidural space contains areolar tissue plus a rich vascular plexus [153]. The anteroposterior width of the epidural space is greatest where the spinal cord is smallest, from approximately T4 to T8 and from L3 to S2 [150,154]. The most common location for an epidural abscess is the posterior midthoracic region. Anterior abscesses are fairly uncommon and usually occur at cervical levels [152]. As there are no anatomical barriers to axial spread of infection, abscesses spread along the epidural space involving an average of 2.8–4.3 segments in axial extent and can occasionally spread over the entire length of the epidural space [152].

Bacteriology

Staphylococus aureus is the causative organism in spinal epidural abscesses that arise from hematogenous dissemination from a skin infection, infection in intravenous lines, or spine surgery. About two-thirds of cases are caused by this organism [155]. A recent review suggested that up to 40% of cases are now caused by MRSA [156]. The other most common causative organisms are aerobic gram-negative bacilli, especially *E. coli* and *Pseudomonas aeruginosa*, as well as streptococci [157–159]. CoNS, although rarely the causative organisms of spinal epidural abscesses, have been reported in cases following epidural catheterization for anesthesia [160]. *Aspergillus* sp., *Mycobacterium tuberculosis*, *Coccidioides immitis*, *Nocardia* sp., and echinococcal cysts have been recovered from patients with chronic abscesses of the epidural space [158,161–163].

Etiology and epidemiology

An epidural abscess develops either by direct extension from a contiguous infection, such as a focus of osteomyelitis in an adjacent vertebral body, or by hematogenous spread of bacteria from a remote site of infection. The latter is the more common cause of acute epidural abscess formation and is the route of infection in about 50% of patients. The most common source of infection for hematogenous spread to the epidural space is a skin infection, such as a furuncle, cellulitis, or infected acne. Skin infections, as well as infections arising in intravenous lines, are a common source of *S. aureus* sepsis leading to spinal epidural abscess. Urinary tract infections, pneumonia, pharyngitis, and dental abscess may also be a source of hematogenous spread of infection to the epidural space [151,152,158]. Vertebral osteomyelitis is particularly common in intravenous drug abusers and is often complicated by the development of an epidural abscess. *Staphylococcus aureus* may also cause vertebral osteomyelitis and associated epidural abscess. In a recent retrospective study, 84% of patients with epidural abscess had associated vertebral osteomyelitis [164]. gram-negative aerobic bacilli are particularly important pathogens in this patient population.

Mild blunt trauma has been reported to precede the development of a spinal epidural abscess in 15–35% of cases. The formation of a small hematoma as a result of the injury provides a *locus minoris resistentiae*, allowing hematogenous seeding of infection [152,165]. Spinal epidural abscesses in children under the age of 12 are almost always the result of hematogenous dissemination of bacteria, most often penicillin-resistant *S. aureus*, from a skin, respiratory, or urinary tract infection [153].

Pathology

The gross pathological changes in the epidural space are those of a collection of pus, demarcated by firm, well-vascularized, thickened epidural fat. In the central portion of the purulent collection, the epidural fat is found in varying stages of disintegration. The gross appearance of the spinal cord at the level of the lesion is usually normal [166]. Microscopically, however, scattered areas of softening and vacuolation of the cord are frequently seen, as well as areas of necrosis with disappearance of cells and disintegration of spinal tracts [167]. The myelomalacia occurring in the spinal cord beneath an epidural abscess is probably secondary to severe impairment of the intrinsic circulation of the cord, as a result of inflammatory thrombosis in the intraspinal vessels [165,168]. These changes, attributable to vascular damage to the cord, are thought to explain the marked neurological dysfunction that has been seen in patients who otherwise had no operative or autopsy evidence of compression deformity of the cord [167,168].

Signs and symptoms

Pain at the level of the affected spine is the most consistent, and usually the first, symptom of spinal epidural abscess. Heusner [169] described a basic clinical pattern of progression of symptoms. Back pain is the initial symptom. Radicular pain in the extremities or girdle pain around the trunk begins within 2–3 days of the onset of back pain. As the disease progresses, the patient experiences paresis of appendicular muscles, loss of sensation below the level of the lesion, and loss of bowel and bladder control. Finally, there is complete paralysis of voluntary muscles and loss of all sensory modalities below the level of the lesion. Nuchal rigidity and the Kernig sign may be elicited [151,152,167,169].

The major clinical features of spinal epidural abscess in adults are not commonly seen in infants and young children. The earliest symptoms in the pediatric age group are nonspecific, and consist of irritability, vomiting, fever, and excessive crying with handling. These symptoms are accompanied by signs of localized spinal tenderness, apparent pain with movement, and a reluctance to lie prone. As a result of the nonspecific presentation of this infection in children, the presence of a spinal epidural abscess is often not recognized until there is evidence of spinal cord compression [153,170].

Differential diagnosis

Major considerations in the differential diagnosis of spinal epidural abscess include acute transverse myelitis, spinal subdural empyema, extradural neoplasm, epidural hematoma, meningitis, disk herniation or infection, and anterior spinal artery syndrome. Acute transverse myelitis is a parainfectious or postvaccinal inflammatory condition of the spinal cord that occurs with a frequency 8–20 times that of epidural abscess, and is often difficult to distinguish, either by history or neurological examination, from an epidural abscess. The clinical presentation of both is similar, except that the absence of back pain favors a diagnosis of acute transverse myelitis and radiographic evidence of osteomyelitis at a level corresponding with the level of neurological impairment suggests an epidural abscess. Osteomyelitis has not been associated with acute transverse myelitis. A typical presentation of spinal subdural empyema consists of backache, fever, and early symptoms of spinal cord compression, with a notable absence of tenderness to percussion over the vertebral column. A neoplasm that has invaded the epidural space produces a slowly evolving clinical syndrome, more suggestive of a chronic, rather than an acute, epidural abscess. Meningitis rarely produces localized spinal tenderness or focal (especially those due to lower motor neuron involvement) neurological deficits. Patients with disk herniations have neurological signs and symptoms referable to a single, or at most a few, spinal nerve roots but are otherwise healthy. The hallmark of an anterior spinal artery syndrome is a dissociated sensory loss. There is bilateral loss of pain and temperature sensation and involvement of the corticospinal tracts and anterior horn cells below the level of the lesion, with preservation of position, vibration, and touch sensation [151,152,171–173].

Diagnosis

MRI is the procedure of choice when a spinal epidural abscess is suspected. MRI visualizes the extension of the epidural abscess in all directions, the degree of spinal cord compression, and the extension of the inflammatory process into the paraspinal tissues [174] (Figure 20.3). An epidural abscess can be readily demonstrated on CT after intrathecal contrast administration; however, this is an invasive procedure. Caution has been urged in performing a lumbar puncture at the site of a possible abscess because of the risk of spread of infection from the epidural to the subarachnoid space. For this reason, when a lumbar abscess is suspected and CT is the procedure for diagnosis, a cisternal or lateral cervical tap is recommended for the intrathecal administration of contrast.

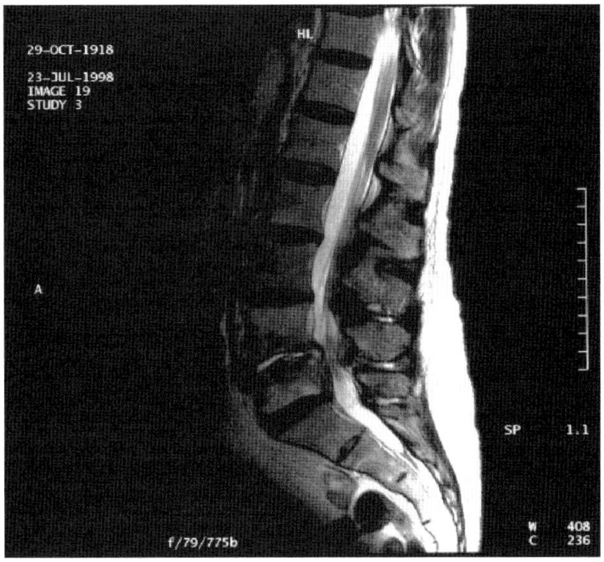

Figure 20.3 Spinal epidural abscess. T2-weighted sagittal MRI shows a severely narrowed L4–L5 disk space with high signal intensity demonstrating fluid content secondary to inflammation within the disk. There is mildly increased signal intensity throughout the L4 and L5 vertebral bodies secondary to reactive edema. The end plates are relatively well preserved. There is a small anterior epidural abscess at the posterior margin of the inflamed disk space. The patient was a 75-year-old woman who presented with back pain. (Image courtesy of Dr Douglas H. Yock Jr, Department of Radiology, Abbott-Northwestern Hospital, Minneapolis, Minnesota, USA.)

Examination of the CSF will be suggestive of a parameningeal focus of infection and may be useful to determine the infecting organism. The protein concentration is usually elevated (> 100 mg/dL) and is markedly elevated in cases with complete spinal block. The glucose concentration is usually normal; glucose levels below 40 mg/dL are evidence of coexistent bacterial meningitis. The CSF pleocytosis is variable, but most marked when frank pus is obtained as a result of penetration of the abscess. Cultures of CSF yield an organism in less than 25% of cases. Plain radiography of the spine may demonstrate osteomyelitis; however, radiographic evidence of osteomyelitis is delayed several weeks after onset of the disease and has been reported in only 30–60% of epidural abscesses associated with vertebral osteomyelitis [150–152,158,167,169,175].

Treatment

Immediate laminectomy with decompression and drainage of the epidural space must be performed to prevent imminent spinal cord necrosis [156]. As *S. aureus* is the etiological agent in the majority of these infections, and given the possibility of MRSA, vancomycin and a third-generation cephalosporin with antipseudomonal activity or meropenem should be initiated preoperatively. If the organism is MSSA, antimicrobial therapy is modified to nafcillin or oxacillin. Parenteral antibiotic therapy is continued for 3–4 weeks in the absence of osteomyelitis, and for 6–8 weeks when vertebral osteomyelitis is present [152,159]. Patients who are not operative candidates may be managed with antibiotic therapy selected by blood culture results or by culture of CT-guided aspirate of the abscess.

Prognosis

Prognosis is usually determined by the length of time paralysis has been present and the degree of loss of sensation at diagnosis and surgical intervention. If the paralysis has been present for less than 24 hours, the chances of either complete or partial recovery are good; however, when the paralysis has been present for more than 36 hours, the chance for recovery is poor. In addition, patients who have complete loss of sensation below the level of the lesion at the time of surgical intervention have very little chance for recovery of meaningful function. Patients with patchy sensory disturbances or no loss of sensation should recover partially or completely [176].

Cranial epidural abscess

Cranial epidural abscess develops in the space between the dura and the inner table of the skull. As the dura is closely apposed to the inner surface of the cranium, an intact dura tends to resist the spread of infection, limiting the size of the abscess as well as minimizing the pressure effects on the brain [167]. The pathophysiology and bacteriology of cranial epidural abscess are very similar to those of subdural empyema. An epidural abscess is usually caused by spread of infection from the frontal sinuses, middle ear, mastoid, or orbit [128]. The abscess may result from direct spread of infection through bone and underlie an osteomyelitis or the infection may reach the epidural space via retrograde spread of thrombophlebitis in the emissary veins that drain these areas [177]. An epidural abscess that arises from frontal sinusitis, middle ear infections, or mastoiditis is usually caused by streptococci or anaerobic organisms. An epidural abscess may also develop as a complication of craniotomy or compound skull fracture and lie contiguous with an area of osteomyelitis [128]. In this setting, *S. aureus* is the most common infecting organism. An epidural infection that develops as a complication of a craniotomy is frequently associated with a subgaleal abscess. This process may also occur in association with other types of intracranial infection, most commonly subdural empyema [126]. In contrast to a spinal epidural abscess, a cranial epidural abscess is rarely the result of hematogenous seeding of the epidural space from a distant site of infection [128].

Signs and symptoms

Intracranial epidural abscess should be suspected when unrelenting headache or persistent fever develop during or after treatment for frontal sinusitis, mastoiditis, or otitis media. If the abscess is large, unilateral headache and mild disturbances of consciousness may occur; however, focal neurological deficits, seizures, and signs of increased ICP do not develop until extension of the infection into the subdural space has occurred, or a deeper intracranial complication has developed [126,128]. Epidural abscesses near the petrous bone are an exception, which may involve the fifth and sixth cranial nerves, and present with ipsilateral facial pain and lateral rectus weakness (Gradenigo syndrome) [126].

Diagnosis

On noncontrast CT, an epidural abscess has the appearance of a poorly defined, lentiform area of low density adjacent to the inner table of the skull. There may be an adjacent area of bone destruction or subgaleal soft tissue mass formation. After contrast administration, the convex inner side of the low-density lesion homogeneously enhances, representing the inflamed dural membrane. On MRI, the appearance of an intracranial epidural abscess is of a lentiform or crescentic purulent fluid collection, which is hyperintense to CSF on T2-weighted images, in the interhemispheric fissure, or overlying a cerebral hemisphere [178]. On both CT and MRI, the underlying brain parenchyma appears normal unless there is an associated intracranial complication [142,177].

Plain radiography of the skull and sinuses may demonstrate an underlying sinusitis or otitis, or changes compatible with osteomyelitis. The changes in the CSF are suggestive of a parameningeal focus of infection, but are nonspecific and include mild pleocytosis, an elevated protein, and a normal glucose. The spinal fluid is usually sterile. There is a danger of tonsillar herniation when a lumbar puncture is performed in this clinical setting [126].

Treatment

Immediate neurosurgical intervention is indicated for drainage of the epidural abscess. At surgery, Gram's stain and culture of the material removed from the epidural space should be performed. Recommendations for choice of antibiotic therapy are the same as described for therapy of subdural empyema. In addition, overlying infected bone or the posterior wall of an infected frontal sinus should be removed. Antibiotics should be continued for at least 3 weeks after surgical drainage. The prognosis for a patient with an epidural abscess, without intracranial complications, is very good [128].

References

1 Morissette I, Gourdeau M, Francoeur J. CSF shunt infections: a fifteen year experience with emphasis on management and outcome. Can J Neurol Sci 1993;20:118–22.

2 Pudenz RH. The ventriculo-atrial shunt. J Neurosurg 1966;25: 602–8.

3 Gardner P, Leipzig T, Phillips P. Infections of central nervous system shunts. Med Clin North Am 1985;69:297–314.

4 Pople IK, Bayston R, Hayward RD. Infection of cerebrospinal fluid shunts in infants: a study of etiological factors. J Neurosurg 1992;77:29–36.

5 Walters BC, Hoffman HF, Hendrick EB, Humphreys RP. Cerebrospinal fluid shunt infection: influences on initial management and subsequent outcome. J Neurosurg 1984;60:1014–21.

6 Forward KR, Ferver HD, Stiver HG. Cerebrospinal fluid shunt infections: a review of 35 infections in 32 patients. J Neurosurg 1983;59:389–94.

7 Frame PT, McLaurin RL. Treatment of CSF shunt infections with intrashunt plus oral antibiotic therapy. J Neurosurg 1984; 60:354–60.

8 Schoenbaum SC, Gardner P, Shillito J. Infections of cerebrospinal fluid shunts: epidemiology, clinical manifestations, and therapy. J Infect Dis 1975;131:543–52.

9 Bayston R. Antibiotic prophylaxis in shunt surgery. Dev Med Child Neurol Suppl 1975;35:99–103.

10 Bayston R, Lari J. A study of the sources of infection in colonised shunts. Dev Med Child Neurol 1974;16(6 suppl 32): 16–22.

11 Brown EM, Edwards RJ, Pople I. Conservative management of patients with cerebrospinal fluid shunt infections. Neurosurgery 2006;58:657–65.
12 Bayston R, Penny SR. Excessive production of mucoid substance in staphylococcus S11A: a possible factor in colonization of Holter shunts. Dev Med Child Neurol Suppl 1972;27:25–8.
13 Schimke RT, Black PH, Mark VH, Swartz MN. Indolent *Staphylococcus albus* or *aureus* bacteraemia after ventriculoatriostomy: role of foreign body in its initiation and perpetuation. N Engl J Med 1961;264:264–70.
14 Borges LF. Cerebrospinal fluid shunts interfere with host defenses. Neurosurgery 1982;10:55–60.
15 Working Party on the Use of Antibiotics in Neurosurgery of the British Society for Antimicrobial Therapy. Treatment of infections associated with shunting for hydrocephalus. Br J Hosp Med 1995;53:368–73.
16 Shurtleff DB, Christie D, Foltz EL. Ventriculo auriculostomy associated infection: a 12-year study. J Neurosurg 1971;35:686–94.
17 Hubschmann OR, Countee RW. Acute abdomen in children with infected ventriculoperitoneal shunts. Arch Surg 1980;115: 305–7.
18 Conen A, Walti LN, Merlo A *et al.* Characteristics and treatment outcome of cerebrospinal fluid shunt-associated infections in adults: a retrospective analysis over an 11-year period. Clin Infect Dis 2008;47:73–82.
19 Black JA, Challacombe DN, Ockenden BG. Nephrotic syndrome associated with bacteraemia after shunt operations for hydrocephalus. Lancet 1965;ii:921–4.
20 Meadow R. Shunt nephritis: renal disease associated with infected ventriculo-atrial shunts. Dev Med Child Neurol 1973;15: 83–4.
21 Rames L, Wise B, Goodman JR, Piel CF. Renal disease with *Staph albus* bacteraemia. JAMA 1970;212:1671–7.
22 Stickler GB, Shin MH, Burke EC *et al.* Diffuse glomerulonephritis associated with infected ventriculoatrial shunt. N Engl J Med 1968;279:1077–82.
23 Bayston R. Serum C-reactive protein test in diagnosis of septic complications of cerebrospinal fluid shunts for hydrocephalus. Arch Dis Child 1979;54:545–8.
24 Deutch S, Dahlberg D, Hedegaard J, Schmidt MB, Moller JK, Ostergaard L. Diagnosis of ventricular drainage-related bacterial meningitis by broad-range real-time polymerase chain reaction. Neurosurgery 2007;61:306–11.
25 Banks JT, Bharara S, Tubbs RS *et al.* Polymerase chain reaction for the rapid detection of cerebrospinal fluid shunt or ventriculostomy infections. Neurosurgery 2005;57:1237–43.
26 Brown EM, Edwards RJ, Pople IK. Conservative management of patients with cerebrospinal fluid shunt infections. Neurosurgery 2008;62(suppl 2):661–9.
27 Wald SL, McLaurin RL. Cerebrospinal fluid antibiotic levels during treatment of shunt infections. J Neurosurg 1980;52:41–6.
28 Keucher TR, Mealey J. Long-term results after ventriculoatrial and ventriculoperitoneal shunting for infantile hydrocephalus. J Neurosurg 1979;50:179–86.
29 Morrice JJ, Young DG. Bacterial colonization of Holter valves: a ten-year survey. Dev Med Child Neurol 1974;16(6 suppl 32): 85–90.
30 James HE, Walsh JW, Wilson HD. Prospective randomized study of therapy in cerebrospinal fluid shunt infections. Neurosurgery 1980;7:459–63.
31 Cook FV, Farrar WE. Vancomycin revisited. Ann Intern Med 1978;88:813–8.
32 Ein ME, Smith NJ, Aruffo JF *et al.* Susceptibility and synergy studies of methicillin-resistant *Staphylococcus epidermidis*. Antimicrob Agents Chemother 1979;16:655–9.
33 O'Brien M, Parent A, Davis B. Management of ventricular shunt infections. Childs Brain 1979;5:304–9.
34 Everett ED, Strausbaugh LJ. Antimicrobial agents and the central nervous system. Neurosurgery 1980;6:691–714.
35 Archer GL. Antimicrobial susceptibility and selection of resistance among *Staphylococcus epidermidis* isolates recovered from patients with infections of indwelling foreign devices. Antimicrob Agents Chemother 1978;14:353–9.
36 Vichyanond P, Olson LC. Staphylococcal CNS infections treated with vancomycin and rifampin. Arch Neurol 1984;41:637–9.
37 Ring JC, Cates KL, Belani KK *et al.* Rifampin for CSF shunt infections caused by coagulase-negative staphylococci. J Pediatr 1979;95:317–9.
38 Osborn JS, Sharp S, Hanson EJ *et al. Staphylococcus epidermidis* ventriculitis treated with vancomycin and rifampin. Neurosurgery 1986;19:824–7.
39 Gombert ME, Landesman SH, Corrado ML *et al.* Vancomycin and rifampin therapy for *Staphylococcus epidermidis* meningitis associated with CSF shunts. J Neurosurg 1981;55:633–6.
40 Eng RHK, Smith SM, Buccini FJ, Cherubin CE. Differences in ability of cell-wall antibiotics to suppress emergence of rifampicin resistance in *Staphylococcus aureus*. J Antimicrob Chemother 1985;15:201–7.
41 Simon GL, Smith RH, Sande MA. Emergence of rifampin-resistant strains of *Staphylococcus aureus* during combination therapy with vancomycin and rifampin: a report of failure. Rev Infect Dis 1983;5:S507–8.
42 Acar JF, Goldstein FW, Duval J. Use of rifampin for the treatment of serious staphylococcal and gram-negative bacillary infections. Rev Infect Dis 1983;5:S502–6.
43 Eymann R, Chehab S, Strowitzki M *et al.* Clinical and economic consequences of antibiotic-impregnated cerebrospinal fluid shunt catheters. J Neurosurg Pediatr 2008;1:444–50.
44 Schlesinger LS, Ross, SC, Schaberg DR. *Staphylococcus aureus* meningitis: a broad-based epidemiologic study. Medicine (Baltimore) 1987;66:148–56.
45 Mulcare RJ, Harter DH. Changing patterns of staphylococcal meningitis. Arch Neurol 1962;7:114–20.
46 Swartz MN, Dodge PR. Bacterial meningitis: a review of selected aspects. N Engl J Med 1965;272:779–87.
47 Studdert TC. Staphylococcal spinal meningitis. BMJ 1958;1: 1457–9.
48 Geiseler PJ, Nelson KE, Levin S *et al.* Community acquired purulent meningitis: a review of 1316 cases during the antibiotic era, 1954–1976. Rev Infect Dis 1980;2:725–45.
49 Roberts FJ, Smith JA, Wagner KR. *Staphylococcus aureus* meningitis: 26 years' experience at Vancouver General Hospital. Can Med Assoc J 1983;128:1418–20.
50 Wellman WE, Senft RA. Bacterial meningitis. III. Infections caused by *Staphylococcus aureus*. Mayo Clin Proc 1964;39:263–9.
51 Carson MJ, Koch R. Management of bacterial meningitis in children. Pediatr Clin North Am 1956;3:377–98.
52 Carpenter RR, Petersdorf RG. Clinical spectrum of bacterial meningitis. Am J Med 1962;33:262–75.

53 Smith ES. Purulent meningitis in infants and children: review of 409 cases. J Pediatr 1954;45:425–36.
54 Kneebone GM. Purulent meningitis in childhood. Med J Aust 1961;2:124–30.
55 Lew D, Southwick FS, Montgomery WW *et al*. Sphenoid sinusitis. A review of 30 cases. N Engl J Med 1983;309:1149–54.
56 Hieber JP, Nelson AJ, McCracken GH. Acute disseminated staphylococcal disease in childhood. Am J Dis Child 1977;131: 181–5.
57 Gordon JJ, Harter DH, Phair JP. Meningitis due to *Staphylococcus aureus*. Am J Med 1985;78:965–70.
58 Musher DM, McKenzie SO. Infections due to *Staphylococcus aureus*. Medicine (Baltimore) 1977;56:383–407.
59 Pedersen M, Benfield TL, Skinhoej P, Jensen AG. Haematogenous *Staphylococcus aureus* meningitis. A 10 year nationwide study of 96 consecutive cases. BMC Infect Dis 2006;6:49.
60 Fisher AM, Wagner HN, Ross RS. Staphylococcal endocarditis. Arch Intern Med 1955;95:427–37.
61 Lerner PI, Weinstein L. Infective endocarditis in the antibiotic era. N Engl J Med 1966;274:199–206.
62 Greenlee JE, Mandell GL. Neurological manifestations of infective endocarditis: a review. Stroke 1973;4:958–63.
63 Mendez-Cashion D, Cordero R. Recurrent meningitis associated with congenital dermal sinus. Ann Intern Med 1961:503–9.
64 Matson DD, Ingraham FD. Intracranial complications of congenital dermal sinuses. Pediatrics 1951;8:463–74.
65 Moise TS. Staphylococcus meningitis secondary to congenital sacral sinus. Surg Gynecol Obstet 1926;42:394–397.
66 Escourolle R, Poirier J. Primary neoplasms. In: Escourolle R, Poirier J, eds. Manual of Basic Neuropathology. Philadelphia: WB Saunders, 1971:46.
67 Schwartz JF, Balentine JD. Recurrent meningitis due to an intracranial epidermoid. Neurology 1978;28:124–9.
68 Gromisch DS, Akbar R, Ubriani R *et al*. Recurrent meningitis due to *Staphylococcus aureus* secondary to a dermoid. Clin Pediatr 1982;21:698–9.
69 Lorber J, Segall M. Bacterial meningitis in spina bifida cystica: review of 37 cases. Arch Dis Child 1962;37:300–8.
70 Groover RV, Sutherland JM, Landing BH. Purulent meningitis of newborn infants: eleven year experience in antibiotic era. N Engl J Med 1961;264:1115–21.
71 Baker CJ. Nosocomial septicemia and meningitis in neonates. Am J Med 1981;70:698–701.
72 Trump DL, Grossman SA, Thompson G, Murray K. CSF infections complicating the management of neoplastic meningitis: clinical features and results of therapy. Arch Intern Med 1982; 142:583–6.
73 Daum RS. Skin and soft-tissue infections caused by methicillin-resistant *Staphylococcus aureus*. N Engl J Med 2007;357:380–90.
74 Centers for Disease Control and Prevention. VISA/VRSA. Vancomycin-intermediate/resistant *Staphylococcus aureus*. Available at http://www.cdc.gov/ncidod/dhqplar_visavrsa.html.
75 Gump DW. Vancomycin for treatment of bacterial meningitis. Rev Infect Dis 1981;3:S289–92.
76 Mamelak AN, Mampalam TJ, Obana WG, Rosenblum ML. Improved management of multiple brain abscesses: a combined surgical and medical approach. Neurosurgery 1995;36:76–85.
77 Jansen C, Frenay HME, Vandertop WP, Visser MR. Intracerebral *Nocardia asteroides* abscess treated by neurosurgical aspiration and combined therapy with sulfadiazine and cefotaxine. Clin Neurol Neurosurg 1991;93:253–5.
78 Coleman JM, Hogg GG, Rosenfeld JV, Waters KD. Invasive central nervous system aspergillosis: cure with liposomal amphotericin B, itraconazole, and radical surgery. Case report and review of the literature. Neurosurgery 1995;36:858–63.
79 Yang S, Zhao C. Review of 140 patients with brain abscess. Surg Neurol 1993;39:290–6.
80 Hagensee ME, Bauwens JE, Kjos B, Bowden RA. Brain abscess following marrow transplantation: experience at the Fred Hutchinson Cancer Research Center, 1984–1992. Clin Infect Dis 1994;19:402–8.
81 Ariza J, Casanova A, Viladrich PF *et al*. Etiological agent and primary source of infection in 42 cases of focal intracranial suppuration. J Clin Microbiol 1986;24:899–902.
82 DeLouvois J. The bacteriology and chemotherapy of brain abscess. J Antimicrob Chemother 1978;4:395–413.
83 McFarlan AM. The bacteriology of brain abscess. BMJ 1943; 2:643–4.
84 Garfield J. Management of supratentorial intracranial abscess: a review of 200 cases. BMJ 1969;2:7–11.
85 Kaplan K. Brain abscess. Med Clin North Am 1985;69:345–60.
86 Garvey G. Current concepts of bacterial infection of the central nervous system: bacterial meningitis and bacterial brain abscess. J Neurosurg 1983;59:735–44.
87 Jadavji T, Humphreys, RP, Prober CG. Brain abscess in infants and children. Pediatr Infect Dis 1985;4:394–8.
88 Brewer NS, MacCarty CS, Wellman WE. Brain abscess: a review of recent experience. Ann Intern Med 1975;82:571–6.
89 DeLouvois J, Gortavi P, Hurley R. Bacteriology of abscesses of the central nervous system: a multicentre prospective study. BMJ 1977;2:981–4.
90 Beller AJ, Sahar A, Praiss I. Brain abscess: review of 89 cases over a period of 30 years. J Neurol Neurosurg Psychiatry 1973;36:757–68.
91 Morgan H, Wood MW, Murphey F. Experience with 88 consecutive cases of brain abscess. J Neurosurg 1973;38:698–704.
92 Yang SY. Brain abscess: a review of 400 cases. J Neurosurg 1981;55:794–9.
93 Hirsh JF, Roux FX, Sainte-Rose C *et al*. Brain abscess in childhood. Childs Brain 1983;10:251–65.
94 Idriss ZH, Gutman LT, Kronfol NM. Brain abscesses in infants and children: current status of clinical findings, management and prognosis. Clin Pediatr 1978;17:738–40.
95 Nielsen H. Cerebral abscess in children. Neuropediatrics 1983; 14:76–80.
96 Waggener JD. The pathophysiology of bacterial meningitis and cerebral abscesses: an anatomical interpretation. Adv Neurol 1974;6:1–17.
97 Kawaga M, Takeshita M, Yato S. Brain abscess in congenital cyanotic heart disease. J Neurosurg 1983;58:913–7.
98 Fischer EG, McLennan JE, Suzuki Y. Cerebral abscess in children. Am J Dis Child 1981;135:746–9.
99 Enzmann DR, Britt RR, Obana WG *et al*. Experimental *Staphylococcus aureus* brain abscess. Am J Neuroradiol 1986;7:395–402.
100 Kerr FWL, King RB, Meagher JN. Brain abscess: a study of forty-seven consecutive cases. JAMA 1958;168:868–72.
101 Chun CH, Johnson JD, Hofstetter M, Raff MJ. Brain abscess: a study of 45 consecutive cases. Medicine (Baltimore) 1986;65: 415–31.

102 Duffy GP. Lumbar puncture in the presence of raised intracranial pressure. BMJ 1969;1:407–9.
103 Carey ME, Chou S, French LA. Experience with brain abscesses. J Neurosurg 1972;36:1–9.
104 Berg L. Focal infections. In: Rowland LP, ed. Merritt's Textbook of Neurology. Philadelphia: Lea & Febiger, 1984:72.
105 Britt RH, Enzmann DR, Yeager AS. Neuropathological and computerized tomographic findings in experimental brain abscess. J Neurosurg 1981;55:590–603.
106 Runge VM, Clanton JA, Price AC *et al.* Evaluation of contrast-enhanced MR imaging in a brain-abscess model. Am J Neuroradiol 1985;6:139–47.
107 Grossman RI, Joseph PM, Wolf G *et al.* Experimental intracranial septic infarction: magnetic resonance enhancement. Radiology 1985;155:649–53.
108 Wispelwey B, Dacey RG, Scheld WM. Brain abscess. In: Scheld WM, Whitley RJ, Durack DT, eds. Infections of the Central Nervous System. Philadelphia: Lippincott Raven, 1991:457.
109 Rosenblum ML, Hoff JT, Normal D *et al.* Nonoperative treatment of brain abscesses in selected high risk patients. J Neurosurg 1980;52:217–25.
110 Frame PT, Watanakunakorn C, McLaurin RL, Khodadad G. Penetration of nafcillin, methicillin and cefazolin into human brain tissue. Neurosurgery 1983;12:142–7.
111 Black P, Graybill JR, Charache P. Penetration of brain abscess by systemically administered antibiotics. J Neurosurg 1973;38:705–9.
112 DeLouvois J, Gortvai P, Hurley R. Antibiotic treatment of abscesses of the central nervous system. BMJ 1977;2:985–7.
113 DeLouvios J, Hurley R. Inactivation of penicillin by purulent exudates. BMJ 1977;1:998–1000.
114 Wispelway B, Scheld WM. Brain abscess. Clin Neuropharmacol 1987;10:483–510.
115 Boom WH, Tuazon CU. Successful treatment of multiple brain abscesses with antibiotics alone. Rev Infect Dis 1985;7:189–99.
116 Rousseaux M, Lesoin F, Destee A *et al.* Developments in the treatment and prognosis of multiple cerebral abscesses. Neurosurgery 1985;16:304–8.
117 Rotherman EB, Kessler LA. Use of computerized tomography in nonsurgical management of brain abscess. Arch Neurol 1979;37:25–6.
118 Kamin M, Biddle D. Conservative management of focal intracerebral infection. Neurology 1981;31:103–6.
119 Sharma R, Mohandas K, Cooke RP. Intracranial abscesses: changes in epidemiology and management over five decades in Merseyside. Infection 2009;37:39–43.
120 Alderson D, Strong AJ, Ingham HR, Selkon JB. Fifteen-year review of the mortality of brain abscess. Neurosurgery 1981; 8:1–6.
121 Northcroft GB, Wyke BD. Seizures following surgical treatment of brain abscesses: a clinical and electroencephalographic study. J Neurosurg 1957;14:249–63.
122 Kaufmann DM, Miller MH, Steigbigel NH. Subdural empyema: analysis of 17 recent cases and review of the literature. Medicine (Baltimore) 1975;54:485–98.
123 Weinman D, Samarasinghe HHR. Subdural empyema. Aust NZ J Surg 1972;41:324–30.
124 Morgan DW, Williams B. Posterior fossa subdural empyema. Brain 1985;108:983–92.
125 Fraser RAR, Ratzan K, Wolpert SM, Weinstein L. Spinal subdural empyema. Arch Neurol 1973;28:235–8.
126 Tunkel AR. Subdural empyema. In: Mandell GL, Bennett JE, Dolin R, eds. Principles and Practice of Infectious Diseases, 6th edn. Philadelphia: Elsevier, 2005:1164–5.
127 Galbraith JG, Barr VW. Epidural abscess and subdural empyema. Adv Neurol 1974;6:257–67.
128 Silverberg AL, DiNubile MJ. Subdural empyema and cranial epidural abscess. Med Clin North Am 1985;69:361–74.
129 Coonrod JD, Dans PE. Subdural empyema. Am J Med 1972; 53:85–91.
130 Farmer TW, Wise GR. Subdural empyema in infants, children and adults. Neurology 1973;23:254–61.
131 Kubik CS, Adams RD. Subdural empyema. Brain 1943;66: 18–43.
132 Kaufman DM, Litman N, Miller MH. Sinusitis: induced subdural empyema. Neurology 1983;33:123–32.
133 List CF. Diagnosis and treatment of acute subdural empyema. Neurology 1955;5:663–70.
134 Jacobson PL, Farmer TW. Subdural empyema complicating meningitis in infants: improved prognosis. Neurology 1981;31:190–3.
135 Bhandari YS, Sarkari NB. Subdural empyema: a review of 37 cases. J. Neurosurg 1970;32:35–9.
136 Courville CB. Subdural empyema secondary to purulent frontal sinusitis: a clinicopathologic study of forty-two cases verified at autopsy. Arch Otolaryngol 1944;39:211–230.
137 McKay RJ, Ingraham FD, Matson DD. Subdural fluid complicating bacterial meningitis. JAMA 1953;152:387–91.
138 Dacey RG, Winn HR, Jane JA, Butler AB. Spinal subdural empyema: report of two cases. Neurosurgery 1978;3:400–3.
139 Schiller F, Shadle OW. Extrathecal and intrathecal suppuration: report of two cases and discussion of the spinal subdural space. Arch Neurol 1962;7:33–6.
140 Weisberg L. Subdural empyema: clinical and computed tomographic correlations. Arch Neurol 1986;43:497–500.
141 Hodges J, Anslow P, Gillett G. Subdural empyema; continuing diagnostic problems in the CT scan era. Q J Med 1986;59: 387–93.
142 Lee SE. Infectious diseases. In: McGraw RP, Boynton SD, Cowell MW, eds. Cranial Computed Tomography. New York: McGraw-Hill, 1983:506.
143 Luken MG, Whelan MA. Recent diagnostic experience with subdural empyema. J Neurosurg 1980;52:764–71.
144 Helfgott DC, Weingarten K, Hartman BJ. Subdural empyema. In: Scheld WM, Whitley RJ, Durack DT, eds. Infections of the Central Nervous System. Philadelphia: Lippincott-Raven, 1991:487.
145 Leys D, Destee A, Petit H, Warot P. Management of subdural intracranial empyemas should not always require surgery. J Neurol Neurosurg Psychiatry 1986;49:635–9.
146 Bannister G, Williams B, Smith S. Treatment of subdural empyema. J Neurosurg 1981;55:82–8.
147 Hockley AD, Williams B. Surgical management of subdural empyema. Childs Brain 1983;10:294–300.
148 LeBeau J, Creissard P, Harispe L, Redondo A. Surgical treatment of brain abscess and subdural empyema. J Neurosurg 1973;38: 198–203.
149 Mauser HW, Tulleken CAF. Subdural empyema: a review of 48 patients. Clin Neurol Neurosurg 1984;86:255–63.
150 D'Angelo CM, Whisler WW. Bacterial infections of the spinal cord and its coverings. In: Vinken PJ, Bruyn GW, Klawans HL, eds. Handbook of Clinical Neurology, vol 33. Amsterdam: North-Holland, 1978:18.

151 Baker AS, Ojemann RG, Swartz MN, Richardson EP. Spinal epidural abscess. N Engl J Med 1975;293:463–8.
152 Verner EF, Musher DM. Spinal epidural abscess. Med Clin North Am 1985;69:375.
153 Baker CJ. Primary spinal epidural abscess. Am J Dis Child 1971;121:377–99.
154 Dandy WE. Abscesses and inflammatory tumors in the spinal epidural space (so-called pachymeningitis externa). Arch Surg 1926;13:477–494.
155 Khan SH, Hussain MS, Griebel RW, Hattingh S. Comparison of primary and secondary spinal epidural abscesses: a retrospective analysis of 29 cases. Surg Neurol 2003;59:28–33.
156 Darouiche RO. Spinal epidural abscess. N Engl J Med 2006;355: 2012–20.
157 Hulme A, Dott NM. Spinal epidural abscess. BMJ 1954;6:64–8.
158 Kaufman DM, Kaplan JG, Litman N. Infectious agents in spinal epidural abscesses. Neurology 1980;30:844–50.
159 Darouiche RO, Hamill RJ, Greensberg SB *et al.* Bacterial spinal epidural abscess: review of 43 cases and literature survey. Medicine (Baltimore) 1992;71:369–85.
160 Ferguson JF, Kirsch WM. Epidural empyema following thoracic extradural block. J Neurosurg 1974;41:762–4.
161 Seres JL, Ono H, Benner EJ. Aspergillosis presenting as spinal cord compression. J Neurosurg 1972;36:221–4.
162 Ingwer I, McLeish KR, Tight RR, White AC. *Aspergillus fumigatus* epidural abscess in a renal transplant recipient. Arch Intern Med 1978;138:153–4.
163 Delaney P, Nieman B. Spinal cord compression by *Coccidioides immitis* abscess. Arch Neurol 1982;39:255–6.
164 Chen WC, Wang JL, Wang JT. Spinal epidural abscess due to *Staphylococcus aureus*: clinical manifestations and outcomes. J Microbiol Immunol Infect 2008;41:215–21.
165 McLaurin RL. Spinal suppuration. Clin Neurosurg 1966;14:314–6.
166 Browder J, Myers R. Pyogenic infections of the spinal epidural space. Surgery 1941;10:296–308.
167 Smith BH. Infections of the dura and its venous sinuses. In: Baker AB, Joynt RJ, eds. Clinical Neurology, vol 2. Philadelphia: Harper & Row, 1986:23.
168 Hancock DO. Study of 49 patients with acute spinal extradural abscess. Paraplegia 1973;10:285–8.
169 Heusner AP. Nontuberculous spinal epidural infections. N Engl J Med 1948;239:845–54.
170 Fischer EG, Greene CS, Winston KR. Spinal epidural abscess in children. Neurosurgery 1981;9:257–60.
171 Altrocchi PH. Acute transverse myelopathy. Arch Neurol 1963; 9:111–9.
172 Altrocchi PH. Acute spinal epidural abscess vs. acute transverse myelopathy. Arch Neurol 1963;9:17–25.
173 Lougheed WM, Hoffman HJ. Spontaneous spinal extradural hematoma. Neurology 1960;10:1059–63.
174 Erntell M, Holtas S, Norlin K *et al.* Magnetic resonance imaging in the diagnosis of spinal epidural abscess. Scand J Infect Dis 1988;20:323–7.
175 Waldvogel FA, Medoff G, Swartz MN. Osteomyelitis: a review of clinical features, therapeutic considerations and unusual aspects: three parts. N Engl J Med 1970;282:198–206.
176 Hakin RN, Burt AA, Cook JB. Acute spinal epidural abscess. Paraplegia 1979;17:330–6.
177 Sharif HS, Ibrahim A. Intracranial epidural abscess. Br J Radiol 1982;55:81–4.
178 Gellin BG, Weingarten K, Gamache FW, Hartman BJ. Epidural abscess. In: Scheld WM, Whitley RJ, Durack DT, eds. Infections of the Central Nervous System. Philadelphia: Lippincott-Raven, 1991:499.

Chapter 21
Diseases of the Eye

Linda A. Ficker
Moorfields Eye Hospital NHS Foundation Trust, London, UK

Introduction

Staphylococcal diseases of the eye include both infections and expression of cell-medicated immunity (CMI) to staphylococcal antigens. The pathogenesis of diseases due to both *Staphylococcus aureus* and coagulase-negative staphylococci (CoNS) has been increasingly well characterized in recent years. This chapter discusses the role of each with respect to ocular anatomy.

Role of staphylococcal colonization of the eyelids

The numbers and pathogenicity of staphylococci colonizing the eyelids influence the risk of infection that may occur in susceptible individuals, including those with ocular surface diseases (e.g., epithelial abnormalities and dry eyes) and those undergoing surgery. Lid colonization also determines the expression of CMI to staphylococcal antigens both in the lids, as blepharitis, and in the cornea, as marginal keratitis or phlyctenulae.

Normal lid colonization has been established using a soluble swab method [1] and may be expressed quantitatively as colony-forming units per milliliter eluate (cfu/mL), the swab having been dissolved in a standard volume of saline. *Staphylococcus aureus* is a transient colonizer of the lids and has been isolated by the soluble swab method from 6% of normal individuals. Normal bacterial counts range from 1 to 10 cfu/mL, while patients with acute folliculitis have yielded counts ranging from 46 to 400 cfu/mL ($P = 0.01$) [2]. Increasingly, methicillin-resistant *S. aureus* (MRSA) has been recognized as a problem in eye disease. Surface colonization is significantly related to carriage in the nares; 78% of patients presenting with ocular surface infections due to MRSA or who were colonized on the ocular surface carry MRSA in the nares compared with only 11% of patients without MRSA in the conjunctiva [3].

CoNS are frequent colonizers of the eyelids, but are not associated with anterior lid margin disease. Some biotypes as identified by the Baird-Parker scheme are more common than others: types II and III are found in 88% and 74% of normal individuals, respectively (bacterial counts not exceeding 1000 cfu/mL) [4]. Both methicillin-resistant *Staphylococcus epidermidis* (MRSE) and MRSA colonization of the ocular surface will determine the likely pathogens and will hence define the virulence of microbial keratitis. MRSE and MRSA were found among patients at risk of carriage, i.e., those receiving long-term antibiotics and steroids and those who were hospitalized. Patients with staphylococcal keratitis were successfully treated with vancomycin, ofloxacin, or arbekacin [5].

Patients with chronic nonulcerative blepharitis are similar to normal individuals, 7% being colonized by *S. aureus* (< 15 cfu/mL) and CoNS isolation being similar with respect to bacterial counts, biotypes, and toxin production [4,6]. However, atopic patients are characterized by significantly increased *S. aureus* colonization of lids and conjunctivae; 80% are colonized and 55% of lid swabs manifest heavy growth [7], as well as increased colonization of the conjunctiva and nasal mucosa.

Staphylococcal blepharitis and associated marginal keratitis

Thygeson [8,9] was the first to classify staphylococcal blepharitis and commented on the association of ulcerative blepharitis and corneal infiltrates that cause significant symptoms: photophobia, pain, and blurred vision. These clinical signs were not frequently unilateral, with associated hordeola, conjunctivitis, and punctate keratopathy (see Plate 21.1). Patients were noted to have dermatological disease such as acne vulgaris and rosacea, as well as impetigo and boils. Microscopic examination of lid margin smears demonstrated staphylococci and leukocytes in affected patients.

Hogan *et al.* [10] determined that the corneal infiltrates in marginal keratitis were usually sterile, although *S. aureus* was isolated from the lids. Typically these peripheral infiltrates are 1–2 mm in diameter and involve the anterior

Staphylococci in Human Disease, 2nd edition. Edited by Kent B. Crossley, Kimberly K. Jefferson, Gordon Archer, Vance G. Fowler, Jr.
 ISBN 978-14051-6332-3.

corneal stroma without ulceration of the epithelium; they are separated from the vascular limbus by clear corneal stroma (see Plate 21.2). Thygeson [8] isolated *S. aureus* from the lids of 133 of 180 patients with acute marginal keratitis; he postulated that bacterial allergy may have caused sterile infiltrates, introducing the concept of *S. aureus* hypersensitivity in the development of corneal disease. Thygeson [11] subsequently explored therapeutic desensitization with staphylococcal toxoid.

Children tend to manifest more central corneal inflammation with vascularization and phlyctenular disease. Phlyctenulae also occur in generalized tuberculosis, in response to circulating antigen, and when the CMI response is modified with survival of bacilli within macrophages. The differential diagnosis of tuberculosis must be investigated. Thygeson noted that children required aggressive therapy to prevent severe recurrent staphylococcal disease; it is interesting that in both children and adults the disease is frequently unilateral (see Plate 21.3). This suggests local CMI in such individuals, which may not be revealed by skin testing until systemic CMI supervenes.

Role of cell-mediated immunity to *S. aureus*

CMI to *S. aureus* was demonstrated by Panton and Valentine in 1929 [12]. Repeated dermal injection of the rabbit with *S. aureus* at different concentrations resulted in delayed-type hypersensitivity. After repeated immunization, the inflammatory response to large inocula of *S. aureus* was considerably reduced, while inocula diluted 100-fold or 1000-fold that were ineffective prior to immunization gave rise to inflammatory lesions. In 1958, Johanovsky [13] demonstrated that this type of immunity was cell-mediated by achieving transfer of immunity from immunized rabbits to normal rabbits. He homogenized the spleen cells of immunized rabbits and injected these into rabbits with negative skin tests. He further demonstrated that immunized rabbits had increased susceptibility to fatal intravenous challenge with live *S. aureus*. In 1949, Boe [14] had previously failed to transfer immunity using serum.

Attempts have been made to desensitize patients with CMI to *S. aureus*, but to date this form of therapy has not been fully investigated. During the pre-antibiotic era, Thygeson [11] attempted desensitization with staphylococcal toxoid in 83 patients. Although the follow-up is not specified, Thygeson observed that patients ($N = 78$) were improved and remained symptom-free, even in the event of recolonization with *S. aureus*. He observed a correlation between the initial hypersensitivity response to intradermal toxoid and clinical improvement. The toxoid preparation was a relatively crude peptic digest and may have contained protein A, which is a candidate antigen for CMI as discussed below.

In 1970, Mudd *et al.* [15] injected patients intradermally with filtered phage lysate. The first injections resulted in hypersensitivity reactions with induration of the skin measuring 19 mm. After the sixth injection this was reduced to 3 mm, but this desensitization was only maintained with repeated injections every 2–4 weeks. It is likely that IgG-blocking antibodies were produced that suppressed antigen expression. The lysate probably included the candidate antigens protein A, peptidoglycan, and teichoic acid.

Rabbit models of staphylococcal blepharitis

In 1962, Hogan *et al.* [10] injected antigen (cell wall/toxic filtrate) into the central corneal stroma of immunized rabbits. An inflammatory response was induced, although this was a mid-peripheral corneal ring and differed from the clinical picture of marginal keratitis. Toxoid was less effective in eliciting this type of response, and nonimmunized control rabbits were not affected.

Exploiting the concept of CMI to *S. aureus*, in 1982 Mondino and Kowalski [16] explored the role of ocular surface challenge with *S. aureus* in immunized rabbits. The rabbits were immunized with either whole-cell vaccines or purified cell walls; subsequently, suspensions of viable *S. aureus* were dropped onto the ocular surface, producing a clinical picture of marginal keratitis with elevated nodular infiltrates (phlyctenulae) and corneal vascularization. Nonimmunized control rabbits did not develop these lesions. Similar experiments in 1987 varied the regimen of immunization and subsequent challenge to produce a clinical picture of acute ulcerative blepharitis [17]. Mondino and Adam [18] were also able to induce CMI to CoNS in the rabbit, although they were unable to cause acute ulcerative blepharitis in immunized animals exposed to live CoNS as for *S. aureus*, suggesting that protein A or some other component unique to *S. aureus* might be an important antigen in the pathogenesis of staphylococcal blepharitis.

Tests of humoral immunity to staphylococci can measure circulating antibodies to staphylococcal toxins or enzymes. Following immunization of the rabbits, Mondino *et al.* [19] identified antibodies to teichoic acid. Such antibodies are variably found in patients with *S. aureus* infections and can be measured in tears using enzyme-linked immunosorbent assay (ELISA) techniques, although only limited quantities of teichoic acid are commercially available [2].

Investigation of cell-mediated immunity in blepharitis

CMI to staphylococcal antigens in patients with chronic blepharitis of various etiologies has been investigated by injecting intradermal suspensions of *S. aureus* (NCTC 6571), *S. epidermidis* (NCTC 7292) and 2.5 ng of protein A [2]. (The normal response to protein A was previously established by White and Nobel [20]; patients with a normal response to protein A were found to give little response to *S. aureus* and none to *S. epidermidis*.) Overall, 40% of 116 patients were found to have enhanced CMI to both *S. aureus* and protein A ($P = 0.001$), but none manifest CMI to CoNS [2]. Patients were not necessarily tested during episodes of active marginal keratitis, nor did all patients have a history of this disease. However, there was a trend suggesting that enhancement of CMI was associated with a history of marginal keratitis requiring treatment with topical steroids. This would be consistent with the concept that CMI plays a role in staphylococcal blepharitis, as postulated by Thygeson. A subgroup of 28% of the patients were atopic, the expected prevalence in the normal population; some of the atopic subjects tested showed total absence of a skin reaction. In 1985, White and Nobel [20] observed that the CMI skin reaction in atopic subjects was reduced compared with normals. All atopic subjects had similar serum IgG and IgE antibodies to *S. aureus* ribitol teichoic acid, and hence neither humoral immunity nor CMI to *S. aureus* appeared to have a role in pathogenesis of chronic allergic conjunctivitis [6,7].

Thygeson's original classification of staphylococcal blepharitis related to anterior lid margin disease due to *S. aureus* colonization or seborrhea, or both [8]. More recently, McCulley and colleagues [21,22] expanded the classification of chronic blepharitis to include posterior lid margin disease, essentially meibomian gland dysfunction with tear film instability. These workers investigated the role of CoNS in generating abnormal meibomian secretions; the relevance of staphylococcal lipase in splitting triglycerides to toxic fatty acids remains speculative.

Blepharitis in immunodeficient patients

Patients, often children, with selective immunodeficiency manifest abnormal responses to *S. aureus*, as observed by Monteil *et al.* [23]. Failure of opsonization and polymorphonuclear leukocyte killing of *S. aureus* results in recurrent staphylococcal infections, which can be successfully treated with normal plasma IgG; others have normal serum inhibition titers and are thought to have defective chemotaxis (Leiner disease) with failure of C5a complement generation or "lazy phagocyte" syndrome (see Plate 21.4). Since these children develop recurrent carbuncles, styes, blepharitis, and marginal keratitis, it is likely that the pathogenesis is enhanced CMI, possibly due to the presence of excessive intracellular (phagocyte, macrophage) antigen [23–25].

Atopic patients with high plasma concentrations of IgE (Job syndrome) also have defective polymorphonuclear leukocyte chemotaxis and develop "cold" staphylococcal abscesses [26]. In these patients, 21% of total IgE was found to bind with *S. aureus* cell wall compared with 2% in normals; only one of these patients had evidence of eye disease.

Treatment of staphylococcal blepharitis and marginal keratitis

Treatment of staphylococcal blepharitis should be targeted at both bacterial colonization and secondary inflammation. Oxytetracycline and fusidic acid are antistaphylococcal but also have well-recognized antiinflammatory properties [27]. A randomized partial crossover study found symptoms to be improved by topical fusidic acid gel in 75% of patients with rosacea and by oral oxytetracycline in 50%. Patients without rosacea did not respond to fusidic acid, and only 25% responded to oxytetracycline [27]. Patients with rosacea are known to have lids that are frequently colonized by *S. aureus*, suggesting that CMI may be a common factor in the pathogenesis of both staphylococcal blepharitis and rosacea [28]. This is consistent with the use of topical steroid, which is effective in treating inflammatory corneal disease, both marginal and phlyctenular keratitis.

The limitation of therapy is the inability to provide adequate prophylaxis against recurrence. Based on the hypothesis that colonization of the eyelids with *S. aureus* elicits a CMI response in susceptible patients, the transient nature of colonization explains recurrent episodes of CMI-induced corneal disease expressed as marginal keratitis. Bacterial resistance precludes long-term antibiotic suppression of lid colonization, but desensitization presents a logical alternative.

Conjunctivitis

Colonization of the conjunctiva

The normal flora of the conjunctiva has been assessed by the soluble swab method [1]. *Staphylococcus aureus* colonizes 1% (6–10 cfu/mL) of the normal population compared with 6% of the normal population for lid margins; CoNS colonize 50% of normal conjunctivae with highly variable counts, sometimes exceeding 100 cfu/mL; micrococci colonize 5% of normal individuals (1–5 cfu/mL).

Staphylococcus aureus is a common cause of purulent conjunctivitis in adults and is often associated with blepharitis. Thygeson reported that this blepharitis is ulcerative, but this is now considered rare. Antibiotic susceptibility among pathogens causing conjunctivitis is changing. Topical fusidic acid gel, polymyxin–trimethoprim (Polytrim), gentamicin, tetracycline, and quinolones were typically effective in the past. There is an increasing incidence of MRSA across different continents. While the clinical disease may be mild, as with methicillin-sensitive *S. aureus* (MSSA), vancomycin has become the therapy of choice in the USA. A recent study of ocular infection caused by MRSA in California found that 100% of 88 isolates were vancomycin susceptible, 97% sulfisoxazole susceptible, 93% tetracycline sensitive, and 64% bacitracin susceptible [29]. Only 15% of isolates were sensitive to ciprofloxacin. Increasing ciprofloxacin resistance has also been reported in Florida [30]: comparing the periods 1990–1995 and 1996–2001, it has increased from 8 to 20.7%. There was a difference between MSSA (5% resistant) and MRSA (55.8% resistant). Gentamicin susceptibility was 99% and 86% respectively. In a study of conjunctival and corneal isolates in Brazil between 1985 and 2000, staphylococcal sensitivity manifested changing trends, with fluoroquinolones generally remaining effective, chloramphenicol demonstrating increased susceptibility, and a drop in the proportion of staphylococci susceptible to cephalothin [31]. A recent study reported that the proportion of *S. aureus* ocular infections caused by MRSA had increased from 30 to 42% between 2000 and 2005 [32]. These studies demonstrate the importance of local knowledge and the value of investigation where appropriate.

Staphylococcal keratitis

Epidemiology

The normal cornea is protected by an intact epithelium and a precorneal tear film containing lysozyme, antibodies, and inflammatory cells. Patients with epithelial loss, ocular surface disease, or tear film deficiency are therefore vulnerable to infection. Infective keratitis is a worldwide problem with different profiles of pathogens in temperate and tropical climates. In Bangladesh, 53.5% of cases were reported to be bacterial, most commonly *Pseudomonas* (24%), and 35.9% fungal [33]. In contrast, in urban Sweden, there were no fungal cases while more than 50% were due to *S. aureus* and *S. epidermidis* [34]. In Baltimore, 28% were due to CoNS and 16% to *S. aureus* infections [35]. In childhood the common pathogens include *Pseudomonas aeruginosa* (34%) and *S. aureus* (20%), in addition to fungi (18%) [36].

The lids of atopic patients are known to be heavily colonized with *S. aureus* and corneal ulceration resulting from atopic keratoconjunctivitis predisposes these patients to secondary *S. aureus* keratitis (see Plate 21.5) [37]. Recurrent keratitis occurs in immunodeficiency in the absence of recognized risk factors such as contact lens wear. Affected patients may be infected by a sequence of different pathogens, including *S. aureus*, CoNS, *Candida* species, and α-hemolytic streptococci, or they may have polymicrobial disease [38]. Collagen-binding adhesin appears to be important for *S. aureus* to achieve corneal adherence and infectivity. A rabbit model of keratitis established that absence of the adhesin reduced the risk of contact lens infection and that reintroduction of the gene restored infectivity [39].

More recently, healthy patients who developed MRSA keratitis after laser refractive surgery were found to have been exposed to healthcare environments. Hence this history is important in the management of such surgery [40].

Clinical presentation

Keratitis typically follows a corneal insult such as trauma, loose surgical sutures, or exposure to contaminated contact lenses. It causes ocular pain with photophobia and blurred vision. Symptoms are related to the epithelial loss and to the inflammatory sequelae including infiltration of the normally clear cornea. The eye is injected with fluorescein staining of the corneal ulceration. Slit-lamp examination reveals white corneal opacification due to inflammation and cells in the anterior chamber. Exotoxin will cause a "Wesley" ring of inflammatory cells, indicating virulent infection and heralding stromal lysis with corneal thinning.

Other manifestations of infection may occur such as "crystalline" keratopathy, which is intrastromal. There is not necessarily epithelial loss as the infection may arise within a suture track. The infiltration has the appearance of a snowflake, in contrast to the typical corneal abscess, which is amorphous. Histopathology reveals a surprising lack of inflammatory cells; these patients are typically using topical steroid medication. This type of keratitis is usually associated with pathogens of lower virulence, such as CoNS or α-hemolytic streptococci.

Diagnosis

Once a clinical diagnosis is made, prompt microbiological investigation is appropriate. A corneal scraping aims to obtain a specimen before prescribing broad-spectrum therapy. The cornea should be anesthetized with unpreserved Benoxinate in order to minimize microbial toxicity. The cornea is scraped with a sterile needle mounted on a syringe. Infiltrated corneal tissue is removed by tangential scraping of the bed of the ulcer and the advancing front, where viable organisms reside. Where there is minimal infiltrate, a calcium alginate swab soaked in broth provides an alternative method preferred by some investigators [41].

Several media should be inoculated primarily, including blood or chocolate agar, Sabouraud agar, thioglycollate broth, and Robertson cooked meat broth, and smears should be prepared for Gram and Giemsa staining. Inevitably, the specimens are extremely small and must be carefully processed to ensure prompt identification of the pathogen. The organism recovered may not be sensitive to the broad-spectrum therapy, which is usually commenced before availability of laboratory results. Early diagnosis permits timely institution of appropriate therapy and optimizes visual recovery.

Microbiological investigations may be considered algorithmically, initially using Gram staining and routine culture media and conditions of incubation (Gram stain and culture results are consistent in more than 60% of cases) [42]. When initial investigations are negative and there is clinical progression, the diagnosis remains that of presumed infection and further investigations are required. The same would apply if a pathogen were identified but the keratitis failed to respond to appropriate antibiotic therapy as indicated by sensitivity tests. Polymicrobial infection or the possibility of emerging resistance must then be considered.

As corneal specimens are of limited size and the patient will have commenced therapy, changing the conditions of incubation of the original plates provides an alternative to cessation of therapy and acquisition of new specimens. This pursues the capnophilic and temperature-sensitive isolates. Washing out the Gram stain and acridine orange presents an opportunity to restain with modified and full Ziehl–Neelsen stains (for *Nocardia* sp. and mycobacteria), which again are reversible and can be washed out for end stains (e.g., Grocott, immunostains, and calcofluor white). Further corneal specimens may be obtained after cessation of therapy for at least 24 hours, either a scrape or a corneal biopsy obtained by lamellar dissection.

Medical treatment

Since fungal infection is rare in temperate climates, bacterial infection is assumed. Intensive hourly broad-spectrum therapy with fortified topical preparations should aim to provide adequate antibiotic concentrations without unnecessary corneal toxicity. Fortified aminoglycosides (e.g., gentamicin or tobramycin) and a cephalosporin (e.g., cefuroxime) have traditionally been recommended and provide combination therapy against *S. aureus* and CoNS, except in the case of MRSA and MRSE. Gentamicin resistance has been reported for both CoNS and *S. aureus* [43]. This finding supports the need for combination therapy with a cephalosporin or with vancomycin. The fluoroquinolones have recently provided a less toxic alternative, but fluoroquinolone resistance in staphylococci is emerging [44–46]. The increasing use of fluoroquinolone wide-spectrum monotherapy has led to fewer corneal scrapes for laboratory investigation among consecutive patients compared over two 12-month periods in 1991 and 1994. Although the spectrum of isolates among those cultured remained unchanged, there appeared to be more severe disease [47]. Vancomycin remains useful in resistant infection, although it is less well tolerated [48].

In addition to antimicrobial agents, cycloplegia and antihypertensive and antiinflammatory therapy are important to minimize complications such as glaucoma and scarring. Topical atropine provides effective and sustained cycloplegia; topical beta-blockers or oral acetazolamide control intraocular pressure. Nonsteroidal antiinflammatory drugs modulate inflammation and pain. Topical steroids may be used judiciously in the absence of fungal coinfection.

Trials of ciprofloxacin have demonstrated good clinical results for monotherapy when compared with conventional fortified gentamicin and cefazolin, with similar times to healing, duration of therapy, and visual outcome [49]. Crystalline deposition may be problematic, especially with ulcers in the visual axis and, on the whole, fluoroquinolones should not be used as first-line therapy for staphylococcal infection.

With respect to methicillin resistance in staphylococcal infections, topical ciprofloxacin 0.3% has been compared in a rabbit model of *S. aureus* keratitis with vancomycin 5.0% and cefazolin 5.0% [50]. For early therapy, instituted within 9 hours of stromal inoculation, ciprofloxacin was found to be significantly more effective in sterilizing the cornea. If therapy was delayed beyond 10 hours, monotherapy did not sterilize the cornea but controlled the infection better than the alternative agents. Clinical experience of MRSA keratitis treated with either ciprofloxacin or vancomycin has been encouraging, with reported cures for recalcitrant disease.

Slime production has been found highly predictive of multidrug resistance and virulence and occurred in 83% of *S. epidermidis*, mostly biotypes I and II, compared with 18% of nonslime producers from ocular isolates causing keratitis [51].

Surgical treatment

Corneal transplantation may be necessary to achieve visual rehabilitation if visually significant scarring persists after 12 months. The prognosis for transplantation in this quiescent postinfective phase is excellent compared with surgery during the acute infection, which is best performed only for emergencies such as corneal perforation [52].

Surgically related endophthalmitis

Infection may supervene after intraocular surgery, most commonly cataract surgery, but it can also follow perforating trauma or may be endogenous in the presence of bacteremia. The incidence of intraocular infection following surgery is estimated to be up to 0.5% and is influenced by the use of lens implants with polypropylene haptics and by perioperative complications [53].

It has been established that adherence of ocular *S. epidermidis* isolates depends on the intercellular adhesin (*ica*) locus, which encodes the antigens mediating adherence to biomaterials. These isolates are therefore more likely to cause infection when introduced into the eye. A further study has described surface modification with a fluoroalkylsilan (Dynasilan), which reduced adherence of common endophthalmitis pathogens, *S. epidermidis* and *Propionibacterium acnes*, on various intraocular lens materials including polymethylmethacrylate, silicone and hydrogel. Hence it may be possible to reduce the infection risk by such means [54,55]. It can be assumed that 10% of perforating injuries with retained intraocular foreign bodies will develop infection; the commonest pathogens reported are *Bacillus* sp. and *Staphylococcus* sp. [56–58]. Patients with endogenous infection usually have systemic disease such as diabetes, with an infective source such as endocarditis. The commonest pathogen is *S. aureus* (25%) [59].

Lens implants are probably contaminated by exposure to ocular surface flora during insertion into the eye; hence if they are isolated from the surface inside an injector this may reduce the risk of infection. A study comparing foldable lens insertion with injected lenses found no difference in anterior chamber contamination among 100 cases without surgical complications. It should be noted that preoperative disinfection with povidone-iodine reduced conjunctival positive cultures from 22% to 4% and the incidence of infection was only 0.1% [60].

Both acute and late-onset chronic infection are recognized [61,62]. Progression of signs and visual dysfunction are related to the virulence of the pathogen. Of all isolates identified in the recent Endophthalmitis Vitrectomy Study, the most common were CoNS (70%) and *S. aureus* (10%) [62]. Early diagnosis and treatment are essential to optimize the visual outcome; ideally, intravitreal antibiotics should be given within 24 hours.

Clinical presentation

Common symptoms of infection are blurred vision, redness, pain, and lid swelling at variable intervals following surgery. The common signs are corneal endothelial inflammatory deposits; intraocular inflammation, which may sediment to form a hypopyon; fibrin in the pupillary aperture; and adhesions between the pupil and lens implant, predisposing to glaucoma. The view of the retina becomes increasingly obscured with progressive inflammation in the vitreous.

Diagnosis

The natural history of infection proceed from inoculation to aqueous infection and subsequent vitreal invasion, with aqueous and vitreous biopsies becoming sequentially positive. Aqueous biopsies tend to be culture negative within about 48 hours of the onset of symptoms; it is therefore important to obtain a simultaneous vitreous biopsy after ultrasound examination.

Characteristic ultrasound findings in endophthalmitis presenting with poor vision and media opacities include retinal detachment, macular detachment, and choroidal detachment [63]. The principal predictor of visual outcome is presenting visual acuity. Ultrasound determines whether these complications influence the biopsy technique and associated risks.

An aqueous biopsy is obtained through a paracentesis incision in the cornea and aspiration into a tuberculin syringe. A vitreous biopsy is obtained by trans-pars plana needle aspiration or with the aid of a vitreous suction cutter. Biopsies should be inoculated immediately into appropriate media and a smear of the material Gram stained (see Plate 21.6). The Gram stain takes an hour because vitreous cannot be heated and has to be air dried and methanol fixed. Gram stain can exclude fungi, particularly yeasts, and will determine the need for intravitreal amphotericin. This drug is not routinely given empirically, as endophthalmitis is usually bacterial and amphotericin is relatively toxic to the retina.

Treatment

The inflammatory response to intraocular infection lags behind the replication of bacteria and determines the final visual outcome. It is therefore essential that treatment be immediate and aggressive, as it cannot be assumed that the endophthalmitis is due to a pathogen of low virulence. Intraocular inflammation can be minimized by early bactericidal and antiinflammatory therapy.

Based on the expected pathogens, mostly staphylococci, the bactericidal broad-spectrum antibiotic combinations that have emerged in recent practice include gentamicin with cefazolin, amikacin with vancomycin, amikacin with cefuroxime, and vancomycin with ceftazidime [64]. These are injected into the vitreal cavity, which is poorly penetrated by many antibiotics. Direct injection overcomes the delay in achieving adequate bactericidal antibiotic levels in the vitreous by oral, intravenous, or subconjunctival administration. Adjunctive intravenous antibiotics prolong the half-life of vitreal drugs by reducing the concentration gradient, which dictates clearance from the vitreous. In the case of β-lactams and ciprofloxacin, probenecid inhibits vitreal clearance. The need for prolonged intravitreal antibiotics probably depends on the severity of the infection, in particular whether there is heavy growth of bacteria. Persistently positive vitreal cultures have occurred with staphylococcal infections and may require repeat intravitreal injections to achieve optimal control of the infection. Inflammation, which may cause a fibrous scar that decreases visual acuity, is targeted with high-dose oral steroid therapy (prednisolone 60 mg/day) and intensive topical steroid drops. Steroids are withheld for fungal infections and if considered life-threatening.

The Endophthalmitis Vitrectomy Study was designed to establish the role of vitrectomy in the management of endophthalmitis [62]. The visual outcome for patients presenting with vision of light perception or worse showed improvement with early vitrectomy, with removal of the infective and inflammatory load. No significant benefit from intravenous antibiotics was demonstrated, but this may not apply to all cases, as two-thirds of patients presenting with endophthalmitis were excluded by the study design.

It is not generally necessary to remove an intraocular lens, in contrast to other infections associated with prostheses. In some cases of chronic infection due to *Propionibacterium* spp., lens implant removal is required to control the endophthalmitis.

It appears from experimental models that have compared animals devoid of complement with controls that the complement system plays an important role in limiting bacterial replication [65]. The severity of inflammation has been correlated with serum IgG antibody levels to CoNS, this being more elevated in more severe infection [66]. Investigation of the immunology of endophthalmitis may refine antiinflammatory strategies in the future.

Coagulase-negative staphylococci

Positive biopsies should not be dismissed as contaminants. These infections are considered low grade and characteristically there is an asymptomatic latent period after surgery, the median diagnostic delay being 7 days with delay greater than 1 month in 12% of cases. CoNS are also associated with chronic infection that manifests a transient response to steroids, with a prolonged course of recurrent inflammation until intravitreal antibiotics are administered. Good visual outcomes are associated with intensive topical steroid during the symptomatic period. Although pain is a common presenting symptom of endophthalmitis, at least 10% of CoNS infections are painless.

The CoNs pathogens have been mostly *S. epidermidis*, but further analysis has revealed about 28% to be other species. The outcome for visual acuity after treatment with vitrectomy and intravitreal antibiotic injection is 20/50 for 38% and 20/400 for 68%, with a retinal detachment rate of 10% compared with 4% for uncomplicated cataract surgery [67,68]. The visual outcome for patients managed with intraocular vancomycin and ceftazidime remains good. In a study of 34 patients, cultures were positive in 79% of which 48% were *S. epidermidis* and 62% achieved 0.1 vision or better [64].

Staphylococcus aureus

Although *S. aureus* is a less common pathogen than CoNS, the infection caused is generally of earlier onset during the postoperative period and tends to be severe and rapidly progressive and results in a relatively poor visual outcome. Early onset of symptoms and signs warrant a high index of suspicion and early consideration of biopsy and intravitreal antibiotic injection [69].

Atopic patients are known to have lid margins heavily colonized with *S. aureus*. This is the most likely pathogen in this subgroup, especially if no preoperative measures were taken to reduce colonization. Increasingly, there are reports of resistant MRSA isolates, and methicillin and other penicillins and cephalosporins have been abandoned as therapy for endophthalmitis.

Endogenous endophthalmitis

Most patients developing endogenous infection have predisposing medical conditions such as diabetes mellitus, gastrointestinal disorders, cardiovascular disease, or malignancy. Common isolates are *S. aureus* and streptococci and both intravitreal and intravenous antibiotic administration are mandatory, given the systemic nature of the infection.

Prophylaxis

Intraocular surgery exposes the eye to contamination from the conjunctival sac and adnexal tissues colonized by diverse microorganisms. Conjunctival colonization tends to be transient and only about 37% of isolates from conjunctival specimens are in concordance with vitreal cultures taken for investigation of postoperative endophthalmitis. Isolates from intraocular biopsies of eyes with endophthalmitis have been identified as belonging to the conjunctival flora by molecular biological techniques [70].

The conjunctival microbial flora has been shown to be more effectively reduced by irrigation of the conjunctival sac with povidone-iodine 5% than by administration of topical broad-spectrum antibiotics as judged by postoperative conjunctival cultures [71]. Lid colonization plays a particular role in atopic patients, who characteristically are heavily colonized with *S. aureus*. As this is a virulent pathogen, prophylaxis with systemic antibiotic is logical for this group for whom the aim is to reduce colonization without the expectation of eradication. It is therefore recommended that, at surgery, both skin preparation with povidone-iodine 15% and irrigation of the conjunctival sac with povidone-iodine 5% be performed. The lids are then isolated by an adhesive plastic drape that enfolds the lid margins. The lacrimal system must be excluded as it is possible source of infection.

There is a threshold inoculum for infection, as demonstrated in animal models in which eyes are injected with logarithmic increments of bacteria. Serial quantitative vitreal cultures define the threshold, but infected eyes are found to remain culture-positive for variable periods. For lower concentrations of inocula, autosterilization occurs by 64 hours; for large inocula the vitreous remains culture-positive, suggesting that the host immune response has been overwhelmed. This suggests that if contamination is minimized, infection does not necessarily supervene.

Current practice in cataract surgery is to include implantation of an intraocular lens. Some materials (e.g., polymethylmethacrylate) have a surface charge that induces bacterial adherence. This can be prevented by coating the implant at surgery with a viscoelastic fluid that has no such electrostatic attraction. Irrigation fluid is normally required for the clearance of cortical lens fibers by an intraocular irrigation–aspiration technique. Excess fluid normally flows out of the anterior chamber through the surgical incision, and it is important that this not pool in the conjunctival sac and recirculate into the anterior chamber, as this is another source of contamination.

Contamination may nonetheless occur, and the aim of postoperative therapy is to prevent intraocular microbial growth. Experimental models have demonstrated that bactericidal levels of antibiotic must be achieved within 3 hours, otherwise infection may supervene even in the presence of bactericidal levels. Penetration of antimicrobials into the anterior chamber has been extensively studied. It has been established that effective concentrations exceeding the minimum inhibitory concentration for most expected pathogens may be achieved using cefuroxime or vancomycin. Cefuroxime 125 mg by subconjunctival injection achieves bactericidal levels in the aqueous partly by leakage into the tear film and reabsorption. Vancomycin is also effective, but probably best used for the treatment of resistant infections. Postoperatively antibiotic drugs (or porcine collagen shields soaked with antibiotics) are often used to prevent wound infections: chloramphenicol in Europe and aminoglycosides (gentamicin or tobramycin) in the USA. These will not inhibit staphylococci, which are already adherent to the polymethylmethacrylate lens implant, since the drugs will not penetrate the cornea and the bacteria are not susceptible within the biofilm.

Atopic patients should be carefully prepared for surgery, especially if there is significant eczematous dermatitis. Chlorhexidine 4% baths (which must not be allowed to get into the eye) and shampooing have a persistent anti-staphylococcal effect and should be performed for 3 days prior to surgery.

Prophylaxis for posttraumatic infection is widely used. Typically, both systemic and local antimicrobial agents are ordered with the drugs selected to provide broad-spectrum coverage. Few data have carefully examined the effectiveness of prophylaxis. In a rabbit model of posttraumatic eye infection, antibiotics were found to be effective when administered early [72].

Conclusion

Staphylococci are pathogenic for both infective and inflammatory eye disease. *Staphylococus aureus* not only causes more virulent infections but may be capable of eliciting CMI due to components in its cell wall. Staphylococci generally cause disease in susceptible individuals by virtue of their colonization of the ocular adnexae and conjunctiva. Treatment depends on understanding and appropriately targeting both the infective and inflammatory mechanisms.

References

1 Badini D, Bron A, Elkington A *et al.* Use of a novel transport method for the quantification of the normal lid flora of the external eye. Microb Ecol Health Dis 1988;1:57–59.

2 Ficker L, Ramakrishnan M, Seal DV *et al.* Role of cell-mediated immunity to staphylococci in blepharitis. Am J Ophthalmol 1991;111:473–9.

3 Kimura N, Sotozono C, Higashihara H *et al.* Relationship between ocular surface infection or colonization of methicillin-resistant *Staphylococcus aureus* and nasal carriage. Nippon Ganka Gakkai Zasshi 2007;111:504–8.

4 Seal DV, Ficker L, Wright P. The role of coagulase negative staphylococci in chronic blepharitis. Microb Ecol Health Dis 1992;5:69–75.

5 Sotozono C, Inagaki K, Fujita A *et al.* Methicillin-resistant *Staphylococcus aureus* and methicillin-resistant *Staphylococcus epidermidis* infections in the cornea. Cornea 2002;21(7 suppl):S94–S101.

6 Seal DV, McGill JT, Jacobs P *et al.* Microbial and immunological investigations of chronic non-ulcerative blepharitis and meibomianitis. Br J Ophthalmol 1985;69:604–611.

7 Tuft SJ, Ramakrishnan M, Seal DV *et al.* The role of *Staphylococcus aureus* in chronic allergic conjunctivitis. Ophthalmology 1992; 9:180–4.

8 Thygeson P. The etiology and treatment of blepharitis: a study in military personnel. *Arch Ophthalmol* 1946;36:445–477.

9 Thygeson P. Marginal corneal infiltrates and ulcers. *Arch Ophthalmol* 1948;39:432–5.

10 Hogan MJ, Diaz-Bonnet V, Okumoto M. Experimental staphylococcal keratitis. Invest Ophthalmol Vis Sci 1962;1:267–72.

11 Thygeson P. Treatment of staphylococci blepharoconjunctivitis with staphylococcus toxoid. Arch Ophthalmol 1941;26:430–434.

12 Panton PN, Valentine FCO. Staphylococcal infection and reinfection. Br J Exp Pathol 1929;10:257–262.

13 Johanovsky J. Role of hypersensitivity in experimental staphylococcal infection. Nature 1958;182:1454.

14 Boe J. Investigation on the importance of bacterial allergy for the development of cutaneous infections due to staphylococci. Acta Derm Venereol 1949;26:111–136.

15 Mudd S, Taubler J, Baker AG. Delayed-type hypersensitivity to *S. aureus* in human subjects. J Reticuloendothel Soc 1970;8: 493–8.

16 Mondino BJ, Kowalski RP. Phlyctenulae and catarrhal infiltrates: occurrence in rabbits immunized with staphylococcal cell walls. Arch Ophthalmol 1982;100:1968–71.

17 Mondino BJ, Caster AI, Dethlefs B. A rabbit model of staphylococcal blepharitis. Arch Ophthalmol 1987;105:409–12.

18 Mondino BJ, Adam S. Ocular immune response to *Staphylococcus epidermidis*. In: Cavanagh DH, ed. The Cornea. Transactions of the World Congress on the Cornea, vol III. Philadelphia: Lippincott-Raven, 1988:431.

19 Mondino BJ, Brawman-Mintzer O, Adamu SA. Corneal antibody levels to ribitol teichoic acid in rabbits immunized with staphylococcal antigens using various routes. Invest Ophthalmol Vis Sci 1987;28:1553–8.

20 White MI, Nobel WC. The cutaneous reaction to staphylococcal protein A in normal subjects and patients with atopic dermatitis or psoriasis. Br J Dermatol 1985;113:179–83.

21 McCulley JP, Dougherty JM, Deneau DG. Classification of chronic blepharitis. Ophthalmology 1982;89:1173–80.

22 Dougherty JM, McCulley JP, Silvany RE, Meyer DR. The role of tetracycline in chronic blepharitis: inhibition of lipase production in staphylococci. Invest Ophthalmol Vis Sci 1991;32: 2970–5.

23 Monteil M, Hobbs J, Citron K. Selective immunodeficiency affecting staphylococcal response. Lancet 1987;ii:880–3.

24 Foroozanfar N, Grohmann PH, Hobbs JR. Abnormal fluorescent actin pattern of lazy phagocyte syndromes. Diagn Immunol 1984;2:25–9.

25 Seal DV, Lightman S. Immunodeficiency, immunity and staphylococcal infection. Lancet 1987;ii:1522.

26 Donabedian H, Gallin J. The hyperimmunoglobulin E recurrent infection (Job's) syndrome. Medicine 1983;62:195–208.

27 Seal DV, Wright P, Ficker L *et al.* Placebo-controlled trial of fusidic acid gel and oxtetracycline for recurrent blepharitis and rosacea. Br J Ophthalmol 1995;79:42–5.

28 Brown S, Shahinian L. Diagnosis and treatment of ocular rosacea. Ophthalmology 1978;85:779–86.

29 Freidlin J, Acharya N, Lietman TM *et al*. Spectrum of eye disease caused by methicillin-resistant *Staphylococcus aureus*. Am J Ophthalmol 2007;144:313–15.
30 Marangon FB, Miller D, Muallem MS *et al*. Ciprofloxacin and levofloxacin resistance among methicillin-sensitive *Staphylococcus aureus* isolates from keratitis and conjunctivitis. Am J Ophthalmol 2004;137:453–8.
31 Chalita MR, Hofling-Lima Al, Paranhos A Jr *et al*. Shifting trends in vitro antibiotic susceptibilities for common ocular isolates during a period of 15 years. Am J Ophthalmol 2004;137:43–51.
32 Asbell PA, Sahm DF, Shaw M *et al*. Increasing prevalence of methicillin resistance in serious ocular infections caused by *Staphylococcus aureus* in the United States: 2000 to 2005. J Cataract Refract Surg 2008;34:814–18.
33 Dunlop AA, Wright ED, Howlander SA *et al*. Suppurative corneal ulceration in Bangladesh. A study of 142 cases examining the microbiological diagnosis, clinical and epidemiological features of bacterial and fungal keratitis. Aust NZ J Ophthalmol 1994;22:105–110.
34 Neumann M, Sjostrand J. Central microbial keratitis in a Swedish city population. A three year prospective study in Gothenburg. Acta Ophthalmol 1993;71:160–4.
35 Wahl JC, Katx HR, Abrams DA. Infectious keratitis in Baltimore. Ann Ophthalmol 1991;23:234–7.
36 Cruz OA, Sabir SM, Capo H, Alfonso EC. Microbial keratitis in childhood. Ophthalmology 1993;100:192–6.
37 Kerr N, Stern GA. Bacterial keratitis associated with vernal keratoconjunctivitis. Cornea 1992;11:355–9.
38 Aristimuno B, Nirankari VS, Hemady RK, Rodrigues MM. Spontaneous ulcerative keratitis in immunocompromised patients. Am J Ophthalmol 1993;115:202–8.
39 Rhem MN, Lech EM, Patti JM *et al*. The collagen-binding adhesin is a virulence factor in *Staphylococcus aureus* keratitis. Infect Immun 2000;68:3776–9.
40 Solomon R, Donnenfeld ED, Perry HD *et al*. Methicillin-resistant *Staphylococcus aureus* infectious keratitis following refractive surgery. Am J Ophthalmol 2007;143:629–34.
41 Benson WH, Lanier JD. Comparison of techniques for culturing corneal ulcers. Ophthalmology 1992;99:800–4.
42 Ficker L, Kirkness CM, Seal DV, McCartney ACE. Microbial keratitis: the false negative. Eye 1991;5:549–59.
43 Mader TH, Maher KL, Stulting RD. Gentamicin resistance in staphylococcal corneal ulcers. Cornea 1991;10:408–10.
44 Insler MS, Fish LA, Silbernagel J *et al*. Successful treatment of methicillin-resistant *Staphylococcus aureus* keratitis with topical ciprofloxacin. Ophthalmology 1991;98:1690–2.
45 Snyder ME, Katz HR. Ciprofloxacin-resistant bacterial keratitis. Am J Ophthalmol 1992;114:336–8.
46 Afshari NA, Ma JJ, Duncan SM *et al*. Trends in resistance to ciprofloxacin, cefazolin, and gentamicin in the treatment of bacterial keratitis. J Ocul Pharmacol Ther 2008;24:217–23.
47 Honig MA, Cohen EJ, Rapuano CJ, Laibson PR. Corneal ulcers and the use of topical fluoroquinolones. CLAO J 1999;25:200–3.
48 Eiferman RA, O'Neill KP, Morrison NA. Methicillin-resistant *Staphylococcus aureus* corneal ulcers. Ann Ophthalmol 1991;23: 414–5.
49 Parks DJ, Abrams DA, Sarfarazi FA, Katz HR. Comparison of topical ciprofloxacin to conventional antibiotic therapy in the treatment of ulcerative keratitis. Am J Ophthalmol 1993; 115:471–7.
50 Callegan MC, Hill JM, Insler MS *et al*. Methicillin-resistant *Staphylococcus aureus* keratitis in the rabbit: therapy with ciprofloxacin, vancomycin and cefazolin. Curr Eye Res 1992;11:1111–9.
51 Nayak N, Satpathy G. Slime production as a virulence factor in *Staphylococcus epidermidis* isolated from bacterial keratitis. Indian J Med Res 2000;111:6–10.
52 Kirkness CM, Ficker LA, Steele AD, Rice NS. The role of penetrating keratoplasty in the management of microbial keratitis. Eye 1991;5:425–31.
53 Menikoff JA, Speaker MG, Marmor M, Raskin EM. A case-control study of risk factors for post-operative endophthalmitis. Ophthalmology 1991;98:1761–8.
54 Pinna A, Sechi LA, Zanetti S *et al*. Adherence of ocular isolates of *Staphylococcus epidermidis* to ACRYSOF intraocular lenses. A scanning electron microscopy and molecular biology study. Ophthalmology 2000;107:2162–6.
55 Kienast A, Kammerer R, Weiss C *et al*. Influence of a new surface modification of intraocular lenses with fluoroalkylsilan on the adherence of endophthalmitis-causing bacteria in vitro. Graefes Arch Clin Exp Ophthalmol 2006;244:1171–7.
56 Alfaro DV, Roth D, Liggett PE. Post-traumatic endophthalmitis. Causative organisms, treatment and prevention. Retina 1994;14: 206–11.
57 Thompson JT, Parver LM, Enger CL *et al*. Infectious endophthalmitis after penetrating injuries with retained intraocular foreign bodies. Ophthalmology 1993;100:1468–74.
58 Seal DV, Kirkness CM. Criteria for intravitreal antibiotics during surgical removal of intraocular foreign bodies. Eye 1992; 6:465–8.
59 Okada AA, Johnson RP, Liles WC *et al*. Endogenous bacterial endophthalmitis. Report of a ten year retrospective study. Ophthalmology 1994;101:832–8.
60 Bausz M, Fodor E, Resch MD, Kristof K. Bacterial contamination in the anterior chamber after povidone-iodine application and the effect of the lens implantation device. J Cataract Refract Surg 2006;32:1691–5.
61 Ficker LA, Wilson LA, Meredith TA *et al*. Chronic bacterial endophthalmitis. Am J Ophthalmol 1987;103:745–8.
62 Endophthalmitis Vitrectomy Study Group. A randomized trial of immediate vitrectomy and of intravenous antibiotics for the treatment of post-operative bacterial endophthalmitis. Results of the Endophthalmitis Vitrectomy Study. Arch Ophthalmol 1995;113:1479–96.
63 Dacey MP, Valencia M, Lee MB *et al*. Echographic findings in infectious endophthalmitis. Arch Ophthalmol 1994;112:1325–33.
64 Versteegh MF, Hooymans JM, De Lavalette VQ, Van Rij G. Acute bacterial endophthalmitis after cataract extraction: results of treatment. Doc Ophthalmol 2000;100:7–15.
65 Giese MJ, Mondino BJ, Glasgow BJ *et al*. Complement system and host defense against staphylococcal endophthalmitis. Invest Ophthalmol Vis Sci 1994;35:1026–32.
66 Pleyer U, Mondino BJ, Adamu SA *et al*. Immune response to *Staphylococcus epidermidis*-induced endophthalmitis in a rabbit model. Invest Ophthalmol Vis Sci 1992;33:2650–63.
67 Maxwell DP, Brent BD, Orillac R *et al*. A natural history study of experimental *Staphylococcus epidermidis* endophthalmitis. Curr Eye Res 1993;100:715–12.
68 Ormerod LD, Ho DD, Becker LE *et al*. Endophthalmitis caused by the coagulase-negative staphylococci: disease spectrum and outcome. Ophthalmology 1993;100:715–23.

69 Mao LK, Flynn HW, Miller D, Pflugfelder SC. Endophthalmitis caused by *Staphylococcus aureus*. Am J Ophthalmol 1993;116: 584–9.

70 Speaker MG, Milch FA, Shah MK *et al*. Role of external bacterial flora in the pathogenesis of acute post-operative endophthalmitis. Ophthalmology 1991;98:639–49.

71 Apt L, Isenberg SJ, Yoshimori R *et al*. The effect of povidone-iodine solution applied at the conclusion of ophthalmic surgery. Am J Ophthalmol 1995;119:701–5.

72 Alfaro DV, Runyan T, Kirkman E *et al*. Intravenouse cefazolin in penetrating eye injuries. Treatment of experimental post-traumatic endophthalmitis. Retina 1993;13:331–4.

Chapter 22
Osteomyelitis and Other Bone and Joint Infections

Odette C. El Helou, Elie F. Berbari and Douglas R. Osmon
Mayo Clinic College of Medicine, Rochester, Minnesota, USA

Osteomyelitis

Osteomyelitis remains one of the most difficult infectious diseases to treat in modern medicine. The hallmark of osteomyelitis is progressive bone destruction, necrosis, and new bone formation. Osteomyelitis is typically due to contiguous spread of infection from adjacent soft tissue structures, hematogenous seeding of the bone, or direct microbial inoculation through trauma or surgery [1]. *Staphylococcus aureus* remains the most frequently encountered pathogen in osteomyelitis. Clinical manifestations are dependent on the bone involved but usually involve pain and swelling in the affected area. Plain film, computed tomography (CT), magnetic resonance imaging (MRI), radionuclide scan, use of biomarkers such as erythrocyte sedimentation rate (ESR) and C-reactive protein (CRP), blood culture, and culture and pathological examination of involved bone are the cornerstones of the diagnostic armamentarium for osteomyelitis. Surgical débridement combined with targeted antimicrobial therapy in the setting of a multidisciplinary approach is often required for successful treatment.

Epidemiology and pathophysiology

There are two major classifications of osteomyelitis. The Waldvogel classification describes three types of osteomyelitis based on the pathogenesis of the illness: (i) secondary to contiguous foci of infection over the involved bone(s); (ii) secondary to hematogenous spread to the bone from infection elsewhere in the body; and (iii) osteomyelitis in the presence of vascular insufficiency (typically in patients with diabetes mellitus or peripheral vascular disease) [2,3]. These types of osteomyelitis are further classified based on the duration of illness (acute versus chronic). Acute osteomyelitis evolves over several days or weeks [4]. Chronic osteomyelitis is characterized by the presence of dead bone (sequestrum) and fistulous tracts, evolving over months to years [4].

The second classification system has been described by Cierny and Mader. In this classification scheme, the treatment of osteomyelitis is influenced by four factors: the condition of the host, the functional impairment caused by the disease, the site of involvement, and the extent of bony necrosis [5]. This classification combines four anatomical types with three physiological classes to define various clinical stages (Table 22.1).

Staphylococcus aureus remains the most common organism causing osteomyelitis, being isolated in more than 50% of cases. The incidence of *S. aureus* osteomyelitis has also

Table 22.1 Staging system of adult osteomyelitis. (Modified from Mader JT, Shirtliff M, Calhoun JH. Staging and staging application osteomyelitis. *Clin Orthop Relat Res.* 2003 Sept;(414):7–24 reproduced with permission.)

Anatomical type of osteomyelitis
Type I: medullary
Type II: superficial
Type III: localized
Type IV: diffuse
Physiological class (host factors)
Class A
Normal host
Class B
B_L: local compromise[1]
B_S: systemic compromise[2]
B_{LS}: both systemic and local compromise
Class C
Treatment more disabling than disease
Clinical stage
Type + class

[1] Local factors affecting immune surveillance, metabolism, and local vascularity: chronic lymphedema, venous stasis, major vessel compromise, arteritis, extensive scarring, radiation fibrosis.
[2] Systemic factors affecting immune surveillance, metabolism, and local vascularity: malnutrition, renal/liver failure, alcohol abuse, immune deficiency, chronic hypoxia, malignancy, diabetes mellitus, extremes of age, steroid therapy, tobacco abuse.

Staphylococci in Human Disease, 2nd edition. Edited by Kent B. Crossley, Kimberly K. Jefferson, Gordon Archer, Vance G. Fowler, Jr.
 ISBN 978-14051-6332-3.

increased secondary to the emergence of community-acquired methicillin-resistant strains [6]. Coagulase-negative staphylococci (CoNS) also account for a significant number of cases, particularly in situations where there has been implantation of a foreign body such as a fracture fixation device. In this subgroup, *Staphylococcus lugdunensis* has emerged as a new pathogen causing osteomyelitis and prosthetic joint infections in both immunocompetent and immunocompromised hosts [7–9]. *Staphylococcus lugdunensis* is more virulent then other CoNS species and clinically can behave similar to *S. aureus*. Some populations have an increased propensity to develop osteomyelitis, such as patients with diabetes mellitus, those with sickle cell disease [10], hemodialysis patients [11], and injection drug users [12].

The virulence factors of *S. aureus* play an important role in the pathogenesis of osteomyelitis and have direct implications for the management of this infection. The virulence of this organism resides in its ability to elaborate several bacterial adhesins that facilitate binding to bone and extracellular matrix protein and its ability to produce a number of factors that promote evasion from host defenses as well as exotoxins that facilitate invasion and tissue penetration [4,13]. Several adhesion molecules have been described and are referred to as MSCRAMMs (microbial surface components recognizing adhesive matrix molecules). These specific adhesion molecules are needed to colonize a particular type of connective tissue and fibers such as elastin, collagen, fibronectin, fibrinogen and bone sialoprotein [4,13,14]. After adhesion to the bone matrix, *S. aureus* elaborates a number of exotoxins that degrade the extracellular matrix and permit bacterial invasion. Furthermore, animal models have shown the ability of this bacterium to be internalized by osteoblasts [13,15]. In these cells, *S. aureus* can survive in a metabolically altered state, which may explain the chronicity of these infections and the higher relapse rates if these infections are treated for short periods of time [4,16,17].

Another major characteristic of *S. aureus* is the ability to form biofilm. In biofilm, bacteria form self-sufficient and self-growing structured colonies that group into communities. These communities are embedded in a hydrated matrix in which bacteria communicate via intercellular signaling called quorum sensing [4,18]. The biofilm-embedded organisms are sealed from the external environment, which renders antimicrobial therapy problematic.

Clinical manifestations

Hematogenous osteomyelitis

Hematogenous osteomyelitis occurs primarily in children at a rate of 1 per 10 000 per year in children younger than 12 years old [19]. Hematogenous osteomyelitis is usually a monomicrobial infection caused by *S. aureus*. Other etiological agents include group A and B streptococci, *Streptococcus pneumoniae*, and *Salmonella* sp. [6,19]. Hematogenous osteomyelitis typically involves the metaphysis of long bones (tibia and femur) in children and adolescents because of the type of vascular supply in this area of the bone. Acute long-bone osteomyelitis can present as local pain, warmth, and tenderness [2]. Fever is a common feature. Erythema and cellulitis can also occur. Bacteremia is present in approximately 50% of cases of acute hematogenous osteomyelitis [3].

There has been an increase in both the severity and frequency of acute osteoarticular infections in children with the emergence of community-acquired methicillin-resistant *S. aureus* (MRSA). In one study [6], the incidence of osteoarticular infections increased from 2.6 to 6.0 per 1000 admissions between 2000 and 2004, with a higher proportion of cases due to MRSA (from 4 to 40%); 71% of patients with MRSA osteomyelitis had periosteal abscess [6].

Although hematogenous long-bone osteomyelitis is uncommon in adults, hematogenous vertebral osteomyelitis does occur. Vertebral osteomyelitis (also known as diskitis, spondylitis, or spondylodiskitis) typically involves the vertebral body and the intervertebral disk and less commonly the posterior elements of the spine. Infection is acquired through hematogenous spread via the arterial blood supply or the venous circulation through the Batson plexus. Another focus of infection (e.g., genitourinary or gastrointestinal) is identified in many cases. The thoracic and lumbar spine is involved in most of the cases. Fever is present in less than 50% of patients, although back and sciatic pain are frequent features [20]. Common risk factors include intravenous drug use, immunocompromise, advanced age, diabetes mellitus, and instrumentation of the spine. The two most common organisms involved in vertebral osteomyelitis are *S. aureus* and CoNS [21,22]. Epidural abscess can also occur with or without vertebral body infection, with a predilection for the cervical spine [21,23].

Hematogenous osteomyelitis can also involve other sites such as the pelvis. In one study performed in Switzerland, 19 (9%) of 220 children with acute hematogenous osteomyelitis had pelvic involvement. These children were significantly older (median age 9.0 years, range 0.04–15.6) than children with hematogenous osteomyelitis manifesting at other anatomical locations. Of the 19 patients, 11 reported minor trauma and all children presented with a limp or refused to walk [24].

Hematogenous osteomyelitis may also involve the sternal and clavicular bones, particularly in association with illicit injection drug use. Osteomyelitis in injection drug users typically has a nonspecific presentation with an insidious onset. Skeletal involvement in injection drug users includes the vertebral column, sternoclavicular joint, sternochondral joint, pubic symphysis, costochondral joint, and sacroiliac joint [25]. Infection of the bone in injection drug users can also result from contiguous spread from organisms present as colonizers of the skin or from the contaminated diluents used to dissolve the drug [12]. *Staphylococcus aureus* is the most frequent isolate in osteomyelitis secondary to injection drug use. Other organisms that are disproportionally isolated are *Pseudomonas* species and *Candida*. Hematogenous osteomyelitis can also occur in patients receiving chronic hemodialysis. Spinal osteomyelitis is the most frequent site in this patient population and *S. aureus* is the most frequent organism recovered [11].

Contiguous focus osteomyelitis

Contiguous focus osteomyelitis usually spreads from neighboring structures such as joints or soft tissue, or from direct inoculation of organisms through trauma or surgery [2]. Osteomyelitis may also occur at a fracture site through inoculation of bacteria at the time of injury or following closed or open fracture fixation in the early postoperative period [21]. Implantation of a fracture fixation device constitutes a risk factor for osteomyelitis, since the foreign body can serve as a substrate for biofilm formation [26]. Cases of implant-related osteomyelitis are often associated with high morbidity requiring prolonged hospitalization and medical therapy as well as recurrent surgical procedures. Risk factors for acquisition of infection following open fracture fixation correlates with the extent of soft tissue damage, the bacterial inoculum, and prior use of antimicrobials [27–34]. The rate of infection following closed fracture fixation is 1.5%, whereas the rate of infectious complications following open fracture fixation is 3–40% [26]. At least 60% of open fractures are contaminated with bacteria at the time of injury [26,35]. Osteomyelitis after an open fracture is usually polymicrobial and often presents as persistent nonunion of the fracture site or delayed wound healing. Systemic and local symptoms such as fever, chills, and erythema are rarely present.

Osteomyelitis in patients with diabetes mellitus or vascular insufficiency

Diabetes mellitus affects approximately 5% of the US population. Of patients with diabetes mellitus, 15% will have a foot problem during their lifetime and 2% per year will develop foot ulcers. Of these, 15% will develop osteomyelitis and 16% will require amputation [36,37]. Diabetic foot infections cause significant morbidity and mortality and are associated with a tremendous financial cost for both the patient and society. Most of the direct cost is related to the inpatient stay and topical treatment [1,38]. Several factors have been associated with increased risk of foot ulceration in patients with diabetes mellitus, including duration of disease for more than 10 years, prior history of a foot ulcer and amputation, limited joint mobility, poor glycemic control, peripheral vascular disease, and neuropathy [21].

Clinical symptoms with this type of osteomyelitis can be subtle, with minimal signs of local inflammation and seldom any systemic manifestations such as fever or chills. The presence of skin ulcerations and soft tissue infection for more than a week should raise concern for osteomyelitis [4]. Diabetic foot ulcers are usually located in the plantar area at sites of high mechanical loading because of repetitive trauma. Impaired arterial perfusion, along with sensory neuropathy, often contribute to the development of skin ulceration. Evaluation for vascular insufficiency with appropriate invasive and noninvasive vascular studies under the direction of a vascular medicine specialist or vascular surgeon should be pursued in these patients.

Chronic diabetic foot infections and osteomyelitis are usually polymicrobial [39]. *Staphylococcus aureus* remains the predominant organism in monomicrobial infections [40,41]. Other major etiological agents are β-hemolytic group B streptococci, enterococci, and facultative Gram-negative bacilli [39]. In one French retrospective study of 48 patients with diabetes mellitus and contiguous osteomyelitis, *S. aureus* (58%) and Gram-negative bacilli (29%) were the most frequent pathogens; 58% of the infections were monomicrobial and 31% of the microorganisms were multidrug resistant, including MRSA [41].

Severe chronic infections are often treated with parenteral broad-spectrum antimicrobials targeting aerobic Gram-positive organisms (including MRSA) and Gram-negative bacteria in addition to anaerobes [42]. Lipsky *et al.* [43] have provided helpful guidelines for the diagnosis, management, and treatment of diabetic foot infections. They offer a step-by-step approach to the management of diabetic foot infection and associated osteomyelitis, discussing the need for surgery, adequate wound care, careful follow-up, and appropriate preventive measures.

Diagnosis

Signs and symptoms

The clinical diagnosis of osteomyelitis is usually suspected based on symptomatology. Chronic osteomyelitis is characterized by the presence of a nonhealing ulcer overlying the involved bone with or without a draining sinus tract [2].

In pedal osteomyelitis, the "probe to bone" test is a simple test that consists of probing through the skin ulcer with a metal probe to try to palpate the bone. If bone is struck, the probe to bone test has been reported to have a positive predictive value of 89% and a negative predictive value of 56% for the diagnosis of osteomyelitis [44]. In a more recent cohort study [45], the probe to bone test had a positive predictive value of only 57%, but the negative predictive value was 98% for the diagnosis of osteomyelitis of the foot in diabetic patients. Patients with diabetes mellitus tend to have minimal signs of inflammation and the diagnosis can be difficult in the presence of Charcot osteoarthropathy.

An acute presentation is common in hematogenous osteomyelitis in children and adolescents. Local pain, warmth, and tenderness constitute the main clinical features in this setting. In adults, however, the clinical presentation of osteomyelitis is rather vague, with subacute to chronic symptoms. Acute osteomyelitis usually evolves over several days or weeks, whereas chronic osteomyelitis develops over months to years. The latter is often characterized by the presence of low-grade inflammation, dead bone, and fistulous tracts [4].

Laboratory studies

The white blood cell count is typically not helpful in the diagnosis of chronic osteomyelitis, with a reported sensitivity of 26% [46]. Both the CRP and ESR values are often elevated in osteomyelitis and are more helpful in the diagnosis of acute hematogenous osteomyelitis. However, ESR can be normal in early disease. In general, CRP is usually more reliable for follow-up of treatment response [4]. These markers of inflammation are nonspecific and are not used solely for diagnostic purposes [47]. Electrolytes such as calcium and phosphate and bone enzymes such as alkaline phosphatase are typically in the normal range [4]. Blood cultures are positive in 50% of cases of acute hematogenous osteomyelitis, but are rarely positive in chronic osteomyelitis [2].

Microbiology

Isolating the microbial pathogen(s) causing a patient's osteomyelitis is crucial for determining adequate antibiotic treatment and avoiding the toxicity and expense of broad-spectrum antimicrobial therapy. Bone cultures should ideally be obtained prior to initiating antimicrobial treatment except when concomitant acute soft tissue infection or sepsis prompt initiation of empirical therapy. Bone biopsy provides the best diagnostic tool for accurately identifying the causative microorganism(s). Tissue specimens that are obtained should be processed for aerobic and anaerobic cultures. Histopathological examination also adds important information since the presence of neutrophils in significant numbers is indicative of osteomyelitis [4]. Swab cultures obtained from draining wounds and sinus tracts are poorly predictive of the infecting organism, but can be useful for infection control purposes [43,48,49]. In the particular case of *S. aureus*, isolation of this microorganism from sinus tract or superficial cultures correlates highly with the recovery of *S. aureus* from surgical specimens [49]. In one prospective study including 21 diabetic patients, two methods for the bacteriological diagnosis of osteomyelitis related to diabetic foot ulcer were evaluated: needle puncture performed across normal skin surrounding the foot ulcer and superficial swabbing of the ulcer. The authors found that the mean number of microorganisms isolated by needle puncture was significantly lower compared with that obtained by superficial swabbing (1.09 vs. 2.04; $P < 0.02$). *Staphylococcus aureus* accounted for 70% of cases when a single bacterial species was obtained by needle puncture. Therefore deep tissue sampling should be emphasized when it can be done safely, particularly when surgical débridement is delayed or contraindicated [50].

Radiographic studies

Radiographic studies remain an important and efficient tool for evaluating patients with suspected osteomyelitis. Plain radiography is usually not sensitive but is inexpensive and readily available as a routine initial test. The sensitivity of plain radiography is 43–75% and the specificity 75–83%. Both depend on the age of the infection and bone involved [51]. Plain radiography can demonstrate lysis of medullary trabeculae, focal loss of cortex, and periosteal reaction with new bone formation [2]. These changes are usually present 10 days after the onset of infection [51]. A negative plain film does not exclude the diagnosis of osteomyelitis.

Three-phase bone scintigraphy is also used in many medical centers for the diagnosis of osteomyelitis. It uses technetium-99m-labeled diphosphonate attached to methylene diphosphonate, which is taken up by metabolically active osteoblasts. This test is widely available, inexpensive, and easily performed. However, three-phase bone scintigraphy lacks specificity in evaluating bone with underlying osseous abnormalities, resulting in greater numbers of false-positive results. The reported specificity and sensitivity in the literature are 46% and 91%, respectively [52]. Other radionuclide techniques that can be used alone or with three-phase bone scintigraphy include gallium scintigraphy and indium-labeled white blood cells (IWBC) [2,51]. Gallium scintigraphy results are often equivocal and require multiple imaging sessions over several days but may be more sensitive and specific than IWBC scanning when combined for the diagnosis of vertebral osteomyelitis. In the specific case of vertebral osteomyelitis, gallium scintigraphy is a helpful diagnostic test that provides information on the surrounding soft tissue [51,53,54]. Radionuclide imaging may be the best test in patients with spine implants or fracture fixation devices because of the degradation of other images caused by orthopedic implants.

Fluorodeoxyglucose positron emission tomography (FDG-PET), which depends on glucose transporters, is also gaining importance in the diagnosis of musculoskeletal infections especially in the spine [51]. One study reported an overall sensitivity and specificity of 100% and 92% for the diagnosis of chronic osteomyelitis [55].

Cross-sectional imaging modalities such as CT and MRI are more accurate than plain radiography in evaluating musculoskeletal infections. These modalities evaluate the bone structure and surrounding soft tissue. Abnormal signal intensity on MRI can be detected as early as 1–2 days after the onset of infection (Figure 22.1). This reflects early changes of inflammatory edema that are seen during the first stages of acute long-bone osteomyelitis. Intravenous gadolinium contrast is useful in assessing soft tissue

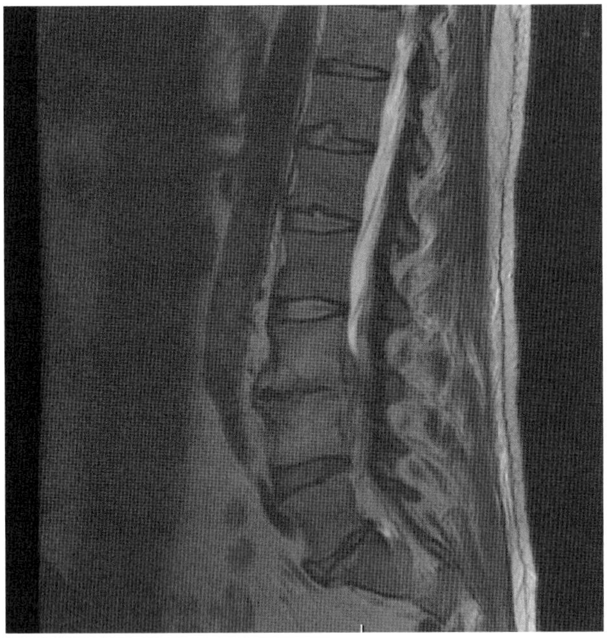

Figure 22.1 MRI of the lumbar spine with intravenous gadolinium. Marked narrowing in the third interspace with end-plate irregularity and enhancement in most of the third and fourth vertebral bodies. Partially enhancing paraspinal tissue and enhancing epidural tissue extending from second through fourth interspaces. Patient diagnosed with methicillin-resistant *S. aureus* disk space infection with associated phlegmon.

abscesses [51]. MRI has 100% negative predictive value for excluding osteomyelitis [51]. It is very useful in the diagnosis of vertebral osteomyelitis and diabetic foot infections [2,56]. Kapoor *et al.* [57] conducted a metaanalysis of 16 studies to determine the diagnostic test performance of MRI for osteomyelitis of the foot and ankle compared with the diagnostic test performance of ^{99m}Tc bone scanning, plain radiography, and white blood cell studies. These investigators found that the diagnostic odds ratio for MRI was consistently better than that for bone scanning (seven studies, 149.9 vs. 3.6), plain radiography (nine studies, 81.5 vs. 3.3), and white blood cell studies (three studies, 120.3 vs. 3.4). In vertebral osteomyelitis, MRI shows marrow edema, loss of vertebral end-plate definition, and fluid in the intervertebral disk [2]. In vertebral osteomyelitis, MRI is the imaging procedure of choice for the diagnosis of diskitis showing marrow edema early in the course of the infection [21]. Follow-up MRI, especially if performed early, is not necessary in every patient with the diagnosis of vertebral osteomyelitis receiving antimicrobials since the radiological images can be misleading and do not necessarily reflect the patient's clinical status [58]. CT is superior to MRI for the detection of sequestra and intraosseous gas. CT is more available than MRI in most medical centers in the USA. CT features of acute osteomyelitis include increased density of the normal fatty medullary canal as it is replaced by infectious edema, blurring fat planes, periosteal reaction, and loss of cortex [51].

Plain radiography is still useful in diabetic foot infections and comparison with previous plain radiography is crucial for determining any acute changes. This is important since significant proportion of patients with diabetes will develop a neuropathic joint characterized by destruction of the bone and joints. When this occurs it is difficult to differentiate from infection. A three-phase bone scan will be unreliable in diagnosing infection specifically in the setting of vascular compromise in diabetic patients. The best and most useful diagnostic tool in this case remains MRI [51]. In diabetic foot osteomyelitis, labeled leukocyte imaging can also be useful in monitoring the response to treatment [59]. In that case the leukocyte scan image intensity will decrease with antimicrobial treatment.

Treatment

The optimal treatment of patients with osteomyelitis often requires the expertise of a multidisciplinary team. A combined surgical and medical approach is the mainstem of treatment in most cases. Appropriate surgical treatment requires extensive débridement of necrotic tissue and soft tissue abscess, dead space management, and adequate soft tissue coverage.

Antimicrobial therapy alone does not arrest osteomyelitis except in the case of acute hematogenous osteomyelitis [4] and selected cases of cortical osteomyelitis. In general, the length of antimicrobial therapy is 4–6 weeks for both acute and chronic osteomyelitis. Two weeks of parenteral antimicrobial therapy for acute hematogenous osteomyelitis is generally sufficient if followed with oral antimicrobial therapy for the rest of the treatment course. Prior studies have shown that relapses rates are higher in patients treated for less than 4 weeks after surgical débridement [60]. Experimental models have shown that 4 weeks of therapy is more effective in sterilizing the bone than 2 weeks [3,61]. For these reasons most experts recommend 4–6 weeks of parenteral antimicrobial therapy for the majority of cases of osteomyelitis.

Oral therapy is also an appealing option for the treatment of osteomyelitis, especially when outpatient parenteral antimicrobial administration becomes an issue. A combination of an oral quinolone with oral rifampin has been evaluated, particularly in the area of staphylococcal orthopedic implant infections [62]. One study has also looked at combination therapy with co-trimoxazole and rifampin in the treatment of staphylococcal osteoarticular infection [63]. In the case of acute hematogenous osteomyelitis affecting children, a shorter course of parenteral antibiotic followed by oral antibiotics has demonstrated high cure rates. In one retrospective study of 39 patients, the median duration of combined therapy was 32 days (range 20–49 days). Parenteral therapy was given for

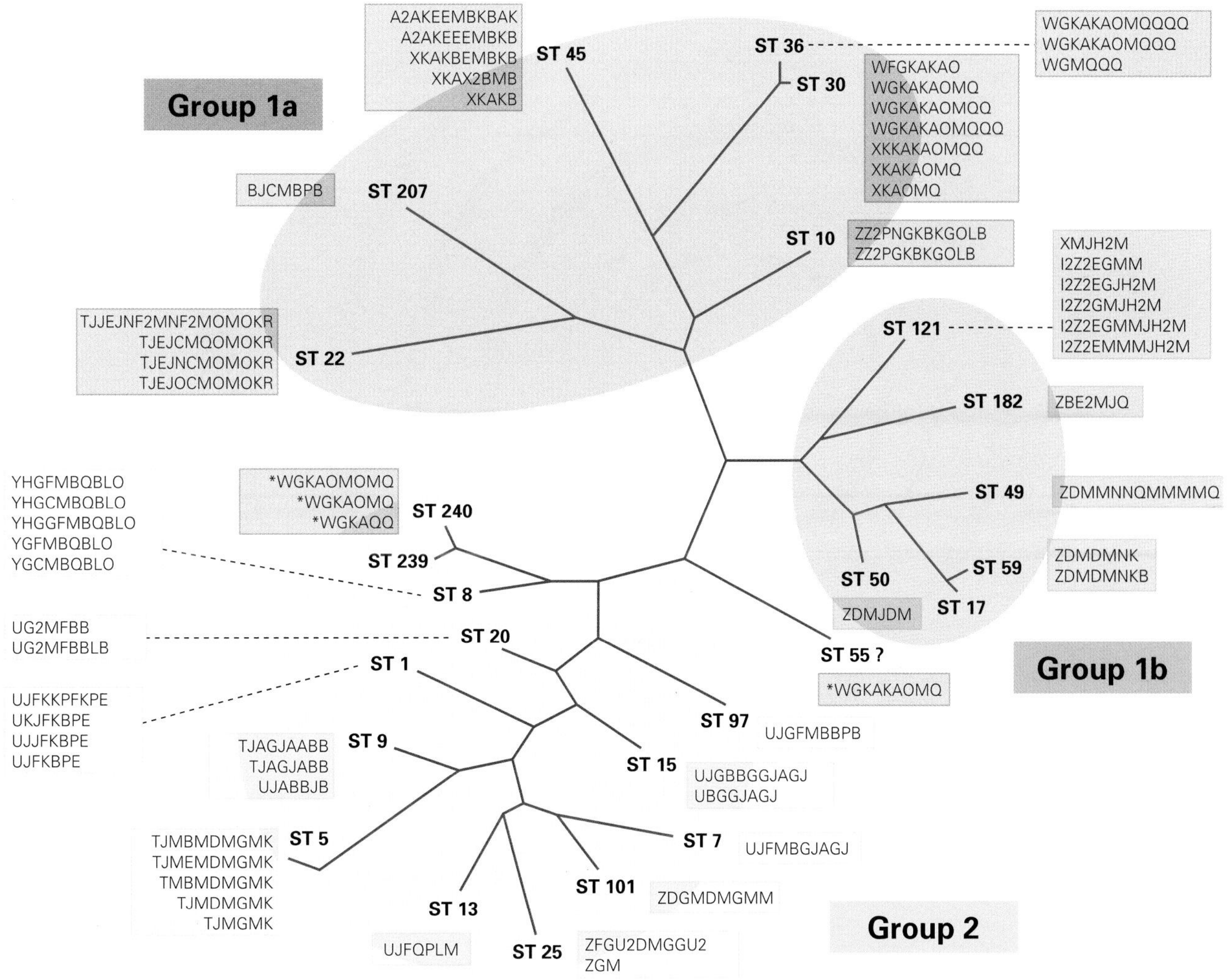

Plate 3.1 Phylogenetic structure (unrooted) of the species *Staphylococcus aureus*, based on Bayesian analysis of 37 genes from 30 representative strains. The three major clusters described by the authors are shaded in blue, green and yellow. *Spa* repeat patterns known to be associated with specific MLST sequence types are indicated in boxes, and shaded according to proposed group affiliation. Two examples of potential recombination are shown (ST239 and ST55) in which the *spa* repeat patterns closely resemble those found in ST30 and ST36. Note that removal of the ambiguously located ST55 may increase the apparent branch length between Groups 1a/1b and Group 2, consistent with previous analyses supporting two major divisions. (Adapted from Cooper JE, Feil EJ. The phylogeny of *Staphylococcus aureus*: which genes make the best intra-species markers? Microbiology 2006;152:1297–305, with permission.)

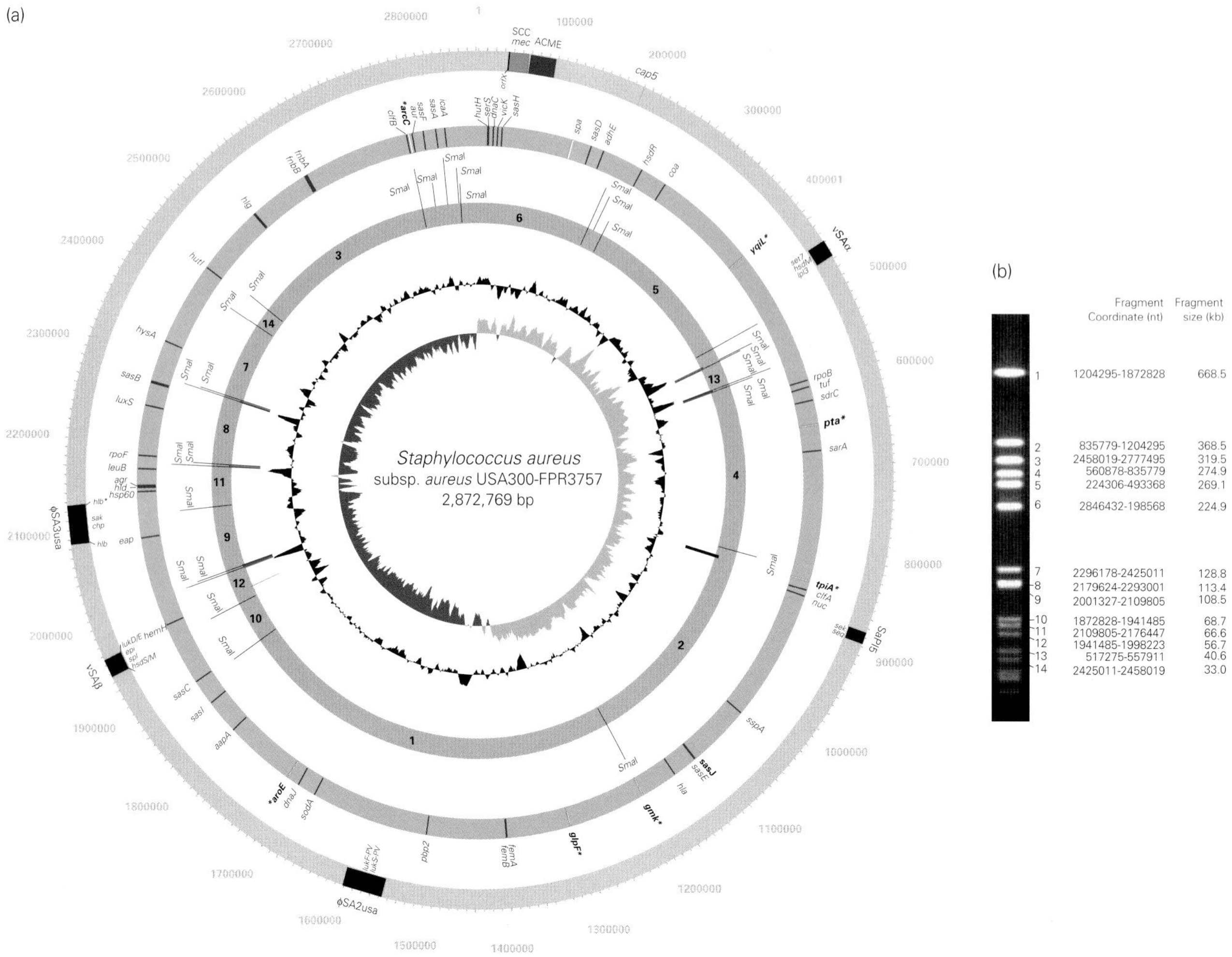

Plate 3.2 (A) Schematic circular diagram of the *Staphylococcus aureus* USA300-FPR3757 genome (141). Concentric circles, from outermost to innermost, are as follows: (a) nucleotide position in 100,000 base-pair intervals; position 1 denotes location of *oriC* (origin of replication); (b) gray circle showing locations of accessory genome elements in clockwise order: SCC*mec*, staphylococcal cassette chromosome *mec*, showing location of *orfX*; ACME, arginine catabolic mobile element; *cap5*, capsular polysaccharide biosynthesis protein operon; genomic island νSAα, containing genes for virulence factors *set7* (superantigen-like protein), *hsdM* (type I restriction-modification system M), and *lpl3* (staphylococcal tandem lipoprotein); SaPI5, *S. aureus* pathogenicity island 5, containing genes for staphylococcal enterotoxins K2 (*sek*) and Q2 (*seq*); prophage ϕSA2usa, containing genes for Panton-Valentine leukocidin (LukF-PV, LukS-PV); genomic island νSAβ, containing genes for *hsdS*/*hsdM* (type I restriction-modification enzymes S and M), *spl* (serine protease Spl operon), *epi* (lantibiotic epidermin operon, also known as bacteriocin *bsa*), and *lukD*/*lukE* (leukotoxins LukD and LukE); prophage ϕSA3usa, containing genes for *chp* (chemotaxis-inhibiting protein CHIPS) and *sak* (staphylokinase), and showing truncation of the *hlb* β-hemolysin gene; (c) light blue circle showing genes pertaining to the core genome (present in all *S. aureus* genomes sequenced thus far), with genes corresponding to the *S. aureus* MLST scheme shown in boldface and labeled with asterisks: *hutH*, histidine ammonia-lyase; *serS*, seryl-tRNA synthetase; *dnaC*, DNA helicase; *vicK*, sensory box histidine kinase; *sasH*, 5′-nucleotidase family protein; *spa*, immunoglobulin G binding protein A precursor; *sasD*, cell wall surface anchor family protein; *adhE*, alcohol dehydrogenase, iron-containing; *hsdR*, type I restriction-modification enzyme R; *coa*, staphylocoagulase; *yqiL*, acetyl-CoA acetyltransferase; *rpoB*, RNA polymerase B; *tuf*, elongation factor EF-Tu; *sdrC*, SdrC protein; *pta*, phosphate acetyltransferase; *sarA*, staphylococcal accessory regulator A; *tpiA*, triose phosphate isomerase; *clfA*, clumping factor A; *nuc*, thermonuclease; *sspA*, V8 protease; *sasJ*, iron transport associated domain protein IsdB; *sasE*, iron transport associated domain protein IsdA; *hla*, alpha-hemolysin precursor; *gmk*, guanylate kinase; *glpF*, glycerol uptake facilitator; *femA*, methicillin resistance protein FemA; *femB*, methicillin resistance protein FemB; *pbp2*, penicillin binding protein 2; *sodA*, superoxide dismutase; *dnaJ*, chaperone protein DnaJ; *aroE*, shikimate 5-dehydrogenase; *aapA*, D-serine/D-alanine/glycine transporter; *sasI*, cell wall surface anchor family protein HarA; *sasC*, cell wall surface anchor family protein; *hemH*, ferrochelatase; *eap*, extracellular adherence protein MAP; *hsp60*, groEL chaperonin; *hld*, delta-hemolysin precursor; *agr*, accessory gene regulator protein operon; *leuB*, 3-isopropylmalate dehydrogenase; *rpoF*, RNA polymerase sigma factor SigB; *luxS*, S-ribosylhomocysteinase/autoinducer 2; *sasB*, truncated protein FmtB; *hysA*, hyaluronidase A; *hutI*, imidazolonepropionase; *hlg*, gamma-hemolysin components HlgA/B/C; *fnbB*, fibronectin binding protein B; *fnbA*, fibronectin binding protein A; *clfB*, clumping factor B; *arcC*, carbamate kinase; *aur*, aureolysin; *sasF*, putative surface anchored protein; *sasA*, LPXTG-motif cell wall surface anchor family; and *icaA*, biofilm-associated polysaccharide intercellular adhesin; (d) light green circle showing *Sma*I restriction sites corresponding to the pulsed-field gel electrophoretic fingerprint of USA300-FPR3757; numbers inside the ring correspond to the 14 largest bands displayed in the gel image shown in part (B); (e) colored bars showing locations of various RNA elements: red bars show locations of ribosomal RNA operons, including the five 16S rRNA genes used in detection and phylogenetic analysis; light blue bars show locations of 55 tRNA genes; black bar shows location of 10Sa tmRNA; (f) dark gray peaks showing percentage of G+C content; and (g) G-C skew [(G − C)/(G + C)] (> 0% olive; < 0% purple). (B) *Sma*I macrorestriction digest of USA300-FPR3757; bands are numbered in decreasing size order, corresponding to numbered fragments in part (A); chromosomal coordinates and fragment sizes are indicated for each band.

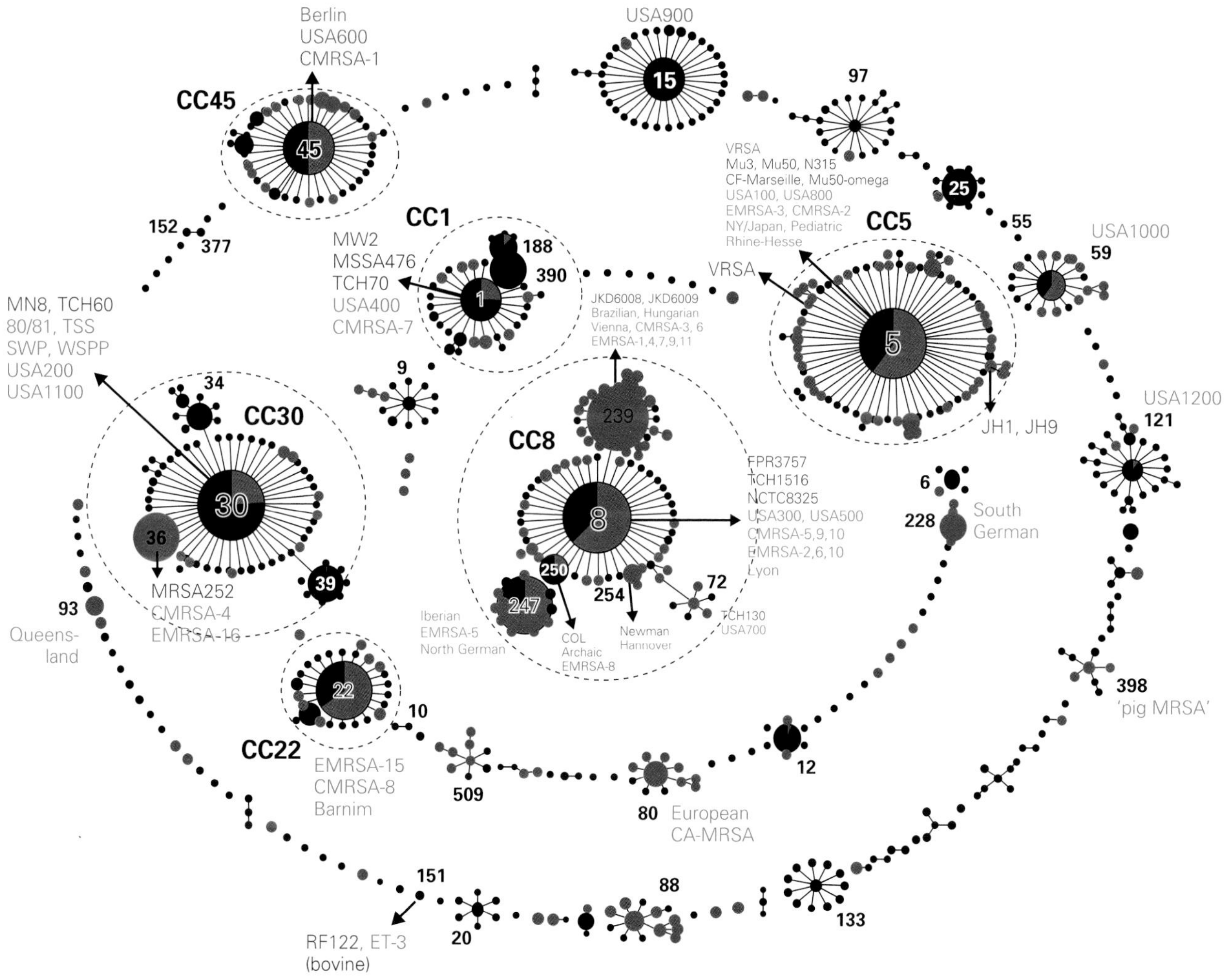

Plate 3.3 Modified "snapshot" of *Staphylococcus aureus* population structure, based on eBURST v3 (107) analysis of the entire MLST database, accessed at http://saureus.mlst.net in January 2008. Minimum number of identical loci for group definition was set to "0" in order to display all available sequence types in a single diagram, and default coloring was changed to black. Each circle represents a unique sequence type (ST); the size of the circle reflects the number of isolates in the database pertaining to that ST. Selected STs are labeled with their sequence type number, inscribed within the circle wherever possible. STs shown alongside clusters refer to the central "hub" or founder (e.g. ST 9, 12, 20, 59), and a handful of singletons are also labeled (ST 10, 55, 93, 151, 152, 377). Clonal complexes (CC) are depicted as clusters of single-locus variants (SLV) and double-locus variants (DLV) surrounding founders (e.g. ST 8, 15, 30, 398) and subgroup founders (e.g. ST 36, 188, 239, 247); major clonal complexes corresponding to pandemic lineages are encircled by dotted lines. Information from the MLST database was utilized to identify all STs in which methicillin-resistance has been reported (MRSA), and the corresponding circles were manually colored in red. All other lineages are assumed to contain only methicillin-susceptible strains (MSSA) and are shown in the default color (black). Principal founders and subgroup founders display the relative frequencies of MRSA in "pie-chart" format. Major extant and historical clones associated with particular STs and CCs are indicated in green letters; genomes are indicated in blue letters (see Table 3.2); known instances of *vanA*+ vancomycin-resistant *S. aureus* (VRSA) are indicated in red letters. Abbreviations: CMRSA, Canadian epidemic MRSA; EMRSA, epidemic MRSA; SWP, Southwest Pacific; TSS, toxic-shock syndrome; WSPP, Western Samoan phage pattern.

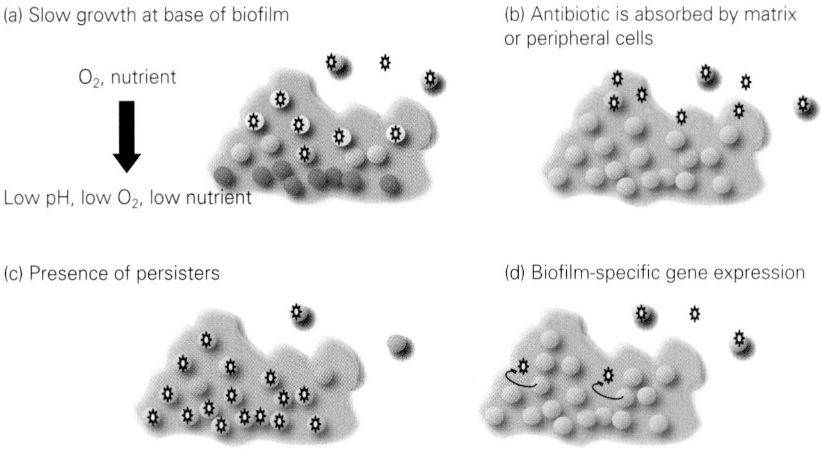

Plate 5.1 Antibiotic resistance in biofilms. The basis for antibiotic resistance is multifactorial: (a) limited levels of nutrients and oxygen result in slow growth deep within the biofilm and this reduces sensitivity to antibiotics that depend on rapid growth to exert their activity; (b) the exopolymeric matrix and peripheral bacteria absorb antibiotics and prevent penetration; (c) persister cells in both biofilm and planktonic populations survive in the presence of antibiotics; (d) biofilm-specific gene expression profiles (e.g., downregulation of permeases) protects bacteria from antibiotic damage.

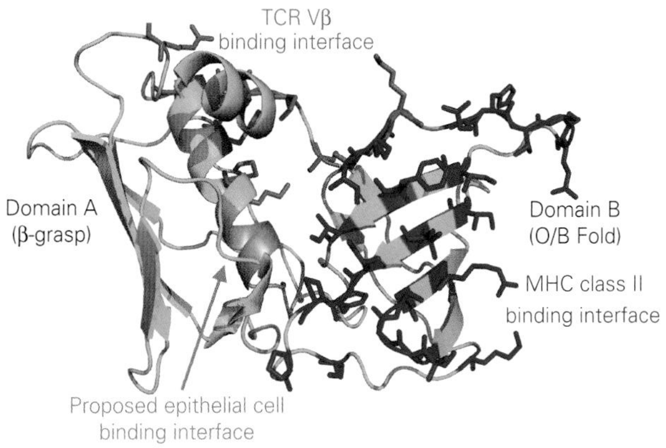

Plate 6.1 Cartoon of the three-dimensional structure of toxic shock syndrome toxin (TSST)-1.

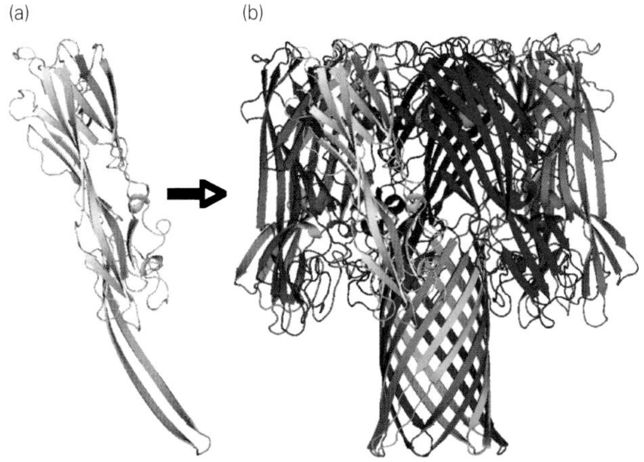

Plate 6.3 Monomeric and heptameric structures of α-toxin.

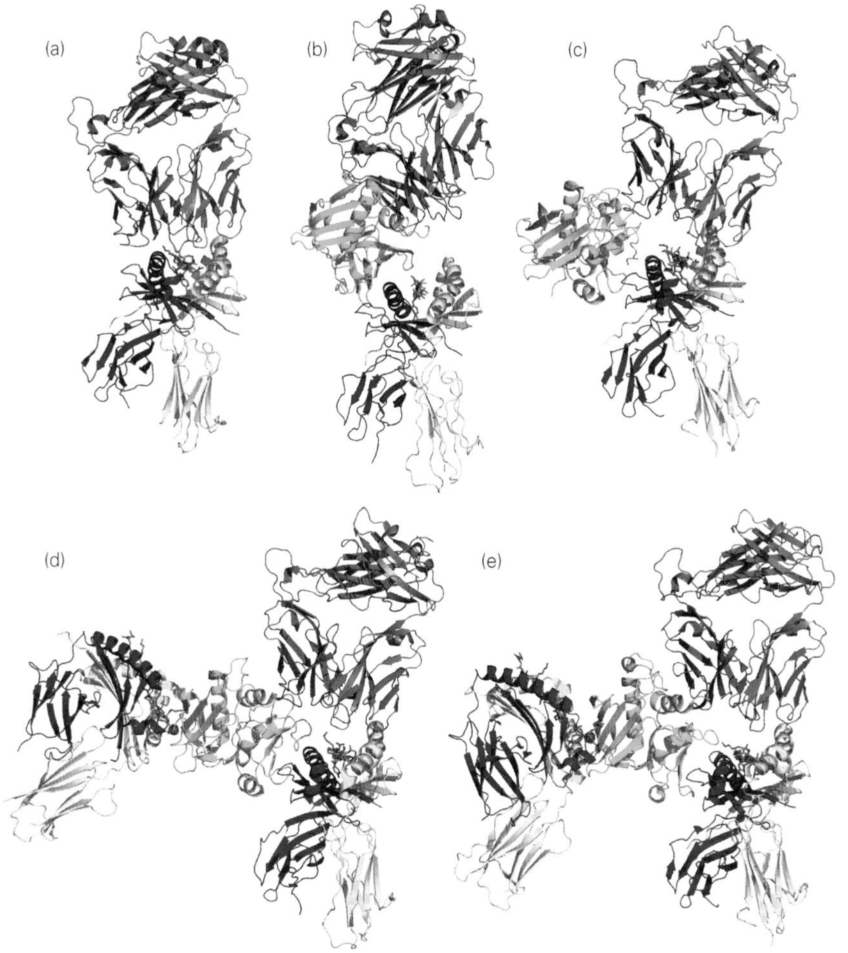

Plate 6.2 Cartoons of superantigen interaction with major histocompatibility complex (MHC) II molecules and variable region β-chain T-cell receptor (TCR). TCR–peptide–MHC is the typical antigenic peptide interaction with MHC II and TCR. (a) Typical peptide recognition by an α/β TCR where both the α- and β-chains of the TCR, in particular the CDR3 loops, recognize the antigenic peptide. (b) The modeled complex for the group I superantigen toxic shock syndrome toxin (TSST)-1 created by superposition of the HLA-DR1–TSST-1 and human Vβ2.1–TSST-1 complexes. Note the displacement of the TCR away from MHC class II such that there are no direct intermolecular contacts between these immune molecules, and how the engagement of MHC class II by TSST-1 encompasses the antigenic peptide. (c) The modeled complex for the group II superantigen SEC3 created by superposition of the HLA-DR1–SEC3 and mouse Vβ8.2–SEC3 complexes. Note how SEC3 forms a "wedge" where the TCR β-chain is displaced away from the MHC class II α-chain and prevents direct contact of the CDR loops with the antigenic peptide; that SEC3 does not contact the antigenic peptide; and how unconventional contacts occur between the TCR α-chain and the MHC class II β-chain that are required to stabilize the complex. (d) The modeled complex for the group III superantigen SEA created by superposition of the low-affinity HLA-DR1–SEA class II and high-affinity zinc-dependent HLA-DR1–SEH complexes. As there is no structural information on how group III superantigens engage the TCR, the SEC3–TCR complex was used to orientate the TCR. (e) The modeled complex for the group V superantigen SEK created by superposition of the human Vβ5.1–SEK and HLA-DR1–SEI complexes. As there is no structural information on how group V superantigens engage MHC class II through a low-affinity interaction, the HLA-DR1–SEA complex was used to orientate this interaction. A representative of the group IV superantigen subclass is not depicted as these are not produced by *S. aureus*, although the activation complex is generally similar to the group III and V models. Colors indicate the following: TCR α- and β-chains are shown in light blue and red, respectively; MHC class II α- and β-chains are shown in dark blue and yellow, respectively; antigenic peptides are shown as grey stick representations; superantigens are shown in green; zinc ion is shown in magenta. The figures were created using Pymol (www.pymol.org).

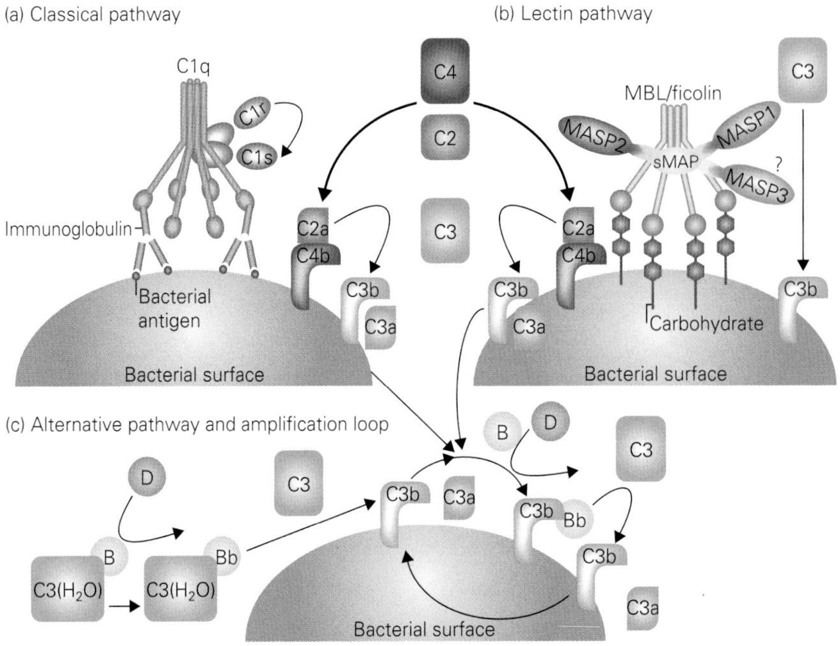

Plate 7.1 Pathways for complement activation. (a) The classical pathway is initiated by the binding of the C1 complex to antibodies bound to antigens on the surface of bacteria. The C1 complex consists of C1q and two molecules each of C1r and C1s. The binding of the recognition subcomponent C1q to the Fc portion of immunoglobulins results in autoactivation of the serine protease C1r. C1r then cleaves and activates C1s, which translates activation of the C1 complex into complement activation through the cleavage of C4 and C2 to form a C4bC2a enzyme complex. C4bC2a acts as a C3 convertase and cleaves C3, which results in products that bind to, and cause the destruction of, invading bacteria. (b) The lectin pathway is initiated by the binding of either mannose-binding lectin (MBL) or ficolin associated with MBL-associated serine protease (MASP)1, MASP2, MASP3, and small MBL-associated protein (sMAP) to an array of carbohydrate groups on the surface of a bacterial cell. Similar to C1s, MASP2 is responsible for the activation of C4 and C2, which leads to the generation of the same C3 convertase (C4bC2a). As in the classical pathway, C3 convertase cleaves C3 to C3b and the chemoattractant peptide C3a. The C3b–C2a–C4b complex then cleaves C5 to C5a and the chemoattractant peptide C5b, which stimulates assembly of factors C6, C7, C8, and C9 (not shown). MASP1 is able to cleave C3 directly. (c) The alternative pathway is initiated by the low-grade activation of C3 by hydrolyzed C3 (C3(H_2O)) and activated factor B (Bb). The activated C3b binds factor B, which is then cleaved into Bb by factor D to form the alternative pathway C3 convertase C3bBb. Once C3b is attached to the cell surface, the amplification loop consisting of the alternative-pathway components is activated, and the C3-convertase enzymes cleave many molecules of C3 to C3b, which bind covalently around the site of complement activation. (From Fujita T. Evolution of the lectin-complement pathway and its role in innate immunity. Nat Rev Immunol 2002;2:346–53, with permission.)

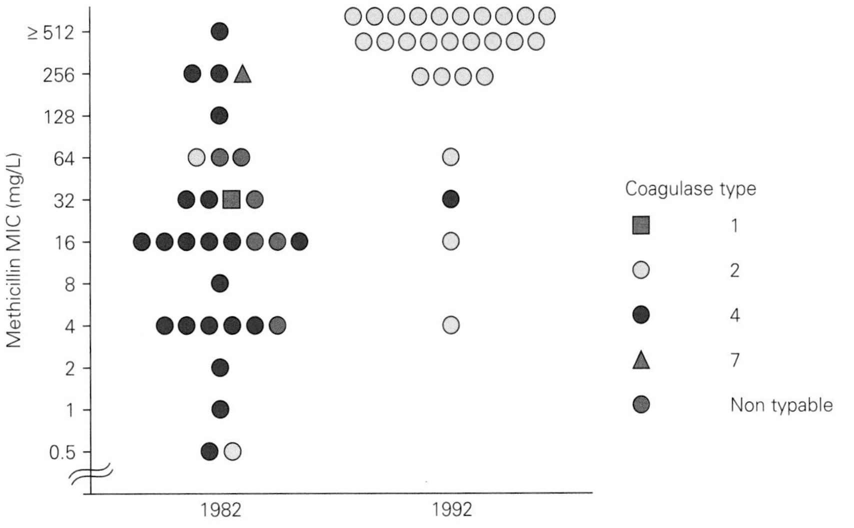

Plate 9.1 Heterotypic to homotypic conversion of methicillin resistance of clonotype II-A MRSA in Japan. The trend for using potent β-lactam antibiotics against MRSA infection drastically changed the epidemiology of MRSA after 1987. By the time of our survey in 1992, almost all the MRSA clonotypes of the 1980s had disappeared from the hospital and a single MRSA clone (clonotype II-A) prevailed; it accounted for 96.3% of all the tested MRSA isolates at the University of Tokyo Hospital in 1992. (From Tanaka T, Okuzumi K, Iwamoto A, Hiramatsu K. A retrospective study on methicillin-resistant *Staphylococcus aureus* clinical strains in Tokyo University Hospital. J Infect Chemother 1995;1:42–51, with permission.)

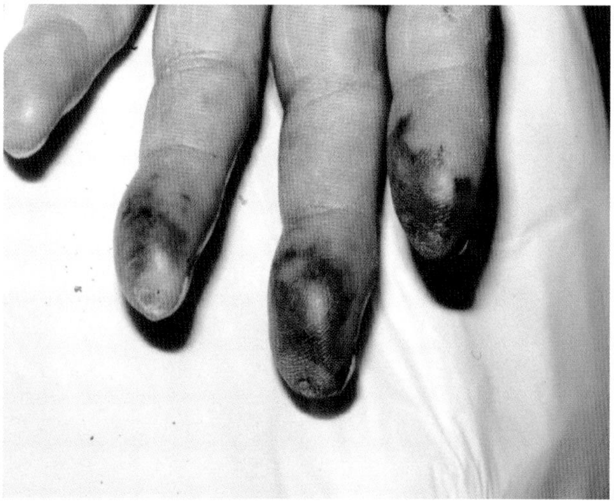

Plate 16.1 Cutaneous infarcts in a patient with *S. aureus* endocarditis.

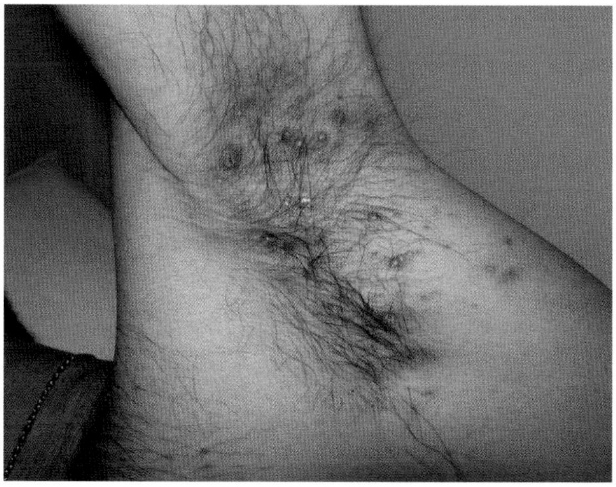

Plate 19.1 Axillary folliculitis due to *S. aureus*. (Courtesy of Dr Fabián Herrera, Division of Infectious Diseases, Centro de Educación Médica e Investigaciones Clínicas, CEMIC, Buenos Aires, Argentina.)

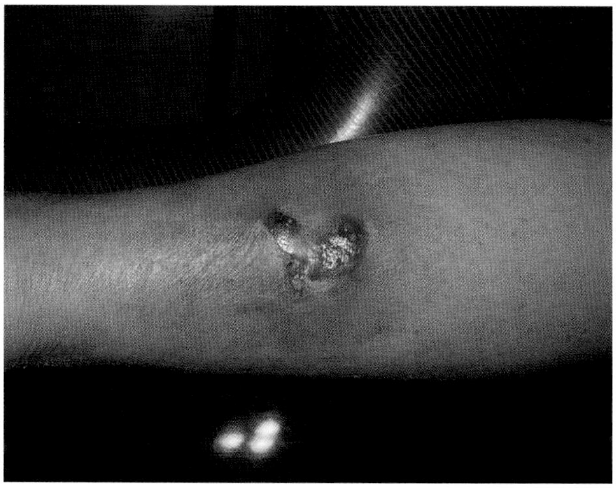

Plate 19.2 Carbuncle due to *S. aureus* in a renal transplant patient. (Courtesy of Dr Fabián Herrera, Division of Infectious Diseases, Centro de Educación Médica e Investigaciones Clínicas, CEMIC, Buenos Aires, Argentina.)

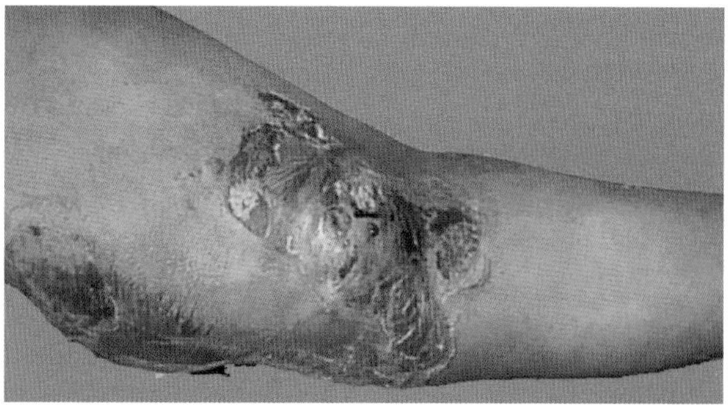

Plate 19.3 Abscess produced by *S. aureus* in a patient undergoing chronic hemodialysis through an arteriovenous fistula. (Courtesy of Dr Carlos Lovesio, Sanatorio Parque, Rosario, Argentina.)

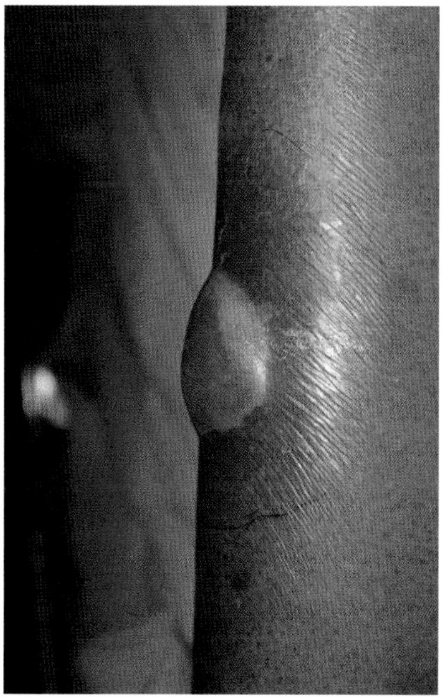

Plate 19.4 Abscess with surrounding cellulitis produced by *S. aureus*. (Courtesy of Dr Claude S. Burton, Division of Dermatology, Duke University Medical Center, Durham, NC, USA.)

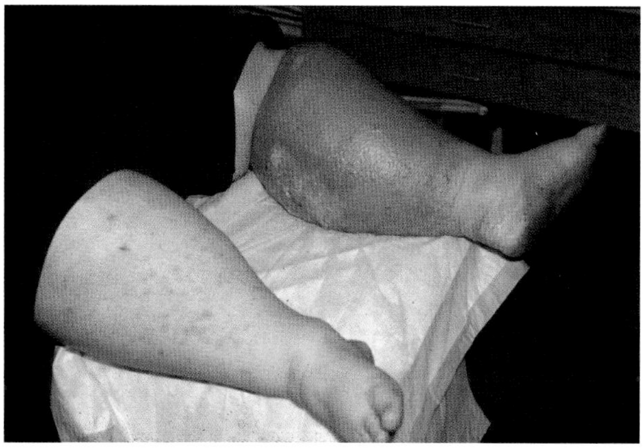

Plate 19.5 Cellulitis of the leg due to methicillin-susceptible *S. aureus* in a patient with morbid obesity. (Courtesy of Dr Claude S. Burton, Division of Dermatology, Duke University Medical Center, Durham, North Carolina, USA.)

(a) (b)

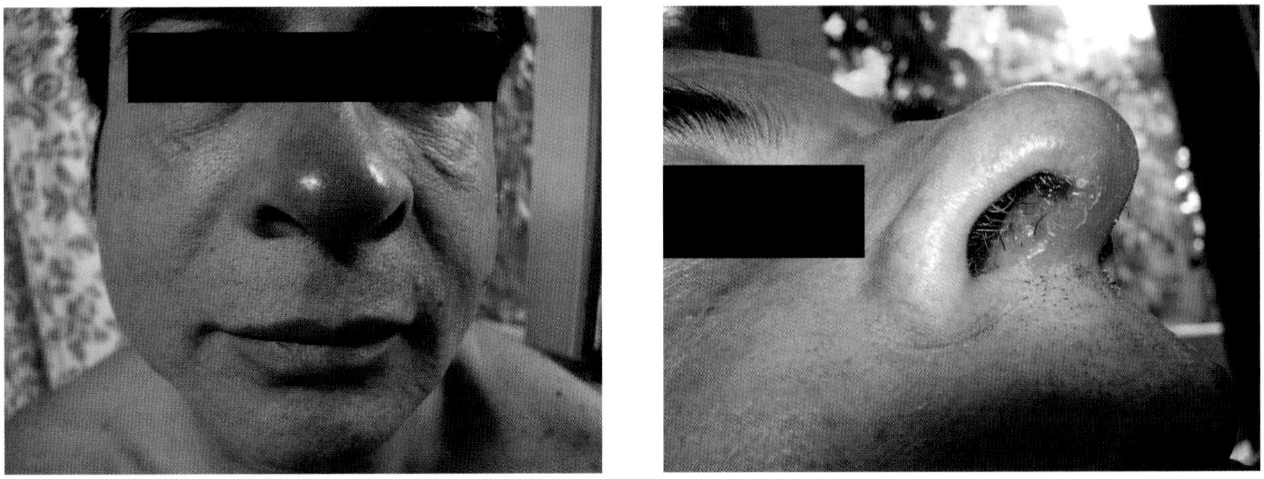

Plate 19.6 (a) Cellulitis of the nose due to methicillin-resistant *S. aureus*; (b) cellulitis of the nose, entry site. (Courtesy of Dr Fabián Herrera, Division of Infectious Diseases, Centro de Educación Médica e Investigaciones Clínicas, CEMIC, Buenos Aires, Argentina.)

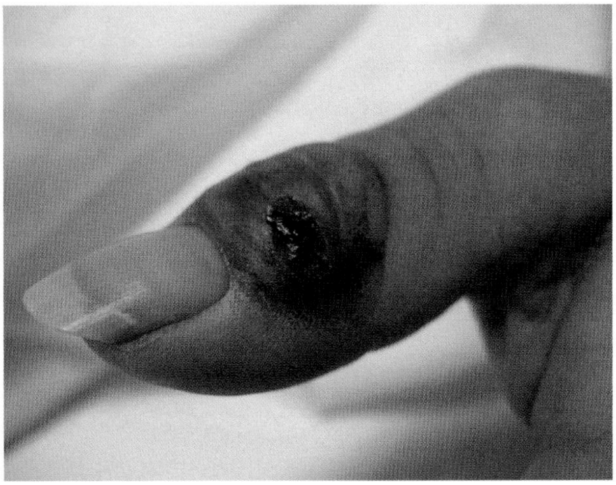

Plate 19.7 Cellulitis of the finger (finger felon) with necrosis produced by methicillin-susceptible *S. aureus* in a bone marrow transplant patient. (Courtesy of Dr Fabián Herrera, Division of Infectious Diseases, Centro de Educación Médica e Investigaciones Clínicas, CEMIC, Buenos Aires, Argentina.)

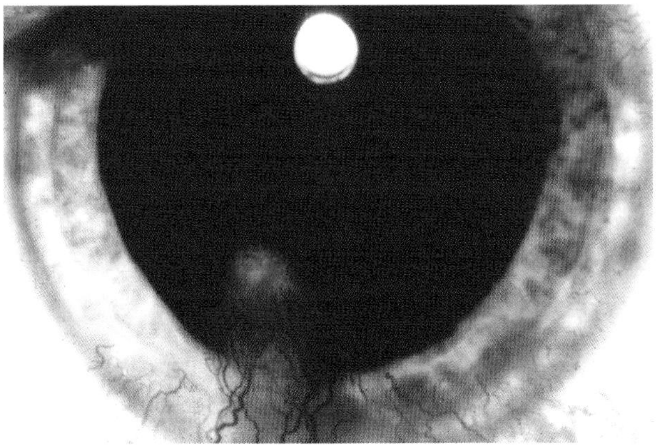

Plate 21.2 Marginal keratitis.

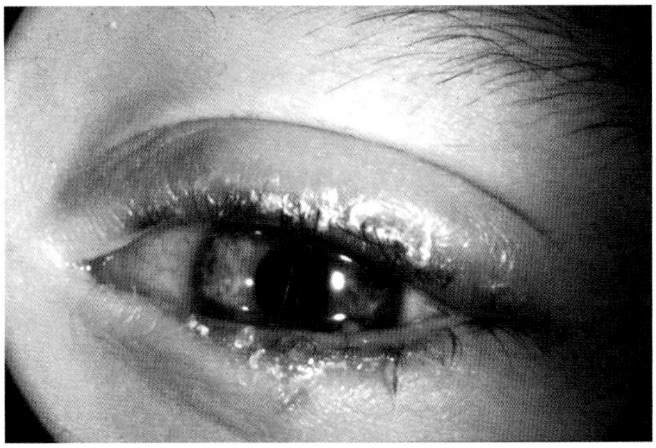

Plate 21.1 Ulcerative blepharitis.

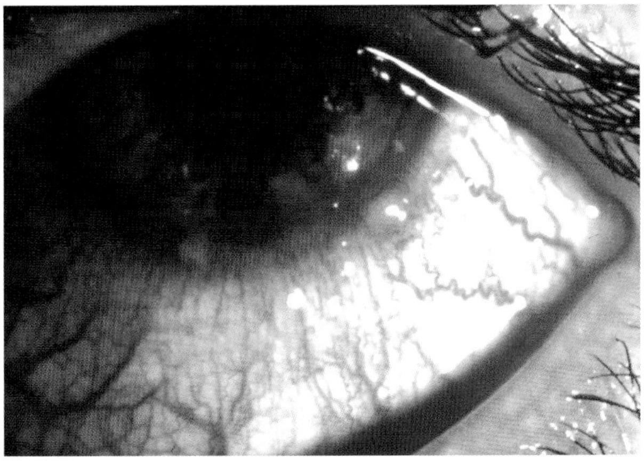

Plate 21.3 Phlyctenular keratitis.

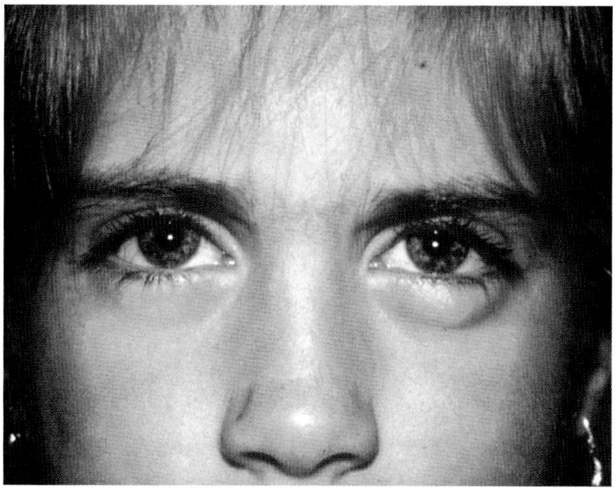

Plate 21.4 Child with lazy phagocyte syndrome showing left lower lid infection. The right cheek is scarred following chronic abscess.

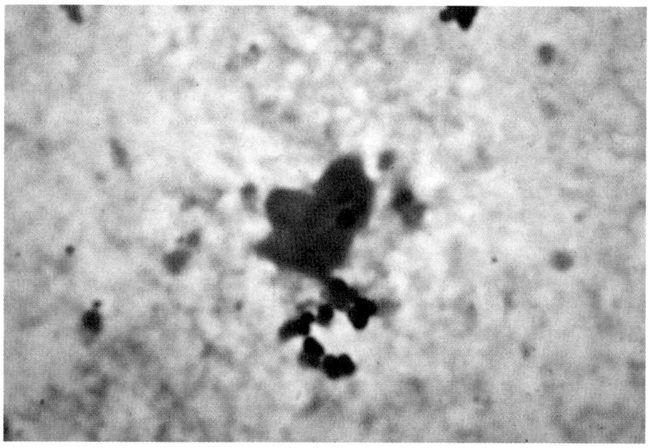

Plate 21.6 Scanty *Staphylococcus epidermidis* organisms typical of Gram stain preparation from vitreous specimen in endophthalmitis.

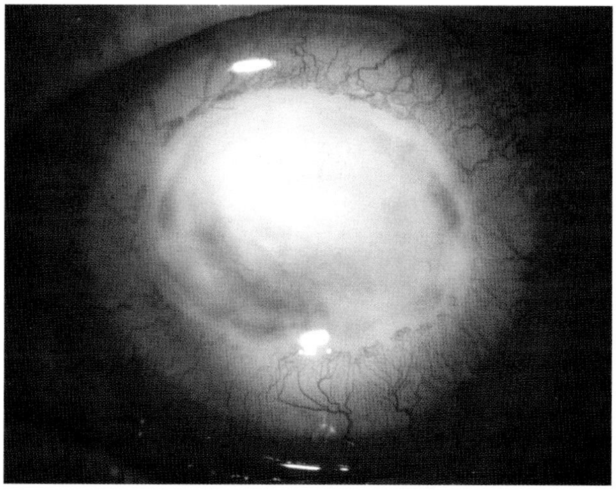

Plate 21.5 *Staphylococus aureus* keratitis in an atopic patient.

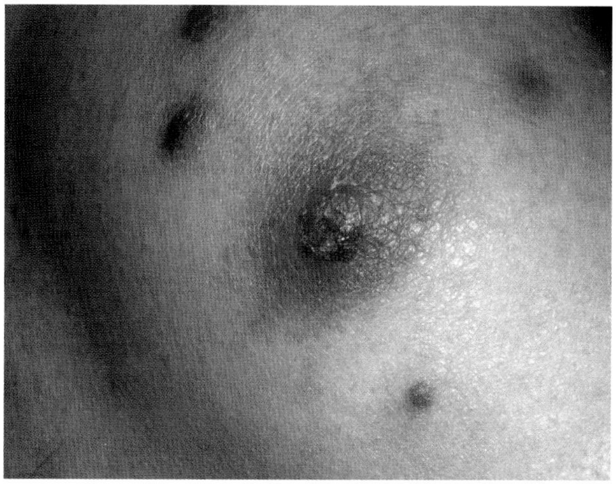

Plate 29.1 A healthy 50-year-old male with a community MRSA furuncle with central necrosis and surrounding erythema mimicking a spider bite. (Photo courtesy of Dr Kelly Cardoro, Department of Dermatology, University of California San Francisco.)

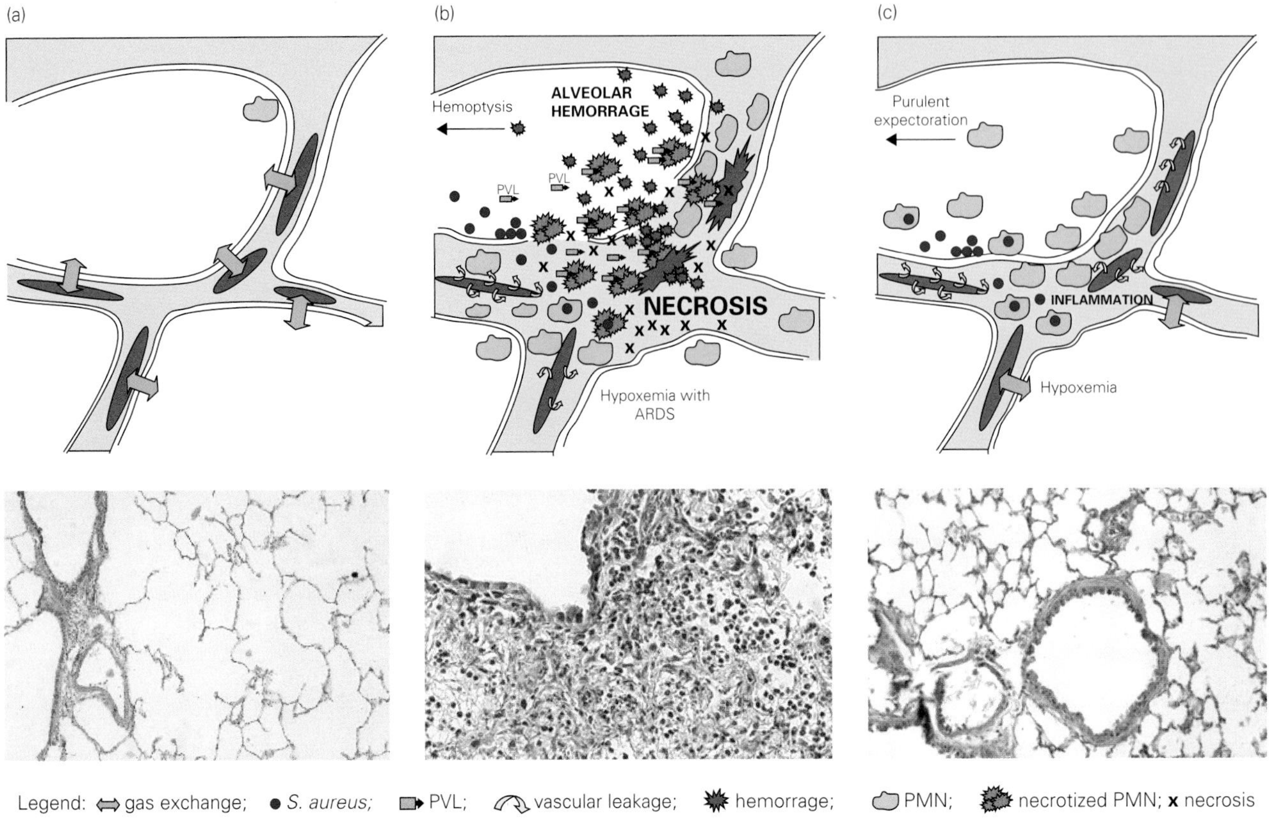

Plate 26.1 Schematic and histopathological views of lung parenchyma in health and in *Staphylococcus aureus* infection. (a) Normal lung parenchyma revealing thin and delicate alveolar septa, with only rare cells (alveolar macrophages) in the airspaces. (b) Mouse lung parenchyma infected by a Panton–Valentine leukocidin (PVL)-positive *S. aureus* isolate, revealing strong neutrophil recruitment, inflammation of the lung parenchyma, tissue necrosis, and alveolar hemorrhage. (c) Mouse lung parenchyma infected by an isogenic *S. aureus* isolate from which the PVL operon had been deleted, revealing normal lung structure with mild leukocyte infiltration and no necrosis or hemorrhage. ARDS, acute respiratory distress syndrome; PMN, polymorphonuclear leukocyte. (Histopathology in (a) courtesy of David Meyronnet, Histopathological Unit, Hospices Civils de Lyon, France; histopathology in (b) and (c) courtesy of Maria Labandeira-Rey and Gabriela Bowden, Center for Extracellular Matrix Biology, Institute of Biosciences and Technology, Houston, Texas, USA.)

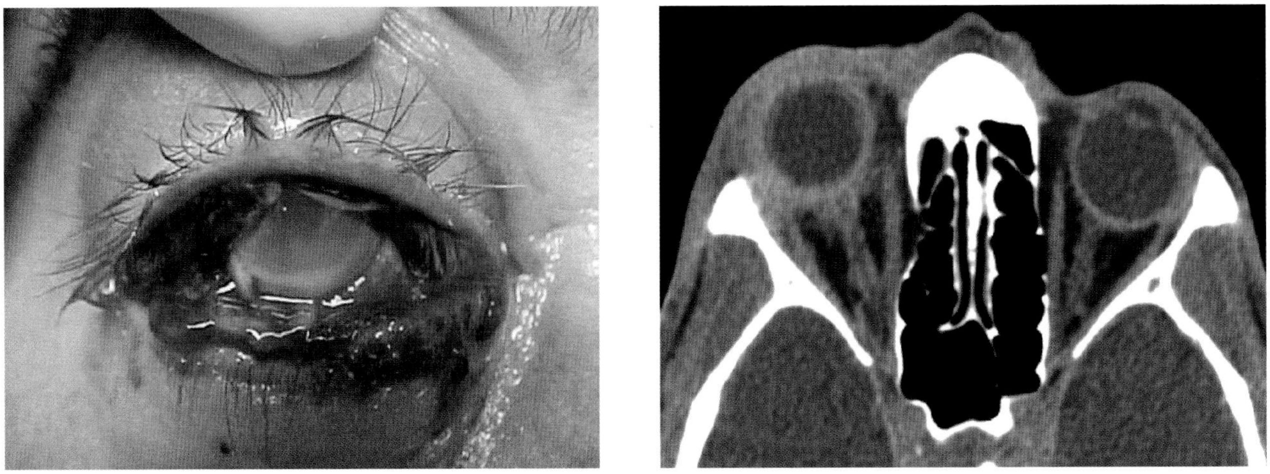

Plate 29.2 (*Left*) Hemorrhagic and chemotic conjunctiva, corneal edema, and a hypopyon. Panophthalmitis due to USA300 clone of MRSA in a 51-year-old injection drug user. (*Right*) Coronal orbital CT scan shows proptosis, periorbital soft tissue swelling, scleral thickening, and retrobulbar fat stranding. (From Rutar T, Chambers HF, Crawford JB *et al*. Ophthalmic manifestations of infections caused by the USA300 clone of community-associated methicillin-resistant *Staphylococcus aureus*. Ophthalmology 2006;113:1455–62, © Elsevier 2006.)

7 days or less. No failures or complications were noted over a median follow-up of 1.5 years [64].

Parenterally administered antimicrobials are most often recommended for staphylococcal osteomyelitis. Guidelines are available for the administration of parenteral antimicrobials in the community setting [65]. Penicillinase-resistant penicillins (such as nafcillin) and cefazolin are the treatment of choice for methicillin-sensitive *S. aureus* (MSSA) or CoNS osteomyelitis. An alternative choice is vancomycin if the patient is allergic to β-lactam antimicrobials. In our practice, we reserve the use of third-generation cephalosporins such as ceftriaxone for penicillin-sensitive staphylococci. Many experts advocate the use of ceftriaxone for MSSA infections [66,67]. The Surveillance Network databases in the USA and Europe assimilate daily antimicrobial susceptibility testing within the USA and certain European countries. This group reported a 99% *in vitro* susceptibility to ceftriaxone in the 2001 MSSA isolates [68]. Ceftriaxone's long half-life permits once-daily dosing, which is convenient in an outpatient setting [4]. Methicillin-resistant staphylococcal infections are most often treated with a glycopeptide. In the USA, vancomycin is the treatment of choice. Teicoplanin, another glycopeptide antibiotic, is widely used in Europe for MRSA and methicillin-resistant CoNS osteomyelitis.

Linezolid, an oxazolidinone, is a bacteriostatic antimicrobial with 100% bioavailability that is also available in a parenteral formulation. It is a good alternative for the treatment of osteomyelitis secondary to MRSA or vancomycin-resistant enterococci (VRE). Pharmacokinetic studies have shown that linezolid achieves concentrations in healthy bone specimens higher than the minimum inhibitory concentrations (MICs) for susceptible Gram-positive cocci [69,70]. The majority of patients usually receive linezolid when other antimicrobials or parenteral therapy are not an option. In one study, linezolid was used for the treatment of osteomyelitis or prosthetic joint infection secondary to either MRSA or VRE and all 11 patients followed prospectively had remission [71]. In a study of 25 cases of serious infection with MRSA with reduced vancomycin susceptibility, all six cases of osteomyelitis or septic arthritis were treated effectively with linezolid in conjunction with surgical debulking [72]. We do not advocate the routine use of linezolid in patients with oxacillin-sensitive staphylococci. In experimental models comparing the use of linezolid for MSSA with cefazolin and no treatment, cefazolin was more effective than linezolid. Treatment with linezolid was not significantly more effective than nontreatment [73]. Although linezolid is an expensive alternative, some studies have shown that the overall cost of linezolid versus vancomycin for outpatients is lower due to lower resource utilization, fewer physician office visits, lower laboratory and pharmacy claims, fewer emergency department visits, and fewer hospitalizations [74]. Side effects associated with long-term use of linezolid include peripheral neuropathy and cytopenias [75]. We limit the use of linezolid to patients intolerant of vancomycin or to osteomyelitis cases secondary to VRE.

Daptomycin, a cyclic lipopeptide antimicrobial agent, has also been recently evaluated as an alternative for treatment of osteomyelitis secondary to Gram-positive bacteria [76,77]. Daptomycin is a convenient bactericidal alternative since it is administered once daily at a dose of 4 mg/kg for the treatment of skin and soft tissue infections. At our institution we currently use a daily dose of 6 mg/kg for the treatment of bone and joint infections. Patients receiving daptomcyin should be monitored for rhabdomyolysis with weekly creatine phosphokinase measurements. Experimental studies in rabbits showed similar results to vancomycin in treating *S. aureus* osteomyelitis. Daptomycin is approved by the Food and Drug Administration (FDA) for the treatment of complicated skin and soft tissue infections or skin-structure infections as well as staphylococcal bacteremias and endocarditis. However, there have been reports of emerging mutational resistance to daptomycin [78,79]. Some of the risk factors implicated are high bacterial inoculum and prior use of vancomycin [79]. Resistance has also been described during treatment for osteomyelitis [80]. Studies evaluating the bone penetration of daptomycin are still lacking.

In the particular case of diabetic foot infection, antimicrobial therapy should target the usual polymicrobial flora. The prescriber should give special consideration to potential risk factors for MRSA or resistant enterococci. Most severe and moderate infections are treated with parenteral therapy whereas mild disease can be managed with oral antimicrobials. Lipsky *et al.* [43] have provided guidelines for the treatment and management of diabetic foot infections based on the severity of the infection. Treatment modalities for the diabetic foot depend on the severity of the infection, such as the extent of tissue involvement, systemic and metabolic signs of infection, and limb ischemia. Early surgical débridement, resection of necrotic soft tissue and bone, and revascularization should be performed when indicated in order to improve outcomes [43,81,82]. The choice between oral versus parenteral antimicrobials depends on the extent of prior surgical débridement and the quality of the remaining soft tissue and bone. Oral antimicrobials with activity against aerobic Gram-positive bacteria, such as first-generation cephalosporins or other narrow-spectrum β-lactam antibiotics (e.g., dicloxacillin), clindamycin or trimethoprim–sulfamethoxazole, are the treatment of choice in mild infections. Broader-spectrum oral antimicrobials with activity against both Gram-positive and Gram-negative bacteria, such as a semisynthetic penicillin with a β-lactamase inhibitor or a combination of tetracycline and a quinolone, should be used for the treatment of moderate infections. Linezolid has also been shown to be as effective as aminopenicillin/β-lactamase inhibitors for the treatment of diabetic foot infection

[83,84]. Long-term use is associated with side effects as mentioned earlier in this chapter. Severe infections require broad-spectrum parenteral antimicrobial therapy with carbapenems or an extended-spectrum semisynthetic penicillin and a β-lactamase inhibitor (e.g., piperacillin–tazobactam). Ertapenem, a carbapenem antibiotic structurally similar to meropenem, is a once-daily outpatient option equivalent to other parenteral antimicrobials such as piperacillin–tazobactam in diabetic foot infection [85].

In all situations, antimicrobial therapy should be modified based on culture results. When monomicrobial resistant Gram-positive infection is present, daptomycin and linezolid constitute alternatives to vancomycin [86]. The duration of therapy depends on the severity of disease and the condition of the underlying viable bone and soft tissue, and varies from 1–2 weeks in mild infections to more than 3 months in severe infections [43].

Outcome

The management of osteomyelitis remains a challenge, with an estimated relapse rate as high as 20–30% [21,43]. In diabetic foot infections, cure rates are high (80–90%) in mild to moderate infection, while 60–80% of severe infections are cured [43]. Patients with *S. aureus* vertebral osteomyelitis achieved an 83% cure rate in one study [87]. Half of those patients achieving cure still had infection-related sequelae such as persistent local or radicular pain, lower extremity weakness, voiding dysfunction, and lower extremity hyporeflexia. Failure rate in osteomyelitis will most likely increase with the increasing frequency of antimicrobial resistance.

Prosthetic joint infection

Infections associated with joint prostheses represent a challenge from both a therapeutic and diagnostic standpoint and result in significant health costs [88]. Infection of a prosthetic joint can also result in significant morbidity leading possibly to limb loss or death. Despite advances in diagnostic techniques, the accurate diagnosis of prosthetic joint infection remains a challenge. Issues related to differentiating chronic low-grade infection from aseptic prosthetic loosening remain problematic. The management of prosthetic joint infection involves a combined medical and surgical approach.

Epidemiology

An improved hospital environment and laminar airflow as well as perioperative antibiotic prophylaxis have resulted in a decreased rate of surgical wound infections in general and implant-related infections following joint arthroplasty in particular [89]. Prosthetic joint infection occurs at a frequency of 1–2% after joint replacement. The rate is usually higher following total knee arthroplasty (TKA) than after total hip arthroplasty (THA) (2.5% vs. 1.5%). The risk of infection increases after revision procedures, with rates of 3.2% and 5.6% for revision THA and TKA respectively [90,91]. The most common organisms causing prosthetic joint infection are CoNS and *S. aureus*, accounting for 30–43% and 12–23% respectively [92]. Less common are streptococci, enterococci, Gram-negative bacilli, anaerobes, polymicrobial and culture-negative infections [92].

Risk factors for the development of prosthetic joint infection have been established in numerous studies [93–97]. In a large case–control study conducted at our institution, the development of a surgical-site infection, a National Nosocomial Infections Surveillance (NNIS) risk index score of 1 or 2, the presence of malignancy, and a history of prior joint arthroplasty were independent risk factors for the development of prosthetic joint infection [98]. Other risk factors that have been identified in uncontrolled retrospective studies include diabetes mellitus, steroid use, obesity, extreme age, poor nutrition, psoriasis, hemophilia, sickle cell hemoglobinopathy, and prolonged preoperative hospitalization [99]. Patients with rheumatoid arthritis have a higher risk of prosthetic joint infections compared to patients with osteoarthritis [99,100]; *S. aureus* is the most common pathogen in this patient population [101].

The risk of prosthetic joint infection in the setting of bacteremia from a distant source is also increased if secondary to *S. aureus* [96,97]. Chu *et al.* [102] found a 42% rate of prosthetic joint infection in the setting of *S. aureus* bacteremia (29 of 71 patients). Another study found that the risk of hematogenous seeding of a joint prosthesis after *S. aureus* bacteremia was 34% (15 of 44 patients) [103].

Pathogenesis

The presence of foreign materials is known to increase the susceptibility to infection. Even a small number of microorganisms is able to colonize surgical implants [97]. CoNS and *S. aureus* are the most common organisms causing biofilm implant infections. In one study, 10^2 colony-forming-units of *S. aureus* were sufficient to infect 95% of subcutaneous implants despite the presence of polymorphonuclear leukocytes [104]. Biofilm is a thick multilayered material composed of an extracellular polysaccharide (polysaccharide intercellular adhesin) that protects the bacteria against phagocytosis and therefore decreases the host's ability to fight the organisms [26,105]. Staphylococci can also adapt rapidly to antibiotic use and, in most cases, *S. aureus* resistance can be acquired by phage transduction or conjugation such as the acquisition of resistance to methicillin and the β-lactam antimicrobials [26,106]. It has also been shown that in certain circumstances, such as the presence of foreign material, staphylococci can show decreased susceptibility to antimicrobials by the phenomenon termed "phenotypic tolerance" [26,106]. *Staphylococcus aureus* also possesses a number of adhesion mechanisms [107].

The cell wall of the bacterium contains specific acids (teichoic acid) that play a role in the formation of biofilm [108].

Some studies have shown that the persistence of an infection may result from the presence of small-colony variants of *S. aureus* [16,109,110]. Those subpopulations of *S. aureus* can be extremely resistant to a variety of antibiotics and can be the cause of chronic longstanding prosthetic joint infection [111]. They usually grow slowly on agar plates and have atypical biochemical and physiological features that makes their identification in the clinical laboratory difficult. Their survival in the host is due to decreased production of toxins and a defect in the electron transport system that permits intracellular location and resistance to host defenses [111].

Staphylococcus lugdunensis has also been increasingly recognized as a cause of joint prosthesis-related infections [9]. *Staphylococcus lugdunensis* is more virulent than other CoNS. It is comparable to *S. aureus* in its clinical presentation.

Clinical presentation

Prosthesis loosening associated with pain and decreased mobility may be the only manifestation of chronic infection. Pain at the implant site is present in more than 90% of cases [99]. Classification schemes for prosthetic joint infection are based on the timing of infection after prosthetic insertion and the presumed mechanism of infection [92]. Classification according to the mechanism of infection divides prosthetic joint infection into infections due to perioperative contamination, hematogenous seeding, or contiguous spread.

Classification categories based on the timing of infection include transmission by perioperative contamination. This at the time of surgery transmission by perioperative contamination occurs at the time of surgery or in the immediate postoperative period. An acute presentation with local signs of cellulitis, erythema, swelling, pain, and delayed wound healing as well as systemic symptoms such as fever and chills is often present in infections that occur within the first postoperative month [97,99]. Purulent drainage and sinus tracts may also be present at the surgical wound site. In the postoperative period, wound healing may not be complete and the implant may not be anatomically separated from the superficial tissues. Thus a superficial wound infection should raise suspicion of subsequent implant involvement [97]. The most common causative organisms in the early postoperative period are *S. aureus*, β-hemolytic streptococci, and aerobic Gram-negative bacteria.

Delayed infection occurs several months to 2 years after prosthesis implantation. It usually presents with subtle symptoms such as chronic pain and implant loosening. In this setting, it is difficult to differentiate from aseptic loosening. However, if there is no mechanical reason for aseptic loosening in the first few years following implantation, the presence of infection should be suspected. The typical microorganisms involved in delayed infection are often less virulent than the pathogens encountered in acute infection (e.g., CoNS and *Propionibacterium* spp.) [89,99]. Early and delayed infections are typically thought to have been acquired during prosthesis implantation.

Late infections (those that occur more than 2 years after prosthesis implantation) are thought to be due to hematogenous seeding but can also be a delayed manifestation of an infection that has been present since the insertion of the prosthesis. Hematogenous infection is often characterized by sudden onset of pain in the setting of concomitant or recent infection occurring elsewhere in the body (e.g., cellulitis, respiratory tract or urinary tract infections) [112]. As mentioned earlier, *S. aureus* bacteremia is a major risk factor for hematogenous seeding of prosthetic material [96]. The risk for hematogenous seeding is higher in knee prostheses [92].

Diagnosis

Clinical history

The accurate diagnosis of prosthetic joint infection is crucial, since management differs from other causes of prosthetic joint failure [113]. The diagnosis is evident when the patient presents with a wound infection or a sinus tract extending to the joint. The diagnosis is more challenging in the presence of a chronic infection presenting only with loosening of the prosthesis. Emphasis should be on gathering information on joint/prosthesis characteristics (e.g., type of prosthesis, date of implantation, past surgeries on the joint), clinical symptoms, drug allergies and intolerances, comorbid conditions, exposure history prior and current antimicrobial therapy including local antimicrobial therapy [113].

Laboratory diagnosis

The peripheral white cell count is not a reliable tool for diagnosing prosthetic joint infection, especially in the setting of low-grade or delayed infection. Nonspecific markers of inflammation such as CRP and ESR can be helpful in establishing the diagnosis and determining a baseline at the time of revision arthroplasty. These markers can be used to assess the response to treatment [114]. Thus, multiple values are more useful than a single value [89]. CRP is more sensitive and specific than ESR in prosthetic joint infection [99].

When considering a preoperative diagnosis of prosthetic joint infection, synovial fluid aspiration is usually performed. Synovial fluid should be submitted for cell count and differential, Gram stain and culture. One study examining synovial fluid analysis and the diagnosis of prosthetic joint infection found that a synovial fluid leukocyte differential of more than 65% neutrophils or a leukocyte count in excess of $1.7 \times 10^3/\mu L$ had 97% and 94% sensitivity, respectively, for detecting an infection in patients without underlying inflammatory joint disease and who were more than 6 months from prosthesis implantation

[115]. Superficial wound culture, sinus tract culture, or swab cultures often reflect the presence of microbial colonization and contamination from adjacent skin [89].

Histopathological examination of periprosthetic tissue also provides useful information and has a relatively high sensitivity (> 80%) and specificity (> 90%) [116]. The degree of inflammation varies among specimens and interpretation can be difficult in patients with underlying inflammatory joint disorders [92]. Culture of periprosthetic tissue provides the most accurate and reliable method for detecting the microorganism causing prosthetic joint infection. Three to six periprosthetic intraoperative samples should be obtained for the optimal diagnosis of prosthetic joint infection [117]. Withholding antimicrobial therapy for at least 2 weeks prior to collecting the specimens increases the yield of recovering an organism [92].

Postoperatively, the surface of the explanted prosthesis can also be cultured for microorganisms. Sonication has been used to dislodge bacteria from the surface of the prosthesis. Trampuz *et al.* [116] showed that sonication increased bacterial recovery. The sensitivity of periprosthetic sonicate-fluid cultures was higher than that of periprosthetic tissue culture for the diagnosis of prosthetic hip and knee infection (78.5% vs. 60.8%; $P < 0.001$) [118]. This new diagnostic technique has gained increasing interest and is now a routine clinical test at our institution. Tissue specimens should still be submitted for fungal and mycobacterial isolation as sonication has not been validated for these types of organisms. Rapid diagnostic tests, such as polymerase chain reaction (PCR), can also be done on sonicate fluid and tissue specimens. These tests are not currently part of the routine clinical microbiology laboratory armamentarium [92].

Imaging studies (Figures 22.2 and 22.3)

Plain radiography is helpful when followed serially after implantation. Plain radiography can show dislocation, lucency at the bone–cement interface, bony erosion, or new subperiosteal bone growth [119,120]. Loosening of the prosthesis does not necessarily indicate infection. The presence of new subperiosteal bone growth is often specific for infection [89]. Cross-sectional imaging modalities such as CT and MRI are not used for the diagnosis of prosthetic joint infection because the images are distorted. MRI can only be used when the implants are composed of titanium or tantalum [99].

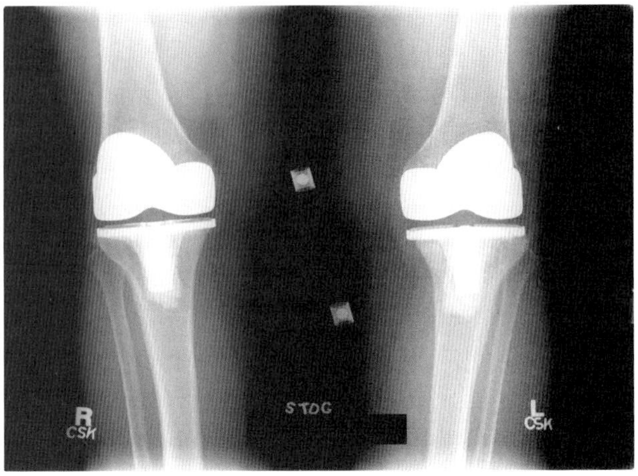

Figure 22.3 Left total knee arthroplasty. Anterior angulation of the tibial component with some lucency of the bone-cement interface of the tibial plateau and lucency of the bone component interface of the tibial stem. Patient diagnosed with methicillin-sensitive *Staphylococcus aureus* left knee arthroplasty infection.

Nuclear medicine tests can be used for the diagnosis of prosthetic joint infection. Combined labeled leukocyte imaging and marrow imaging is the procedure of choice since it has an overall accuracy of 88–98% [51]. Multiple types of tracers have been studied; those most commonly used are labeled with indium (^{111}In-oxyquinoline) or technetium (^{99m}Tc-hexamethylpropyleneamine oxime). A new type of tracer, ^{99m}Tc-UBI 29-41, which binds preferentially to bacteria, is under investigation in animal models of

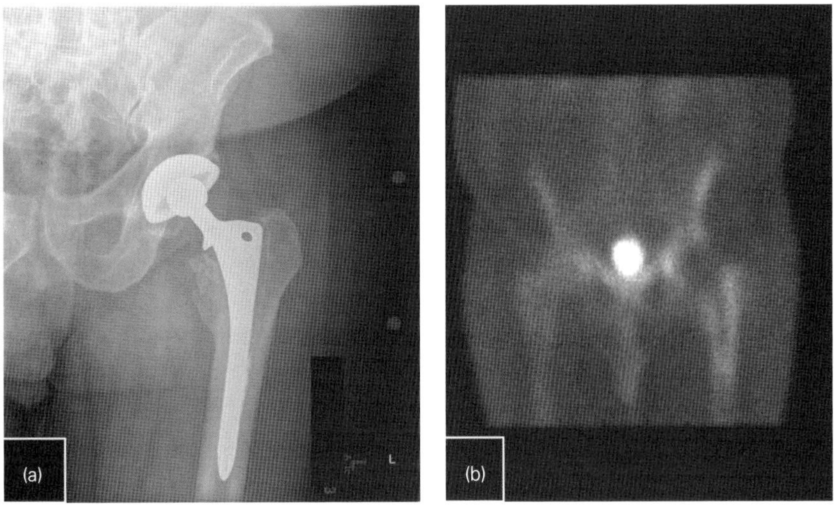

Figure 22.2 (a) Anteroposterior view of a left hip showing an uncemented total hip arthroplasty with a wide area of lucency about the femoral stem, worrisome for component loosening. (b) Combined labeled leukocyte imaging and marrow imaging in the same patient demonstrating discordant ^{111}In-labeled white blood cell activity around the proximal left femoral prosthesis, more marked anteriorly. Patient found to have a methicillin-resistant coagulase-negative staphylococcal hip arthroplasty infection.

Table 22.2 Classification scheme of orthopedic device infections. (Modified from Tsukayama *et al.* [127] with permission.)

Definition	Timing	Treatment
Positive intraoperative culture	Intraoperatively	Intravenous antibiotics ± chronic suppression
Early postoperative infection	First month	Débridement, salvage attempt
Acute hematogenous infection	Late acute onset	Débridement, salvage attempt
Late (chronic) infection	Chronic clinical course	Prosthesis removal ± staged exchange

S. aureus prosthetic joint infection and has an estimated sensitivity of 100% [121,122]. Leukocyte imaging is helpful in differentiating aseptic loosening from infection since neutrophils are usually present in the setting of a prosthetic infection but absent in aseptic loosening. FDG-PET, which depends on glucose uptake that is typically increased in infections, is not very helpful at differentiating infected prostheses from aseptic loosening. In one study the reported sensitivity and specificity of FDG-PET for the diagnosis of periprosthetic hip infections were 95% and 93%, respectively [123]. FDG-PET can provide false-positive results in knee prostheses and is more helpful in hip prostheses [124].

Treatment

The management of prosthetic joint infection involves both medical and surgical approaches. The team of physicians should include orthopedic and plastic surgeons as well as infectious disease specialists. The goal of treatment is to achieve adequate mobility and a painless joint as well as to cure the infection. Multiple factors need to be taken into account prior to defining treatment options, such as host factors (including the functional impairment related to the joint and the underlying medical condition and immune system status), the virulence of the infecting organism, the presence of biofilm, and the condition and viability of the surrounding soft tissue and bone.

In general, early postoperative or hematogenous infections are treated with prosthesis retention. Patients with chronic infections or a loose prosthesis often require removal of the infected prosthesis if the patient's overall medical condition permits [99]. As mentioned earlier, the most frequent organisms causing prosthetic joint infections are *S. aureus* and CoNS [92]. The formation of biofilm in staphylococcal infections renders most antimicrobials ineffective [26]. Bacteria within a biofilm are protected from phagocytosis and antibiotics unless antimicrobials active against microorganisms in biofilm can be utilized [125]. The increasing rate of methicillin-resistant strains from both the community and healthcare setting constitute an additional treatment challenge. In one recent study reviewing 137 patients with prosthetic joint infections between 1995 and 2004, 33% of the episodes were secondary to *S. aureus* and 9% of the isolates were methicillin resistant. In selected studies, the presence of methicillin-resistant strains was associated with a higher risk of treatment failure compared with methicillin-sensitive strains [hazard ratio 9.2, 95% confidence interval (CI) 2.40–35.46] [126].

There are no prospective, randomized, controlled clinical trials comparing the different surgical modalities and evaluating the appropriate length of medical therapy. Decisions about treatment regimens are based on combined data from many case series and a few recent randomized trials comparing different medical therapies, on the experience of physicians caring for the patient, and on the individual circumstances of each case. A classification scheme based on when the infection occurs following joint implantation has been previously described and is shown in Table 22.2 [127,128].

Medical therapy

Antimicrobial therapy should be guided by adequate periprosthetic tissue or sonicate culture results. Antimicrobials should be withheld when possible until specimens are obtained. Empirical treatment should target *S. aureus* and CoNS, the most frequent organisms encountered. Risk factors for the possibility of healthcare- or community-acquired MRSA should also be assessed. Risk factors for MRSA include recent hospitalization, outpatient visit, nursing home admission, antibiotic exposure, chronic illness, injection drug use, and close contact with a person with risk factors [129]. Other populations at risk are soldiers, prisoners, homeless persons, intravenous drug users, men who have sex with men, certain ethnic groups such as Pacific Islanders, Native Americans/Alaska Natives, Pacific and Canadian aboriginal people, and competitive athletes, specifically those who participate in contact sports such as rugby, football, and wrestling [130–133].

Once periprosthetic specimens are collected, empirical therapy can be initiated. A first-generation cephalosporin or vancomycin should be used as initial treatment in the majority of cases. The antibiotic therapy is then modified according to culture results and *in vitro* susceptibility testing. The length of parenteral antimicrobial therapy depends on the surgical treatment and the organism. Vancomycin is preferred if there is a history of immediate hypersensitivity reaction to a penicillin or cephalosporin or there are risk factors for MRSA; vancomycin is the drug of choice for MRSA. Teicoplanin is another glycopeptide antibiotic, mainly used in Europe, with similar activity to vancomycin. If the patient is hypersensitive to, or intolerant of, vancomycin or if the organism is not highly susceptible, other options need to be considered.

Linezolid is an attractive alternative because of its high bioavailability and activity against Gram-positive organisms. In one review, 11 patients with osteomyelitis and prosthetic joint infection were followed. Linezolid was given for a mean of 10 weeks and all patients had clinical and radiological cure. Most of the pathogens isolated were MRSA [134]. In another report, 20 patients with orthopedic infections including eight prosthetic joint infections were reviewed. Most of the patients had a resection arthroplasty followed by linezolid therapy for a median of 32 days; 55% achieved clinical cure at a mean follow-up of 276 days [135]. Long-term use of linezolid is associated with reversible myelosuppression, reversible optic neuropathy, and irreversible peripheral neuropathy [134].

Daptomycin is a cyclic glycopeptide recently approved by the FDA for the treatment of soft tissue and skin infections secondary to Gram-positive bacteria including MRSA. Daptomycin is a bactericidal agent active against organisms in biofilm [136,137]. A systematic review of the safety and effectiveness of daptomycin in the treatment of bone and joint infections found that eradication of infection was achieved in 43 of 53 cases (81.1%) [138].

Combination therapy with highly bioavailable orally administered antimicrobials has been described for orthopedic implants infected with staphylococci [63,139–143]. Rifampin in combination with other antimicrobials has been extensively studied in both experimental models and clinical studies. Rifampin is a bactericidal agent that has excellent activity against staphylococci, and is active against biofilm-producing organisms [89,144]. However, rifampin should not be used alone because of the potential for rapid emergence of resistance [139]. Combination therapy has used rifampin with a quinolone (ciprofloxacin, levofloxacin), fusidic acid, β-lactam antibiotics, or trimethoprim–sulfamethoxazole [139,142,143]. Quinolones are usually used in combination therapy, since monotherapy is associated with a low eradication rate and the potential for emergence of resistance [92,145]. In one study that examined the outcome of staphylococcal prosthetic joint infection treated with débridement and long-term levofloxacin and rifampin, 60 patients (age 74.6 ± 8.4 years) with staphylococcal prosthetic joint infections were reviewed. Success of this conservative management was higher in patients with shorter duration of symptoms, hip infections, and methicillin susceptibility [146]. Similar results were seen in one study comparing rifampin combined with fusidic acid or ofloxacin for the treatment of implant infections due to staphylococci [140]. Combination therapy is mainly used in situations where the infected prosthesis is retained after initial débridement [139,140,143,145]. Newer rifamycin derivatives are also being investigated in combination therapy for the treatment of implant-associated infections caused by *S. aureus* in experimental models. The newer rifamycins are associated with fewer drug–drug interactions [146].

Long-term, oral, suppressive antimicrobial therapy is typically used when the prosthetic joint is retained after débridement. [147]. Although utilized frequently, there are no prospective data supporting its use and the available retrospective information is limited [148–152]. In one review, 2 of 20 patients with staphylococcal prosthetic joint infections treated with surgical débridement and prosthesis retention followed by a combination of rifampicin and fusidic acid had treatment failure. The cumulative risk of treatment failure after 1 year was 11.76% (95% CI 3.08–39.40). Of 11 patients with infections involving MRSA, 10 had successful outcomes [143]. In our institution, we analyzed the outcome of 99 episodes of prosthetic joint infection treated with débridement and component retention followed by chronic suppression with a rifampin-free regimen. Chronic suppression was used in 89% of the cases; 55% were secondary to *S. aureus* and CoNS. The 2-year survival rate free of treatment failure was 60% (95% CI 50–71) [150]. Other studies have produced similar results [148]. The optimal antimicrobial regimen for chronic suppression in staphylococcal prosthetic joint infection treated with débridement and component retention has not been established. Some of the antimicrobials used as agents for chronic suppression are first-generation cephalosporins, minocycline, or trimethoprim–sulfamethoxazole [99]. The goal of suppressive therapy is to maintain a pain-free functional prosthesis. Table 22.3 summarizes the different antimicrobial agents used for each type of surgical intervention.

Antimicrobial-impregnated devices

Use of antimicrobial-impregnated polymethylmethacrylate (PMMA) cement is widespread in the prophylaxis and treatment of staphylococcal prosthetic joint infection. It is used in the form of antibiotic-impregnated spacers or for fixation at the time of reimplantation arthroplasty when staged surgery is used to treat prosthetic joint infection. There are six commercially available low-dose FDA-approved products for use in the second-stage surgery of a two-stage procedure [153]. The most commonly used antibiotics in PMMA cement are aminoglycosides (tobramycin or gentamicin) in combination with vancomycin. Daptomycin can also be used but clinical experience with this antimicrobial is limited [154]. Aminoglycosides are used consistently despite reports of high-level resistance to both tobramycin and gentamicin among staphylococci. In one study of staphylococcal prosthetic joint infection [155], 41% and 66% of staphylococcal isolates were found to be resistant *in vitro* to gentamicin and tobramycin respectively. The rate of resistance was higher in MRSA [155]. The β-lactam antibiotics such as penicillin and cephalosporins can also be used, but are usually avoided because of the risk of hypersensitivity reactions [99]. The use of antibiotic-impregnated cement at the time of reimplantation arthroplasty increases the rate of successful cure of the infection in both one-stage and two-stage exchange procedures [156].

The use of antibiotic-impregnated spacers in two-stage revisions has become the standard of care in the USA. Antibiotic-impregnated spacers will prevent soft tissue contractures and joint instability and might facilitate

Table 22.3 Medical therapy based on surgical modalities for staphylococcal prosthetic joint infection.

Type of surgical modality	Methicillin-susceptible *S. aureus* or CoNS	Methicillin-resistant *S. aureus* or CoNS
Two-stage exchange	Nafcillin sodium or oxacillin sodium 1.5–2 g i.v. every 4 hours for 4–6 weeks or cefazolin 1–2 g i.v. every 8 hours for 4–6 weeks[1,2] • 6–8 week delay for TKA reimplantation • 3-month delay for THA reimplantation	Vancomycin 15 mg/kg i.v. every 12 hours or daptomycin 6 mg/kg i.v. every 24 hours or linezolid 600 mg i.v./p.o. every 12 hours for 4–6 weeks • 6–8 week delay for TKA reimplantation • 3-month delay for THA reimplantation
Débridement and retention of the components	Nafcillin sodium or oxacillin sodium 1.5–2 g i.v. every 4 hours for 2–6 weeks or cefazolin 1–2 g i.v. every 8 hours for 2–6 weeks *plus* oral rifampin 300–450 mg b.i.d. Followed by a quinolone or first-generation cephalosporin or TMP–SMX or minocycline *plus* rifampin for 6–8 weeks (THA) or 20–22 weeks (TKA) Followed by chronic oral suppression: first-generation cephalosporin or oral antistaphylococcal penicillin or TMP–SMX or minocycline Alternative (if β-lactam allergy) for parenteral antimicrobial: vancomycin, daptomycin or linezolid	Vancomycin 15 mg/kg i.v. every 12 hours or daptomycin 6 mg/kg i.v. every 24 hours or linezolid 600 mg i.v./p.o. every 12 hours for 2–6 weeks *plus* oral rifampin 300 mg t.i.d. or 400 mg b.i.d. Followed by a quinolone or TMP–SMX or minocycline *plus* rifampin for 6–8 weeks (THA) or 20–22 weeks (TKA) Followed by chronic oral suppression: TMP–SMX or minocycline
One-stage exchange	Nafcillin sodium or oxacillin sodium 1.5–2 g i.v. every 4 hours for 4–6 weeks or cefazolin 1–2 g i.v. every 8 hours for 4–6 weeks followed by chronic suppression[3] Alternative (if β-lactam allergy) for parenteral antimicrobial: vancomycin, daptomycin or linezolid	Vancomycin 15 mg/kg i.v. every 12 hours or daptomycin 6 mg/kg i.v. every 24 hours or linezolid 600 mg i.v./p.o. every 12 hours for 4–6 weeks followed by chronic suppression
Resection arthroplasty	Nafcillin sodium or oxacillin sodium 1.5–2 g i.v. every 4 hours for 4–6 weeks or cefazolin 1–2 g i.v. every 8 hours for 4–6 weeks followed by chronic suppression Alternative (if β-lactam allergy) for parenteral antimicrobial: vancomycin, daptomycin or linezolid	Vancomycin 15 mg/kg i.v. every 12 hours or daptomycin 6 mg/kg i.v. every 24 hours or linezolid 600 mg i.v./p.o. every 12 hours for 4–6 weeks

[1] *Staphylococcus aureus* is usually treated for 6 weeks.
[2] Antimicrobial dosage varies depending on creatinine clearance, drug intolerances, hepatic function, and drug interactions.
[3] The use of rifampin is optional. The use of chronic suppression is also dictated by individual patient circumstances.
CoNS, coagulase-negative staphylococci; TKA, total knee arthroplasty; THA, total hip arthroplasty; TMP–SMX, trimethoprim–sulfamethoxazole.

reimplantation surgery [157]. There are two types of spacers: articulating and nonarticulating. The latter are static and deliver high concentrations of antimicrobial locally (but are associated with reduction in the range of motion). Articulating spacers are FDA approved and are becoming more popular since they allow more interim joint mobility and function [157,158].

Surgical therapy

Four main surgical options are usually used in conjunction with systemic and local antimicrobial therapy. The type of surgical modality usually depends on when the infection occurs after initial prosthesis implantation, the stability of the implant, the host's medical condition, the quality of the surrounding soft tissue, and the organism isolated. Other factors such as previous surgeries on the same joint, previous revision arthroplasties, comorbid host conditions, and patient and surgeon preferences are also taken into consideration as well.

Débridement and retention of the prosthesis

Débridement and retention of the prosthesis is an appealing modality when dealing with patients with well-fixed prostheses, especially if the infection is secondary to a nonvirulent organism [159]. Patients with early and late acute-onset hematogenous infection can also benefit from this type of approach [92]. The likelihood of treatment success is higher with shorter duration of symptoms (< 2 weeks), absence of a sinus tract or loosening of the prosthesis, early débridement within 2–5 days of onset of symptoms, and presence of a susceptible organism. Treatment failure is higher if the infection is secondary to *S. aureus* or if a rifampin-containing regimen is not used [89,127,149,150,160–162]. In one randomized controlled trial conducted by Zimmerli *et al.* [139], patients with orthopedic implant-related staphylococcal infections were treated with débridement and retention combined with ciprofloxacin plus placebo or rifampin. Cure rate was 100% in patients treated for 3–6 months with rifampin–ciprofloxacin, compared with 58% in the ciprofloxacin–placebo group [89]. The suggested duration of intravenous antimicrobial therapy is 2–6 weeks, followed by 3 months of oral therapy for hip prostheses and 6 months for knee prostheses [99]. The 2-year cumulative probability of success without treatment failure has been reported to be in the 60% range in one study that examined the outcome of staphylococcal prosthetic joint infection treated with débridement and retention [150].

Two-stage replacement arthroplasty

The two-stage exchange procedure for THA or TKA infection involves removal of the infected prosthesis with débridement of all infected tissue followed by administration of antimicrobial therapy, and subsequent delayed reimplantation of a second prosthesis. The surgical techniques and the duration of antimicrobial therapy varies between institutions. Two-stage exchange is usually the procedure of choice in the treatment of chronic prosthetic joint infections or those associated with loosening of the prosthesis. In addition, this approach is recommended if compromised soft tissue, sinus tracts, deep abscess formation, and infections with virulent organisms are present [89,99]. Sia *et al.* [99] reviewed studies involving 1077 prostheses treated by two-stage exchange and found an overall success of 87%. In another review, the reported success rate was 98% for *S. aureus* prosthetic joint infections treated with prosthesis removal and delayed reimplantation arthroplasty [163]. The type and duration of parenteral antimicrobial therapy are described in Table 22.3. At Mayo Clinic, we advocate a 6–8 week delay for TKA reimplantation and a 3-month delay for THA.

One-stage replacement arthroplasty

One-stage replacement arthroplasty or direct exchange involves the removal of infected prosthetic material, débridement of the surrounding bone and soft tissue, followed by implantation of a new prosthesis during the same surgery. Parenteral antimicrobial therapy follows the surgical procedure. One-stage exchange surgery is usually performed for infections involving a THA and usually follows some strict criteria: healthy patients, a favorable soft tissue envelope, preoperative identification of the causative organism, a microorganism that is "antibiotic sensitive," and minimal femoral osseous defects after prosthesis removal [164,165]. Direct exchange is also performed with antibiotic-impregnated bone cement. The success rates of a one-stage exchange for infected hip and infected knee are 86–100% and 75–100% [164,166–171]. In these studies, the number of prosthetic joint infections with knee prostheses was small compared with the case series involving hip prostheses. This procedure usually requires prolonged postsurgical antimicrobial therapy for better success rates; however, it might carry the risk of recurrence with residual microorganisms [99,172].

Resection arthroplasty, arthrodesis, and amputation

Resection arthroplasty and arthrodesis are performed in patients with severe immunodeficiency, in active intravenous drug users, and in patients for whom a joint replacement will not provide additional functional benefit [89]. Resection arthroplasty is the definitive removal of the infected prosthetic material and soft tissue without subsequent delayed reimplantation of a new prosthesis. It is usually followed by 4–6 weeks of antimicrobial therapy. Patients who undergo this type of procedure have poor functional outcome.

Arthrodesis is an adequate salvage procedure when further surgeries are not possible for patients with TKA infection. The goal is to achieve a painless stable joint. Arthrodesis can be performed using internal fixation, with a plate or an intramedullary nail, or external fixation. In some cases, bone grafting is required to achieve union. Arthrodesis is performed when there is poor bone stock, or recurrent infection or infection with a virulent organism that failed multiple procedures [173]. Amputation is a consideration when salvage procedures are not successful. It is indicated in the case of uncontrollable pain or in the presence of severe bone loss and vascular insufficiency [174].

Septic arthritis

Septic arthritis is a medical and orthopedic emergency. If not promptly recognized and treated, it can lead to rapid joint destruction, cartilage loss, and joint malfunction. Septic arthritis is a relatively uncommon disease, with a peak incidence of 6 per 100 000 per year [175]. The incidence is higher for patients less than 15 and above 55 years of age. The most common joints involved are the hip and the knee. Risk factors include underlying inflammatory joint disease such as rheumatoid arthritis. The incidence of septic arthritis in patients with rheumatoid arthritis is 70 per 100 000 per year [176].

Epidemiology and pathogenesis

Systemic as well as local factors are known to increase the risk for septic arthritis [177]. Systemic disorders that increase the risk of developing septic arthritis include rheumatoid arthritis, diabetes mellitus, chronic liver disease, chronic renal failure/hemodialysis, malignancies, alcoholism, and psoriasis. Patients with underlying joint disease have an increased risk of developing septic arthritis, such as those with rheumatoid arthritis, gout, pseudogout, or osteoarthritis. A history of recent trauma or surgical procedure can also increase the risk of septic arthritis [177]. Dubost *et al.* found that septic arthritis occurred in patients with rheumatoid arthritis of longer duration (mean 15 years); one-third of infected joints involved the knee with more frequent involvement of the elbows and wrists. *Staphylococcus aureus* was recovered in 80% and 60% of patients with and without rheumatoid arthritis, respectively. Staphylococcal infection and polyarticular infection were associated with higher mortality rates (35% and 49%, respectively). CoNS and β-hemolytic group A, B and G streptococci, mainly *Streptococcus pyogenes*, are also frequent pathogens causing bacterial arthritis [176].

Neisseria gonorrhoeae and *Neisseria meningitidis* account for at least 20% of septic arthritis cases [176]. MRSA has recently emerged as an important cause of septic arthritis. In one retrospective review of hematogenous septic arthritis cases, 34% of patients had an infection secondary to MRSA. Patients with MRSA septic arthritis were more likely to be older, with a predilection for the glenohumeral joint [178]. The mechanisms of infection in septic arthritis are similar to the ones described for osteomyelitis. Bacteria can infect the joint through hematogenous spread, contiguous infection, or direct inoculation secondary to trauma or a surgical procedure.

Clinical presentation

It is of extreme importance to exclude the possibility of septic arthritis in a patient presenting with a swollen and painful joint. This is especially true if this clinical presentation follows an intervention involving the joint, such as arthroscopy or intraarticular injection. In a recent meta-analysis of 14 studies, 653 cases of adult septic arthritis were analyzed [179]. The main aim of the study was to evaluate the accuracy of clinical presentation in patients with septic arthritis. The most frequent symptoms identified were joint pain, joint swelling, and fever. Sweating and rigors were not reported frequently. In general, MRSA septic arthritis presents more frequently with fever compared with MSSA [178]. Septic arthritis is typically a monoarticular disease. Polyarticular disease is seen in patients with overwhelming sepsis, especially in the case of septic arthritis secondary to MRSA. The upper extremity joints are less frequently involved, but septic arthritis can involve the interphalangeal joints, wrist, elbow, or shoulder [180]. The hip is more commonly involved in children [177]. Younger adults usually have obvious symptomatology, with a painful joint, swelling, and fever. Prompt intervention is crucial to avoid joint complications and loss of function. When septic arthritis occurs in patients at the extremes of age, other foci of infection are likely to be found [181].

Diagnosis

Laboratory diagnosis

In general, most laboratory parameters are of limited diagnostic value for the diagnosis of septic arthritis. The diagnostic value of peripheral white cell count, ESR, and CRP is low [182–184]. One should not solely rely on these tests to rule out the possibility of an infection. Blood cultures obtained prior to initiation of antimicrobial therapy are positive in 30–50% of patients with infectious arthritis [178,182].

The diagnosis of septic arthritis most often relies on synovial fluid examination. Aspiration of the synovial fluid in the presence of an effusion should be performed in order to obtain a prompt diagnosis and to determine optimal antimicrobial therapy. The Gram stain is positive in 50–70% of cases [178]. The synovial fluid white cell count has a reported sensitivity and specificity of 64% and 88% respectively [182,183]. In one review of 202 patients with a synovial fluid white cell count higher than $2000/mm^3$, a synovial fluid white cell count in excess of $50\,000/mm^3$ was observed in 70% of patients with septic arthritis, with a majority of cases secondary to *S. aureus* [184]. One systematic review found that the likelihood of septic arthritis is increased if the percentage of synovial polymorphonuclear cells is at least 90% (likelihood ratio 3.4, 95% CI 2.8–4.2) and the synovial fluid white cell count is higher than $100\,000/mm^3$ (likelihood ratio 28.0, 95% CI 12.0–66.0) [179]. The synovial fluid should be sent for cell count and differential, Gram stain, and anaerobic and aerobic bacterial culture. Other types of specific cultures will need to be requested based on the clinical context and the host's immune condition. PCR has also been evaluated, with promising results for the detection of pathogens causing septic arthritis [18,185].

Imaging

Plain radiography can show soft tissue swelling, effacement of the fat planes, and joint distension. Ultrasound is useful for evaluating joint effusion although not always indicative of septic arthritis. Ultrasound is also useful for performing arthrocentesis [51,175]. Cross-sectional imaging modalities are useful in evaluating the surrounding soft tissue and bone and assessing for possible periarticular osteomyelitis. Radionuclide studies are not very helpful in the diagnosis of septic arthritis.

Treatment

The choice of empirical antimicrobial therapy is guided by the clinical context and results of the Gram stain when positive. Because of the high risk of rapid joint destruction, initiation of antimicrobials should not be delayed whenever the diagnosis of septic arthritis is suspected. Appropriate antimicrobial therapy should be initiated until definitive culture results are obtained. A careful history and review of epidemiological risk factors should be performed in order to assess the risk of MRSA infection. When Gram-positive cocci are documented on Gram stains, an antistaphylococcal antimicrobial should be administered. Vancomycin is the drug of choice if the patient is allergic to β-lactam antibiotics or in the presence of MRSA risk factors. Cefazolin is adequate empirical therapy in selected patients when the Gram stain is inconclusive or if the patient is not critically ill or does not have any documented β-lactam allergy or any risk factors for resistant organisms. An antipseudomonal agent should be added in septic arthritis secondary to intravenous drug injection.

The duration of antimicrobial therapy is not well defined and varies by institution. Many factors are usually taken into consideration, such as joint location, the presence of a contiguous focus of osteomyelitis, host factors, adequate drainage of the synovial fluid, and the type and virulence of the infecting organism. Uncomplicated *S. aureus* septic arthritis is usually treated for 3 weeks with parenteral antimicrobials. Some authors recommend intravenous therapy for at least 1 week followed by 4–6 weeks of oral therapy [178]. CoNS septic arthritis following an intra-articular injection or arthroscopy is usually treated for 2 weeks after the procedure [43]. Narrowing the antimicrobial therapy will need to be done once the synovial culture yields a positive result. Since a major inflammatory response leading to purulent synovial fluid occurs in septic arthritis, some authors have suggested a course of corticosteroids in combination with antimicrobial therapy. In a double-blind, randomized, placebo-controlled study in children with hematogenous septic arthritis, the addition of steroids improved the functionality of the joint [186].

Different surgical techniques can be performed for the drainage of a septic joint in order to sterilize the synovial space and achieve joint decompression. Repetitive joint aspirations are usually combined with sterile physiological saline irrigation. The type of drainage performed (surgery or arthroscopy) depends on joint location and the feasibility of the procedure [135,187]. The infected joint will need to be mobilized as soon as possible, if symptoms permit, in order to avoid muscle contracture and atrophy [178].

Outcome

The mortality and morbidity resulting from septic arthritis are not negligible. The sequelae arising from infection involving weight-bearing joints have significant impact on the quality of life and are often associated with decreased functionality. The reported mortality of septic arthritis related to systemic infection ranges from 5 to 20% [176]. Older age, polyarticular infection, infection secondary to *S. aureus*, septic arthritis of the hip, infection of a prosthetic joint, and preexisting joint disease are negative prognostic factors [176,188]. Septic arthritis will continue to be a challenge for the clinician with the increasing prevalence of multidrug-resistant microorganisms, especially *S. aureus*, and the increasing need for subsequent joint replacement for joint damage.

References

1 Tennvall G, Apelqvist J, Eneroth M. Costs of deep foot infections in patients with diabetes mellitus. PharmacoEconomics 2000;18:225–38.

2 Davis JS. Management of bone and joint infections due to *Staphylococcus aureus*. Intern Med J 2005;35(suppl 2):S79–S96.

3 Waldvogel FA, Medoff G, Swartz MN. Osteomyelitis: a review of clinical features, therapeutic considerations and unusual aspects. 3. Osteomyelitis associated with vascular insufficiency. N Engl J Med 1970;282:316–22.

4 Lew DP, Waldvogel FA. Osteomyelitis. Lancet 2004;364:369–79.

5 Cierny G III, Mader JT, Penninck JJ. A clinical staging system for adult osteomyelitis. Clin Orthop Relat Res 2003;414:7–24.

6 Arnold SR, Elias D, Buckingham SC *et al.* Changing patterns of acute hematogenous osteomyelitis and septic arthritis: emergence of community-associated methicillin-resistant *Staphylococcus aureus*. J Pediatr Orthop 2006;26:703–8.

7 Greig JM, Wood MJ. *Staphylococcus lugdunensis* vertebral osteomyelitis. Clin Microbiol Infect 2003;9:1139–41.

8 Thomas S, Hoy C, Capper R. Osteomyelitis of the ear canal caused by *Staphylococcus lugdunensis*. J Infect 2006;53:e227–e229.

9 Sampathkumar P, Osmon DR, Cockerill FR III. Prosthetic joint infection due to *Staphylococcus lugdunensis*. Mayo Clin Proc 2000;75:511–12.

10 M'Bappe P, Girot R. [Osteo-articular complications of sickle-cell-anemia in adult.] Rev Prat 2004;54:1568–9, 1571–2.

11 Nicholls A, Edward N, Catto GR. Staphylococcal septicaemia, endocarditis, and osteomyelitis in dialysis and renal transplant patients. Postgrad Med J 1980;56:642–8.

12 Kak V, Chandrasekar PH. Bone and joint infections in injection drug users. Infect Dis Clin North Am 2002;16:681–95.

13 Hudson MC, Ramp WK, Nicholson NC, Williams AS, Nousiainen MT. Internalization of *Staphylococcus aureus* by cultured osteoblasts. Microb Pathog 1995;19:409–19.

14 Patti JM, Jonsson H, Guss B *et al.* Molecular characterization and expression of a gene encoding a *Staphylococcus aureus* collagen adhesin. J Biol Chem 1992;267:4766–72.

15 Ellington JK, Reilly SS, Ramp WK, Smeltzer MS, Kellam JF, Hudson MC. Mechanisms of *Staphylococcus aureus* invasion of cultured osteoblasts. Microb Pathog 1999;26:317–23.

16 Proctor RA, van Langevelde P, Kristjansson M, Maslow JN, Arbeit RD. Persistent and relapsing infections associated with small-colony variants of *Staphylococcus aureus*. Clin Infect Dis 1995;20:95–102.

17 Baumert N, von Eiff C, Schaaff F, Peters G, Proctor RA, Sahl HG. Physiology and antibiotic susceptibility of *Staphylococcus aureus* small colony variants. Microb Drug Resist 2002;8:253–60.

18 Trampuz A, Osmon DR, Hanssen AD, Steckelberg JM, Patel R. Molecular and antibiofilm approaches to prosthetic joint infection. Clin Orthop Relat Res 2003;414:69–88.

19 Dahl LB, Høyland AL, Dramsdahl H, Kaaresen PI. Acute osteomyelitis in children: a population-based retrospective study 1965 to 1994. Scand J Infect Dis 1998;30:573–7.

20 Maiuri F, Iaconetta G, Gallicchio B, Manto A, Briganti F. Spondylodiscitis. Clinical and magnetic resonance diagnosis. Spine 1997;22:1741–6.

21 Sia IG, Berbari EF. Infection and musculoskeletal conditions: osteomyelitis. Best Pract Res Clin Rheumatol 2006;20:1065–81.

22 Carragee EJ. Pyogenic vertebral osteomyelitis. J Bone Joint Surg Am 1997;79:874–80.

23 Hadjipavlou AG, Mader JT, Necessary JT, Muffoletto AJ. Hematogenous pyogenic spinal infections and their surgical management. Spine 2000;25:1668–79.

24 Weber-Chrysochoou C, Corti N, Goetschel P, Altermatt S, Huisman TA, Berger C. Pelvic osteomyelitis: a diagnostic challenge in children. J Pediatr Surg 2007;42:553–7.

25 Roca RP, Yoshikawa TT. Primary skeletal infections in heroin users: a clinical characterization, diagnosis and therapy. Clin Orthop Relat Res 1979;144:238–48.

26 Harris LG, Richards RG. Staphylococci and implant surfaces: a review. Injury 2006;37(suppl 2):S3–S14.

27 Merritt K. Factors increasing the risk of infection in patients with open fractures. J Trauma 1988;28:823–7.

28 DeLong WG Jr, Born CT, Wei SY, Petrik ME, Ponzio R, Schwab CW. Aggressive treatment of 119 open fracture wounds. J Trauma 1999;46:1049–54.

29 Puno RM, Grossfeld SL, Henry SL, Seligson D, Harkess J, Tsai TM. Functional outcome of patients with salvageable limbs with grades III-B and III-C open fractures of the tibia. Microsurgery 1996;17:167–73.

30 Sterett WI, Ertl JP, Chapman MW, Moehring HD. Open tibia fractures in the splenectomized trauma patient: results of treatment with locking, intramedullary fixation. J Trauma 1995;38:639–41.

31 Holcombe SJ, Schneider RK, Bramlage LR, Embertson RM. Use of antibiotic-impregnated polymethyl methacrylate in horses with open or infected fractures or joints: 19 cases (1987–1995). J Am Vet Med Assoc 1997;211:889–93.

32 Ostermann PA, Seligson D, Henry SL. Local antibiotic therapy for severe open fractures. A review of 1085 consecutive cases. J Bone Joint Surg Br 1995;77:93–7.

33 Henry SL, Ostermann PA, Seligson D. The prophylactic use of antibiotic impregnated beads in open fractures. J Trauma 1990; 30:1231–8.

34 Worlock P, Slack R, Harvey L, Mawhinney R. The prevention of infection in open fractures. An experimental study of the effect of antibiotic therapy. J Bone Joint Surg Am 1988;70:1341–7.

35 Faisham WI, Nordin S, Aidura M. Bacteriological study and its role in the management of open tibial fracture. Med J Malaysia 2001;56:201–6.

36 Caputo GM, Cavanagh PR, Ulbrecht JS, Gibbons GW, Karchmer AW. Assessment and management of foot disease in patients with diabetes. N Engl J Med 1994;331:854–60.

37 Ramsey SD, Newton K, Blough D *et al.* Incidence, outcomes, and cost of foot ulcers in patients with diabetes. Diabetes Care 1999;22:382–7.

38 Ragnarson Tennvall G, Apelqvist J. Health-economic consequences of diabetic foot lesions. Clin Infect Dis 2004;39 (suppl 2):S132–S139.

39 Calhoun JH, Overgaard KA, Stevens CM, Dowling JP, Mader JT. Diabetic foot ulcers and infections: current concepts. Adv Skin Wound Care 2002;15:31–42; quiz 44–5.

40 Yoga R, Khairul A, Sunita K, Suresh C. Bacteriology of diabetic foot lesions. Med J Malaysia 2006;61(suppl A):14–16.

41 Couret G, Desbiez F, Thieblot P *et al.* [Emergence of monomicrobial methicillin-resistant *Staphylococcus aureus* infections in diabetic foot osteomyelitis (retrospective study of 48 cases).] Presse Med 2007;36:851–8.

42 Lipsky BA. Empirical therapy for diabetic foot infections: are there clinical clues to guide antibiotic selection? Clin Microbiol Infect 2007;13:351–3.

43 Lipsky BA, Berendt AR, Deery HG *et al.* Diagnosis and treatment of diabetic foot infections. Clin Infect Dis 2004;39:885–910.

44 Grayson ML, Gibbons GW, Balogh K, Levin E, Karchmer AW. Probing to bone in infected pedal ulcers. A clinical sign of underlying osteomyelitis in diabetic patients. JAMA 1995;273:721–3.

45 Lavery LA, Armstrong DG, Peters EJ, Lipsky BA. Probe-to-bone test for diagnosing diabetic foot osteomyelitis: reliable or relic? Diabetes Care 2007;30:270–4.

46 Peters KM, Koberg K, Rosendahl T, Haubeck HD. PMN elastase in bone and joint infections. Int Orthop 1994;18:352–5.

47 Jones NS, Anderson DJ, Stiles PJ. Osteomyelitis in a general hospital. A five-year study showing an increase in subacute osteomyelitis. J Bone Joint Surg Br 1987;69:779–83.

48 Perry CR, Pearson RL, Miller GA. Accuracy of cultures of material from swabbing of the superficial aspect of the wound and needle biopsy in the preoperative assessment of osteomyelitis. J Bone Joint Surg Am 1991;73:745–9.

49 Mackowiak PA, Jones SR, Smith JW. Diagnostic value of sinus-tract cultures in chronic osteomyelitis. JAMA 1978;239:2772–5.

50 Kessler L, Piemont Y, Ortega F *et al.* Comparison of microbiological results of needle puncture vs. superficial swab in infected diabetic foot ulcer with osteomyelitis. Diabet Med 2006;23:99–102.

51 Palestro CJ, Love C, Miller TT. Infection and musculoskeletal conditions: imaging of musculoskeletal infections. Best Pract Res Clin Rheumatol 2006;20:1197–218.

52 Wrobel JS, Connolly JE. Making the diagnosis of osteomyelitis. The role of prevalence. J Am Podiatr Med Assoc 1998;88:337–43.

53 Love C, Patel M, Lonner BS, Tomas MB, Palestro CJ. Diagnosing spinal osteomyelitis: a comparison of bone and Ga-67 scintigraphy and magnetic resonance imaging. Clin Nucl Med 2000;25:963–77.

54 Palestro CJ, Torres MA. Radionuclide imaging in orthopedic infections. Semin Nucl Med 1997;27:334–45.

55 Guhlmann A, Brecht-Krauss D, Suger G *et al.* Chronic osteomyelitis: detection with FDG PET and correlation with histopathologic findings. Radiology 1998;206:749–54.

56 Modic MT, Feiglin DH, Piraino DW *et al.* Vertebral osteomyelitis: assessment using MR. Radiology 1985;157:157–66.

57 Kapoor A, Page S, Lavalley M, Gale DR, Felson DT. Magnetic resonance imaging for diagnosing foot osteomyelitis: a meta-analysis. Arch Intern Med 2007;167:125–32.

58 Kowalski TJ, Layton KF, Berbari EF *et al.* Follow-up MR imaging in patients with pyogenic spine infections: lack of correlation with clinical features. AJNR Am J Neuroradiol 2007;28:693–9.

59 Newman LG, Waller J, Palestro CJ *et al.* Unsuspected osteomyelitis in diabetic foot ulcers. Diagnosis and monitoring by leukocyte scanning with indium 111 oxyquinoline. JAMA 1991; 266:1246–51.

60 Norden CW, Shinners E, Niederriter K. Clindamycin treatment of experimental chronic osteomyelitis due to *Staphylococcus aureus*. J Infect Dis 1986;153:956–9.

61 Berbari E, Steckelberg J, Osmon D. Osteomyelitis. In: Mandell GL, Bennett JE, Dolin R, eds. Principles and Practice of Infectious Diseases, 6th edn. Philadelphia: Churchill Livingstone, 2005:1322–31.

62 Drancourt M, Stein A, Argenson JN, Zannier A, Curvale G, Raoult D. Oral rifampin plus ofloxacin for treatment of *Staphylococcus*-infected orthopedic implants. Antimicrob Agents Chemother 1993;37:1214–8.

63 Sanchez C, Matamala A, Salavert M *et al.* [Cotrimoxazole plus rifampicin in the treatment of staphylococcal osteoarticular infection.] Enferm Infecc Microbiol Clin 1997;15:10–13.

64 Bachur R, Pagon Z. Success of short-course parenteral antibiotic therapy for acute osteomyelitis of childhood. Clin Pediatr 2007;46:30–5.

65 Tice AD, Rehm SJ, Dalovisio JR *et al.* Practice guidelines for outpatient parenteral antimicrobial therapy. IDSA guidelines. Clin Infect Dis 2004;38:1651–72.
66 Esposito S, Leone S, Noviello S *et al.* Outpatient parenteral antibiotic therapy for bone and joint infections: an Italian multicenter study. J Chemother 2007;19:417–22.
67 Tice A. The use of outpatient parenteral antimicrobial therapy in the management of osteomyelitis: data from the Outpatient Parenteral Antimicrobial Therapy Outcomes Registries. Chemotherapy 2001;47(suppl 1):5–16.
68 Jones ME, Karlowsky JA, Draghi DC, Thornsberry C, Sahm DF, Nathwani D. Epidemiology and antibiotic susceptibility of bacteria causing skin and soft tissue infections in the USA and Europe: a guide to appropriate antimicrobial therapy. Int J Antimicrob Agents 2003;22:406–19.
69 Lovering AM, Zhang J, Bannister GC *et al.* Penetration of linezolid into bone, fat, muscle and haematoma of patients undergoing routine hip replacement. J Antimicrob Chemother 2002;50:73–7.
70 Rana B, Butcher I, Grigoris P, Murnaghan C, Seaton RA, Tobin CM. Linezolid penetration into osteo-articular tissues. J Antimicrob Chemother 2002;50:747–50.
71 Rao N, Ziran BH, Hall RA, Santa ER. Successful treatment of chronic bone and joint infections with oral linezolid. Clin Orthop Relat Res 2004;427:67–71.
72 Howden BP, Ward PB, Charles PG *et al.* Treatment outcomes for serious infections caused by methicillin-resistant *Staphylococcus aureus* with reduced vancomycin susceptibility. Clin Infect Dis 2004;38:521–8.
73 Patel R, Piper KE, Rouse MS, Steckelberg JM. Linezolid therapy of *Staphylococcus aureus* experimental osteomyelitis. Antimicrob Agents Chemother 2000;44:3438–40.
74 McKinnon PS, Carter CT, Girase PG, Liu LZ, Carmeli Y. The economic effect of oral linezolid versus intravenous vancomycin in the outpatient setting: the payer perspective. Manag Care Interface 2007;20:23–34.
75 Waldrep TW, Skiest DJ. Linezolid-induced anemia and thrombocytopenia. Pharmacotherapy 2002;22:109–12.
76 Finney MS, Crank CW, Segreti J. Use of daptomycin to treat drug-resistant Gram-positive bone and joint infections. Curr Med Res Opin 2005;21:1923–6.
77 Holtom PD, Zalavras CG, Lamp KC, Park N, Friedrich LV. Clinical experience with daptomycin treatment of foot or ankle osteomyelitis: a preliminary study. Clin Orthop Relat Res 2007;461:35–9.
78 Boucher HW, Sakoulas G. Perspectives on daptomycin resistance, with emphasis on resistance in *Staphylococcus aureus*. Clin Infect Dis 2007;45:601–8.
79 Hawkey PM. Pre-clinical experience with daptomycin. J Antimicrob Chemother 2008;62(suppl 3):iii7–iii14.
80 Vikram HR, Havill NL, Koeth LM, Boyce JM. Clinical progression of methicillin-resistant *Staphylococcus aureus* vertebral osteomyelitis associated with reduced susceptibility to daptomycin. J Clin Microbiol 2005;43:5384–7.
81 Henke PK, Blackburn SA, Wainess RW *et al.* Osteomyelitis of the foot and toe in adults is a surgical disease: conservative management worsens lower extremity salvage. Ann Surg 2005;241:885–92, discussion 892–4.
82 Tan JS, Friedman NM, Hazelton-Miller C, Flanagan JP, File TM Jr. Can aggressive treatment of diabetic foot infections reduce the need for above-ankle amputation? Clin Infect Dis 1996;23:286–91.
83 Lipsky BA, Itani K, Norden C. Treating foot infections in diabetic patients: a randomized, multicenter, open-label trial of linezolid versus ampicillin-sulbactam/amoxicillin-clavulanate. Clin Infect Dis 2004;38:17–24.
84 Armstrong DG, Lipsky BA. Advances in the treatment of diabetic foot infections. Diabetes Technol Ther 2004;6:167–77.
85 Lipsky BA, Armstrong DG, Citron DM, Tice AD, Morgenstern DE, Abramson MA. Ertapenem versus piperacillin/tazobactam for diabetic foot infections (SIDESTEP): prospective, randomised, controlled, double-blinded, multicentre trial. Lancet 2005;366:1695–703.
86 Lipsky BA, Stoutenburgh U. Daptomycin for treating infected diabetic foot ulcers: evidence from a randomized, controlled trial comparing daptomycin with vancomycin or semi-synthetic penicillins for complicated skin and skin-structure infections. J Antimicrob Chemother 2005;55:240–5.
87 Priest DH, Peacock JE Jr. Hematogenous vertebral osteomyelitis due to *Staphylococcus aureus* in the adult: clinical features and therapeutic outcomes. South Med J 2005;98:854–62.
88 Darouiche RO. Treatment of infections associated with surgical implants. N Engl J Med 2004;350:1422–9.
89 Zimmerli W, Trampuz A, Ochsner PE. Prosthetic-joint infections. N Engl J Med 2004;351:1645–54.
90 Hanssen AD, Rand JA. Evaluation and treatment of infection at the site of a total hip or knee arthroplasty. Instr Course Lect 1999;48:111–22.
91 Lentino JR. Prosthetic joint infections: bane of orthopedists, challenge for infectious disease specialists. Clin Infect Dis 2003;36:1157–61.
92 Trampuz A, Zimmerli W. Prosthetic joint infections: update in diagnosis and treatment. Swiss Med Wkly 2005;135:243–51.
93 Poss R, Thornhill TS, Ewald FC, Thomas WH, Batte NJ, Sledge CB. Factors influencing the incidence and outcome of infection following total joint arthroplasty. Clin Orthop Relat Res 1984;182:117–26.
94 Ragni MV, Crossett LS, Herndon JH. Postoperative infection following orthopaedic surgery in human immunodeficiency virus-infected hemophiliacs with CD4 counts ≤ $200/mm^3$. J Arthroplasty 1995;10:716–21.
95 Wilson MG, Kelley K, Thornhill TS. Infection as a complication of total knee-replacement arthroplasty. Risk factors and treatment in sixty-seven cases. J Bone Joint Surg Am 1990;72:878–83.
96 Ainscow DA, Denham RA. The risk of haematogenous infection in total joint replacements. J Bone Joint Surg Br 1984;66:580–2.
97 Zimmerli W. Infection and musculoskeletal conditions: prosthetic-joint-associated infections. Best Pract Res Clin Rheumatol 2006;20:1045–63.
98 Berbari EF, Hanssen AD, Duffy MC *et al.* Risk factors for prosthetic joint infection: case–control study. Clin Infect Dis 1998;27:1247–54.
99 Sia IG, Berbari EF, Karchmer AW. Prosthetic joint infections. Infect Dis Clin North Am 2005;19:885–914.
100 Robertsson O, Knutson K, Lewold S, Lidgren L. The Swedish Knee Arthroplasty Register 1975–1997: an update with special emphasis on 41,223 knees operated on in 1988–1997. Acta Orthop Scand 2001;72:503–13.

101 Berbari EF, Osmon DR, Duffy MC *et al*. Outcome of prosthetic joint infection in patients with rheumatoid arthritis: the impact of medical and surgical therapy in 200 episodes. Clin Infect Dis 2006;42:216–23.

102 Chu VH, Crosslin DR, Friedman JY *et al*. *Staphylococcus aureus* bacteremia in patients with prosthetic devices: costs and outcomes. Am J Med 2005;118:1416.

103 Murdoch DR, Roberts SA, Fowler VG Jr *et al*. Infection of orthopedic prostheses after *Staphylococcus aureus* bacteremia. Clin Infect Dis 2001;32:647–9.

104 Zimmerli W, Waldvogel FA, Vaudaux P, Nydegger UE. Pathogenesis of foreign body infection: description and characteristics of an animal model. J Infect Dis 1982;146:487–97.

105 Mack D, Haeder M, Siemssen N, Laufs R. Association of biofilm production of coagulase-negative staphylococci with expression of a specific polysaccharide intercellular adhesin. J Infect Dis 1996;174:881–4.

106 Vaudaux P, Lew DP. Tolerance of staphylococci to bactericidal antibiotics. Injury 2006;37(suppl 2):S15–S19.

107 Herrmann M, Vaudaux PE, Pittet D *et al*. Fibronectin, fibrinogen, and laminin act as mediators of adherence of clinical staphylococcal isolates to foreign material. J Infect Dis 1988;158: 693–701.

108 Gross M, Cramton SE, Götz F, Peschel A. Key role of teichoic acid net charge in *Staphylococcus aureus* colonization of artificial surfaces. Infect Immun 2001;69:3423–6.

109 Proctor RA, Kahl B, von Eiff C, Vaudaux PE, Lew DP, Peters G. Staphylococcal small colony variants have novel mechanisms for antibiotic resistance. Clin Infect Dis 1998;27(suppl 1):S68–S74.

110 von Eiff C, Proctor RA, Peters G. Small colony variants of staphylococci: a link to persistent infections. Berl Munch Tierarztl Wochenschr 2000;113:321–5.

111 von Eiff C, Peters G, Becker K. The small colony variant (SCV) concept: the role of staphylococcal SCVs in persistent infections. Injury 2006;37(suppl 2):S26–S33.

112 Maderazo EG, Judson S, Pasternak H. Late infections of total joint prostheses. A review and recommendations for prevention. Clin Orthop Relat Res 1988;229:131–42.

113 Patel R, Osmon D, Hanssen A. The diagnosis of prosthetic joint infections. Current techniques and emerging technologies. Clin Orthop Relat Res 2005;437:55–8.

114 Spangehl MJ, Masri BA, O'Connell JX, Duncan CP. Prospective analysis of preoperative and intraoperative investigations for the diagnosis of infection at the sites of two hundred and two revision total hip arthroplasties. J Bone Joint Surg Am 1999;81: 672–83.

115 Trampuz A, Hanssen AD, Osmon DR, Mandrekar J, Steckelberg JM, Patel R. Synovial fluid leukocyte count and differential for the diagnosis of prosthetic knee infection. Am J Med 2004;117:556–62.

116 Trampuz A, Piper KE, Hanssen AD *et al*. Sonication of explanted prosthetic components in bags for diagnosis of prosthetic joint infection is associated with risk of contamination. J Clin Microbiol 2006;44:628–31.

117 Atkins BL, Athanasou N, Deeks JJ *et al*. Prospective evaluation of criteria for microbiological diagnosis of prosthetic-joint infection at revision arthroplasty. The OSIRIS Collaborative Study Group. J Clin Microbiol 1998;36:2932–9.

118 Trampuz A, Piper KE, Jacobson MJ *et al*. Sonication of removed hip and knee prostheses for diagnosis of infection. N Engl J Med 2007;357:654–63.

119 Cuckler JM, Star AM, Alavi A, Noto RB. Diagnosis and management of the infected total joint arthroplasty. Orthop Clin North Am 1991;22:523–30.

120 Stumpe KD, Nötzli HP, Zanetti M *et al*. FDG PET for differentiation of infection and aseptic loosening in total hip replacements: comparison with conventional radiography and three-phase bone scintigraphy. Radiology 2004;231:333–41.

121 Akhtar MS, Qaisar A, Irfanullah J *et al*. Antimicrobial peptide ^{99m}Tc-ubiquicidin 29–41 as human infection-imaging agent: clinical trial. J Nucl Med 2005;46:567–73.

122 Akhtar MS, Iqbal J, Khan MA *et al*. ^{99m}Tc-labeled antimicrobial peptide ubiquicidin (29–41) accumulates less in *Escherichia coli* infection than in *Staphylococcus aureus* infection. J Nucl Med 2004;45:849–56.

123 Parvizi J, Ghanem E, Menashe S, Barrack RL, Bauer TW. Periprosthetic infection: what are the diagnostic challenges? J Bone Joint Surg Am 2006;88(suppl 4):138–47.

124 Sampedro MF, Patel R. Infections associated with long-term prosthetic devices. Infect Dis Clin North Am 2007;21:785–819, x.

125 Hoyle BD, Costerton JW. Bacterial resistance to antibiotics: the role of biofilms. Prog Drug Res 1991;37:91–105.

126 Salgado CD, Dash S, Cantey JR, Marculescu CE. Higher risk of failure of methicillin-resistant *Staphylococcus aureus* prosthetic joint infections. Clin Orthop Relat Res 2007;461:48–53.

127 Tsukayama DT, Estrada R, Gustilo RB. Infection after total hip arthroplasty. A study of the treatment of one hundred and six infections. J Bone Joint Surg Am 1996;78:512–23.

128 Segawa H, Tsukayama DT, Kyle RF, Becker DA, Gustilo RB. Infection after total knee arthroplasty. A retrospective study of the treatment of eighty-one infections. J Bone Joint Surg Am 1999;81:1434–45.

129 Beam JW, Buckley B. Community-acquired methicillin-resistant *Staphylococcus aureus*: prevalence and risk factors. J Athl Train 2006;41:337–40.

130 Centers for Disease Control and Prevention. Community-associated methicillin-resistant *Staphylococcus aureus* infections in Pacific Islanders, Hawaii, 2001–2003. MMWR 2004;53: 767–70.

131 Centers for Disease Control and Prevention. Methicillin-resistant *Staphylococcus aureus* infections among competitive sports participants: Colorado, Indiana, Pennsylvania, and Los Angeles County, 2000–2003. MMWR 2003;52:793–5.

132 Centers for Disease Control and Prevention. Methicillin-resistant *Staphylococcus aureus* infections in correctional facilities: Georgia, California, and Texas, 2001–2003. MMWR 2003;52: 992–6.

133 Klevens RM, Morrison MA, Fridkin SK *et al*. Community-associated methicillin-resistant *Staphylococcus aureus* and health-care risk factors. Emerg Infect Dis 2006;12:1991–3.

134 Rao N, Hamilton CW. Efficacy and safety of linezolid for Gram-positive orthopedic infections: a prospective case series. Diagn Microbiol Infect Dis 2007;59:173–9.

135 Razonable RR, Osmon DR, Steckelberg JM. Linezolid therapy for orthopedic infections. Mayo Clin Proc 2004;79:1137–44.

136 Edmiston CE Jr, Goheen MP, Seabrook GR *et al*. Impact of selective antimicrobial agents on staphylococcal adherence to biomedical devices. Am J Surg 2006;192:344–54.

137 Laplante KL, Mermel LA. In vitro activity of daptomycin and vancomycin lock solutions on staphylococcal biofilms in a central venous catheter model. Nephrol Dial Transplant 2007;22: 2239–46.
138 Falagas ME, Giannopoulou KP, Ntziora F, Papagelopoulos PJ. Daptomycin for treatment of patients with bone and joint infections: a systematic review of the clinical evidence. Int J Antimicrob Agents 2007;30:202–9.
139 Zimmerli W, Widmer AF, Blatter M, Frei R, Ochsner PE. Role of rifampin for treatment of orthopedic implant-related staphylococcal infections: a randomized controlled trial. Foreign-Body Infection (FBI) Study Group. JAMA 1998;279:1537–41.
140 Drancourt M, Stein A, Argenson JN, Roiron R, Groulier P, Raoult D. Oral treatment of *Staphylococcus* spp. infected orthopaedic implants with fusidic acid or ofloxacin in combination with rifampicin. J Antimicrob Chemother 1997;39:235–40.
141 Stein A, Bataille JF, Drancourt M *et al.* Ambulatory treatment of multidrug-resistant *Staphylococcus*-infected orthopedic implants with high-dose oral co-trimoxazole (trimethoprim–sulfamethoxazole). Antimicrob Agents Chemother 1998;42: 3086–91.
142 Widmer AF, Gaechter A, Ochsner PE, Zimmerli W. Antimicrobial treatment of orthopedic implant-related infections with rifampin combinations. Clin Infect Dis 1992;14:1251–3.
143 Aboltins CA, Page MA, Buising KL *et al.* Treatment of staphylococcal prosthetic joint infections with débridement, prosthesis retention and oral rifampicin and fusidic acid. Clin Microbiol Infect 2007;13:586–91.
144 Costerton JW, Stewart PS, Greenberg EP. Bacterial biofilms: a common cause of persistent infections. Science 1999;284:1318–22.
145 Schwank S, Rajacic Z, Zimmerli W, Blaser J. Impact of bacterial biofilm formation on in vitro and in vivo activities of antibiotics. Antimicrob Agents Chemother 1998;42:895–8.
146 Trampuz A, Murphy CK, Rothstein DM, Widmer AF, Landmann R, Zimmerli W. Efficacy of a novel rifamycin derivative, ABI-0043, against *Staphylococcus aureus* in an experimental model of foreign-body infection. Antimicrob Agents Chemother 2007; 51:2540–5.
147 Steckelberg J, Osmon D. Prosthetic joint infection. In: Waldovgel F, Bisno A, eds. Infections Associated With Indwelling Medical Devices. Washington, DC: ASM Press, 2000:173–209.
148 Rao N, Crossett LS, Sinha RK, Le Frock JL. Long-term suppression of infection in total joint arthroplasty. Clin Orthop Relat Res 2003;414:55–60.
149 Brandt CM, Sistrunk WW, Duffy MC *et al. Staphylococcus aureus* prosthetic joint infection treated with débridement and prosthesis retention. Clin Infect Dis 1997;24:914–19.
150 Marculescu CE, Berbari EF, Hanssen AD *et al.* Outcome of prosthetic joint infections treated with débridement and retention of components. Clin Infect Dis 2006;42:471–8.
151 Tsukayama DT, Wicklund B, Gustilo RB. Suppressive antibiotic therapy in chronic prosthetic joint infections. Orthopedics 1991;14:841–4.
152 Goulet JA, Pellicci PM, Brause BD, Salvati EM. Prolonged suppression of infection in total hip arthroplasty. J Arthroplasty 1988;3:109–16.
153 Jiranek WA, Hanssen AD, Greenwald AS. Antibiotic-loaded bone cement for infection prophylaxis in total joint replacement. J Bone Joint Surg Am 2006;88:2487–500.
154 Hall EW, Rouse MS, Jacofsky DJ *et al.* Release of daptomycin from polymethylmethacrylate beads in a continuous flow chamber. Diagn Microbiol Infect Dis 2004;50:261–5.
155 Anguita-Alonso P, Hanssen AD, Osmon DR, Trampuz A, Steckelberg JM, Patel R. High rate of aminoglycoside resistance among staphylococci causing prosthetic joint infection. Clin Orthop Relat Res 2005;439:43–7.
156 Garvin KL, Hanssen AD. Infection after total hip arthroplasty. Past, present, and future. J Bone Joint Surg Am 1995;77:1576–88.
157 Cui Q, Mihalko WM, Shields JS, Ries M, Saleh KJ. Antibiotic-impregnated cement spacers for the treatment of infection associated with total hip or knee arthroplasty. J Bone Joint Surg Am 2007;89:871–82.
158 Mabry TM, Hanssen AD. Articulating antibiotic spacers: a matter of personal preference. Orthopedics 2007;30:783–5.
159 Barberán J, Aguilar L, Carroquino G *et al.* Conservative treatment of staphylococcal prosthetic joint infections in elderly patients. Am J Med 2006;119:993 e7–10.
160 Marculescu C, Berbari E, Hanssen A, and 2003. Significance of acute inflammation in joint tissue at reimplantation arthroplasty in patients with prosthetic joint infection treated with two-stage exchange. Infections Diseases Society of America Annual Meeting. San Diego 2003; abstract 283.
161 Tattevin P, Crémieux AC, Pottier P, Huten D, Carbon C. Prosthetic joint infection: when can prosthesis salvage be considered? Clin Infect Dis 1999;29:292–5.
162 Burger RR, Basch T, Hopson CN. Implant salvage in infected total knee arthroplasty. Clin Orthop Relat Res 1991;273:105–12.
163 Brandt CM, Duffy MC, Berbari EF, Hanssen AD, Steckelberg JM, Osmon DR. *Staphylococcus aureus* prosthetic joint infection treated with prosthesis removal and delayed reimplantation arthroplasty. Mayo Clin Proc 1999;74:553–8.
164 Ure KJ, Amstutz HC, Nasser S, Schmalzried TP. Direct-exchange arthroplasty for the treatment of infection after total hip replacement. An average ten-year follow-up. J Bone Joint Surg Am 1998;80:961–8.
165 Jackson WO, Schmalzried TP. Limited role of direct exchange arthroplasty in the treatment of infected total hip replacements. Clin Orthop Relat Res 2000;381:101–5.
166 Hope PG, Kristinsson KG, Norman P, Elson RA. Deep infection of cemented total hip arthroplasties caused by coagulase-negative staphylococci. J Bone Joint Surg Br 1989;71:851–5.
167 Raut VV, Siney PD, Wroblewski BM. One-stage revision of infected total hip replacements with discharging sinuses. J Bone Joint Surg Br 1994;76:721–4.
168 Callaghan JJ, Katz RP, Johnston RC. One-stage revision surgery of the infected hip. A minimum 10-year followup study. Clin Orthop Relat Res 1999;369:139–43.
169 Bengston S, Knutson K. The infected knee arthroplasty: a 6-year follow-up of 357 cases. Acta Orthop Scand 1991;62: 301–11.
170 Goksan SB, Freeman MA. One-stage reimplantation for infected total knee arthroplasty. J Bone Joint Surg Br 1992;74:78–82.
171 Freeman MA, Sudlow RA, Casewell MW, Radcliff SS. The management of infected total knee replacements. J Bone Joint Surg Br 1985;67:764–8.
172 Wilde AH. Management of infected knee and hip prostheses. Curr Opin Rheumatol 1994;6:172–6.

173 Manzotti A, Pullen C, Deromedis B, Catagni MA. Knee arthrodesis after infected total knee arthroplasty using the Ilizarov method. Clin Orthop Relat Res 2001;389:143–9.
174 Isiklar ZU, Landon GC, Tullos HS. Amputation after failed total knee arthroplasty. Clin Orthop Relat Res 1994;299:173–8.
175 Nade S. Septic arthritis. Best Pract Res Clin Rheumatol 2003;17:183–200.
176 Tarkowski A. Infection and musculoskeletal conditions: infectious arthritis. Best Pract Res Clin Rheumatol 2006;20:1029–44.
177 Garcia-De La Torre I. Advances in the management of septic arthritis. Infect Dis Clin North Am 2006;20:773–88.
178 Dubost JJ, Fis I, Soubrier M, Lopitaux R, Ristori JM, Bussiere JL and Sauvezie B. Septic arthritis in rheumatoid polyarthritis. 24 cases and review of the literature. *Rev Rhum Ed Fr* 1994;61:153–165.
179 Margaretten ME, Kohlwes J, Moore D, Bent S. Does this adult patient have septic arthritis? JAMA 2007;297:1478–88.
180 Mehta P, Schnall SB, Zalavras CG. Septic arthritis of the shoulder, elbow, and wrist. Clin Orthop Relat Res 2006;451:42–5.
181 Goldenberg DL. Septic arthritis. Lancet 1998;351:197–202.
182 Li SF, Cassidy C, Chang C, Gharib S, Torres J. Diagnostic utility of laboratory tests in septic arthritis. Emerg Med J 2007;24:75–7.
183 Li SF, Henderson J, Dickman E, Darzynkiewicz R. Laboratory tests in adults with monoarticular arthritis: can they rule out a septic joint? Acad Emerg Med 2004;11:276–80.
184 Coutlakis PJ, Roberts WN, Wise CM. Another look at synovial fluid leukocytosis and infection. J Clin Rheumatol 2002;8:67–71.
185 Lin S, Mariani B, Johnson J, Sinha R, Tuan R. The use of molecular genetic testing for the detection of septic arthritis. Orthop Trans 1997;21:552–3.
186 Odio CM, Ramirez T, Arias G *et al.* Double blind, randomized, placebo-controlled study of dexamethasone therapy for hematogenous septic arthritis in children. Pediatr Infect Dis J 2003;22:883–8.
187 Acosta FL Jr, Chin CT, Quiñones-Hinojosa A, Ames CP, Weinstein PR, Chou D. Diagnosis and management of adult pyogenic osteomyelitis of the cervical spine. Neurosurg Focus 2004;17:E2.
188 Kaandorp CJ, Krijnen P, Moens HJ, Habbema JD, van Schaardenburg D. The outcome of bacterial arthritis: a prospective community-based study. Arthritis Rheum 1997;40:884–92.

Chapter 23
Staphylococcal Pneumonia

Ethan Rubinstein[1] *and Marin H. Kollef*[2]
[1] Section of Infectious Diseases, Faculty of Medicine, University of Manitoba, Winnipeg, Canada
[2] Washington University School of Medicine, St Louis, Missouri, USA

Introduction

Pneumonia caused by *Staphylococcus aureus* has until recently been regarded as an infrequent infection that was seen primarily as a complication of viral respiratory infections, particularly influenza. During the last decade, staphylococcal pneumonia has emerged as an important clinical problem. This is the result of the dissemination of MRSA in both healthcare settings and the community.

Epidemiology and pathogenesis

Epidemiology

Until the 1990s, staphylococcal pneumonia was considered an uncommon form of community-acquired pneumonia (CAP), accounting for 2–5% of all CAP and occurring primarily in patients with influenza [1–3]. In addition, *S. aureus* was recognized as an important but infrequent cause of nosocomial pneumonia, especially in pregnant women and in the elderly [4,5].

Hospital-associated pneumonia

However, in the past two decades, the epidemiology of staphylococcal pneumonia has changed dramatically. *Staphylococcus aureus* now accounts for 20–40% of all hospital-acquired pneumonia (HAP) and ventilator-associated pneumonia (VAP). Methicillin-resistant *S. aureus* (MRSA) containing the staphylococcal cassette chromosome (SCC)*mec* types I–III is the predominant organism. A survey of 59 hospitals in the USA involving 4543 patients with culture-positive pneumonia between January 2002 and January 2004 identified MRSA as a frequent potential pathogen in CAP (8.9%), healthcare-associated pneumonia (26.5%), HAP (22.9%), and VAP (14.6%) [6]. Indeed, *S. aureus* was identified as the only pathogen independently associated with mortality by logistic regression analysis [6].

In Europe the changes were even more striking. The incidence of nosocomial staphylococcal pneumonia increased from 2% in 1974 to about 50% in 1997 in Spain and France [7,8]. In the same period MRSA as a cause of VAP increased 3.1-fold and rivaled Gram-negative pathogens such as *Pseudomonas aeruginosa* [9]. In contrast, in 19 Canadian intensive care units (ICUs), MRSA accounted for only 4.7% of respiratory tract pathogens [10].

Community-acquired pneumonia

Similarly, community-acquired staphylococcal pneumonia has resurfaced as an important infection. Necrotizing CAP secondary to *S. aureus* and involving previously healthy young men was first described during the 1914–1918 Spanish influenza epidemic [2]. However, until the late 1990s this disease was seen quite infrequently. A milestone publication by Gillet *et al.* [11] in 2002 from France described 16 cases of CAP caused by a new *S. aureus* strain, now labeled community-associated (CA)-MRSA, that contained the SCC*mec* IV gene as well as Panton–Valentine leukocidin (PVL). In this series the patients were young (median age 14.8 years), the pneumonia was frequently preceded by an influenza-like illness, the disease course was stormy, and the 48-hour hospital mortality was 63%. Similar data from the USA confirmed the lethal potential of this post-influenza pneumonia. A recent report from the USA described 10 patients coinfected with influenza virus and *S. aureus* in December 2006 and January 2007 [12]. In 2006–2007, influenza-associated pediatric mortality in the USA increased in frequency over prior years. Isolation of *S. aureus* from a sterile site or endotracheal tube culture increased markedly over this period. In the 2006–2007 influenza season, 64% of these *S. aureus* isolates were methicillin resistant [13].

In recent years, isolates with the characteristics of CA-MRSA have increasingly been recovered from healthcare settings. This migration has been variable among hospitals, regions, and countries and has made differentiation of CA-MRSA and hospital-associated (HA)-MRSA particularly difficult. For example, in a retrospective surveillance study of all patients with nosocomial MRSA infections in Los Angeles, it was found that CA-MRSA (defined as isolates with SCC*mec* IV) increased from 17 to 56% between

Staphylococci in Human Disease, 2nd edition. Edited by Kent B. Crossley, Kimberly K. Jefferson, Gordon Archer, Vance G. Fowler, Jr.

Table 23.1 Factors associated with community-associated (CA)-MRSA infection [77].

Children less than 2 years old
Athletes (mainly contact-sport participants)
Injection drug users
Men who have sex with men
Military personnel
Inmates of correctional facilities, residential homes or shelters
Veterinarians, pet owners, and pig farmers
Post-influenza like illness and/or severe pneumonia
Recent or concurrent colonization or infection with CA-MRSA

1999 and 2004; among respiratory MRSA isolates, 29% were CA-MRSA [14]. In contrast, between 1990 and 2004, researchers in San Diego found a 19% increase in HA-MRSA respiratory isolates but only a 0.4% increase in sputum CA-MRSA isolates [15].

Risk factors

Risk factors for HAP/VAP caused by MRSA have been identified and include previous receipt of antibiotics, older age, prolonged hospital stay, recent hospital stay, nursing home residence, diabetes mellitus, hemodialysis, and head trauma [16,17].

Risk factors specific for CA-MRSA pneumonia are not clearly identified. One could propose that generic risk factors for CA-MRSA (Table 23.1) would be reasonable considerations, although a recent influenza-like illness followed by severe pneumonia, or the presence of concurrent or recent skin and soft tissue infection with CA-MRSA may be the most important clues to the etiology of pneumonia. Interestingly, a recent European report supported the notion that owning dogs, cats, or horses might also be a risk factor for CA-MRSA pneumonia [18]. In a report from Canada, a fatal case of CA-MRSA pneumonia following influenza in a youngster was described with subsequent CA-MRSA spread to other family members, emphasizing the contagious potential of this pathogen [19].

Pathogenesis

Staphylococcal pneumonia develops following introduction of these organisms into the lower respiratory tract in the absence of effective host defenses. This may occur by inhalation of the organism or by a hematogenous route.

Pneumonia that results from hematogenous spread may be seen in patients with tricuspid valve endocarditis. Patients usually present with chest pain and/or dyspnea. Usually these patients are intravenous drug abusers and have multiple nodular opacities on chest radiography. Patients with soft tissue infection and osteomyelitis may present with pulmonary opacities that cavitate. Pneumothorax (as a result of rupture of a pneumatocele) occurs and empyema may also develop. Evidence of pleural involvement is present in up to 50% of patients with staphylococcal pneumonia [20].

Inhalation of *S. aureus* or contamination of the airway with staphylococci may also result in pneumonia. Because pharyngeal colonization with *S. aureus* is common, the organism may enter the lungs with aspiration of oropharyngeal contents [20]. Contaminated hands of healthcare workers manipulating endotracheal tubes, oral secretions draining onto tracheostomy dressings and endotracheal suctioning are other routes for entry of the organism into the lungs.

Host and bacterial factors

Pulmonary factors that may protect against staphylococcal colonization and infection include alveolar lining fluid containing surfactant, immunoglobulins, complement, free fatty acids, iron-binding proteins, and inflammatory cytokines such as tumor necrosis factor, interleukin (IL)-1 and IL-8; alveolar macrophages; polymorphonuclear neutrophils; and functional cell-mediated immunity. A recent study demonstrated marked immune response by 6 hours after intranasal inoculation of *S. aureus* in mice. A dramatic release of proteins involved in coagulation and inflammation was noted [21]. The staphylococcal factors that may help in establishing pneumonia are described in Chapters 4–6.

PVL has gained considerable attention as a marker of CA-MRSA, but it also has an important function as a white blood cell lysing factor. In a recent study it was found that PVL directly targeted mitochondrial *Bax*-independent apoptosis of human neutrophils following incubation, and mitochondrial membrane changes were visible within 5 min of exposure [22]. In patients with CA-MRSA pneumonia, pulmonary cells with fragmented DNA were visible along with one of the components of PVL, LukS-PVL [22].

Recently, clinical isolates of isogenic PVL-negative and PVL-positive *S. aureus* strains, as well as purified PVL, were used in a mouse acute pneumonia model. PVL alone was found to be sufficient to cause pneumonia, and the expression of PVL induced global changes in transcriptional levels of genes encoding secreted and cell wall-anchored staphylococcal proteins, including the lung inflammatory factor staphylococcal protein A (Spa). Although this suggests that PVL may play an important role in mediating CA-MRSA pneumonia [23], the issue remains unresolved [24]. In addition, staphylococcal adhesion protein (CNA) allows *S. aureus* colonization of the respiratory epithelium. This process is facilitated by viral damage to the respiratory epithelium. After attachment, staphylococci produce α-hemolysin and possibly β- and γ-hemolysins, which may lead to epithelial necrosis, vascular damage, and further lung damage [11].

Differences in the virulence of various staphylococcal strains associated with community-acquired infection have been suggested by observations of disease severity and

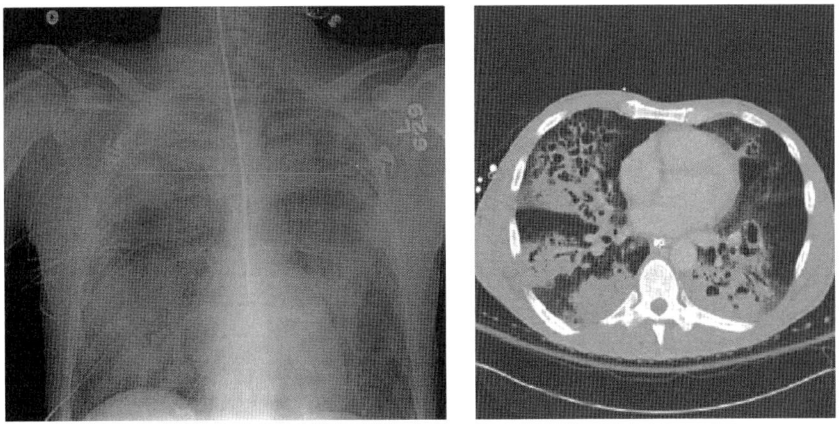

Figure 23.1 Chest radiography and computed tomography of the chest of a young patient with community-associated MRSA.

mortality. Montgomery *et al.* [25] recently demonstrated increased mortality in a rat model of pneumonia when USA300 isolates were compared with USA400. The authors suggested that this was the result of increased expression of regulatory systems that resulted in enhanced output of key virulence factors.

These pathophysiological factors are evident at autopsy of patients who die from CA-MRSA pneumonia, revealing extensive necrotic ulcerations of the tracheal and bronchial mucosa, massive hemorrhagic necrosis of the interalveolar septa, and a high density of staphylococci adhering to the epithelium extending from the larynx to the lobar bronchi. In addition, staphylococcal staphylokinase, a plasminogen activator capable of inactivating neutrophil α-defensins and impairing phagocytosis, was found to be bound *in vitro* by cathelicidin, an antimicrobial peptide. This interaction enables cathelicidin to facilitate fibrinolysis and spread of the infection [26].

Clinical features

Community-acquired pneumonia

Methicillin-susceptible *S. aureus* (MSSA) has been well documented as a cause of CAP. These infections have traditionally been regarded as uncommon and usually occur after a viral respiratory tract infection [1–4]. In general, these infections are of acute onset, usually associated with marked toxicity and, in some cases, with pneumatoceles [1].

Children and young adults are often infected, with neonates comprising a significant proportion of cases [1]. In recent years, CA-MRSA has been increasingly documented as a cause of staphylococcal pneumonia. Pneumonia in young healthy adults with a preceding influenza-like illness, severe respiratory symptoms, hemoptysis, high fever, leukopenia, very high C-reactive protein (> 400 mg/L), hypotension, and a chest radiograph showing multilobular cavitating alveolar infiltrates should lead one to suspect CA-MRSA infection [27,28]. A published review of 25 cases of PVL-positive CA-MRSA pneumonia [29], other case reports [30,31], and an additional case series of 17 patients from the USA [27] supports this clinical presentation (Figure 23.1).

Young age (median 14.8 years) was a remarkable feature of CA-MRSA pneumonia in the Gillet *et al.* series of 16 European patients [11]. In the USA, median age in one study was 21 years [27]. In a study of pediatric patients, there was no difference in the median ages of those with MRSA or MSSA infection [32]. In contrast, the mean age of 36 European patients with hospital-acquired PVL-negative MRSA pneumonia was 70.1 years (range 59.2–81.4) [11].

Underlying disorders have been described in 7 of 44 (16%) of the recently reported cases and preceding documented influenza or clinical respiratory viral infection was present in 83% of the recent US cases [27–31] and in 12 of 16 (75%) of the European cases [11]. Fever of 39°C or more, heart rate 140 bpm or more, hemoptysis and pleural effusion, and leukopenia were significantly more common in PVL-positive patients in the European cases [11]. Hemoptysis has also been frequently described in patients with CA-MRSA pneumonia [27–29,32,33]. In the series described by Gillet *et al.* [11], the survival rate at 48 hours was 63% for PVL-positive patients compared with 94% for PVL-negative patients ($P = 0.007$) (Figure 23.2).

Patients with CA-MRSA pneumonia were often seriously ill and frequently had complications. In the series reported by Hageman *et al.* [27], 81% of hospitalized patients needed admission to the ICU, 62% required intubation, and 46% had chest tube placement. The mortality in this series was 29%. In a recent review of cases of community-acquired *Staphyloccus aureus* pneumonia, the overall mortality in case series published from 1999 to 2007 was 43%.

A report reviewing the factors associated with mortality due to necrotizing CAP caused by PVL-positive MRSA (i.e., CA-MRSA) in 50 patients from Europe found that the overall mortality was 56% and the median survival was 10 days. All deaths were secondary to refractory shock and/or respiratory failure. Fatal outcome was associated with the classical severity factors (need for mechanical ventilation, inotrope use, and acute respiratory distress

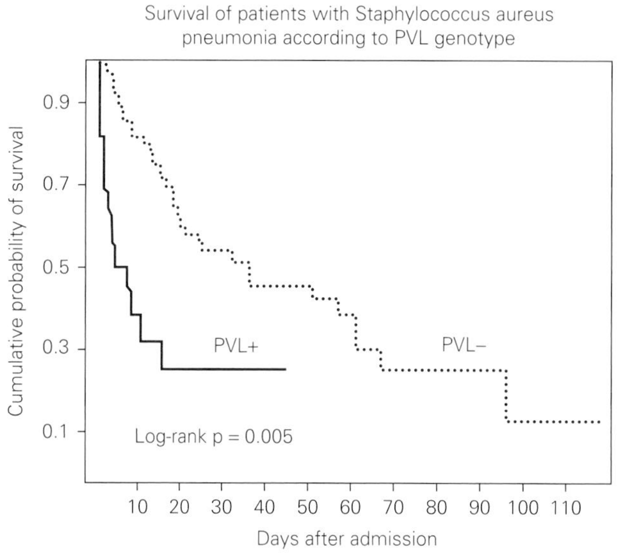

Figure 23.2 Survival of patients with *S. aureus* pneumonia according to Panton–Valentine leukocidin (PVL) genotype. (From Gillet *et al.* [11] with permission.)

syndrome) but in addition with airway bleeding, and with leukopenia and erythroderma occurring within the first 24 hours after admission to the hospital [35].

Hospital-acquired pneumonia

Staphylococcus aureus (both methicillin-susceptible and -resistant) is a common cause of HAP. Isolation of MRSA from the sputum, often without evident signs of clinical pneumonia, is a common and challenging clinical problem. Data from several sources suggest that the incidence of nosocomial staphylococcal pneumonia has been steadily increasing over the last two decades [36]. Unfortunately, there are no distinguishing features of staphylococcal HAP or VAP. Kay *et al.* [20] reported that multilobe involvement, lower lobe disease, and pleural involvement were common findings.

Staphylococcus aureus was reported to cause some 21% of cases of VAP in a French study based on cultural data from bronchoalveolar lavage (BAL) completed a decade ago [9]. In a more recent study, Shorr *et al.* [37] reviewed a database comprising information from 59 US acute-care hospitals and identified 499 clinically diagnosed cases of VAP [37]. Because of the design of the database, these were all early-onset cases of VAP. *Staphylococcus aureus* was the leading cause and was responsible for 154 cases; 59 of these were MRSA. Patients with MRSA were noted to be older than those with susceptible isolates and to have longer hospital stays and greater costs for their care. It is not clear if MRSA pneumonia is associated with increased mortality compared with MSSA pneumonia. Two recent studies of VAP found no difference in mortality in patients with MRSA pneumonia compared with those with methicillin-susceptible infection [38,39].

Diagnosis

The diagnosis of staphylococcal pneumonia may at times be obvious, for example as an infection complicating influenza. Nevertheless, differentiation needs to be made from pneumococcal pneumonia, and Gram stain and sputum culture should be able to differentiate between the two etiologies. On other occasions the exact diagnosis may be obscure. Identifying patients with CA-MRSA requires focusing on epidemiological risk factors combined with a characteristic clinical and radiological presentation. Isolates from blood, other sterile sites, and respiratory secretions should be typed and tested for the presence of PVL.

There are many hurdles in diagnosing the etiology of nosocomial pneumonia accurately. The first is that chest radiography misses 26% of VAP; when compared with autopsy, radiography has a diagnostic accuracy of only 68% [40]. The second is that positive blood cultures accompany only 5–15% of HAP and 24–36% of VAP and are thus of limited diagnostic value [41,42]. Another problem is that endotracheal microbiological sampling has only 40% agreement with lung biopsy [43], and only 15% of the samples meet adequacy criteria (≥ 25 white blood cells/field and ≤ 10 epithelial cells/field) [40,43]. Invasive diagnostic procedures also have their problems. The threshold of bacterial concentration (set at $\geq 10^3$/mL for protected brush specimens and $> 10^4$/mL for BAL) is complicated by antibiotic use and by the timing of the procedure and the need to refrigerate the samples overnight that cannot be processed immediately for (semi)quantitative culture. A recent randomized trial comparing the diagnostic utility of BAL plus quantitative cultures with endotracheal aspiration plus nonquantitative cultures found similar clinical outcomes [44].

A soluble triggering receptor expressed on myeloid cells has recently emerged as a possible candidate test for the diagnosis of VAP [45]. This test has an acceptable degree of specificity, but its value still has to be confirmed in larger studies. A microarray-based technique for the detection of PVL components, and possibly staphylococcal enterotoxins and superantigens, may also in the future prove to be useful in the diagnosis of CA-MRSA pneumonia [46]. Recently, Bouza *et al.* [47] applied E-test strips directly on agar and were able to predict the pathogen's susceptibility and minimum inhibitory concentration (MIC) in 75.4% of the patients within 24 hours. Assays to measure polymerase chain reaction (PCR) and reverse transcriptase (RT)-PCR of PVL, *mec*A, and type IV cassette are under development. It is conceivable that in the not too distant future rapid diagnostic methods will become available for a more timely diagnosis of MRSA pneumonia. Still unknown is the contribution of these diagnostic methods to improvement in care and reduction in mortality of patients with MRSA pneumonia.

At present we suggest the following diagnostic pathway. For patients with suspected staphylococcal pneumonia,

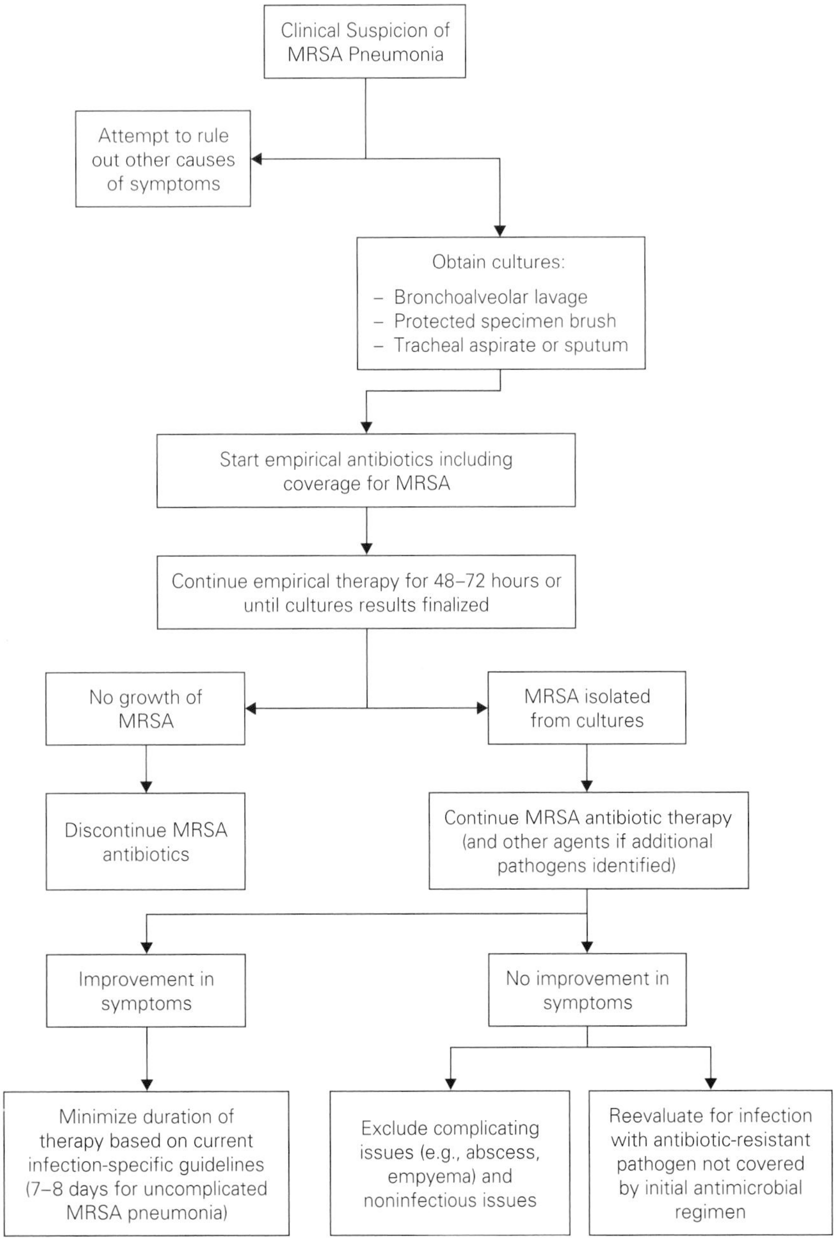

Figure 23.3 Management of suspected staphylococcal pneumonia in the healthcare setting (non-CA-MRSA).

obtain sputum Gram stain and cultures of blood, sputum and pleural fluid (when present) within the shortest possible time. Severe pneumonia in the community should be suspected to be caused by CA-MRSA if the following key features are present: influenza-like prodrome, hemoptysis [48], erythroderma, severe respiratory symptoms, high fever, leukopenia, hypotension [35], and a chest radiograph showing multilobular infiltrates that may cavitate [12]. Additional laboratory testing of the staphylococcal isolate should include assays for the presence of PVL, type IV cassette, and superantigens and enterotoxins. Patients with suspected MRSA pneumonia need to be isolated until susceptibility results become available and treatment should be started within 4 hours [49].

In patients suspected of having healthcare-associated pneumonia (i.e., not CA-MRSA), we use the algorithm shown in Figure 23.3. For those likely to have CA-MRSA, we obtain assays for those factors (e.g., PVL) that will help identify these infections.

Therapy

Timeliness

The first, and perhaps the most important, concept concerning treatment of staphylococcal pneumonia is the need for rapid institution of appropriate antibiotic therapy. This has been repeatedly recognized. For example, Kollef and Ward [50] found that when adequate therapy was instituted, the hospital mortality from VAP decreased from 60.8% to 33.3%. And Kumar *et al.* [51] demonstrated that in septic patients each hour delay in therapy was associated with an increase in mortality of 6.3%. In the recent cases from Georgia and Louisiana in the USA, it was also demonstrated that the median time from onset of symptoms to death was only 3.5 days (range 2–25 days). Of the six patients who received a β-lactam antibiotic and a macrolide, four died [12]. Thus it is clear that appropriate antibiotic therapy must be administered as *early as possible* to minimize short-term mortality from HAP and VAP.

Vancomycin

At present, the Food and Drug Administration (FDA) has approved two agents for use in MRSA pneumonia, vancomycin and linezolid. In addition, newly developed antibiotics are undergoing clinical trials in staphylococcal pneumonia. For years vancomycin was the only antibiotic available for the treatment of MRSA pneumonia. Unfortunately, the cure rate was disappointing. Bacteremia with staphylococcal pneumonia occurs late (mean 9 days) in the course of patients who suffer from HAP/VAP [16] and is associated with an all-cause mortality of 55.5% despite early and appropriate therapy. Vancomycin was associated with more unfavorable outcome compared with β-lactam antibiotics (although the difference was not statistically significant in this relatively small series) [16]. The results of this study are in accord with those of Gonzalez *et al.* [52], which showed inferior therapeutic results with vancomycin compared with β-lactam antibiotics in bacteremic *S. aureus* pneumonia. MRSA and MSSA pneumonia treated with vancomycin had 50% and 47% mortality, respectively, when treated with vancomycin while MSSA pneumonia treated with β-lactams had only 5% mortality [52,53].

The reason for the unsatisfactory results of vancomycin are multifactorial (see Chapter 32 for a detailed discussion of this drug). First, the vancomycin molecule is relatively large (molecular weight 1449.25) and thus penetrates poorly into the alveolar lining fluid (ALF) and into alveolar macrophages. As a result levels attained in ALF are only one-sixth of the plasma concentration [54]. In a clinical trial, 36% of patients had ALF levels of 4 mg/L or less [54], which is below the breakpoint of vancomycin resistance for *S. aureus*. As a result of these findings there have been differing opinions as to whether higher vancomycin trough levels of 15–20 μg/mL would result in better therapeutic outcomes than conventional trough levels of 5–15 μg/mL, although present experience does not suggest that this is the case. Patients having high vancomycin trough serum levels and high serum vancomycin area under the concentration–time curve (AUC) seemed to have similar outcome to those with lower vancomycin serum levels and significantly more nephrotoxicity when vancomycin was combined with other nephrotoxic agents [55–57]. The definitive study to address this issue is still awaited.

A second explanation for the poor performance of vancomycin in patients with CA-MRSA pneumonia may lie in its inability to influence PVL and other toxin production. A recent *in vitro* study evaluating the effect of vancomycin, nafcillin, clindamycin, and linezolid on clinical isolates of MSSA and MRSA has shown that antibiotics have differing effects on the expression of toxins by staphylococci [58]. Clindamycin and linezolid markedly suppressed the formation of PVL, α-hemolysin, and toxic shock syndrome toxin (TSST)-1 (by suppressing translation, but not transcription). On the other hand, nafcillin stimulated toxin production, and toxin levels with vancomycin were comparable to control samples not exposed to antibiotics [58]. Suppression of toxins correlates with improved outcomes, suggesting that neither vancomycin nor nafcillin may be the ideal treatments for toxin-producing *S. aureus*.

It is the general impression of experienced clinicians that vancomycin should not be used as single-agent treatment in CA-MRSA pneumonia. It is unknown at the present time if antibiotic combinations containing rapidly bactericidal agents combined with a toxin-suppressing agent might be associated with improved clinical outcome.

Linezolid

The other therapeutic option for the treatment of MRSA pneumonia is linezolid. Linezolid, unlike vancomycin, has favorable pharmacokinetics in ALF: AUC/MIC, ~ 120; maximum concentration/MIC, 16.1; and time above MIC, 100% [59]. In addition, linezolid, similarly to clindamycin, may reduce staphylococcal exotoxin production [58] and thus diminish proinflammatory cytokine production in the infected lung. It remains to be proven whether the bacteriostatic activity of linezolid against MRSA is beneficial in pneumonia.

Two large, prospective, randomized clinical trials have been completed comparing vancomycin with linezolid. In the first trial conducted by Rubinstein *et al.* [60], patients were randomized to receive either linezolid (600 mg i.v. every 12 hours) plus aztreonam (1–2 g i.v. every 8 hours) or vancomycin (1 g i.v. every 12 hours) plus aztreonam (1–2 g every 8 hours). Of the 396 included in the intention-to-treat analyses, 203 patients received linezolid–aztreonam and 193 received vancomycin–aztreonam. However, only 32 patients were diagnosed with MRSA. Among clinically evaluable patients, cure rates were 66% for linezolid-treated patients and 68% for vancomycin-treated patients. In a second identical trial [61], 623 patients were enrolled. The clinical cure rate in the clinically evaluable population was 68% for patients receiving linezolid ($N = 168$) and 65% for patients receiving vancomycin ($N = 171$). The eradication rate for the microbiologically evaluable population with MRSA (42 patients in total with MRSA) was 63% for linezolid-treated patents ($N = 19$) and 43% for vancomycin-treated patients ($N = 23$) (95% CI –8 to 28.6; P = nonsignificant).

In an analysis of the results of these two pooled trials [60,61] comparing linezolid to vancomycin in HAP and VAP, Wunderink *et al.* [62] were able to obtain statistical significance favoring the use of linezolid in MRSA-infected patients. However, this analysis was criticized on methodological grounds (nonprespecified subgroup analysis, heterogeneity of results in the separate studies, and the small numbers of patients infected with MRSA). As a result, a new industry-sponsored study is underway to clarify whether linezolid is superior to vancomycin.

There are other criticisms of previous antibiotic studies in MRSA pneumonia including the fact that many of these studies were not strictly controlled and included patients with various comorbidities. In addition, MICs were not performed on all isolates in all the studies, vancomycin levels were often not reported, and patients were not stratified according to vancomycin MIC data. Also, most studies were performed before 2000 (i.e., before the upsurge in CA-MRSA), and most studies were performed prior to the gradual upward shift of vancomycin MIC (from < 1 μg/mL to about 2.0 μg/mL) for *S. aureus*. Finally, rigorous testing for vancomycin-heteroresistant *S. aureus* was not performed. Taken together, it is obvious that additional studies of new agents for MRSA pneumonia are urgently needed.

Newer antistaphylococcal agents such as tigecycline, telavancin, and ceftibiprole are presently undergoing clinical trials in HAP/VAP and in CAP. Tigecycline was submitted for approval by the FDA for the therapy of CAP based on two phase III clinical trials that showed equivalence to levofloxacin. However, for the treatment of VAP, tigecycline was inferior to imipenem–cilastatin and equal to this agent in HAP (Wyeth News Release July 6, 2007 http://www.wyeth.com/news).

Treatment considerations for CA-MRSA

Despite the presence and growing importance of MRSA and CA-MRSA as the causative agents of CAP, most existing guidelines do not address this issue specifically, except for the recent Canadian guidelines [50]. This systematic review of the literature should be considered the current definitive recommendations for these infections [50]. The review suggests that severe pneumonia in the community should be suspected to be caused by CA-MRSA if the following key features are present: influenza-like prodrome, hemoptysis, fever, shock, leukopenia, pneumatoceles, abscesses, consolidation, and respiratory failure. Management principles should include culture of blood, sputum, and pleural specimens, infectious disease consultation, ICU admission, chest drainage (if appropriate), and parenteral antibiotic treatment including vancomycin 1 g i.v. every 12 hours or linezolid 600 mg i.v. every 12 hours (which these guidelines consider superior to vancomycin). This treatment needs to be guided by an infectious disease consultant as other options, such as adding rifampicin, may also be considered. Finally, respiratory infection control measures are important as the potential for *S. aureus* to disperse during a concurrent respiratory tract illness where sneezing and coughing are common (the so-called "cloud phenomenon") remains a source of concern for secondary infection [63].

Intravenous immunoglobulin has been shown to neutralize the damaging pore-forming effect of PVL on polymorphonuclear neutrophils [64]. The mechanism of this action is not entirely clear and the role of intravenous immunoglobulin in treating CA-MRSA pneumonia still awaits clinical confirmation. As mentioned earlier, the role of clindamycin and linezolid as therapeutic measures that neutralize staphylococcal toxins [58] needs to be assessed clinically in appropriate trials.

Duration and modification of therapy

After an initial broad-spectrum antibiotic regimen is prescribed, modification of the regimen using a deescalation strategy should be based on the patient's clinical response as well as microbiological results (especially quantitative lower respiratory cultures) and change in the clinical pulmonary infection score (CPIS) [65]. Modification should include decreasing the number and/or spectrum of antibiotics, shortening the duration of therapy in patients who have uncomplicated infections and who are demonstrating signs of clinical improvement, and discontinuing antibiotics altogether in patients who have a noninfectious etiology identified (see Figure 23.3). Prolonged administration of antibiotics to hospitalized patients has been shown to be the most important risk factor for the emergence of colonization and infection with antibiotic-resistant bacteria [9,66]. Therefore, attempts have been made to reduce the duration of antibiotic treatment for specific bacterial infections. Several clinical trials have found that 7–8 days of antibiotic treatment is acceptable for most nonbacteremic patients with VAP [67]. However, with regard to VAP caused by MRSA and certainly for CA-MRSA pneumonia, additional consideration is required as the studies that evaluated a standardized regimen of treatment and the duration of therapy [67,68] contained a limited number of patients with VAP due to MRSA. Thus the optimal antibiotic regimen and its duration in patients with MRSA pneumonia remains unknown.

A recent metaanalysis of four randomized trials demonstrated that the use of quantitative bacterial cultures obtained from the lower respiratory tract may facilitate deescalation of empirical broad-spectrum antibiotics and reduce drug-specific antibiotic days of treatment [69]. Similarly, Kollef *et al.* [6] found that patients with clinical suspicion of VAP but culture-negative BAL results for a major pathogen could have antimicrobial therapy safely discontinued within 72 hours. Interestingly, the mean modified CPIS (a diagnostic algorithm that relies on readily available clinical, radiographic, and microbiological criteria, thus making it an attractive alternative for diagnosing VAP) of these same patients on day 3 was approximately 6, suggesting that this quantitative clinical assessment of the risk for VAP could have been employed to discontinue antibiotics. [65]. As a result, several recently published guidelines for the antibiotic management of nosocomial pneumonia and severe sepsis currently recommend the discontinuation of empirical antibiotic therapy after 48–72 hours if

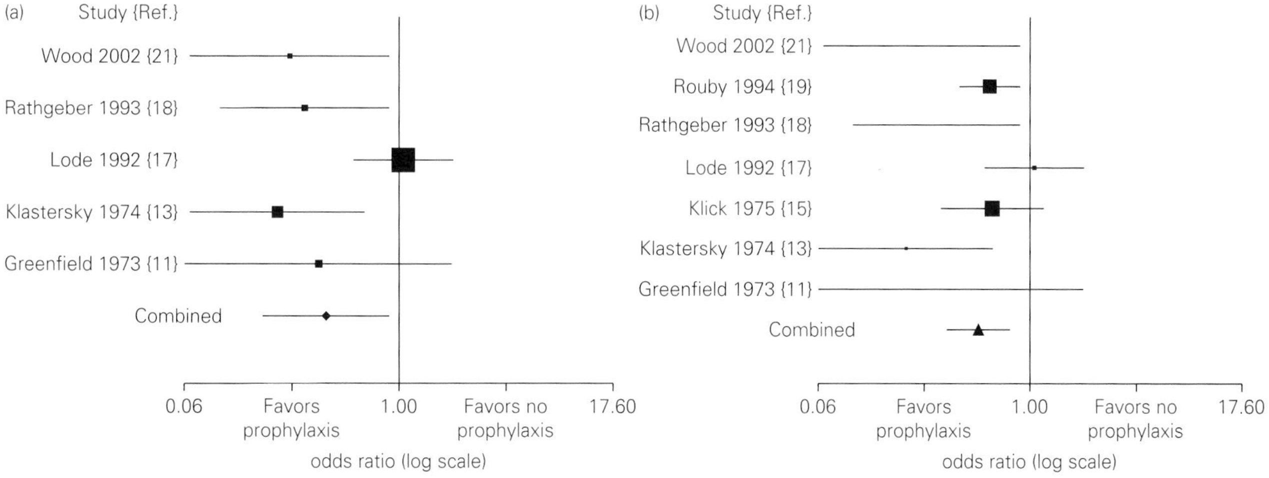

Figure 23.4 Metaanalysis of the effect of intratracheal antibiotics on acquired pneumonia: (a) randomized controlled trials only; (b) secondary analysis including nonrandomized studies. (From Falagas *et al.* [72] with permission.)

cultures are negative or the signs of infection have resolved [70,71]. In the future, more specific markers for the presence of bacterial infection (e.g., sTREM1, procalcitonin levels) may allow shorter courses of empirical antibiotic administration in patients without identified bacterial infections [45].

The management of a patient with suspected staphylococcal pneumonia is depicted in Figure 23.3. Combination therapy for patients with severe pneumonia in the community seems warranted, especially during the influenza season. Use of linezolid for MRSA pneumonia in the ICU setting may well result in better outcomes than standard therapy.

Prophylaxis

Falagas *et al.* [72] performed a metaanalysis on the use of intratracheal antibiotics in preventing HAP but the analysis did not specifically address MRSA. The analysis found a slight nonsignificant preventive effect when randomized controlled trials were analyzed (although the largest study in this analysis found no beneficial effect). When nonrandomized trials were included in their analysis, a small nonsignificant beneficial effect was found. Nevertheless, in this analysis too there was no effect on mortality (Figure 23.4).

In a metaanalysis (including four studies) to determine the effect of oral decontamination with chlorhexidine on the incidence of nosocomial pneumonia (without particular reference to MRSA pneumonia), Pineda *et al.* [73] found a risk reduction for the development of nosocomial pneumonia (odds ratio 0.53, 95% CI 0.27–1.05) but no effect on overall mortality. Another recent investigation found a reduction in the tracheal flora and development of VAP in intubated patients when chlorhexidine or chlorhexidine/colistin were used, with the difference becoming statistically significant in patients with longer-term intubation ($\geq$ 4 days) [74]. There was no significant reduction in *S. aureus* VAP in this study as a result of the oral decontamination.

The use of other topical antistaphylococcal agents like mupirocin has yet to be evaluated as prophylaxis for MRSA pneumonia. A silver-coated endotracheal tube has been tried clinically with results that suggest it contributes to a decreased incidence of pneumonia [75].

Conclusions

The incidence of both HA-MRSA and CA-MRSA pneumonia is increasing. A recent study on the outcomes of VAP demonstrated that MRSA pneumonia was associated with significant prolongation of mechanical ventilation compared with pneumonia caused by other organisms [76].

CA-MRSA pneumonia is associated with an influenza-like illness often affecting young healthy individuals and results in an acute infection with a stormy course, numerous complications, and high mortality rates. HA-MRSA is also a frequently fatal illness that infects the lungs of older debilitated patients, especially those on ventilatory support. A high level of suspicion, aggressive diagnostic measures, and rapid institution of therapy are essential if we are to change the mortality of these diseases. Unfortunately, early diagnosis is often difficult and relies on a careful epidemiological history as well as invasive techniques. Since the rapid determination of the etiology of severe pneumonia is possible only in a limited number of cases, broad-spectrum antibiotics that cover MRSA should be instituted early. Therapy with vancomycin for MRSA (and MSSA) pneumonia has been disappointing for various microbiological, pharmacokinetic, pharmacodynamic, and clinical reasons. Linezolid may be a better choice in the future, although testing in more patients with both HA-MRSA and CA-MRSA pneumonia is essential. The role of adjuvant therapy remains unclear. Protocols aimed at reducing the incidence of VAP through the use of oral chlorhexidine, coated endotracheal tubes, and other prophylactic measures deserve serious consideration.

References

1 Rebhan AW, Edwards HE Staphylococcal pneumonia: a review of 329 cases. Can Med Asoc J 1960;82:513–17.

2 Chickering HT, Park JH Jr. *Staphylococcus aureus* pneumonia. JAMA 1919;72:617:

3 Hausmann W. Karlish AJ. Staphylococcal pneumonia in adults. BMJ 1956;2:845–7.

4 Oswald NC, Shooter RA, Curwen MP. Pneumonia complicating Asian influenza. BMJ 1958;2:1305–11.

5 Schwarzmann SW, Adler JL, Sullivan RJ Jr, Marine WM. Bacterial pneumonia during the Hong Kong influenza epidemic of 1968–1969. Arch Intern Med 1971;127:1037–41.

6 Kollef MH, Shorr A, Tabak YP, Gupta V, Liu LZ, Johannes RS. Epidemiology and outcomes of health-care-associated pneumonia: results from a large US database of culture-positive pneumonia. Chest 2005;128:3854–62.

7 Germaud P, Caillet S, Caillon J, Allenet MC. [Community-acquired pneumonia caused by *Staphylococcus aureus* in non-HIV infected adult patients.] Rev Pneumol Clin 1999;55:83–7.

8 Pujol M, Corbella X, Pena C *et al.* Clinical and epidemiological findings in mechanically-ventilated patients with methicillin-resistant *Staphylococcus aureus* pneumonia. Eur J Clin Microbiol Infect Dis 1998;17:622–8.

9 Trouillet JL, Chastre J, Vuagnat A *et al.* Ventilator-associated pneumonia caused by potentially drug-resistant bacteria. Am J Respir Crit Care Med 1998;157:531–9.

10 Zhanel GG, Decorby M, Laing N *et al.* Activity of tigecycline against 3807 pathogens obtained from Canadian intensive care units: results of the Canadian National Intensive Care Unit (CAN-ICU) Study. Abstract 262, presented at the 46th Annual Meeting of the Interscience Conference on Antimicrobial Agents and Chemotherapy (ICAAC), September 27–30, 2006, San Francisco, CA.

11 Gillet Y, Issartel B, Vanhems P *et al.* Association between *Staphylococcus aureus* strains carrying gene for Panton–Valentine leukocidin and highly lethal necrotising pneumonia in young immunocompetent patients. Lancet 2002;359:753–9.

12 Centers for Disease Control and Prevention. Severe methicillin-resistant *Staphylococcus aureus* community-acquired pneumonia associated with influenza: Louisiana and Georgia, December 2006 to January 2007. MMWR 2007;56:325–9.

13 Finelli L, Fiore A, Dhara R *et al.* Influenza-associated pediatric mortality in the United States: increases of *Staphylococcus aureus* coinfection. Pediatrics 2008;122:805–11.

14 Miller LG, Perdreau-Remington F, Rieg G *et al.* Necrotizing fasciitis caused by community-associated methicillin-resistant *Staphylococcus aureus* in Los Angeles. N Engl J Med 2005;352:1445–53.

15 Crum NF, Lee RU, Thornton SA *et al.* Fifteen-year study of the changing epidemiology of methicillin-resistant *Staphylococcus aureus.* Am J Med 2006;119:943–51.

16 DeRyke CA, Lodise TP Jr, Rybak MJ, McKinnon PS. Epidemiology, treatment, and outcomes of nosocomial bacteremic *Staphylococcus aureus* pneumonia. Chest 2005;128:1414–22.

17 Jeffres MN, Isakow W, Doherty JA *et al.* Predictors of mortality for methicillin-resistant *Staphylococcus aureus* health-care-associated pneumonia: specific evaluation of vancomycin pharmacokinetic indices. Chest 2006;130:947–55.

18 Witte W, Strommenger B, Stanek C, Cuny C. Methicillin-resistant *Staphylococcus aureus* ST398 in humans and animals, Central Europe. Emerg Infect Dis 2007;13:255–8.

19 Adam H, McGeer A, Simor A. A fatal case of post-influenza, community-associated MRSA pneumonia in an Ontario teenager with subsequent familial transmission. Can Commun Dis Rep 2007;33:45–8.

20 Kay MG, Fox MJ, Bartlett JG *et al.* The clinical spectrum of *Staphylococcus aureus* pulmonary infection. Chest 1990;97:788–92.

21 Ventura CL, Higdon R, Hohmann L *et al. Staphylococcus aureus* elicits marked alterations in the airway proteome during early pneumonia. Infect Immun 2008;76:5862–72.

22 Genestier AL, Michallet MC, Prevost G *et al. Staphylococcus aureus* Panton–Valentine leukocidin directly targets mitochondria and induces Bax-independent apoptosis of human neutrophils. J Clin Invest 2005;115:3117–27.

23 Labandeira-Rey M, Couzon F, Boisset S *et al. Staphylococcus aureus* Panton–Valentine leukocidin causes necrotizing pneumonia. Science 2007;315:1130–3.

24 Bubeck Wardenburg J, Palazzolo-Balance AM, Otto M *et al.* Panton–Valentine leukocidin is not a virulence determinant in murine models of community-associated methicillin-resistant *Staphylococcus aureus* disease. J Infect Dis 2008;198:1166–70.

25 Montgomery CP, Boyle-Vavra S, Adem PV *et al.* Comparison of virulence in community-associated methicillin-resistant *Staphylococcus aureus* pulsotypes USA300 and USA400 in a rat model of pneumonia. J Infect Dis 2008;198:561–70.

26 Braff MH, Jones AL, Skerrett SJ, Rubens CE. *Staphylococcus aureus* exploits cathelicidin antimicrobial peptides produced during early pneumonia to promote staphylokinase-dependent fibronilysis. J Infect Dis 2007;195:1365–72.

27 Hageman JC, Uyeki TM, Francis JS *et al.* Severe community-acquired pneumonia due to *Staphylococcus aureus*, 2003–04 influenza season. Emerg Infect Dis 2006;12:894–9.

28 Morgan M. *Staphylococcus aureus*, Panton–Valentine leukocidin, and necrotising pneumonia. BMJ 2005;331:793–4.

29 Wargo KA, Eiland EH III. Appropriate antimicrobial therapy for community-acquired methicillin-resistant *Staphylococcus aureus* carrying the Panton–Valentine leukocidin genes. Clin Infect Dis 2005;40:1376–8.

30 Monaco M, Antonucci R, Palange P, Venditti M, Pantosti A. Methicillin-resistant *Staphylococcus aureus* necrotizing pneumonia. Emerg Infect Dis 2005;11:1647–8.

31 Peleg AY, Munckhof WJ. Fatal necrotising pneumonia due to community-acquired methicillin-resistant *Staphylococcus aureus* (MRSA). Med J Aust 2004;181:228–9.

32 Bodi M, Ardanuy C, Rello J. Impact of Gram-positive resistance on outcome of nosocomial pneumonia. Crit Care Med 2001;29(4 suppl):N82–N86.

33 Micek ST, Dunne M, Kollef MH. Pleuropulmonary complications of Panton–Valentine leukocidin-positive community-acquired methicillin-resistant *Staphylococcus aureus*: importance

of treatment with antimicrobials inhibiting exotoxin production. Chest 2005;128:2732–8.

34 Hidron AI, Low CE, Honig EG, Blumberg HM. Emergence of community-acquired meticillin-resistant *Staphylococus aureus* strain community-onset pneumonia. *Lancet Infect Dis* 2009;9: 384–92.

35 Gillet Y, Venhems P, Lina G *et al*. Factors predicting mortality in community-acquired pneumonia caused by *Staphylococcus aureus* containing Panton–Valentine leukocidin. Clin Infect Dis 2007; 45:315–21.

36 Lynch JP III. Hospital-acquired pneumonia: risk factors, microbiology and treatment. Chest 2001;119:373S–384S.

37 Shorr AF, Tabak YP, Gupta V *et al*. Morbidity and cost burden of methicillin-resistant *Staphylococcus aureus* in early onset ventilator-associated pneumonia. Crit Care 2006;10:R97.

38 Combes A, Luyt CE, Fagon JY *et al*. Impact of methicillin resistance on outcome of *Staphylococcus aureus* ventilator-associated pneumonia. Am J Respir Crit Care Med 2004;170:786–92.

39 Zahar JR, Clec'h C, Tafflet M *et al*. Is methicillin resistance associated with a worse prognosis in *Staphylococcus aureus* ventilator-associated pneumonia? Clin Infect Dis 2005;41:1224–31.

40 Kollef MH. Diagnosis of ventilator-associated pneumonia. N Engl J Med 2006;355:2691–3.

41 Fagon JY, Chastre J, Hance AJ *et al*. Detection of nosocomial lung infection in ventilated patients. Use of a protected specimen brush and quantitative culture techniques in 147 patients. Am Rev Respir Dis 1988;138:110–16.

42 Seidenfeld JJ, Pohl DF, Bell RC, Harris GD, Johanson WG Jr. Incidence, site, and outcome of infections in patients with the adult respiratory distress syndrome. Am Rev Respir Dis 1986;134:12–16.

43 Torres A, Martos A, Puig de la Bellacasa J *et al*. Specificity of endotracheal aspiration, protected specimen brush, and bronchoalveolar lavage in mechanically ventilated patients. Am Rev Respir Dis 1993;147:952–7.

44 Canadian Critical Care Trials Group. A randomized trial of diagnostic techniques for ventilator-associated pneumonia. N Engl J Med 2006;355:2619–30.

45 Gibot S, Cravoisy A, Levy B, Bene MC, Faure G, Bollaert PE. Soluble triggering receptor expressed on myeloid cells and the diagnosis of pneumonia. N Engl J Med 2004;350:451–8.

46 Monecke S, Slickers P, Hotzel H *et al*. Microarray-based characterisation of a Panton–Valentine leukocidin-positive community-acquired strain of methicillin-resistant *Staphylococcus aureus*. Clin Microbiol Infect 2006;12:718–28.

47 Bouza E, Torres MV, Radice C *et al*. Direct E-test (AB Biodisk) of respiratory samples improves antimicrobial use in ventilator-associated pneumonia. Clin Infect Dis 2007;44:382–7.

48 Barton-Forbes M, Hawkes M, Moore D *et al*. Guidelines for the prevention and management of community associated methicillin resistant *Staphyococcus aureus* (CA-MRSA): a perspective for Canadian health care practitioners. Can J Infect Dis Med Microbiol 2006;17(suppl C):1B–24B.

49 Houck PM, Bratzler DW, Nsa W, Ma A, Bartlett JG. Timing of antibiotic administration and outcomes for Medicare patients hospitalized with community-acquired pneumonia. Arch Intern Med 2004;164:637–44.

50 Kollef MH, Ward S. The influence of mini-BAL cultures on patient outcomes: implications for the antibiotic management of ventilator-associated pneumonia. Chest 1998;113:412–20.

51 Kumar A, Roberts D, Wood KE *et al*. Duration of hypotension before initiation of effective antimicrobial therapy is the critical determinant of survival in human septic shock. Crit Care Med 2006;34:1589–96.

52 Gonzalez C, Rubio M, Romero-Vivas J, Gonzalez M, Picazo JJ. Bacteremic pneumonia due to *Staphylococcus aureus*: a comparison of disease caused by methicillin-resistant and methicillin-susceptible organisms. Clin Infect Dis 1999;29:1171–7.

53 Rello J, Torres A, Ricart M *et al*. Ventilator-associated pneumonia by *Staphylococcus aureus*. Comparison of methicillin-resistant and methicillin-sensitive episodes. Am J Respir Crit Care Med 1994;150:1545–9.

54 Scheetz MH, Wunderink RG, Postelnick MJ, Noskin GA. Potential impact of vancomycin pulmonary distribution on treatment outcomes in patients with methicillin-resistant *Staphylococcus aureus* pneumonia. Pharmacotherapy 2006;26:539–50.

55 Hidayat LK, Hsu DI, Quist R, Shriner KA, Wong-Beringer A. High-dose vancomycin therapy for methicillin-resistant *Staphylococcus aureus* infections: efficacy and toxicity. Arch Intern Med 2006;166:2138–44.

56 Jeffres MN, Isakow W, Doherty JA *et al*. Predictors of mortality for methicillin-resistant *Staphylococcus aureus* health-care-associated pneumonia: specific evaluation of vancomycin pharmacokinetic indices. Chest 2006;130:947–55.

57 Jeffres MN, Isakow W, Doherty JA *et al*. A retrospective analysis of possible renal toxicity associated with vancomycin in patients with health care-associated methicillin-resistant *Staphylococcus aureus* pneumonia. Clin Ther 2007;29:1107–15.

58 Stevens DL, Ma Y, Salmi DB, McIndoo E, Wallace RJ, Bryant AE. Impact of antibiotics on expression of virulence-associated exotoxin genes in methicillin-sensitive and methicillin-resistant *Staphylococcus aureus*. J Infect Dis 2007;195:202–11.

59 Conte JE Jr, Golden JA, Kipps J, Zurlinden E. Intrapulmonary pharmacokinetics of linezolid. Antimicrob Agents Chemother 2002;46:1475–80.

60 Rubinstein E, Cammarata S, Oliphant T, Wunderink R. Linezolid (PNU-100766) versus vancomycin in the treatment of hospitalized patients with nosocomial pneumonia: a randomized, double-blind, multicenter study. Clin Infect Dis 2001;32:402–12.

61 Wunderink RG, Cammarata SK, Oliphant TH, Kollef MH. Continuation of a randomized, double-blind, multicenter study of linezolid versus vancomycin in the treatment of patients with nosocomial pneumonia. Clin Ther 2003;25:980–92.

62 Wunderink RG, Rello J, Cammarata SK, Croos-Dabrera RV, Kollef MH. Linezolid vs vancomycin: analysis of two double-blind studies of patients with methicillin-resistant *Staphylococcus aureus* nosocomial pneumonia. Chest 2003;124:1789–97.

63 Bischoff WE, Wallis ML, Tucker BK *et al*. "Gesundheit!" sneezing, common colds, allergies, and *Staphylococcus aureus* dispersion. J Infect Dis 2006;194:1119–26.

64 Gauduchon V, Cozon G, Vandenesch F *et al*. Neutralization of *Staphylococcus aureus* Panton Valentine leukocidin by intravenous immunoglobulin in vitro. J Infect Dis 2004;189:346–53.

65 Luna CM, Blanzaco D, Niederman MS *et al*. Resolution of ventilator associated pneumonia: prospective evaluation of clinical pulmonary infection score as an early clinical predictor of outcome. Crit Care Med 2003;31:676–82.

66 Kollef MH, Fraser VJ. Antibiotic resistance in the intensive care unit. Ann Intern Med 2001;134:298–314.

67 Chastre J, Wolff M, Fagon JY *et al.* Comparison of 8 vs 15 days of antibiotic therapy for ventilator-associated pneumonia in adults: a randomized trial. JAMA 2003;290:2588–98.

68 Ibrahim EH, Ward S, Sherman G, Schaiff R, Fraser VJ, Kollef MH. Experience with a clinical guideline for the treatment of ventilator-associated pneumonia. Crit Care Med 2001;29:1109–15.

69 Shorr AF, Sherner JH, Jackson WL, Kollef MH. Invasive approaches to the diagnosis of ventilator-associated pneumonia: a meta-analysis. Crit Care Med 2005;33:46–53.

70 American Thoracic Society (ATS), Infectious Diseases Society of America (IDSA). Guidelines for the management of adults with hospital-acquired, ventilator-associated, and healthcare-associated pneumonia. Am J Respir Crit Care Med 2005;171:388–416.

71 Chastre J, Fagon JY. Ventilator-associated pneumonia. Am J Respir Crit Care Med 2002;165:867–903.

72 Falagas ME, Siempos II, Bliziotis IA, Michalopoulos A. Administration of antibiotics via the respiratory tract for the prevention of ICU-acquired pneumonia: a meta-analysis of comparative trials. Crit Care 2006;10:R123.

73 Pineda LA, Saliba RG, El Solh AA. Effect of oral decontamination with chlorhexidine on the incidence of nosocomial pneumonia: a meta-analysis. Crit Care 2006;10:R35.

74 Koeman M, van der Vwn AJ, Hak E *et al.* Oral decontamination with chlorhexidine reduces the incidence of ventilator-associated pneumonia. Am J Respir Crit Care Med 2006;173:1348–55.

75 Rello J, Kollef M, Diaz E *et al.* Reduced burden of bacterial airway colonization with a novel silver-coated endotracheal tube in a randomized multiple-center feasibility study. Crit Care Med 2006;34:2766–72.

76 Vidaur L, Planas K, Sierra R *et al.* Ventilator-associated pneumonia: impact of organisms on clinical resolution and medical resources utilization. Chest 2008;133:625–32.

77 Hawkes M, Barton M, Conly J, Nicolle L, Barry C, Ford-Jones EL. Community-associated MRSA: superbug at our doorstep. Can Med Assoc J 2007;176:54–56.

Chapter 24
Urinary Tract Infections

S. Gatermann[1] *and Kent B. Crossley*[2]
[1] Abt. Med. Microbiologie, Ruhr-Universitaet Bochum, Bochum, Germany
[2] University of Minnesota Medical School, Veterans Administration Medical Center, Minneapolis, Minnesota, USA

Introduction

Urinary tract infection (UTI) is one of the most common disorders caused by bacteria. These infections may be frequent and relatively trivial, as in cystitis in normal woman, or severe and potentially life-threatening, as in bacteremic infections originating within the kidney. Surprisingly, staphylococci are not commonly thought of as causes of UTI. *Staphylococcus saprophyticus* is one of the most common causes of UTI in normal young women. Other coagulase-negative staphylococci (CoNS) are occasionally implicated in infection, particularly in individuals with obstruction or disordered urinary tract anatomy. *Staphylococcus aureus* may also be encountered in these situations.

The bulk of this chapter is devoted to a discussion of the nature of UTI caused by *S. saprophyticus*. The relatively limited information available about UTIs caused by other staphylococci is also discussed.

Staphylococcus saprophyticus

The organism

Staphylococcus saprophyticus is a coagulase-negative, novobiocin-resistant staphylococcus. It usually grows in slightly convex, sometimes slimy, unpigmented or yellowish colonies with a diameter of 4–9 mm [1]. The genomic sequence of the type strain ATCC15305 (CCM883) has been determined. It consists of 2.5 Mb and contains a large number of genes that may be involved in osmotic homeostasis [2]. Most strains do not reduce nitrate or produce phosphatase, although an inducible phosphatase of low activity has been described [3]. Clinical isolates usually produce a surface-associated lipase [4], although the type strain is lipase-negative. *Staphylococcus saprophyticus* does not ferment mannose and its growth is inhibited by the presence of this sugar, which can be used for identification of the organism [5]. The basis for this phenomenon is currently unknown. The great majority of strains are resistant to cadmium [6] and arsenate (S. Gatermann, unpublished data). Association of the organism with human disease was first noted in 1962, when Torres-Pereira [7] reported the isolation of closely related CoNS from the urine of 40 women suffering from acute UTI. All isolates possessed antigen 51, as determined by conventional serological techniques. Later, the organism was found to belong to the *Micrococcus* subgroup 3 (later called *S. saprophyticus* subgroup 3) [8–10] of the Baird-Parker scheme and was reclassified as *S. saprophyticus* in 1975 [1].

Clinical manifestations

Staphylococcus saprophyticus almost exclusively causes UTIs in young female outpatients. Bacteriuria in hospitalized patients is only rarely caused by *S. saprophyticus* [11–13], as is UTI in males [9,10]. In the report by Torres-Pereira [7], most isolates were from females. Maskell [8] found 82 infections in women but only one in a male patient, and Digranes and Oeding [11] reported that 59 of 60 of their isolates were from women. Jordan *et al.* [14] found that many patients with *S. saprophyticus* UTI reported to the emergency room of their hospital, corroborating the predilection of *S. saprophyticus* for outpatients. In women aged 16–25 years, *S. saprophyticus* is a common cause of UTIs, accounting for up to 42.3% of all infections [12].

Hematuria, pyuria, and flank pain are common symptoms of UTI caused by *S. saprophyticus* [10,15–17]. Renal involvement is not uncommon and is indicated by a reduced renal concentrating capacity that returns to normal after appropriate treatment [18–20] and by the frequent detection of antibody-coated bacteria [21,22]. Reports of isolation of *S. saprophyticus* from renal calculi [23] also suggest that the kidneys may be infected. However, systemic infection, e.g., septicemia [24,25] or endocarditis [26], is a rare complication of *S. saprophyticus* UTI. As with UTI caused by other organisms, recurrences are common [12,18].

In contrast to the situation seen in women, UTI with *S. saprophyticus* in men occurs mainly in patients with predisposing conditions such as indwelling urinary catheters or obstructions [27]. Hovelius *et al.* [27] reported that men with infection caused by this organism were older and many of them (21 of 51, 41%) were hospitalized. In men

Staphylococci in Human Disease, 2nd edition. Edited by Kent B. Crossley, Kimberly K. Jefferson, Gordon Archer, Vance G. Fowler, Jr.
 ISBN 978-14051-6332-3.

Characteristics	*S. saprophyticus*	Other staphylococci
Patients	Young sexually active females Outpatients without predispositions	Elderly, debilitated, hospitalized men and women
Acquistion	Contamination/colonization of skin and mucous membranes	Often ascends along catheters
Seasonal predilection	Late summer and early fall	None
Catheter present	No	Yes
Reservoir	Animals	Skin of patient
Symptoms	Severe	Usually mild
Involvement of upper urinary tract	Common	Rare
Adhesion to uroepithelia	Yes	No
Antibiotic resistance	Unusual	Common

Table 24.1 Comparison of urinary tract infections caused by *S. saprophyticus* and other staphylococci.

without predisposing conditions, the symptoms were very similar to those observed in women. According to a Swedish report [28], supported by others [29] and by our own observations, there is a second peak of incidence in boys aged 5–15 years. *Staphylococcus saprophyticus* may be a cause of urethritis in men [30] and has been discussed as a cause of prostatitis [31]; however, it is not clear whether it is the causative organism or merely a colonizer, because the organism was recovered during treatment and then disappeared after therapy without additional treatment [32] (Table 24.1).

Infections other than UTI, such as pneumonia [33] or infections associated with port catheters [34], have been described but appear to be very uncommon.

Epidemiology

UTIs with *S. saprophyticus* occur more often during late summer and fall [8,12,21], which parallels the incidence of sexually transmitted diseases [35]. During this part of the year, urethral and rectal cultures contain the organism more often [36,37]. In cases of acute UTI, the mucous membranes of the urogenital tract or the rectum are regularly colonized with *S. saprophyticus* [14,36,38,39], suggesting that infection with *S. saprophyticus* proceeds via the same route as with other urinary pathogens. This notion is supported by the finding that plasmid profiles of isolates from the rectum of infected patients were similar to those of isolates from the urinary tract [38]. However, in a prospective study of 19 female subjects colonized by *S. saprophyticus*, Rupp *et al.* [36] failed to identify any progression to symptomatic UTI. Factors predisposing to UTIs with *S. saprophyticus* include prior outdoor swimming and an occupation in meat processing or meat production [17]. The most significant factor, however, is probably recent sexual intercourse [36,40]. Hormonal influences may also play a role, as infected women tend to have had their menstrual periods more recently and have a concurrent diagnosis of vaginal candidosis [36].

As normal human skin is infrequently colonized with *S. saprophyticus* [41], the source of infection remains unclear. The association of infection with sexual intercourse, peak incidence in late summer and fall, and isolation of the organism from cases of urethritis would suggest sexual transmission, although this has never been conclusively proven. *Staphylococcus saprophyticus* can be isolated from the carcasses of slaughtered animals [38], from the gloves of meat handlers [38], from rectal swabs, udders and fodder of pigs, cattle, and goats [39,42,43], and from processed food such as cheese [44] and sausages [45]. Hedman *et al.* [46] therefore suggested that the ingestion of contaminated raw or undercooked meat precedes colonization and infection with *S. saprophyticus*; however, infections in vegetarians are not exceptionally rare [17]. Recently, using pulsed-field gel electrophoresis (PFGE), the molecular epidemiology of *S. saprophyticus* isolates from Sweden and Germany was studied by Widerström *et al.* [47]. The authors found striking similarities among strains isolated from geographically different areas over an 11-year period. The PFGE analysis noted a uniform banding pattern suggesting a stable genome.

Therapy

Staphylococcus saprophyticus is generally susceptible to most antibiotics, including penicillins, trimethoprim, and aminoglycosides. Although there has been a report of β-lactamase production in *S. saprophyticus*, the minimum inhibitory concentrations of those strains are clinically attainable very easily and the clinical implication of this finding has not been assessed [48]. Therapeutic failures with sulfonamides, nitrofurantoin, and enoxacin have been reported [15,49]. In contrast, the organism is susceptible to most modern inhibitors of DNA gyrase, although less so to fleroxacin [50]. The activity of fosfomycin is weaker than against other staphylococci [51] and erythromycin-resistant strains occur. Thus, most common agents used to treat UTI are active against *S. saprophyticus*. Some reports suggest that the failure rates of short-course regimens are higher than in Gram-negative bacteria [52,53].

Recently, a few isolates carrying mecA have also been described [180,181].

Pathogenesis of *S. saprophyticus* infections

Adhesion to human tissue is an accepted prerequisite for microbial infections. It was known from the work of Hovelius *et al.* [18] that in infected urine *S. saprophyticus* typically adheres to exfoliated epithelial cells and to hyaline or cellular casts. This observation prompted studies on adherence of *S. saprophyticus* to various eukaryotic cells and to extracellular material. The organism was found to cause direct agglutination of sheep erythrocytes [54], to attach to various epithelial cells [55–57], and to exhibit a hydrophobic surface [58]. As *S. saprophyticus* was isolated from the renal pelvis of a patient with urinary calculi [18], it was pointed out that the organism produces the enzyme urease, which had been implicated in the pathogenesis of UTI by *Proteus* sp. [59]. Many of these properties have been studies in detail by various groups.

Virulence factors

Adherence to eukaryotic cells

In urine infected with *S. saprophyticus*, clusters of staphylococci adhering to exfoliated epithelial cells and to hyaline or cellular casts are a typical observation [18]. It was therefore suggested that, similar to uropathogenic *Escherichia coli*, adherence might be a virulence trait of *S. saprophyticus*. *Staphylococcus saprophyticus* adheres in higher numbers to exfoliated uroepithelial cells than to cells from other sources, such as skin or buccal epithelium [56]. It also attached to tissue cultures of human urethra [60]. These data show that *S. saprophyticus* possesses the ability to adhere to human uroepithelial cells; data from other studies indicate that adherence of *S. saprophyticus* to uroepithelial cells is stronger than that of *E. coli*, *Enterobacter aerogenes*, or *Staphylococcus epidermidis* [55,61]. We have recently shown that *S. saprophyticus* ATCC15305 is internalized in human bladder cancer cells [62].

In vitro, permanent eukaryotic cell lines such as HEp2, HeLa, Vero, MDCK, and LLC-PK_1 have been used as targets [57,61,63,64]. Marked variation of adherence capabilities among clinical isolates of *S. saprophyticus* was observed in these experiments [61,63]. Differing adherence phenotypes may indicate differential expression of the structure responsible for this property or may result from the presence of alternate adhesins. It has also been shown that growth under anaerobic conditions increases adhesion of *S. saprophyticus* [65]. In contrast, Teti *et al.* [66] showed that lipoteichoic acids isolated from *S. saprophyticus* partially inhibited binding to exfoliated uroepithelial cells, suggesting that more than one bacterial structure is involved in adhesion.

Some groups have tried to identify structures on the eukaryotic cell that may be targets for adhesins of *S. saprophyticus*. Binding to serum proteins deposited on polyetherurethane disks [67] or to renal tubular cells (LLC-PK_1) derived from pig [64] could be inhibited by *N*-acetyl-D-galactosamine. However, another study suggests that *S. saprophyticus* possesses a surface receptor that recognizes *N*-acetyl-D-glucosamine [68]. In this context it is of interest that surface structures containing *N*-acetyl-D-galactosamine or *N*-acetyl-D-glucosamine are present on urothelial cells [69].

Surface hydrophobicity

Hydrophobic interactions are thought to play a role during the early phases of bacterial attachment. Studies using the BATH (bacterial adhesion to hydrocarbons) test found that many (79 of 100) strains of *S. saprophyticus* isolated from UTIs exhibited a hydrophobic surface [58]; only 2 of 100 were not hydrophobic. Surface hydrophobicity of *S. saprophyticus* is probably mediated by a protein [70], because it can be reduced by protease treatment. Interestingly, some strains express a hydrophobic surface regardless of the growth conditions, whereas in others expression of this property can be affected by appropriate culture conditions [70]. Thus it can be assumed that many strains of *S. saprophyticus* possess the propensity to exhibit a hydrophobic surface that may play a role in adherence of the organism.

Hemagglutination and fibronectin binding

Because adhesion of *E. coli* to epithelial cells is associated with agglutination of erythrocytes [71], the hemagglutination ability of *S. saprophyticus* was also tested. Hovelius and Mårdh [54] reported hemagglutination of sheep erythrocytes in a large proportion (28 of 30) of strains of *S. saprophyticus*. Hemagglutination is heat labile (86°C, 10 min) and sensitive to trypsin and to treatment with trichloracetic acid. These data indicate that the molecule responsible for hemagglutination is a protein.

Clinical isolates of *S. saprophyticus* may show substantially different hemagglutination titers [61,63]. This may be an indication of differential expression of the hemagglutinin; alternatively, there may be more the one hemagglutinin involved in erythrocyte binding. The results of Beuth *et al.* [72] point to the latter conclusion. This group described two subsets of strains, one that agglutinated horse and one that agglutinated rabbit erythrocytes. However, it has been shown that anaerobic growth conditions increase hemagglutination titers and induce hemagglutination in strains that had been characterized as hemagglutination negative [65]. This finding is important, considering that hemagglutination-negative strains can be isolated from clinically overt infections [54,61] and thus would challenge the notion that the hemagglutinin is important in the pathogenesis of *S. saprophyticus* UTI. It also offers an explanation for the observation that expression of the hemagglutinin requires growth in broth, whereas agar-grown bacteria do not hemagglutinate [54]: growth on agar facilitates access to oxygen, whereas broth-grown bacteria likely encounter a more anaerobic atmosphere.

The hemagglutinating strain CCM883 was used for visualization of fibrillar surface structures by electron microscopy [73]. From cells of this strain, a protein with an approximate molecular mass of 160 kDa was purified. Immunogold staining with an antiserum raised to this protein revealed its presence on the cells. The antiserum was also used to inhibit hemagglutination, suggesting that the 160-kDa surface polypeptide is the hemagglutinin of *S. saprophyticus*. Predictably, the amount of surface-associated 160-kDa protein is increased by anaerobic growth [65], the increase being most pronounced in strains that were reputedly hemagglutination negative.

Because many hemagglutinins of Gram-negative bacteria bind to structures on the red cell that contain carbohydrates, a carbohydrate specificity of the *S. saprophyticus* hemagglutinin was sought. Gunnarsson *et al.* [74] found that structures containing terminal β-D-galactose-*p*-(1-4)-β-D-2-acetamido-2-deoxyglucose-*p*-(1-) were good inhibitors of hemagglutination (at concentrations of 200–300 µg/mL). However, other authors [72] reported activity of a combination of *N*-acetylgalactosamine and *N*-acetylglucosamine or *N*-acetylneuraminic acid (sialic acid) and *N*-acetylglucosamine, but not of *N*-acetyl-lactosamine. Others have found that mannose, lactose and, in some strains, *N*-acetyl-lactosamine inhibited hemagglutination [63]. These authors used much higher concentrations of the carbohydrates (5 mg/mL or 0.1 mol/L) than Gunnarsson *et al.* [74]. In our group, we were not able to show any inhibition by these sugars or combinations thereof. Later it was shown that the receptor on erythrocytes is proteinaceous in nature rather than a carbohydrate [75], although the exact receptor has not been identified.

Although it is unclear whether the hemagglutinin binds to carbohydrates, it was found that the molecule binds human fibronectin [76]. Switalski *et al.* [77] had shown earlier that fibronectin binds to CoNS, including *S. saprophyticus*, but did not identify the structures associated with this property. Fibronectin binding is saturable and can be inhibited by fibronectin, the purified hemagglutinin, and antibody to the hemagglutinin [76]. Although the target on the fibronectin molecule for binding by the hemagglutinin is currently unknown, it is clear that the domain on the hemagglutinin/fibronectin-binding protein responsible for fibronectin binding is different from that mediating hemagglutination [76]. The carbohydrate side chains of fibronectin are probably not targets of the bacterial molecule, because deglycosylation does not inhibit the interaction.

Because strains can be found that do not cause hemagglutination but adhere to epithelial cells [61,63], it appears that adhesion and hemagglutination are mediated by different structures. However, nonhemagglutinating strains adhere in low numbers only [61]. Comparison of hemagglutination titers with adherence to epithelial cells yielded conflicting results: in a study that used HEp2 cells [61], no correlation was found, whereas a good correlation between hemagglutination titers and adherence to human ureteral epithelium was seen [78]. These contradictory results may reflect expression of different surface structures on cells of various origins. It has now been shown that the hemagglutinin is involved in adherence to uroepithelial cells [79].

Collagen binding

When studying the surface-associated lipase, Ssp, Sakinc *et al.* [4] found that many strains of *S. saprophyticus* bind to collagen; however, the type strain does not. Previously, only one study had reported collagen binding of *S. saprophyticus* [80].

Autolysin/adhesin of S. saprophyticus

Hell *et al.* [81] used an expression library constructed in *E. coli* to identify a surface protein that reacted with an antiserum raised against the 160-kDa protein described as the fibronectin-binding protein also involved in hemagglutination and adherence. Unexpectedly, the deduced protein sequence showed similarities to the major autolysin of *S. aureus*, Atl [82]. The staphylococcal autolysins are composed of two enzymatic domains that are interconnected by three 150-amino-acid repeats that contain GW motifs [83] which are thought to mediate noncovalent attachment to the cell wall [84]. In contrast to other staphylococcal autolysins, Aas (autolysin/adhesin of *S. saprophyticus*) shows a deletion of about half of the central repeat. Interestingly, expressed peptides derived from Aas bound fibronectin only if at least one of the central repeats was present. A similar situation has been described for *S. epidermidis* AtlE, an autolysin responsible for primary attachment to plastic, where the interconnecting repeats are necessary for binding [85]. In keeping with the proposed function of the GW repeat motifs present in the three long repeats, autolytic activity of the recombinant amidase depended on presence in *cis* of at least one of the long repeats [86]. In addition, autolytic activity could be inhibited by the presence of expressed repeats or by fibronectin [86], indicating that the sequences needed for cell wall binding are also those necessary for fibronectin binding. In the first description of Aas it had also been shown that this protein bound to membrane proteins of erythrocytes that had been immobilized on nitrocellulose membranes [81], thus corroborating its role in hemagglutination.

Surface-associated protein, a surface-associated lipase, of S. saprophyticus

Hemagglutination or adhesion to eukaryotic cells is often mediated by distinct bacterial surface structures. In

Gram-negative organisms these surface organelles are usually heteropolymers of small subunits that have distinct functions such as structural integrity or adherence. Some Gram-positive bacteria also express proteinaceous surface appendages. These proteins are usually larger and possess several domains with different functions. A paradigm is the fibrillar M protein of the group A streptococci that mediates adhesion to eukaryotic cells and to matrix proteins, and plays a role in the pathogenesis of sequelae associated with *Streptococcus pyogenes* infections [79]. Other examples include fimbriae and fibrillae of *Streptococcus sanguis* [87], the aggregation substance of *Enterococcus faecalis* [88], and several surface proteins of *S. aureus*.

Until 1989, there were only a few reports that indicated surface appendages on *S. saprophyticus* might exist [89,90]. In none of these studies, however, was it attempted to isolate or characterize the molecules associated with the observed structures. In 1989, we discovered that unusual culture conditions, i.e., growth on dialysis membranes placed on top of brain heart infusion agar, were needed for efficient expression of a previously undescribed surface protein of *S. saprophyticus* [91]. The protein can be released from the bacteria by mild shearing. It possesses an apparent molecular mass of 95 kDa when run under reducing conditions and exhibits a native molecular mass of about 500 kDa under nonreducing conditions in the presence of 8 mol/L urea. The protein is present in most clinical isolates of *S. saprophyticus* (> 98%) [92]. The surface of bacteria producing this protein is covered with copious amounts of surface-associated material [91]. The appendages are similar in length (50–75 nm) but have no determinable width and thus match the definition of fibrils. They are most conspicuous between adjacent cells and are more prominent on the "old" cell wall, whereas the septation areas of dividing cells are not covered, a situation similar to that seen with the aggregation substance of *E. faecalis*. The protein, designated Ssp (*S. saprophyticus* surface-associated protein), binds to tubular epithelial cells (LLC-PK_1) in a concentration-dependent manner [93] and thus may function as an adhesin of *S. saprophyticus*.

Since we did not find any target for binding of Ssp, its function remained largely elusive for many years. In the new millennium we used primers derived from the N-terminus of the native protein and another derived from the N-terminus of an Ssp fragment derived by proteolytic digestion to identify its genetic sequence. Unexpectedly, the sequence showed high similarities to lipases, especially to those of other staphylococci [4]. In keeping with this observation we found that virtually all clinical isolates of *S. saprophyticus* express lipolytic activity and possess *ssp*; however, the sequenced type strain does not express this enzyme due to a mutation in its structural gene. Since collagen binding had been described for another surface-associated lipase of *S. epidermidis*, GehD [94], we tested this property for the wild type, a specific lipase-negative mutant, and the complemented mutant and did not find any evidence for participation of the surface-bound enzyme in collagen binding. Lipases have been thought to contribute to virulence by detoxification of toxic lipids released by the host, alone or in combination with another enzyme termed FAME (fatty acid-modifying enzyme) [95]. Very few attempts have been made to associate virulence with expression of lipases and we are not aware of any proposed function in UTIs. However, in a recent preliminary work using an infection model in mice, we were able to show that Ssp may contribute to virulence in the urinary tract [96].

Very similar to other staphylococcal lipases, Ssp prefers short-chain fatty acids although long-chain substrates are cleaved too, justifying its classification as a true lipase [97]. The protein binds calcium ions, similar to the other staphylococcal lipases; withstands boiling for 15 min, preserving 30% of its initial activity; and shows a pH optimum of about 6.

Collagen-binding SdrI

When screening a library of *S. saprophyticus* 7108 DNA with an antiserum directed toward Ssp, we obtained a reactive clone whose DNA encoded a protein belonging to the MSCRAMMs (microbial surface components recognizing adhesive matrix molecules) [98]. The protein shows the typical structural properties of SD repeat proteins, a subgroup of Gram-positive surface proteins that possess the typical properties of cell wall-associated proteins, such as a cell wall-anchoring motif (LPXTG), but additionally show a region characterized by repeats rich in serine and arginine, hence the name SD proteins [99]. The SdrI of *S. saprophyticus* 7108 possesses the longest SD repeat region described so far, 834 amino acids in total. The exact function of the SD repeats is unknown, although in ClfA, the fibrinogen-binding clumping factor of *S. aureus*, a minimal length is required for function [100]. By using a specific *sdr*I mutant, we could show that SdrI is the collagen-binding adhesin of *S. saprophyticus*. Preliminary work using an *in vivo* infection model in mice suggested that SdrI is involved in the pathogenesis of UTIs [96]. In *E. coli* it has been shown that collagen binding by the Dr adhesin is needed for efficient internalization of the bacteria into host cells [101].

Hemagglutinin/adhesin UafA

The genomic sequence of *S. saprophyticus* ATCC15305 revealed the presence of only one cell wall-bound surface protein, UafA [2]. A deletion mutant no longer hemagglutinated sheep erythrocytes and did not adhere to a human T24 bladder carcinoma cell line. These functions were reinstituted by introducing *uaf*A into the mutant. Although these data seemed to indicate that *S. saprophyticus* possesses fewer surface proteins than other staphylococci [2], our data on *sdr*I, which is not present in the sequenced strain, and on Ssp, which is not expressed by the type strain, suggest that similar to other staphylococci, adhesion is redundantly encoded in *S. saprophyticus*.

Miscellaneous virulence factors

Expression of several other properties that may contribute to virulence has been described. These include production of an extracellular slime substance, whose expression requires the presence of urea but is repressed by alkaline pH [102]. However, the significance of slime production during clinical infections remains unclear because action of the urease will cause alkalization of the urine during infection and because other authors [103], using Congo red agar to detect slime production, found slime production in only 11% of clinical isolates.

Other properties include the presence of a capsule [104], extracellular products with T-cell mitogenic activity [105], invasiveness into Hep2 cells [106], and binding to nasal mucin [107]. The chemical composition of these factors and their possible relevance during infections is largely unknown. Interestingly, the presence of various sugars or periodate treatment of mucin did not decrease binding of *S. saprophyticus*, whereas trypsin treatment significantly decreased attachment [107].

Toxic products

Staphylococcus saprophyticus has been generally described as a nonhemolytic species [1]. No hemolysis is observed after growth on agar containing sheep, rabbit, ox, or human erythrocytes. However, one group has reported that some strains (9 of 14) produced a δ-toxin-like extracellular compound that exhibits hemolytic activity toward human and guinea-pig erythrocytes [108,109] and caused damage to mouse fibroblasts [109]. Although the *agr* system of *S. saprophyticus* has been cloned and sequenced and was found to possess and produce an RNAIII [110], this molecule does not code for δ-toxin activity.

Urease

Staphylococcus saprophyticus has been isolated from urinary stones and from the pelvic urine of a patient with a ureteral concretion [23]. Urinary concretions may form during infection with urease-producing bacteria [111]; interestingly, all clinical isolates of *S. saprophyticus* produce urease. The enzyme hydrolyzes urea, yielding ammonia and carbon dioxide. In aqueous environments ammonium ions are formed, which leads to alkalization. This in turn causes precipitation of salts like struvite ($MgNH_4PO_4$) or carbonate apatite [$Ca_{10}(PO_4CO_3OH)_6(OH)_2$] [112]. In addition, the alkaline pH and ammonia as well as ammonium ions can exert direct toxic effects toward the eukaryotic cell and may modulate the immune responses of polymorphonuclear neutrophils [113,114].

The native urease of *S. saprophyticus* has a molecular mass of 420 kDa and consists of three different subunits of 72.4, 20.4, and 13.9 kDa [115]. The enzyme's K_m is 6.64 mmol/L and V_{max} 4.59 μmol/min per mg [116]. About 5.3 kb of DNA that code for the structural subunits and several auxiliary peptides are required for expression of enzyme activity. This is in agreement with findings for many other microbial ureases. The additional peptides are necessary, for example, for nickel incorporation or regulation [117]. Interestingly, the ureases of *S. saprophyticus* and the related *S. xylosus* contain threonine instead of the usually highly conserved cysteine in the active center [115,118].

To assess the contribution of the enzyme to virulence of *S. saprophyticus*, a urease-negative mutant was generated by chemical mutagenesis [119]. In addition, the urease genes were cloned and reintroduced into the urease-negative mutant [116]. Virulence of the parent and the mutant strain was assessed in a rat model of ascending unobstructed UTI. Organs of animals infected with the parent strain yielded higher bacterial counts and were larger than those challenged with the mutant. The strain carrying the cloned urease gene showed bacterial counts similar to those of the urease-positive parent strain. Moreover, urinary calculi consisting of struvite were only seen in animals infected with the urease-positive strains. Differences in kidney bacterial counts and kidney weights were not statistically significant but differences in bladder bacterial counts and weights were. It was therefore concluded that the urease of *S. saprophyticus* contributes mainly to cystopathogenicity.

These experiments therefore established that urease functions as the major virulence factor during UTI with *S. saprophyticus*. The enzyme is responsible for the tissue damage seen in experimental infections and may therefore contribute to tissue invasiveness.

Hypothetical events during infections with *S. saprophyticus*

The most important step during infection is probably colonization by the microorganism. As *S. saprophyticus* is not a common member of the resident microbial flora of the human skin, colonization requires acquisition of the organism, e.g., through ingestion of contaminated food. Sexual transmission may play a role in some situations. If one accepts that rectal colonization usually precedes infection, it is safe to assume that *S. saprophyticus* encounters anaerobic conditions at this site. Anaerobic conditions increase the amount of surface-exposed hemagglutinin/adhesin of *S. saprophyticus* and may thus increase the propensity of a given strain to cause infection. Host factors, like previous sexual intercourse, prior outdoor swimming, or a particular hormonal status, may serve as additional predisposing conditions. This is suggested not only by an epidemiological study [36] but also by *in vitro* data that showed a higher susceptibility to adherence by the vaginal epithelium during the postmenstrual phase [120]. Once *S. saprophyticus* has entered the urinary tract, Aas, SdrI and UafA may function as adhesins. It is unclear which target these proteins bind to, since intact uroepithelia do not express surface-exposed fibronectin [121]. It is also interesting to note that *S. saprophyticus*, when grown under conditions that facilitate expression of the hemagglutinin, shows a relative preference for kidney colonization in experimental infections [61]. This corresponds to the frequent kidney involvement in clinical infections. The eukaryotic targets for binding of *S. saprophyticus* are probably surface proteins, because experiments with mucin [107] or fibronectin [76] did not find a major role for protein–carbohydrate interactions. After a microcolony has been established, toxic products generated by urease might accumulate and cause tissue damage, giving rise to the rather severe symptoms seen in clinical infections. Ssp, which is produced by cells grown on a solid support, might play a role as an intercellular adhesin or provide a matrix for crystal formation effected by urease activity.

It is clear from clinical as well as experimental data that urease, the hemagglutinin, SdrI, and Ssp are expressed during infection with *S. saprophyticus* [96]. An anaerobic atmosphere and a liquid environment, which both facilitate expression of the hemagglutinin, are likely to be encountered in the human host. There is also room in this concept for fibronectin binding: it may come into play after some tissue damage has been caused, which would expose subepithelial tissues and give rise to fibronectin secretion. Secreted host proteins, cellular debris, extracellular bacterial proteins, slime, and urease-generated precipitation of salts may form concretions with embedded bacteria that would facilitate reinfection, contribute to tissue damage and, in rare cases, lead to persistence of the organism. Binding to collagen, mediated by SdrI, might contribute to pathogenesis and persistence by a mechanism similar to that in *E. coli* [101].

Other coagulase-negative staphylococci

UTIs with CoNS other than *S. saprophyticus* present with a different clinical picture and a distinct epidemiology (see Table 24.1). These bacteria are most often isolated from hospitalized patients with predisposing conditions such as indwelling catheters, instrumentation, or anatomical abnormalities [9,11,19,108,122]. In addition, the patients are usually older than those with *S. saprophyticus* UTI [123] and there is no predilection for women [124]. In this clientele, contamination or colonization of the urinary tract is common, causing severe problems in interpretation of a positive urine culture [125]. Moreover, infections with CoNS often present with few symptoms [126], which aggravates the diagnostic difficulties. In outpatients, contamination and infection can usually be discriminated by taking a second sample [127]; unfortunately, this did not hold true for inpatients.

Virulence factors of CoNS have been studied most extensively for device-associated infections caused by *S. epidermidis*, whereas data on properties associated with virulence in UTI is scant, probably because it is difficult to establish experimental infections with CoNS. Similar to the situation in humans, successful induction of experimental infection with *S. epidermidis* usually requires the presence of a foreign body, such as a catheter. Although one can be tempted to assume that the pathogenesis of UTI by *S. epidermidis* or other CoNS may rely on the same virulence factors as discussed for device-associated infections, this view would be challenged by a report that *S. epidermidis* strains from patients with infection or colonization did not differ in putative virulence factors [125]. Since that study, many new virulence factors have been discovered and these properties need to be assessed. In addition, even with CoNS, there is some species restriction in clinical UTIs: *S. epidermidis*, *S. haemolyticus*, and *S. warneri* predominate [123], although other species have also been described [128,129]. This may be due to the relative predominance of these three species on the human skin or may indicate a propensity to cause infection.

Staphylococcus lugdunensis has been associated with a variety of serious infections in humans. Haile *et al.* [130] found that 6% of 500 isolates of CoNS isolated from consecutive urine cultures were *S. lugdunensis*. The organism was never isolated alone, but only as part of mixed flora. Only one-third of the patients were treated with antibiotics. More recently, a child from whom this organism was isolated in urine was reported [131]. The organism was isolated in pure culture and a renal scan showed focal defects consistent with pyelonephritis.

Virulence factors of coagulase-negative staphylococci other than *S. saprophyticus*

If one assumes that the steps in the pathogenesis of UTI with CoNS are similar to those of device-associated infections, colonization of an artificial device, such as an indwelling catheter, would be the first step. In contrast to *S. saprophyticus*, *S. epidermidis* and *S. haemolyticus* are abundant on the human skin and most strains causing infections are probably endogenous. Devices introduced into the body are contaminated during the insertion process or are colonized from external contaminated sites such as the catheter hub or, in urinary catheters, from the meatus [124]. It is generally accepted that the most important virulence factor of CoNS is their ability to adhere to and form biofilms on artificial devices. In earlier reports, formation of a biofilm was labeled slime production. However, current opinion is that biofilm formation can be separated into two phases: primary attachment and accumulation. Earlier authors did not recognize this differentiation and measured only the ultimate outcome, namely biofilm formation. For this reason, it is not clear whether an observation of absence of slime (or biofilm) was due to reduced attachment or inability to form a multilayered colony. In recent years, techniques that differentiate these phases have become available. Care should be exercised when interpreting the results of older studies.

Primary attachment

In the very early phase of attachment, unspecific forces such as Van der Waals forces, electrochemical forces, or hydrophobic interactions are thought to play a major role [132]. Specific mechanisms, such as receptor-mediated adherence, ensue. Several adhesins are thought to function during this phase. Tojo *et al.* described a large (> 500 kDa) polysaccharide adhesin (PS/A) that mediates attachment but is not responsible for formation of a multilayered colony [133,134]. The antigen inhibits binding of PS/A-positive strains to catheters and is crucial in the pathogenesis of device-associated infections because Tn*917* insertions abolishing expression of the molecule reduce virulence [135]. In addition, immunization with PS/A results in protection from infection [136]. However, some strains do not produce PS/A, but still attach and form biofilms [133,137]. The hemagglutinin of *S. epidermidis*, described by Rupp and Archer [138], could be the additional adhesin implicated by this finding. Hemagglutination is associated with adherence as measured by biofilm production and is probably mediated by a different cell surface carbohydrate [139].

Although most surface antigens described for *S. epidermidis* consist mainly of carbohydrates, there is evidence that proteins may also be involved. Timmermann *et al.* [140] raised monoclonal antibodies to whole cells of *S. epidermidis* and identified an antibody that inhibited adherence to polystyrene. This antibody recognized a surface-associated protein that appears in two forms: a 280-kDa and a 250-kDa product. Production of the 280-kDa polypeptide is associated with the expression of adherence, whereas strains producing the 250-kDa protein are nonadherent. Switch between the two forms is apparently effected by proteolytic cleavage of the 280-kDa product [141].

Comparatively little is known about the genetics of adhesion. Recently, Heilmann *et al.* [142] identified Tn*917* mutants that lacked expression of four cell surface proteins and showed decreased primary adhesion but were able to form multilayered colonies [142]. A cloned 60-kDa protein complemented the adhesion phenotype.

There have been only a very few reports on adhesion of CoNS to uroepithelia. Most often other CoNS species were used as controls in experiments with *S. saprophyticus*. Adherence of *S. epidermidis* was unequivocally less avid than that of *S. saprophyticus*.

Formation of multilayered cell clusters

Staphylococci usually form cell clusters and hence posses means for intercellular interaction. The typical appearance of catheters colonized with *S. epidermidis* is that of multilayered colonies or bacterial films embedded in an extracellular matrix. Production of this extracellular material occurs only after prolonged incubation, suggesting a role for additional factors prior to this phase. Owing to the impressive appearance of the slime layer, a considerable amount of work focused on this property. Several attempts were made to purify and characterize this material. Ludwicka *et al.* [143] used ion-exchange chromatography to separate their slime preparation into four fractions, of which three contained galactose as the major component while one contained mainly mannose. Later work, by Drewry *et al.* [144] and Hussain *et al.* [145], indicated that the galactose of slime preparations probably originates from agar. Preparations from media solidified without agar did not contain significant galactose but yielded glucose and glucosamine as the major components [145]. Christensen *et al.* [134] described a slime-associated antigen (SAA) that was present in extracts prepared from biofilm-producing strains but not in nonbiofilm-producing mutants. The antigen is probably a carbohydrate, because it is heat resistant and resistant to protease treatment. It consists mainly of glucose and contains galactose in only small amounts. The SAA status of a given strain predicts its ability to produce biofilm, whereas the PS/A status predicts its ability to adhere to plastic.

Apparently, there are several antigens involved in biofilm formation. Mack *et al.* [146] described a polysaccharide intercellular adhesin that is associated with accumulative growth. Mutants, generated by Tn*917* mutagenesis, were no longer able to produce biofilm but showed no significant difference from the parent in primary attachment experiments [147]. Later, the structure of this polysaccharide was determined [148]. Heilmann *et al.* [142] characterized a Tn*917* mutant that no longer showed accumulative growth but still adhered to polystyrene, and Schumacher-Perdreau *et al.* [149] used chemical mutagenesis to generate an accumulation-negative mutant that lacked expression of two extracellular proteins [149].

Biological effects of biofilm production

Growth of staphylococci in a biofilm interferes with the action of commonly used antibiotics [150,151] as well as with phagocytosis of the adhering bacteria [152]. The biology of both phenomena is not well understood; however, most slime-producing *S. epidermidis* are less hydrophobic than their counterparts that do not produce slime and a hydrophilic surface makes a particle less prone to phagocytosis. It has also been noted that *S. epidermidis* adhering to polyurethanes express increased levels of urease and degrade the artificial substratum [153].

Enzymes, toxins, and inhibition of neutrophils

Staphylococcus aureus is known to produce and secrete a plethora of virulence factors. Although presence of extracellular virulence factors is less common in CoNS, enzymes such as nucleases or proteases, hemolysins, toxins, and factors inhibiting the action of neutrophils have been described. Many clinical isolates of *S. epidermidis* produce an extracellular elastase [154]. The enzyme is a cysteine protease that degrades human immunoglobulins, fibronectin, albumin, and fibrinogen [155] and may therefore contribute to invasiveness of the organism. Other extracellular enzymes are less well characterized and their contribution to pathogenesis is rather speculative.

Staphylococcus epidermidis elaborates a hemolysin with similarities to the δ-toxin of *S. aureus* [156]. Strains isolated from infants with neonatal necrotizing enterocolitis produced high levels of this toxin and were more likely to be resistant to multiple antibiotics [157]. Production of enterotoxins or a substance like toxic shock syndrome toxin has been described [158,159] but appears to be very uncommon. Noble *et al.* [160] described a neutrophil-inhibitory factor secreted by some strains of *S. epidermidis*. The substance inhibits neutrophil bactericidal activity and consists of two fractions with high (> 300 kDa) and low (20–40 kDa) molecular mass of unknown chemical composition.

Interplay of virulence factors during UTI with coagulase-negative staphylococci

CoNS other than *S. saprophyticus* seem to require impaired host defense mechanisms to establish infection. Since these bacteria are usually less adherent than *S. saprophyticus*, indwelling devices or anatomical abnormalities may provide routes for access and niches for survival. Once a biofilm has been formed, the protective functions of the extracellular material hamper eradication of the bacteria by therapeutic or immunological means. Bacteria that detach from the biofilm can grow to high densities in the static planktonic phase that is typical of urinary tracts with catheters or anatomical abnormalities and facilitate colonization by an organism with lower inherent virulence. In this situation, even the scarce extracellular virulence factors of *S. epidermidis* may gain some importance.

Admittedly, this sequence of events and the role outlined for the various virulence properties is rather speculative; however, it would explain the lack of symptoms in most patients and the preference for the debilitated host who has undergone urinary instrumentation or manipulations.

Urinary tract infections caused by *Staphylococcus aureus*

Staphylococcus aureus may also cause UTI. The infections range from asymptomatic bacteriuria to those that are severe and associated with bacteremia. Given the frequency with which the perineal area is colonized with *S. aureus*, it is perhaps surprising that this organism is relatively uncommonly recovered as a cause of UTI [161]. In two community-based studies in Britain and France, 0.5 and 1.3% of isolates from urine cultures were *S. aureus* [162,163]. Demuth *et al.* [164] found that *S. aureus* was isolated from about 1% of positive urine cultures in a study conducted in a municipal hospital and in a veterans' hospital. Arpi and Renneberg [165] reported that 3.3% of positive urine culutures performed between 1977 and 1981 at a Danish hospital yielded *S. aureus*.

Table 24.2 Symptoms at presentation among 33 patients with *S. aureus* urinary tract infection.[1]

Symptom	No. (%) of patients
Fever (> 38.5°C)	24 (73)
Change in mental status	7 (21)
Hematuria	11 (33)
Dysuria	4 (12)
Suprapubic pain	4 (12)
Flank pain	1 (3)

[1] Defined as > 10^5 organisms/mL from a voided specimen or 10^4 organisms/mL from a catheter specimen, no clinical evidence of a site of infection outside the urinary tract, and at least two of the following: temperature > 38.5°C, change in mental status, gross hematuria, suprapubic discomfort, dysuria, or flank pain [177].

In both Demuth and Arpi's studies, elderly men were the group that most frequently had *S. aureus* bacteriuria. Demuth *et al.* [164] reported that 71% of their patients had pyuria and only 39% had urinary tract symptoms or fever. In both studies, indwelling catheters, urinary tract obstruction, instrumentation or surgery were frequent (45–66% of patients). Demuth's group found 55% of cases to be nosocomial; in Arpi's study 81% were hospital-acquired. Secondary bacteremias occurred in 5.5% and 8.3% of patients, respectively, in the two studies.

Considerable other data make it clear that *S. aureus* may cause serious UTI at any age. Fortunov *et al.* [166] reported three UTIs among a group of 12 neonates with invasive community-acquired *S. aureus* infections. In older patients, this organism may cause clinical UTI and perinephric or renal abscess (Table 24.2). In a series of prostatic abscesses published 20 years ago, 6 of 99 were caused by *S. aureus* [167]. While there is no comparable recent review, case reports published in the last 5 years are all of methicillin-resistant infections [168–171]. These abscesses are most commonly the result of bacteremia.

In nursing homes, *S. aureus* bacteremia may be seen as a complication of *S. aureus* UTI. Lesse and Mylotte [172] noted that the urinary tract was the most common source for bacteremic infection in a group of nursing home patients and accounted for 18% of episodes. Sapico *et al.* [173] reported 11 patients with methicillin-resistant *S. aureus* (MRSA) bacteriuria. Most of these patients had had indwelling urinary catheters or urological operations. Bacteriuria was documented to last up to 14 weeks. Coll *et al.* [174] examined risk factors for MRSA bacteriuria in a skilled care nursing home. Urinary catheter and antibiotic use were significantly associated with MRSA bacteriuria.

Lee *et al.* [175] studied the relationship between *S. aureus* bacteremia and bacteriuria over a 5-year period. These investigators found that among 59 patients with *S. aureus* bacteremia who had a urine culture within 48 hours of a positive blood culture, 27% had more than 10^5 *S. aureus* recovered from the urine in pure culture. In 6 of these 16 patients, staphylococcal UTI was apparently the source of the bacteremia. In the balance of the subjects, there was no explanation for the bacteriuria.

Three additional studies have examined the relationship between *S. aureus* bacteremia and bacteriuria. Sheth and DiNubile [176] identified all patients with *S. aureus* in urine cultures over a 1-year period in a 550-bed university medical center. They found that 40 of 45 patients with *S. aureus* in the urine were not bacteremic and that in only one of these patients was a distant infection later diagnosed. Muder *et al.* [177] noted that, of 102 patients with *S. aureus* bacteriuria, 13 were bacteremic. These authors observed that urinary tract colonization is often followed by symptomatic infection and bacteremia. In a more recent study, 2 of 79 bacteremic patients had *S. aureus* bacteriuria in the absence of clinical signs of a UTI [178]. Taken together, these results indicate that *S. aureus* bacteremia may develop from a urinary tract site. It is also likely, at least in a small percentage of patients, that bacteriuria may be a consequence of bacteremia. In patients with no indwelling catheter and no urinary tract symptoms, bacteriuria may be associated with a distant and undiagnosed focus of staphylococcal infection. The data suggest this does not occur frequently. One study has examined the occurrence of mortality in patients with concomitant *S. aureus* bacteremia and bacteriuria [179]. These authors found that the simultaneous presence of both conditions was a significant risk for both intensive-care admission and death.

References

1 Schleifer KH, WE Kloos. Isolation and characterization of staphylococci from human skin. I. Amended descriptions of *Staphylococcus epidermidis* and *Staphylococcus saprophyticus* and description of three new species: *S. cohnii*, *S. haemolyticus*, *S. xylosus*. Int J Syst Bacteriol 1975;25:60–1.

2 Kuroda M, Yamashita A, Hirakawa H *et al.* Whole genome sequence of *Staphylococcus saprophyticus* reveals the pathogenesis of uncomplicated urinary tract infection. Proc Natl Acad Sci USA 2005;102:13272–7.

3 Soro O, Grazi G, Varaldo PE, Satta G. Phosphatase activity of staphylococci is constitutive in some species and repressed by phosphates in others. J Clin Microbiol 1990;28:2707–10.

4 Sakinc T, Woznowski M, Ebsen M, Gatermann SG. The surface-associated protein of *Staphylococcus saprophyticus* is a lipase. Infect Immun 2005;73:6419–28.

5 Pereira AT, Cristino JAGM. The characterization of *Staphylococcus saprophyticus* and its biological distinction from other novobiocin-resistant staphylococci. Zentralbl Bakteriol Suppl 1985;14:137–43.

6 Cristino JA, Pereira AT, Andrade LG. Diversity of plasmids in *Staphylococcus saprophyticus* isolated from urinary tract infections in women. Epidemiol Infect 1989;102:413–19.

7 Torres Pereira A. Coagulase-negative strains of staphylococcus possessing antigen 51 as agents of urinary infection. J Clin Pathol 1962;15:252–3.

8 Maskell R. Importance of coagulase-negative staphylococci as pathogens in the urinary tract. Lancet 1974;i:1155–8.

9 Meers PD, Whyte W, Sandys G. Coagulase-negative staphylococci and micrococci in urinary tract infections. J Clin Pathol 1975;28:270–3.

10 Mitchell RG. Classification of *Staphylococcus albus* strains isolated from the urinary tract. J Clin Pathol 1968;21:93–6.

11 Digranes A, Oeding P. Characterization of Micrococcaceae from the urinary tract. Acta Pathol Microbiol Scand B 1975;83: 373–81.

12 Wallmark G, Arremark I, Telander B. *Staphylococcus saprophyticus*: a frequent cause of acute urinary tract infection among female outpatients. J Infect Dis 1978;138:791–7.

13 Marrie TJ, Kwan C, Noble MA, West A, Duffield L. *Staphylococcus saprophyticus* as a cause of urinary tract infections. J Clin Microbiol 1982;16:427–31.

14 Jordan PA, Irvani A, Richard GA, Baer H. Urinary tract infections caused by *Staphylococcus saprophyticus*. J Infect Dis 1980;142:510–15.

15 Hovelius B, Mårdh PA. *Staphylococcus saprophyticus* as a common cause of urinary tract infections. Rev Infect Dis 1984;6:328–37.

16 Kerr H. Urinary infections caused by Micrococcus subgroup 3. J Clin Pathol 1973;26:918–20.

17 Hedman P, Ringertz O. Urinary tract infections caused by *Staphylococcus saprophyticus*. A matched case control study. J Infect 1991;23:145–53.

18 Hovelius B, Mårdh PA, Bygren P. Urinary tract infections caused by *Staphylococcus saprophyticus*: recurrences and complications. J Urol 1979;122:645–7.

19 Lewis JF, Brake SR, Anderson DJ, Vredeveld GN. Urinary tract infection due to coagulase-negative *Staphylococcus*. Am J Clin Pathol 1982;77:736–9.

20 Stattin Norinder B, Sandberg T, Norrby R. Renal concentrating capacity in female outpatients with symptomatic urinary tract infection. Scand J Urol Nephrol 2005;39:483–7.

21 Latham RH, Running K, Stamm WE. Urinary tract infections in young adult women caused by *Staphylococcus saprophyticus*. JAMA 1983;250:3063–6.

22 Hovelius B, Mårdh PA. Antibody-coating and haemagglutination by *Staphylococcus saprophyticus*. Acta Pathol Microbiol Immunol Scand B 1985;93:37–40.

23 Fowler JE. *Staphylococcus saprophyticus* as the cause of infected urinary calculus. Ann Intern Med 1985;102:342–3.

24 Golledge C. *Staphylococcus saprophyticus* bacteremia. J Infect Dis 1988;157:215.

25 Lee W, Carpenter RJ, Phillips LE, Faro S. Pyelonephritis and sepsis due to *Staphylococcus saprophyticus*. J Infect Dis 1987;155: 1079–80.

26 Singh VR, Raad I. Fatal *Staphylococcus saprophyticus* native valve endocarditis in an intravenous drug addict. J Infect Dis 1990;162:783–4.

27 Hovelius B, Colleen S, Mårdh PA. Urinary tract infections in men caused by *Staphylococcus saprophyticus*. Scand J Infect Dis 1984;16:37–41.

28 Hedman P. *Staphylococcus saprophyticus*: epidemiological and clincal aspects. Dissertation, Department of Clinical Bacteriology, Karolinska Institute, Stockholm, Sweden, 1992.

29 Schille R, Sierig G, Spencker FB, Handrick W. Harnwegsinfektionen durch *Staphylococcus saprophyticus* bei einem Kind. Klin Padiatr 2000;212:126–8.

30 Hovelius B, Thelin I, Mårdh PA. *Staphylococcus saprophyticus* in the aetiology of nongonococcal urethritis. Br J Vener Dis 1979;55:369–374.

31 Carson CC, McGraw VD, Zwadyk P. Bacterial prostatitis caused by *Staphylococcus saprophyticus*. Urology 1982;19:576–8.

32 Bergman B, Wedren H, Holm SE. *Staphylococcus saprophyticus* in males with symptoms of chronic prostatitis. Urology 1989; 34:241–5.

33 Hell W, Kern T, Klouche M. *Staphylococcus saprophyticus* as an unusual agent of nosocomial pneumonia. Clin Infect Dis 1999; 29:685–6.

34 Choi SH, Woo JH, Jeong JY *et al.* Clinical significance of *Staphylococcus saprophyticus* identified on blood culture in a tertiary care hospital. Diagn Microbiol Infect Dis 2006;56: 337–9.

35 Wright R, Judson FN. Relative and seasonal incidences of the sexually transmitted diseases. Br J Vener Dis 1978;54:433–40.

36 Rupp ME, Soper DE, Archer GL. Colonization of the female genital tract with *Staphylococcus saprophyticus*. J Clin Microbiol 1992;30:2975–9.

37 Ringertz O, Torssander J. Prevalence of *Staphylococcus saprophyticus* in patients in a veneral disease clinic. Eur J Clin Microbiol 1987;5:358–61.

38 Hedman P, Ringertz O, Olsson K, Wollin R. Plasmid-identified *Staphylococcus saprophyticus* isolated from the rectum of patients with urinary tract infections. Scand J Infect Dis 1991;23:569–72.

39 Mårdh PA, Hovelius B, Hovelius K, Nilsson PO. Coagulase-negative, novobiocin-resistant staphylococci on the skin of animals and man, on meat and in milk. Acta Vet Scand 1978; 19:243–53.

40 Gillespie WA, Sellin MA, Gill P, Stephens M, Tuckwell LA, Hilton AL. Urinary tract infection in young women, with special reference to *Staphylococcus saprophyticus*. J Clin Pathol 1978; 31:348–50.

41 Kloos WE. Ecology of human skin. In: Mårdh PA, Schleifer KH, eds. Coagulase-negative Staphylococci. Stockholm: Almqvist & Wiksell, 1986:37–50.

42 Hedman P, Ringertz O, Lindström M, Olsson K. The origin of *Staphylococcus saprophyticus* from cattle and pigs. Scand J Infect Dis 1993;25:57–60.

43 Valle J, Piriz S, de la Fuente R, Vadillo S. Staphylococci isolated from healthy goats. *Zentralbl Veterinarmed B* 1991;38:81–89.

44 Mounier J, Gelsomino R, Goerges S *et al.* Surface microflora of four smear-ripened cheeses. Appl Environ Microbiol 2005;71: 6489–500.

45 Samelis J, Metaxopoulos J, Vlassi M, Pappa A. Stability and safety of traditional Greek salami: a microbiological ecology study. Int J Food Microbiol 1998;44:69–82.

46 Hedman P, Ringertz O, Eriksson B *et al. Staphylococcus saprophyticus* found to be a common contaminant of food. J Infect 1990;21:11–19.

47 Widerström M, Wiström J, Ferry S, Karlsson C, Monsen T. Molecular epidemiology of *Staphylococcus saprophyticus* isolated from women with uncomplicated community-acquired urinary tract infection. J Clin Microbiol 2007;45:1561–4.

48 Latham RH, Zeleznik D, Minshew BH, Schoenknecht FD, Stamm W. *Staphylococcus saprophyticus* β-lactamase production and disk diffusion susceptibility testing for three β-lactam antimicrobial agents. Antimicrob Agents Chemother 1984;26: 670–2.

49 Bailey RR, Gorrie SI, Peddie BA, Davies PR. Double blind, randomised trial comparing single dose enoxacin and trimethoprim for treatment of bacterial cystitis. NZ Med J 1987;100:618–19.

50 Bannerman TL, Wadiak DL, Kloos WE. Susceptibility of *Staphylococcus* species and subspecies to fleroxacin. Antimicrob Agents Chemother 1991;35:2135–9.

51 Loulergue J, Pinon G, Laudat P, Audurier A. La résistance à la fosfomycine chez *Staphylococcus saprophyticus* et chez les autres espèces de staphylocoques coagulase négative (Fosfomycin susceptibility of *Staphylococcus saprophyticus* and other coagulase negative staphylococci). Ann Microbiol 1984;135A:239–47.

52 Osterberg E, Aberg H, Hallander HO, Kallner A, Lundin A. Efficacy of single-dose versus seven-day trimethoprim treatment of cystitis in women: a randomized double-blind study. J Infect Dis 1990;161:942–7.

53 Neringer R, Forsgren A, Hansson C, Ode B. Lomefloxacin versus norfloxacin in the treatment of uncomplicated urinary tract infections: three-day versus seven-day treatment. The South Swedish Lolex Study Group. Scand J Infect Dis 1992;24:773–80.

54 Hovelius B, Mårdh PA. Haemagglutination by *Staphylococcus saprophyticus* and other staphylococcal species. Acta Pathol Microbiol Immunol Scand B 1979;87:45–50.

55 Mårdh PA, Colleen S, Hovelius B. Attachment of bacteria to exfoliated cells from the urogenital tract. Invest Urol 1979;15: 367–71.

56 Colleen S, Hovelius B, Wieslander A, Mårdh PA. Surface properties of *Staphylococcus saprophyticus* and *Staphylococcus epidermidis* as studied by adherence tests and two-polymer aqueous phase systems. Acta Pathol Microbiol Immunol Scand B 1979;87:321–8.

57 Almeida RJ, Jorgensen JH. Comparison of adherence and urine growth rate properties of *Staphylococcus saprophyticus* and *Staphylococcus epidermidis*. Eur J Clin Microbiol 1984;3:542–5.

58 Schneider PF, Riley TV. Cell-surface hydrophobicity of *Staphylococcus saprophyticus*. Epidemiol Infect 1991;106:71–5.

59 Musher DM, Griffith DP, Yawn D, Rossen RD. Role of urease in pyelonephritis resulting from urinary tract infection with *Proteus*. J Infect Dis 1975;131:177–81.

60 Colleen S, Mårdh PA. Bacterial colonization of human urethral mucosa. Scand J Urol Nephrol 1981;15:181–7.

61 Gatermann S, Marre R, Heesemann J, Henkel W. Hemagglutinating and adherence properties of *Staphylococcus saprophyticus*: epidemiology and virulence in experimental urinary tract infection of rats. FEMS Microbiol Immunol 1988;47:179–86.

62 Szabados F, Kleine B, Anders A *et al. Staphylococcus saprophyticus* ATCC 15305 is internalized into human urinary bladder carcinoma cell line 5637. FEMS Microbiol Lett 2008;285:163–9.

63 Milagres LG, Melles CA. Differencias nas propriedades adesivas de *Staphylococcus saprophyticus* a céllulas HEp-2 e eritrócitos (Differences in the adhesive properties of *Staphylococcus saprophyticus* to HEp-2 cells and erythrocytes). Rev Inst Med Trop Sao Paulo 1992;34:315–21.
64 Gatermann S, Kretschmar M, Kreft B, Straube E, Schmidt H, Marre R. Adhesion of *Staphylococcus saprophyticus* to renal tubular epithelial cells is mediated by an *N*-acetyl-galactosamine-specific structure. Zentralbl Bakteriol 1991;275:358–63.
65 Gatermann S, Meyer HGW. Expression of *Staphylococcus saprophyticus* surface properties is modulated by the atmosphere. Med Microbiol Immunol 1995;184:81–5.
66 Teti G, Chiofalo MS, Tomasello F, Fava C, Mastroeni P. Mediation of *Staphylococcus saprophyticus* adherence to uroepithelial cells by lipoteichoic acid. Infect Immun 1987;55:839–42.
67 Jansen B, Beuth J, Ko HL. Evidence for lectin-mediated adherence of *S. saprophyticus* and *P. aeruginosa* to polymers. Zentralbl Bakteriol 1990;272:437–42.
68 Morioka H, Tachibana M. Agglutination of *Staphylococcus saprophyticus*: a structural and cytochemical study. FEMS Microbiol Lett 1995;132:101–5.
69 Ward GK, Stewart SS, Price GB, Mackillop WJ. Cellular heterogeneity in normal human urothelium: quantitative studies of lectin binding. Histochem J 1987;19:337–44.
70 Meyer HGW, Gatermann S. Surface properties of *Staphylococcus saprophyticus*: Hydrophobicity, haemagglutination and *Staphylococcus saprophyticus* surface-associated protein (Ssp) represent distinct entities. APMIS 1994;102:538–44.
71 Donnenberg MS, Welch RA. Virulence determinants of uropathogenic *Escherichia coli*. In: Mobley HLT, Warren JW, eds. Urinary Tract Infections: Molecular Pathogenesis and Clinical Maganement. Washington, DC: ASM Press, 1996:135–74.
72 Beuth J, Ko L, Schumacher-Perdrau F, Peters G, Heczko P, Pulverer G. Hemagglutination by *Staphylococcus saprophyticus* and other coagulase-negative staphylococci. Microb Pathog 1988;4:379–83.
73 Gatermann S, Meyer HGW, Wanner G. *Staphylococcus saprophyticus* hemagglutinin is a 160-kD surface polypeptide. Infect Immun 1992;60:4127–32.
74 Gunnarsson A, Mårdh PA, Lundblad A, Svensson S. Oligosaccharide structures mediating agglutination of sheep erythrocytes by *Staphylococcus saprophyticus*. Infect Immun 1984;45: 41–6.
75 Meyer HG, Muthing J, Gatermann SG. The hemagglutinin of *Staphylococcus saprophyticus* binds to a protein receptor on sheep erythrocytes. Med Microbiol Immunol 1997;186:37–43.
76 Gatermann S, Meyer HGW. *Staphylococcus saprophyticus* hemagglutinin binds fibronectin. Infect Immun 1994;62:4556–63.
77 Switalski LM, Rydén C, Rubin K, Ljungh A, Höök M, Wadström T. Binding of fibronectin to *Staphylococcus* strains. Infect Immun 1983;42:628–33.
78 Fujita K, Yokota T, Oguri T, Fujime M, Kitagawa R. In vitro adherence of *Staphylococcus saprophyticus*, *Staphylococcus epidermidis*, *Staphylococcus haemolyticus*, and *Staphylococcus aureus* to human ureter. Urol Res 1992;20:399–402.
79 Fischetti VA. Streptococcal protein M. Molecular design and biological behavior. Clin Microbiol Rev 1989;2:285–314.
80 Paulsson M, Ljungh A, Wadstrom T. Rapid identification of fibronectin, vitronectin, laminin, and collagen cell surface binding proteins on coagulase-negative staphylococci by particle agglutination assays. J Clin Microbiol 1992;30:2006–12.
81 Hell W, Meyer HG, Gatermann SG. Cloning of aas, a gene encoding a *Staphylococcus saprophyticus* surface protein with adhesive and autolytic properties. Mol Microbiol 1998;29:871–81.
82 Oshida T, Sugai M, Komatsuzawa H, Hong YM, Suginaka H, Tomasz A. A *Staphylococcus aureus* autolysin that has an *N*-acetylmuramoyl-L-alanine amidase domain and an endo-beta-*N*-acetylglucosaminidase domain: cloning, sequence analysis, and characterization. Proc Natl Acad Sci USA 1995;92:285–9.
83 Braun L, Dramsi S, Dehoux P, Bierne H, Lindahl G, Cossart P. InlB: an invasion protein of *Listeria monocytogenes* with a novel type of surface association. Mol Microbiol 1997;25:285–94.
84 Baba T, Schneewind O. Targeting of muralytic enzymes to the cell division site of Gram-positive bacteria: repeat domains direct autolysin to the equatorial surface ring of *Staphylococcus aureus*. EMBO J 1998;17:4639–46.
85 Heilmann C, Hussain M, Peters G, Götz F. Evidence for autolysin-mediated primary attachment of *Staphylococcus epidermidis* to a polystyrene surface. Mol Microbiol 1997;24:1013–24.
86 Hell W, Reichl S, Anders A, Gatermann S. The autolytic activity of the recombinant amidase of *Staphylococcus saprophyticus* is inhibited by its own recombinant GW repeats. FEMS Microbiol Lett 2003;227:47–51.
87 Handley PS, Carter PL, Fielding J. *Streptococcus salivarius* strains carry either fibrils or fimbriae on the cell surface. J Bacteriol 1984;157:64–72.
88 Galli D, Wirth R, Wanner G. Identification of aggregation substances of *Enterococcus faecalis* cells after induction by sex pheromones. An immunological and ultrastructural investigation. Arch Microbiol 1989;151:486–90.
89 Schmidt H, Naumann G, Putzke HP. Detection of different fimbriae-like structures on the surface of *Staphylococcus saprophyticus*. Zentralbl Bakteriol Hyg A 1988;268:228–37.
90 Christiansen G, Mårdh PA. Electron microscopy of negative-stained *Staphylococcus saprophyticus* reveals filamentous surface protrusions. In: Mårdh PA, Schleifer KH, eds. Cogulase-negative Staphylococci. Stockholm: Almqvist & Wicksell, 1986:145–7.
91 Gatermann S, Kreft B, Marre R, Wanner G. Identification and characterization of a surface-associated protein (Ssp) of *Staphylococcus saprophyticus*. Infect Immun 1992;60:1055–60.
92 Gatermann S. Virulence factors of *Staphylococcus saprophyticus*, *Staphylococcus epidermidis*, and enterococci. In: Mobley HLT, Warren JW, eds. Urinary Tract Infections: Molecular Pathogenesis and Clinical Management. Washington, DC: ASM Press, 1996:313–40.
93 Gatermann S, Meyer HGW, Marre R, Wanner G. Identification and characterization of surface proteins from *Staphylococcus saprophyticus*. Zentralbl Bakteriol 1993;278:258–74.
94 Bowden MG, Visai L, Longshaw CM, Holland KT, Speziale P, Hook M. Is the GehD lipase from *Staphylococcus epidermidis* a collagen binding adhesin? J Biol Chem 2002;277:43017–23.
95 Mortensen JE, Shryock TR, Kapral FA. Modification of bactericidal fatty acids by an enzyme of *Staphylococcus aureus*. J Med Microbiol 1992;36:293–8.
96 Sakinc T, Kline KA, Ingersoll MA, Hultgren SJ, Gatermann SG. Contribution of the lipase Ssp and the SdrI of *Staphylococcus saprophyticus* to virulence in experimental urinary tract infections of mice. Abstract B411 presented at the 107th General

Meeting of the American Society for Microbiology, May 21–25, 2007, Toronto, Canada.

97 Sakinc T, Kleine B, Gatermann SG. Biochemical characterization of the surface-associated lipase of *Staphylococcus saprophyticus*. FEMS Microbiol Lett 2007;274:335–41.

98 Patti JM, Allen BL, McGavin MJ, Hook M. MSCRAMM-mediated adherence of microorganisms to host tissues. Annu Rev Microbiol 1994;48:585–617.

99 McCrea KW, Hartford O, Davis S *et al.* The serine-aspartate repeat (Sdr) protein family in *Staphylococcus epidermidis*. Microbiology 2000;146:1535–46.

100 Hartford O, Francois P, Vaudaux P, Foster TJ. The dipeptide repeat region of the fibrinogen-binding protein (clumping factor) is required for functional expression of the fibrinogen-binding domain on the *Staphylococcus aureus* cell surface. Mol Microbiol 1997;25:1065–76.

101 Selvarangan R, Goluszko P, Singhal J *et al.* Interaction of Dr adhesin with collagen type IV is a critical step in *Escherichia coli* renal persistence. Infect Immun 2004;72:4827–35.

102 Hjelm E, Lundell-Etherden I. Slime production by *Staphylococcus saprophyticus*. Infect Immun 1991;59:445–8.

103 Riley TV, Schneider PF. Infrequency of slime production by urinary isolates of *Staphylococcus saprophyticus*. J Infect 1992;24:63–6.

104 Hancock IC. Encapsulation of coagulase-negative staphylococci. Int J Med Microbiol 1989;272:11–18.

105 Hjelm E, Lundell-Etherden I. Effects of extracellular products from *Staphylococcus saprophyticus* on human lymphocytes. APMIS 1989;97:935–40.

106 Schmidt H, Bukholm G, Holberg-Petersen M. Adhesiveness and invasiveness of staphylococcal species in a cell culture model. APMIS 1989;97:655–60.

107 Sanford BA, Thomas VL, Ramsay MA. Binding of staphylococci to mucus in vivo and in vitro. Infect Immun 1989;57:3735–42.

108 Gemmell CG. Extracellular toxins and enzymes of coagulase-negative staphylococci. In: Easmon CSF, Adlam C, eds. Staphylococci and Staphylococcal Infections. London: Academic Press, 1983:809–27.

109 Gemmell CG, Thelestam M. Toxinogenicity of clinical isolates of coagulase-negative staphylococci towards various animal cells. Acta Pathol Microbiol Immunol Scand B 1981;89:417–21.

110 Sakinc T, Kulczak P, Henne K, Gatermann SG. Cloning of an agr homologue of *Staphylococcus saprophyticus*. FEMS Microbiol Lett 2004;237:157–61.

111 Mobley HLT, Hausinger RP. Microbial ureases: significance, regulation, and molecular characterization. Microbiol Rev 1989;53:85–108.

112 Griffith DP, Musher DM, Itin C. Urease, the primary cause of infection-induced urinary stones. Invest Urol 1976;13:346–50.

113 Gordon AH, D'Arcy Hart P, Young MR. Ammonia inhibits phagosome–lysosome fusion in macrophages. Nature 1980;286:79–80.

114 Brunkhorst B, Niederman R. Ammonium decreases human polymorphonuclear leukocyte cytoskeletal actin. Infect Immun 1991;59:1378–86.

115 Schäfer UK, Kaltwasser H. Urease from *Staphylococcus saprophyticus*: purification, characterization and comparison to *Staphylococcus xylosus* urease. Arch Microbiol 1994;161:393–9.

116 Gatermann S, Marre R. Cloning and expression of *Staphylococcus saprophyticus* urease gene sequences in *Staphylococcus carnosus* and contribution of the enzyme to virulence. Infect Immun 1989;57:2998–3002.

117 Mobley HLT, Island MD, Hausinger RP. Molecular biology of microbial ureases. Microbiol Rev 1995;59:451–80.

118 Jose J, Schäfer UK, Kaltwasser H. Threonine is present instead of cysteine at the active site of urease from *Staphylococcus xylosus*. Arch Microbiol 1994;161:384–92.

119 Gatermann S, John J, Marre R. *Staphylococcus saprophyticus* urease: characterization and contribution to uropathogenicity in unobstructed urinary tract infection of rats. Infect Immun 1989;57:110–16.

120 Forslin L, Danielsson D. In vitro studies of the adherence of *Neisseria gonorrhoeae* and other urogenital bacteria to vaginal and uroepithelial cells, with special regard to the menstrual cycle. Gynecol Obstet Invest 1980;11:327–40.

121 Westerlund B, Korhonen TK. Bacterial proteins binding to the mammalian extracellular matrix. Mol Microbiol 1993;9:687–94.

122 Nicolle LE, Hoban SA, Harding GKM. Characterization of coagulase-negative staphylococci from urinary tract specimens. J Clin Microbiol 1983;17:267–71.

123 Leighton PM, Little JA. Identification of coagulase-negative staphylococci isolated from urinary tract infections. Am J Clin Pathol 1986;85:92–5.

124 Larsen RA, Burke JP. The epidemiology and risk factors for nosocomial catheter-associated bacteriuria caused by coagulase-negative staphylococci. Infect Control 1986;7:212–15.

125 Rimland D, Alexander W. Absence of factors associated with significant urinary tract infections caused by coagulase-negative staphylococci. Diagn Microbiol Infect Dis 1989;12:123–7.

126 Rupp ME, Archer GL. Coagulase-negative staphylococci: pathogens associated with medical progress. Clin Infect Dis 1994;19:231–43.

127 McGuckin MB, Tomasco J, MacGregor RR. Significance of bacteriuria with presumed non-pathogenic organisms. J Urol 1980;124:240–1.

128 Orrett FA, Shurland SM. Significance of coagulase-negative staphylococci in urinary tract infections in a developing country. Conn Med 1998;62:199–203.

129 Stepanovic S, Jezek P, Vukovic D, Dakic I, Petrás P. Isolation of members of the *Staphylococcus sciuri* group from urine and their relationship to urinary tract infections. J Clin Microbiol 2003;41:5262–4.

130 Haile D, Hughes J, Vetter E *et al.* Frequency of isolation of *Staphylococcus lugdunensis* in consecutive urine cultures and relationship to urinary tract infection. J Clin Microbiol 2002;40:654–6.

131 Casanova-Roman M, Sanchez-Porto A, Casanova-Bellido M. Urinary tract infection due to *Staphylococcus lugdunensis* in a healthy child. Scand J Infect Dis 2004;36:149–57.

132 Gristina AG. Biomaterial-centered infection: microbial adhesion versus tissue integration. Science 1987;237:1588–95.

133 Tojo M, Yamashita N, Goldman DA, Pier GB. Isolation and characterization of a capsular polysaccharide adhesin from *Staphylococcus epidermidis*. J Infect Dis 1988;157:713–22.

134 Christensen GD, Barker LP, Mawhinney TP, Baddour LM, Simpson WA. Identification of an antigenic marker of slime

production for *Staphylococcus epidermidis*. Infect Immun 1990; 58:2906–11.

135 Shiro H, Muller E, Gutierrez N *et al.* Transposon mutants of *Staphylococcus epidermidis* deficient in elaboration of capsular polysaccharide/adhesin and slime are avirulent in a rabbit model of endocarditis. J Infect Dis 1994;169:1042–9.

136 Kojima Y, Tojo M, Goldmann DA, Tosteson TD, Pier GB. Antibody to the capsular polysaccharide adhesin protects rabbits against catheter-related bacteremia due to coagulase-negative staphylococci. J Infect Dis 1990;162:435–41.

137 Muller E, Takeda S, Shiro H, Goldmann D, Pier GB. Occurrence of capsular polysaccharide adhesin among clinical isolates of coagulase-negative staphylococci. J Infect Dis 1993;168:1211–18.

138 Rupp ME, Archer GL. Hemagglutination and adherence to plastic by *Staphylococcus epidermidis*. Infect Immun 1992;60:4322–7.

139 Rupp ME, Sloot N, Meyer HGW, Han J, Gatermann S. Characterization of the hemagglutinin of *Staphylococcus epidermidis*. J Infect Dis 1995;172:1509–18.

140 Timmermann CP, Fleer A, Besnier JM, DeGraaf L, Cremers F, Verhoef J. Characterization of a proteinaceous adhesin of *Staphylococcus epidermidis* which mediates attachment to polystyrene. Infect Immun 1991;59:4187–92.

141 Veenstra GJ, Cremers FF, van Dijk H, Fleer A. Ultrastructural organization and regulation of biomaterial adhesin of *Staphylococcus epidermidis*. J Bacteriol 1996;178:537–41.

142 Heilmann C, Gerke C, Perdreau-Remington F, Götz F. Characterization of Tn917 insertion mutants of *Staphylococcus epidermidis* affected in biofilm formation. Infect Immun 1996; 64:277–82.

143 Ludwicka A, Uhlenbruck G, Peters G *et al.* Investigations on extracellular slime substance produced by *Staphylococcus epidermidis*. Zentralbl Bakteriol Hyg A 1984;258:256–67.

144 Drewry DT, Galbraith L, Wilkinson BJ, Wilkinson SG. Staphylococcal slime: a cautionary tale. J Clin Microbiol 1990; 28:1292–6.

145 Hussain M, Wilcox MH, White PJ. The slime of coagulase-negative staphylococci: biochemistry and relation to adherence. FEMS Microbiol Rev 1993;104:191–208.

146 Mack D, Siemsen N, Laufs R. Parallel induction by glucose of adherence and a polysaccharide antigen specefic for plastic-adherent *Staphylococcus epidermidis*: evidence for functional relation to intercellular adhesion. Infect Immun 1992;60:2048–57.

147 Mack D, Nedelmann M, Krokotsch A, Schwarzkopf A, Heesemann J, Laufs R. Characterization of transposon mutants of biofilm-producing *Staphylococcus epidermidis* impaired in the accumulative phase of biofilm production: genetic identification of a hexosamine-containing polysaccharide intercellular adhesin. Infect Immun 1994;62:3244–53.

148 Mack D, Fischer W, Krokotsch A *et al.* The intercellular adhesin involved in biofilm formation of *Staphylococcus epidermidis* is a linear beta 1,6 linked glucosaminoglycan: purification and structural analysis. J Bacteriol 1996;178:175–83.

149 Schumacher-Perdreau F, Heilmann C, Peters G, Götz F, Pulverer G. Comparative analysis of a biofilm-forming *Staphylococcus epidermidis* strain and its adhesion-positive, accumulation-negative mutant m7. FEMS Microbiol Lett 1994;117:71–8.

150 Gristina AG, Jennings RA, Naylor PT, Myrvik QN, Webb LX. Comparative in vitro antibiotic resistance of surface-colonizing coagulase-negative staphylococci. Antimicrob Agents Chemother 1989;33:813–16.

151 Gristina AG, Hobgood CD, Webb LX, Myrvik QN. Adhesive colonization of biomaterials and antibiotic resistance. Biomaterials 1987;8:423–6.

152 Rodgers J, Phillips F, Olliff C. The effects of extracellular slime from *Staphylococcus epidermidis* on phagocytic ingestion and killing. FEMS Immunol Med Microbiol 1994;9:109–15.

153 Jansen B, Schumacher-Perdreau F, Peters G, Pulverer G. Evidence for degradation of synthetic polyurethanes by *Staphylococcus epidermidis*. Zentralbl Bakteriol 1991;276:36–45.

154 Janda JM. Elastolytic activity among staphylococci. J Clin Microbiol 1986;24:945–6.

155 Sloot N, Thomas M, Marre R, Gatermann S. Purification and characterisation of elastase from *Staphylococcus epidermidis*. J Med Microbiol 1992;37:201–5.

156 Mckevitt AI, Bjornson GL, Mauracher CA, Scheifele DW. Amino acid sequence of a deltalike toxin from *Staphylococcus epidermidis*. Infect Immun 1990;58:1473–5.

157 Scheifele DW, Bjornson GL. Delta toxin activity in coagulase-negative staphylococci from the bowels of neonates. J Clin Microbiol 1988;26:279–82.

158 Breckinridge JC, Bergdoll MS. Outbreak of food-borne gastroenteritis due to a coagulase-negative enterotoxin-producing staphylococcus. N Engl J Med 1971;284:541–3.

159 Crass BA, Bergdoll MS. Involvement of coagulase-negative staphylococci in toxic shock syndrome. J Clin Microbiol 1986; 23:43–5.

160 Noble MA, Grant SK, Hajen E. Characterization of a neutrophil-inhibitory factor from clinically significant *Staphylococcus epidermidis*. J Infect Dis 1990;162:909–13.

161 Jarvis WR. The epidemiology of colonization. Infect Control Hosp Epidemiol 1996;17:47–52.

162 Barret SP, Savage MA, Rebec MP, Guyot A, Andrews N, Shrimptom SB. Antibiotic sensitivity of bacteria associated with community-acquired urinary tract infection in Britain. J Antimicrob Chemother 1999;44:359–65.

163 Goldstein FW. Antibiotic susceptibility of bacterial strains isolated from patients with community-acquired urinary tract infections in France. Eur J Clin Microbiol Infect Dis 2000;19: 112–17.

164 Demuth PJ, Gerding DN, Crossley K. *Staphylococcus aureus* bacteriuria. Arch Intern Med 1979;139:78–80.

165 Arpi M, Renneberg J. The clinical significance of *Staphylococcus aureus* bacteriuria. J Urol 1984;132:697–700.

166 Fortunov RM, Hulten KG, Hammerman WA, Mason EO Jr, Kaplan SL. Community-acquired *Staphylococcus aureus* infections in term and near-term previously healthy neonates. Pediatrics 2006;118:871–81.

167 Weinberger M, Cytron S, Servadio C *et al.* Prostatic abscess in the antibiotic era. Rev Infect Dis 1988;10:239–49.

168 Fraser TG, Smith ND, Noskin GA. Persistent methicillin-resistance *Staphylococcus aureus* bacteremia due to a prostatic abscess. Scand J Infect Dis 2003;35:273–4.

169 Baker SD, Horger DC, Keane TE. Community-acquired methicillin-resistant *Staphylococcus aureus* prostatic abcess. Urology 2004;64:808–10.

170 Tobian AA, Ober SK. Dual perinephric and prostatic abscesses from methicillin-resistant *Staphylococcus aureus*. South Med J 2007;100:515–16.

171 Pierce JR Jr, Saeed Q, Davis WR. Prostatic abscess due to community-acquired methicillin-resistant *Staphylococcus aureus*. Am J Med Sci 2008;335:154–6.

172 Lesse AJ, Mylotte JM. Clinical and molecular epidemiology of nursing home-associated *Staphylococcus aureus* bacteremia. Am J Infect Control 2006;34:642–50.

173 Sapico FL, Montgomerie JZ, Canawati HN, Aeilts G. Methicillin-resistant *Staphylococcus aureus* bacteriuria. Am J Med Sci 1981;281:101.

174 Coll PP, Crabtree BF, O'Connor PJ, Klenzak S. Clinical risk factors for methicillin-resistant *Staphylococcus aureus* bacteriuria in a skilled-care nursing home. Arch Fam Med 1994;3:357–360.

175 Lee BK, Crossley K, Gerding DN. The association between *Staphylococcus aureus* bacteremia and bacteriuria. Am J Med 1978;65:303–306.

176 Sheth S, DiNubile MJ. Clinical significance of *Staphylococcus aureus* bacteriuria without concurrent bacteremia. Clin Infect Dis 1997;24:1268–9.

177 Muder RR, Brennen C, Rihs JD *et al.* Isolation of *Staphylococcus aureus* from the urinary tract: association of isolation with symptomatic urinary tract infection and subsequent staphylococcal bacteremia. Clin Infect Dis 2006;42:46–50.

178 Ekkelenkamp MB, Verhoef J, Bonten MJ. Quantifying the relationship between *Staphylococcus aureus* bacteremia and *S. aureus* bacteruria: a retrospective analysis in a tertiary care hospital. Clin Infect Dis 2007;44:1457–9.

179 Huggan PJ, Murdoch DR, Gallagher K, Chambers ST. Concomitant *Staphylococcus aureus* bacteriuria is associated with poor clinical outcome in adults with *S. aureus* bacteraemia. J Hosp Infect 2008;69:345–9.

180 Higashide M, Kuroda M, Ohkawa S, Ohta T. Evaluation of a cefoxitin disk diffusion test for the detection of mecA-positive methicillin-resistant Staphylococcus saprophyticus. *Int J Antimicrob Agents* 2006 June; 27(6):500–4.

181 Söderquist B, Berglund C. Methicillin-resistant Staphylococcus saprophyticus in Sweden carries various types of staphylococcal cassette chromosome mec (SCCmec). *Clin Microbiol Infect* 2009 May 16. [Epub ahead of print].

Chapter 25
Toxic Shock Syndrome

Aaron DeVries
Infectious Disease Epidemiology, Prevention, and Control Section, Minnesota Department of Health and University of Minnesota School of Medicine, St Paul, Minnesota, USA

Introduction

Staphylococcal toxic shock syndrome (TSS) is a systemic illness resulting from the production of unique toxins called superantigens. When superantigens are produced by *Staphylococcus aureus* and absorbed into the body, a severe illness culminating in shock and multisystem organ failure can result. Over the last 30 years, much has been learned about the pathophysiology, associated morbidity, risk factors, clinical features, and therapeutics of this syndrome.

Epidemiology and pathogenesis

Early case descriptions

The earliest description of TSS was published in 1927 by Stevens who described three children with a scarlatiniform rash, erythematous throat, and desquamation related to staphylococcal infection [1]. One year later in Australia, a batch of diphtheroid antitoxin was contaminated with *S. aureus* and an illness occurred in many of those who received the injections. Afflicted individuals developed fevers, vomiting, diarrhea, hypotension, and a rash similar to Stevens' description [2,3]. Other case reports of rash, systemic illness, and desquamation related to staphylococci were described in subsequent years [4,5]. In 1978, Todd *et al.* [6] first used the term "toxic shock syndrome" to describe seven children with fever, confusion, headache, conjunctival hyperemia, scarlatiniform rash, edema, vomiting, diarrhea, hepatic abnormalities, acute renal failure, disseminated intravascular coagulation, shock, and desquamation associated with *S. aureus*.

Epidemiology

By early 1980, 55 cases of this newly described syndrome had been reported from 13 states to the Centers for Disease Control and Prevention (CDC) [7]. While Todd's case series included children of both genders, the cases reported to CDC were 95% female and had a median age of 25 years. To further investigate these cases, a highly specific case definition was developed that comprised early as well as late clinical manifestations (Table 25.1) [8]. Early case–control studies quickly revealed a close relationship between TSS and tampon use during menstruation [9–11]. High-absorbency tampon use was strongly correlated with TSS, with Rely brand tampons having a significantly higher relative risk compared with other tampon brands (7.7, 99% confidence interval 2.1–27.9) [8,12]. The company voluntarily removed Rely from the market in September 1980. By 1985, polyacrylate-containing high-absorbency tampons were also removed from sale.

From the earliest description of TSS, cases unrelated to menstruation were also identified in nonmenstruating women, men, and children [6,13]. *Staphylococcus aureus* infection and a toxin that certain strains produce emerged as an important common link between menstrual and nonmenstrual cases [13,14]. Nonmenstrual cases were identified in persons with skin infections, surgical wounds, adenitis, bursitis, postpartum vaginal infections, and primary bacteremia [14–16]. Unlike menstrual cases, nonmenstrual TSS cases ranged in age from neonates to the elderly and were from a relatively broad racial and ethnic background [14,17].

Surveillance by several methods in the early 1980s identified incidence rates of 6.2–12.3 per 100 000 women, with 15–24 year olds being the highest incidence age group at 13.9–16 per 100 000 [18–20]. There were wide differences in incidence among various states, ranging from 2.4 per 100 000 women in northern California to 16 per 100 000 women in Colorado [20–22]. Some of these regional differences resulted from variability in surveillance methods. Racial and ethnic variability was also an independent factor, with whites having more than twice the incidence compared with nonwhites (0.58 vs. 0.22 per 100 000) [20,23].

Eventually, there was a significant decrease in the incidence among young women, from about 15 per 100 000 in 1980 to 1.0 per 100 000 in 1986 [21,23]. A combination of factors, including the removal of highly absorbent tampons from the market, an extensive public campaign, women seeking care earlier, and decreased tampon use, likely

Staphylococci in Human Disease, 2nd edition. Edited by Kent B. Crossley, Kimberly K. Jefferson, Gordon Archer, Vance G. Fowler, Jr.
 ISBN 978-14051-6332-3.

Table 25.1 Current CDC surveillance case definition for toxic shock syndrome (last updated 1997). (From Centers for Disease Control and Prevention [102].)

Clinical criteria

Fever
Temperature ≥ 38.9°C (102.0°F)

Rash
Diffuse macular erythroderma

Desquamation
1–2 weeks after onset of illness, particularly on the palms and soles

Hypotension
Systolic blood pressure ≤ 90 mmHg for adults or less than fifth percentile by age for children aged < 16 years; orthostatic drop in diastolic blood pressure ≥ 15 mmHg from lying to sitting, orthostatic syncope, or orthostatic dizziness

Multisystem involvement
Three or more of the following:
- Gastrointestinal: vomiting or diarrhea at onset of illness
- Muscular: severe myalgia or creatine phosphokinase level at least twice the upper limit of normal (ULN)
- Mucous membrane: vaginal, oropharyngeal, or conjunctival hyperemia
- Renal: blood urea nitrogen or creatinine at least twice ULN for laboratory or urinary sediment with pyuria (≥ 5 white blood cells per high-power field) in the absence of urinary tract infection
- Hepatic: total bilirubin, alanine aminotransferase (ALT), or asparate aminotransferase (AST) levels at least twice ULN for laboratory
- Hematological: platelets < 100×10^9/L
- Central nervous system: disorientation or alterations in consciousness without focal neurological signs when fever and hypotension are absent

Laboratory criteria

Negative results on the following tests, if obtained:
- Blood, throat, or cerebrospinal fluid cultures (blood culture may be positive for *S. aureus*)
- Rise in titer to Rocky Mountain spotted fever, leptospirosis, or measles

Case classification

Probable case
Meets the laboratory criteria and four of the five clinical findings described above are present

Confirmed case
Meets the laboratory criteria and all five of the clinical findings described above are present, including desquamation, unless the patient dies before desquamation occurs

brought about the decrease in incidence [24]. From 1986 through 1996, the number of cases of TSS reported passively to CDC remained stable (Figure 25.1) [25]. Given the limitations of the national passive surveillance system, it is possible that significant changes in disease rates could have gone undetected.

Pathogenesis

TSS involves a unique interplay between toxins made by *S. aureus*, host susceptibility, and a profound host immune response. Some *S. aureus* strains produce toxins with unique properties called superantigens. These can be absorbed across mucosal membranes or introduced directly through a wound into a typically sterile site [26,27]. Superantigens bind to the exterior surface of the major histocompatibility complex class II (MHC II) receptor on antigen-presenting cells and to the Vβ variable region on the T-cell receptor (TCR) away from the typical antigen-binding site [27–30]. With exposure to a typical antigen, only 0.01–0.03% of the total T-cell population is activated. In contrast, with superantigen exposure, the nonspecific MHC II and TCR binding results in enormous nonspecific T-cell activation where up to 20% of all T cells in the body are activated at one time. This massive T-cell activation leads to substantial cytokine production, including tumor necrosis factor (TNF)-α/β, interferon (IFN)-γ, and interleukin (IL)-2 [27–29,31]. Without appropriate regulation, these cytokines cause the multiple clinical signs and symptoms associated with TSS, including fever, hypotension, multiorgan failure, rash, desquamation, and mucous membrane inflammation [27,32].

Multiple unique *S. aureus* superantigens can cause TSS. Toxic shock syndrome toxin (TSST)-1 was the first *S. aureus* superantigen described and causes almost all menstrual-associated TSS [27,29]. In cases not associated with menstruation, a large number of other superantigens in addition

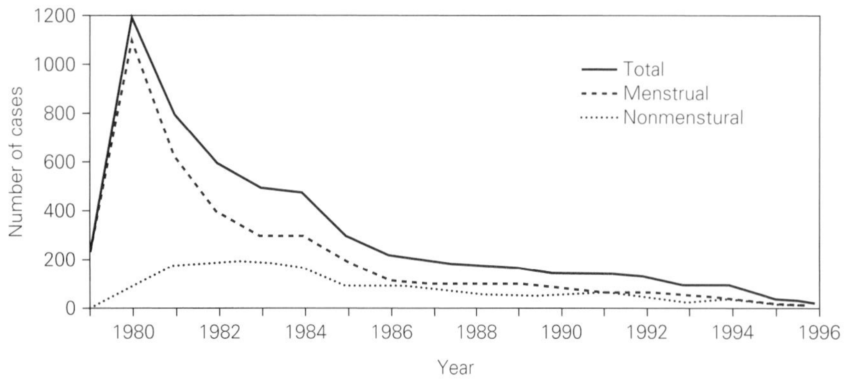

Figure 25.1 Number of cases of toxic shock syndrome reported to CDC annually from 1979 through 1996. Solid line, total number of cases; dashed line, menstrual cases; dotted line, nonmenstrual cases. (Adapted from Hajjeh *et al.* [25] with permission.)

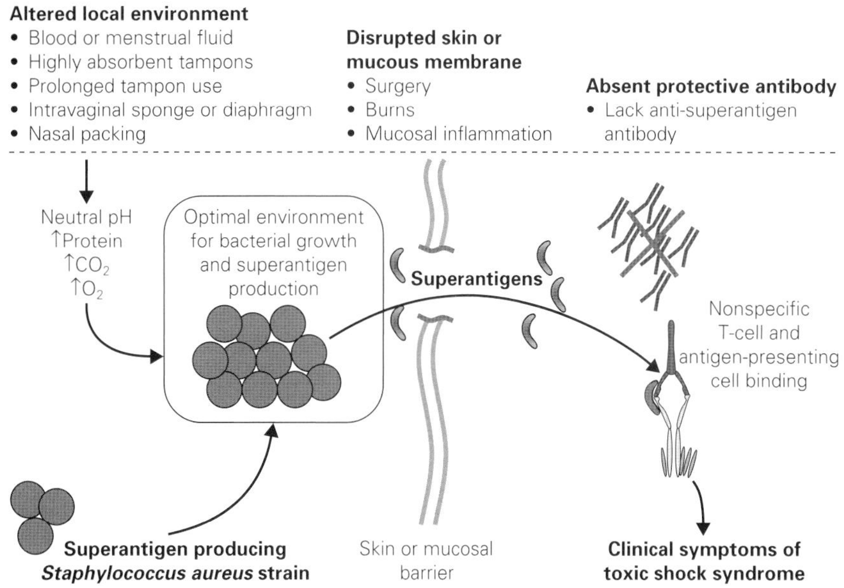

Figure 25.2 Risk factors associated with toxic shock syndrome (TSS). In the presence of an *S. aureus* strain that produces superantigens, an altered local host environment, disruption in the skin or mucous membranes, and absent protective antibody can lead to the clinical symptoms of TSS.

to TSST-1 have been identified as the cause of TSS, including staphylococcal enterotoxin B (SEB), staphylococcal enterotoxin C (SEC), staphylococcal enterotoxin G (SEG), staphylococcal enterotoxin I (SEI) and rarely others [27, 33,34]. This difference in the range of causative superantigens between menstrual and nonmenstrual TSS is thought to be due to the relative ease with which TSST-1 is absorbed across mucosal surfaces [27]. In contrast, other superantigens are poorly absorbed across mucous membranes and require direct inoculation into a sterile site [27]. The evolutionary purpose of these proteins is unclear as their expression frequently results in illness or death to the host with no appreciable improvement in dispersion or replication of the organism [31]. For a more in-depth discussion of superantigens, see Chapter 6.

Risk factors

There are several factors that are important in the process of developing TSS, including (i) the presence of a staphylococcal strain that produces superantigens, (ii) a local environment which favors the production of superantigens by *S. aureus*, (iii) disruption in the skin or mucous membranes, and (iv) a lack of antibody against superantigens (Figure 25.2). Typically, a combination of these factors is required to result in the clinical syndrome of TSS.

Staphylococcal strain

One required risk factor in the development of TSS is the presence of an *S. aureus* strain that produces a superantigen capable of causing TSS. While many *S. aureus* strains carry superantigen genes, isolates from patients with TSS produce high levels of superantigens compared with isolates from patients without TSS as measured by an *in vitro* assay of superantigen production [35]. Superantigen-producing strains may be either present as a colonizing organism or found at the site of a clinically significant infection.

Recently, the point prevalence of *S. aureus* colonization in the anterior nares, perianal region, or vagina among menstruating women was found to be 25% [36]. Of all participants, 6% were found to be colonized with *S. aureus* and 25% of these strains were found to have the gene for TSST-1. Strains of community-acquired methicillin-resistant *S. aureus* (CA-MRSA) that combine increased resistance to β-lactam antibiotics with increased virulence have emerged in the last 10 years and are becoming increasingly prevalent. In one study, TSST-1-positive methicillin-sensitive *S. aureus* (MSSA) and MRSA isolates compared by pulsed-field gel electrophoresis were identical, with the exception of the band representing the methicillin-resistance element [37]. Additional studies of CA-MRSA strains have identified those with both TSST-1 and other superantigen genes [38,39]. As strains of *S. aureus* increase and decrease in prevalence over time, one result may be that the incidence of TSS may change accordingly [40–42].

Local environment

Environment suitable for toxin production

Changes in body microenvironments where *S. aureus* can live alter the rate of growth and the amount of superantigen produced. The presence of a protein-rich substrate provides a suitable culture media to promote replication and colony growth [31,43,44]. A relatively neutral pH, between 6.5 and 8.0, was also found to promote superantigen expression [43]. Additionally, the presence of both increased carbon dioxide and increased oxygen levels increases superantigen production [45,46]. A combination of these factors promotes an increase in superantigen absorption and an increased likelihood of TSS.

Tampons and TSS

During menses, the vagina becomes a highly suitable environment for promotion of bacterial growth and toxin production. Blood and menstrual fluid are rich in protein substrates and cause the typically acidic vaginal environment to become more neutral. When tampons are used, there is the additional effect of changing a usually anaerobic environment to one that is more aerobic while maintaining higher carbon dioxide levels [31,47].

Certain materials in tampons were identified as associated with a higher risk of TSS compared with other products. Early epidemiological studies identified use of Rely brand tampons as highly correlated with TSS compared with women not using Rely [8,12,48]. This product contained a combination of materials, including a polyester foam, carboxymethylcellulose, and a surfactant used as a binding agent, that were found to promote TSST-1 production [49]. Polyacrylate rayon appeared to also promote TSST-1 production but to a lesser degree [48]. Highly absorbent tampons containing polyester foam and carboxymethylcellulose were removed from the market in 1980 and polyacrylate rayon tampons followed in 1985. The removal of these products likely made a substantial contribution to the decrease in incidence of TSS observed in that time period [25]. More recently, studies of cotton and cotton-rayon tampons did not find an increase in the *in vitro* production of superantigens [49,50].

Both *in vitro* and epidemiological studies identified use of high-absorbency tampons as more important than the specific tampon material [48–53]. In response, the Food and Drug Administration began regulating absorbency of tampons and established standardized absorbency labeling. In 1994 five absorbency classifications were introduced (light, regular, super, super-plus, and ultra) to provide consumers with standardization across brands. Additionally, continuous use of tampons for greater than 24 hours may also be an independent risk factor for TSS [11,53]. Therefore, it is recommended that the lowest absorbency tampon be used during menstruation and that the tampon be changed at least every 8 hours.

In the past, tampon use was more prevalent among young white women, with significant variation among other racial and ethnic groups [53]. A population-based assessment of tampon use practices across age and racial/ethnic groups has not been publicly reported recently. In a convenience sample survey of 713 female conference attendees in 2000, 80% of women less than 40 years of age reported using tampons on a regular basis, whereas other estimates have indicated that only 50% of women use them at some point during menstruation [36,54]. Changes in tampon use practices compared with the 1980s, including new products and how they are used, may be important reemerging risk factors for TSS.

Intravaginal sponge, diaphragm, and cervical cap use

Other intravaginal products such as contraceptive devices have been linked to TSS cases unrelated to menstruation. Intravaginal contraceptive sponges likely increase the risk of TSS [55] and TSS cases have been reported among users of diaphragms and cervical caps [56]. Taken together, barrier contraceptive users have significantly higher odds of TSS compared with users of nonbarrier contraceptives [56]. For intravaginal sponges, the increased risk is likely due to factors similar to those associated with tampons (e.g., changes in pH and oxygen and carbon dioxide concentrations). The connection between TSS and use of cervical caps and diaphragm is less clear.

Nasal packing

Following surgical manipulation or episodes of significant nasal bleeding, packing is inserted into the nose to tamponade disrupted blood vessels and prevent additional blood loss. The material used in nasal packing is similar to that in tampons and likely presents the same potential risk for TSS as do tampons. The first case report of nasal packing linked to TSS was published in 1983 [57]. Additional cases have been identified following endonasal sinus surgery without nasal packing [58]. One estimate of TSS incidence among nasal surgery patients for 1980–1983 was calculated at 16 per 100 000, which was higher than the estimated incidence of menstrual cases at that time [59].

Post partum

TSS has also been described following both vaginal and cesarean section delivery in women not using vaginally inserted contraceptive barrier devices or tampons [14,60–62]. In the weeks following delivery, the vaginal environment is very similar to that during menstruation and provides an environment which promotes *S. aureus* growth and toxin production [27].

Disruption in skin or mucous membranes

Nonmenstrual cases of TSS likely represent about half of all cases [13,14,23,25]. Disruption of the skin or mucosal surface allows organisms to enter the body where bacterial multiplication and superantigen absorption can occur. As discussed above, TSST-1 can be absorbed across mucosal surfaces, whereas other superantigens cannot. Almost all menstrual TSS cases are associated with TSST-1, whereas nonmenstrual cases with disruption of the skin or mucosal surface are due to not only TSST-1 but also SEB, SEC, SEG, and SEI [27,33,34].

Of nonmenstrual cases, most are due to postoperative wound infections or other skin and soft tissue infections [14,63]. In one review of all surgeries performed over a 13-year period, the incidence of TSS was 3 per 100 000 surgeries [64]. Burn victims also appear to be at higher risk even with minimal total body surface area involvement [65]. In one pediatric burn unit, 6 of 71 (8%) patients developed TSS over a 15-month period of observation [66]. Adult burn patients with TSS are typically rare, with the difference possibly due to higher levels of protective anti-superantigen antibody [67]. Varicella-zoster lesions have also been described as a primary site of *S. aureus* superinfection resulting in TSS [68].

Lack of anti-superantigen antibody

Antibodies against staphylococcal superantigens are typically protective against TSS and their absence is a significant risk factor leading to an increased chance of developing TSS [69–71]. Recently, Kansal *et al.* [72] identified antibodies directed against TSST-1 as specific IgG1 and IgG4; no IgM or IgA antibodies were detected. Anti-TSST-1 antibodies, as well as anti-SEB and anti-SEC antibodies, are typically acquired early in life, with up to 30% of all 2 year olds and 90% of 25 year olds having protective serum levels [27]. These antibodies are likely formed in response to low levels of *S. aureus* superantigen exposure early in life [27,73]. In contrast, more than 90% of patients who develop TSS lack protective antibody at the time of their illness, and only 50% develop protective levels by 2 months after their illness [74]. This is the major reason why up to one-third of TSS patients have at least one recurrence of TSS [75].

Recently, among 3012 North American menstruating women between the ages of 13 and 40, 81% had anti-TSST-1 antibody, with 25% colonized vaginally, nasally, or rectally with *S. aureus* [36]. There was a significantly lower prevalence of protective anti-TSST-1 antibody levels among black participants (78%) compared with white participants (86%; $P < 0.01$). The seroprevalence among Hispanic and Asian participants was similar (84% for both groups) and was not significantly different from that of whites [36]. There are no seroprevalence data on anti-SEB, anti-SEC, and anti-SEQ antibodies.

Clinical manifestations

Classic TSS

A complex interplay between *S. aureus* and the host's immune response leads to the manifestations of TSS. The pathophysiology of this disease begins with *S. aureus* colonization or infection followed by bacterial superantigen production and absorption into the body (Figure 25.3). Antecedent symptoms prior to the onset of the classic syndrome may be absent (as in colonization of the vaginal mucosa) or may be very mild (e.g., at the site of a benign-appearing wound). Typically, in wound or other skin infections, the localized symptoms are minimal and often missed at the time of presentation to healthcare providers [63]. Nonmenstrual cases will also often present with TSS symptoms later than menstrual cases (7 vs. 3 days) from the onset of the antecedent event such as menstruation or a surgical procedure. This may be partly due to differences in the causative superantigens [63].

Nausea and vomiting, fever, myalgias, and headaches are usually the first symptoms observed (Figure 25.4) [76]. Progression is typically rapid and can occur despite appropriate supportive and antimicrobial therapy. Within the next 24–48 hours hypotension, diarrhea, and the classic rash develop, with multisystem organ failure following [63,76,77]. A recent description of the clinical findings in TSS is shown in Table 25.2 [63,78].

Following superantigen binding, T cells are activated, releasing a wide range of cytokines. The direct effect of these cytokines on vascular endothelium causes capillary leak, with a resulting decreased intravascular hydrostatic pressure. The resulting intravascular volume depletion is similar to endotoxin-mediated shock [27]. Hypotension results from the decreased intravascular volume and, if prolonged, results in cholestatic hepatitis and prerenal azotemia. Increased interstitial fluid can lead to peripheral limb edema and pulmonary edema as well as acute respiratory distress syndrome. In the central nervous system, the increased interstitial fluid can cause cerebral edema, altered mental status, and seizures [79]. Erythrodermic

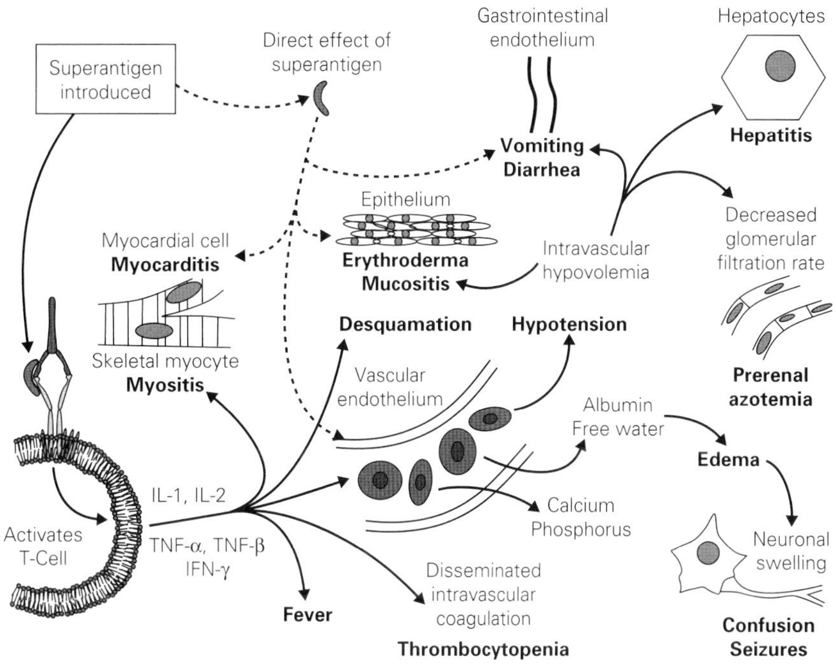

Figure 25.3 Pathophysiology of symptoms of toxic shock syndrome (TSS). Superantigens activate T cells and the release of cytokines. A combination of unregulated cytokine release and the direct effect of superantigens lead to the symptoms of TSS. IFN, interferon; IL, interleukin; TNF, tumor necrosis factor.

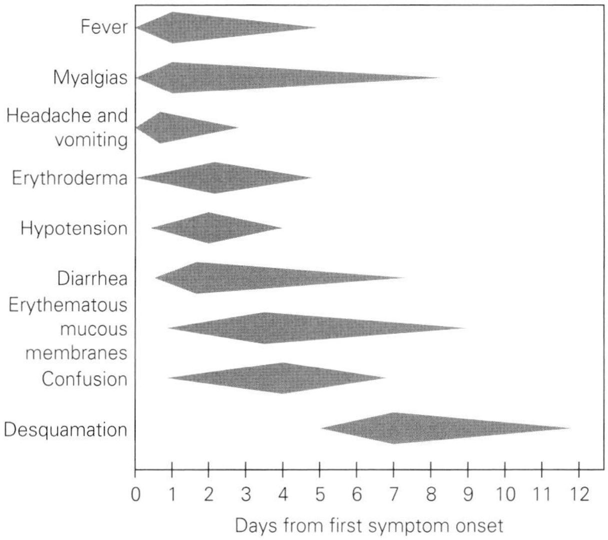

Figure 25.4 Typical progression of symptoms in classic toxic shock syndrome. (Adapted from Chesney *et al.* [76] and Wiesenthal & Todd [77] with permission.)

rash, mucous membrane inflammation, and diarrhea are also caused in part by the capillary leak [63,79]. As illness progresses, mucous membrane ulcers and a maculopapular rash may occur [76]. In a process that is not completely understood, superantigen may also bind directly to other tissues including myocytes, epithelium, gastrointestinal endothelium [27,80], and vascular endothelium, mediating some of the observed symptoms [27,31,79,81–84].

In skeletal muscle, IL-1 releases prostaglandins, which cause proteolysis, elevated creatine phosphokinase, and muscle pain [79]. Cardiac muscle can also be affected, with decreased systolic function, acute arrhythmias and, rarely, the development of myocarditis [80,85–87]. TNF-α, IL-1, and IL-6 release can lead to disseminated intravascular coagulation with platelet consumption, thrombocytopenia, and petechiae [88].

IFN-γ is thought to mediate desquamation through the inhibition of an epidermal protein called predesquamin. Desquamation typically occurs between 1 and 3 weeks after the first symptom. When stimulated by IFN-γ, predesquamin inhibits attachment and growth of normal keratinocytes and promotes the cleavage of mature cells [89]. Hypotension and hypoperfusion may also play a role in this process.

Broad clinical spectrum of illness

The pathophysiology of TSS results in a continuum of symptoms from very mild to severe [90–92]. The most severe cases have profound alteration in hemodynamics resulting in multisystem organ failure and death. Normally, symptoms are less severe and many patients frequently lack some of the clinical findings, such as hemodynamic instability and organ failure [75,92]. Early intervention often decreases the likelihood of progression to severe illness and possibly the chance of long-term sequelae. It has been suggested that milder disease and early intervention may prevent a long-lasting antibody response resulting in an increased chance for recurrence of TSS [31,93,94].

Fever and erythroderma are often early symptoms in TSS [95]. Of 56 pediatric patients presenting to an emergency room with fever and erytheroderma, 51 (91%) required hospitalization, 23 (41%) had hypotension, and 18

Table 25.2 Characteristics of staphylococcal toxic shock syndrome (TSS) 2000–2003. (From DeVries *et al.* [78] with permission.)

Characteristics	All TSS cases (N = 44) (range or percent of total)	Menstrual TSS (N = 23) (range or percent of total)	Nonmenstrual TSS (N = 21) (range or percent of total)
All six criteria	11 (25%)	9 (39%)	2 (10%)[1]
Temperature ≥ 38.9°C (102.0°F)	43 (98%)	23 (100%)	20 (95%)
Hypotension[2]	43 (98%)	23 (100%)	20 (95%)
Rash consistent with erythroderma	44 (100%)	23 (100%)	21 (100%)
Desquamation	14 (32%)	9 (39%)	5 (24%)
Multisystem involvement[3]	43 (98%)	23 (100%)	20 (95%)
Gastrointestinal involvement	36 (82%)	20 (87%)	16 (76%)
Vomiting	33 (75%)	20 (87%)	13 (62%)
Diarrhea	25 (58%)	14 (64%)	11 (52%)
Mucous membrane involvement	31 (70%)	16 (70%)	15 (71%)
Muscular involvement	32 (73%)	20 (87%)	12 (57%)[1]
No. with myalgias	23 (58%)	18 (78%)	5 (29%)[4]
Median CPK	270 (6–13 451) (N = 29)	98 (20–4430) (N = 15)	446 (6–13 451) (N = 14)
Renal involvement	36 (82%)	20 (87%)	16 (76%)
Median BUN	27.5 (7–69)	24 (7–69)	32 (7–57)
Median creatinine	1.7 (0.3–6.8)	1.3 (0.9–5.8)	1.9 (0.3–6.8)
Pyuria	27 (77%) (N = 35)	19 (95%) (N = 20)	8 (53%) (N = 15)[4]
Hepatic involvement	22 (50%)	11 (48%)	11 (52%)
AST	49 (13–14 904) (N = 41)	33 (14–937) (N = 21)	70 (13–14904) (N = 20)
ALT	50 (6–4602) (N = 41)	45.5 (6–311) (N = 21)	53 (16–4602) (N = 20)
Total bilirubin	1.8 (0.3–9.4) (N = 39)	2.1 (0.3–7.4) (N = 21)	1.6 (0.3–9.4) (N = 18)
Hematological involvement	22 (50%)	10 (43%)	12 (57%)
Lowest platelet count	99 (4–401)	106 (18–266)	90 (4–401)
Central nervous system involvement	10 (23%)	4 (17%)	6 (29%)
Cases due to MRSA[5]	3 (9%) (N = 31)	1 (5%) (N = 19)	2 (15%) (N = 13)
Cases with positive blood culture	3 (7%)	1 (4%)	2 (9%)

[1] Comparison between menstrual and nonmenstrual cases ($P < 0.05$).
[2] Hypotension defined as orthostatic hypotension or syncope, or systolic blood pressure ≤ 90 mmHg if age ≥ 16 years, ≤ 5th percentile for age if < 16 years.
[3] Mulitsystem involvement as defined as abnormality in three or more organ systems including gastrointestinal, muscular, mucous membranes, central nervous system, hematological, hepatic, or renal. See Table 25.1.
[4] Comparison between menstrual and nonmenstrual cases ($P < 0.01$).
[5] N indicates number of isolates.
ALT (Units/L), alanine aminotransferase; AST (Units/L), asparate aminotransferase; BUN (mg/dL), blood urea nitrogen; CPK (Units/L), creatine phosphokinase, CREATININE (mg/dL), PLATELET COUNT (/mm^3).

(32%) required intensive care unit admission. Of the 56 patients, 16 (29%) had TSS and 13 (81%) of these developed hypotension [95]. Fever and erythroderma occur during a time of hemodynamic compensation and represents a window during which appropriate therapeutic interventions may prevent progression to hypotension and multisystem organ failure.

Immunodeficiency may play a limited role in altering the typical clinical presentation of TSS. Patients with AIDS have been noted to rarely develop a prolonged clinical course consistent with TSS, with severe and persistent desquamation referred to as recalcitrant erythematous desquamating disorder (RED) [96]. Conversely, rabbits given very high doses of cyclosporine appear to be protected from the effects of superantigen exposure [97]. There are few reported cases of TSS among immunosuppressed patients. One report describes a series of patients with multiple myeloma who lacked rash, mucosal findings, or desquamation but whom the authors felt had a clinical syndrome consistent with TSS [98]. As the other clinical manifestations of TSS (hypotension and multisystem organ failure) can be found in many forms of septic shock, it is unclear if these cases represented TSS.

Late sequelae

Persistent morbidity following TSS occurs frequently and is related to both the severity of the initial illness and the timing of appropriate interventions. In one review of 22 menstrual and nonmenstrual cases prospectively followed for up to 3 years, Kain *et al.* [63] reported that 92% of menstrual cases and 78% of nonmenstrual cases had at least one late sequela. Long-term morbidity can range from mild and short term to severe, persistent, and life-altering. Dermatological complications include a late-onset papular rash, persistent desquamation, alopecia, and nail loss in up to half of patients [63,99]. Neuropsychiatric morbidity with long-term memory loss, chronic headaches, impaired concentration, neuromyasthenias, anorexia, and persistent abnormal electroencephalography has also been identified in up to half of patients [63,100]. Cardiovascular impairment including recurrent syncope, cardiomyopathy, abnormal electrocardiography, and persistent delayed capillary refill with limb hypoperfusion occurs in as many as one-quarter of cases [63,85]. A persistent skeletal muscle myopathy has also been described [99]. About one-third of women experience persistent menstrual irregularity and menorrhagia [63].

Recurrence of TSS can occur in patients who fail to mount an appropriate anti-superantigen antibody response following their first exposure. Recurrent episodes can occur in either menstrual or nonmenstrual cases and are usually milder than the primary episode. The lack of an appropriate immune response may be the result of superantigens causing a predominantly helper T cell type 1 response over helper T cell type 2 response, leading to increased B-cell apoptosis [31]. Both the rates of persistent morbidity and recurrence of TSS are reduced when appropriate antistaphylococcal antibiotics are given during the acute phase of illness [63,75,79].

Table 25.3 Differential diagnosis of toxic shock syndrome.

Infectious
Group A streptococcal toxic shock syndrome
Clostridium sordellii toxic shock syndrome
Streptococcus suis toxis shock syndrome
Meningococcemia and meningococcal meningitis
Staphylococcal scalded skin syndrome
Streptobacillus moniliformis (rat bite fever)
Capnocytophaga canimorsus (dog bite)
Hantavirus pulmonary syndrome
Invasive salmonella infection
Influenza
Brucellosis
Adenovirus
Ehrlichiosis
Measles
Leptospirosis
Rickettsia rickettsii (Rocky Mountain spotted fever)
Other sepsis (Gram negative/Gram positive)
Noninfectious
Kawasaki disease
Systemic lupus erythematosus
Erythema multiforme
Toxic epidermal necrolysis
Drug intoxication or drug immune reaction
Phenytoin
Cocaine
Pseudoephedrine
Aerosolized mercury
Quinidine
Salicylates
Sulfamonamide
β-Lactam antibiotics
Quinolone antibiotics
Cutaneous T-cell lymphoma
Pityriasis rubra pilaris

Diagnosis

Differential diagnosis

Despite a clear understanding of many of the pathological processes, TSS remains a clinical diagnosis. No single laboratory test or combination of tests confirms the diagnosis. It is only with assembly of epidemiological risk factors, clinical symptoms, signs, laboratory information, and a high index of suspicion that the diagnosis is made. Depending on the grouping of symptoms, the differential diagnosis is extremely broad. While TSS is a unique syndrome, there is significant overlap with other infectious and noninfectious syndromes and careful consideration is needed to assess and eliminate alternative diagnoses. Table 25.3 provides a list of infectious and noninfectious diseases with clinical manifestations that overlap with the TSS clinical syndrome.

Clinical diagnosis

Following the modern description of TSS by Todd *et al.*, a standardized epidemiological case definition was established [6,8]. This definition was designed to be highly specific so that similar cases could be compared with control groups for the purpose of identifying risk factors. It was observed that many less severe cases lacked some of the multisystem organ dysfunction criteria, and did not develop desquamation, especially in circumstances where medical care was instituted early [90]. To help address this greater breadth of illness severity (and diagnostic certainty), "possible" and "confirmed" categories of TSS were created [17,90]. Since then, several alternative and simplified case definitions have been proposed, but no change has been adopted widely [101]. The current CDC case definition in Table 25.1 is largely unchanged from the original 1980 definition [102].

As this definition was designed for epidemiological purposes, caution should be used in its application as a diagnostic tool. For instance, if a clinician waits for more severe symptoms such as hypotension or organ failure to develop, a worse clinical outcome could occur if appropriate interventions are delayed. It is important to be attuned to the associated epidemiological risk factors and the early symptoms such as erythrodermic rash, fever, vomiting, and diarrhea and have a high index of suspicion for TSS so that targeted treatment can be initiated early. As the clinical syndrome progresses in the first 48 hours of illness, symptoms and laboratory findings become increasingly consistent with the definition. Table 25.2 outlines the typical frequency of laboratory and clinical abnormalities in a recent case series [78].

Additional supportive testing

If *S. aureus* is isolated, testing for superantigen production can be performed by some research and references laboratories. Anti-superantigen antibody testing performed during the acute illness may be helpful in the diagnosis of TSS if the antibodies are absent [74]. A measurable antibody response typically develops within 1–6 weeks following illness [74]. Documenting a difference between acute and convalescent anti-superantigen antibody titers can be of aid particularly in difficult or complicated cases. In these settings, lack of seroconversion likely identifies a patient who is at risk for recurrence, warranting interventions to prevent a second episode. Caution should be used in interpreting antibody results without knowing the implicated superantigen from the clinical isolate. If a case of TSS is caused by SEB, testing for anti-SEB antibody and not anti-TSST-1 would be necessary to document an effective protective antibody level.

Recently, testing for Vβ2-positive T cells by flow cytometry has been suggested as a method of diagnosing TSS [103]. While Vβ2 T cells stimulated by TSST-1 are important in the pathogenesis of TSS [30,104], other types of T cells are stimulated with other superantigens (Vβ3, Vβ12, and Vβ5.1 in SEB for instance) [105]. Additionally, the level of Vβ2 T cells has not been established in other similar syndromes such as Gram-negative septic shock, and therefore its positive predictive value for TSS is unknown.

Treatment

There are four important principles in the management of TSS: (i) identifying and treating the source of infection or colonization, (ii) using targeted antimicrobial therapy, (iii) rapidly initiating supportive care, and (iv) considering indications for adjunctive therapy such as intravenous immunoglobulin (IVIG) (Table 25.4).

Table 25.4 Principles of treatment of toxic shock syndrome.

Identify and treat source of infection
Remove foreign materials such as tampons
Drain all abscesses
Irrigate all open wounds
Aggressive early goal-directed therapy
Endotracheal intubation, if necessary
Intravenous fluids
Vasoactive medications as needed
Initiate appropriate antimicrobial therapy
Effective antistaphylococcal antimicrobials
Antimicrobials targeting protein synthesis
Consider adjunctive therapies
Intravenous immunoglobulin
Activated protein C infusion

Source control

A key factor in the pathophysiology of TSS is the ongoing production and circulation of superantigens. Making a meticulous effort to identify and remove the source of infection, if possible, is the first and most important aspect of treatment. All foreign bodies that may harbor *S. aureus* should be removed. Tampon removal in menstrual TSS cases is vital in order to prevent worsening of symptoms. Wounds, particularly in the perioperative period, may be a focus of infection with minimal or no signs of inflammation. Wound irrigation and bandage changes, even if the wounds appear uninvolved, can prevent further bacterial growth and superantigen absorption. If an abscess or loculated fluid collection exists, drainage and culture of the fluid is crucial.

Antimicrobial therapy

There are two main factors in selecting an appropriate antimicrobial or combination of antimicrobials to treat a patient with TSS: (i) the drug should be highly efficacious at killing *S. aureus* and (ii) the drug should inhibit ongoing superantigen production.

Bactericidal antimicrobials with activity against the cell wall have been the preferred empirical therapeutic agents. These antibiotics are typically β-lactamase-resistant antistaphylococcal penicillins and cephalosporins. There are some data to support concern that low levels of penicillins may actually increase superantigen production, and it is therefore important to ensure adequate drug dosing [106]. Since 2000, there have been growing reports of TSS resulting from MRSA strains, particularly in patients with a skin or soft tissue source [103,107–109]. In one review MRSA was associated with 9% of all cases during 2000–2003 [78]. The use of agents active against MRSA as an empirical antibiotic choice is becoming increasingly necessary. There are only case reports and *in vitro* data supporting the efficacy of vancomycin, linezolid, teicoplanin, or daptomycin in TSS; however, these drugs are becoming increasingly used to treat this illness [108,110,111].

Antimicrobials that target protein synthesis such as clindamycin have been shown to inhibit superantigen production [112]. Similar findings have been confirmed with linezolid and gentamicin [110,113,114]. However, protein synthesis inhibitors are considered bacteriostatic, with a relatively longer time to kill than cell wall-active agents. There is no comparison of cell wall-active drugs with protein synthesis inhibitors in staphylococcal TSS. In streptococcal TSS, there appears to be evidence that protein synthesis inhibitor-containing regimens do better than cell wall-active agents alone [115]. Therefore, in mild cases of TSS, and depending on local antimicrobial sensitivity profiles, it is recommended that either a cell wall-active agent such as a β-lactamase-resistant antistaphylococcal penicillin or clindamycin be used for MSSA and vancomycin or linezolid for MRSA. In more severe cases, the combination of a cell wall-active agent and protein synthesis inhibitor is recommended.

Supportive care

Many of the same principles established for other forms of shock apply to TSS. Early goal-directed therapy for patients with systemic inflammatory response syndrome and hypotension is likely key during the acute management of shock [116]. Early and aggressive fluid resuscitation, use of vasoactive agents, and endotracheal intubation have been demonstrated to significantly increase survival in patients with septic shock and can be practically applied in real-world settings during resuscitation [116,117]. In considering the similar pathophysiology, the same therapeutic principles should apply to TSS. Aggressive supportive care is a key component in the treatment of TSS.

Adjunctive therapy

The replacement of anti-superantigen antibody by IVIG has been used during the acute phase of illness. Anti-superantigen antibodies are thought to bind directly to superantigens, preventing them from activating T cells. The efficacy of anti-TSST-1 antibodies has been confirmed in rabbit models [118]. There is reasonable clinical evidence to support the use of IVIG in streptococcal TSS; however, similar data are not available to confirm the benefit in staphylococcal TSS [119,120]. There is also significant variation in the amount of anti-superantigen antibodies present in different IVIG preparations, which makes the level of benefit in staphylococcal TSS difficult to determine [121]. There is typically a 5–10% risk of mild infusion reactions and a much lower frequency of severe reactions [122]. Given the relatively low risk of infusion reactions and the potential benefit, IVIG is a reasonable adjunctive therapy in patients who are severely ill or who are not responding to initial therapies.

In patients with severe sepsis, infusions of drotrecogin alfa, also known as activated protein C, have demonstrated a survival benefit compared with placebo [123]. There have been several case reports of its use in TSS [107,124] and it was used in 14% of TSS patients in the Minneapolis–St Paul metropolitan area during 2000–2003 [78]. Recently, drotrecogin alfa use was studied in patients with sepsis, single organ failure, and APACHE II scores less than 25. This trial was stopped early as drotrecogin alfa did not provide appreciable mortality benefit and participants receiving the infusion were twice as likely to have severe bleeding complications [125]. Drotrecogin alfa should therefore be used with extreme caution in patients with mild to moderate illness and be reserved for TSS patients who are seriously ill.

Primary and secondary prophylaxis

Prolonged prophylactic antimicrobials are used routinely following sinonasal procedures, particularly when nasal packing is used. While no randomized trials exist regarding the use of antimicrobials in this setting, two-thirds of otolaryngologists reported in a survey that they routinely use prophylactic antimicrobials following septoplasty procedures [126]. With the incidence of TSS without prophylactic antimicrobials at 16 per 100 000 [59] and the incidence of *Clostridium difficile* diarrhea per outpatient antibiotic prescription at 10 per 100 000 [127] (10–100 times higher among hospitalized patients [128,129]), this practice may result in more complications than the number of TSS cases it prevents.

Among burn patients, there appears to be an increased incidence of TSS [66]. A group in Ireland observed a decrease in the rate of TSS among children with burns, from 8% of all admissions to no confirmed TSS cases following a single dose of an antistaphylococcal β-lactam antibiotic on admission [130]. No study has confirmed this observation. The risk of complications from a single antimicrobial dose is substantially less than multiple days of therapy and this strategy may be reasonable.

Consideration of secondary prophylaxis is appropriate in patients with recurrent TSS. Patients who use high-absorbency tampons or use them continuously for at least 1 day during their menstrual cycle are at increased risk of developing TSS [48,53]. With recurrent episodes, observed in up to one-third of patients with menstrual TSS [63,75,79], it is recommended that tampons be avoided and the least absorbent product be used [51,131]. Additionally, it may be appropriate to check for anti-superantigen antibodies among persons with recurrent TSS and, if absent, these individuals should avoid use of tampons indefinitely.

Related morbidity and mortality

Most patients recover fully following appropriate and timely treatment of TSS. Illness may persist in certain individuals, with most of the late sequelae being relatively mild and reversible. Desquamation occurs 7–14 days following onset of symptoms. As described above, there are TSS cases in persons with AIDS who have persistent desquamation [96]. Typically, however, desquamation resolves without significant complication. Involvement of other integumental structures can be persistent, with alopecia or nail loss in up to 50% [63].

Central nervous complications have also been regularly observed, with about half of patients having difficulty with long- or short-term memory, recurrent headaches, electroencephalographic abnormalities, or difficulty with concentration [63,100]. Also, cardiovascular complications, including recurrent syncope, electrocardiographic abnormalities, or a protracted cardiomyopathy, are seen in one-quarter of cases [63,80,87].

Early recognition of TSS by clinicians and early effective supportive care decreases mortality. The case fatality rate prior to 1980 was 10%. During 1980–1981 it decreased to 3.1% and by 1983 was 2.6% [17,132]. It has remained approximately at this level since then [25]. Typically, increased age, a nonmenstrual primary source, and multiple comorbidities are associated with increased mortality [23,25,133].

References

1 Stevens FA. The occurrence of *Staphylococcus aureus* infection with a scarlitiniform rash. JAMA 1927;88:1957–8.
2 Goodman JS. Toxic-shock syndrome and the Bundaberg disaster. N Engl J Med 1980;303:1417.
3 Report of the Royal Commisson on the fatalities at Bundaberg. Med J Aust 1928;2:2–31.
4 Aranow H, Wood WB. Staphylococcal infection simulating scarlet fever. JAMA 1942;119:1491–5.
5 McCloskey RV. Scarlet fever and necrotizing fasciitis caused by coagulase-positive hemolytic *Staphylococcus aureus*, phage type 85. Ann Intern Med 1973;78:85–7.
6 Todd J, Fishaut M, Kapral F, Welch T. Toxic-shock syndrome associated with phage-group-I Staphylococci. Lancet 1978;ii: 1116–18.
7 Toxic shock syndrome. MMWR CDC Surveill Summ 1980;29: 229–30.
8 Follow up on toxic shock syndrome. MMWR CDC Surveill Summ 1980;29:441–5.
9 Davis JP, Chesney PJ, Wand PJ, LaVenture M. Toxic-shock syndrome: epidemiologic features, recurrence, risk factors, and prevention. N Engl J Med 1980;303:1429–35.
10 Follow up on toxic shock syndrome. MMWR CDC Surveill Summ 1980;29:297–9.
11 Shands KN, Schmid GP, Dan BB *et al.* Toxic-shock syndrome in menstruating women: association with tampon use and *Staphylococcus aureus* and clinical features in 52 cases. N Engl J Med 1980;303:1436–42.
12 Schlech WF III, Shands KN, Reingold AL *et al.* Risk factors for development of toxic shock syndrome. Association with a tampon brand. JAMA 1982;248:835–9.
13 Reingold AL, Dan BB, Shands KN, Broome CV. Toxic-shock syndrome not associated with menstruation. A review of 54 cases. Lancet 1982;i:1–4.
14 Reingold AL, Hargrett NT, Dan BB, Shands KN, Strickland BY, Broome CV. Nonmenstrual toxic shock syndrome: a review of 130 cases. Ann Intern Med 1982;96:871–4.
15 Bartlett P, Reingold AL, Graham DR *et al.* Toxic shock syndrome associated with surgical wound infections. JAMA 1982;247: 1448–50.
16 Bracero L, Bowe E. Postpartum toxic shock syndrome. Am J Obstet Gynecol 1982;143:478–9.
17 Reingold AL, Hargrett NT, Shands KN *et al.* Toxic shock syndrome surveillance in the United States, 1980 to 1981. Ann Intern Med 1982;96:875–80.
18 Latham RH, Kehrberg MW, Jacobson JA, Smith CB. Toxic shock syndrome in Utah: a case-control and surveillance study. Ann Intern Med 1982;96:906–8.
19 Osterholm MT, Forfang JC. Surveillance of toxic shock syndrome in Minnesota: comments on national surveillance. Ann Intern Med 1982;96:887–90.
20 Broome CV. Epidemiology of toxic shock syndrome in the United States: overview. Rev Infect Dis 1989;11(suppl 1):S14–S21.
21 Todd JK, Wiesenthal AM, Ressman M, Caston SA, Hopkins RS. Toxic shock syndrome. II. Estimated occurrence in Colorado as influenced by case ascertainment methods. Am J Epidemiol 1985;122:857–67.
22 Petitti DB, Reingold A, Chin J. The incidence of toxic shock syndrome in Northern California. 1972 through 1983. JAMA 1986;255:368–72.
23 Gaventa S, Reingold AL, Hightower AW *et al.* Active surveillance for toxic shock syndrome in the United States, 1986. Rev Infect Dis 1989;11(suppl 1):S28–S34.
24 Centers for Disease Control and Prevention. Reduced incidence of menstrual toxic-shock syndrome: United States, 1980–1990. MMWR 1990;39:421–3.
25 Hajjeh RA, Reingold A, Weil A, Shutt K, Schuchat A, Perkins BA. Toxic shock syndrome in the United States: surveillance update, 1979–1996. Emerg Infect Dis 1999;5:807–10.
26 Rajagopalan G, Smart MK, Murali N, Patel R, David CS. Acute systemic immune activation following vaginal exposure to staphylococcal enterotoxin B: implications for menstrual shock. J Reprod Immunol 2007;73:51–9.
27 Dinges MM, Orwin PM, Schlievert PM. Exotoxins of *Staphylococcus aureus*. Clin Microbiol Rev 2000;13:16–34.
28 Schlievert PM. Role of superantigens in human disease. J Infect Dis 1993;167:997–1002.
29 Schlievert PM, Shands KN, Dan BB, Schmid GP, Nishimura RD. Identification and characterization of an exotoxin from *Staphylococcus aureus* associated with toxic-shock syndrome. J Infect Dis 1981;143:509–16.
30 Moza B, Varma AK, Buonpane RA *et al.* Structural basis of T-cell specificity and activation by the bacterial superantigen TSST-1. EMBO J 2007;26:1187–97.
31 McCormick JK, Yarwood JM, Schlievert PM. Toxic shock syndrome and bacterial superantigens: an update. Annu Rev Microbiol 2001;55:77–104.
32 Kotb M, Norrby-Teglund A, McGeer A *et al.* An immunogenetic and molecular basis for differences in outcomes of invasive group A streptococcal infections. Nat Med 2002;8: 1398–404.
33 Jarraud S, Cozon G, Vandenesch F, Bes M, Etienne J, Lina G. Involvement of enterotoxins G and I in staphylococcal toxic shock syndrome and staphylococcal scarlet fever. J Clin Microbiol 1999;37:2446–9.
34 Fey PD, Said-Salim B, Rupp ME *et al.* Comparative molecular analysis of community- or hospital-acquired methicillin-resistant *Staphylococcus aureus*. Antimicrob Agents Chemother 2003;47:196–203.
35 Schlievert PM, Osterholm MT, Kelly JA, Nishimura RD. Toxin and enzyme characterization of *Staphylococcus aureus* isolates

from patients with and without toxic shock syndrome. Ann Intern Med 1982;96:937–40.
36 Parsonnet J, Hansmann MA, Delaney ML *et al.* Prevalence of toxic shock syndrome toxin 1-producing *Staphylococcus aureus* and the presence of antibodies to this superantigen in menstruating women. J Clin Microbiol 2005;43:4628–34.
37 Durand G, Bes M, Meugnier H *et al.* Detection of new methicillin-resistant *Staphylococcus aureus* clones containing the toxic shock syndrome toxin 1 gene responsible for hospital- and community-acquired infections in France. J Clin Microbiol 2006;44:847–53.
38 Ferry T, Bes M, Dauwalder O *et al.* Toxin gene content of the Lyon methicillin-resistant *Staphylococcus aureus* clone compared with that of other pandemic clones. J Clin Microbiol 2006;44:2642–4.
39 Diep BA, Carleton HA, Chang RF, Sensabaugh GF, Perdreau-Remington F. Roles of 34 virulence genes in the evolution of hospital- and community-associated strains of methicillin-resistant *Staphylococcus aureus*. J Infect Dis 2006;193:1495–503.
40 Seybold U, Kourbatova EV, Johnson JG *et al.* Emergence of community-associated methicillin-resistant *Staphylococcus aureus* USA300 genotype as a major cause of health care-associated blood stream infections. Clin Infect Dis 2006;42:647–56.
41 Fitzgerald JR, Sturdevant DE, Mackie SM, Gill SR, Musser JM. Evolutionary genomics of *Staphylococcus aureus*: insights into the origin of methicillin-resistant strains and the toxic shock syndrome epidemic. Proc Natl Acad Sci USA 2001;98:8821–6.
42 Moran GJ, Krishnadasan A, Gorwitz RJ *et al.* Methicillin-resistant *S. aureus* infections among patients in the emergency department. N Engl J Med 2006;355:666–74.
43 Schlievert PM, Blomster DA. Production of staphylococcal pyrogenic exotoxin type C: influence of physical and chemical factors. J Infect Dis 1983;147:236–42.
44 Todd JK, Todd BH, Franco-Buff A, Smith CM, Lawellin DW. Influence of focal growth conditions on the pathogenesis of toxic shock syndrome. J Infect Dis 1987;155:673–81.
45 Ross RA, Onderdonk AB. Production of toxic shock syndrome toxin 1 by *Staphylococcus aureus* requires both oxygen and carbon dioxide. Infect Immun 2000;68:5205–9.
46 Yarwood JM, Schlievert PM. Oxygen and carbon dioxide regulation of toxic shock syndrome toxin 1 production by *Staphylococcus aureus* MN8. J Clin Microbiol 2000;38:1797–803.
47 Wagner G, Bohr L, Wagner P, Petersen LN. Tampon-induced changes in vaginal oxygen and carbon dioxide tensions. Am J Obstet Gynecol 1984;148:147–50.
48 Osterholm MT, Davis JP, Gibson RW *et al.* Tri-state toxic-state syndrome study. I. Epidemiologic findings. J Infect Dis 1982; 145:431–40.
49 Parsonnet J, Modern PA, Giacobbe KD. Effect of tampon composition on production of toxic shock syndrome toxin-1 by *Staphylococcus aureus* in vitro. J Infect Dis 1996;173:98–103.
50 Schlievert PM. Comparison of cotton and cotton/rayon tampons for effect on production of toxic shock syndrome toxin. J Infect Dis 1995;172:1112–14.
51 Berkley SF, Hightower AW, Broome CV, Reingold AL. The relationship of tampon characteristics to menstrual toxic shock syndrome. JAMA 1987;258:917–20.
52 Petitti DB, Reingold A. Tampon characteristics and menstrual toxic shock syndrome. JAMA 1988;259:686–7.
53 Reingold AL, Broome CV, Gaventa S, Hightower AW. Risk factors for menstrual toxic shock syndrome: results of a multistate case-control study. Rev Infect Dis 1989;11(suppl 1):S35–S41.
54 Czerwinski BS. Variation in feminine hygiene practices: as a function of age. J Obstet Gyn Neonat Nursing 2000;29:625–33.
55 Faich G, Pearson K, Fleming D, Sobel S, Anello C. Toxic shock syndrome and the vaginal contraceptive sponge. JAMA 1986; 255:216–18.
56 Schwartz B, Gaventa S, Broome CV *et al.* Nonmenstrual toxic shock syndrome associated with barrier contraceptives: Report of a case-control study. Rev Infect Dis 1989;11(suppl 1):S43–S48.
57 Hull HF, Mann JM, Sands CJ, Gregg SH, Kaufman PW. Toxic shock syndrome related to nasal packing. Arch Otolaryngol 1983;109:624–6.
58 Younis RT, Lazar RH. Delayed toxic shock syndrome after functional endonasal sinus surgery. Arch Otolaryngol Head Neck Surg 1996;122:83–5.
59 Jacobson JA, Kasworm EM. Toxic shock syndrome after nasal surgery. Case reports and analysis of risk factors. Arch Otolaryngol Head Neck Surg 1986;112:329–32.
60 Petitti DB, Reingold AL. Update through 1985 on the incidence of toxic shock syndrome among members of a prepaid health plan. Rev Infect Dis 1989;11(suppl 1):S22–S26; discussion S26–S27.
61 Andrews MM, Parent EM, Barry M, Parsonnet J. Recurrent nonmenstrual toxic shock syndrome: clinical manifestations, diagnosis, and treatment. Clin Infect Dis 2001;32:1470–9.
62 Davis D, Gash-Kim TL, Heffernan EJ. Toxic shock syndrome: case report of a postpartum female and a literature review. J Emerg Med 1998;16:607–14.
63 Kain KC, Schulzer M, Chow AW. Clinical spectrum of nonmenstrual toxic shock syndrome (TSS): comparison with menstrual TSS by multivariate discriminant analyses. Clin Infect Dis 1993;16:100–6.
64 Graham DR, O'Brien M, Hayes JM, Raab MG. Postoperative toxic shock syndrome. Clin Infect Dis 1995;20:895–9.
65 Frame JD, Eve MD, Hackett ME *et al.* The toxic shock syndrome in burned children. Burns Incl Therm Inj 1985;11:234–41.
66 Brown AP, Khan K, Sinclair S. Bacterial toxicosis/toxic shock syndrome as a contributor to morbidity in children with burn injuries. Burns 2003;29:733–8.
67 Withey SJ, Carver N, Frame JD, Walker CC. Toxic shock syndrome in adult burns. Burns 1999;25:659–62.
68 Jacobson JA, Burke JP, Benowitz BA, Clark PV. Varicella zoster and staphylococcal toxic shock syndrome in a young man. JAMA 1983;249:922–3.
69 Bergdoll MS, Crass BA, Reiser RF *et al.* An enterotoxin-like protein in *Staphylococcus aureus* strains from patients with toxic shock syndrome. Ann Intern Med 1982;96:969–71.
70 Bonventre PF, Linnemann C, Weckbach LS *et al.* Antibody responses to toxic-shock-syndrome (TSS) toxin by patients with TSS and by healthy staphylococcal carriers. J Infect Dis 1984;150:662–6.
71 Schlievert PM. Alteration of immune function by staphylococcal pyrogenic exotoxin type C: possible role in toxic-shock syndrome. J Infect Dis 1983;147:391–8.
72 Kansal R, Davis C, Hansmann MA *et al.* Structural and functional properties of antibodies to the superantigen TSST-1 and their relationship to menstrual toxic shock syndrome. J Clin Immunol 2007;27:327–38.

73 Vergeront JM, Stolz SJ, Crass BA, Nelson DB, Davis JP, Bergdoll MS. Prevalence of serum antibody to staphylococcal enterotoxin F among Wisconsin residents: implications for toxic-shock syndrome. J Infect Dis 1983;148:692–8.
74 Stolz SJ, Davis JP, Vergeront JM *et al.* Development of serum antibody to toxic shock toxin among individuals with toxic shock syndrome in Wisconsin. J Infect Dis 1985;151:883–9.
75 Davis JP, Osterholm MT, Helms CM *et al.* Tri-state toxic-shock syndrome study. II. Clinical and laboratory findings. J Infect Dis 1982;145:441–8.
76 Chesney PJ, Davis JP, Purdy WK, Wand PJ, Chesney RW. Clinical manifestations of toxic shock syndrome. JAMA 1981;246:741–8.
77 Wiesenthal AM, Todd JK. Toxic shock syndrome in children aged 10 years or less. Pediatrics 1984;74:112–17.
78 DeVries A, Lesher L, Lynfield R. Staphylococcal toxic shock syndrome, Minnesota, 2000–2003. Presented at the 44th Annual Meeting of Infectious Disease Society of America, Toronto, Canada, 2006.
79 Chesney PJ. Clinical aspects and spectrum of illness of toxic shock syndrome: overview. Rev Infect Dis 1989;11(suppl 1):S1–S7.
80 Crews JR, Harrison JK, Corey GR, Steenbergen C, Bashore TM. Stunned myocardium in the toxic shock syndrome. Ann Intern Med 1992;117:912–13.
81 Parsonnet J, Gillis ZA. Production of tumor necrosis factor by human monocytes in response to toxic-shock-syndrome toxin-1. J Infect Dis 1988;158:1026–33.
82 Fisher CJ Jr, Horowitz Z, Albertson TE. Cardiorespiratory failure in toxic shock syndrome: effect of dobutamine. Crit Care Med 1985;13:160–5.
83 Parsonnet J, Hickman RK, Eardley DD, Pier GB. Induction of human interleukin-1 by toxic-shock-syndrome toxin-1. J Infect Dis 1985;151:514–22.
84 Parsonnet J. Mediators in the pathogenesis of toxic shock syndrome: overview. Rev Infect Dis 1989;11(suppl 1):S263–S269.
85 Rolston RD, Yabek SM, Florman AL, Berman W Jr, Fripp RR, Paul DA. Severe cardiac conduction abnormalities associated with atypical toxic shock syndrome. J Pediatr 1990;117:89–92.
86 Olson RD, Stevens DL, Melish ME. Direct effects of purified staphylococcal toxic shock syndrome toxin 1 on myocardial function of isolated rabbit atria. Rev Infect Dis 1989;11(suppl 1): S313–S315.
87 Burns JR, Menapace FJ. Acute reversible cardiomyopathy complicating toxic shock syndrome. Arch Intern Med 1982;142: 1032–4.
88 Zeerleder S, Hack CE, Wuillemin WA. Disseminated intravascular coagulation in sepsis. Chest 2005;128:2864–75.
89 Brysk MM, Bell T, Tyring SK, Rajaraman S. Cytokines modulate terminal differentiation and the expression of predesquamin in cultured keratinocytes. Exp Cell Res 1994;211:49–52.
90 Tofte RW, Williams DN. Toxic shock syndrome. Evidence of a broad clinical spectrum. JAMA 1981;246:2163–7.
91 Chesney PJ, Slama SL, Hawkins RL *et al.* Outpatient diagnosis and management of toxic-shock syndrome. N Engl J Med 1981;304:1426.
92 Bass JW, Harden LB, Peixotto JH. Probable toxic shock syndrome without shock and multisystem involvement. Pediatrics 1982;70:279–81.
93 Bergdoll MS, Crass BA, Reiser RF, Robbins RN, Davis JP. A new staphylococcal enterotoxin, enterotoxin F, associated with toxic-shock-syndrome *Staphylococcus aureus* isolates. Lancet 1981;i:1017–21.
94 Chesney PJ, Bergdoll MS, Davis JP, Vergeront JM. The disease spectrum, epidemiology, and etiology of toxic-shock syndrome. Annu Rev Microbiol 1984;38:315–38.
95 Byer RL, Bachur RG. Clinical deterioration among patients with fever and erythroderma. Pediatrics 2006;118:2450–60.
96 Cone LA, Woodard DR, Byrd RG, Schulz K, Kopp SM, Schlievert PM. A recalcitrant, erythematous, desquamating disorder associated with toxin-producing staphylococci in patients with AIDS. J Infect Dis 1992;165:638–43.
97 Dinges MM, Gregerson DS, Tripp TJ, McCormick JK, Schlievert PM. Effects of total body irradiation and cyclosporin A on the lethality of toxic shock syndrome toxin-1 in a rabbit model of toxic shock syndrome. J Infect Dis 2003;188:1142–5.
98 Kamel NS, Banks MC, Dosik A, Ursea D, Yarilina AA, Posnett DN. Lack of muco-cutaneous signs of toxic shock syndrome when T cells are absent: *S. aureus* shock in immunodeficient adults with multiple myeloma. Clin Exp Immunol 2002;128:131–9.
99 Chesney PJ, Crass BA, Polyak MB *et al.* Toxic shock syndrome: management and long-term sequelae. Ann Intern Med 1982; 96:847–51.
100 Rosene KA, Copass MK, Kastner LS, Nolan CM, Eschenbach DA. Persistent neuropsychological sequelae of toxic shock syndrome. Ann Intern Med 1982;96:865–70.
101 Wiesenthal AM, Ressman M, Caston SA, Todd JK. Toxic shock syndrome. I. Clinical exclusion of other syndromes by strict and screening definitions. Am J Epidemiol 1985;122:847–56.
102 Centers for Disease Control and Prevention. Toxic shock syndrome: 1997 case definition. http://www.cdc.gov/epo/dphsi/casedef/toxicsscurrent.htm. Accessed October 2003.
103 Matsuda Y, Kato H, Yamada R *et al.* Early and definitive diagnosis of toxic shock syndrome by detection of marked expansion of T-cell-receptor VBeta2-positive T cells. Emerg Infect Dis 2003;9:387–9.
104 Llewelyn M, Sriskandan S, Terrazzini N, Cohen J, Altmann DM. The TCR Vbeta signature of bacterial superantigens spreads with stimulus strength. Int Immunol 2006;18:1433–41.
105 Brogan PA, Shah V, Klein N, Dillon MJ. Vbeta-restricted T cell adherence to endothelial cells: a mechanism for superantigen-dependent vascular injury. Arthritis Rheum 2004;50:589–97.
106 Parsonnet J. Nonmenstrual toxic shock syndrome: new insights into diagnosis, pathogenesis, and treatment. Curr Clin Top Infect Dis 1996;16:1–20.
107 Haddadin D, Samnani I, Moorman J. Drotrecogin alfa (activated) for nonmenstrual toxic shock syndrome associated with methicillin resistant *Staphylococcus aureus* infection. South Med J 2006;99:1295–6.
108 Jamart S, Denis O, Deplano A *et al.* Methicillin-resistant *Staphylococcus aureus* toxic shock syndrome. Emerg Infect Dis 2005; 11:636–7.
109 Cui L, Kasegawa H, Murakami Y, Hanaki H, Hiramatsu K. Postoperative toxic shock syndrome caused by a highly virulent methicillin-resistant *Staphylococcus aureus* strain. Scand J Infect Dis 1999;31:208–9.
110 Stevens DL, Wallace RJ, Hamilton SM, Bryant AE. Successful treatment of staphylococcal toxic shock syndrome with linezolid: a case report and in vitro evaluation of the production of

toxic shock syndrome toxin type 1 in the presence of antibiotics. Clin Infect Dis 2006;42:729–30.

111 Denis O, Deplano A, Nonhoff C *et al.* In vitro activities of ceftobiprole, tigecycline, daptomycin, and 19 other antimicrobials against methicillin-resistant *Staphylococcus aureus* strains from a national survey of Belgian hospitals. Antimicrob Agents Chemother 2006;50:2680–5.

112 Schlievert PM, Kelly JA. Clindamycin-induced suppression of toxic-shock syndrome: associated exotoxin production. J Infect Dis 1984;149:471.

113 Bernardo K, Pakulat N, Fleer S *et al.* Subinhibitory concentrations of linezolid reduce *Staphylococcus aureus* virulence factor expression. Antimicrob Agents Chemother 2004;48:546–55.

114 van Langevelde P, van Dissel JT, Meurs CJ, Renz J, Groeneveld PH. Combination of flucloxacillin and gentamicin inhibits toxic shock syndrome toxin 1 production by *Staphylococcus aureus* in both logarithmic and stationary phases of growth. Antimicrob Agents Chemother 1997;41:1682–5.

115 Zimbelman J, Palmer A, Todd J. Improved outcome of clindamycin compared with beta-lactam antibiotic treatment for invasive *Streptococcus pyogenes* infection. Pediatr Infect Dis J 1999;18:1096–100.

116 Rivers E, Nguyen B, Havstad S *et al.* Early goal-directed therapy in the treatment of severe sepsis and septic shock. N Engl J Med 2001;345:1368–77.

117 Trzeciak S, Dellinger RP, Abate NL *et al.* Translating research to clinical practice: a 1-year experience with implementing early goal-directed therapy for septic shock in the emergency department. Chest 2006;129:225–32.

118 Scott DF, Best GK, Kling JM, Thompson MR, Adinolfi LE, Bonventre PF. Passive protection of rabbits infected with toxic shock syndrome-associated strains of *Staphylococcus aureus* by monoclonal antibody to toxic shock syndrome toxin 1. Rev Infect Dis 1989;11(suppl 1):S214–S217.

119 Kaul R, McGeer A, Norrby-Teglund A *et al.* Intravenous immunoglobulin therapy for streptococcal toxic shock syndrome: a comparative observational study. Clin Infect Dis 1998;28:800–7.

120 Darenberg J, Ihendyane N, Sjolin J *et al.* Intravenous immunoglobulin G therapy in streptococcal toxic shock syndrome: a European randomized, double-blind, placebo-controlled trial. Clin Infect Dis 2003;37:333–40.

121 Schrage B, Duan G, Yang LP, Fraser JD, Proft T. Different preparations of intravenous immunoglobulin vary in their efficacy to neutralize streptococcal superantigens: implications for treatment of streptococcal toxic shock syndrome. Clin Infect Dis 2006;43:743–6.

122 Negi V, Elluru S, Siberil S *et al.* Intravenous immunoglobulin: an update on the clinical use and mechanisms of action. J Clin Immunol 2007;27:233–45.

123 Bernard GR, Vincent J-L, Laterre P-F *et al.* Efficacy and safety of recombinant human activated protein C for severe sepsis. N Engl J Med 2001;344:699–709.

124 Kravitz GR, Dries DJ, Peterson ML, Schlievert PM. Purpura fulminans due to *Staphylococcus aureus*. Clin Infect Dis 2005;40: 941–7.

125 Abraham E, Laterre P-F, Garg R *et al.* Drotrecogin alfa (activated) for adults with severe sepsis and a low risk of death. N Engl J Med 2005;353:1332–41.

126 Rechtweg JS, Paolini RV, Belmont MJ, Wax MK. Postoperative antibiotic use of septoplasty: a survey of practice habits of the membership of the American Rhinologic Society. Am J Rhinol 2001;15:315–20.

127 Hirschhorn L, Trnka Y, Onderdonk A, Lee M, Platt R. Epidemiology of community-acquired *Clostridium difficile*-associated diarrhea. J Infect Dis 1994;169:127–33.

128 Dallal R, Harbrecht B, Boujoukas A *et al.* Fulminant *Clostridium difficile*: an underappreciated and increasing cause of death and complications. Ann Surg 2002;235:363–72.

129 Berild D, Smaabrekke L, Halvorsen DS, Lelek M, Stahlsberg EM, Ringertz SH. *Clostridium difficile* infections related to antibiotic use and infection control facilities in two university hospitals. J Hosp Infect 2003;54:202–6.

130 Rashid A, Brown AP, Khan K. On the use of prophylactic antibiotics in prevention of toxic shock syndrome. Burns 2005;31:981–5.

131 Reingold AL. Toxic shock syndrome: an update. Am J Obstet Gynecol 1991;165:1236–9.

132 Reingold AL. Epidemiology of toxic-shock syndrome, United States, 1960–1984. MMWR CDC Surveill Summ 1984;33:19SS–22SS.

133 Reingold AL. Toxic shock syndrome and the contraceptive sponge. JAMA 1986;255:242–3.

Chapter 26
Toxin-mediated Syndromes

Tristan Ferry and Jerome Etienne
INSERM U851 and Centre National de Référence des Staphylocoques, Université Lyon, Lyon, France

Introduction

Staphylococcus aureus can produce multiple virulence factors, including toxins [1,2]. Among the various families of *S. aureus* toxins, some (hemolysins, most of the bicomponent synergohymenotropic toxins) promote tissue invasion and facilitate, with other produced virulence factors such as enzymes, the occurrence of classical suppurative infections [1–3]. Others have particular targeted effects [such as Panton–Valentine leukocidin (PVL), a bicomponent synergohymenotropic toxin] or particular mechanisms of action (superantigenic and exfoliative toxins), promoting local and/or systemic clinical manifestations that define toxin-mediated syndromes [1,2,4–6].

A syndrome consists of a combination of several clinically recognizable features, which often occur together. Most syndromes include one or more characteristics that are essential for diagnosis, plus minor features that may be present or absent. Staphylococcal toxin-mediated syndromes may be due to the single action of a toxin or to the combined effects of a toxin and one or several other virulence factors [2]. Staphylococcal superantigenic toxins can cause food poisoning, toxic shock syndrome and, possibly, purpura fulminans [2,7,8]. Exfoliative toxins are responsible for bullous impetigo and staphylococcal scalded skin syndrome (SSSS) [2,9]. PVL aggravates skin and musculoskeletal infections and is associated with necrotizing pneumonia [2,10].

Why is it important?

Staphylococcal toxin-mediated syndromes vary widely in their frequency and severity. In some (e.g., food poisoning), cases are common and death infrequent. For others (e.g., purpura fulminans), the syndrome is uncommon but mortality is high. Rapid ongoing changes in the causative strains, usually to community-acquired methicillin-resistant *S. aureus* (CA-MRSA) that produces PVL, of some diseases (e.g., bone and joint infection) has significantly altered the epidemiology, severity, and management of these conditions. Initiation of appropriate antistaphylococcal treatment may eradicate a focus of infection and/or block the production or action of a toxin. Identifying and characterizing the organism allows control of the strain in hospital or community outbreaks.

Specific topics with illustrations

Syndromes associated with superantigenic toxins

The toxins

To date, 21 superantigenic toxins produced by *S. aureus* have been described, comprising toxic shock syndrome toxin (TSST)-1 and 20 staphylococcal enterotoxin (SE) or staphylococcal enterotoxin-like (SEl) toxins with emetic properties in monkeys (SEA, SEB, SEC, SED, SEE, SEG, SEH, SEI, SElJ, SElK, SElL, SElM, SElN, SElO, SEP, SElQ, SElR, SElU, SElU2, SElV [1,11,12]. These superantigenic toxins are usually produced in the postexponential growth phase, although some that are weakly produced (e.g., SEA) are thought to be made in the exponential phase [1]. They are heat-stable and potent mitogens. They bypass normal antigen presentation by cross-linking the Vβ domain of the T-cell receptor with major histocompatibility complex class II molecules on antigen-presenting cells. A given superantigenic toxin thereby selectively stimulates and expands one or several Vβ subsets, leading to massive T-cell proliferation and to the release of proinflammatory cytokines [1,12,13].

Staphylococcal food poisoning

Pathogenesis

Staphylococcal food poisoning is due to ingestion of food containing a staphylococcal enterotoxin [8]. The main source of contamination is human and handlers contaminate the food via manual contact or via the respiratory tract by coughing and/or sneezing [8]. Contamination may occur before or after the heat treatment of the food and cold-chain failure is one of the main facilitators of *S. aureus* growth with neutral pH [8,14]. Pasteurization kills *S. aureus* but has no noteworthy effect on preformed

Staphylococci in Human Disease, 2nd edition. Edited by Kent B. Crossley, Kimberly K. Jefferson, Gordon Archer, Vance G. Fowler, Jr.

enterotoxins [1,8]. Many different foods may favor the production of enterotoxins (e.g., milk and cream, butter, ham, cheeses, sausage, cooked meals including poultry-based meals, fish and shellfish, eggs, and sandwich fillings) and the origin of staphylococcal food poisoning differs widely among countries due to differences in consumption and food habits [15–17]. The amount of toxin required to cause staphylococcal food poisoning in humans is estimated to be about 100 ng [18].

Little is known about how enterotoxins cause food poisoning. They probably affect the gastrointestinal tract in multiple ways [8]. Firstly, they may activate the sympathetic nervous system by stimulating the vagus nerve, as denervation of the abdominal viscera blocks emesis in monkeys challenged with enterotoxin by mouth [19]. Enterotoxins may also have a direct effect on the intestinal epithelium, inducing secretion of water and electrolytes into the bowel lumen and inhibiting their reabsorption [20,21]. Enterotoxins may also activate intraepithelial lymphocytes after crossing epithelial cell membranes by a facilitated transcytotic mechanism [22]. Finally, enterotoxins may interact with mast cells, leading to histamine and leukotriene release, followed by nausea and vomiting [23]. Overall, digestive troubles observed during staphylococcal food poisoning may be explained by sympathetic activation coupled with production of cytokines and mediators in response to enterotoxins [8].

Epidemiology

Staphylococcus aureus is the most frequent cause of toxin-mediated food-borne disease, and the second most frequent cause (after *Salmonella*) of all food-borne diseases [8,24,25]. Most of these *S. aureus* isolates are susceptible to methicillin [8]. Regular microbiological surveys have revealed that about one-quarter of strains contaminating prepared food and raw ingredients are enterotoxigenic [8]. Nevertheless, estimations vary considerably from one food to another and from one report to another. Older studies do not take into account newly described enterotoxins (such as those belonging to the *egc* locus) [16,26,27]. SEA, SEB, and SED are the enterotoxins most frequently responsible for outbreaks of staphylococcal food poisoning [8,16]. The involvement of enterotoxins encoded by the *egc* locus is unclear. This locus is frequently detected in isolates responsible for food poisoning, but it is mainly associated with genes encoding classical enterotoxins such as SEA [8,16,27]. There is good correlation between the presence of genes encoding classical enterotoxins and their production *in vitro*, whereas most isolates harboring the *seg* and *sei* genes (belonging to the *egc* locus) do not produce detectable SEG or SEI [28,29]. Finally, in animal models, SEG has different emetic activities compared with SEI as higher doses of SEG are required [30]. Quantitative studies of *egc*-encoded enterotoxins in foods would help to demonstrate their involvement in staphylococcal food poisoning.

Clinical syndrome

Staphylococcal food poisoning is defined by the onset of an acute illness with gastrointestinal symptoms affecting two or more people who shared a meal in the previous 6 hours. The onset of symptoms is acute and rapid (sometimes only 30 min after the meal), and most patients recover spontaneously within 24 hours. The symptoms include nausea, violent vomiting, abdominal cramps, and liquid diarrhea [31].

Differential diagnosis

Various bacteria can cause food poisoning, but rapid onset (< 6 hours) is usually associated with preformed toxins. *Bacillus cereus* causes vomiting 30 min to 6 hours after the consumption of contaminated food (milk products and cereals, including cooked rice and pasta) due to a heat-stable low-molecular-weight toxin [32]. However, *B. cereus* food poisoning is three to four times less frequent than staphylococcal food poisoning in the USA and Europe [8,24]. *Clostridium perfringens* can also cause toxin-mediated food poisoning. The toxin is not preformed in foods but produced in the gut and symptoms thus occur at least 8 hours after ingestion of contaminated food [33]. Salmonellae, the leading cause of food poisoning in the USA and Europe (about 1.4 million cases annually in the USA), can also cause sudden-onset nausea and abdominal cramping [8,24]. As *Salmonella* food poisoning is not mediated by a toxin, the incubation period is longer and generally ranges from 12 to 72 hours. Salmonella food poisoning, as is true of that caused by other invasive enteric pathogens, can also be associated with fever and mucus-containing and/or bloody diarrhea, which are lacking in staphylococcal food poisoning.

Diagnosis

Staphylococcal food poisoning is confirmed by at least one of the following: (i) recovery of more than 10^5 *S. aureus* per gram of food remnants; (ii) detection of enterotoxins in food remnants; and (iii) isolation of *S. aureus* strains with the same phage type from both vomit and food remnants [8]. Enterotoxins can be detected directly in food using a commercial kit based on rapid reverse passive latex agglutination, although this method is only suitable for classical enterotoxins (SEA, SEB, SEC, and SED) [29].

Treatment

Symptomatic treatment such as hydration and management of gastrointestinal symptoms is usually sufficient. Antibiotics are not beneficial, as the source of the disorder is a preformed toxin.

Prevention

The first preventive measure is the application of appropriate hygienic procedures and enforcement of the cold chain. Microbial risk assessment in the case of staphylococcal food poisoning relies on the identification and quantification of coagulase-positive isolates in end products, and on assessment of enterotoxin production [8].

Staphylococcal purpura fulminans

Pathogenesis

Classic purpura fulminans consists of necrotizing inflammatory skin lesions provoked by endotoxins (produced by Gram-negative bacteria), as demonstrated by the Shwartzman-like reaction in animal models [34]. Gram-positive bacteria such as streptococci and staphylococci, which do not produce endotoxin, may also cause purpura fulminans but the virulence factors involved are unclear [35]. Kravitz *et al.* [7] have described five cases of *S. aureus* septic shock with purpura fulminans directly associated with strains that produced large amounts of TSST-1, SEB, or SEC *in vitro*. Staphylococcal purpura fulminans may represent an overlap between toxic shock and septic shock resulting from coproduction of superantigenic toxins and other virulence factors (capsule or cell-wall components, α-toxin, etc.). The former would enhance the proinflammatory response and create a "cytokine storm" leading to disseminated intravascular coagulation and dermal vascular thrombosis [7,36].

Patients with fulminant meningococcemia have markedly reduced plasma levels of activated protein C, owing to dysfunction of the endothelial protein C activation pathway. Activated protein C is not only an anticoagulant but is also an important modulator of the inflammatory response. Meningococcemia is generally far more likely than other types of bacteremia to disrupt the activated protein C pathway [37]. Reduction of activated protein C may play a role in the pathogenesis of staphylococcal purpura fulminans.

Epidemiology

Because *S. aureus*-induced illnesses are not notifiable, we do not know the precise frequency of purpura fulminans caused by this organism. Kravitz *et al.* [7] recorded five cases in a 4-year period in the Minneapolis–St Paul area of the USA. Staphylococcal purpura fulminans is considered a newly emerging illness associated with superantigen production. One of the cases described by Kravitz *et al.* was related to the major American CA-MRSA clone, and the incidence of this syndrome may therefore increase in future.

Clinical syndrome

Like patients with *Neisseria meningitidis* purpura fulminans, patients with staphylococcal purpura fulminans present with the four cardinal features, namely large purpuric skin lesions, fever, hypotension, and disseminated intravascular coagulation. The cutaneous lesions appear early in the disease and are characterized by petechiae and purpura mainly located on the trunk and extremities, and sometimes over the entire body. The purpuric lesions are initially small, irregular, slightly elevated, and painful. Large hemorrhagic lesions then appear rapidly, together with disseminated intravascular coagulation and multiple organ failure [7,37]. Meningococcemia is by far the most common infection associated with purpura fulminans, followed by streptococcal infection [35,37,38]. Differential diagnoses of purpura fulminans include Rocky Mountain spotted fever, endocarditis, and thrombotic thrombocytopenic purpura (which may be associated with leptospirosis). However, the purpura progresses less rapidly in these latter conditions than during meningococcal or staphylococcal purpura fulminans [38].

Diagnosis

Staphylococcal purpura fulminans is diagnosed when the described clinical syndrome is present and *S. aureus* is recovered in cultures of blood or respiratory secretions (especially when necrotizing pneumonia is also present [7]). Ideally, the detection of *in vivo* production of superantigenic toxins should be required to demonstrate the involvement of these toxins during the process of the disease.

Treatment

Treatment of patients with staphylococcal purpura fulminans includes symptomatic management of organ dysfunction and classical antistaphylococcal chemotherapy [7]. As during fulminant meningococcemia, early administration of activated protein C (drotrecogin) may help to minimize purpuric skin injury and downregulate the inflammatory cascade before irreparable tissue injury occurs [7,35]. Specific treatment that blocks the production and/or activity of superantigenic toxins may be indicated [7,36].

How to detect superantigenic toxins *in vivo*

Superantigenic toxins can be detected in vomit in cases of staphylococcal food poisoning, but identifying the toxin in the suspect food is more useful for identifying and eradicating the source of contamination [8,29,31].

It is not currently possible to detect superantigenic toxins directly in blood or other biological fluids or tissues in patients with staphylococcal purpura fulminans or toxic shock syndrome. Implication of the superantigenic toxins is mainly based on detection of the corresponding genes or by testing *in vitro* toxin production by the clinical isolate [6,7]. During menstrual and nonmenstrual toxic shock syndrome, detecting the Vβ signature of a superantigenic toxin is a first approach to obtaining an early biological marker that may facilitate the timely introduction of antitoxin agents [39–41].

How to block the effect of superantigenic toxins

Specific treatment of purpura fulminans, as toxic shock syndrome, may include antibiotics such as clindamycin and linezolid that block toxin production, and administration of intravenous immunoglobulin (IVIG) that blocks superantigenic activity *in vitro* [42,43].

Syndromes associated with exfoliative toxins

The toxins

Staphylococcus aureus exfoliative toxins (ETs) are serine proteases that do not possess significant enzymatic activity in their native state [1,4]. They specifically target desmoglein-1, one of the main cell–cell adhesion molecules of the epidermis. Three-dimensional structural analysis of ETs suggests that binding of the N-terminal α-helix to desmoglein-1 results in a conformational change that reveals the active site of the toxin and allows it to cleave the extracellular domain of desmoglein-1 ("key-in-lock" mechanism), thereby disrupting cell–cell adhesion [1,4]. Early studies of ETs suggested they might have superantigenic properties, but recent *in vitro* analyses have failed to confirm this and uncertainty about this issue remains [44,45]. There are three ET serotypes, designated ETA, ETB, and ETD [9,46,47]. ETA is the predominant isoform in Europe and the USA, whereas ETB is the most frequent in Japan [9,48,49]. Each ET serotype may also contribute to regional differences in ET-associated diseases [51]. The *eta* gene is chromosomal, whereas *etb* is carried on plasmids [9,46]. Isolates dually positive for *etd* and PVL can cause deep-seated infections such as furuncles, cutaneous abscesses, and finger pulp infection [52]. Most syndromes associated with ETs mainly affect children.

Bullous impetigo

Impetigo is caused by group A β-hemolytic streptococci and/or by *S. aureus*. It is the most frequent contagious pediatric skin infection. Bullous impetigo accounts for 10–30% of cases of *S. aureus* impetigo and is associated with intraepidermic ET production after local bacterial invasion [46]. Some authors see a continuum of disease, with differing exotoxin involvement, from staphylococcal nonbullous impetigo to bullous impetigo and abscesses [46,53].

Pathogenesis

Bullous impetigo is a suppurative superficial skin infection associated with ET-positive staphylococci. The epidemic *S. aureus* strain is easily transmitted by skin contact and by handling objects such as toys and furniture. As during impetigo, *S. aureus* invades the skin, sometimes after minor trauma, and infects the horny layer (stratum corneum) of the epidermis due to the production of cytotoxins and enzymes that damage the skin and cause inflammation [4,46]. Local ET production cleaves cell–cell links and promotes blister formation (Figure 26.1). Specific cleavage of cells in the stratum spinosum and stratum granulosum depends on which of the four desmoglein isoforms are present (see Figure 26.1) [4,46]. In bullous impetigo the skin damage is restricted to the site of infection. A recent survey showed that *S. aureus* isolates responsible for nonbullous impetigo (also called crusted impetigo) may also harbor genes encoding ETA and/or ETB, suggesting that bullous and nonbullous *S. aureus* impetigo may be part of the same disease [53].

Epidemiology

ETA seems to be more specifically linked to bullous impetigo, as a recent study has revealed that 60% of

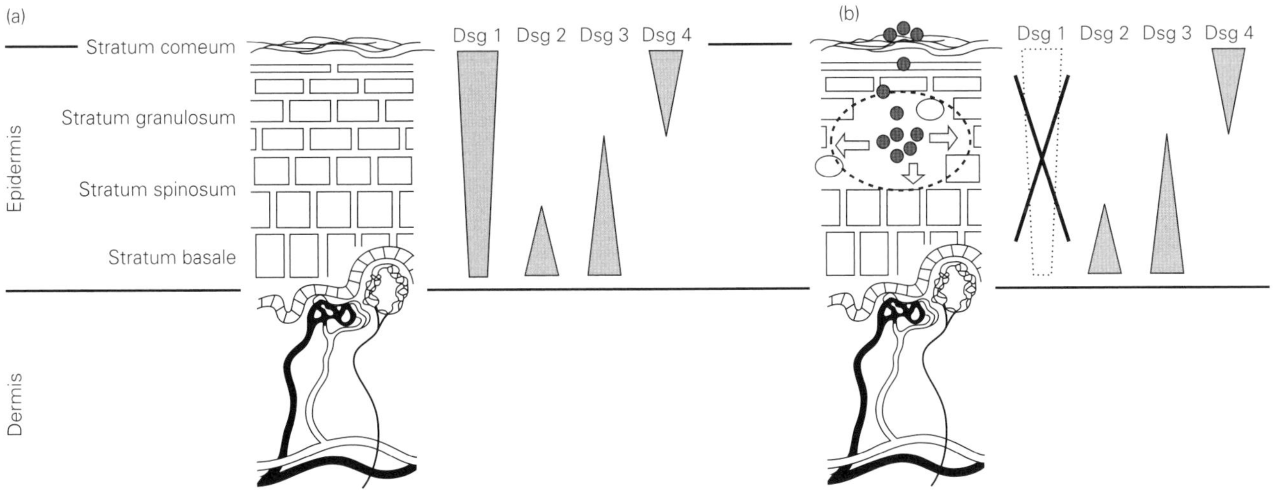

Figure 26.1 (a) Distribution of desmoglein isoforms in human epidermis. Desmoglein-1 is expressed throughout the human epidermis, whereas desmoglein-3 expression is restricted to the basal and immediate suprabasal layers. Desmoglein-2 and desmoglein-4 expression are restricted to the basal layer and just below the horny layer, respectively. (b) Pathophysiology of intraepidermal blisters caused by exfoliative toxins during bullous impetigo. Specific cleavage of desmoglein-1 by exfoliative toxins causes blisters in the stratum spinosum and stratum granulosum, where the loss of desmoglein-1 function is not compensated for by the other desmoglein isoforms.

S. aureus isolates responsible for bullous impetigo are positive for *eta* whereas only 5% are positive for *etb* [51]. Outbreaks of impetigo have been described, mainly in nurseries. A CA-MRSA clone harboring *eta* was detected in Japan in 2002, and more recently in Switzerland [54,55].

Clinical syndrome

Bullous impetigo starts with small or large (usually > 5 mm in diameter) superficial and fragile bullae on the trunk, face and/or extremities. Often, only the remnants of ruptured bullae are left by the time the patient is seen by a physician, in the form of eroded plaques surrounded by scales and sometimes covered with crusts. Bullous impetigo is not associated with lymphadenopathy [46].

Diagnosis

Clinical diagnosis of bullous impetigo is usually simple. Isolation from an intact bulla of an *S. aureus* strain producing an ET or harboring an ET gene confirms the diagnosis. Differential diagnoses include thermal burns and herpes simplex virus infection, characterized by clustered vesicles on an erythematous base (usually on the lips) [46].

Treatment

Management of bullous impetigo includes improved hygiene. Treatment may also include total body washing with soap and water and cleansing of the affected area with antiseptic lotion. Systemic antistaphylococcal antibiotics are usually recommended. Even if bullous impetigo appears to be less contagious than nonbullous impetigo, outbreaks have been reported in schools and in nurseries and requiring infected students to remain at home may limit dissemination of the epidemic strain [56].

Staphylococcal scalded skin syndrome

Pathogenesis

SSSS, also known as Ritter disease, is the generalized form of bulllous impetigo, with disseminated flaccid blisters and desquamation [9,46]. ETs spread through the bloodstream from a focal site of colonization (such as the nose or pharynx) or from a site of infection (lungs, urinary tract, etc.), causing remote epidermal damage (Figure 26.2) [9,46]. Similarities have been noted between the pathogenesis of SSSS and an autoimmune blistering skin disease called pemphigus foliaceus, which is associated with IgG autoantibodies targeting desmoglein-1 [46]. As during pemphigus foliaceus, epidermal blistering occurs during SSSS and the mucosae are not involved, even though they also contain desmoglein-1.

The "desmoglein compensation" hypothesis may explain why the stratum spinosum and stratum granulosum are blistered by ETs during SSSS while the mucosa is spared [4,9,46]. In humans, four desmoglein isoforms with tissue-specific distributions have been identified. Desmoglein-1 is expressed throughout the epidermis (most intensely in superficial layers) but exclusively in superficial layers of

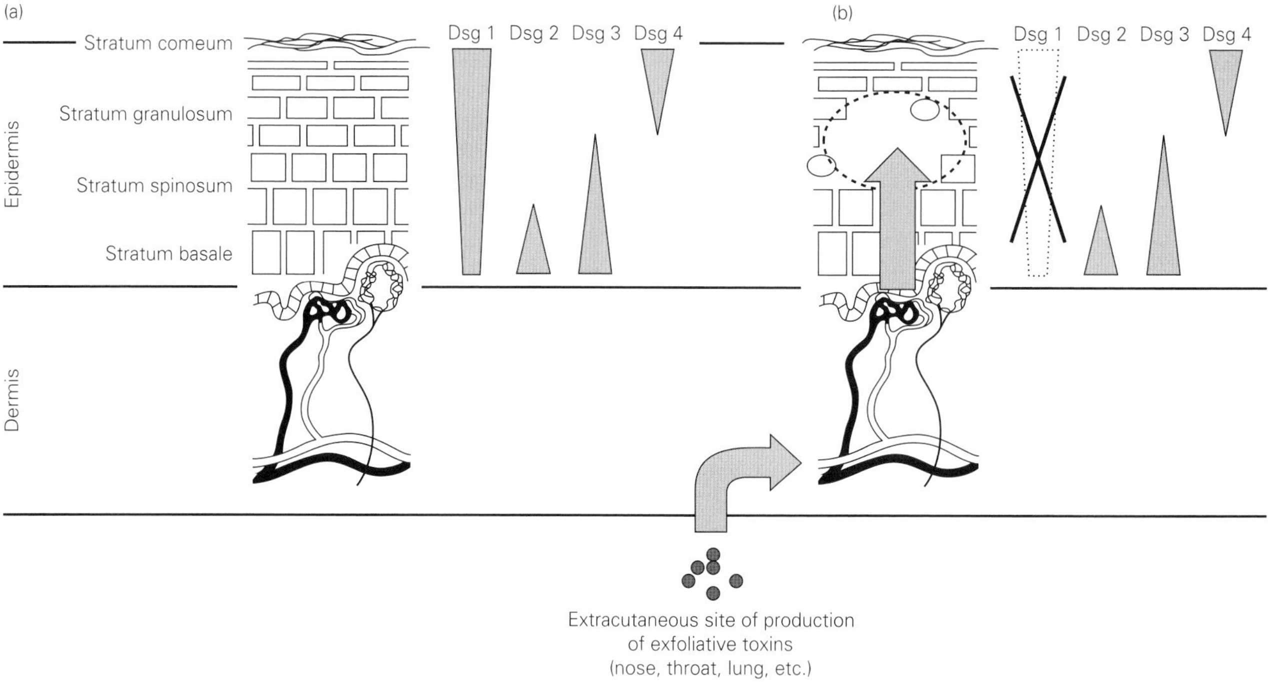

Figure 26.2 (a) Distribution of desmoglein isoforms in human epidermis. (b) Pathophysiology of intraepidermal blisters caused by exfoliative toxins during staphylococcal scalded skin syndrome. Specific cleavage of desmoglein-1 by exfoliative toxins that spread throughout the body from a distant site of production causes blisters in the stratum spinosum and stratum granulosum, where the loss of desmoglein-1 function is not compensated for by the other desmoglein isoforms.

mucosae. Desmoglein-3 is expressed in the basal and immediate suprabasal layers of the epidermidis and throughout the mucosal epithelia. Thus, when desmoglein-1 is the target of staphylococcal ETs, blisters occur exclusively in the superficial epidermis (see Figure 26.2), as desmoglein-3 maintains cell–cell adhesion in the mucosa [4,9,46].

Epidemiology

Newborns and young children (< 5 years) are most commonly affected by SSSS [9,46]. Adults might be protected as they are more likely than children to produce antibodies that neutralize ETs [9,46]. SSSS in adults is often associated with immunosuppression or renal failure, as the kidneys are critical for clearing ETs from the bloodstream [9,46,57–59]. SSSS seems to be more strongly associated with ETB than with ETA [9,50,51]. The rare cases of generalized SSSS reported in young immunocompetent adults have been associated with *etb*-harboring strains [51,60]. Most *S. aureus* isolates responsible for sporadic SSSS are susceptible to methicillin [9,51,61]. Nosocomial outbreaks of SSSS due to both methicillin-susceptible *S. aureus* (MSSA) and MRSA have been described in European hospitals [62,63]. No cases of SSSS due to CA-MRSA have so far been described. Few data are available on the incidence of SSSS. In Germany, the population-based registry of severe skin reactions suggests a low overall incidence of 0.009–0.13 per million inhabitants per year [58].

Clinical syndrome

The primary infection usually begins in the conjunctiva, nasopharynx, ear, urinary tract, or skin. The clinical picture of SSSS begins with acute systemic signs such as fever and malaise, associated with faint macules, predominantly around the eyes, nose or mouth in children, rapidly followed by a generalized erythematous scarlatiniform eruption that is more pronounced in skinfolds. Large sheets of epidermis detach within about 24–48 hours, mainly in skinfolds and around orifices, and the Nikolsky sign is positive (i.e., an intact blister spreads when lateral pressure is applied to its edge). Disseminated highly fragile flaccid bullae are also present. The mucous membranes are respected. The resulting desquamation reveals an erythematous base that heals rapidly. Severity ranges from localized blisters to exfoliation of the entire body surface. Most children recover with appropriate care, but SSSS is fatal in up to 60% of adults, who usually have an underlying illness and frequently develop bacteremia and pneumonia, implying a bad prognosis [9,38,46].

Diagnosis

The diagnosis of SSSS is based on the clinical appearance (widespread blistering of the epidermis without mucosal damage), the characteristic histopathology (midepidermal splitting at the level of the zona granulosa), and isolation of an *S. aureus* strain from a site of colonization or infection that produces ETA or ETB *in vitro* or that harbors an ET-encoding gene [9,38,46]. In contrast to bullous impetigo, the blister fluid is sterile and the *S. aureus* strain responsible for the disease is more difficult to isolate. The main differential diagnosis is toxic epidermal necrolysis (Lyell syndrome), which usually involves the mucosae and in which subepidermal cleavage is associated with epidermal necrosis [38,64].

Treatment

Like patients with widespread burns, patients with SSSS have poor temperature control, lose large amounts of fluids, and are very susceptible to secondary infections. Hospitalization is necessary and management consists of fluid resuscitation, local treatment (barrier creams and compresses), and systemic antibiotics to eradicate the focus of infection [9,38,64].

How to detect exfoliative toxins *in vivo*

There is currently no simple test for ETs in bulla fluid or serum that is suitable for use in hospital laboratories. Recently, however, Ladhani *et al.* [65] developed a system that detects picogram amounts of ETA directly in serum.

How to block the effect of exfoliative toxins

Antibiotics such as clindamycin that inhibit the production of other exotoxins, such as α-toxin, PVL and superantigenic toxins, are not known to block ET production and are not recommended for the treatment of SSSS.

Syndromes associated with Panton–Valentine leukocidin

The toxin

PVL is a bicomponent synergohymenotropic toxin that targets the outer membrane of polymorphonuclear cells (PMNs), monocytes, and macrophages. Membrane attack begins on contact with the first PVL component, LukS, followed by oligomerization with the second component, LukF, thus creating a pore. This induces calcium channels to open, leading to calcium influx, massive release of inflammatory mediators, and apoptosis or necrosis of the cell, depending on the PVL concentration. In humans, the contribution of PVL to the severity of *S. aureus* infection is unclear as our understanding is mainly based on the association of genes encoding PVL and clinical symptoms. Animal models are useful for studying the role of PVL in PVL-associated diseases, and the influence of the PVL phage on the expression of other virulence factors [66–68].

Skin and soft tissue infection

Pathogenesis

Staphylococcus aureus is one of the main pathogens responsible for skin and soft tissue infections, combining the expression of various virulence factors such as adhesins (microbial surface components recognizing adhesive matrix molecules, or MSCRAMMs) (see Chapter 4) with the production of toxins and enzymes that promote skin invasion [2,69]. PVL is not required to induce skin and soft tissue infection, as most *S. aureus* isolates responsible for these infections do not harbor the phage that encodes PVL. However, skin and soft tissue infections due to *S. aureus* strains that harbor the PVL phage are usually more severe. Hence, PVL may enhance the virulence of *S. aureus* strains. PVL has a direct proinflammatory and dermonecrotic effect: when injected intradermally to rabbits, PVL induces severe inflammatory lesions with capillary dilation, chemotaxis, PMN infiltration, and skin necrosis [70]. The degree of necrosis depends on the dose of PVL. None of these effects occur in rabbits immunized against LukS and LukF [70].

Epidemiology

The epidemiology of skin and soft tissue infections is changing with the spread of CA-MRSA clones that harbor the PVL phage [71]. Up to now, most PVL-positive *S. aureus* skin and soft tissue infections have been due to unrelated MSSA strains [10]. However, in a recent survey, Moran *et al.* [72] showed that the predominant CA-MRSA clone in the USA (USA300) is now the most common identifiable cause of skin and soft tissue infections among patients presenting to emergency departments in 11 cities [72]. In Europe, the prevalence is generally lower (about 1–7%), but some countries such as Greece are reporting much higher rates [73,74]. The incidence of skin and soft tissue infections due to CA-MRSA could potentially increase rapidly all over Europe in coming years. Incarcerated persons, intravenous drug users, native Americans, Pacific Islanders, athletes, men who have sex with men, soldiers, and children are groups that have been identified as being at risk for CA-MRSA infections, although many patients with CA-MRSA infection have none of these risk factors [71,75].

Clinical syndrome

Skin and soft tissue infections associated with PVL-positive *S. aureus* strains seem to be more severe than those caused by their PVL-negative counterparts. Necrotic skin lesions are a common presentation of PVL-positive *S. aureus* infections. Superficial skin lesions include furuncle-associated infections or glabrous skin abscesses that are often incorrectly attributed to insect bites [69,71,75]. Furuncles caused by PVL-positive *S. aureus* strains are associated with more rapidly progressive infection, a more frequent need for surgical drainage, and the occurrence of concomitant multiple sites of infection [71,76,77]. Abscesses of the glabrous skin associated with PVL-positive *S. aureus* (mainly CA-MRSA) infections may involve various parts of the skin such as a limb, the buttock, the umbilicus, the neck, or the face [75]. Sometimes, rapid extension of the infection may occur and lead to life-threatening soft tissue infection. Rutar *et al.* [78] reported an orbital cellulitis with bilateral loss of vision and cavernous sinus thrombosis following a mistreated USA300 CA-MRSA facial furuncle.

Necrotizing fasciitis with PVL-positive *S. aureus* strains has been previously described, but was infrequent until the spread of the CA-MRSA USA300 clone [79]. At present, monomicrobial *S. aureus* necrotizing fasciitis is an emerging severe soft tissue infection in the USA. Miller *et al.* [80] reported 14 cases in the Los Angeles area in 2005. Like necrotizing fasciitis of other origins, CA-MRSA necrotizing fasciitis often begins with pain that appears disproportionate to the appearance of the skin lesion, followed by alarming clinical changes such as altered mental status, septic shock, gray-blue skin color with ill-defined patches, and sometimes violaceous bullae [38,79,80]. Again, like necrotizing fasciitis of other origins, underlying comorbidities such as diabetes mellitus and cancer are often present. However, CA-MRSA necrotizing fasciitis can affect young injecting drug users, with or without HIV or hepatitis C virus infection. In these cases the necrotizing fasciitis may be located in the upper limbs. Serious late complications are frequent, sometimes requiring lengthy intensive care and reconstructive surgery [80].

Diagnosis

The diagnosis of PVL-positive *S. aureus* skin and soft tissue infections is based on isolation of the responsible strain and detection of the genes encoding PVL. However, multiple furuncles requiring surgical drainage, or severe infections such as necrotizing fasciitis, especially in a geographical area with a high prevalence of CA-MRSA, should make PVL-positive *S. aureus* infection a consideration [71,75,77,80]. CA-MRSA necrotizing fasciitis cannot be distinguished from polymicrobial or group A streptococcal necrotizing fasciitis on clinical grounds alone [80].

Treatment

The treatment of PVL-associated infections depends on assessment of the severity of the clinical presentation and the type of skin and soft tissue infection [75]. Management of uncomplicated CA-MRSA skin and soft tissue infections consists primarily of incision and drainage of fluctuant lesions [81]. Antimicrobial chemotherapy has only a moderate impact on clinical outcome of these infections and may be reserved for patients with abscesses larger than 5 cm in length (although this definition may not be appropriate for infections in infants), for patients with systemic signs of infection such as fever and tachycardia, and/or for patients with a suboptimal response to surgery [75,81].

Oral β-lactam antibiotics may be used for outpatients infected with a methicillin-susceptible strain but can no longer be considered reliable as empirical treatment in areas with a high prevalence of CA-MRSA [75]. Results of susceptibility testing of CA-MRSA and clinical experience provide support for the use of oral clindamycin, trimethoprim–sulfamethoxazole, or tetracyclines. Management of CA-MRSA severe skin and soft tissue infections may require intravenous therapy with vancomycin, clindamycin, quinupristin–dalfopristin, or linezolid. Newer drugs such as daptomycin and tigecycline may be effective, but are not recommended in children [75]. Moreover, the need to monitor creatine phosphokinase levels limits the use of daptomycin when necrotizing fasciitis is suspected [82].

Clinical necrotizing fasciitis requires early intravenous broad-spectrum antimicrobial therapy covering susceptible and resistant Gram-positive, Gram-negative, and anaerobic organisms before CA-MRSA is identified [38]. Necrotizing fasciitis also requires extensive surgical débridement (fasciotomy) to remove necrotic tissues [38,80]. As during group A streptococcal fasciitis associated with shock, the prognosis may be improved by drugs such as clindamycin and linezolid, which inhibit ribosomal translation of streptococcal superantigenic toxins and PVL, and by IVIG (which blocks the activity of streptococcal superantigenic toxins and PVL *in vitro*) [42,43,83].

Severe pediatric bone and joint infections

Pathogenesis

Staphylococcus aureus is classically responsible for osteoarticular infections in both children and adults [84–86]. Few *S. aureus* isolates in this setting harbor the PVL phage. However, bone and joint infections due to PVL-positive *S. aureus* strains are increasingly frequent in children and are usually more severe [87,88]. Acute hematogeneous osteomyelitis and septic arthritis are the most frequent bone and joint infections in children. The metaphyses of long bones, particularly of the tibia and femur, are the most common sites of acute hematogeneous osteomyelitis, as blood flow in the sinusoidal vessels of these areas is lower in children [86,89]. PVL production in the intramedullary cavity is suspected of causing local complications by enhancing the inflammatory response, reducing the blood supply to the cortex, and favoring the formation of bone abscess and sequestrum. In the same way, PVL production in joint fluid may enhance the proinflammatory response, PMN recruitment, and clinical signs of arthritis [90,91].

Epidemiology

Staphylococcus aureus is one of the most frequent causes of acute hematogeneous osteomyelitis and septic arthritis in children, along with *Streptococcus pneumoniae*, *Haemophilus influenzae* type b (now less frequent because of widespread vaccination), and *Kingella kingae* [86,89,92,93]. PVL-positive *S. aureus* strains responsible for severe bone and joint infections may be either susceptible or resistant to methicillin [90,91]. In parts of the USA where the incidence of CA-MRSA infection is high, most severe bone and joint infections are now associated with these strains [87,88].

Clinical syndrome

Compared with PVL-negative forms, PVL-positive *S. aureus* osteomyelitis and arthritis are characterized by more acute onset of symptoms (hospital admission within 24 hours after the first symptom), more frequent association with septic shock, a longer time to defervescence, longer hospitalization, and higher rates of early and late complications. PVL-positive *S. aureus* osteomyelitis is more likely to involve bone abscesses, sequestra, and bone destruction. Early local complications such as subperiosteal abscess, myositis, pyomyositis, and necrotizing fasciitis are more frequent (Figure 26.3) [87,88,90,91,94,95]. Venous thrombosis is also more common and may facilitate the onset of septic emboli and multifocal bilateral pneumonia [96]. Late complications such as pathological fracture, leg-length discrepancies, and radiographic bone abnormalities (bone condensation or geodes) are also more frequent than in PVL-negative forms [91,97].

Diagnosis

The diagnosis of PVL-associated *S. aureus* osteoarticular infection is based on the isolation of a PVL-positive *S. aureus* strain by culture of blood or osteoarticular samples [88,90,91]. Severe osteoarticular infections in children, with early local complications detected by magnetic resonance imaging, especially in countries with a high CA-MRSA prevalence, may also suggest the diagnosis (see Figure 26.3) [88].

Treatment

Treatment of osteoarticular infections involves lengthy antimicrobial chemotherapy, plus surgical incision and débridement of the affected bone in selected cases [86, 91,98]. Clindamycin has excellent bone and joint penetration, and subinhibitory concentrations of this drug downregulate PVL release *in vitro* [43,99,100]. Moreover, as most CA-MRSA strains (contrary to hospital-acquired MRSA) are susceptible *in vitro* to clindamycin, this drug may be a useful option for osteoarticular CA-MRSA infections [71,88,101]. However, many CA-MRSA strains are resistant to macrolides, by means of *msrA*-mediated efflux or an *erm* gene that provides an MLS_Bi phenotype (the strain is susceptible to clindamycin but resistant to erythromycin, with a positive D-zone test) [102]. In the latter case, lengthy use of clindamycin may induce clindamycin resistance and negatively affect clinical outcome [103]. The addition of a glycopeptide, rifampicin or a fluoroquinolone (for adults only) may prevent such resistance. Linezolid is of limited utility, as lengthy therapy with this drug is associated with hematotoxicity and neurotoxicity [104,105]. Surgical treatment is frequently required for PVL-positive *S. aureus* osteorarticular infections. Early, extensive and repeated surgical drainage and/or excision of necrotic tissue leads to faster resolution of symptoms and better final outcome [91].

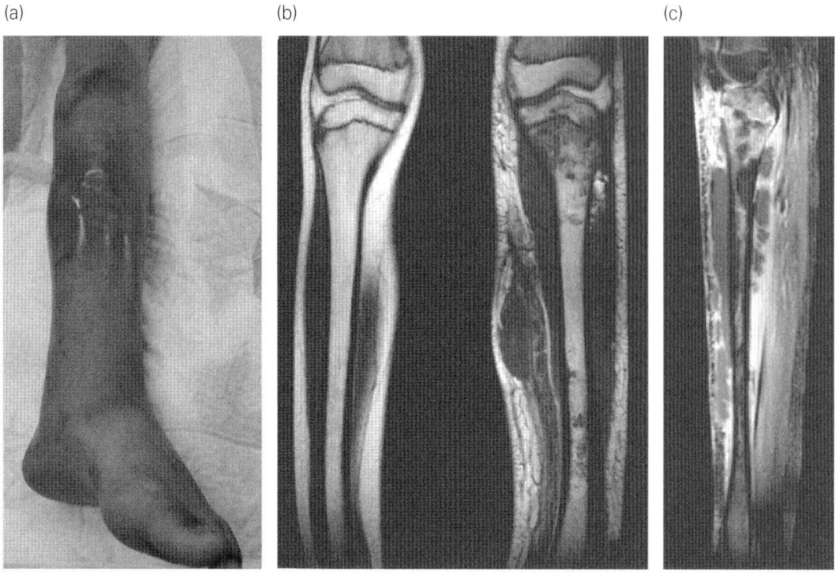

Figure 26.3 Osteomyelitis of the left tibia due to PVL-positive methicillin-susceptible *S. aureus* in a 12-year-old child. (a) Note the severe inflammatory response with visible and palpable abscesses. Magnetic resonance imaging without gadolinium (b) and with gadolinium (c) revealed severe bone involvement, with bone abscesses, subperiosteal abscesses, and necrotizing myositis. (Images courtesy of Bruno Dohin, Pediatric Surgical Unit, Pavillon T bis, Hôpital Edouard Herriot, Lyon, France.)

Necrotizing pneumonia

Community-onset necrotizing pneumonia due to PVL-positive *S. aureus* is a worrying emerging infection with a frequently fatal outcome [71].

Pathogenesis

PVL-positive *S. aureus* strains usually infect the lungs via the airways. Influenza often precedes the onset of *S. aureus* necrotizing pneumonia, causing airway epithelial damage that impairs ciliary function and bacterial clearance, and exposing type I and IV collagens and laminin [71,106,107]. PVL-positive *S. aureus* strains often harbor the gene encoding collagen-binding protein, which promotes *S. aureus* adhesion to basal cells of the respiratory epithelium [106]. Moreover, PVL-positive *S. aureus* strains may overexpress protein A, which activates tumor necrosis factor α receptors on the surface of respiratory epithelial cells, thereby triggering PMN recruitment [108,109]. Given the capacity of PVL to cause PMN necrosis and apoptosis *in vitro*, PVL may play a major role in the observed inflammation and necrosis of the respiratory epithelium and parenchyma in this setting [110]. A major role for PVL was recently shown in a mouse model of acute pneumonia (Plate 26.1) [66].

Epidemiology

Cases occur sporadically in the USA and Europe. In Europe, especially in France, most cases of necrotizing pneumonia are due to unrelated MSSA strains. Few are due to the CA-MRSA clone that predominates in Europe [107]. The incidence of necrotizing pneumonia in the USA is unknown, but many reports describe cases related to the CA-MRSA USA300 clone [71].

Clinical syndrome

Most published cases involve children and teenagers. Necrotizing pneumonia is a rapidly progressive form of extensive pneumonia leading to acute respiratory distress, with or without pleural effusion, hemoptysis and leukopenia [71,107]. In a survey, 67% of patients had influenza-like symptoms before hospital admission. Most patients also developed respiratory distress necessitating mechanical ventilation. Airway bleeding did not occur in all the patients, but when it did occur outcome was usually fatal. Severe leukopenia, which may reflect the abundance of *in situ* PVL production, is also predictive of a fatal outcome. Some patients in this survey had a generalized rash, a feature that had not previously been reported, and all of them died [106]. Necrotizing pneumonia can also be associated with skin and soft tissue infections and/or with osteoarticular infections. In such cases the lungs are infected via the bloodstream by means of septic emboli. Computed tomography of the chest shows multilobular consolidation in the lungs, pleural effusion, cavitations, and destruction of the pulmonary parenchyma [71,94,107]. Differential diagnoses include acute lung abscesses due to anaerobes (secondary to aspiration pneumonia after generalized seizures for example), *Fusobacterium necrophorum* postanginal bacteremia (Lemmiere syndrome), or to highly virulent *Klebsiella pneumoniae* strains that are endemic in Taiwan and the USA [111,112]. Pulmonary cavities associated with hemoptysis may also occur in tuberculosis (but the symptoms are not as acute as in necrotizing pneumonia) and in coccidioidomycosis (valley fever) [113,114]. This latter fungal disease is usually associated in its early stages with an influenza-like illness, with fever, cough, and pulmonary infiltrates. Cavitation and hemoptysis can occur in disseminated cases. Return from an endemic area (southwestern USA and northern Mexico), in association with eosinophilia, should raise the possibility of this diagnosis [113].

Diagnosis

Diagnosis is based on the isolation of a PVL-positive

S. aureus strain by culture of blood and/or respiratory samples. The diagnosis is also strongly suggested by a severe respiratory illness associated with abscess formation, hemoptysis, and leukopenia especially following an influenza-like illness [71,107].

Treatment

Treatment of necrotizing pneumonia is based first on intensive supportive care, as most patients develop respiratory distress and septic shock. Extracorporeal membrane oxygenation may be useful in particular cases [115]. The use of activated protein C is limited, owing to the risk of severe hemoptysis. Early antibiotic therapy appears to be crucial [94]. Intravenous vancomycin can be combined with clindamycin. Linezolid, which shows good lung penetration, may serve as an alternative to vancomycin; like clindamycin it downregulates PVL production *in vitro*, although the clinical relevance of this effect is unclear [43,99,100]. Linezolid or clindamycin have to be administered as soon as the diagnosis is clinically suspected (in case of extensive community-acquired pneumonia with leukopenia). As subinhibitory concentrations of oxacillin enhance PVL production by CA-MRSA *in vitro*, empirical therapy with oxacillin during CA-MRSA necrotizing pneumonia may enhance the production of PVL *in vivo* if administred alone [99,100]. Daptomycin is not indicated in this setting, as its activity is inhibited by pulmonary surfactants [82]. Finally, IVIG may possibly be beneficial, but controlled studies are hindered by the frequently rapid fatal outcome [42].

How to detect PVL *in vivo*

It is theoretically possible to detect PVL directly in respiratory samples. In the future, PVL detection and quantification *in situ* could serve as a prognostic marker [116].

How to block the production and action of PVL

As noted above, subinhibitory concentrations of clindamycin and linezolid inhibit PVL production *in vitro* whereas vancomycin has little if any effect [43,99]. IVIG, which contains PVL-specific antibodies, can inhibit pore formation and the cytopathic effect of PVL *in vitro* [42]. The clinical impact of agents that block the production and action of PVL remains to be tested.

Conclusion

Staphylococcal toxin-mediated syndromes are numerous and heterogeneous. Each toxin may act directly or indirectly, and alone or in combination with other virulence factors. The emergence and spread of MRSA that produce particular toxins, such as exfoliative toxins, superantigenic toxins and PVL, is modifying the epidemiology and treatment of these syndromes.

References

1 Dinges MM, Orwin PM, Schlievert PM. Exotoxins of *Staphylococcus aureus*. Clin Microbiol Rev 2000;13:16–34.

2 Lowy FD. *Staphylococcus aureus* infections. N Engl J Med 1998; 339:520–32.

3 Essmann F, Bantel H, Totzke G *et al. Staphylococcus aureus* alpha-toxin-induced cell death: predominant necrosis despite apoptotic caspase activation. Cell Death Differ 2003;10:1260–72.

4 Ladhani S. Understanding the mechanism of action of the exfoliative toxins of *Staphylococcus aureus*. FEMS Immunol Med Microbiol 2003;39:181–9.

5 Miles G, Jayasinghe L, Bayley H. Assembly of the bi-component leukocidin pore examined by truncation mutagenesis. J Biol Chem 2006;281:2205–14.

6 Stevens DL. The toxic shock syndromes. Infect Dis Clin North Am 1996;10:727–46.

7 Kravitz GR, Dries DJ, Peterson ML, Schlievert PM. Purpura fulminans due to *Staphylococcus aureus*. Clin Infect Dis 2005;40: 941–7.

8 Le Loir Y, Baron F, Gautier M. *Staphylococcus aureus* and food poisoning. Genet Mol Res 2003;2:63–76.

9 Ladhani S. Recent developments in staphylococcal scalded skin syndrome. Clin Microbiol Infect 2001;7:301–7.

10 Lina G, Piemont Y, Godail-Gamot F *et al*. Involvement of Panton–Valentine leukocidin-producing *Staphylococcus aureus* in primary skin infections and pneumonia. Clin Infect Dis 1999; 29:1128–32.

11 Lina G, Bohach GA, Nair SP, Hiramatsu K, Jouvin-Marche E, Mariuzza R. Standard nomenclature for the superantigens expressed by *Staphylococcus*. J Infect Dis 2004;189:2334–6.

12 Thomas D, Chou S, Dauwalder O, Lina G. Diversity in *Staphylococcus aureus* enterotoxins. Chem Immunol Allergy 2007;93: 24–41.

13 Holtfreter S, Broker BM. Staphylococcal superantigens: do they play a role in sepsis? Arch Immunol Ther Exp (Warsz) 2005;53:13–27.

14 Regassa LB, Novick RP, Betley MJ. Glucose and nonmaintained pH decrease expression of the accessory gene regulator (agr) in *Staphylococcus aureus*. Infect Immun 1992;60:3381–8.

15 Genigeorgis CA. Present state of knowledge on staphylococcal intoxication. Int J Food Microbiol 1989;9:327–60.

16 Kerouanton A, Hennekinne JA, Letertre C *et al*. Characterization of *Staphylococcus aureus* strains associated with food poisoning outbreaks in France. Int J Food Microbiol 2007;115: 369–75.

17 Wieneke AA, Roberts D, Gilbert RJ. Staphylococcal food poisoning in the United Kingdom, 1969–90. Epidemiol Infect 1993; 110:519–31.

18 Evenson ML, Hinds MW, Bernstein RS, Bergdoll MS. Estimation of human dose of staphylococcal enterotoxin A from a large outbreak of staphylococcal food poisoning involving chocolate milk. Int J Food Microbiol 1988;7:311–16.

19 Sugiyama H, Hayama T. Abdominal viscera as site of emetic action for staphylococcal enterotoxin in the monkey. J Infect Dis 1965;115:330–6.

20 Iandolo JJ, Tweten RK. Purification of staphylococcal enterotoxins. Methods Enzymol 1988;165:43–52.

21 Kent TH. Staphylococcal enterotoxin gastroenteritis in rhesus monkeys. Am J Pathol 1966;48:387–407.

22 Hamad AR, Marrack P, Kappler JW. Transcytosis of staphylococcal superantigen toxins. J Exp Med 1997;185:1447–54.

23 Scheuber PH, Denzlinger C, Wilker D, Beck G, Keppler D, Hammer DK. Cysteinyl leukotrienes as mediators of staphylococcal enterotoxin B in the monkey. Eur J Clin Invest 1987;17: 455–9.

24 Centers for Disease Control and Prevention. Surveillance for foodborne disease outbreaks: United States, 1993–1997. MMWR 2000;49(SS01):1–51.

25 Scallan E. Activities, achievements, and lessons learned during the first 10 years of the Foodborne Diseases Active Surveillance Network: 1996–2005. Clin Infect Dis 2007;44:718–25.

26 Akineden O, Annemuller C, Hassan AA, Lammler C, Wolter W, Zschock M. Toxin genes and other characteristics of *Staphylococcus aureus* isolates from milk of cows with mastitis. Clin Diagn Lab Immunol 2001;8:959–64.

27 Rosec JP, Gigaud O. Staphylococcal enterotoxin genes of classical and new types detected by PCR in France. Int J Food Microbiol 2002;77:61–70.

28 Omoe K, Ishikawa M, Shimoda Y, Hu DL, Ueda S, Shinagawa K. Detection of seg, seh, and sei genes in *Staphylococcus aureus* isolates and determination of the enterotoxin productivities of *S. aureus* isolates harboring seg, seh, or sei genes. J Clin Microbiol 2002;40:857–62.

29 Thompson NE, Razdan M, Kuntsmann G, Aschenbach JM, Evenson ML, Bergdoll MS. Detection of staphylococcal enterotoxins by enzyme-linked immunosorbent assays and radioimmunoassays: comparison of monoclonal and polyclonal antibody systems. Appl Environ Microbiol 1986;51:885–90.

30 Hu DL, Omoe K, Shimoda Y, Nakane A, Shinagawa K. Induction of emetic response to staphylococcal enterotoxins in the house musk shrew (*Suncus murinus*). Infect Immun 2003;71: 567–70.

31 Tranter HS. Foodborne staphylococcal illness. Lancet 1990;336: 1044–6.

32 McKillip JL. Prevalence and expression of enterotoxins in *Bacillus cereus* and other *Bacillus* spp., a literature review. Antonie Van Leeuwenhoek 2000;77:393–9.

33 Brynestad S, Granum PE. *Clostridium perfringens* and foodborne infections. Int J Food Microbiol 2002;74:195–202.

34 Movat HZ, Burrowes CE, Cybulsky MI, Dinarello CA. Acute inflammation and a Shwartzman-like reaction induced by interleukin-1 and tumor necrosis factor. Synergistic action of the cytokines in the induction of inflammation and microvascular injury. Am J Pathol 1987;129:463–76.

35 Rintala E, Kauppila M, Seppala OP *et al.* Protein C substitution in sepsis-associated purpura fulminans. Crit Care Med 2000; 28:2373–8.

36 Chambers HF. Staphylococcal purpura fulminans: a toxin-mediated disease? Clin Infect Dis 2005;40:948–50.

37 Rosenstein NE, Perkins BA, Stephens DS, Popovic T, Hughes JM. Meningococcal disease. N Engl J Med 2001;344:1378–88.

38 Ramos-e-Silva M, Pereira AL. Life-threatening eruptions due to infectious agents. Clin Dermatol 2005;23:148–56.

39 Matsuda Y, Kato H, Yamada R *et al.* Early and definitive diagnosis of toxic shock syndrome by detection of marked expansion of T-cell-receptor Vβ 2-positive T cells. Emerg Infect Dis 2003;9:387–9.

40 Ferry T, Thomas D, Bouchut JC *et al.* Early diagnosis of staphylococcal toxic shock syndrome by detection of the TSST-1 Vbeta signature in peripheral blood of a 12-year-old boy. Pediatr Infect Dis J 2008;27:274–7.

41 Ferry T, Thomas D, Perpoint T *et al.* Analysis of superantigenic toxin Vbeta T-cell signatures during cases of staphylococcal toxic shock syndrome and septic shock. Clin Microb Infect 2008;14: 546–54.

42 Gauduchon V, Cozon G, Vandenesch F *et al.* Neutralization of *Staphylococcus aureus* Panton Valentine leukocidin by intravenous immunoglobulin in vitro. J Infect Dis 2004;189:346–53.

43 Stevens DL, Ma Y, Salmi DB, McIndoo E, Wallace RJ, Bryant AE. Impact of antibiotics on expression of virulence-associated exotoxin genes in methicillin-sensitive and methicillin-resistant *Staphylococcus aureus*. J Infect Dis 2007;195:202–11.

44 Tokura Y, Heald PW, Yan SL, Edelson RL. Stimulation of cutaneous T-cell lymphoma cells with superantigenic staphylococcal toxins. J Invest Dermatol 1992;98:33–7.

45 Vath GM, Earhart CA, Rago JV *et al.* The structure of the superantigen exfoliative toxin A suggests a novel regulation as a serine protease. Biochemistry 1997;36:1559–66.

46 Stanley JR, Amagai M. Pemphigus, bullous impetigo, and the staphylococcal scalded-skin syndrome. N Engl J Med 2006;355: 1800–10.

47 Yamaguchi T, Nishifuji K, Sasaki M *et al.* Identification of the *Staphylococcus aureus* etd pathogenicity island which encodes a novel exfoliative toxin, ETD, and EDIN-B. Infect Immun 2002; 70:5835–45.

48 Bailey CJ, de Azavedo J, Arbuthnott JP. A comparative study of two serotypes of epidermolytic toxin from *Staphylococcus aureus*. Biochim Biophys Acta 1980;624:111–20.

49 de Azavedo J, Arbuthnott JP. Prevalence of epidermolytic toxin in clinical isolates of *Staphylococcus aureus*. J Med Microbiol 1981;14:341–4.

50 Kondo I, Sakurai S, Sarai Y, Futaki S. Two serotypes of exfoliatin and their distribution in staphylococcal strains isolated from patients with scalded skin syndrome. J Clin Microbiol 1975;1:397–400.

51 Yamasaki O, Yamaguchi T, Sugai M *et al.* Clinical manifestations of staphylococcal scalded-skin syndrome depend on serotypes of exfoliative toxins. J Clin Microbiol 2005;43:1890–3.

52 Yamasaki O, Tristan A, Yamaguchi T *et al.* Distribution of the exfoliative toxin D gene in clinical *Staphylococcus aureus* isolates in France. Clin Microbiol Infect 2006;12:585–8.

53 Durupt F, Mayor L, Bes M *et al.* Prevalence of *Staphylococcus aureus* toxins and nasal carriage in furuncles and impetigo. Br J Dermatol 2007;157:1161–7.

54 Liassine N, Auckenthaler R, Descombes MC, Bes M, Vandenesch F, Etienne J. Community-acquired methicillin-resistant *Staphylococcus aureus* isolated in Switzerland contains the Panton–Valentine leukocidin or exfoliative toxin genes. J Clin Microbiol 2004;42:825–8.

55 Yamaguchi T, Yokota Y, Terajima J *et al.* Clonal association of *Staphylococcus aureus* causing bullous impetigo and the emergence of new methicillin-resistant clonal groups in Kansai district in Japan. J Infect Dis 2002;185:1511–16.

56 Nakashima AK, Allen JR, Martone WJ *et al.* Epidemic bullous impetigo in a nursery due to a nasal carrier of *Staphylococcus aureus*: role of epidemiology and control measures. Infect Control 1984;5:326–31.

57 Decleire PY, Blondiaux G, Delaere B, Glupczynski Y. Staphyloccocal scalded skin syndrome in an adult. Acta Clin Belg 2004;59:365–8.

58 Mockenhaupt M, Idzko M, Grosber M, Schopf E, Norgauer J. Epidemiology of staphylococcal scalded skin syndrome in Germany. J Invest Dermatol 2005;124:700–3.

59 Plano LR, Adkins B, Woischnik M, Ewing R, Collins CM. Toxin levels in serum correlate with the development of staphylococcal scalded skin syndrome in a murine model. Infect Immun 2001;69:5193–7.

60 Opal SM, Johnson-Winegar AD, Cross AS. Staphylococcal scalded skin syndrome in two immunocompetent adults caused by exfoliatin B-producing *Staphylococcus aureus*. J Clin Microbiol 1988;26:1283–6.

61 Noguchi N, Nakaminami H, Nishijima S, Kurokawa I, So H, Sasatsu M. Antimicrobial agent of susceptibilities and antiseptic resistance gene distribution among methicillin-resistant *Staphylococcus aureus* isolates from patients with impetigo and staphylococcal scalded skin syndrome. J Clin Microbiol 2006; 44:2119–25.

62 El Helali N, Carbonne A, Naas T *et al*. Nosocomial outbreak of staphylococcal scalded skin syndrome in neonates: epidemiological investigation and control. J Hosp Infect 2005;61:130–8.

63 O'Connell N, Mannix M, Philip R *et al*. Infant staphylococcal scalded skin syndrome, Ireland, 2007: preliminary outbreak report. Euro Surveillance 2007;12:E070614.5. Available from http://www.eurosurveillance.org/ew/2007/.asp#5

64 Coleman JC, Dobson NR. Diagnostic dilemma: extremely low birth weight baby with staphylococcal scalded-skin syndrome or toxic epidermal necrolysis. J Perinatol 2006;26:714–16.

65 Ladhani S, Robbie S, Garratt RC, Chapple DS, Joannou CL, Evans RW. Development and evaluation of detection systems for staphylococcal exfoliative toxin A responsible for scalded-skin syndrome. J Clin Microbiol 2001;39:2050–4.

66 Labandeira-Rey M, Couzon F, Boisset S *et al*. *Staphylococcus aureus* Panton–Valentine leukocidin causes necrotizing pneumonia. Science 2007;315:1130–3.

67 Voyich JM, Otto M, Mathema B *et al*. Is Panton–Valentine leukocidin the major virulence determinant in community-associated methicillin-resistant *Staphylococcus aureus* disease? J Infect Dis 2006;194:1761–70.

68 Diep BA, Palazzo-Balance AM, Tattevin P *et al*. Contribution of Panton–Valentine leukocidin in community-associated methicillin-resistant *Staphylococcus aureus* pathogenesis. PLoS ONE 2008;3:e3198.

69 Iwatsuki K, Yamasaki O, Morizane S, Oono T. Staphylococcal cutaneous infections: invasion, evasion and aggression. J Dermatol Sci 2006;42:203–14.

70 Cribier B, Prevost G, Couppie P, Finck-Barbancon V, Grosshans E, Piemont Y. *Staphylococcus aureus* leukocidin: a new virulence factor in cutaneous infections? An epidemiological and experimental study. Dermatology 1992;185:175–80.

71 Zetola N, Francis JS, Nuermberger EL, Bishai WR. Community-acquired meticillin-resistant *Staphylococcus aureus*: an emerging threat. Lancet Infect Dis 2005;5:275–86.

72 Moran GJ, Krishnadasan A, Gorwitz RJ *et al*. Methicillin-resistant *S. aureus* infections among patients in the emergency department. N Engl J Med 2006;355:666–74.

73 Chini V, Petinaki E, Foka A, Paratiras S, Dimitracopoulos G, Spiliopoulou I. Spread of *Staphylococcus aureus* clinical isolates carrying Panton–Valentine leukocidin genes during a 3-year period in Greece. Clin Microbiol Infect 2006;12:29–34.

74 Robert J, Etienne J, Bertrand X. Methicillin-resistant *Staphylococcus aureus* producing Panton–Valentine leukocidin in a retrospective case series from 12 French hospital laboratories, 2000–2003. Clin Microbiol Infect 2005;11:585–7.

75 Daum RS. Clinical practice. Skin and soft-tissue infections caused by methicillin-resistant *Staphylococcus aureus*. N Engl J Med 2007;357:380–90.

76 Issartel B, Tristan A, Lechevallier S *et al*. Frequent carriage of Panton–Valentine leucocidin genes by *Staphylococcus aureus* isolates from surgically drained abscesses. J Clin Microbiol 2005; 43:3203–7.

77 Yamasaki O, Kaneko J, Morizane S *et al*. The association between *Staphylococcus aureus* strains carrying Panton–Valentine leukocidin genes and the development of deep-seated follicular infection. Clin Infect Dis 2005;40:381–5.

78 Rutar T, Chambers HF, Crawford JB *et al*. Ophthalmic manifestations of infections caused by the USA300 clone of community-associated methicillin-resistant *Staphylococcus aureus*. Ophthalmology 2006;113:1455–62.

79 Lee YT, Chou TD, Peng MY, Chang FY. Rapidly progressive necrotizing fasciitis caused by *Staphylococcus aureus*. J Microbiol Immunol Infect 2005;38:361–4.

80 Miller LG, Perdreau-Remington F, Rieg G *et al*. Necrotizing fasciitis caused by community-associated methicillin-resistant *Staphylococcus aureus* in Los Angeles. N Engl J Med 2005;352: 1445–53.

81 Ruhe JJ, Smith N, Bradsher RW, Menon A. Community-onset methicillin-resistant *Staphylococcus aureus* skin and soft-tissue infections: impact of antimicrobial therapy on outcome. Clin Infect Dis 2007;44:777–84.

82 Eisenstein BI. Lipopeptides, focusing on daptomycin, for the treatment of Gram-positive infections. Expert Opin Investig Drugs 2004;13:1159–69.

83 Stevens DL. Streptococcal toxic shock syndrome. Clin Microbiol Infect 2002;8:133–6.

84 Lew DP, Waldvogel FA. Osteomyelitis. Lancet 2004;364:369–79.

85 Sia IG, Berbari EF. Infection and musculoskeletal conditions: osteomyelitis. Best Pract Res Clin Rheumatol 2006;20:1065–81.

86 Vazquez M. Osteomyelitis in children. Curr Opin Pediatr 2002; 14:112–15.

87 Arnold SR, Elias D, Buckingham SC *et al*. Changing patterns of acute hematogenous osteomyelitis and septic arthritis: emergence of community-associated methicillin-resistant *Staphylococcus aureus*. J Pediatr Orthop 2006;26:703–8.

88 Martinez-Aguilar G, Avalos-Mishaan A, Hulten K, Hammerman W, Mason EO Jr, Kaplan SL. Community-acquired, methicillin-resistant and methicillin-susceptible *Staphylococcus aureus* musculoskeletal infections in children. Pediatr Infect Dis J 2004;23:701–6.

89 Kao HC, Huang YC, Chiu CH *et al*. Acute hematogenous osteomyelitis and septic arthritis in children. J Microbiol Immunol Infect 2003;36:260–5.

90 Bocchini CE, Hulten KG, Mason EO Jr, Gonzalez BE, Hammerman WA, Kaplan SL. Panton–Valentine leukocidin genes are associated with enhanced inflammatory response and local disease in acute hematogenous *Staphylococcus aureus* osteomyelitis in children. Pediatrics 2006;117:433–40.

91 Dohin B, Gillet Y, Kohler R *et al.* Pediatric bone and joint infections due to Panton–Valentine leukocidin-positive *Staphylococcus aureus*. Pediatr Infect Dis J 2007;26:1042–8.

92 Chometon S, Benito Y, Chaker M *et al.* Specific real-time polymerase chain reaction places *Kingella kingae* as the most common cause of osteoarticular infections in young children. Pediatr Infect Dis J 2007;26:377–81.

93 Stott NS. Review article: paediatric bone and joint infection. J Orthop Surg (Hong Kong) 2001;9:83–90.

94 Gonzalez BE, Martinez-Aguilar G, Hulten KG *et al.* Severe staphylococcal sepsis in adolescents in the era of community-acquired methicillin-resistant *Staphylococcus aureus*. Pediatrics 2005;115:642–8.

95 Sdougkos G, Chini V, Papanastasiou DA *et al.* Methicillin-resistant *Staphylococcus aureus* producing Panton–Valentine leukocidin as a cause of acute osteomyelitis in children. Clin Microbiol Infect 2007;13:651–4.

96 Gonzalez BE, Teruya J, Mahoney DH Jr *et al.* Venous thrombosis associated with staphylococcal osteomyelitis in children. Pediatrics 2006;117:1673–9.

97 Gelfand MS, Cleveland KO, Heck RK, Goswami R. Pathological fracture in acute osteomyelitis of long bones secondary to community-acquired methicillin-resistant *Staphylococcus aureus*: two cases and review of the literature. Am J Med Sci 2006;332:357–60.

98 Darville T, Jacobs RF. Management of acute hematogenous osteomyelitis in children. Pediatr Infect Dis J 2004;23:255–7.

99 Dumitrescu O, Boisset S, Badiou C *et al.* Effect of antibiotics on *Staphylococcus aureus* producing Panton–Valentine leukocidin. Antimicrob Agents Chemother 2007;51:1515–19.

100 Dumitrescu O, Badiou C, Bes M et. al. Effect of antibiotics alone and in combination, on Panton–Valentine leukocidin production by a *Staphylococcus aureus* reference strain. Clin Microbiol Infect 2008;14:384–8.

101 Martinez-Aguilar G, Hammerman WA, Mason EO Jr, Kaplan SL. Clindamycin treatment of invasive infections caused by community-acquired, methicillin-resistant and methicillin-susceptible *Staphylococcus aureus* in children. Pediatr Infect Dis J 2003;22:593–8.

102 Lewis JS II, Jorgensen JH. Inducible clindamycin resistance in staphylococci: should clinicians and microbiologists be concerned? Clin Infect Dis 2005;40:280–5.

103 Siberry GK, Tekle T, Carroll K, Dick J. Failure of clindamycin treatment of methicillin-resistant *Staphylococcus aureus* expressing inducible clindamycin resistance in vitro. Clin Infect Dis 2003;37:1257–60.

104 Ferry T, Ponceau B, Simon M *et al.* Possibly linezolid-induced peripheral and central neurotoxicity: report of four cases. Infection 2005;33:151–4.

105 Perry CM, Jarvis B. Linezolid: a review of its use in the management of serious Gram-positive infections. Drugs 2001;61: 525–51.

106 de Bentzmann S, Tristan A, Etienne J, Brousse N, Vandenesch F, Lina G. *Staphylococcus aureus* isolates associated with necrotizing pneumonia bind to basement membrane type I and IV collagens and laminin. J Infect Dis 2004;190:1506–15.

107 Gillet Y, Vanhems P, Lina G *et al.* Factors predicting mortality in necrotizing community-acquired pneumonia caused by *Staphylococcus aureus* containing Panton–Valentine leukocidin. Clin Infect Dis 2007;45:315–21.

108 Gomez MI, Lee A, Reddy B *et al. Staphylococcus aureus* protein A induces airway epithelial inflammatory responses by activating TNFR1. Nat Med 2004;10:842–8.

109 Kahl BC, Peters G. Microbiology. Mayhem in the lung. Science 2007;315:1082–3.

110 Genestier AL, Michallet MC, Prevost G *et al. Staphylococcus aureus* Panton–Valentine leukocidin directly targets mitochondria and induces Bax-independent apoptosis of human neutrophils. J Clin Invest 2005;115:3117–27.

111 Dykhuizen RS, Olson ES, Clive S, Douglas JG. Necrobacillosis (Lemmiere's syndrome): a rare cause of necrotizing pneumonia. Eur Respir J 1994;7:2246–8.

112 Wang JL, Chen KY, Fang CT, Hsueh PR, Yang PC, Chang SC. Changing bacteriology of adult community-acquired lung abscess in Taiwan: *Klebsiella pneumoniae* versus anaerobes. Clin Infect Dis 2005;40:915–22.

113 DiCaudo DJ. Coccidioidomycosis: a review and update. J Am Acad Dermatol 2006;55:929–42.

114 Frieden TR, Sterling TR, Munsiff SS, Watt CJ, Dye C. Tuberculosis. Lancet 2003;362:887–99.

115 Stroud MH, Okhuysen-Cawley R, Jaquiss R, Berlinski A, Fiser RT. Successful use of extracorporeal membrane oxygenation in severe necrotizing pneumonia caused by *Staphylococcus aureus*. Pediatr Crit Care Med 2007;8:282–7.

116 Badiou C, Dumitrescu O, Croze M *et al.* Panton–Valentine leukocidin is expressed at toxic levels in human skin abscesses. Clin Microbiol Infect 2008;14:1180–3.

Chapter 27
Staphylococcal Diarrhea and Enterocolitis

Mark H. Wilcox
Department of Microbiology, University of Leeds and Leeds Teaching Hospitals, Leeds, UK

Introduction

Clostridium difficile is widely acknowledged to be the most common cause of antibiotic-associated diarrhea (AAD) and most cases of antibiotic-associated colitis (AAC) and pseudomembranous colitis (PMC). However, *C. difficile* cannot be recovered from a substantial proportion of AAD cases (and from occasional AAC and PMC cases), and thus direct antibiotic-mediated activity on gut flora or gut motility or alternative infective or noninfective (e.g., inflammatory) causes must account for these. Alternative potential infective causes of AAD include *Clostridium perfringens*, *Klebsiella* spp., *Candida* spp., and *Staphylococcus aureus* [1–3].

Prior to the identification of the role of *C. difficile* in diarrhea and colitis, first documented in the late 1970s [4,5], a large number of reports claimed that *S. aureus* was the primary cause of PMC [6–18]. These reports decreased from the mid-1960s, from which we may infer that either the earlier diagnoses implicating *S. aureus* in cases of colitis were erroneous (i.e., *C. difficile* was not sought or recognized) or that the epidemiology of infective AAD and AAC changed. It is possible, for example, that the introduction of new antibiotics, including antistaphylococcal agents (e.g., semisynthetic penicillins and vancomycin), provided a selective pressure for the emergence of hitherto uncommon pathogens, such as *C. difficile*, at the expense of *S. aureus*. Notably, the epidemiology of nosocomial *S. aureus* infection changed dramatically, particularly with the introduction of sequential new antibiotics between 1950 and 1990. Epidemic *S. aureus* strains circulating in the 1950s became much less prevalent in following decades. Methicillin-resistant *S. aureus* (MRSA) clones have since become predominant in varied healthcare settings and, most recently, community-associated strains have spread rapidly. Similarly, the epidemiology of *C. difficile* infection has recently undergone dramatic changes, with major alterations in the clinical presentation and outcome of cases, notably associated with the emergence of a newly recognized clone (ribotype 027, NAP 1). It is unlikely that we will ever know the answer to the conundrum of why *S. aureus* enterocolitis now appears to be much less common than it was in the early antibiotic era. It is clear, however, that *S. aureus* is a cause of some AAD cases and occasional cases of AAC (including enterocolitis). Furthermore, because routine laboratory investigation of such cases now rarely includes specific testing for *S. aureus*, the true extent of its involvement may be underappreciated.

Staphylococci in Human Disease, 2nd edition. Edited by Kent B. Crossley, Kimberly K. Jefferson, Gordon Archer, Vance G. Fowler, Jr.

Staphylococcal enterocolitis in the early antibiotic era

The early cases of staphylococcal enterocolitis that were reported at the start of the antibiotic era were primarily, but not always [11], in the perioperative setting [13,14,19]. The cases typically presented in the first 2 weeks after surgery and were notable for the often severe and rapidly progressive circulatory collapse. The cases were unresponsive to antibiotic therapy (although of course the options available were very limited) and usually fatal. Diarrhea was not always seen, but mild abdominal pain and distension were present in most patients and preceded circulatory collapse by only a few hours. Tetracycline and chloramphenicol were the most commonly implicated antibiotics [11,12]. The reported macroscopic and histological changes predominantly affected the colon and would later become recognized as typical of the changes seen in AAC and PMC. However, the small intestine was grossly congested in autopsy specimens from two of five patients reported by Reiner *et al.* [12], one of whom showed a diffuse mononuclear cellular infiltration of the mucosa and submucosa. The other cases had focal enteritis that was largely healed.

Investigators continued to implicate *S. aureus* in the etiology of pseudomembranous enterocolitis in the early 1950s [8–10,14]. Sommers and colleagues reported three fatal cases of membranous enteritis associated with *S. aureus* [8,9]. The first patient was a 43-year-old man who had

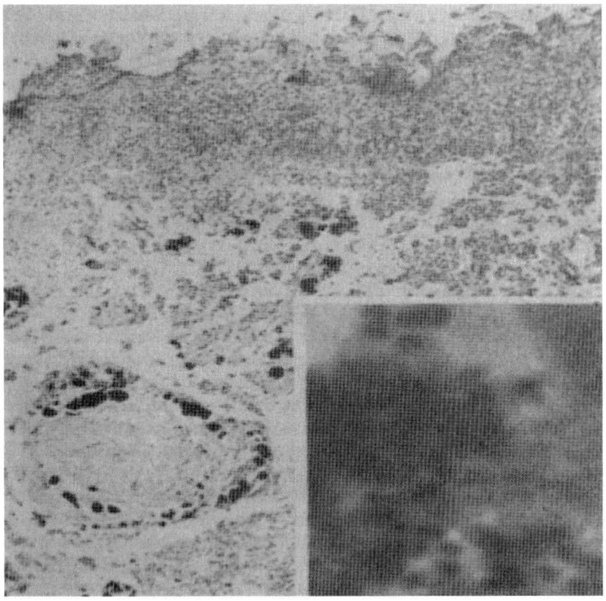

Figure 27.1 Portion of "pseudodiphtheritic" cast seen in the jejunum and ileum at autopsy of a 43-year-old man with an ileostomy who underwent a colectomy and developed shock and diarrhea after receiving penicillin, oxytetracycline, and sulfisoxazole postoperatively. Gram stain demonstrating colonies of staphylococci as dark clumps (×50), and details of staphylococci (×3000). Stool cultures grew *Staphylococcus aureus* and *Pseudomonas*. (From Brown *et al.* [8] with kind permission of Springer Science and Business Media.)

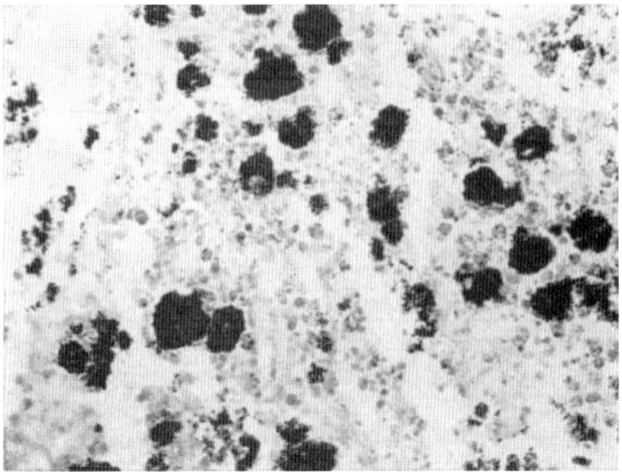

Figure 27.2 Gram stain demonstrating numerous colonies of staphylococci in enteric cast of a patent with pseudomembranous enteritis (×171). (From Wakefield & Sommers [9] with permission.)

undergone a subtotal colectomy and ileosigmoidostomy years before because of ulcerative colitis. He presented with fever and the presumed diagnosis of acute ulcerative sigmoid colitis and was treated with chloramphenicol, penicillin, and a sulphonamide before operation for completion of the colectomy, leaving the ileostomy intact. Oxytetracycline and streptomycin were begun postoperatively, but his course was marked by fever, copious watery discharges from the ileostomy, and profound shock leading to death. The jejunum and ileum were found at autopsy to be lined by a continuous "pseudodiphtheritic" cast from which *S. aureus* and pseudomonads were cultured; Gram stain of the membrane revealed many clusters of Gram-positive cocci buried in fibrin (Figures 27.1 and 27.2). Heart blood also grew *S. aureus*. The second patient was a 62-year-old woman who had received chlortetracycline preoperatively and then oxytetracycline, penicillin, streptomycin, and chlortetracycline following a laparotomy. She developed fever and progressive circulatory insufficiency and died 3 days later. The significant autopsy findings were a soft, wrinkled, tan-pink fibrinous membrane that could easily be peeled from the mucosa beginning 10 cm below the gastrojejunostomy and extending distally throughout the entire small intestine, and a penetrating duodenal ulcer. Microscopically, the small bowel showed severe acute and chronic inflammation with very little remaining epithelium. Attached to the intestinal surface was a thick membrane composed of fibrin and leukocytes and Gram stain of the exudates revealed "many colonies of staphylococci," similar to those shown in Figure 27.1. The colon was not abnormal. Cultures of heart blood yielded *S. aureus* and *Streptococcus* spp. The third patient was a 46-year-old man who had a partial gastric resection and was given penicillin, streptomycin, oxytetracycline, and a sulphonamide. He developed diarrhea, fever, and shock and died. At autopsy, the mucosa of the small bowel was covered with a yellow-brown membrane; microscopically, the upper half of the mucosa was replaced by necrosis and a membranous exudate composed of fibrin, leukocytes, and "colonies of staphylococci" (Figure 27.3). A necrotizing pneumonia was also present and *S. aureus* resistant to penicillin, streptomycin, and oxtytetracycline was found in post-mortem cultures of the lung and blood. It is noteworthy that the intestinal pathology found in these patients was confined to the small intestine (although one patient had undergone a total colectomy prior to the onset of the enteritis), typical pseudomembranous enteritis was seen in the jejunum and ileum of all three cases, *S. aureus* was isolated from the intestinal membrane in two of the three cases, from heart blood of all three and "identified by Gram stain in large numbers in the intestinal fibrinous casts," and all received perioperative antibiotics.

In 1953, Dearing and Heilman [10] presented evidence that *S. aureus* (*Micrococcus pyogenes*) strains that had grown resistant to antibiotics prescribed in the hospital could produce gastrointestinal and indeed systemic reactions when they were present in the intestinal tract in large numbers. They cited other recent reports implicating oxytetracycline in diarrhea [11,20,21], believed that diarrhea was an indication to discontinue administration of

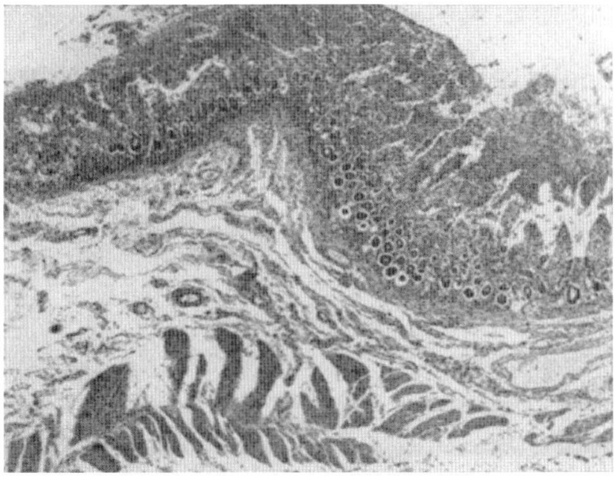

Figure 27.3 Membranous staphylococcal enteritis found at autopsy of a 46-year-old man who underwent a partial gastric resection and gastroenterostomy because of a penetrating and partially obstructing peptic ulcer. He developed staphylococcal pneumonia postoperatively and was treated with penicillin, streptomycin, sulfisoxazole, and oxytetracycline. One week later he developed fever, vomiting, diarrhea, confusion, and shock and died. The upper half of the small intestinal mucosa was replaced by necrosis and a membranous exudate containing granulocytes and colonies of staphylococci. The gland crypts show focal necrosis and granulocytic infiltrates. Cultures of the membranes, blood and lung grew *S. aureus* resistant to penicillin, streptomycin, and oxytetracycline. (From Wakefield & Sommers [9] with permission.)

this antibiotic, and went on to show that erythromycin could be used therapeutically in such cases. In 44 hospitalized patients, cultures were taken intraoperatively from the intestinal lumen of those patients who had received oxytetracycline before surgery. If staphylococci were found, the patient either received erythromycin prophylactically the day after operation or was observed to see whether symptoms would develop in the absence of erythromycin; if they did, erythromycin was then administered orally. Patients who developed diarrhea after antibiotic therapy had cultures of stools or swabs of the mucous membranes of freshly resected intestinal specimens to determine whether *S. aureus* was present. Importantly, selective media and coagulase and susceptibility tests were used to detect antibiotic-resistant *S. aureus* strains. The results showed that those patients whose cultures yielded few staphylococci had no diarrheal symptoms. When patients had predominant cultures of *S. aureus* (after oxytetracycline was discontinued) and they were given erythromycin, no diarrhea was experienced and staphylococci disappeared from their stools. All patients who had staphylococci isolated in pure culture at operation and who were simply observed after the discontinuation of oxytetracycline experienced "rather severe gastrointestinal and systemic reactions" that subsided after the administration of erythromycin. Another group of patients with staphylococci in their stools developed diarrhea while receiving antibiotics, and both symptoms and staphylococci disappeared after erythromycin was begun. Five patients died with severe diarrhea and shock without treatment with erythromycin after use of a tetracycline. Necropsies showed pseudomembranous ileocolitis and pure cultures of staphylococci in stools of four of five patients. In 1954, Pettet *et al.* [22] described autopsy findings in 107 cases of pseudomembranous enterocolitis. Pseudomembranes were seen throughout the intestine, generally were loosely adherent and thus easily separated from the mucosa, but were restricted to the small intestine in approximately half of the cases. Peritonitis was also present in two-thirds of the cases with extensive pseudomembranes. Fecal cultures were not routinely performed, but high *S. aureus* counts were seen in five cases.

Dearing and Heilman's studies in particular are persuasive of a staphylococcal etiology in some cases of enteritis. These authors found *S. aureus* in large numbers in the feces of patients with mild to extremely severe antibiotic-related diarrhea that could be treated or prevented by administration of erythromycin. Notably, they showed a strong association between severe untreated diarrhea, pure cultures of *S. aureus* in stools, and death from enterocolitis. However, as Dearing and Heilman [10] cautioned, the number of patients they studied who had enterocolitis was small. They also pointed out that one of their patients who was not treated with erythromycin and who died with pseudomembranous enterocolitis did not have intestinal contents positive for staphylococci on selective media at either operation or necropsy. It is entirely possible, of course, that this patient died of *C. difficile* colitis. Two patients with colitis in this study were said to have both enteritis and colitis. Strickler and Rice [17] also concluded that pseudomembranous colitis and staphylococcal enterocolitis were two distinct as well as different entities. They noted those cases in which staphylococci were not found in stool cultures from patients with pseudomembranous enterocolitis, but they also stressed that staphylococci will not grow well on the media used routinely at that time for culturing stools for common Gram-negative enteropathogens. More recent reports, discussed below, have further clarified that *S. aureus* enteritis and *C. difficile* colitis are distinct infections [2,23–26].

In 1955, Surgalla and Dack [27] conducted studies to determine whether staphylococci from the stools of patients with enteritis after antibiotic therapy produced enterotoxin. Despite the fact that their patients with enteritis had a high mortality rate, as compared with patients with an acute episode of food poisoning following ingestion of a single dose of enterotoxin, these investigators reasoned that if an enterotoxin were produced continuously by ingested staphylococci (because competing organisms in the intestines were inhibited by the antibiotics the patients had received), a more severe, protracted, and disastrous illness than food poisoning might result. *Staphylococcus aureus* was isolated often as a heavy and/or pure growth from 33 patients. Two of 18 patients they studied had diarrhea on admission to the hospital after receiving antibiotics, and most of the remaining 16 patients developed diarrhea within 1 week after antibiotic therapy. Tests for enterotoxin production were made by feeding 50-mL culture supernates to each of four young rhesus monkeys through a stomach tube. Emesis within the next 5 hours in at least two of the four animals was considered a positive test for the presence of an enterotoxin. Of 33 coagulase-positive isolates tested, 30 produced such an enterotoxin.

A series of 109 cases of staphylococcal enterocolitis, most associated with perioperative antibiotics (especially chloramphenicol, neomycin, or a sulphonamide), was reported in 1966 [6]. Vancomycin, combined with fluid and electrolyte replacement and discontinuation of the offending antibiotics, was successful in the treatment of staphylococcal enterocolitis. None of 45 patients treated with oral vancomycin (0.5 g every 4–6 hours for 3–5 days) died because of the infection; conversely, 8 of 54 (15%) who received other antibiotics died with enterocolitis. Diarrhea usually began 3–9 days after the start of antibiotic therapy; copious green watery stools were common, while blood and mucus were noted in the feces of only 12 patients. Shock was observed in 16 of 109 patients (15%). In the great majority of patients, heavy growth of coagulase-positive staphylococci was obtained in fecal cultures.

In 1963, Altemeier *et al.* [18] reported on 155 patients who were thought to have staphylococcal enterocolitis following antibiotic therapy. Most of these patients had preexisting gastrointestinal disorders. Their report was limited to patients whose stool cultures on selective media revealed *S. aureus*; about half of the isolates were susceptible to erythromycin. Interestingly, 44 of their patients had received neomycin prior to developing diarrhea (32 in preparation for surgery); 66% of the isolates were non-typable, and the authors therefore concluded that this was a new strain of *S. aureus*.

Staphylococcal enterocolitis in the post-penicillin era

Relatively few studies were published concerning staphylococcal pseudomembranous enterocolitis during the 1960s, and those that were tended to question the role played by staphylococci [28–30]. Enterocolitis following the use of antibiotics appeared to become an uncommon disease following the introduction and wide clinical use of vancomycin and semisynthetic penicillinase-resistant β-lactam antibiotics. In the mid-1970s large numbers of cases of PMC began to be recognized, particularly following the use of clindamycin, cephalosporins, or ampicillin. Staphylococci were rarely found in the diarrheal stools of these patients, but the illness was successfully treated with oral vancomycin, to which staphylococci were uniformly susceptible. This paradox was resolved when vancomycin-susceptible *C. difficile* isolates were found to be the cause of the disease in 1977 and 1978 [4,5]. Consequently, staphylococci became ignored as a causative agent of serious and life-threatening nosocomial AAD syndromes. This was despite the possibility that a proportion of AAD cases could be caused by *S. aureus*, particularly since the great majority (70–80%) of such patients are not found to be *C. difficile* toxin positive. Endoscopic examination and/or specific microbiological testing for *S. aureus* in such cases are uncommon, indicating that this etiological explanation is usually not considered. Subsequently, however, a number of reports have provided further evidence that *S. aureus* enterocolitis is a distinct entity, especially as *C. difficile* infection has been considered and excluded.

Staphylococcus aureus enterocolitis in the *Clostridium difficile* era

In 1980, Batts *et al.* [31] described three cases of staphylococcal enterocolitis with interesting supplementary information. The first case was a 3-year-old boy who presented with severe vomiting and profuse diarrhea following ampicillin treatment for a sore throat; despite aggressive supportive treatment he died. Fecal cultures showed a heavy growth of *S. aureus*, and at autopsy enteritis was observed from the jejunum to the ileocecal valve. Mucosal scrapings were positive in Walker rat carcinoma cell cultures for a cytotoxin that appeared to be distinct to that produced by *C. difficile* as it was not neutralized by either *C. difficile* or *C. sordellii* antitoxins; the toxin was not detected in fibroblast cell cultures. A 41-year-old woman with sigmoidoscopy evidence of colitis without pseudomembranes had fecal cultures that yielded a heavy growth of *S. aureus* but which were negative for *C. difficile*. Similarly, fecal filtrates were negative for *C. difficile* cytotoxin B in fibroblast cell cultures, but were positive in Walker cells for a cytotoxin. She was treated with oral vancomycin and recovered promptly. A third case also had sterile fecal filtrates that were positive for a cytotoxin identical to those implicated in the first two patients. Two of the *S. aureus* isolates were available for study and were shown not to produce staphylococcal enterotoxins A–E by gel-diffusion techniques. However, sterile culture supernatants produced cytopathic effects in Walker cell cultures identical to those seen with the stool filtrates. None of the cytotoxin fecal filtrates was neturalized by *C. sordellii* antitoxin, and they were not heat labile or lethal for hamsters when given intraperitoneally; also, they did not enhance capillary permeability when injected into the skin of rabbits, as would be expected with *C. difficile* toxin B. These results suggest that *S. aureus* produces a cytotoxin that may cause a severe form of diarrhea and enteritis, and that Walker rat carcinoma cell lines (but not fibroblast cells) may be useful for further studies.

In 1982, McDonald *et al.* [23] described 10 cases of AAD thought to be caused by MRSA over a 12-month period at the Royal Melbourne Hospital, Australia. All the cases had received multiple broad-spectrum antibiotics. The diagnoses were made according to Gram-stain appearances of fecal smears, heavy predominant growth of MRSA in fecal cultures, and the absence of other bowel pathogens including toxigenic *C. difficile*. Diarrhea usually responded to treatment with vancomycin or bacitracin, and in those who improved the stools cleared of staphylococci.

A report of 34 patients (seven of whom died) with presumed MRSA enterocolitis occurred in 1991 [32]. Notably, both *C. difficile* and MRSA were isolated from half of these cases, raising the possibility of coinfection. Inamatsu *et al.* [33] also attempted to isolate both *S. aureus* and *C. difficile* from 150 fecal samples from patients with AAD. *Staphylococcus aureus* alone was isolated from 21% of samples, *C. difficile* alone from 34%, and both from 15%. Intriguingly, in 2004 Froberg *et al.* [24] reported a case of simultaneous infection with *C. difficile* and MRSA. These were associated with discrete colonic pseudomembranes typical of *C. difficile* infection, and confluent loosely adherent pseudomembranes in the small bowel that showed good evidence of MRSA infection. The 64-year-old man had chronic obstructive pulmonary disease and was admitted to hospital with worsening respiratory status. He received oral trimethoprim–sulfamethoxazole as part of the management of his respiratory disease. After 1 week he developed a distended abdomen with decreased bowel sounds, and required intubation and mechanical ventilation. His peripheral white blood cell count was 32 000/mm^3. Empirical therapy with intravenous ceftizoxime and metronidazole was initiated for treatment of a presumed perforated viscus and abdominal infection. Oral neomycin was also administered. Despite initial improvement, intravenous vancomycin, metronidazole, and amikacin were also subsequently commenced. The patient's condition gradually deteriorated, and he developed intermittent fevers and started passing liquid green stools. MRSA was the predominant organism noted on stool culture. All therapeutic interventions were eventually stopped, and the patient died 2 months after hospital admission. An autopsy was conducted 4 hours after death. A colonic perforation was found with 4 L of multiloculated purulent fluid in the abdominal cavity that grew MRSA, *Proteus mirabilis*, *Escherichia coli*, and *Enterococcus* spp. Blood culture yielded MRSA. A stool specimen was culture- and cytotoxin-positive for *C. difficile*, but culture-negative for other conventional enteric pathogens. The mucosal surfaces of the duodenum, jejunum, and ileum had multiple patches of well-organized yellowish-green pseudomembrane that was minimally adherent to the underlying villi. Histopathological examination of the small bowel showed extensive pseudomembranes comprising fibrin, inflammatory cells, and necrotic debris containing large numbers of polymorphonuclear cells (many of which contained phagocytosed bacteria) and clusters of Gram-positive cocci adjacent to the luminal border. Pseudomembrane tissue was positive for MRSA using polymerase chain reaction. In contrast, the cecum and sections of ascending, transverse, and descending colon had multiple, discrete, yellow-colored, tightly adherent pseudomembranes typical of *C. difficile* PMC. This case clearly supports the hypothesis that *S. aureus* can be responsible for pseudomembranous small bowel pathology that is distinct from the characteristic lesions found in *C. difficile* PMC.

In 1999, Gravet *et al.* [25] reported that *S. aureus* was isolated as the predominant or only isolate from fecal cultures of 60 patients during a 2-year study in a French university hospital; diarrhea occurred in 90% of these patients. During the same period, 460 samples were culture and/or toxin positive for *C. difficile*, giving positivity rates of 1.7% and 13.4%, respectively. Of the *S. aureus* culture-positive cases, 98% had received antibiotics in the month before diarrhea. *Staphylococcus aureus* was not isolated as the predominant isolate in fecal cultures from 57 control patients without diarrhea who received antimicrobial treatment for more than 5 days; 92% of the *S. aureus* isolates from cases were methicillin resistant. The DNA pulse types always matched for multiple *S. aureus* isolates from a single patient, including when these included blood culture strains. Production of both enterotoxin A and the bicomponent leukotoxin LukE-LukD by the *S. aureus* isolates was significantly more common than in randomly collected isolates.

In 2005, Boyce and Havill [26] prospectively examined patients with nosocomial diarrhea for heavy growth of MRSA in their stool, while excluding other bacterial, parasitic, and viral known pathogens. Over 18 months, 11 patients were identified with nosocomial AAD associated with enterotoxin-producing MRSA strains. Quantitative cultures showed that the majority of affected patients had in excess of 1.0×10^8 cfu of MRSA per gram of feces (Table 27.1). In a retrospective analysis of these cases, patients had a greater number of days of diarrhea than 34 patients without MRSA in their stool ($P < 0.001$) or 16 randomly selected patients colonized or infected with enterotoxin-negative MRSA ($P < 0.001$).

In 2006, a UK study compared the relative frequency of *C. difficile*, *C. perfringens*, and *S. aureus* AAD [2]. During 11 months, 4659 inpatient fecal specimens were tested for *C. difficile* cytotoxin, *C. perfringens* enterotoxin, and *S. aureus* by Vero cell assay, enzyme-linked immunosorbent assay, and growth on fresh blood agar, respectively. In AAD cases, the prevalences of *C. difficile* cytotoxin, *C. perfringens* enterotoxin, and *S. aureus* were 12.7%, 3.3%, and 0.2%,

Table 27.1 Characteristics of MRSA-associated diarrhea in 11 patients. (From Boyce & Havill [26] with permission.)

Case	Enterotoxin of stool	MRSA (cfu/g) stool	Days diarrhea detected[1]	Maximum no. of BMs per 24 hours	Maximum volume of stool (mL) per 24 hours	No. of *C. difficile* toxin assays
1	A, B, E	6.5×10^8	14	12	8250	4
2	A, B	1.7×10^8	7	8	2150	1
3	D	3.2×10^8	3	5	475	3
4	A, B	2.6×10^7	5	–[2]	3100	4
5	QNS	1.6×10^8	4	10	2425	4
6	D	3.0×10^7	12	9	1700	3
7	QNS	Not done	7	10	–	2
8	D	2.3×10^8	4	6	–	3
9	A, B	2.6×10^9	8	7	1000	3
10	Indeterminate	2.1×10^8	7	7		7
11	A, B	1.0×10^9	10	7	3150	3

[1] Days with three or more loose/liquid stools per 24 hours.
[2] Colostomy.
BM, bowel movements; QNS, quantity not sufficient.

respectively (15.8% overall). Thus, *C. difficile* AAD was approximately four and 60 times more common than *C. perfringens* AAD and *S. aureus* AAD, respectively. All 10 *S. aureus* isolates were methicillin resistant; five were enterotoxin C producers, one produced enterotoxins C and D, two produced enterotoxin A and toxic shock syndrome toxin (TSST)-1, and two were nonenterotoxigenic. Unlike the earlier French study [25], none of the *S. aureus* isolates produced detectable Panton–Valentine leukocidin, LukE-LukD, LukM-LukF′-PV-like, or exfoliative toxins A and B. The MRSA isolates were distributed among three genotypes. A nonfecal *S. aureus* isolate was obtained from three AAD patients (one wound swab sample, one urine specimen, and one sputum specimen). Each of these isolates showed 100% DNA band homology with the corresponding fecal isolate. Phage typing results identified the two enterotoxin A-producing isolates as UK epidemic strains (EMRSA-16); all remaining isolates were EMRSA-15. These results were consistent with the molecular epidemiology of MRSA strains in the study institution. These three more recent studies [2,25,26] show that while *S. aureus* is less common than *C. difficile* (and possibly *C. perfringens*) as a cause of AAD, unless specific testing is carried out it is likely that such cases will continue to remain undiagnosed. It is possible that antibiotic pressures that have selected for MRSA may in turn lead to *S. aureus* AAD in some patients for reasons that as yet remain undetermined.

Methicillin-resistant *Staphylococcus aureus* enteritis in Japan

MRSA enteritis was prevalent in Japan in the early 1990s, gradually declining in the second half of that decade. A survey of 144 Japanese hospitals reported 831 cases of MRSA enteritis between 1990 and 1992 [34], with an associated mortality ranging from 1.3 to 24% [35,36]. Cases had high fever and watery diarrhea, sometimes leading to severe dehydration and shock, and were associated with gastrointestinal tract surgery [34,37,38], histamine H_2-receptor antagonists [38,39], and broad-spectrum antimicrobial agents [40,41]. A favored treatment included intravenous minocycline, to which the MRSA strains were often susceptible and was associated with good response.

Takesue *et al.* [42,43] investigated the production of staphylococcal enterotoxins and TSST-1 in patients with postoperative MRSA enteritis. Nine of 10 isolates from the feces of patients with enteritis were staphylococcal enterotoxin (SE)A and SEC coproducing strains, and all those that produced SEC also produced TSST-1. The coincidence in time of the prevalence of MRSA enteritis and the isolation of SEA and SEC coproducing strains suggested that these strains were the cause of MRSA enteritis. Strains that produced SEB without TSST-1 were also common. The authors concluded that strains which produced both SEA and SEC tended to cause enteritis associated with TSST-like symptoms, possibly because of the high titers of these toxins. A recent report from Japan [44] found that 8 of 12 historical MRSA isolates from patients with enteritis produced high levels of SEA and TSST-1 but not SEC. Of 186 nonenteritis contemporaneous MRSA isolates, 157 produced SEC and TSST-1 but not SEA. Only 7 of 186 nonenteritis isolates had pulsed-field gel electrophoresis (PFGE) patterns indistinguishable from those of the enteritis isolates, and these did not produce SEA and showed relatively low levels of TSST-1 production. These findings suggest that the disappearance of MRSA enteritis resulted from the decreased incidence of enteritis-causing clones and phenotypic changes in prevalent isolates.

There is considerable evidence that staphylococcal enterotoxins cause diarrhea in animals [45–47] and humans [48–50]. However, given the multitude of exotoxins and other virulence determinants produced by *S. aureus* it is not surprising that a single toxin phenotype or genotype has not been identified as being associated with *S. aureus* enterocolitis. A fundamental issue here remains whether isolates shown to have particular toxin genes present *in vitro* actually express these *in vivo*. Clearly, a model system to examine the behavior of *S. aureus* isolates with putative enterocolitis potential would be advantageous to delineate the pathogenesis of this condition. It is clear that while the incidence of *S. aureus* enterocolitis may have changed through the antibiotic era, this is not a disease of historical interest alone.

Staphylococcus aureus toxic shock syndrome

Vomiting and diarrhea are prominent manifestations of the staphylococcal toxic shock syndrome; *S. aureus* strains that produce TSST-1 often also produce staphylococcal enterotoxins [15,16,51,52]. In addition, both TSST-1 and staphylococcal enterotoxins are superantigens that stimulate monocytes and macrophages to produce various cytokines that may contribute to the clinical manifestations. Paris *et al.* [53] described lesions found at autopsy in 12 fatal cases, but most of their attention was focused on the vagina, cervix, lung, liver, and kidney. Gastrointestinal tissues were reported as normal in five of the nine patients studied. Two patients had acute gastric ulceration and three had intestinal lymphoid hyperplasia. Larkin *et al.* [54] reported their pathological observations in nine fatal cases and saw various degrees of surface denudation of the entire gastrointestinal tract, but neither pseudomembranes nor bowel infarcts were found. It appears therefore that enterocolitis is not a frequent feature of toxic shock syndrome. The absence of intestinal lesions and abnormalities suggests that the diarrheal symptoms occurring in *S. aureus* toxic shock syndrome are a consequence of pronounced vasodilation in the gastrointestinal tract, mirroring that seen peripherally, with rapid movement of serum proteins and fluids from intravascular to extravascular compartments and ultimately into the intestinal lumen.

References

1 Beaugerie L, Petit JC. Microbial–gut interactions in health and disease. Antibiotic-associated diarrhoea. Best Pract Res Clin Gastroenterol 2004;18:337–52.

2 Asha NJ, Tompkins D, Wilcox MH. Comparative analysis of prevalence, risk factors, and molecular epidemiology of antibiotic-associated diarrhea due to *Clostridium difficile*, *Clostridium perfringens*, and *Staphylococcus aureus*. J Clin Microbiol 2006;44:2785–91.

3 Högenauer C, Langner C, Beubler E *et al.* *Klebsiella oxytoca* as a causative organism of antibiotic-associated hemorrhagic colitis. N Engl J Med 2006;355:2418–26.

4 Rifkin GD, Silva J, Fekety FR. Antibiotic-induced colitis. Implication of a toxin neutralised by *Clostridium sordellii* antitoxin. Lancet 1977;310:1103–6.

5 Bartlett JG, Chang TW, Gurwith M *et al.* Antibiotic-associated pseudomembranous colitis due to toxin producing clostridia. N Engl J Med 1978;298:531–6.

6 Khan MY, Hall WH. Staphylococcal enterocolitis: treatment with oral vancomycin. Ann Intern Med 1966;65:1–8.

7 Terplan K, Paine JR, Sheffer J *et al.* Fulminating gastroenterocolitis caused by staphylococci. Its apparent connection with antibiotic medication. Gastroenterology 1953;24:476–509.

8 Brown WJ, Winston R, Sommers SC. Membranous staphylococcal enteritis after antibiotic therapy: report of two cases. Am J Dig Dis 1953;20:73–5.

9 Wakefield RH, Sommers SC. Fatal membranous staphylococcal enteritis in surgical patients. Ann Surg 1953;138:249–52.

10 Dearing WH, Heilman FR. Micrococcic (staphylococci) enteritis as a complication of antibiotic therapy: its response to erythromycin. Proc Mayo Clin 1953;28:121.

11 Jackson GG, Haight TH, Kass EH *et al.* Terramycin therapy of pneumonia: clinical and bacteriological studies in 91 cases. Ann Intern Med 1951;35:1175–202.

12 Reiner L, Schlesinger MJ, Miller GM. Pseudomembranous colitis following aureomycin and chloramphenicol. Arch Pathol 1952;54:39–67.

13 Dixon CF, Weissmann RE. Acute pseudomembranous enteritis or enterocolitis: a complication following intestinal surgery. Surg Clin North Am 1948;28:999.

14 Hansbro GL, Ferrell TF. Acute pseudomembranous enterocolitis simulating acute surgical diseases of the abdomen. Am J Surg 1953;19:82–6.

15 Williams E. Staphylococcal pseudomembranous enterocolitis complicating treatment with aureomycin. Lancet 1954;264:999–1000.

16 Kleckner MS, Bargen JA, Baggenstoss AH. Pseudomembranous enterocolitis: clinicopathologic study of fourteen cases in which the disease was not preceded by an operation. Gastroenterology 1952;212–22.

17 Strickler JH, Rice CO. Pseudomembranous enterocolitis: a comparison with staphylococcal colitis. Minn Med 1966;49:899–904.

18 Altemeier WA, Hummel RP, Hill EO. Staphylococcal enterocolitis following antibiotic therapy. Ann Surg 1963;157:847–58.

19 Penner A, Bernheim AI. Acute postoperative enterocolitis, study of pathologic nature of shock. Arch Pathol 1939;27:966.

20 Janbon M, Bertrand L, Salvaing J, Labauge R. Le syndrome choleriforme de la terramycin. Montpellier Med 1952;41–42:312–23.

21 Haight TH, Finland M. Laboratory and clinical studies on erythromycin. N Engl J Med 1952;247:227–32.

22 Pettet JD, Baggenstoss AH, Dearing WH, Judd ES. Postoperative pseudomembranous enterocolitis. Surg Gynecol Obstet 1954;98:546–52.

23 McDonald M, Ward P, Harvey K. Antibiotic-associated diarrhoea and methicillin-resistant *Staphylococcus aureus*. Med J Aust 1982;1:462–4.

24 Froberg MK, Palavecino E, Dykoski R, Gerding DN, Peterson LR, Johnson S. *Staphylococcus aureus* and *Clostridium difficile* cause distinct pseudomembranous intestinal diseases. Clin Infect Dis 2004;39:747–50.

25 Gravet A, Rondeau M, Harf-Monteil C *et al*. Predominant *Staphylococcus aureus* isolated from antibiotic-associated diarrhea is clinically relevant and produces enterotoxin A and bicomponent toxin LukE-LukD. J Clin Microbiol 1999;37:4012–19.

26 Boyce JM, Havill NL. Nosocomial antibiotic-associated diarrhea associated with enterotoxin-producing strains of methicillin-resistant *Staphylococcus aureus*. Am J Gastroenterol 2005;100: 1828–34.

27 Surgalla MJ, Dack GM. Enterotoxin produced by micrococci from cases of enteritis after antibiotic therapy. JAMA 1955;158:649–50.

28 Cohen LS, Fekety FR, Cluff LE. Studies on the epidemiology of staphylococcal infection, the changing ecology of hospital staphylococci. N Engl J Med 1962;266:367–72.

29 Borriello S, Larson E, Welch A *et al*. Enterotoxigenic *Clostridium perfringens*: a possible cause of antibiotic-associated diarrhoea. Lancet 1984;323:305–7.

30 McBride M. Antibiotic-associated pseudomembranous enteritis due to *Clostridium difficile*. Clin Infect Dis 1995;21:455.

31 Batts D, Silva J, Fekety R. Staphylococcal enterocolitis. In: Current Chemotherapy and Infectious Diseases. Proceedings of the 11th International Conference on Chemotherapy and the 19th Interscience Conference on Antimicrobial Agents and Chemotherapy. Washington, DC: ASM Press, 1980:994.

32 Matsuo S, Aihara M, Takahashi H. Clinical and pathological study of 34 patients with isolation of methicillin-resistant *Staphylococcus aureus* in stool culture. Kansenshogaku Zasshi 1991; 65:1394–402.

33 Inamatsu T, Ooshima H, Masuda Y *et al*. Clinical spectrum of antibiotic associated enterocolitis due to methicillin resistant *Staphylococcus aureus*. Nippon Rinsho 1992;50:1087–92.

34 Ochiai M, Tanimura H, Umemoto Y *et al*. Current occurrence and infection control of MRSA enteritis for surgical patients in Japan (first report) [Japanese with English summary]. Kansenshogaku Zasshi 1995;69:262–71.

35 Hori K, Yura J, Shinagawa N *et al*. Postoperative enterocolitis and current status of MRSA enterocolitis: the result of a questionnaire survey in Japan [Japanese with English summary]. Kansenshogaku Zasshi 1989;63:701–7.

36 Shinagawa N, Koide H. A questionnaire survey on postoperative MRSA enterocolitis [Japanese with English summary]. Nippon Geka Kansensho Kenkyu 1997;8:101–7.

37 Kodama T, Santo T, Yokoyama T *et al*. Postoperative enteritis caused by methicillin-resistant *Staphylococcus aureus*. Surg Today 1997;27:816–25.

38 Takeuchi K, Tsuzuki Y, Ando T *et al*. Clinical studies of enteritis caused by methicillin-resistant *Staphylococcus aureus*. Eur J Surg 2001;167:293–6.

39 Shigeta K, Tanaka S, Nomura K. Relation of sputum and feces and methicillin-resistant *Staphylococcus aureus* (MRSA) detection [Japanese with English summary]. Kansenshogaku Zasshi 1996;70:1062–7.

40 Han SJ, Jung PM, Kim H *et al*. Multiple intestinal ulcerations and perforations secondary to methicillin-resistant *Staphylococcus aureus* enteritis in infants. J Pediatr Surg 1999;34:381–6.

41 Schiller B, Chiorazzi N, Farber BF. Methicillin-resistant staphylococcal enterocolitis. Am J Med 1998;105:164–6.

42 Takesue Y, Yokoyama T, Kodama T *et al*. Toxin involvement in methicillin-resistant *Staphylococcus aureus* enteritis in gastroenterological surgery. Gastroenterol Jpn 1991;26:716–20.

43 Takesue Y, Yokoyama T, Kodama T *et al*. A study on postoperative enteritis caused by methicillin resistant *Staphylococcus aureus*. Surg Today 1993;23:4–8.

44 Okii K, Hiyama E, Takesue Y, Kodaira M, Sueda T, Yokoyama T. Molecular epidemiology of enteritis-causing methicillin-resistant *Staphylococcus aureus*. J Hosp Infect 2006;62:37–43.

45 Tan T-L, Drake CT, Jacobson MJ *et al*. The experimental development of pseudomembranous enterocolitis. Surg Gynecol Obstet 1959;108:415–20.

46 Kakamura Y, Aramaki Y, Kakiuchi T. A mouse model for postoperative fatal enteritis due to *Staphylococcus* infection. J Surg Res 2001;96:35–43.

47 Bergdoll MS. Monkey feeding test for staphylococcal enterotoxins. Methods Enzymol 1988;165:324–33.

48 Eisenberg MS, Gaarslev K, Brown W *et al*. Staphylococcal food poisoning aboard a commercial aircraft. Lancet 1975;ii: 595–9.

49 Holmberg SD, Blake PA. Staphylococcal food poisoning in the United States. JAMA 1984;251:487–9.

50 Raj HD, Bergdoll MS. Effect of enterotoxin B on human volunteers. J Bacteriol 1969;98:833–4.

51 Altemeier W, Lewis S, Schlievert P *et al*. *Staphylococcus aureus* associated with toxic shock syndrome, phage typing and toxin capability testing. Ann Intern Med 1982;96:978–82.

52 Bergdoll M, Crass B, Reiser R *et al*. Enterotoxin-like protein in *Staphylococcus aureus* strains from patients with toxic shock syndrome. Ann Intern Med 1982;96:969–71.

53 Paris AL, Herwaldt LA, Blum D *et al*. Pathological findings in twelve fatal cases of toxic shock syndrome. Ann Intern Med 1982;96:852–7.

54 Larkin S, Williams D, Osterholm M *et al*. Toxic shock syndrome: clinical, laboratory, and pathologic findings in nine fatal cases. Ann Intern Med 1982;96:858–64.

Chapter 28
Infections in Immunocompromised Patients

Lisa E. Davidson and Helen W. Boucher
Division of Geographic Medicine and Infectious Diseases, Tufts Medical Center, Boston, Massachusetts, USA

Introduction

One of the major accomplishments of modern medicine has been the discovery of life-saving and life-prolonging therapies for conditions that were once fatal. Patients with malignancy and immune disorders and those in need of organ transplants now have multiple options for disease treatment and management with immunosuppressive therapy. However, these life-saving therapies come with a cost – higher risk of infection. In particular, as the number of immunocompromised patients (who have prolonged survival) continues to increase, so does the rate of infections in this population [1,2]. Chronic medical conditions associated with an altered immune response to infection (such as diabetes and chronic kidney disease) have become more common as the population ages and life expectancy increases. Another great accomplishment in the last 100 years, the advancement of antimicrobial therapy, has been met with the development of resistant organisms that are widely spread in the hospital environment and now the community. These risk factors are not mutually exclusive. In any one patient they may represent a "triple threat": underlying disease resulting in a suppressed immune system, use of immunosuppressive therapies to manage disease, and colonization or infection with resistant bacteria.

Epidemiology

The staphylococci have emerged as predominant pathogens for these triple-threat patients. In the USA, *Staphylococcus aureus* is reported as a diagnosis in approximately 290 000 discharges per year [3,4]. Infections with *S. aureus* are associated with a significant increase in hospital length of stay and in-hospital mortality [4,5]. In 2005, approximately 19 000 deaths were attributed to invasive methicillin-resistant *S. aureus* (MRSA) infection [6]. In a large surveillance survey of nosocomial bloodstream infections, the staphylococci were the most common organisms isolated from blood cultures of infected patients, causing over 50% of all bloodstream infections [7]. Several large studies have shown that diseases associated with chronic immunosuppression (e.g., cirrhosis, dialysis, and HIV), malignancy, and old age are associated with increased risk of infection from *S. aureus* [2,3,8–10]. In addition, risk factors that are often associated with immunosuppression or the immunocompromised host such as prolonged hospitalization, previous antimicrobial therapy, intensive care unit (ICU) or burn unit admission, surgical-site infection, chronic dermatosis, mucositis, intestinal breakdown, and pulmonary mucosal alterations have all been associated with increased rates of staphylococcal infection [9,11–14]. In a prospective study of infective endocarditis, rates of hemodialysis dependence, immunosuppression, and *S. aureus* infection all significantly increased over a 6-year period [15]. By far the greatest risk factors for *S. aureus* infection in the immunocompromised host are nasal colonization and catheter-associated infection. These two topics are discussed in depth later in this chapter.

The most common method of acquisition of staphylococcal infection in the immunocompromised host is nosocomial transmission. The staphylococci in general and MRSA in particular have become a leading cause of nosocomial pneumonia, surgical wound infection, endocarditis, and bloodstream infections [16–22]. For example, data from the National Nosocomial Infections Surveillance System show that MRSA now accounts for more than 60% of *S. aureus* isolates in US hospital ICUs [23,24]. Patients acquiring MRSA infection as a consequence of healthcare contact are more likely to have a number of comorbid conditions, including advanced age, implanted medical devices, or recent hospitalization [25]. Several reports have documented the emergence of the USA300 clone, the predominant strain of MRSA acquired in the community, among patients with traditional risk factors for hospital-associated MRSA [26]. In a study of 132 MRSA bloodstream infections in one hospital in urban Atlanta, 107 (92%) MRSA-infected patients had contact with the healthcare system in the previous year and 49 (42%) met the criteria

Staphylococci in Human Disease, 2nd edition. Edited by Kent B. Crossley, Kimberly K. Jefferson, Gordon Archer, Vance G. Fowler, Jr.
 ISBN 978-14051-6332-3.

for a nosocomial infection [27]. Genetic analyses showed that 34% of the MRSA isolates were pulsed-field type USA300, including 28% of the healthcare-associated infections as well as 20% of the nosocomial bloodstream infections. The mixing of hospital- and community-acquired (CA)-MRSA has also been observed in ICU infections [28]. In patients with end-stage renal disease there is an increasing proportion of infections with CA-MRSA strains, particularly inpatients undergoing dialysis [29]. In particular, demographic characteristics, risk factors, and outcomes were similar between community- and hospital-acquired strains.

Reasons staphylococci are so effective in causing infections in immunocompromised patients

The pathogenesis of staphylococcal infections in immunocompromised hosts is related to a number of defects in host defense systems. This includes breakdown in nonspecific host defenses (including skin and mucosal barriers) and abnormal response to the acute inflammation typically characterized by staphylococcal infection. In the immunocompromised host, more than one mechanism may be impaired, leading to more severe infection.

Colonization

The skin is the most important mechanism of defense against staphylococcal infection in the immunocompromised patient. Approximately 30–50% of normal individuals are colonized with *S. aureus* and 10–20% remain persistently colonized [30]. Data from the NHANES survey in 2003–2004 documented a decrease in colonization rates with *S. aureus*, from 32.4% in 2001–2002 to 28.6% in 2003–2004 [31]. However, the prevalence of colonization with MRSA increased from 0.8 to 1.5%. Colonization with MRSA was independently associated with healthcare exposure in males, age greater than 60 years, and diabetes. In 2003–2004, a total of 19.7% [95% confidence interval (CI) 12.4–28.8] of MRSA-colonized persons carried a pulsed-field gel electrophoresis (PFGE) type associated with community transmission [32]. The anterior nares are the most common reservoir of *S. aureus* infection, but other body sites, including the axilla, perineum, and sites of skin or mucous membrane disruption, can also be a source of staphylococcal infection [33–35]. Colonization rates are markedly increased in several immunocompromised populations, including those with diabetes, cirrhosis [36,37] or chronic renal failure, injection drug users, and patients receiving dialysis. HIV infection has also been documented as a risk factor for colonization [38,39]. Carriage of staphylococci, particularly MRSA, has been associated with an increased risk of infection in dialysis, HIV, nosocomial bacteremia, cirrhosis, and solid organ transplants [34,37,40–43].

Central venous catheters

Perhaps the greatest risk factor for staphylococcal infection in immunocompromised hosts is the presence of a central venous catheter (CVC). Coagulase-negative staphylococci (CoNS) and *S. aureus* are the most common bacteria in catheter-related infection [23]. The presence of a CVC is significantly associated with hospital-acquired *S. aureus* bacteremia [44]. Neutropenia, HIV, and hematological malignancy have all been significantly associated as risk factors for CVC-related infection [45]. Age over 65 years has also been shown to be a risk factor for CVC-related infection [45]. In a study of patients with cancer, catheter-related *S. aureus* bacteremia was associated with an attributable mortality rate of 12% and a complication rate of 40% [46]. In patients with neutropenia, the most prevalent risk factor for bloodstream infection is the presence of a CVC and bloodstream infection is associated with a crude mortality rate of 36% [1]. In patients with HIV and bloodstream infection, CVCs are the most common predisposing factor for bloodstream infections, *S. aureus* and CoNS the most common isolates, and attributable mortality is 10–20% in a number of recent epidemiological studies [47–50]. Similarly, CVC use is associated with *S. aureus* infection in cirrhotic and liver transplant patients [36,37,43].

Pathogenesis

Staphylococci stimulate a nonspecific acute inflammatory response that is characterized by the infiltration of a large number of polymorphonuclear leukocytes (PMNs) at the site of invasion. Therefore, any disease affecting the recruitment or function of PMNs may predispose the host to infection. Today the most common neutrophil dysfunction in the immunocompromised host is neutropenia (circulating neutrophils $< 500/\text{mm}^3$). There are several primary disorders characterized by neutropenia, including Kostmann syndrome (congenital neutropenia), glycogen storage disease type Ib, and failure of release of neutrophils from the marrow. More commonly, medical conditions associated with bone marrow failure such as acute leukemia, myleodysplastic syndromes, HIV, and primary immunodeficiency syndromes (e.g., X-linked hyper-IgM, X-linked agammaglobulinemia, and reticular dysgenesis) are associated with neutropenia.

Defects in the migration and adhesion of leukocytes can also predispose the host to staphylococcal infections. Hyper-IgE syndrome, leukocyte adhesion defects type I and II, and Shwachman syndrome are all associated with defects of neutrophil migration [51]. Defects of migration have also been associated with diabetes mellitus, metabolic storage disease, malnutrition, immaturity, and burns. Disorders of phagocytic killing ability include chronic granulomatous disease, glycogen storage disease type Ib, Chédiak–Higashi syndrome, and specific granule deficiency

[51]. Chronic granulomatous disease is characterized by genetic defects in the ability of phagocytes to generate reactive oxygen intermediates from molecular oxygen. This results in decreased ability of PMNs to kill invading organisms, particularly *S. aureus* [52]. Treatment options include interferon (IFN)-γ to decrease opportunistic infections, allogeneic stem-cell transplantation, and experimental gene therapy [53].

While the pathogenesis of staphylococcal infections is strongly associated with nonspecific host defense systems, the humoral and cell-mediated immune systems play an important secondary role. Patients with either T-cell- or B-cell-mediated diseases often develop staphylococcal infections as a consequence of frequent hospitalization resulting in increased colonization, intravascular access, and interventions that may predispose them to infection [30,54]. The major exception to this has been the well-documented association between HIV and staphylococcal infection. Although HIV is typically thought of as a T-cell-mediated disease, the increased incidence of staphylococcal infection may also be attributed to the impairment in neutrophil function, decreased activation of macrophages, and decreased maturation of B cells. In addition, staphylococcal superantigens have been shown to induce HIV replication in monocytes and CD4 cells [55–58].

Diseases with multifactorial host defense defects

Diabetes mellitus

Patients with diabetes mellitus have a number of host defense abnormalities that may predispose them to staphylococcal infection. Impaired glucose control has been associated with defects in adherence, chemotaxis and phagocytosis of PMNs and impaired T-cell function [59,60]. In addition, microvascular disease resulting in poor tissue perfusion, neuropathy, frequent use of intravascular lines, and frequent hospitalization are all risk factors that predispose diabetics to infection. These disruptions in host defense result in important susceptibility to infections due to a variety of pathogens, including *S. aureus*. Diabetic mice are more susceptible to hindpaw infections with *S. aureus* than nondiabetic mice [60]. Once an infection is acquired, diabetes is a risk factor for poor outcome. For example, diabetes, as well as infection due to *S. aureus*, were independent predictors of mortality in patients with infective endocarditis [61].

Increased rates of *S. aureus* colonization have been shown in patients with insulin-dependent diabetes or poor glycemic control [62–68]. However, several studies have shown conflicting results about the risk of *S. aureus* carriage in noninsulin-dependent diabetics [62–68]. Although the staphylococci are common causes of bacteremia in diabetic patients [8,59], surprisingly few studies have specifically evaluated the frequency of staphylococcal bacteremia in diabetic compared with nondiabetic patients. In a study of nosocomial *S. aureus* bacteremia in nasal carriers versus noncarriers, diabetes was not found to be a significant risk factor for bacteremia [41]. A recent survey of NHANES data demonstrated that diabetic patients colonized with *S. aureus* are more likely to have an MRSA isolate [69]. Diabetes has also been found to be a risk factor for developing persistent *S. aureus* bacteremia [70].

The staphylococci are the predominant organisms responsible for skin and soft tissue infections in diabetic patients [71]. In particular, MRSA accounts for 40–80% of all *S. aureus* skin and soft tissue infections in diabetic patients [72–74]. Hospitalization, prolonged antibiotic exposure, and nasal colonization are risk factors for diabetic wound colonization with MRSA [72,74]. Although MRSA infection in the diabetic wound is usually hospital or healthcare acquired, community-associated MRSA is becoming an increasingly important source of skin and soft tissue infection in diabetic patients [75,76].

Chronic renal failure

Patients with chronic kidney disease have many factors which make them susceptible to infection, including uremia (which affects phagocyte, B-cell and T-cell function), iron overload, nutrition, anemia, poor skin integrity, presence of diabetes mellitus, advanced age, and frequent hospitalization [77–81]. Once patients require dialysis, the rates of infection with staphylococci increase dramatically. Nasal carriage occurs in 40–80% of patients on dialysis and has been shown to increase the risk of infection in both continuous ambulatory peritoneal dialysis (CAPD) and hemodialysis [34,77,82–84]. In a recent study of 120 patients on hemodialysis, 40 (33%) were colonized with *S. aureus* and 26 (65%) were colonized with MRSA [85]. Among the 26 MRSA isolates, 10 (38.5%) carried staphylococcal cassette chromosome (SCC)*mec* type IV (i.e., CA-MRSA), and seven of these ten carried the genes for Panton–Valentine leukocidin (PVL). Among 10 patients who presented with or developed an *S. aureus* infection, eight were colonized with *S. aureus*, seven with MRSA, and three with SCC*mec* type IV strains [85]. The predominant mode of staphylococcal infection is bacteremia due to migration of pathogenic bacteria from skin to the bloodstream via the catheter hub and lumen. The risk of bacteremia is related to the type of vascular access [86]. The incidence of *S. aureus* bacteremia in hemodialysis patients ranges from 5 to 27% [78]. However, in those patients with MRSA infection, the incidence of infection is much greater (100-fold) than the normal population [87]. *Staphylococcus aureus* bacteremia in dialysis patients is associated with a high rate of complications, including endocarditis, septic arthritis, thrombophlebitis, abscess, osteomyelitis, and sepsis [88–90]. Although CoNS were traditionally the most common pathogen causing catheter-related infection in

CAPD, *S. aureus* is now the predominant cause of bacteremia and peritonitis [82,84,91–93].

Cirrhosis

Patients with cirrhosis can have immune deficits that include impaired phagocytosis and chemotaxis, decreased complement levels, and poor opsonization [94]. In the past, Gram-negative organisms were the predominant source of infection in cirrhotic patients. However, due to selective pressures from the wide use of prophylactic antibiotics and increased spread of nosocomial infections, the staphylococci are becoming increasingly important causes of infection in cirrhotics. Patients with cirrhosis have higher rates of *S. aureus* colonization, particularly with MRSA [36,37,42,95]. Nasal carriers are more likely to develop *S. aureus* infections, have higher Child–Pugh scores, and increased mortality [36,37,42]. In hospitalized cirrhotic patients, the staphylococci are the most common cause of bacteremia [96,97]. The staphylococci are also a significant cause of spontaneous bacterial peritonitis, pneumonia, and bacteriuria [42,96–98]. Infection with staphylococci in patients with cirrhosis is significantly associated with higher mortality [96,97].

Human immunodeficiency virus

Staphylococcus aureus has become an increasingly important pathogen in patients infected with HIV. Although considered primarily a disease of cell-mediated immunity, infection with HIV affects all arms of the immune system. HIV-infected patients may have impaired neutrophil chemotaxis and phagocytosis, impaired production of oxygen species, reduced expression of adhesion molecules, and accelerated apoptosis of neutrophils [99]. In addition, patients may experience treatment-related causes of neutrophil dysfunction as a result of antibiotics and antiviral medications.

Until recently, the majority of staphylococcal infections in HIV patients were associated with CVCs and nasal carriage [39,100–102]. In a study of 443 HIV-positive patients, 29.6% were persistent *S. aureus* carriers [103]. However, rates of colonization with MRSA in HIV-positive patients may be higher than in the non-HIV population or in previous studies of HIV-infected patients [104]. Bloodstream infection is the most common cause of nosocomial infection in HIV patients and *S. aureus* is the most common pathogen [47,49,50,105]. Compared with the era before highly active antiretroviral therapy, the incidence of *S. aureus* bacteremia in HIV patients has significantly decreased, from 3.7 episodes per 100 person-years (1991–1996) to 2.78 episodes per 100 person-years (1997–2000) [105]. MRSA accounts for 30–50% of isolates and is significantly associated with low CD4 count, β-lactam use, and previous hospitalization [105,106]. A recent study in HIV-infected children demonstrated increased carriage of MRSA that was significantly associated with administration of trimethoprim-sulfamethoxazole (TMP-SMX) [107]. This differs from studies in adults, which have shown (TMP-SMX) to be be protective of MRSA colonization [104].

In HIV-infected patients, *S. aureus* primarily causes bacteremia and soft tissue infections. *Staphylococcus aureus* is also a common cause of bacterial pneumonia in HIV patients [108–111]. However, *S. aureus* is often an under-recognized pathogen and in advanced disease may be less obvious than other opportunistic infections [108,112]. Staphylococcal septic arthritis, pyomyositis, pericarditis, mastitis, epidural abscess, and liver abscess have all been reported in patients with HIV [111,113–120].

Recent data suggest that CA-MRSA may be a more common pathogen causing necrotizing skin and soft tissue infections in patients with HIV [38,106]. In a case–control study of HIV-positive men who have sex with men, CA-MRSA skin infections were associated with high-risk sex and drug-using behaviors [121]. In another study of skin and soft tissue infections in an HIV outpatient clinic, 93% of skin and soft tissue infections were due to MRSA and approximately 50% of patients had nonhealthcare-associated risk factors for infection (prior incarceration, chronic dermatoses, homelessness, intravenous drug use, alcohol abuse) [122]. Most of these isolates were USA300, demonstrating the importance of this emerging pathogen among this immunocompromised patient population.

Staphylococcal infections in patients with malignancy and organ transplantation

Until the early 1980s, Gram-negative pathogens were the predominant infecting bacteria in patients with malignancy and disease- or chemotherapy-associated neutropenia. However, Gram-positive organisms are now the predominant pathogens. This can be attributed to several factors: the practice of routine prophylaxis for Gram-negative infections, increasing nosocomial transmission of Gram-positive bacteria, and changes in the conditioning and treatment regimens for many hematological malignancies.

Malignancy

CoNS and *S. aureus* are the most common sources of bloodstream infection in patients with malignancy, usually due to the presence of intravascular devices [123]. In patients with cancer, catheter-related infection with *S. aureus* is associated with high rates of complicating infections, including metastatic infections, venous thrombosis, endocarditis, and septic shock [46,123]. Solid tumors are more likely to be associated with intravascular complications such as septic thrombophlebitis and endocarditis, while hematological malignancies are more likely to be associated with extravascular complications such as septic emboli, abscess, and septic shock [46,124]. In patients with stem-cell transplants, bacteremia is most commonly caused by CoNS and usually occurs during the pre-engraftment period [125,126]. Mucositis and damage to the skin are the common predisposing factors for infection in bone marrow transplant patients [127,128]. Although less common than *S. aureus*, there are case report of CoNS causing invasive infections such as endocarditis, septic arthritis, and meningitis [129].

Neutropenia

CoNS are the most common cause of bloodstream infection in neutropenic patients [7,126,130,131]. While previously a less common pathogen, the rates of *S. aureus* infection in neutropenic patients have increased dramatically over the last 20 years [1,7,132]. Acute leukemia, oral mucositis, CVCs, and bacteremia of unknown origin are all risk factors for developing *S. aureus* infection in the neutropenic patient [1,133]. Neutropenic patients with *S. aureus* bacteremia (particularly MRSA bacteremia) have higher rates of mortality and adverse events than do those with bacteremia due to other pathogens.

Solid organ transplantation

Solid organ transplant patients are subject to a number of risk factors that contribute to an increased risk of infection: immunodeficiency from underlying diseases, frequent hospitalizations and antimicrobial use, and immunosuppressive regimens post transplant. In transplant recipients, staphylococcal infections are a common cause of bacterial infection in the acute period (30 days) as a result of colonization with bacteria and the presence of intravascular devices [134,135]. The staphylococci are a more common source of infection in liver and cardiac transplant patients and an infrequent source of infection in kidney transplant patients despite the high rate of colonization in patients undergoing CAPD and hemodialysis prior to transplantation. There are several case reports of CA-MRSA causing infection in solid organ transplant patients, including recurrent cellulitis, abscess, osteomyelitis, and necrotizing fasciitis [136].

In contrast to the immunocompetent population, liver transplant recipients are more commonly colonized by MRSA than methicillin-sensitive *S. aureus* (MSSA) [40,43,137]. Colonization with MRSA is associated with higher MELD scores and an increased risk of infection after transplant [40,43,137,138]. Colonized transplant patients have an increased risk of posttransplant complications and longer ICU stays [40,138–140]. In a series of patients undergoing living related donor transplants, preoperative MRSA colonization, preoperative use of antimicrobials, operation time (≥ 16 hours), and postoperative apheresis independently predicted postoperative MRSA infection. Bloodstream infections, pneumonia, and abdominal and wound infections with *S. aureus* are common causes of infection in liver transplant recipients [139–143]. Primary cytomegalovirus infection has also been associated with an increase in MRSA infection [140]. Because of their prolonged and frequent hospitalizations and long-term immunosuppression, liver transplant patients are also at risk for acquiring staphylococcal carriage in the posttransplant period [141,144]. There is also ongoing research to determine if high hepatic iron at the time of transplantation is a risk factor for *S. aureus* bacteremia [145].

Cardiac transplant candidates often require the use of ventricular assist devices (VAD) as a bridge to transplantation. CoNS and *S. aureus* are the most common organisms causing VAD-associated infection [146–148]. Removal of the device is often curative and patients with VAD infections do not seem to have increased morbidity and mortality after transplantation [135,149]. Although the risk of mediastinitis after cardiac transplant is low (2.5–2.9%), the most common pathogens causing mediastinitis are *S. aureus* and CoNS [135,150–152]. Mediastinitis is usually associated with underlying comorbidities, nasal carriage, and intravascular infection [150–153].

In addition, transplant patients may be at risk for acquiring staphylococcal infections from the donor. In a case series of liver and kidney transplants from cadaveric donors with endocarditis, *S. aureus* and CoNS were the most commons sources of donor endocarditis [154]. Infective endocarditis has been reported in kidney transplant recipients due to previous infection of intravascular devices and arteriovenous grafts [155–158]. However, studies have demonstrated no reduction in patient or graft survival [154,159]. More concerning may be the increase in CA-MRSA in the donor population. In a case of living related donor liver transplant, fatal CA-MRSA necrotizing pneumonia occurred in a previously uncolonized liver transplant recipient [160]. The same strain of CA-MRSA was detected in the living donor.

Trauma and burns

Staphylococcus aureus may be considered an "opportunistic" pathogen in burn and trauma patients [161]. In both cases, patients who have survived the initial injury have a high rate of morbidity and mortality due to colonizing bacteria. *Staphylococus aureus* is the most common pathogen isolated from burn and trauma patients, which likely reflects infection from endogenous bacteria or nosocomially acquired infection [162,163]. Nasal colonization at the time of severe head trauma has been associated with increased risk of *S. aureus* pneumonia and infection [164]. Aggressive wound management with early débridement, wound grafting, and silver-based dressings have decreased wound infection in the acute phase of burn recovery. However, large burns (> 30%) have been associated with increased rates of infection and mortality due to systemic immunosuppression [163,165]. Large burn wounds provide an ideal culture medium for bacteria as they have

Table 28.1 Drugs that predispose immunocompromised patients to staphylococcal infection.

Pathology	Drug
Alteration of host nasal and mucosal defense systems	Antibiotics Glucocorticoids
Depression or abnormal function of polymorphonuclear leukocytes	Glucocorticoids Antivirals (zidovudine, ganciclovir) Antibiotics (β-lactams, TMP–SMX, vancomycin, linezolid) Cytotoxic and marrow suppressive agents (cyclosporine, azathioprine)
Alteration of cytokine responses that may predispose host to infection	TNF-α inhibitors Glucocorticoids Cyclosporine, FK-506 (tacrolimus)
Antiproliferative effects on T-cell and B-cell responses	Mycophenolate mofetil, antithymocyte globulins, antilymphocyte globulins

TMP–SMX, trimethoprim–sulfamethoxazole; TNF, tumor necrosis factor.

abundant necrotic tissue. Patients with burn wounds also have compromised innate immune responses and decreased cellular and humoral immune system activation [166]. In addition, *S. aureus* produces collagenases and hyaluronidase, exotoxins, toxic shock syndrome toxin (TSST)-1, and enterotoxins, which predispose burn patients to toxic shock syndrome [167]. Finally, MRSA is a major cause of infection in burn units [163,168].

Drugs that predispose immunocompromised patients to staphylococcal infection

Therapy with a number of immunosuppressive drugs has been associated with increased rates of staphylococcal infection. In many cases, these medications are used as disease-modifying agents in patients already immunocompromised due to the nature of their underlying disease (Table 28.1).

Glucocorticoids

The administration of glucocorticoids has profound effects on the immune function of macrophages and granulocytes. Glucocorticoids decrease the adhesion and recruitment of phagocytes, inhibit the transcription of cytokines, and decrease inflammatory response. However, there are few studies documenting a significant association between the use of glucocorticoids and increased rates of infection with *S. aureus*. An evaluation of over 16 000 patients with rheumatoid arthritis within the National Databank for Rheumatic Diseases found that prednisone was associated with an increased risk of hospitalization for pneumonia (hazard ratio 1.7, 95% CI 1.5 – 2.0) [169]. In a study of pulmonary infiltrates in patients on long-term glucocorticoid therapy, the staphylococci were the most common cause of bacterial infection [170]. In a study of *S. aureus* bacteremia in neutropenic versus nonneutropenic patients, neutropenic patients were significantly more likely to be receiving glucocorticoid therapy [124]. However, there was no statistically significant association between glucocorticoid use and development of bacteremia. There have been case reports in the literature of *S. aureus* abscesses secondary to steroid injection, although it is unclear if this is due to the use of steroids or introduction of colonizing skin bacteria into a sterile space in an immunocompromised host [171]. Some *in vitro* studies have suggested that TSST-1 induced by *S. aureus* infection attenuates the clinical efficacy of glucocorticoids [172,173]. Further investigation into the association of glucocorticoids and risk of infection with *S. aureus* is needed.

Antimicrobials

Often therapies that are employed to treat or prevent infection can cause profound neutropenia and make an already compromised host even more susceptible. Several classes of antimicrobials including sulfonamides, penicillins, cephalosporins, oxazolidinones, and vancomycin have been associated with neutropenia.

Immunomodulatory drugs

Staphylococcus aureus is a potent inducer of tumor necrosis factor (TNF)-α and TNF-α is important in promoting neutrophil killing of *S. aureus*. The use of anti-TNF-α for the treatment of rheumatoid arthritis and inflammatory bowel disease has raised concerns about the increased risk of staphylococcal infection. *Staphylococcus aureus* is a significant cause of infection in patients treated with anti-TNF-α [174–176]. In particular, patients treated with anti-TNF-α and methotrexate have a higher rate of colonization with *S. aureus* [174]. Moreover, in a recent meta-analysis of the risk for serious infection among patients with rheumatoid arthritis receiving anti-TNF antibody therapy in nine randomized controlled trials, the pooled odds ratio for serious infection among anti-TNF recipients was 2.0 (95% CI 1.3–2.1) [177]. Importantly, most serious infections were bacterial. Combination treatment with multiple disease-modifying agents has been associated with complicated *S. aureus* infections such as pericarditis [178], myositis [179], and necrotizing fasciitis [180].

Clinical manifestations and diagnosis

Infections in the immunocompromised host may be difficult to diagnose. Traditional symptoms such as fever and production of purulent secretions may be blunted due to absence or malfunction of PMNs. Since regular signs of acute infection are unreliable, a thorough medical history, review of systems, and physical examination may be the key to diagnosis. In particular, a patient report of focal symptoms or new physical examination findings should be given particular attention. However, the absence of physical examination findings should not rule out any source of infection [181]. The past medical history may also be an important clue to identifying the source of infection. Comorbidities, previous wound infection, previous indwelling catheter or nonremovable hardware, and hospitalization in the last 6 months have all been associated with increased risk of staphylococcal infection [9,30,59,89].

Routine laboratory assessment for the immunocompromised patient with suspicion of infection should include complete blood count with differential, liver function tests, electrolytes, and blood cultures. Blood cultures are crucial to the diagnosis of bloodstream infection in an immunocompromised host. It is recommended that at least two sets of cultures be obtained. In patients with an intravascular catheter, one set of blood cultures should be drawn peripherally and one set from the central venous line [182,183]. In an immunocompromised patient, the report of a single positive blood culture should be the signal for initiation of empirical treatment of staphylococcal infections (see discussion below). This is particularly true for *S. aureus* infections. In patients with a single positive blood culture for CoNS who are clinically asymptomatic and afebrile, it is important to obtain multiple follow-up blood cultures from the indwelling line and peripherally. A single isolated culture may represent a contaminant but multiple positive cultures from the catheter likely indicate catheter infection. Blood cultures should be repeated for persistent fevers or rigors. Positive blood cultures 48–96 hours after the initial positive blood culture have been associated with development of complicated infection [184].

Patients with *S. aureus* infection, particularly bacteremia, have a high incidence of metastatic infection [184–186]. In addition to a careful physical examination, radiographic studies and echocardiography are important diagnostic tools for identifying areas of infection and should be initiated promptly. Primary infection can also occur in any organ system, particularly the lungs, urine, and soft tissue. Samples should be obtained from the involved organ system whenever possible and evaluated for analysis and culture. In patients with mental status changes, a lumbar puncture should be performed and Gram stain and culture of the cerebrospinal fluid should be evaluated. Especially in cases of skin and soft tissue infection, prompt surgical débridement may be required and surgical evaluation should be initiated early.

Life-threatening clinical syndromes may present atypically in the immunocompromised host. These patients may quickly develop systemic inflammatory response syndrome and sepsis due to a suppressed response to tissue injury and uncontrolled inflammation. This is commonly in response to bacterial infection, but may be related to noninfectious causes as well [187]. Because of suppression of T-cell responses, patients may lack the typical mucocutaneous symptoms characterizing toxic shock syndromes [188–190]. Necrotizing fasciitis due to CA-MRSA has been associated with injection drug use, diabetes, cirrhosis, cancer, and HIV [76]. *Staphylococcus aureus* may also be a source of enteritis in patients with malignancy [191].

Treatment and prevention

Options for the treatment of staphylococcal infections are covered in detail in chapter 31. Therefore, we attempt to limit this discussion to topics pertinent to the immunocompromised host.

Glycopeptides

Vancomycin is the most commonly used agent for treatment of staphylococcal infections in immunocompromised patients. In particular, it has been considered the first-line antibiotic for treatment of MRSA infections. In patients who require long outpatient antibiotic therapy, particularly patients with end-stage renal disease, vancomycin is often used because of its easy dosing schedule. However, studies comparing vancomycin with β-lactam antibiotics for invasive MSSA infections have demonstrated more microbiological failure, persistent bacteremia, and clinical relapse with vancomycin therapy, suggesting that β-lactam antibiotics are superior for these infections [185,192].

There is a large body of investigation evaluating the use of glycopeptides for the empirical treatment of neutropenic fever. Patients with a hematopoietic stem-cell transplant or high-intensity chemotherapy regimen are at increased risk for developing infection due to neutropenia and mucosal damage from immunosuppressive medications. Early institution of broad-spectrum empirical therapy has significantly decreased the mortality from

Table 28.2 Indications for empirical therapy of staphylococcal infection in patients with neutropenic fever.[1]

Clinically apparent, serious catheter-related infection
Blood culture positive for Gram-positive bacteria prior to final identification and susceptibility testing
Known colonization with MRSA
Hypotension or septic shock
Soft tissue infection

[1] Based on recommendations from the National Comprehensive Cancer Network [128] and Infectious Disease Society of America [182].

Gram-negative infection. However, most of these regimens do not provide appropriate empirical therapy for Gram-positive organisms. Several trials have attempted to evaluate the use of vancomycin or glycopeptides at the onset of neutropenic fever or as rescue therapy [193–197]. These trials have not shown a reduction in mortality, but have shown increased costs and adverse reactions with the addition of empirical Gram-positive coverage compared with placebo. Therefore, the routine use of empirical antistaphylococcal coverage for neutropenic fever is not currently recommended [128,182]. Instead, empirical Gram-positive coverage should be reserved for patients with a high risk of staphylococcal infection (Table 28.2).

In order to avoid the development of resistant pathogens, therapy should be reassessed within 2–3 days; if a Gram-positive pathogen is not identified, empirical therapy should be discontinued. Clinicians are often reticent to discontinue antibiotics in immunocompromised patients even when there is no clear evidence of staphylococcal infection. The judicious use of antistaphylococcal antibiotics in immunocompromised patients cannot be stressed enough. The high rate of MRSA colonization combined with overexposure or long-term use of glycopeptides has led to the development of vancomycin-intermediate *S. aureus* (VISA) and vancomycin-resistant *S. aureus* (VRSA), particularly in patients with end-stage renal disease requiring hemodialysis [198–201]. In addition, heterogeneous glycopeptide-intermediate *S. aureus* may play an increasing role in the development of VISA and VRSA in the immunocompromised host [201,202]. Treatment failure of MRSA infection with standard therapy, especially in patients with previous vancomycin exposure, should alert the physician to the possibility of a VISA or VRSA strain. Particular care is required for the evaluation of these organisms.

Linezolid

Much less data have been reported in the literature on the use of linezolid in the immunocompromised host. One study evaluating vancomycin and linezolid in patients with febrile neutropenia found clinical outcomes to be equivalent, but fewer drug-related adverse outcomes were reported in the linezolid group [203]. Linezolid has also been shown to be well tolerated in patients undergoing solid organ transplantation [204]. Patients treated with linezolid are at risk of developing thrombocytopenia [205]. In two studies of neutropenic cancer patients, linezolid was not associated with an increase in the risk of thrombocytopenia or decreased myeloid recovery [203,206]. Linezolid has been increasingly used in the treatment of skin and soft tissue infections, especially in diabetic patients [73,207–209]. Linezolid resistance has been reported in immunocompromised patients, particularly when used for prophylaxis of Gram-positive infections [210]. It is important to note that linezolid is not approved for the treatment of catheter-related bloodstream infections. In March 2007, the Food and Drug Administration issued a warning to physicians regarding the use of linezolid for the treatment of catheter-related bloodstream infections [211]. In an open-label randomized study, linezolid was found to be inferior to standard of care and associated with more deaths among patients infected with Gram-negative organisms alone, among those with both Gram-positive and Gram-negative organisms, and in those who had no infection when they entered the study [211].

Daptomycin

Daptomycin is a new treatment for drug-resistant Gram-positive infections with concentration-dependent bactericidal activity against staphylococci, including MRSA and glycopeptide intermediate-resistant *S. aureus*. However, few studies have specifically examined the use of daptomycin in the immunocompromised host. In a study of diabetic foot infections caused by Gram-positive pathogens, the safety and clinical efficacy of daptomycin were similar to standard antibiotics [212]. Of note, daptomycin-resistant *S. aureus* has been reported in immunocompromised patients with cirrhosis and diabetes [213,214].

Prevention of infection

Since colonization with *S. aureus* increases the risk of subsequent infection, eradication of nasal carriage has been an area of intense investigation. A short course of treatment with nasal mupirocin ointment has been shown to be highly effective in eradicating colonization and decreasing infection, particularly in patients with end-stage renal disease requiring dialysis, HIV, and liver transplant [215–217]. However, strategies using mupirocin for prophylaxis of infection and recurrence of colonization have demonstrated no significant benefit [215,217–219]. In addition, these studies have also demonstrated that serious adverse events and development of antimicrobial resistance can result from therapy. The exception to these findings is the use of mupirocin to decrease colonization and prevent exit-site infections in patients undergoing peritoneal dialysis [220,221]. Mupirocin has also been used in conjunction with infection control strategies to prevent outbreaks of MRSA in ICUs and burn units [222,223]. With the emergence of CA-MRSA, studies are reexamining multifaceted approaches for decolonization including chlorhexidine washes, intranasal mupirocin, and oral antistaphylococcal antibiotics [224].

Prevention of catheter-related infection in the immunocompromised host is extremely important. Appropriate aseptic techniques, skin antisepsis, appropriate catheter dressings, and location of catheter placement have all been shown to decrease rates of infection [225]. In particular, using 2% chlorhexidine preparation for skin prophylaxis, maximal sterile barrier precautions during insertion, avoiding routine replacement of CVCs, and appropriate use of short-term antibiotic-impregnated catheters should be emphasized [225]. Stringent infection control strategies are also a key element in preventing colonization and infection [226,227].

The removal of catheters in the immunocompromised host with bloodstream infection is often a difficult clinical decision. Studies have clearly documented that removal of a central venous line is essential for clearance and resolution of complicated staphylococcal infection [183]. If the patient has erythema or purulence overlying the exit site, a complicated tunnel infection, or clinical signs of sepsis, then the catheter should be removed and cultured [128,183]. However, in patients who require ongoing, long-term vascular access, frequent replacement of indwelling lines has significant morbidity and mortality. If the infection is caused by *S. aureus*, catheter removal is generally recommended and systemic antimicrobial therapy given for 10–14 days or longer in cases of complicated infection [128,183]. However, in cases where there is no other venous access site, some studies have documented the use of a combination of systemic antimicrobials and antibiotic-lock therapy [228–230]. Catheter salvage is generally more successful in patients with CoNS infection, although salvage of catheters in neutropenic patients with *S. aureus* bacteremia has been demonstrated [231]. In a metaanalysis of studies of high-risk patients (including malignancy) with long-term central indwelling devices, prophylactic use of vancomycin lock solution has been shown to reduce the risk of bloodstream infection [232]. The use of antibiotic lock therapy and catheter salvage in immunocompromised patients requires greater study before further recommendations can be made.

Outcome, morbidity, and mortality

Infection due to *S. aureus* imposes a high and increasing burden on utilization of healthcare resources, morbidity, and mortality. Although the overall mortality from *S. aureus* bacteremia has decreased over the last 25 years, the incidence rates have doubled [2]. Healthcare costs for all patients with *S. aureus* bacteremia in the presence of indwelling devices are increased, and are twice as high among patients with hospital-acquired *S. aureus* bacteremia [233].

Cancer patients with *S. aureus* infection have higher rates of metastatic infection and mortality [123,133]. Mortality from staphylococcal bloodstream infection in patients with malignancy ranges from 17.6 to 33% [1]. In patients on hemodialysis, *S. aureus* bacteremia was associated with increases in mortality, the risk of complications, and length of stay [234]. Bloodstream infection after hematopoietic stem-cell transplantation is associated with increased mortality [126]. *Staphylococcus aureus* infection increases the rates of posttransplant complications and mortality in solid organ transplant recipients [139,143]. Infection with *S. aureus* in burn unit patients has been associated with increased risk of death, increased length of stay, and hospital costs [4]. Comorbidities and older age may also be contributing risk factors for increased mortality.

Future directions

As the population of immunocompromised patients grows, so does the need for novel therapies to treat staphylococcal infections in this high-risk population. Immunocompromised patients are at the greatest risk of infection but are often the most difficult group to study. These individuals are often excluded from clinical trials due to their underlying disease. However, these patients are often the first to use novel therapies due to the life-threatening nature of staphylococcal infection and the high risk of resistant infection. New antimicrobials are under evaluation for the treatment of MRSA infection (including dalbavancin, telavancin, ceftibiprole) and may provide important treatment options. In particular, immunocompromised patients with increased risk of staphylococcal infections may benefit from either active or passive prevention of *S. aureus* infection. Monoclonal antibodies for the treatment of *S. aureus* infection are currently undergoing clinical trials [235,236]. Development of an active immunization strategy also continues to be an area of intense investigation [237].

References

1 Wisplinghoff H, Seifert H, Wenzel RP, Edmond MB. Current trends in the epidemiology of nosocomial bloodstream infections in patients with hematological malignancies and solid neoplasms in hospitals in the United States. Clin Infect Dis 2003;36:1103–10.

2 Benfield T, Espersen F, Frimodt-Moller N *et al.* Increasing incidence but decreasing in-hospital mortality of adult *Staphylococcus aureus* bacteraemia between 1981 and 2000. Clin Microbiol Infect 2007;13:257–63.

3 Kuehnert MJ, Hill HA, Kupronis BA, Tokars JI, Solomon SL, Jernigan DB. Methicillin-resistant-*Staphylococcus aureus* hospitalizations, United States. Emerg Infect Dis 2005;11:868–72.
4 Noskin GA, Rubin RJ, Schentag JJ *et al.* The burden of *Staphylococcus aureus* infections on hospitals in the United States: an analysis of the 2000 and 2001 Nationwide Inpatient Sample Database. Arch Intern Med 2005;165:1756–61.
5 Rubin RJ, Harrington CA, Poon A, Dietrich K, Greene JA, Moiduddin A. The economic impact of *Staphylococcus aureus* infection in New York City hospitals. Emerg Infect Dis 1999; 5:9–17.
6 Klevens RM, Morrison MA, Nadle J *et al.* Invasive methicillin-resistant *Staphylococcus aureus* infections in the United States. JAMA 2007;298:1763–71.
7 Wisplinghoff H, Bischoff T, Tallent SM, Seifert H, Wenzel RP, Edmond MB. Nosocomial bloodstream infections in US hospitals: analysis of 24 179 cases from a prospective nationwide surveillance study. Clin Infect Dis 2004;39:309–17.
8 Breen JD, Karchmer AW. *Staphylococcus aureus* infections in diabetic patients. Infect Dis Clin North Am 1995;9:11–24.
9 Musher DM, Lamm N, Darouiche RO, Young EJ, Hamill RJ, Landon GC. The current spectrum of *Staphylococcus aureus* infection in a tertiary care hospital. Medicine 1994;73:186–208.
10 Laupland KB, Church DL, Mucenski M, Sutherland LR, Davies HD. Population-based study of the epidemiology of and the risk factors for invasive *Staphylococcus aureus* infections. J Infect Dis 2003;187:1452–9.
11 Boyce JM. Methicillin-resistant *Staphylococcus aureus*. Detection, epidemiology, and control measures. Infect Dis Clin North Am 1989;3:901–13.
12 Fishbain JT, Lee JC, Nguyen HD *et al.* Nosocomial transmission of methicillin-resistant *Staphylococcus aureus*: a blinded study to establish baseline acquisition rates. Infect Control Hosp Epidemiol 2003;24:415–21.
13 Thompson RL, Cabezudo I, Wenzel RP. Epidemiology of nosocomial infections caused by methicillin-resistant *Staphylococcus aureus*. Ann Intern Med 1982;97:309–17.
14 Zetola N, Francis JS, Nuermberger EL, Bishai WR. Community-acquired meticillin-resistant *Staphylococcus aureus*: an emerging threat. Lancet Infect Dis 2005;5:275–86.
15 Cabell CH, Jollis JG, Peterson GE *et al.* Changing patient characteristics and the effect on mortality in endocarditis. Arch Intern Med 2002;162:90–4.
16 Diekema DJ, Pfaller MA, Schmitz FJ *et al.* Survey of infections due to *Staphylococcus* species: frequency of occurrence and antimicrobial susceptibility of isolates collected in the United States, Canada, Latin America, Europe, and the Western Pacific region for the SENTRY Antimicrobial Surveillance Program, 1997–1999. Clin Infect Dis 2001;32(suppl 2):S114–S132.
17 Cosgrove SE, Sakoulas G, Perencevich EN, Schwaber MJ, Karchmer AW, Carmeli Y. Comparison of mortality associated with methicillin-resistant and methicillin-susceptible *Staphylococcus aureus* bacteremia: a meta-analysis. Clin Infect Dis 2003;36:53–9.
18 Whitby M, McLaw ML, Berry G. Mortality rates associated with methicillin-resistant and -susceptible *Staphylococcus aureus* infections. Clin Infect Dis 2003;37:459; author reply 459–60.
19 Fowler VG Jr, Miro JM, Hoen B *et al. Staphylococcus aureus* endocarditis: a consequence of medical progress. JAMA 2005;293: 3012–21.
20 Miro JM, Anguera I, Cabell CH *et al. Staphylococcus aureus* native valve infective endocarditis: report of 566 episodes from the International Collaboration on Endocarditis Merged Database. Clin Infect Dis 2005;41:507–14.
21 Hoban DJ, Biedenbach DJ, Mutnick AH, Jones RN. Pathogen of occurrence and susceptibility patterns associated with pneumonia in hospitalized patients in North America: results of the SENTRY Antimicrobial Surveillance Study (2000). Diagn Microbiol Infect Dis 2003;45:279–85.
22 Steinberg JP, Clark CC, Hackman BO. Nosocomial and community-acquired *Staphylococcus aureus* bacteremias from 1980 to 1993: impact of intravascular devices and methicillin resistance. Clin Infect Dis 1996;23:255–9.
23 National Nosocomial Infections Surveillance (NNIS) System Report. Data summary from January 1992 through June 2004, issued October 2004. Am J Infect Control 2004;32:470–85.
24 Centers for Disease Control and Prevention. Methicillin (oxacillin)-resistant Staphylococcus aureus (MRSA) Among ICU Patients, 1995–2004 Available from http://www.cdc.gov/ncidod/dhqp/pdf/ar/ICU_RESTrend1995–2004.pdf. Accessed July 31, 2007.
25 Crum NF, Lee RU, Thornton SA *et al.* Fifteen-year study of the changing epidemiology of methicillin-resistant *Staphylococcus aureus*. Am J Med 2006;119:943–51.
26 Maree CL, Daum RS, Boyle-Vavra S, Matayoshi K, Miller LG. Community-associated methicillin-resistant *Staphylococcus aureus* isolates causing healthcare-associated infections. Emerg Infect Dis 2007;31:236–42.
27 Seybold U, Kourbatova EV, Johnson JG *et al.* Emergence of community-associated methicillin-resistant *Staphylococcus aureus* USA300 genotype as a major cause of health care-associated blood stream infections. Clin Infect Dis 2006;42:647–56.
28 Klevens RM, Edwards JR, Tenover FC, McDonald LC, Horan T, Gaynes R. Changes in the epidemiology of methicillin-resistant *Staphylococcus aureus* in intensive care units in US hospitals, 1992–2003. Clin Infect Dis 2006;42:389–91.
29 Johnson LB, Venugopal AA, Pawlak J, Saravolatz LD. Emergence of community-associated methicillin-resistant *Staphylococcus aureus* infection among patients with end-stage renal disease. Infect Control Hosp Epidemiol 2006;27:1057–62.
30 Lowy FD. *Staphylococcus aureus* infections. N Engl J Med 1998;339:520–32.
31 Gorwitz RJ, Kruszon-Moran D, McAllister SK *et al.* Changes in the prevalence of nasal colonization with *Staphylococcus aureus* in the United States, 2001–2004. J Infect Dis 2008;197:1226–34.
32 Kuehnert MJ, Kruszon-Moran D, Hill HA *et al.* Prevalence of *Staphylococcus aureus* nasal colonization in the United States, 2001–2002. J Infect Dis 2006;193:172–9.
33 Squier C, Rihs JD, Risa KJ *et al. Staphylococcus aureus* rectal carriage and its association with infections in patients in a surgical intensive care unit and a liver transplant unit. Infect Control Hosp Epidemiol 2002;23:495–501.
34 Kluytmans J, van Belkum A, Verbrugh H. Nasal carriage of *Staphylococcus aureus*: epidemiology, underlying mechanisms, and associated risks. Clin Microbiol Rev 1997;10:505–20.
35 von Eiff C, Becker K, Machka K, Stammer H, Peters G. Nasal carriage as a source of *Staphylococcus aureus* bacteremia. N Engl J Med 2001;344:11–16.
36 Chang FY, Singh N, Gayowski T, Wagener MM, Marino IR. *Staphylococcus aureus* nasal colonization in patients with cirrhosis:

prospective assessment of association with infection. Infect Control Hosp Epidemiol 1998;19:328–32.
37 Campillo B, Dupeyron C, Richardet JP. Epidemiology of hospital-acquired infections in cirrhotic patients: effect of carriage of methicillin-resistant *Staphylococcus aureus* and influence of previous antibiotic therapy and norfloxacin prophylaxis. Epidemiol Infect 2001;127:443–50.
38 Mathews WC, Caperna JC, Barber RE *et al.* Incidence of and risk factors for clinically significant methicillin-resistant *Staphylococcus aureus* infection in a cohort of HIV-infected adults. J Acquir Immune Defic Syndr 2005;40:155–60.
39 Weinke T, Schiller R, Fehrenbach FJ, Pohle HD. Association between *Staphylococcus aureus* nasopharyngeal colonization and septicemia in patients infected with the human immunodeficiency virus. Eur J Clin Microbiol Infect Dis 1992;11:985–9.
40 Desai D, Desai N, Nightingale P, Elliott T, Neuberger J. Carriage of methicillin-resistant *Staphylococcus aureus* is associated with an increased risk of infection after liver transplantation. Liver Transplant 2003;9:754–9.
41 Wertheim HF, Vos MC, Ott A *et al.* Risk and outcome of nosocomial *Staphylococcus aureus* bacteraemia in nasal carriers versus non-carriers. Lancet 2004;364:703–5.
42 Dupeyron C, Campillo SB, Mangeney N, Richardet JP, Leluan G. Carriage of *Staphylococcus aureus* and of Gram-negative bacilli resistant to third-generation cephalosporins in cirrhotic patients: a prospective assessment of hospital-acquired infections. Infect Control Hosp Epidemiol 2001;22:427–32.
43 Chang FY, Singh N, Gayowski T, Drenning SD, Wagener MM, Marino IR. *Staphylococcus aureus* nasal colonization and association with infections in liver transplant recipients. Transplantation 1998;65:1169–72.
44 Jensen AG, Wachmann CH, Poulsen KB *et al.* Risk factors for hospital-acquired *Staphylococcus aureus* bacteremia. Arch Intern Med 1999;159:1437–44.
45 Tacconelli E, Tumbarello M, Pittiruti M *et al.* Central venous catheter-related sepsis in a cohort of 366 hospitalised patients. Eur J Clin Microbiol Infect Dis 1997;16:203–9.
46 Ghanem GA, Boktour M, Warneke C *et al.* Catheter-related *Staphylococcus aureus* bacteremia in cancer patients: high rate of complications with therapeutic implications. Medicine (Baltimore) 2007;86:54–60.
47 Nicastri E, Petrosillo N, Viale P, Ippolito G. Catheter-related bloodstream infections in HIV-infected patients 1. Ann NY Acad Sci 2001;946:274–90.
48 Senthilkumar A, Kumar S, Sheagren JN. Increased incidence of *Staphylococcus aureus* bacteremia in hospitalized patients with acquired immunodeficiency syndrome. Clin Infect Dis 2001;33: 1412–16.
49 Stroud L, Srivastava P, Culver D *et al.* Nosocomial infections in HIV-infected patients: preliminary results from a multicenter surveillance system (1989–1995). Infect Control Hosp Epidemiol 1997;18:479–85.
50 Petrosillo N, Viale P, Nicastri E *et al.* Nosocomial bloodstream infections among human immunodeficiency virus-infected patients: incidence and risk factors 1. Clin Infect Dis 2002;34: 677–85.
51 Lekstrom-Himes JA, Gallin JI. Immunodeficiency diseases caused by defects in phagocytes. N Engl J Med 2000;343:1703–14.
52 Malech HL, Hickstein DD. Genetics, biology and clinical management of myeloid cell primary immune deficiencies: chronic granulomatous disease and leukocyte adhesion deficiency. Curr Opin Hematol 2007;14:29–36.
53 International Chronic Granulomatous Disease Cooperative Study Group. A controlled trial of interferon gamma to prevent infection in chronic granulomatous disease. N Engl J Med 1991;324:509–16.
54 Donnelly JP, de Pauw BE. Infections in the immunocompromised host: general principles. In: Mandel GL, Bennett JE, Dolin R, eds. Principles and Practice of Infectious Diseases, 6th edn. Philadelphia: Elsevier, 2005:3421–32.
55 Brinchmann JE, Gaudernack G, Thorsby E, Vartdal F. Staphylococcal exotoxin superantigens induce human immunodeficiency virus type 1 expression in naturally infected $CD4^+$ T cells. J Virol 1992;66:5924–8.
56 Goujard C, Wallon C, Rudent A, Boue F, Barre-Sinoussi F, Delfraissy JF. Staphylococcal superantigens activate HIV-1 replication in naturally infected monocytes. Aids 1994;8:1397–404.
57 Hashimoto K, Shigeta S, Baba M. Superantigen toxic shock syndrome toxin-1 (TSST-1) enhances the replication of HIV-1 in peripheral blood mononuclear cells through selective activation of $CD4^+$ T lymphocytes. J Acquir Immune Defic Syndr Hum Retrovirol 1995;10:393–9.
58 Juffermans NP, Paxton WA, Dekkers PE *et al.* Up-regulation of HIV coreceptors CXCR4 and CCR5 on CD4(+) T cells during human endotoxemia and after stimulation with (myco)bacterial antigens: the role of cytokines. Blood 2000;96:2649–54.
59 Joshi N, Caputo GM, Weitekamp MR, Karchmer AW. Infections in patients with diabetes mellitus. N Engl J Med 1999;341: 1906–12.
60 Rich J, Lee JC. The pathogenesis of *Staphylococcus aureus* infection in the diabetic NOD mouse. Diabetes 2005;54:2904–10.
61 Chu VH, Cabell CH, Benjamin DK Jr *et al.* Early predictors of in-hospital death in infective endocarditis. Circulation 2004; 109:1745–9.
62 Tamer A, Karabay O, Ekerbicer H. *Staphylococcus aureus* nasal carriage and associated factors in type 2 diabetic patients. Jpn J Infect Dis 2006;59:10–14.
63 Ahluwalia A, Sood A, Sood A, Lakshmy R, Kapil A, Pandey RM. Nasal colonization with *Staphylococcus aureus* in patients with diabetes mellitus. Diabet Med 2000;17:487–8.
64 Chandler PT, Chandler SD. Pathogenic carrier rate in diabetes mellitus. Am J Med Sci 1977;273:259–65.
65 Smith JA, O'Connor JJ. Nasal carriage of *Staphylococcus aureus* in diabetes mellitus. Lancet 1966;ii:776–7.
66 Tuazon CU, Perez A, Kishaba T, Sheagren JN. *Staphylococcus aureus* among insulin-injecting diabetic patients. An increased carrier rate. JAMA 1975;231:1272.
67 Boyko EJ, Lipsky BA, Sandoval R *et al.* NIDDM and prevalence of nasal *Staphylococcus aureus* colonization. San Luis Valley Diabetes Study. Diabetes Care 1989;12:189–92.
68 Lipsky BA, Pecoraro RE, Chen MS, Koepsell TD. Factors affecting staphylococcal colonization among NIDDM outpatients. Diabetes Care 1987;10:483–6.
69 Graham PL III, Lin SX, Larson EL. A U.S. population-based survey of *Staphylococcus aureus* colonization. Ann Intern Med 2006;144:318–25.
70 Khatib R, Johnson LB, Sharma M, Fakih MG, Ganga R, Riederer K. Persistent *Staphylococcus aureus* bacteremia: incidence and outcome trends over time. Scand J Infect Dis 2009;41:4–9.

71 Tentolouris N, Jude EB, Smirnof I, Knowles EA, Boulton AJ. Methicillin-resistant *Staphylococcus aureus*: an increasing problem in a diabetic foot clinic. Diabet Med 1999;16:767–71.

72 Hartemann-Heurtier A, Robert J, Jacqueminet S *et al.* Diabetic foot ulcer and multidrug-resistant organisms: risk factors and impact. Diabet Med 2004;21:710–15.

73 Lipsky BA, Berendt AR, Deery HG *et al.* Diagnosis and treatment of diabetic foot infections. Clin Infect Dis 2004;39:885–910.

74 Roghmann MC, Siddiqui A, Plaisance K, Standiford H. MRSA colonization and the risk of MRSA bacteraemia in hospitalized patients with chronic ulcers. J Hosp Infect 2001;47:98–103.

75 Eady EA, Cove JH. Staphylococcal resistance revisited: community-acquired methicillin resistant *Staphylococcus aureus*. An emerging problem for the management of skin and soft tissue infections. Curr Opin Infect Dis 2003;16:103–24.

76 Miller LG, Perdreau-Remington F, Rieg G *et al.* Necrotizing fasciitis caused by community-associated methicillin-resistant *Staphylococcus aureus* in Los Angeles. N Engl J Med 2005;352: 1445–53.

77 Sexton DJ. Vascular access infections in patients undergoing dialysis with special emphasis on the role and treatment of *Staphylococcus aureus*. Infect Dis Clin North Am 2001;15:731–42, vii.

78 Marr KA. *Staphylococcus aureus* bacteremia in patients undergoing hemodialysis. Semin Dial 2000;13:23–9.

79 Powe NR, Jaar B, Furth SL, Hermann J, Briggs W. Septicemia in dialysis patients: incidence, risk factors, and prognosis. Kidney Int 1999;55:1081–90.

80 Perazella MA, Brewster UC, Perazella MA. Intravenous iron and the risk of infection in end-stage renal disease patients. Semin Dial 2004;17:57–60.

81 Haag-Weber M, Dumann H, Horl WH. Effect of malnutrition and uremia on impaired cellular host defence. Miner Electrolyte Metab 1992;18:174–85.

82 Vychytil A, Lorenz M, Schneider B, Horl WH, Haag-Weber M. New strategies to prevent *Staphylococcus aureus* infections in peritoneal dialysis patients. J Am Soc Nephrol 1998;9:669–76.

83 Yu VL, Goetz A, Wagener M *et al. Staphylococcus aureus* nasal carriage and infection in patients on hemodialysis. Efficacy of antibiotic prophylaxis. N Engl J Med 1986;315:91–6.

84 Piraino B, Perlmutter JA, Holley JL, Bernardini J. *Staphylococcus aureus* peritonitis is associated with *Staphylococcus aureus* nasal carriage in peritoneal dialysis patients. Perit Dial Int 1993; 13(suppl 2):S332–S334.

85 Johnson LB, Jose J, Yousif F, Pawlak J, Saravolatz LD. Prevalence of colonization with community-associated methicillin-resistant *Staphylococcus aureus* among end-stage renal disease patients and healthcare workers. Infect Control Hosp Epidemiol 2009;30:4–8.

86 Klevens RM, Tokars JI, Andrus M. Electronic reporting of infections associated with hemodialysis. Nephrol News Issues 2005;19:37–8, 43.

87 Centers for Disease Control and Prevention. Invasive methicillin-resistant *Staphylococcus aureus* infections among dialysis patients: United States, 2005. MMWR 2007;56:197–9.

88 Abbott KC, Agodoa LY. Etiology of bacterial septicemia in chronic dialysis patients in the United States. Clin Nephrol 2001;56:124–31.

89 Marr KA, Kong L, Fowler VG *et al.* Incidence and outcome of *Staphylococcus aureus* bacteremia in hemodialysis patients. Kidney Int 1998;54:1684–9.

90 Nissenson AR, Dylan ML, Griffiths RI *et al.* Clinical and economic outcomes of *Staphylococcus aureus* septicemia in ESRD patients receiving hemodialysis. Am J Kidney Dis 2005;46: 301–8.

91 Bernardini J, Holley JL, Johnston JR, Perlmutter JA, Piraino B. An analysis of ten-year trends in infections in adults on continuous ambulatory peritoneal dialysis (CAPD). Clin Nephrol 1991;36:29–34.

92 Leigh DA. Peritoneal infections in patients on long-term peritoneal dialysis before and after human cadaveric renal transplantation. J Clin Pathol 1969;22:539–44.

93 Szeto CC, Leung CB, Chow KM *et al.* Change in bacterial aetiology of peritoneal dialysis-related peritonitis over 10 years: experience from a centre in South-East Asia. Clin Microbiol Infect 2005;11:837–9.

94 Rajkovic IA, Williams R. Abnormalities of neutrophil phagocytosis, intracellular killing and metabolic activity in alcoholic cirrhosis and hepatitis. Hepatology 1986;6:252–62.

95 Chapoutot C, Pageaux GP, Perrigault PF *et al. Staphylococcus aureus* nasal carriage in 104 cirrhotic and control patients. A prospective study. J Hepatol 1999;30:249–53.

96 Campillo B, Richardet JP, Kheo T, Dupeyron C. Nosocomial spontaneous bacterial peritonitis and bacteremia in cirrhotic patients: impact of isolate type on prognosis and characteristics of infection. Clin Infect Dis 2002;35:1–10.

97 Thulstrup AM, Sorensen HT, Schonheyder HC, Moller JK, Tage-Jensen U. Population-based study of the risk and short-term prognosis for bacteremia in patients with liver cirrhosis. Clin Infect Dis 2000;31:1357–61.

98 Rabinovitz M, Prieto M, Gavaler JS, Van Thiel DH. Bacteriuria in patients with cirrhosis. J Hepatol 1992;16:73–6.

99 Kuritzkes DR. Neutropenia, neutrophil dysfunction, and bacterial infection in patients with human immunodeficiency virus disease: the role of granulocyte colony-stimulating factor. Clin Infect Dis 2000;30:256–60.

100 Mukau L, Talamini MA, Sitzmann JV, Burns RC, McGuire ME. Long-term central venous access vs other home therapies: complications in patients with acquired immunodeficiency syndrome. JPEN J Parenter Enteral Nutr 1992;16:455–9.

101 Nguyen MH, Kauffman CA, Goodman RP *et al.* Nasal carriage of and infection with *Staphylococcus aureus* in HIV-infected patients. Ann Intern Med 1999;130:221–5.

102 Frank U, Daschner FD, Schulgen G, Mills J. Incidence and epidemiology of nosocomial infections in patients infected with human immunodeficiency virus. Clin Infect Dis 1997;25:318–20.

103 Melles DC, Pauw E, van den Boogaard L *et al.* Host–microbe interplay in persistent *Staphylococcus aureus* nasal carriage in HIV patients. Microbes Infect 2008;10:151–8.

104 Cenizal MJ, Hardy RD, Anderson M, Katz K, Skiest DJ. Prevalence of and risk factors for methicillin-resistant *Staphylococcus aureus* (MRSA) nasal colonization in HIV-infected ambulatory patients. J Acquir Immune Defic Syndr 2008;48:567–71.

105 Tumbarello M, de Gaetano DK, Tacconelli E *et al.* Risk factors and predictors of mortality of methicillin-resistant *Staphylococcus aureus* (MRSA) bacteraemia in HIV-infected patients. J Antimicrob Chemother 2002;50:375–82.

106 Senthilkumar A, Kumar S, Sheagren JN. Increased incidence of *Staphylococcus aureus* bacteremia in hospitalized patients with acquired immunodeficiency syndrome 1. Clin Infect Dis 2001;33:1412–16.

107 Cotton MF, Wasserman E, Smit J, Whitelaw A, Zar HJ. High incidence of antimicrobial resistant organisms including extended spectrum beta-lactamase producing Enterobacteriaceae and methicillin-resistant *Staphylococcus aureus* in nasopharyngeal and blood isolates of HIV-infected children from Cape Town, South Africa. BMC Infect Dis 2008;8:40.

108 Afessa B, Green B. Bacterial pneumonia in hospitalized patients with HIV infection: the Pulmonary Complications, ICU Support, and Prognostic Factors of Hospitalized Patients with HIV (PIP) Study. Chest 2000;117:1017–22.

109 Salami AK, Olatunji PO, Oluboyo PO, Akanbi AA, Fawibe EA. Bacterial pneumonia in the AIDS patients. West Afr J Med 2006;25:1–5.

110 Soubani AO, Michelson MK, Karnik A. Pleural fluid findings in patients with the acquired immunodeficiency syndrome: correlation with concomitant pulmonary disease. South Med J 1999;92:400–3.

111 Dicpinigaitis PV, Levy DE, Gnass RD, Bernstein RG. Pneumonia due to *Staphylococcus aureus* in a patient with AIDS: review of incidence and report of an atypical roentgenographic presentation. South Med J 1995;88:586–90.

112 Tumbarello M, Tacconelli E, Lucia MB, Cauda R, Ortona L. Predictors of *Staphylococcus aureus* pneumonia associated with human immunodeficiency virus infection. Respir Med 1996;90: 531–7.

113 Smith NP, Nelson MR, Moore D, Gazzard BG. Cerebral abscesses in a patient with AIDS caused by methicillin-resistant *Staphylococcus aureus* (MRSA). Int J STD AIDS 1997;8:459–60.

114 Gunnarsson G, Friedman LS, Wanke C. Liver abscesses due to *Staphylococcus aureus* in a patient with AIDS who underwent small bowel biopsy: case report and review. Clin Infect Dis 1994;18:802–4.

115 Grant A, Pitkin AD, Buscombe JR, Corcoran GD, Miller RF. *Staphylococcus aureus* pericarditis in a patient with AIDS. Genitourin Med 1993;69:324–5.

116 Rivera J, Monteagudo I, Lopez-Longo J, Sanchez-Atrio A. Septic arthritis in patients with acquired immunodeficiency syndrome with human immunodeficiency virus infection. J Rheumatol 1992;19:1960–2.

117 Nelson MR, Daniels D, Dean R, Barton S, Gazzard BG. *Staphylococcus aureus* psoas abscess in a patient with AIDS. Int J STD AIDS 1992;3:294.

118 Schwartzman WA, Lambertus MW, Kennedy CA, Goetz MB. Staphylococcal pyomyositis in patients infected by the human immunodeficiency virus. Am J Med 1991;90:595–600.

119 Pirofski L, Casadevall A. Mixed staphylococcal and cryptococcal epidural abscess in a patient with AIDS. Rev Infect Dis 1990;12:964–5.

120 Buskila D, Tenenbaum J. Septic bursitis in human immunodeficiency virus infection. J Rheumatol 1989;16:1374–6.

121 Lee NE, Taylor MM, Bancroft E *et al.* Risk factors for community-associated methicillin-resistant *Staphylococcus aureus* skin infections among HIV-positive men who have sex with men. Clin Infect Dis 2005;40:1529–34.

122 Skiest D, Brown K, Hester J *et al.* Community-onset methicillin-resistant *Staphylococcus aureus* in an urban HIV clinic. HIV Medicine 2006;7:361–8.

123 Gopal AK, Fowler VG Jr, Shah M *et al.* Prospective analysis of *Staphylococcus aureus* bacteremia in nonneutropenic adults with malignancy. J Clin Oncol 2000;18:1110–15.

124 Shah MA, Sanders L, Lanclos K *et al. Staphylococcus aureus* bacteremia in patients with neutropenia. South Med J 2002;95: 782–4.

125 Salazar R, Sola C, Maroto P *et al.* Infectious complications in 126 patients treated with high-dose chemotherapy and autologous peripheral blood stem cell transplantation. Bone Marrow Transplant 1999;23:27–33.

126 Poutsiaka DD, Price LL, Ucuzian A, Chan GW, Miller KB, Snydman DR. Blood stream infection after hematopoietic stem cell transplantation is associated with increased mortality. Bone Marrow Transplant 2007;40:63–70.

127 Blijlevens NM, Donnelly JP, de Pauw BE. Microbiologic consequences of new approaches to managing hematologic malignancies. Rev Clin Exp Hematol 2005;9:E2.

128 Freifeld AG, Segal BH. Prevention and treatment of cancer-related infection. National Comprehensive Cancer Network. http://www.nccn.org/professionals/physician_gls/PDF/infections.pdf. Accessed July 31, 2007.

129 Choi G, van den Borne MP, Visser CE, Kersten MJ, Kater AP. Invasive infections with a coagulase-negative staphylococcus in an immunocompromised patient: case report and review of the literature. Ann Hematol 2008;87:771–2.

130 Wisplinghoff H, Cornely OA, Moser S *et al.* Outcomes of nosocomial bloodstream infections in adult neutropenic patients: a prospective cohort and matched case–control study. Infect Control Hosp Epidemiol 2003;24:905–11.

131 Seifert H, Cornely O, Seggewiss K *et al.* Bloodstream infection in neutropenic cancer patients related to short-term nontunnelled catheters determined by quantitative blood cultures, differential time to positivity, and molecular epidemiological typing with pulsed-field gel electrophoresis. J Clin Microbiol 2003;41:118–23.

132 Morris PG, Hassan T, McNamara M *et al.* Emergence of MRSA in positive blood cultures from patients with febrile neutropenia: a cause for concern. Support Care Cancer 2008;16:1085–8.

133 Gonzalez-Barca E, Carratala J, Mykietiuk A, Fernandez-Sevilla A, Gudiol F. Predisposing factors and outcome of *Staphylococcus aureus* bacteremia in neutropenic patients with cancer. Eur J Clin Microbiol Infect Dis 2001;20:117–19.

134 Miller LW, Naftel DC, Bourge RC *et al.* Infection after heart transplantation: a multiinstitutional study. Cardiac Transplant Research Database Group. J Heart Lung Transplant 1994;13: 381–92.

135 Montoya JG, Giraldo LF, Efron B *et al.* Infectious complications among 620 consecutive heart transplant patients at Stanford University Medical Center. Clin Infect Dis 2001;33:629–40.

136 Adeyemi OA, Qi C, Zembower TR *et al.* Invasive infections with community-associated methicillin-resistant *Staphylococcus aureus* after kidney transplantation. J Clin Microbiol 2008;46: 2809–13.

137 Bert F, Bellier C, Lassel L *et al.* Risk factors for *Staphylococcus aureus* infection in liver transplant recipients. Liver Transplant 2005;11:1093–9.

138 Woeste G, Zapletal C, Wullstein C, Golling M, Bechstein WO. Influence of methicillin-resistant *Staphylococcus aureus* carrier status in liver transplant recipients. Transplant Proc 2005;37: 1710–12.

139 Schneider CR, Buell JF, Gearhart M *et al.* Methicillin-resistant *Staphylococcus aureus* infection in liver transplantation: a matched controlled study. Transplant Proc 2005;37:1243–4.

140 Singh N, Paterson DL, Chang FY *et al.* Methicillin-resistant *Staphylococcus aureus*: the other emerging resistant Gram-positive coccus among liver transplant recipients. Clin Infect Dis 2000;30:322–7.
141 Santoro-Lopes G, de Gouvea EF, Monteiro RC *et al.* Colonization with methicillin-resistant *Staphylococcus aureus* after liver transplantation. Liver Transplant 2005;11:203–9.
142 Singh N, Gayowski T, Wagener MM, Marino IR. Bloodstream infections in liver transplant recipients receiving tacrolimus. Clin Transplant 1997;11:275–81.
143 Torre-Cisneros J, Herrero C, Canas E, Reguera JM, De La Mata M, Gomez-Bravo MA. High mortality related with *Staphylococcus aureus* bacteremia after liver transplantation. Eur J Clin Microbiol Infect Dis 2002;21:385–8.
144 Hashimoto M, Sugawara Y, Tamura S *et al.* Impact of new methicillin-resistant *Staphylococcus aureus* carriage postoperatively after living donor liver transplantation. Transplant Proc 2007;39:3271–5.
145 Singh N, Wannstedt C, Keyes L *et al.* Hepatic iron content and the risk of *Staphylococcus aureus* bacteremia in liver transplant recipients. Prog Transplant 2007;17:332–6.
146 Monkowski DH, Axelrod P, Fekete T, Hollander T, Furukawa S, Samuel R. Infections associated with ventricular assist devices: epidemiology and effect on prognosis after transplantation. Transpl Infect Dis 2007;9:114–20.
147 Springer WE, Wasler A, Radovancevic B *et al.* Retrospective analysis of infection in patients undergoing support with left ventricular assist systems. ASAIO J 1996;42:M763–M765.
148 Schmid C, Schneider M, Etz C, Scheld HH. Heart transplantation in a patient with a left ventricular assist device and methicillin-resistant *Staphylococcus aureus* infection. Ann Thorac Surg 2004;78:1820–1.
149 Goldstein DJ, Oz MC, Rose EA. Implantable left ventricular assist devices. N Engl J Med 1998;339:1522–33.
150 Baldwin RT, Radovancevic B, Sweeney MS, Duncan JM, Frazier OH. Bacterial mediastinitis after heart transplantation. J Heart Lung Transplant 1992;11:545–9.
151 Stolf NA, Fiorelli AI, Bacal F *et al.* Mediastinitis after cardiac transplantation. Arq Bras Cardiol 2000;74:419–30.
152 Senechal M, LePrince P, Tezenas du MS *et al.* Bacterial mediastinitis after heart transplantation: clinical presentation, risk factors and treatment. J Heart Lung Transplant 2004;23:165–70.
153 Dodds Ashley ES, Carroll DN, Engemann JJ *et al.* Risk factors for postoperative mediastinitis due to methicillin-resistant *Staphylococcus aureus*. Clin Infect Dis 2004;38:1555–60.
154 Caballero F, Lopez-Navidad A, Perea M, Cabrer C, Guirado L, Sola R. Successful liver and kidney transplantation from cadaveric donors with left-sided bacterial endocarditis. Am J Transplant 2005;5:781–7.
155 Nassar GM, Ayus JC. Infectious complications of old nonfunctioning arteriovenous grafts in renal transplant recipients: a case series. Am J Kidney Dis 2002;40:832–6.
156 D'Cunha PT, Davenport DS, Fisher KA. Successful treatment of *Staphylococcus aureus* bacterial endocarditis in a renal transplant recipient. Transplant Infect Dis 2003;5:144–6.
157 Bishara J, Robenshtok E, Weinberger M, Yeshurun M, Sagie A, Pitlik S. Infective endocarditis in renal transplant recipients. Transplant Infect Dis 1999;1:138–43.
158 Paterson DL, Dominguez EA, Chang FY, Snydman DR, Singh N. Infective endocarditis in solid organ transplant recipients. Clin Infect Dis 1998;26:689–94.
159 Angelis M, Cooper JT, Freeman RB. Impact of donor infections on outcome of orthotopic liver transplantation. Liver Transplant 2003;9:451–62.
160 Obed A, Schnitzbauer AA, Bein T, Lehn N, Linde HJ, Schlitt HJ. Fatal pneumonia caused by Panton–Valentine leucocidin-positive methicillin-resistant *Staphylococcus aureus* (PVL-MRSA) transmitted from a healthy donor in living-donor liver transplantation. Transplantation 2006;81:121–4.
161 Villavicencio RT, Wall MJ Jr. The pathogenesis of *Staphylococcus aureus* in the trauma patient and potential future therapies 1. Am J Surg 1996;172:291–6.
162 Croce MA, Fabian TC, Stewart RM *et al.* Empiric monotherapy versus combination therapy of nosocomial pneumonia in trauma patients. J Trauma 1993;35:303–9.
163 Edwards-Jones V, Greenwood JE. What's new in burn microbiology? James Laing Memorial Prize Essay 2000. Burns 2003; 29:15–24.
164 Campbell W, Hendrix E, Schwalbe R, Fattom A, Edelman R. Head-injured patients who are nasal carriers of *Staphylococcus aureus* are at high risk for *Staphylococcus aureus* pneumonia. Crit Care Med 1999;27:798–801.
165 Vindenes H, Bjerknes R. The frequency of bacteremia and fungemia following wound cleaning and excision in patients with large burns. J Trauma 1993;35:742–9.
166 Bauer GJ, Yurt RW. Burns. In: Mandel GL, Bennett JE, Dolin R, eds. Principles and Practice of Infectious Diseases, 6th edn. Philadelphia: Elsevier, 2005:3547–52.
167 Edwards-Jones V, Dawson MM, Childs C. A survey into toxic shock syndrome (TSS) in UK burns units. Burns 2000;26:323–33.
168 Kimura A, Mochizuki T, Nishizawa K, Mashiko K, Yamamoto Y, Otsuka T. Trimethoprim–sulfamethoxazole for the prevention of methicillin-resistant *Staphylococcus aureus* pneumonia in severely burned patients. J Trauma 1998;45:383–7.
169 Wolfe F, Caplan L, Michaud K. Treatment for rheumatoid arthritis and the risk of hospitalization for pneumonia: associations with prednisone, disease-modifying antirheumatic drugs, and anti-tumor necrosis factor therapy. Arthritis Rheum 2006;54:628–34.
170 Agusti C, Rano A, Filella X *et al.* Pulmonary infiltrates in patients receiving long-term glucocorticoid treatment: etiology, prognostic factors, and associated inflammatory response. Chest 2003;123:488–98.
171 Koka VK, Potti A. Spinal epidural abscess after corticosteroid injections 1. South Med J 2002;95:772–4.
172 Konno O, Hirano T, Katsuyama K, Oka K, Matsuno N, Nagao T. Bacterial superantigen TSST-1 attenuates suppressive efficacy of glucocorticoids and calcineurin inhibitors against blastogenesis of peripheral blood mononuclear cells from patients with chronic renal failure on hemodialysis treatment. Transpl Immunol 2007;17:187–92.
173 Fukushima H, Hirano T, Oka K. *Staphylococcus aureus*-superantigen decreases FKBP51 mRNA expression and cell-response to suppressive efficacy of a glucocorticoid in human peripheral blood mononuclear cells: possible implication of mitogen-activated protein kinase pathways. Eur J Pharmacol 2007;570:222–8.
174 Bassetti S, Wasmer S, Hasler P *et al.* *Staphylococcus aureus* in patients with rheumatoid arthritis under conventional and anti-tumor necrosis factor-alpha treatment 1. J Rheumatol 2005;32:2125–9.
175 Ferraccioli G, Mecchia F, Di Poi E, Fabris M. Anticardiolipin antibodies in rheumatoid patients treated with etanercept or

conventional combination therapy: direct and indirect evidence for a possible association with infections. Ann Rheum Dis 2002;61:358–61.

176 Kroesen S, Widmer AF, Tyndall A, Hasler P. Serious bacterial infections in patients with rheumatoid arthritis under anti-TNF-alpha therapy. Rheumatology 2003;42:617–21.

177 Bongartz T, Sutton AJ, Sweeting MJ, Buchan I, Matteson EL, Montori V. Anti-TNF antibody therapy in rheumatoid arthritis and the risk of serious infections and malignancies: systematic review and meta-analysis of rare harmful effects in randomized controlled trials. JAMA 2006;295:2275–85.

178 Sweet DD, Isac G, Morrison B, Fenwick J, Dhingra V. Purulent pericarditis in a patient with rheumatoid arthritis treated with etanercept and methotrexate. CJEM 2007;9:40–2.

179 Oda S, Fujinaga H, Takahashi K. Infectious myositis involving the piriformis in a patient with rheumatoid arthritis. Mod Rheumatol 2006;16:260–3.

180 Fitch PG, Cron RQ. Septic abscess in a child with juvenile idiopathic arthritis receiving anti-tumor necrosis factor-alpha. J Rheumatol 2006;33:825–7.

181 Fowler VG Jr, Li J, Corey GR *et al.* Role of echocardiography in evaluation of patients with *Staphylococcus aureus* bacteremia: experience in 103 patients. J Am Coll Cardiol 1997;30:1072–8.

182 Hughes WT, Armstrong D, Bodey GP *et al.* 2002 guidelines for the use of antimicrobial agents in neutropenic patients with cancer. Clin Infect Dis 2002;34:730–51.

183 Mermel LA, Farr BM, Sherertz RJ *et al.* Guidelines for the management of intravascular catheter-related infections. Clin Infect Dis 2001;32:1249–72.

184 Fowler VG Jr, Olsen MK, Corey GR *et al.* Clinical identifiers of complicated *Staphylococcus aureus* bacteremia. Arch Intern Med 2003;163:2066–72.

185 Chang FY, Peacock JE Jr, Musher DM *et al. Staphylococcus aureus* bacteremia: recurrence and the impact of antibiotic treatment in a prospective multicenter study. Medicine (Baltimore) 2003; 82:333–9.

186 Libman H, Arbeit RD. Complications associated with *Staphylococcus aureus* bacteremia. Arch Intern Med 1984;144:541–5.

187 Bone RC. The pathogenesis of sepsis. Ann Intern Med 1991;115: 457–69.

188 Kamel NS, Banks MC, Dosik A, Ursea D, Yarilina AA, Posnett DN. Lack of muco-cutaneous signs of toxic shock syndrome when T cells are absent: *S. aureus* shock in immunodeficient adults with multiple myeloma. Clin Exp Immunol 2002;128:131–9.

189 Goldberg NS, Ahmed T, Robinson B, Ascensao J, Horowitz H. Staphylococcal scalded skin syndrome mimicking acute graft-vs-host disease in a bone marrow transplant recipient. Arch Dermatol 1989;125:85–7.

190 Huseyin TS, Maynard JP, Leach RD. Toxic shock syndrome in a patient with breast cancer and systemic lupus erythematosus. Eur J Surg Oncol 2001;27:330–1.

191 Takeuchi F, Watanabe S, Baba T *et al.* Whole-genome sequencing of *Staphylococcus haemolyticus* uncovers the extreme plasticity of its genome and the evolution of human-colonizing staphylococcal species. J Bacteriol 2005;187:7292–308.

192 Stryjewski ME, Szczech LA, Benjamin DK Jr *et al.* Use of vancomycin or first-generation cephalosporins for the treatment of hemodialysis-dependent patients with methicillin-susceptible *Staphylococcus aureus* bacteremia. Clin Infect Dis 2007;44:190–6.

193 European Organization for Research and Treatment of Cancer (EORTC) International Antimicrobial Therapy Cooperative Group and the National Cancer Institute of Canada Clinical Trials Group. Vancomycin added to empirical combination antibiotic therapy for fever in granulocytopenic cancer patients. J Infect Dis 1991;163:951–8.

194 Paul M, Borok S, Fraser A, Vidal L, Leibovici L. Empirical antibiotics against Gram-positive infections for febrile neutropenia: systematic review and meta-analysis of randomized controlled trials. J Antimicrob Chemother 2005;55:436–44.

195 Vardakas KZ, Samonis G, Chrysanthopoulou SA, Bliziotis IA, Falagas ME. Role of glycopeptides as part of initial empirical treatment of febrile neutropenic patients: a meta-analysis of randomised controlled trials. Lancet Infect Dis 2005;5:431–9.

196 Cometta A, Kern WV, De Bock R *et al.* Vancomycin versus placebo for treating persistent fever in patients with neutropenic cancer receiving piperacillin–tazobactam monotherapy. Clin Infect Dis 2003;37:382–9.

197 Erjavec Z, de Vries-Hospers HG, Laseur M, Halie RM, Daenen S. A prospective, randomized, double-blinded, placebo-controlled trial of empirical teicoplanin in febrile neutropenia with persistent fever after imipenem monotherapy. J Antimicrob Chemother 2000;45:843–9.

198 Sieradzki K, Roberts RB, Haber SW, Tomasz A. The development of vancomycin resistance in a patient with methicillin-resistant *Staphylococcus aureus* infection. N Engl J Med 1999;340:517–23.

199 Chang S, Sievert DM, Hageman JC *et al.* Infection with vancomycin-resistant *Staphylococcus aureus* containing the vanA resistance gene. N Engl J Med 2003;348:1342–7.

200 Centers for Disease Control and Prevention. *Staphylococcus aureus* resistant to vancomycin: United States, 2002. MMWR 2002;51:565–7.

201 Fridkin SK. Vancomycin-intermediate and -resistant *Staphylococcus aureus*: what the infectious disease specialist needs to know. Clin Infect Dis 2001;32:108–15.

202 Bert F, Clarissou J, Durand F *et al.* Prevalence, molecular epidemiology, and clinical significance of heterogeneous glycopeptide-intermediate *Staphylococcus aureus* in liver transplant recipients. J Clin Microbiol 2003;41:5147–52.

203 Jaksic B, Martinelli G, Perez-Oteyza J, Hartman CS, Leonard LB, Tack KJ. Efficacy and safety of linezolid compared with vancomycin in a randomized, double-blind study of febrile neutropenic patients with cancer. Clin Infect Dis 2006;42:597–607.

204 Odakowska-Jedynak U, Paczek L, Krawczyk M *et al.* Resistance of Gram-positive pathogens to antibiotics is a therapeutic challenge after liver transplantation: clinical experience in one center with linezolid. Transplant Proc 2003;35:2304–6.

205 Shorr AF, Kunkel MJ, Kollef M. Linezolid versus vancomycin for *Staphylococcus aureus* bacteraemia: pooled analysis of randomized studies. J Antimicrob Chemother 2005;56:923–9.

206 Smith PF, Birmingham MC, Noskin GA *et al.* Safety, efficacy and pharmacokinetics of linezolid for treatment of resistant Gram-positive infections in cancer patients with neutropenia. Ann Oncol 2003;14:795–801.

207 Itani KM, Weigelt J, Li JZ, Duttagupta S. Linezolid reduces length of stay and duration of intravenous treatment compared with vancomycin for complicated skin and soft tissue infections due to suspected or proven methicillin-resistant *Staphylococcus aureus* (MRSA). Int J Antimicrob Agents 2005;26:442–8.

208 Weigelt J, Itani K, Stevens D *et al.* Linezolid versus vancomycin in treatment of complicated skin and soft tissue infections. Antimicrob Agents Chemother 2005;49:2260–6.

209 Lipsky BA, Itani K, Norden C. Treating foot infections in diabetic patients: a randomized, multicenter, open-label trial of linezolid versus ampicillin–sulbactam/amoxicillin–clavulanate. Linezolid Diabetic Foot Infections Study Group. Clin Infect Dis 2004;38:17–24.
210 Roberts SM, Freeman AF, Harrington SM, Holland SM, Murray PR, Zelazny AM. Linezolid-resistant *Staphylococcus aureus* in two pediatric patients receiving low-dose linezolid therapy. Pediatr Infect Dis J 2006;25:562–4.
211 Information for Healthcare Professionals: Linezolid (marketed as Zyvox). Center for Drug Evaluation and Research, US Food and Drug Administration, March 16, 2007. http://www.fda.gov/cder/drug/infopage/linezolid/default.htm. Accessed July 31, 2007.
212 Lipsky BA, Stoutenburgh U. Daptomycin for treating infected diabetic foot ulcers: evidence from a randomized, controlled trial comparing daptomycin with vancomycin or semi-synthetic penicillins for complicated skin and skin-structure infections. J Antimicrob Chemother 2005;55:240–5.
213 Mangili A, Bica I, Snydman DR, Hamer DH. Daptomycin-resistant, methicillin-resistant *Staphylococcus aureus* bacteremia. Clin Infect Dis 2005;40:1058–60.
214 Skiest DJ. Treatment failure resulting from resistance of *Staphylococcus aureus* to daptomycin. J Clin Microbiol 2006;44:655–6.
215 Laupland KB, Conly JM. Treatment of *Staphylococcus aureus* colonization and prophylaxis for infection with topical intranasal mupirocin: an evidence-based review. Clin Infect Dis 2003;37:933–8.
216 Tacconelli E, Carmeli Y, Aizer A, Ferreira G, Foreman MG, D'Agata EM. Mupirocin prophylaxis to prevent *Staphylococcus aureus* infection in patients undergoing dialysis: a meta-analysis. Clin Infect Dis 2003;37:1629–38.
217 Paterson DL, Rihs JD, Squier C, Gayowski T, Sagnimeni A, Singh N. Lack of efficacy of mupirocin in the prevention of infections with *Staphylococcus aureus* in liver transplant recipients and candidates. Transplantation 2003;75:194–8.
218 Loeb M, Main C, Walker-Dilks C, Eady A. Antimicrobial drugs for treating methicillin-resistant *Staphylococcus aureus* colonization. Cochrane Database Syst Rev 2003;4:CD003340.
219 Wertheim HF, Vos MC, Ott A *et al.* Mupirocin prophylaxis against nosocomial *Staphylococcus aureus* infections in nonsurgical patients: a randomized study. Ann Intern Med 2004;140: 419–25.
220 Strippoli GF, Tong A, Johnson D, Schena FP, Craig JC. Antimicrobial agents for preventing peritonitis in peritoneal dialysis patients. Cochrane Database Syst Rev 2004;4:CD004679.
221 Perez-Fontan M, Rosales M, Rodriguez-Carmona A, Falcon TG, Valdes F. Mupirocin resistance after long-term use for *Staphylococcus aureus* colonization in patients undergoing chronic peritoneal dialysis. Am J Kidney Dis 2002;39:337–41.
222 Safdar N, Marx J, Meyer NA, Maki DG. Effectiveness of preemptive barrier precautions in controlling nosocomial colonization and infection by methicillin-resistant *Staphylococcus aureus* in a burn unit. Am J Infect Control 2006;34:476–83.
223 Sandri AM, Dalarosa MG, Ruschel de Alcantara L, da Silva Elias L, Zavascki AP. Reduction in incidence of nosocomial methicillin-resistant *Staphylococcus aureus* (MRSA) infection in an intensive care unit: role of treatment with mupirocin ointment and chlorhexidine baths for nasal carriers of MRSA. Infect Control Hosp Epidemiol 2006;27:185–7.
224 Simor AE, Phillips E, McGeer A *et al.* Randomized controlled trial of chlorhexidine gluconate for washing, intranasal mupirocin, and rifampin and doxycycline versus no treatment for the eradication of methicillin-resistant *Staphylococcus aureus* colonization. Clin Infect Dis 2007;44:178–85.
225 O'Grady NP, Alexander M, Dellinger EP *et al.* Guidelines for the prevention of intravascular catheter-related infections. Infect Control Hosp Epidemiol 2002;23:759–69.
226 Muto CA, Jernigan JA, Ostrowsky BE *et al.* SHEA guideline for preventing nosocomial transmission of multidrug-resistant strains of *Staphylococcus aureus* and enterococcus. Infect Control Hosp Epidemiol 2003;24:362–86.
227 Singh N, Squier C, Wannstedt C, Keyes L, Wagener MM, Cacciarelli TV. Impact of an aggressive infection control strategy on endemic *Staphylococcus aureus* infection in liver transplant recipients. Infect Control Hosp Epidemiol 2006;27:122–6.
228 Raad I, Hachem R, Tcholakian RK, Sherertz R. Efficacy of minocycline and EDTA lock solution in preventing catheter-related bacteremia, septic phlebitis, and endocarditis in rabbits. Antimicrob Agents Chemother 2002 Feb;46:327–32.
229 Carratala J, Niubo J, Fernandez-Sevilla A *et al.* Randomized, double-blind trial of an antibiotic-lock technique for prevention of Gram-positive central venous catheter-related infection in neutropenic patients with cancer. Antimicrob Agents Chemother 1999;43:2200–4.
230 Chatzinikolaou I, Zipf TF, Hanna H *et al.* Minocycline–ethylenediaminetetraacetate lock solution for the prevention of implantable port infections in children with cancer. Clin Infect Dis 2003;36:116–19.
231 Kim SH, Kang CI, Kim HB *et al.* Outcomes of Hickman catheter salvage in febrile neutropenic cancer patients with *Staphylococcus aureus* bacteremia. Infect Control Hosp Epidemiol 2003;24: 897–904.
232 Safdar N, Maki DG. Use of vancomycin-containing lock or flush solutions for prevention of bloodstream infection associated with central venous access devices: a meta-analysis of prospective, randomized trials. Clin Infect Dis 2006;43:474–84.
233 Chu VH, Crosslin DR, Friedman JY *et al.* *Staphylococcus aureus* bacteremia in patients with prosthetic devices: costs and outcomes. Am J Med 2005;118:1416.
234 Engemann JJ, Friedman JY, Reed SD *et al.* Clinical outcomes and costs due to *Staphylococcus aureus* bacteremia among patients receiving long-term hemodialysis. Infect Control Hosp Epidemiol 2005;26:534–9.
235 Weems JJ Jr, Steinberg JP, Filler S *et al.* Phase II, randomized, double-blind, multicenter study comparing the safety and pharmacokinetics of tefibazumab to placebo for treatment of *Staphylococcus aureus* bacteremia. Antimicrob Agents Chemother 2006;50:2751–5.
236 Domanski PJ, Patel PR, Bayer AS *et al.* Characterization of a humanized monoclonal antibody recognizing clumping factor A expressed by *Staphylococcus aureus*. Infect Immun 2005;73: 5229–32.
237 Shinefield H, Black S, Fattom A *et al.* Use of a *Staphylococcus aureus* conjugate vaccine in patients receiving hemodialysis. N Engl J Med 2002;346:491–6.

Chapter 29
Clinical Manifestations of Community-acquired MRSA Infections

Brian S. Schwartz[1] *and Henry F. Chambers*[1,2]

[1] University of California San Francisco and [2] Division of Infectious Diseases, San Francisco General Hospital, San Francisco, California, USA

Introduction

History

The first recognized case of methicillin-resistant *Staphylococcus aureus* (MRSA) infection was reported in 1961 shortly after the introduction of methicillin as an agent active against penicillin-resistant *S. aureus* [1]. MRSA remained chiefly a nosocomial pathogen, with a steady rise in infection rates over the next three decades [2]. Initial cases of MRSA from the community occurred in individuals with identifiable hospital-associated risk factors: prior exposure to healthcare facilities, hospitalization with prolonged stay in the intensive care unit, prolonged antimicrobial therapy, surgical procedures, and close proximity to other patients with MRSA [3–8].

In the late 1990s, the epidemiology of MRSA changed dramatically. The majority of infections began to be seen in young healthy individuals lacking any exposure to the healthcare setting or other identifiable risk factors for MRSA [2,9–11]. In 1998, a retrospective study of MRSA infections in children in Chicago revealed a marked increase in incidence of MRSA infections in those without any predisposing risk factors, from 10 cases per 100 000 admissions during 1988–1990 to 259 cases per 100 000 admissions during 1993–1995 [12]. Shortly thereafter, reports emerged from communities throughout the USA of individuals with MRSA infections without classic risk factors. These cases included healthy children presenting with severe MRSA infections (septic arthritis, bacteremia/septic shock, and necrotizing pneumonia) [13], previously healthy adults with MRSA skin and soft tissue infections (SSTIs) [14], and outbreaks of infection in childcare centers [15] and among athletes [16,17].

MRSA has now become a predominant community pathogen throughout many communities in the USA [18] and abroad [19–21]. In the USA a single clone of MRSA, USA300 [multilocus sequence type (ST)8], has become the most prevalent cause of staphylococcal SSTI in many communities [22,23].

Community MRSA: a clinical definition

Accurately defining community MRSA is problematic. Different groups have used different terms, including "community-acquired," "community-onset," "community-associated," and "community" MRSA. These terms have all aimed to describe several clonal strains of MRSA that were acquired in patients lacking "classical" risk factors for acquisition of nosocomial isolates of MRSA. Most early studies based their definitions on time of isolate collection relative to time of hospital admission, classifying isolates collected within 24–72 hours of hospital admission as of community origin and those collected after 72 hours as hospital-acquired [24]. Other studies have further narrowed their cohorts to exclude patients with classic risk factors for MRSA infection, such as hospitalization, surgery, dialysis, residence in a long-term care facility within 1 year of enrollment, or presence of invasive medical devices [25]. The present Centers for Disease Control and Prevention (CDC) Active Bacterial Core Surveillance Program defines a CA-MRSA case as follows [26]:

> A patient with an MRSA infection and no history of the following: surgery, hospitalization, or residence in a long-term care facility within the year before infection, presence of a percutaneous device or indwelling catheter, dialysis within the previous year, hospitalization > 48 h before MRSA culture, or previous MRSA infection or colonization.

A more recent CDC study evaluating invasive MRSA infections divided these into healthcare-associated and community-associated based on the risk factors for healthcare-associated acquisition listed above. The authors then subdivided the healthcare-associated disease into community-onset versus hospital-onset, determined by whether the culture was collected less than or more than 48 hours into the hospitalization [27]. Because *S. aureus* can persist as a colonizer for months to years, misclassification

Staphylococci in Human Disease, 2nd edition. Edited by Kent B. Crossley, Kimberly K. Jefferson, Gordon Archer, Vance G. Fowler, Jr.
 ISBN 978-14051-6332-3.

of the source of an infection is common [28,29]. As discussed further below, it may be more accurate to define strain origin by molecular characteristics and genotype. Several studies have suggested that the distinction between community- and hospital-acquired MRSA is blurring as molecular typing methods have indicated that strains of community origin, specifically the USA300 clone, are emerging in the healthcare setting and causing nosocomial infections [30–33]. In this chapter we use the term "CA-MRSA" to indicate strains likely belonging to USA300 and USA400 (MW2) clones. We use the term "HA-MRSA" to refer to strains likely from classical nosocomial lineages, which have their roots in the healthcare setting.

Community MRSA: a microbiological/molecular definition

CA-MRSA strains differ from HA-MRSA strains in several important ways: (i) antibiotic resistance phenotype, (ii) presence of a staphylococcal cassette chromosome (SCC)*mec* type IV element, (iii) enhanced fitness, (iv) enhanced virulence, and (v) genotype.

HA-MRSA strains are generally resistant to multiple antibiotic classes. However, community MRSA strains are typically resistant only to β-lactams and one or two other drug classes [11]. This is partly due to the type IV SCC*mec* element, which lacks resistance genes other than *mecA*, the gene that encodes the low-affinity penicillin-binding protein PBP2a, which confers class resistance to β-lactams. The type II and type III SCC*mec* elements classically found in nosocomial MRSA contain multiple antibiotic resistance determinants in addition to *mecA*.

CA-MRSA strains are fit. They grow at similar rates to methicillin-susceptible *S. aureus* (MSSA) strains and faster than HA-MRSA [34]. Lee *et al.* [35] demonstrated *in vitro* that *S. aureus* isolates transformed with SCC*mec* type I exhibited increased glucose consumption and ATP demand and decreased cell yield. However, transformation with SCC*mec* type IV had no adverse energetic effects. Given this enhanced fitness, CA-MRSA have been able to successfully compete in a wide array of geographical locations and within diverse populations [33,36–42].

In addition to being fit, community MRSA strains are virulent. Numerous reports describe otherwise healthy individuals with invasive disease accompanied by high rates of bacteremia [40], bone and joint infections [40,43], pyomyositis [44], necrotizing pneumonia [39,45], necrotizing fasciitis [42,46], and death [13]. Panton–Valentine leukocidin (PVL) is present in the majority of CA-MRSA isolates and may play a role in virulence, although this is still controversial. Other recently discovered genes may also encode virulence factors [47].

MRSA strains are strikingly clonal. The original CA-MRSA strains were members of the USA400 (MW2) clone (ST1) [48–50], which were unrelated to any of the five common nosocomial clones [51]. USA300 is ST8, clonal cluster (CC)8 genotype, a common hospital lineage. USA300 is very closely related to the CC8 COL strain, the original 1961 MRSA isolate [51]. First identified from outbreaks in jails in Los Angeles and San Francisco in 2001 [36,52], USA300 is by far the predominant CA-MRSA clone in the USA, largely replacing USA400 [18,22,53].

Epidemiology and pathogenesis

Epidemiology

Prevalence/burden of disease

Not only has the prevalence of MRSA in the community increased, so has the overall burden of *S. aureus* disease [40,53,54]. This increase has been primarily due to the increase in CA-MRSA cases, with stable rates or less significant increases in the burden of MSSA strains [53,55–57]. Thus, community MRSA strains compete successfully against other *S. aureus* strains, whether methicillin resistant or susceptible, in both the community and the hospital. As mentioned above, the increasing prevalence of CA-MRSA was first described in 1998 [12], and over the following decade other studies have supported this finding in both pediatric [56] and adult populations [10,52,54]. Increased incidence of CA-MRSA disease has also been reported in military recruits [58–60], prisoners [52,61,62], and individuals presenting to emergency rooms [18,63]. Increased colonization rates have also been documented in similar populations. Of recent note, the prevalence of CA-MRSA is also increasing among hospitalized patients [31,37,64].

Risk factors and at-risk populations

The factors governing CA-MRSA transmission have not been well defined but seem to fall into two main categories: (i) increased exposure of the host to a culture-positive source and (ii) host factors that increase the risk for infection. Factors that increase exposure are intimate contact with infected persons, colonized persons, or exposure to contaminated environments. Risk factors that make a host susceptible to infection include disruption of normal skin integrity and abnormal immunity, especially that due to altered neutrophil function and poor hygiene. Documented groups with outbreaks of CA-MRSA infection are listed in Table 29.1 and risk factors from published studies are listed in Table 29.2.

Exposure to infected persons or an environment frequented by infected persons is an important risk factor for infection. Studies of adults [10,18], athletes [41,65,66], prisoners [36,52,58], military personnel [58–60], rural Alaskans [67], and HIV-positive men who have sex with men (MSM) [68] all revealed that direct or close contact with infected individuals (locker proximity, field position, shared household, sexual activity) or intimate contact with a shared environment with infected persons (sports

Table 29.1 Groups reported in CA-MRSA outbreaks.

Athletes (football, rugby, wrestling, fencing) [16,17,41,65,66,203]
Healthy adults [14]
Healthy children [12,13,15]
HIV-positive men who have sex with men [57,68]
Household contacts of persons with CA-MRSA SSTI [72–75]
Hospitalized patients [33]
Homeless/urban poor [53,77,146,204]
Persons infected with influenza [39,45,130,205]
Intravenous drug users [26,33,42,77,133,146,204,206]
Institutionalized adults with developmental disabilities [207]
Military recruits [58–60,81,208]
Native Americans [49,209]
Newborns and postpartum mothers [37,210]
Pacific Islanders [211]
Prisoners [38,52,53,58,61,76,77]
Recipients of tattoos [208]
Rural Alaskans [67,209]

SSTI, skin and soft tissue infection.

Table 29.2 Risk factors associated with CA-MRSA infection or colonization.

Direct contact[1] with a person or shared environment[2] with a person with CA-MRSA skin and soft tissue infection [10,18,36,41,52,58–60,65–75]
Abnormalities of skin: skin wounds, body shaving, dermatological diseases (eczema, psoriasis) [11,41,65,66,76]
Intravenous drug use [33,77,78]
Homelessness [146]
Obesity [76]
Prior hospitalization [80]
Prior antibiotic use [10,18,67,81,82]
Poor hygiene [76]
Immune suppression, e.g., patients receiving immunosuppressive medications or who have HIV or diabetes mellitus [80]

[1] Direct contact includes routine (household contacts), sexual (heterosexual or men who have sex with men), contact sports.
[2] Shared environment includes use of hot tub, whirlpool, or sauna; sports equipment; towels; hygiene products.

equipment, personal hygiene products, towels, hot tubs, whirlpools, saunas) increase the risk of disease acquisition. Smaller outbreak studies have also supported the importance of direct or close contact, as seen by clusters of infections in heterosexual couples [69,70], postpartum mothers and their neonates [71], and nuclear families without other obvious risk factors [72–75].

Disruption of skin integrity is an additional important factor in development of CA-MRSA infections, likely due to the absence of important defense mechanisms present in intact skin. In studies of football players, "turf burns" and body shaving were risk factors for infection [41,65,66]. Additionally, in healthy children, healthy adults, and prison inmates, abnormal skin conditions (infection, dermatitis, and eczema) were significant risk factors for CA-MRSA disease [11,76]. Intravenous drug use has been identified in several studies as a risk factor for CA-MRSA infection [33,77,78], although the relative contributions of needle-sharing that results in close contact and of disruption in skin integrity are difficult to separate. Interestingly, one study demonstrated that use of snorted or smoked illicit drugs was a risk factor for CA-MRSA infection, whereas injection drug use was not, suggesting that close contact is a significant factor in transmission [79]. In addition, HIV disease is associated with increased risk for CA-MRSA colonization [80], and CD4 counts below 50/μL in HIV-positive MSM have been linked to CA-MRSA infection [57].

Prolonged antibiotic use is a well-defined risk factor for HA-MRSA [5], although it is uncertain whether prior antibiotic use predisposes patients to CA-MRSA infection or colonization. Five studies examining risk factors for CA-MRSA infection or colonization found prior antibiotic use a positive risk factor [10,18,67,81,82]. However, three studies of mixed-age populations with CA-MRSA infections and colonization did not support these findings [33,79,80]. These conflicting data likely reflect that early in the spread of CA-MRSA antibiotics may play a role in its ability to establish a niche. However, given its equivalent fitness to MSSA, once it becomes established it is easily able to maintain its position as the predominant clone regardless of antibiotic pressure [34,35].

Staphylococcus aureus colonization is a significant risk factor for subsequent *S. aureus* infection [83]. Colonization with CA-MRSA may further increase risk of infection. In one large study of 812 military recruits, 24 (3%) were colonized with CA-MRSA and 229 (28%) were colonized with MSSA. Nine (38%) individuals colonized with CA-MRSA developed SSTI compared with only eight (3%) of those colonized with MSSA ($P < 0.001$) [81]. An outbreak investigation of CA-MRSA SSTI in rural Alaska and one of football players supported the notion that colonization is associated with infection [65,67]; however, two other outbreak investigations of football players with CA-MRSA SSTI have not [41,66].

CA-MRSA in the healthcare setting

CA-MRSA isolates have recently become predominant strains of *S. aureus* in some hospitals and in some groups of nonhospitalized patients with healthcare-associated risk factors [30,64]. Nosocomial outbreaks of strains of CA-MRSA have been reported in the USA [32,33,37,64], Europe [84], and Australia [85]. Outbreaks have been reported in newborns [37,86], postpartum women [37], patients undergoing prosthetic joint replacement [32], and in a heterogeneous population of hospitalized patients [33]. Clinical manifestations of nosocomial CA-MRSA disease have included SSTI, pneumonia, prosthetic joint infections, and bacteremia [31–33,37,84–87]. In San Francisco, USA300 has become the predominant cause of healthcare-associated MRSA infections [88].

Pathogenesis

Virulence factors

Staphylococcus aureus produces a wide array of virulence factors. PVL is the virulence factor that is epidemiologically most strongly associated with CA-MRSA strains and it may be an important factor in determining clinical manifestations of infections caused by CA-MRSA.

As the name implies, PVL is toxic for leukocytes. It is a member of a family of closely related two-component (S and F components, each encoded by a different gene), heptameric, cytolytic pore-forming staphylococcal toxins that also includes γ-hemolysin and leukocidin [89,90]. PVL targets and lyses human and rabbit granulocytes and provokes a potent dermonecrotic reaction in rabbits [91], but is not lethal when injected intravenously [92]. In their original papers, Panton and Valentine observed an association between strains producing leukotoxin and severe disease [92,93]. Severe and recurrent skin infections, necrotizing pneumonia, and necrotizing fasciitis have all been associated with PVL-positive strains [42,94,95].

In investigations of clinical isolates of CA-MRSA, PVL genes were present in 69–100% of isolates [10,11,18,38,40, 63,96]. The prevalence of PVL among *S. aureus* isolates other than CA-MRSA is low, about 1–5% [11,96–98]. USA300 and USA400 both have PVL genes. Despite the strong epidemiological association between PVL, virulence, and emergence of CA-MRSA, considerable controversy remains about the role of PVL.

Voyich *et al.* [99] examined nine PVL-positive and PVL-negative *S. aureus* clinical isolates representing a variety of genotypes in a mouse sepsis model and hairless mouse cutaneous abscess model. Among the strains tested were a PVL-positive USA300 strain and a USA400 strain. PVL-negative deletion mutants were just as lethal in mice as PVL-positive parents, produced comparable skin infections, and were indistinguishable in neutrophil lysis and bacterial killing assays. These investigators concluded that PVL was not a major virulence determinant. The strength of these experiments is that wild-type strains were used, so that the genetic context is relevant. A potential weakness is that the mouse may not be the best model species because it is relatively insensitive to the biological effects of PVL [100,101].

In contrast to these results are those of Labandeira-Ray *et al.* [102]. These investigators found that instillation into the lung of large amounts of purified toxin (≥ 3 μg) or a large inoculum of a laboratory strain of *S. aureus* which overexpressed PVL induced inflammatory changes in the lungs in a mouse pneumonitis model. A puzzling result was that expression of PVL was also associated with global changes in transcriptional levels of 119 genes in stationary-phase cells (26 of which have a role in pathogenesis) and 27 genes in exponential-phase cells (nine of which are involved in pathogenesis), including staphylococcal protein A (10–50 fold increase in transcription). In hind-sight, use of RN6390 as a PVL host is problematic because its 8325 genetic background is defective in the accessory sigma factor, sigma B [103], which controls stress response and is an important regulator of virulence gene expression, including *agr*. Such profound effects on gene expression raise the possibility that the experimental outcome is not due to the presence of PVL genes but a consequence of major genetic perturbations.

Other than PVL, CA-MRSA carries multiple exotoxin genes that are unique when compared with HA-MRSA isolates and which may be important factors in severity of clinical disease [23]. In addition, the arginine catabolic mobile element (ACME) is a recently identified gene cluster that appears to be unique to the USA300 clone of CA-MRSA [47]. It is a possible virulence factor involved in colonization and pathogenesis [104].

Clinical manifestations

Skin and soft tissue infections

SSTIs are the most common clinical manifestation of CA-MRSA disease (77–97%) [10,25,26,55,56]. In fact CA-MRSA has become a major, and perhaps predominant, cause of SSTIs in the USA [18,22]. Although there is variability in the manifestations of CA-MRSA SSTIs (Table 29.3), abscesses with or without surrounding cellulitis account for 46–70% of disease [25,26,63,77,105,106]. Cellulitis is present in 4–42% of cases [25,26,63,77,105,106]. The frequency of cellulitis as the sole manifestation of CA-MRSA is not well defined. In only one study have authors defined "pure cellulitis" as a clinical manifestation of CA-MRSA SSTI. In this study of 137 patients presenting to the emergency room, 13% of cases were defined as pure cellulitis [63]. However, in a study of 531 cases of CA-MRSA SSTI, cellulitis was present in 116 (22%), all of which were associated with a focal lesion [105]. Other cutaneous lesions account for the remainder of disease: furuncles 5–14% [63,77,106], wound infections 5–10% [25,26,63], folliculitis 5–7% [25,26], and impetigo 2–9% [25,26,106]. Furuncles are frequently reported in outbreaks [63,65,67].

Community MRSA SSTIs are most commonly found on the extremities (lower more than upper) but also in the perineal or perirectal regions, trunk, and face [10,105,106]. These lesions are often accompanied by central necrosis and surrounding cellulitis and may be mistaken for spider bites (see Plate 29.1) [18,36,61,107,108]. In an outbreak of CA-MRSA SSTI in a prison in Los Angeles County, exterminators were called in for eradication of suspected spiders, but none were found [36,109]. Signs of systemic inflammation are infrequent in isolated CA-MRSA SSTIs. Studies have shown fever to be present in 25–48% of

Table 29.3 Reported clinical manifestations of CA-MRSA infections.

Skin and soft tissue infections	
Impetigo [25,26,106]	
Folliculitis [25,26]	
Cellulitis [25,26,63,77,105,106]	
Furuncle [63,77,106]	
Abscess [25,26,63,77,105,106]	
Wound infection [25,26,63]	
Omphalitis [37,71]	
Mastitis with or without breast abscess [37,71,210]	
Systemic disease with cutaneous manifestations	
Staphylocccal toxic shock syndrome [116]	
Staphylococcal scalded skin syndrome [116]	
Purpura fulminans with or without Waterhouse–Friderichsen syndrome [117,118]	
Musculoskeletal infections	
Bursitis [25,77]	
Septic arthritis [26,77,119]	
Prosthetic joint infections [32]	
Pyomyositis and myositis [44]	
Osteomyelitis [26,119]	
Necrotizing fasciitis [42,46]	
Head and neck infections	
Acute sinusitis [10]	
Otitis media [11,82]	
Lymphadenitis [55,56]	
Orbital cellulitis [125]	
Panophthalmitis [125]	
Lid abscess [125]	
Endogenous endophthalmitis [125]	
Venous sinus thrombosis [125–127]	
Meningitis [25]	
Brain abscess (authors' personal experience)	
Pulmonary infections	
Pneumonia (often necrotizing) [11,12,25,26,33,39,45,96,130–132]	
Septic pulmonary embolus [45,123]	
Lung abscess [45,71,130]	
Empyema [45,71,130]	
Urinary tract infections [11,25,71,210]	
Bloodstream/cardiac infections	
Bacteremia [10,11,22,25,26,53,55,56,111,136]	
Infective endocarditis [126,133]	
Septic thrombophlebitis [45,123]	
Infection of myocardium and/or epicardium without valvular infection [40]	

patients presenting with CA-MRSA SSTIs [63,110] and an abnormal leukocyte count in only 28% of patients [105].

Recurrence of CA-MRSA SSTI is very common and may be related to colonization of close contacts and the individual's environment [18,61,63,65,111]. HIV-infected individuals have recurrence rates of 21–45%, which is much higher than rates reported in the general population [10,18,111–115]. Hospitalization of adult patients with CA-MRSA SSTI ranges from 16 to 41% of cases [10,22,26, 63,105]. In a series that included patients presenting with invasive CA-MRSA disease, the admission rate ranged from 16 to 75% [10,25]. In one pediatric medical center the incidence of CA-MRSA infection peaked at 277 cases per 10 000 admissions between 2002 and 2003 [55]. Despite the fact that CA-MRSA has become the predominant cause of *S. aureus* SSTIs in certain areas, the rate of invasive disease or rehospitalization in this group appears to be similar to the rates seen in patients with MSSA SSTIs [56,111].

Infrequently, strains of CA-MRSA can produce systemic syndromes with cutaneous manifestations such as staphylococcal scalded skin syndrome [116], staphylococcal toxic shock syndrome [116], purpura fulminans [117,118], and Waterhouse–Friderichsen syndrome [118].

Invasive musculoskeletal disease

Severe infections of deep skin and soft tissues as well as bone and joint have been reported with CA-MRSA. These include pyomyositis and myositis, necrotizing fasciitis, septic arthritis, and osteomyelitis [42–44,46,119]. *Staphylococcus aureus* is the most common pathogen associated with pyomyositis [120] and has been reported as a cause of myositis as well [121]. Pannaraj *et al.* [44] reported a marked increase in cases at a US pediatric hospital between 2000 and 2005, with CA-MRSA as the leading pathogen. Patients with pyomyositis or myositis presented with pain, fever, limp, and swelling and those with CA-MRSA required surgical drainage more frequently than those with other pathogens.

Since *S. aureus* is a common cause of both osteomyelitis and septic arthritis, it is no surprise that CA-MRSA is being increasingly reported as a cause of these infections [119]. Acute osteomyelitis due to PVL-positive CA-MRSA results in a more significant elevation and prolongation of elevation in inflammatory markers (erythrocyte sedimentation rate and C-reactive protein) compared with patients infected with MSSA or PVL-negative strains of *S. aureus* [43,122]. Children with acute osteomyelitis due to CA-MRSA may be at increased risk for concomitant venous thromboses, septic thrombophlebitis, and septic pulmonary emboli [45,123].

Necrotizing fasciitis is a severe life-threatening disease not thought to be caused by *S. aureus* alone. Empirical coverage for MRSA was not routinely recommended in the past but now should be included in initial therapy [124]. In 2005, Miller *et al.* [42] reported 14 cases of a subacute form of necrotizing fasciitis caused by MRSA in adults who were predominantly intravenous drug users. One-third of these patients had no predisposing risk factors for necrotizing fasciitis and all patients survived. All isolates genotyped were USA300 clones and PVL positive. Additionally, one case of CA-MRSA necrotizing fasciitis has been reported in a previously healthy 5-day-old child [46].

Head and neck infections

Although the extremities are most commonly involved in CA-MRSA SSTIs, the structures of the head and neck may be involved as well [10,105,106]. Numerous clinical series of CA-MRSA disease have included cases of acute sinusitis, otitis interna, and lymphadenitis [10,11,25,55,56]. Ocular infections have also been prominently reported and have included orbital cellulitis, endogenous endophthalmitis, panophthalmitis, and lid abscesses (see Plate 29.2) [125]. Additionally, several cases of ocular infections have resulted in venous sinus thromboses, a life-threatening complication [125–127].

Respiratory tract infections

Staphylococcus aureus is isolated in 3–5% of cases of community-acquired pneumonia (CAP) in the USA [128] and MRSA is one of the most common causes of hospital-acquired pneumonia [129]. However, MRSA was not associated with CAP in patients without classical risk factors for MRSA until the late 1990s, when it was reported in several cases of otherwise healthy children [12,13]. Since then, numerous cases of children and adults with severe pulmonary disease have been reported [11,12,25,26,33,39,45, 96,130–132] and pulmonary disease now accounts for 2–6% of cases of CA-MRSA [11,25,55,77]. The incidence of CA-MRSA CAP and prevalence of CA-MRSA among CAP cases has not been defined.

Two different mechanisms of pulmonary disease have been described: primary pulmonary disease and secondary disease from septic thrombophlebitis or right-sided infective endocarditis [45,133]. Concomitant infection with influenza has been closely associated with CA-MRSA pulmonary disease in both adult and pediatric populations [39,45,130]. Radiographic findings in this population may reveal single-lobe or multilobe disease, cavitation, necrosis, pneumatoceles, diffuse airspace disease, effusions, and/or empyema (Figure 29.1) [45,130]. Necrosis with cavitation is a prominent feature in many of these cases [39,45,130,131]. PVL may play a role in the pathogenesis of necrotizing pulmonary disease. However, since almost all isolates of CA-MRSA carry PVL, it is difficult to determine if PVL is indeed an important factor. In a mixed population of patients with PVL-positive MSSA or MRSA necrotizing pneumonia, independent risk factors for death in a multivariate analysis were leukopenia and erythroderma within 24 hours of admission [134]. Growth of bacteria from blood and sputum is common in these cases and the mortality rate for patients with CA-MRSA necrotizing pneumonia has been reported to be 25–100% [39,130,131]. Given the increasing prevalence of CA-MRSA CAP, the Infectious Diseases Society of America/American Thoracic Society 2007 guidelines for the treatment of CAP now recommend consideration of antimicrobial coverage of this pathogen in patients with severe pneumonia and influenza and/or cavitary lung disease [135].

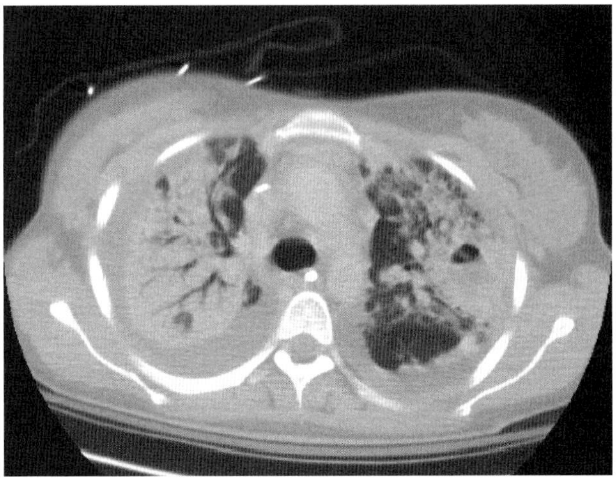

Figure 29.1 Noncontrast-enhanced chest CT of a 29 year-old previously healthy woman with bilateral dense consolidations and a 3 × 2 cm air-filled cavity in the left-upper lobe. Her blood and sputum cultures grew CA-MRSA.

Bloodstream and cardiac infections

Between 0.2 and 6% of patients with CA-MRSA disease will present with concomitant bacteremia [10,11,22,25, 26,53,55,56,111,136]. However, bacteremia is present in 50–93% of patients presenting with invasive CA-MRSA disease [26,40]. CA-MRSA is a major cause of *S. aureus* bacteremia in patients with or without healthcare-associated risk factors, including nosocomial bloodstream infections [33,87,137]. Patients with CA-MRSA bacteremia have similar outcomes to patients with HA-MRSA or CA-MSSA disease even when controlling for other comorbidities [87,138].

Cases of infective endocarditis due to CA-MRSA are now being reported [126,133]. In the largest series to date, which included only seven patients, all patients were intravenous drug users and 71% had right-sided disease [133]. Other cardiac manifestations may include myocardial and endocardial infection in the absence of valvular disease, which was described at autopsy of two patients with disseminated CA-MRSA infection [40].

Diagnosis

The identification of CA-MRSA requires isolation of the organism in culture from sterile sites (blood, material from a surgically drained abscess, synovial fluid, or bone aspirate) or nonsterile sites such as sputum culture in the proper clinical setting (severe pneumonia). However, these tests do not discriminate between CA-MRSA and HA-MRSA isolates. Several strategies may be considered in order to make this distinction: (i) epidemiological analysis, (ii) review of antimicrobial susceptibility patterns, or (iii) molecular analysis. As described earlier, prolonged colonization and the emergence of CA-MRSA in the healthcare setting prevent epidemiological data from being sensitive or specific for the identification of CA-MRSA. The unique antimicrobial susceptibility patterns of CA-MRSA may be a useful tool. However, antimicrobial susceptibilities are not uniform and as CA-MRSA isolates become established in the healthcare setting they may acquire other resistance genes. Popovich *et al.* [139] formed a set of phenotypic prediction rules and found that ciprofloxacin sensitivity alone had a 90% positive predictive value for the identification of CA-MRSA. However, the addition of any other antimicrobial susceptibility or epidemiological information did not improve the prediction model.

Pulsed-field gel electrophoresis (PFGE) is currently the gold standard for molecular identification of CA-MRSA. Other molecular studies, including sequencing of the protein A gene polymorphic region (*spa*-typing) and polymerase chain reaction (PCR) testing for SCC*mec* type IV, PVL or ACME, may be alternative approaches. However, these techniques can be tedious and prolonged turnround times limit their clinical utility. Moreover, the clinical relevance of determining whether an MRSA isolate is a community clone is not clear. Several groups are presently working on rapid PCR assays for detection of PVL and multilocus sequence typing for more rapid detection [140–142].

Treatment

Skin and soft tissue infections

The present epidemic of CA-MRSA disease has presented clinicians with the dilemma of choosing new treatments for a wide array of *S. aureus* infections, especially SSTIs. Unfortunately, no randomized, well-controlled, clinical trials exist to define the optimal antimicrobial treatment of CA-MRSA SSTIs or the role antibiotics play in the management of drainable cutaneous abscesses. Presently, two large trials, sponsored by the National Institutes of Health, are in progress to address these questions.

Surgical drainage

Incision and drainage was the treatment of choice for most cutaneous abscesses prior to the era of CA-MRSA [124,143]. Between 63 and 90% of patients with MRSA-associated abscesses will require incision and drainage of these lesions [18,105,110,144] and the lack of timely incision and drainage is associated with poor outcomes [111]. Three studies have directly evaluated whether incision and drainage alone is adequate therapy for skin abscesses during the era of CA-MRSA [105,110,145]. A study of children (mean age 5.5 years) with CA-MRSA SSTI did not reveal any benefit to antimicrobial therapy over incision and drainage alone; however, the authors found that a lesion more than 5 cm in diameter was a significant predictor for hospitalization [110]. A retrospective observational study demonstrated a small but statistically significant increase in cure rate with the addition of an active antimicrobial agent following surgical drainage [105]. Additionally, a randomized, double-blind, placebo-controlled trial was conducted comparing cefalexin to placebo for adults with surgically drained purulent CA-MRSA SSTI. Not surprisingly, the study found no benefit of cefalexin therapy but did report a 90% cure rate in the placebo group [145]. Several other studies have also been unable to find a benefit of active antimicrobial therapy in the treatment of CA-MRSA SSTI following surgical drainage [25,111,146]. Despite these data, a survey of primary-care physicians revealed that 87% of physicians treat abscesses with antimicrobial therapy and 80% of these physicians do not use antimicrobials active against MRSA [147]. At this time, in coordination with the recommendations of CDC, we would not routinely recommend antibiotic therapy following drainage of CA-MRSA abscesses unless the patient has one or more of the conditions listed in Table 29.4, which include severe disease, abnormal host immunity, or a lesion difficult to drain completely [148].

Antimicrobial therapy

The empirical antimicrobial treatment of suspected staphylococcal infections should be guided by local rates of methicillin resistance. Some experts recommended using a 10–15% prevalence rate of MRSA in the community to trigger use of anti-MRSA empirical therapy [149]. However, in patients with moderate to severe infections due to suspected staphylococcal disease, treatment with antimicrobials active for MRSA is recommended regardless of community prevalence. The oral antimicrobial agents with the most consistent activity against CA-MRSA include clindamycin, the long-acting tetracyclines, trimethoprim–sulfamethoxazole, rifampin, and linezolid (Table 29.5).

Table 29.4 Situations for considering adjuvant antimicrobial therapy following incision and débridement of a CA-MRSA skin and soft tissue infection. (Adapted from Gorwitz *et al.* [148] with permission.)

Severe or extensive disease and/or rapid progression in presence of associated cellulitis
Signs and symptoms of systemic illness
Associated comorbidities or immune suppression (diabetes mellitus, HIV/AIDS, neoplastic disease)
Extremes of age
Abscess in area difficult to drain
Associated septic phlebitis
Lack of response to treatment with incision and drainage alone

Table 29.5 Oral antimicrobial agents for treatment of CA-MRSA infections.

Antimicrobial agent	Resistance rates	Recommended adult dosing	Comment
Clindamycin	3–24%	300–450 mg t.i.d. to q.i.d.	Increasing resistance rates in the community. Standard testing does not evaluate for inducible resistance, so D-test must be performed. Good activity against groups A–G β-hemolytic streptococci
Long-acting tetracyclines	9–24%		Doxycycline and minocycline may be active against tetracycline-resistant strains
Doxycycline		100 mg b.i.d.	
Minocycline		100 mg b.i.d.	
Trimethoprim–sulfamethoxazole	0–10%	1–2 double-strength tablets (160/800 mg) b.i.d.	Low resistance rates in community. Reasonable option for empirical therapy
Rifampin	0–4%	300–450 mg b.i.d.	Must be used in combination with second active agent otherwise rapid development of resistance. Potent inducer of CYP3A4
Fluoroquinolones	18–43%		Levofloxacin and moxifloxacin have lower MICs than ciprofloxacin. Should not be used alone since resistance may develop when used as monotherapy; consider combination with rifampin
Ciprofloxacin		750 mg b.i.d.	
Levofloxacin		750 mg q.d.	
Moxifloxacin		400 mg q.d.	
Linezolid	0–4%	600 mg b.i.d.	Only oral agent approved by FDA for treatment of MRSA infection. Very costly

Oral agents

Clindamycin

Clindamycin is a lincosamide that acts by binding at the 50S ribosomal subunit resulting in inhibition of protein synthesis. The Food and Drug Administration (FDA) approved clindamycin for the treatment for serious infectious due to *S. aureus*, although it is not specifically approved for MRSA infections [148]. In addition to activity against MRSA it has activity against group A streptococci, another common cause of SSTI [150]. Clindamycin has been used with success in the treatment of CA-MRSA infections, primarily SSTIs [151,152]. CA-MRSA isolates have been sensitive to clindamycin in 76–97% of cases over the last decade [10,12,25,26,55,56,79,136]. However, clindamycin resistance may be increasing and a multidrug-resistant strain of CA-MRSA carrying the pUSA03 plasmid, which codes for constitutive clindamycin resistance, has been found in increasing prevalence in Boston and San Francisco [56,153–156].

While standard broth microdilution methods evaluate for constitutive resistance to clindamycin, they do not detect inducible resistance. Inducible resistance to clindamycin, referred to as macrolide lincosamide streptogramin B inducible resistance (MLS_Bi), results from induction of the *erm* gene, which expresses a methylase that modifies the binding site for clindamycin (as well as macrolides) at the 23S rRNA of the 50S bacterial ribosome [157]. This inducible phenotype is reported in 0–7% of CA-MRSA isolates [23,153,158] but some experts report higher rates [159]. The presence of MLS_Bi is not evident by standard techniques and a D-test is required for detection [157]. The D-test is performed by plating a standardized quantity of organism on an agar plate with clindamycin and

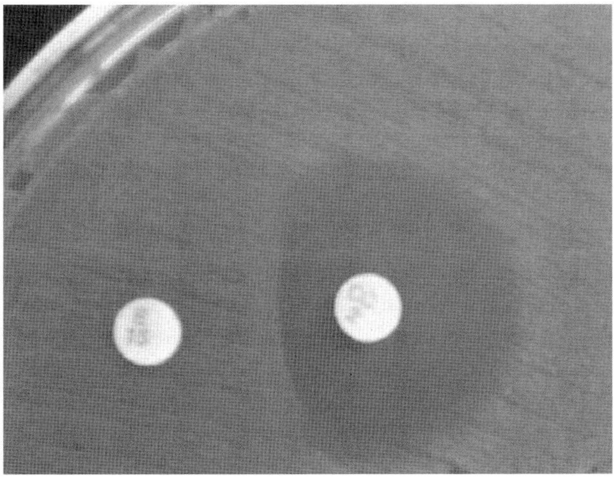

Figure 29.2 Positive D-test. Blunting of the clindamycin zone of inhibition (left side) suggests the presence of the *erm* gene in the test isolate that is inducible by erythromycin. E, erythromycin; CC, clindamycin. (Photo courtesy of Dr Barbara Haller, Department of Laboratory Medicine, San Francisco General Hospital.)

erythromycin disks in close proximity. An MLS_Bi strain will express *erm* in the presence of erythromycin, resulting in blunting of the clindamycin zone of inhibition on the zone margin closest to the erythromycin disk, resulting in the presence of a "D" pattern (Figure 29.2). Whether the presence of MLS_Bi results in treatment failure is unclear [157,160]. However, there are reports of emergence of constitutive resistance and clindamycin treatment failure in patients with moderate to severe infections [157,161–163]. The impact of MLS_Bi on the treatment outcomes of a patient receiving clindamycin for uncomplicated SSTI may be less as these patients are often cured with incision and drainage alone. At this time, a D-test is recommended for all erythromycin-resistant, clindamycin-sensitive isolates when clindamycin therapy is considered. Patients with uncomplicated infections with MLS_Bi strains may not need to undergo a change in therapy if clindamycin has already been initiated and there is a good clinical response, but for moderate to severe infections with MLS_Bi strains an alternative agent may be preferred until more data are available.

Tetracyclines

The tetracycline class of antimicrobials includes the long-acting tetracyclines, doxycycline, and minocycline, which are most commonly used in the treatment of CA-MRSA disease. These agents are bacteriostatic against *S. aureus* and inhibit protein synthesis by binding to the 30S ribosome. Doxycycline and minocycline have enhanced anti-staphylococcal activity compared with tetracycline [164]. They are FDA approved for treatment of SSTIs due to *S. aureus* though not specifically for methicillin-resistant strains [148].

Doxycycline and minocycline appear to be effective in the treatment of MRSA SSTIs [165,166] but may be less efficacious in the treatment of severe MRSA infections [166]. Of CA-MRSA isolates, 76–100% are susceptible to tetracycline [10,25,26,55,79,136]. However, much like clindamycin, resistance rates are increasing in some regions [153]. Tetracycline resistance in *S. aureus* is conferred by the presence of the *tetK* or *tetM* genes. The *tetK* gene encodes for an efflux pump which confers resistance to tetracycline, may cause a small increase in the minimum inhibitory concentration (MIC) of doxycycline, but has no effect on the MIC of minocycline [167]. Tetracycline resistance conferred via the *tetM* gene results in high-level resistance to all tetracyclines via alteration of the drug-binding site [148,166,168]. To date, the *tetK* gene, but not the *tetM* gene, has been described in the genome of some isolates of USA300 [23,153]. Tetracyclines are not recommended for pregnant women or children under the age of 8 years.

Trimethoprim–sulfamethoxazole

The combination agent trimethoprim–sulfamethoxazole (TMP–SMX) affects sequential steps in the biosynthetic pathway of tetrahydrofolic acid and is nearly 100% bioavailable. TMP–SMX is not FDA approved for the treatment of staphylococcal infection [148]. However, *in vitro* this combination has bactericidal activity against sensitive *S. aureus* isolates [169] and TMP–SMX is active against 90–100% of CA-MRSA isolates [10,12,25,26,55,136]. Data about the efficacy of TMP–SMX for the treatment of MRSA infections is limited [106,170–172]. In 1992, Markowitz *et al.* [172] conducted a randomized trial to evaluate the efficacy of TMP–SMX versus vancomycin for a mix of moderate to severe *S. aureus* infections in hospitalized intravenous drug users; 47% of isolates were MRSA. Treatment with TMP–SMX resulted in equivalent cure rates in patients with MRSA infections, although it was inferior to vancomycin in patients with MSSA infections. A recent study reported increased cure rates for SSTI after a change in empirical antimicrobial therapy from β-lactams to TMP–SMX in an area with high rates of CA-MRSA [173]. Although *in vitro* antagonism between rifampin and TMP–SMX been described for MRSA [169,174], a small study of patients with CA-MRSA SSTI reported improved efficacy with the addition of rifampin to TMP–SMX [106]. TMP–SMX prophylaxis may decrease the risk of CA-MRSA infections in HIV-positive men [68]. TMP–SMX may be a reasonable first-line oral agent for the treatment of a suspected CA-MRSA SSTI requiring antimicrobial therapy. Caution is advised when treating a patient with TMP–SMX if group A streptococcus is a possible pathogen, given the limited data on its activity against this organism [175]. TMP–SMX in not recommended for treatment of women during the third trimester of pregnancy.

Rifampin

Rifampin has excellent antistaphylococcal activity but resistance develops quickly when used as a single agent [176]. CA-MRSA isolates are highly susceptible (96–100%) to rifampin [25,26,55,79,136]. Presently, rifampin is indicated in the treatment of MRSA prosthetic valve infective endocarditis [177] and may have efficacy in the treatment of staphylococcal prosthetic joint infections [178]. One study of patients with MRSA infective endocarditis demonstrated a trend toward prolonged duration of bacteremia in patients receiving rifampin in combination with vancomycin when compared with vancomycin alone [179]. Studies have not evaluated the efficacy of rifampin in the treatment of CA-MRSA infections. Despite the lack of data, rifampin is regularly used in the treatment of CA-MRSA infections [159,180]. When studied *in vitro* rifampin may be antagonistic when added to TMP–SMX [169,174], synergistic if added to minocycline [181], and may decrease the rate of fluoroquinolone resistance [182]. Rifampin is a potent inducer of the cytochrome P450 enzymes and has many drug–drug interactions. Its role in the treatment of CA-MRSA infections is not clear at this time.

Fluoroquinolones

The fluoroquinolone antimicrobials ciprofloxacin, levofloxacin, and moxifloxacin are FDA approved for the treatment SSTIs due to *S. aureus* [148]. However, CA-MRSA isolates are resistant in 18–43% of cases [25,26,55,79,136] and resistance rates as high as 85% have been reported [153]. Fluoroquinolone resistance develops quickly in *S. aureus* isolates [183,184]. We do not recommend fluoroquinolones for empirical treatment of suspected CA-MRSA infections. However, if susceptibility to a fluoroquinolone has been demonstrated and a clinician chooses to treat a susceptible CA-MRSA isolate with a fluoroquinolone, the addition of rifampin is recommended to minimize the development of resistance during treatment [182].

Macrolides

The macrolides (erythromycin, azithromycin, and clarithromycin) are all approved for treatment of SSTIs due to *S. aureus* [148] but no clinical data exist for the use of these agents against MRSA infections. Moreover, resistance rates range between 56 and 91% [10,12,25,26,55,136] and consequently they should not be used empirically and are rarely used for the treatment of CA-MRSA infections.

Linezolid

Linezolid is an oxazolidinone with good antistaphylococcal activity and excellent bioavailability. It is FDA approved for the treatment of complicated SSTIs and nosocomial pneumonia in adults due to MRSA [148]. Linezolid is a bacteriostatic agent that is active against 96–100% of CA-MRSA isolates [25,26,79,111]. The efficacy of linezolid for treatment of MRSA has been demonstrated in two open-label randomized controlled trials. The studies both used vancomycin as the comparison and one study of MRSA SSTI suggested that linezolid may be superior to vancomycin based on analysis of secondary outcomes [185,186]. A large study of patients with diabetic foot infections, including osteomyelitis, found linezolid equivalent to vancomycin plus an aminopenicillin/β-lactamase inhibitor combination in the subgroup of patients with MRSA infections [187]. Linezolid has been evaluated in pediatric populations with MRSA SSTI [188,189]. Linezolid-resistant *S. aureus* isolates, though rare, have been reported in the literature [190]. Most isolates develop resistance via changes at the ribosomal binding site [191]. Experts have expressed concern over the rapid emergence of linezolid resistance and caution against overuse [190]. Linezolid is significantly more expensive than the other oral agents mentioned. Linezolid can result in myelosuppression [192] as well as mitochondrial toxicity, resulting in peripheral neuropathy, optic neuritis, and lactic acidosis [193,194].

Intravenous therapy

Vancomycin is the first-line intravenous agent for severe MRSA infections. However, other intravenous antimicrobials such as daptomycin [195] and tigecycline [196] have demonstrated efficacy and are FDA approved for the treatment of MRSA SSTIs. Quinupristin–dalfopristin has *in vitro* activity against MRSA but does not have a specific MRSA indication from the FDA. In addition, clindamycin, the long-acting tetracyclines, TMP–SMX, fluoroquinolones, rifampin, and linezolid are all available in intravenous formulation. Many new agents with activity against MRSA are currently in the late stages of development and will likely be available in the next several years.

Vancomycin

Vancomycin has been the most extensively studied antibiotic in clinical trials involving patients with SSTIs. It has served as the comparator group in evaluating the efficacy of linezolid, daptomycin, and tigecycline. In four clinical trials, over 400 patients with MRSA were treated with vancomycin and the cure rates for patients with MRSA SSTI ranged from 67 to 75% [185,186,195,196]. However, the efficacy of vancomycin for severe MRSA infections has recently come into question as vancomycin MICs for MRSA have been gradually increasing [197,198]. CA-MRSA with intermediate resistance to vancomycin has recently been reported as well [199]. While the optimal therapy for severe CA-MRSA infections is currently unknown, vancomycin remains a drug of first choice for empirical therapy of suspected MRSA infection in which a parenteral agent is indicated.

Decolonization

CA-MRSA nasal colonization is an identified risk factor for *S. aureus* infection [81] and one could therefore speculate that elimination of CA-MRSA nasal carriage may prevent both primary and secondary infections. However, in the present era of CA-MRSA, studies have failed to show a benefit of intranasal mupirocin in the prevention of primary or secondary SSTIs. A randomized controlled trial of healthy military recruits with CA-MRSA nasal colonization revealed that a 5-day course of intranasal mupirocin had no effect on the rate of CA-MRSA skin and skin-structure infections (SSSIs) at 16 weeks following treatment [200]. A second, retrospective study of 61 MSM with CA-MRSA SSSIs and MRSA nasal colonization found that individuals who received intranasal mupirocin still had a 32% recurrence rate [201]. These results suggest that a positive nasal culture for CA-MRSA does not accurately define patients at risk for recurrent disease nor is intranasal mupirocin efficacious for preventing subsequent disease. One potential explanation is that CA-MRSA is able to colonize nonnasal sites. This hypothesis is supported by a recent study of patients with *S. aureus* infection which showed that patients with CA-MRSA SSSI were more likely to be colonized in nonnasal sites (axilla, inguinal region, and/or rectum) when compared with those infected with either HA-MRSA or MSSA [202]. In addition, a mupirocin-resistant strain of the USA300 clone of CA-MRSA has been increasing in prevalence in Boston and San Francisco [156]. These findings together suggest that intranasal mupirocin would not be an effective strategy for eradication of CA-MRSA colonization or prevention of recurrent CA-MRSA SSSI. However, the most successful means for CA-MRSA decolonization is unknown but a strategy able to act on multiple body sites would likely be most effective. At present, CDC does not recommend routine decolonization [148]. (See Chapter 30 for additional information on decolonization.)

References

1 Jevons MP, Coe AW, Parker MT. Methicillin resistance in staphylococci. Lancet 1963;i:904–7.
2 Chambers HF. The changing epidemiology of *Staphylococcus aureus*? Emerg Infect Dis 2001;7:178–82.
3 Saravolatz LD, Markowitz N, Arking L, Pohlod D, Fisher E. Methicillin-resistant *Staphylococcus aureus*. Epidemiologic observations during a community-acquired outbreak. Ann Intern Med 1982;96:11–16.
4 Saravolatz LD, Pohlod DJ, Arking LM. Community-acquired methicillin-resistant *Staphylococcus aureus* infections: a new source for nosocomial outbreaks. Ann Intern Med 1982;97:325–9.
5 Thompson RL, Cabezudo I, Wenzel RP. Epidemiology of nosocomial infections caused by methicillin-resistant *Staphylococcus aureus*. Ann Intern Med 1982;97:309–17.
6 Boyce JM. Are the epidemiology and microbiology of methicillin-resistant *Staphylococcus aureus* changing? JAMA 1998;279:623–4.
7 Graffunder EM, Venezia RA. Risk factors associated with nosocomial methicillin-resistant *Staphylococcus aureus* (MRSA) infection including previous use of antimicrobials. J Antimicrob Chemother 2002;49:999–1005.
8 Lodise TP Jr, McKinnon PS, Rybak M. Prediction model to identify patients with *Staphylococcus aureus* bacteremia at risk for methicillin resistance. Infect Control Hosp Epidemiol 2003;24:655–61.
9 Deresinski S. Methicillin-resistant *Staphylococcus aureus*: an evolutionary, epidemiologic, and therapeutic odyssey. Clin Infect Dis 2005;40:562–73.
10 Crum NF, Lee RU, Thornton SA *et al.* Fifteen-year study of the changing epidemiology of methicillin-resistant *Staphylococcus aureus*. Am J Med 2006;119:943–51.
11 Naimi TS, LeDell KH, Como-Sabetti K *et al.* Comparison of community- and health care-associated methicillin-resistant *Staphylococcus aureus* infection. JAMA 2003;290:2976–84.
12 Herold BC, Immergluck LC, Maranan MC *et al.* Community-acquired methicillin-resistant *Staphylococcus aureus* in children with no identified predisposing risk. JAMA 1998;279:593–8.
13 Centers for Disease Control and Prevention. Four pediatric deaths from community-acquired methicillin-resistant *Staphylococcus aureus*: Minnesota and North Dakota, 1997–1999. JAMA 1999;282:1123–5.
14 Gorak EJ, Yamada SM, Brown JD. Community-acquired methicillin-resistant *Staphylococcus aureus* in hospitalized adults and children without known risk factors. Clin Infect Dis 1999;29:797–800.
15 Adcock PM, Pastor P, Medley F, Patterson JE, Murphy TV. Methicillin-resistant *Staphylococcus aureus* in two child care centers. J Infect Dis 1998;178:577–80.
16 Lindenmayer JM, Schoenfeld S, O'Grady R, Carney JK. Methicillin-resistant *Staphylococcus aureus* in a high school wrestling team and the surrounding community. Arch Intern Med 1998;158:895–9.
17 Stacey AR, Endersby KE, Chan PC, Marples RR. An outbreak of methicillin resistant *Staphylococcus aureus* infection in a rugby football team. Br J Sports Med 1998;32:153–4.
18 Moran GJ, Krishnadasan A, Gorwitz RJ *et al.* Methicillin-resistant *S. aureus* infections among patients in the emergency department. N Engl J Med 2006;355:666–74.
19 Grundmann H, Aires-de-Sousa M, Boyce J, Tiemersma E. Emergence and resurgence of meticillin-resistant *Staphylococcus aureus* as a public-health threat. Lancet 2006;368:874–85.
20 Larsen A, Stegger M, Goering R, Sorum M, Skov R. Emergence and dissemination of the methicillin resistant *Staphylococcus aureus* USA300 clone in Denmark (2000–2005). Euro Surveillance 2007;12(2).
21 Cohen PR. Community-acquired methicillin-resistant *Staphylococcus aureus* skin infections: a review of epidemiology, clinical features, management, and prevention. Int J Dermatol 2007;46: 1–11.
22 King MD, Humphrey BJ, Wang YF, Kourbatova EV, Ray SM, Blumberg HM. Emergence of community-acquired methicillin-resistant *Staphylococcus aureus* USA 300 clone as the predominant cause of skin and soft-tissue infections. Ann Intern Med 2006;144:309–17.
23 Tenover FC, McDougal LK, Goering RV *et al.* Characterization of a strain of community-associated methicillin-resistant *Staphylococcus aureus* widely disseminated in the United States. J Clin Microbiol 2006;44:108–18.
24 Salgado CD, Farr BM, Calfee DP. Community-acquired methicillin-resistant *Staphylococcus aureus*: a meta-analysis of prevalence and risk factors. Clin Infect Dis 2003;36:131–9.
25 Fridkin SK, Hageman JC, Morrison M *et al.* Methicillin-resistant *Staphylococcus aureus* disease in three communities. N Engl J Med 2005;352:1436–44.
26 Buck JM, Como-Sabetti K, Harriman KH *et al.* Community-associated methicillin-resistant *Staphylococcus aureus*, Minnesota, 2000–2003. Emerg Infect Dis 2005;11:1532–8.
27 Klevens RM, Morrison MA, Nadle J *et al.* Invasive methicillin-resistant *Staphylococcus aureus* infections in the United States. JAMA 2007;298:1763–71.
28 Sanford MD, Widmer AF, Bale MJ, Jones RN, Wenzel RP. Efficient detection and long-term persistence of the carriage of methicillin-resistant *Staphylococcus aureus*. Clin Infect Dis 1994; 19:1123–8.
29 Scanvic A, Denic L, Gaillon S, Giry P, Andremont A, Lucet JC. Duration of colonization by methicillin-resistant *Staphylococcus aureus* after hospital discharge and risk factors for prolonged carriage. Clin Infect Dis 2001;32:1393–8.
30 Klevens RM, Morrison MA, Fridkin SK *et al.* Community-associated methicillin-resistant *Staphylococcus aureus* and health-care risk factors. Emerg Infect Dis 2006;12:1991–3.
31 Otter JA, French GL. Nosocomial transmission of community-associated methicillin-resistant *Staphylococcus aureus*: an emerging threat. Lancet Infect Dis 2006;6:753–5.
32 Kourbatova EV, Halvosa JS, King MD, Ray SM, White N, Blumberg HM. Emergence of community-associated methicillin-resistant *Staphylococcus aureus* USA 300 clone as a cause of health care-associated infections among patients with prosthetic joint infections. Am J Infect Control 2005;33:385–91.
33 Seybold U, Kourbatova EV, Johnson JG *et al.* Emergence of community-associated methicillin-resistant *Staphylococcus aureus* USA300 genotype as a major cause of health care-associated blood stream infections. Clin Infect Dis 2006;42:647–56.
34 Okuma K, Iwakawa K, Turnidge JD *et al.* Dissemination of new methicillin-resistant *Staphylococcus aureus* clones in the community. J Clin Microbiol 2002;40:4289–94.
35 Lee SM, Ender M, Adhikari R, Smith JM, Berger-Bachi B, Cook GM. Fitness cost of staphylococcal cassette chromosome mec

in methicillin-resistant *Staphylococcus aureus* by way of continuous culture. Antimicrob Agents Chemother 2007;51:1497–9.

36 Centers for Disease Control and Prevention. Outbreaks of community-associated methicillin-resistant *Staphylococcus aureus* skin infections: Los Angeles County, California, 2002–2003. MMWR 2003;52:88.

37 Bratu S, Eramo A, Kopec R *et al.* Community-associated methicillin-resistant *Staphylococcus aureus* in hospital nursery and maternity units. Emerg Infect Dis 2005;11:808–13.

38 Diep BA, Sensabaugh GF, Somboona NS, Carleton HA, Perdreau-Remington F. Widespread skin and soft-tissue infections due to two methicillin-resistant *Staphylococcus aureus* strains harboring the genes for Panton–Valentine leucocidin. J Clin Microbiol 2004;42:2080–4.

39 Francis JS, Doherty MC, Lopatin U *et al.* Severe community-onset pneumonia in healthy adults caused by methicillin-resistant *Staphylococcus aureus* carrying the Panton–Valentine leukocidin genes. Clin Infect Dis 2005;40:100–7.

40 Gonzalez BE, Martinez-Aguilar G, Hulten KG *et al.* Severe staphylococcal sepsis in adolescents in the era of community-acquired methicillin-resistant *Staphylococcus aureus*. Pediatrics 2005;115:642–8.

41 Kazakova SV, Hageman JC, Matava M *et al.* A clone of methicillin-resistant *Staphylococcus aureus* among professional football players. N Engl J Med 2005;352:468–75.

42 Miller LG, Perdreau-Remington F, Rieg G *et al.* Necrotizing fasciitis caused by community-associated methicillin-resistant *Staphylococcus aureus* in Los Angeles. N Engl J Med 2005;352:1445–53.

43 Bocchini CE, Hulten KG, Mason EO Jr, Gonzalez BE, Hammerman WA, Kaplan SL. Panton–Valentine leukocidin genes are associated with enhanced inflammatory response and local disease in acute hematogenous *Staphylococcus aureus* osteomyelitis in children. Pediatrics 2006;117:433–40.

44 Pannaraj PS, Hulten KG, Gonzalez BE, Mason EO Jr, Kaplan SL. Infective pyomyositis and myositis in children in the era of community-acquired, methicillin-resistant *Staphylococcus aureus* infection. Clin Infect Dis 2006;43:953–60.

45 Gonzalez BE, Hulten KG, Dishop MK *et al.* Pulmonary manifestations in children with invasive community-acquired *Staphylococcus aureus* infection. Clin Infect Dis 2005;41:583–90.

46 Dehority W, Wang E, Vernon PS, Lee C, Perdreau-Remington F, Bradley J. Community-associated methicillin-resistant *Staphylococcus aureus* necrotizing fasciitis in a neonate. Pediatr Infect Dis J 2006;25:1080–1.

47 Diep BA, Gill SR, Chang RF *et al.* Complete genome sequence of USA300, an epidemic clone of community-acquired methicillin-resistant *Staphylococcus aureus*. Lancet 2006;367:731–9.

48 Baba T, Takeuchi F, Kuroda M *et al.* Genome and virulence determinants of high virulence community-acquired MRSA. Lancet 2002;359:1819–27.

49 Groom AV, Wolsey DH, Naimi TS *et al.* Community-acquired methicillin-resistant *Staphylococcus aureus* in a rural American Indian community. JAMA 2001;286:1201–5.

50 Fey PD, Said-Salim B, Rupp ME *et al.* Comparative molecular analysis of community- or hospital-acquired methicillin-resistant *Staphylococcus aureus*. Antimicrob Agents Chemother 2003;47:196–203.

51 Enright MC, Robinson DA, Randle G, Feil EJ, Grundmann H, Spratt BG. The evolutionary history of methicillin-resistant *Staphylococcus aureus* (MRSA). Proc Natl Acad Sci USA 2002;99:7687–92.

52 Pan ES, Diep BA, Carleton HA *et al.* Increasing prevalence of methicillin-resistant *Staphylococcus aureus* infection in California jails. Clin Infect Dis 2003;37:1384–8.

53 Hota B, Ellenbogen C, Hayden MK, Aroutcheva A, Rice TW, Weinstein RA. Community-associated methicillin-resistant *Staphylococcus aureus* skin and soft tissue infections at a public hospital: do public housing and incarceration amplify transmission? Arch Intern Med 2007;167:1026–33.

54 Carleton HA, Diep BA, Charlebois ED, Sensabaugh GF, Perdreau-Remington F. Community-adapted methicillin-resistant *Staphylococcus aureus* (MRSA): population dynamics of an expanding community reservoir of MRSA. J Infect Dis 2004;190:1730–8.

55 Purcell K, Fergie J. Epidemic of community-acquired methicillin-resistant *Staphylococcus aureus* infections: a 14-year study at Driscoll Children's Hospital. Arch Pediatr Adolesc Med 2005;159:980–5.

56 Kaplan SL, Hulten KG, Gonzalez BE *et al.* Three-year surveillance of community-acquired *Staphylococcus aureus* infections in children. Clin Infect Dis 2005;40:1785–91.

57 Mathews WC, Caperna JC, Barber RE *et al.* Incidence of and risk factors for clinically significant methicillin-resistant *Staphylococcus aureus* infection in a cohort of HIV-infected adults. J Acquir Immune Defic Syndr 2005;40:155–60.

58 Aiello AE, Lowy FD, Wright LN, Larson EL. Meticillin-resistant *Staphylococcus aureus* among US prisoners and military personnel: review and recommendations for future studies. Lancet Infect Dis 2006;6:335–41.

59 Campbell KM, Vaughn AF, Russell KL *et al.* Risk factors for community-associated methicillin-resistant *Staphylococcus aureus* infections in an outbreak of disease among military trainees in San Diego, California, in 2002. J Clin Microbiol 2004;42:4050–3.

60 Zinderman CE, Conner B, Malakooti MA, LaMar JE, Armstrong A, Bohnker BK. Community-acquired methicillin-resistant *Staphylococcus aureus* among military recruits. Emerg Infect Dis 2004;10:941–4.

61 Centers for Disease Control and Prevention. Methicillin-resistant *Staphylococcus aureus* infections in correctional facilities: Georgia, California, and Texas, 2001–2003. MMWR 2003;52:992–6.

62 Centers for Disease Control and Prevention. Methicillin-resistant *Staphylococcus aureus* skin or soft tissue infections in a state prison: Mississippi, 2000. MMWR 2001;50:919–22.

63 Frazee BW, Lynn J, Charlebois ED, Lambert L, Lowery D, Perdreau-Remington F. High prevalence of methicillin-resistant *Staphylococcus aureus* in emergency department skin and soft tissue infections. Ann Emerg Med 2005;45:311–20.

64 Maree CL, Daum RS, Boyle-Vavra S, Matayoshi K, Miller LG. Community-associated methicillin-resistant *Staphylococcus aureus* isolates causing healthcare-associated infections. Emerg Infect Dis 2007;13:236–42.

65 Nguyen DM, Mascola L, Brancoft E. Recurring methicillin-resistant *Staphylococcus aureus* infections in a football team. Emerg Infect Dis 2005;11:526–32.

66 Begier EM, Frenette K, Barrett NL *et al.* A high-morbidity outbreak of methicillin-resistant *Staphylococcus aureus* among players on a college football team, facilitated by cosmetic body shaving and turf burns. Clin Infect Dis 2004;39:1446–53.

67 Baggett HC, Hennessy TW, Rudolph K *et al.* Community-onset methicillin-resistant *Staphylococcus aureus* associated with antibiotic use and the cytotoxin Panton–Valentine leukocidin during a furunculosis outbreak in rural Alaska. J Infect Dis 2004;189: 1565–73.

68 Lee NE, Taylor MM, Bancroft E *et al.* Risk factors for community-associated methicillin-resistant *Staphylococcus aureus* skin infections among HIV-positive men who have sex with men. Clin Infect Dis 2005;40:1529–34.

69 Cook HA, Furuya EY, Larson E, Vasquez G, Lowy FD. Heterosexual transmission of community-associated methicillin-resistant *Staphylococcus aureus*. Clin Infect Dis 2007;44:410–13.

70 Roberts JR, McCawley L, Laxton M, Trumbo H. Genital community-associated methicillin resistant *Staphylococcus aureus* infection can be a sexually transmitted disease. Ann Emerg Med 2007;50:93–4.

71 Fortunov RM, Hulten KG, Hammerman WA, Mason EO Jr, Kaplan SL. Community-acquired *Staphylococcus aureus* infections in term and near-term previously healthy neonates. Pediatrics 2006;118:874–81.

72 Jones TF, Creech CB, Erwin P, Baird SG, Woron AM, Schaffner W. Family outbreaks of invasive community-associated methicillin-resistant *Staphylococcus aureus* infection. Clin Infect Dis 2006;42:e76–e78.

73 Huijsdens XW, van Santen-Verheuvel MG, Spalburg E *et al.* Multiple cases of familial transmission of community-acquired methicillin-resistant *Staphylococcus aureus*. J Clin Microbiol 2006; 44:2994–6.

74 L'Heriteau F, Lucet JC, Scanvic A, Bouvet E. Community-acquired methicillin-resistant *Staphylococcus aureus* and familial transmission. JAMA 1999;282:1038–9.

75 Faden H, Ferguson S. Community-acquired methicillin-resistant *Staphylococcus aureus* and intrafamily spread of pustular disease. Pediatr Infect Dis J 2001;20:554–5.

76 Turabelidze G, Lin M, Wolkoff B, Dodson D, Gladbach S, Zhu BP. Personal hygiene and methicillin-resistant *Staphylococcus aureus* infection. Emerg Infect Dis 2006;12:422–7.

77 Gilbert M, MacDonald J, Gregson D *et al.* Outbreak in Alberta of community-acquired (USA300) methicillin-resistant *Staphylococcus aureus* in people with a history of drug use, homelessness or incarceration. Can Med Assoc J 2006;175:149–54.

78 Huang H, Flynn NM, King JH, Monchaud C, Morita M, Cohen SH. Comparisons of community-associated methicillin-resistant *Staphylococcus aureus* (MRSA) and hospital-associated MSRA infections in Sacramento, California. J Clin Microbiol 2006;44: 2423–7.

79 Miller LG, Perdreau-Remington F, Bayer AS *et al.* Clinical and epidemiologic characteristics cannot distinguish community-associated methicillin-resistant *Staphylococcus aureus* infection from methicillin-susceptible *S. aureus* infection: a prospective investigation. Clin Infect Dis 2007;44:471–82.

80 Hidron AI, Kourbatova EV, Halvosa JS *et al.* Risk factors for colonization with methicillin-resistant *Staphylococcus aureus* (MRSA) in patients admitted to an urban hospital: emergence of community-associated MRSA nasal carriage. Clin Infect Dis 2005;41:159–66.

81 Ellis MW, Hospenthal DR, Dooley DP, Gray PJ, Murray CK. Natural history of community-acquired methicillin-resistant *Staphylococcus aureus* colonization and infection in soldiers. Clin Infect Dis 2004;39:971–9.

82 Dietrich DW, Auld DB, Mermel LA. Community-acquired methicillin-resistant *Staphylococcus aureus* in southern New England children. Pediatrics 2004;113:e347–e352.

83 Muder RR, Brennen C, Wagener MM *et al.* Methicillin-resistant staphylococcal colonization and infection in a long-term care facility. Ann Intern Med 1991;114:107–12.

84 Linde H, Wagenlehner F, Strommenger B *et al.* Healthcare-associated outbreaks and community-acquired infections due to MRSA carrying the Panton–Valentine leucocidin gene in southeastern Germany. Eur J Clin Microbiol Infect Dis 2005;24: 419–22.

85 O'Brien FG, Pearman JW, Gracey M, Riley TV, Grubb WB. Community strain of methicillin-resistant *Staphylococcus aureus* involved in a hospital outbreak. J Clin Microbiol 1999;37:2858–62.

86 Healy CM, Hulten KG, Palazzi DL, Campbell JR, Baker CJ. Emergence of new strains of methicillin-resistant *Staphylococcus aureus* in a neonatal intensive care unit. Clin Infect Dis 2004;39: 1460–6.

87 Popovich KJ, Weinstein RA, Hota B. Are community-associated methicillin-resistant *Staphylococcus aureus* (MRSA) strains replacing traditional nosocomial MRSA strains? Clin Infect Dis 2008;46:787–94.

88 Liu C, Graber CJ, Karr M *et al.* A population-based study of the incidence and molecular epidemiology of methicillin-resistant *Staphylococcus aureus* disease in San Francisco, 2004–2005. Clin Infect Dis 2008;46:1637–46.

89 Kaneko J, Kamio Y. Bacterial two-component and hetero-heptameric pore-forming cytolytic toxins: structures, pore-forming mechanism, and organization of the genes. Biosci Biotechnol Biochem 2004;68:981–1003.

90 Guillet V, Roblin P, Werner S *et al.* Crystal structure of leucotoxin S component: new insight into the staphylococcal beta-barrel pore-forming toxins. J Biol Chem 2004;279:41028–37.

91 Gravet A, Colin DA, Keller D, Girardot R, Monteil H, Prevost G. Characterization of a novel structural member, LukE-LukD, of the bi-component staphylococcal leucotoxins family. FEBS Lett 1998;436:202–8.

92 Panton PN, Valentine FCO. Staphylococcal toxin. Lancet 1932; 222:506–8.

93 Valentine FCO. Further observations on the role of toxin in staphylococcal infection. Lancet 1936;230:526–31.

94 Lina G, Piemont Y, Godail-Gamot F *et al.* Involvement of Panton–Valentine leukocidin-producing *Staphylococcus aureus* in primary skin infections and pneumonia. Clin Infect Dis 1999;29:1128–32.

95 Gillet Y, Issartel B, Vanhems P *et al.* Association between *Staphylococcus aureus* strains carrying gene for Panton–Valentine leukocidin and highly lethal necrotising pneumonia in young immunocompetent patients. Lancet 2002;359:753–9.

96 Vandenesch F, Naimi T, Enright MC *et al.* Community-acquired methicillin-resistant *Staphylococcus aureus* carrying Panton–Valentine leukocidin genes: worldwide emergence. Emerg Infect Dis 2003;9:978–84.

97 Prevost G, Couppie P, Prevost P *et al.* Epidemiological data on *Staphylococcus aureus* strains producing synergohymenotropic toxins. J Med Microbiol 1995;42:237–45.

98 Kuehnert MJ, Kruszon-Moran D, Hill HA *et al.* Prevalence of *Staphylococcus aureus* nasal colonization in the United States, 2001–2002. J Infect Dis 2006;193:172–9.

99 Voyich JM, Otto M, Mathema B *et al.* Is Panton–Valentine leukocidin the major virulence determinant in community-associated methicillin-resistant *Staphylococcus aureus* disease? J Infect Dis 2006;194:1761–70.
100 Gladstone GP, van Heyningen WE. Staphylococcal leukocidins. Br J Exp Pathol 1957;38:123–37.
101 Szmigielski S, Prevost G, Monteil H, Colin DA, Jeljaszewicz J. Leukocidal toxins of staphylococci. Zentralbl Bakteriol 1999; 289:185–201.
102 Labandeira-Rey M, Couzon F, Boisset S *et al.* *Staphylococcus aureus* Panton–Valentine leukocidin causes necrotizing pneumonia. Science 2007;315:1130–3.
103 Horsburgh MJ, Aish JL, White IJ, Shaw L, Lithgow JK, Foster SJ. sigma B modulates virulence determinant expression and stress resistance: characterization of a functional rsbU strain derived from *Staphylococcus aureus* 8325–4. J Bacteriol 2002; 184:5457–67.
104 Goering RV, McDougal LK, Fosheim GE, Bonnstetter KK, Wolter DJ, Tenover FC. Epidemiologic distribution of the arginine catabolic mobile element among selected methicillin-resistant and methicillin-susceptible *Staphylococcus aureus* isolates. J Clin Microbiol 2007;45:1981–4.
105 Ruhe JJ, Smith N, Bradsher RW, Menon A. Community-onset methicillin-resistant *Staphylococcus aureus* skin and soft-tissue infections: impact of antimicrobial therapy on outcome. Clin Infect Dis 2007;44:777–84.
106 Iyer S, Jones DH. Community-acquired methicillin-resistant *Staphylococcus aureus* skin infection: a retrospective analysis of clinical presentation and treatment of a local outbreak. J Am Acad Dermatol 2004;50:854–8.
107 Dominguez TJ. It's not a spider bite, it's community-acquired methicillin-resistant *Staphylococcus aureus*. J Am Board Fam Pract 2004;17:220–6.
108 Fagan SP, Berger DH, Rahwan K, Awad SS. Spider bites presenting with methicillin-resistant *Staphylococcus aureus* soft tissue infection require early aggressive treatment. Surg Infect (Larchmt) 2003;4:311–15.
109 Miller LG, Spellberg B. Spider bites and infections caused by community-associated methicillin-resistant *Staphylococcus aureus*. Surg Infect (Larchmt) 2004;5:321–2; author reply 322.
110 Lee MC, Rios AM, Aten MF *et al.* Management and outcome of children with skin and soft tissue abscesses caused by community-acquired methicillin-resistant *Staphylococcus aureus*. Pediatr Infect Dis J 2004;23:123–7.
111 Miller LG, Quan C, Shay A *et al.* A prospective investigation of outcomes after hospital discharge for endemic, community-acquired methicillin-resistant and -susceptible *Staphylococcus aureus* skin infection. Clin Infect Dis 2007;44:483–92.
112 Anderson EJ, Hawkins C, Bolon MK, Palella FJ Jr. A series of skin and soft tissue infections due to methicillin-resistant *Staphylococcus aureus* in HIV-infected patients. J Acquir Immune Defic Syndr 2006;41:125–7.
113 Skiest D, Brown K, Hester J *et al.* Community-onset methicillin-resistant *Staphylococcus aureus* in an urban HIV clinic. HIV Med 2006;7:361–8.
114 Crum-Cianflone NF, Burgi AA, Hale BR. Increasing rates of community-acquired methicillin-resistant *Staphylococcus aureus* infections among HIV-infected persons. Int J STD AIDS 2007; 18:521–6.
115 Shastry L, Rahimian J, Lascher S. Community-associated methicillin-resistant *Staphylococcus aureus* skin and soft tissue infections in men who have sex with men in New York City. Arch Intern Med 2007;167:854–7.
116 Chi CY, Wang SM, Lin HC, Liu CC. A clinical and microbiological comparison of *Staphylococcus aureus* toxic shock and scalded skin syndromes in children. Clin Infect Dis 2006;42:181–5.
117 Kravitz GR, Dries DJ, Peterson ML, Schlievert PM. Purpura fulminans due to *Staphylococcus aureus*. Clin Infect Dis 2005;40: 941–7.
118 Adem PV, Montgomery CP, Husain AN *et al.* *Staphylococcus aureus* sepsis and the Waterhouse–Friderichsen syndrome in children. N Engl J Med 2005;353:1245–51.
119 Arnold SR, Elias D, Buckingham SC *et al.* Changing patterns of acute hematogenous osteomyelitis and septic arthritis: emergence of community-associated methicillin-resistant *Staphylococcus aureus*. J Pediatr Orthop 2006;26:703–8.
120 Chiedozi LC. Pyomyositis. Review of 205 cases in 112 patients. Am J Surg 1979;137:255–9.
121 Adamski GB, Garin EH, Ballinger WE, Shulman ST. Generalized nonsuppurative myositis with staphylococcal septicemia. J Pediatr 1980;96:694–7.
122 Sdougkos G, Chini V, Papanastasiou DA *et al.* Methicillin-resistant *Staphylococcus aureus* producing Panton–Valentine leukocidin as a cause of acute osteomyelitis in children. Clin Microbiol Infect 2007;13:651–4.
123 Gonzalez BE, Teruya J, Mahoney DH Jr *et al.* Venous thrombosis associated with staphylococcal osteomyelitis in children. Pediatrics 2006;117:1673–9.
124 Stevens DL, Bisno AL, Chambers HF *et al.* Practice guidelines for the diagnosis and management of skin and soft-tissue infections. Clin Infect Dis 2005;41:1373–406.
125 Rutar T, Chambers HF, Crawford JB *et al.* Ophthalmic manifestations of infections caused by the USA300 clone of community-associated methicillin-resistant *Staphylococcus aureus*. Ophthalmology 2006;113:1455–62.
126 Bahrain M, Vasiliades M, Wolff M, Younus F. Five cases of bacterial endocarditis after furunculosis and the ongoing saga of community-acquired methicillin-resistant *Staphylococcus aureus* infections. Scand J Infect Dis 2006;38:702–7.
127 Rutar T, Zwick OM, Cockerham KP, Horton JC. Bilateral blindness from orbital cellulitis caused by community-acquired methicillin-resistant *Staphylococcus aureus*. Am J Ophthalmol 2005;140:740–2.
128 Bartlett JG, Mundy LM. Community-acquired pneumonia. N Engl J Med 1995;333:1618–24.
129 Chastre J, Fagon JY. Ventilator-associated pneumonia. Am J Respir Crit Care Med 2002;165:867–903.
130 Hageman JC, Uyeki TM, Francis JS *et al.* Severe community-acquired pneumonia due to *Staphylococcus aureus*, 2003–04 influenza season. Emerg Infect Dis 2006;12:894–9.
131 Dufour P, Gillet Y, Bes M *et al.* Community-acquired methicillin-resistant *Staphylococcus aureus* infections in France: emergence of a single clone that produces Panton–Valentine leukocidin. Clin Infect Dis 2002;35:819–24.
132 Mongkolrattanothai K, Boyle S, Kahana MD, Daum RS. Severe *Staphylococcus aureus* infections caused by clonally related community-acquired methicillin-susceptible and methicillin-resistant isolates. Clin Infect Dis 2003;37:1050–8.

133 Haque NZ, Davis SL, Manierski CL *et al*. Infective endocarditis caused by USA300 methicillin-resistant *Staphylococcus aureus* (MRSA). Int J Antimicrob Agents 2007;30:72–7.

134 Gillet Y, Vanhems P, Lina G *et al*. Factors predicting mortality in necrotizing community-acquired pneumonia caused by *Staphylococcus aureus* containing Panton–Valentine leukocidin. Clin Infect Dis 2007;45:315–21.

135 Mandell LA, Wunderink RG, Anzueto A *et al*. Infectious Diseases Society of America/American Thoracic Society consensus guidelines on the management of community-acquired pneumonia in adults. Clin Infect Dis 2007;44(suppl 2):S27–S72.

136 Naimi TS, LeDell KH, Boxrud DJ *et al*. Epidemiology and clonality of community-acquired methicillin-resistant *Staphylococcus aureus* in Minnesota, 1996–1998. Clin Infect Dis 2001;33:990–6.

137 Murray RJ, Lim TT, Pearson JC, Grubb WB, Lum GD. Community-onset methicillin-resistant *Staphylococcus aureus* bacteremia in Northern Australia. Int J Infect Dis 2004;8:275–83.

138 Wang JL, Chen SY, Wang JT *et al*. Comparison of both clinical features and mortality risk associated with bacteremia due to community-acquired methicillin-resistant *Staphylococcus aureus* and methicillin-susceptible *S. aureus*. Clin Infect Dis 2008;46: 799–806.

139 Popovich K, Hota B, Rice T, Aroutcheva A, Weinstein RA. Phenotypic prediction rule for community-associated methicillin-resistant *Staphylococcus aureus*. J Clin Microbiol 2007;45: 2293–5.

140 Berglund C, Molling P, Sjoberg L, Soderquist B. Multilocus sequence typing of methicillin-resistant *Staphylococcus aureus* from an area of low endemicity by real-time PCR. J Clin Microbiol 2005;43:4448–54.

141 Johnsson D, Molling P, Stralin K, Soderquist B. Detection of Panton–Valentine leukocidin gene in *Staphylococcus aureus* by LightCycler PCR: clinical and epidemiological aspects. Clin Microbiol Infect 2004;10:884–9.

142 McDonald RR, Antonishyn NA, Hansen T *et al*. Development of a triplex real-time PCR assay for detection of Panton–Valentine leukocidin toxin genes in clinical isolates of methicillin-resistant *Staphylococcus aureus*. J Clin Microbiol 2005;43:6147–9.

143 Llera JL, Levy RC. Treatment of cutaneous abscess: a double-blind clinical study. Ann Emerg Med 1985;14:15–19.

144 Cohen PR, Kurzrock R. Community-acquired methicillin-resistant *Staphylococcus aureus* skin infection: an emerging clinical problem. J Am Acad Dermatol 2004;50:277–80.

145 Rajendran PM, Young D, Maurer T *et al*. Randomized, double-blind, placebo-controlled trial of cephalexin for treatment of uncomplicated skin abscesses in a population at risk for community methicillin-resistant *Staphylococcus aureus* infection. Antimicrob Agents Chemother 2007;51:4044–8.

146 Young DM, Harris HW, Charlebois ED *et al*. An epidemic of methicillin-resistant *Staphylococcus aureus* soft tissue infections among medically underserved patients. Arch Surg 2004;139: 947–51; discussion 951–3.

147 Rajendran PM, Young DM, Maurer T, Chambers HF, Jacobson MA, Harris HW. Antibiotic use in the treatment of soft tissue abscesses: a survey of current practice. Surg Infect (Larchmt) 2007;8:237–8.

148 Gorwitz RJ, Powers JH, Jernigan JA, and Participants in the CDC-Convened Experts' Meeting on Management of MRSA in the Community. Strategies for clinical management of MRSA in the community: summary of a meeting convened by the Centers for Disease Control and Prevention, 2006. http://www.cdc.gov/ncidod/dhqp/pdf/ar/CAMRSA_ExpMtgStrategies.pdf.

149 Kaplan SL. Treatment of community-associated methicillin-resistant *Staphylococcus aureus* infections. Pediatr Infect Dis J 2005;24:457–8.

150 Swartz MN. Clinical practice. Cellulitis. N Engl J Med 2004;350: 904–12.

151 Martinez-Aguilar G, Hammerman WA, Mason EO Jr, Kaplan SL. Clindamycin treatment of invasive infections caused by community-acquired, methicillin-resistant and methicillin-susceptible *Staphylococcus aureus* in children. Pediatr Infect Dis J 2003;22:593–8.

152 Frank AL, Marcinak JF, Mangat PD *et al*. Clindamycin treatment of methicillin-resistant *Staphylococcus aureus* infections in children. Pediatr Infect Dis J 2002;21:530–4.

153 Han LL, McDougal LK, Gorwitz RJ *et al*. High frequencies of clindamycin and tetracycline resistance in methicillin-resistant *Staphylococcus aureus* pulsed-field type USA300 isolates collected at a Boston ambulatory health center. J Clin Microbiol 2007;45:1350–2.

154 Braun L, Craft D, Williams R, Tuamokumo F, Ottolini M. Increasing clindamycin resistance among methicillin-resistant *Staphylococcus aureus* in 57 northeast United States military treatment facilities. Pediatr Infect Dis J 2005;24:622–6.

155 Hulten KG, Kaplan SL, Gonzalez BE *et al*. Three-year surveillance of community onset health care-associated *Staphylococcus aureus* infections in children. Pediatr Infect Dis J 2006;25:349–53.

156 Diep BA, Chambers HF, Graber CJ *et al*. Emergence of multidrug-resistant, community-associated, methicillin-resistant *Staphylococcus aureus* clone USA300 in men who have sex with men. Ann Intern Med 2008;148:249–57.

157 Lewis JS II, Jorgensen JH. Inducible clindamycin resistance in staphylococci: should clinicians and microbiologists be concerned? Clin Infect Dis 2005;40:280–5.

158 Chavez-Bueno S, Bozdogan B, Katz K *et al*. Inducible clindamycin resistance and molecular epidemiologic trends of pediatric community-acquired methicillin-resistant *Staphylococcus aureus* in Dallas, Texas. Antimicrob Agents Chemother 2005;49:2283–8.

159 Daum RS. Clinical practice. Skin and soft-tissue infections caused by methicillin-resistant *Staphylococcus aureus*. N Engl J Med 2007;357:380–90.

160 Panagea S, Perry JD, Gould FK. Should clindamycin be used as treatment of patients with infections caused by erythromycin-resistant staphylococci? J Antimicrob Chemother 1999;44:581–2.

161 Siberry GK, Tekle T, Carroll K, Dick J. Failure of clindamycin treatment of methicillin-resistant *Staphylococcus aureus* expressing inducible clindamycin resistance in vitro. Clin Infect Dis 2003;37:1257–60.

162 Watanakunakorn C. Clindamycin therapy of *Staphylococcus aureus* endocarditis. Clinical relapse and development of resistance to clindamycin, lincomycin and erythromycin. Am J Med 1976;60:419–25.

163 Levin TP, Suh B, Axelrod P, Truant AL, Fekete T. Potential clindamycin resistance in clindamycin-susceptible, erythromycin-resistant *Staphylococcus aureus*: report of a clinical failure. Antimicrob Agents Chemother 2005;49:1222–4.

164 Minuth JN, Holmes TM, Musher DM. Activity of tetracycline, doxycycline, and minocycline against methicillin-susceptible and -resistant staphylococci. Antimicrob Agents Chemother 1974;6:411–14.
165 Ruhe JJ, Menon A. Tetracyclines as an oral treatment option for patients with community-onset methicillin-resistant *Staphylococcus aureus* skin and soft-tissue infections. Antimicrob Agents Chemother 2007;51:3298–303.
166 Ruhe JJ, Monson T, Bradsher RW, Menon A. Use of long-acting tetracyclines for methicillin-resistant *Staphylococcus aureus* infections: case series and review of the literature. Clin Infect Dis 2005;40:1429–34.
167 Trzcinski K, Cooper BS, Hryniewicz W, Dowson CG. Expression of resistance to tetracyclines in strains of methicillin-resistant *Staphylococcus aureus*. J Antimicrob Chemother 2000; 45:763–70.
168 Bismuth R, Zilhao R, Sakamoto H, Guesdon JL, Courvalin P. Gene heterogeneity for tetracycline resistance in *Staphylococcus* spp. Antimicrob Agents Chemother 1990;34:1611–14.
169 Kaka AS, Rueda AM, Shelburne SA III, Hulten K, Hamill RJ, Musher DM. Bactericidal activity of orally available agents against methicillin-resistant *Staphylococcus aureus*. J Antimicrob Chemother 2006;58:680–3.
170 Cenizal MJ, Skiest D, Luber S *et al.* Prospective randomized trial of empiric therapy with trimethoprim–sulfamethoxazole or doxycycline for outpatient skin and soft tissue infections in an area of high prevalence of methicillin-resistant *Staphylococcus aureus*. Antimicrob Agents Chemother 2007;51:2628–30.
171 Szumowski JD, Cohen DE, Kanaya F, Mayer KH. Treatment and outcomes of infections by methicillin-resistant *Staphylococcus aureus* at an ambulatory clinic. Antimicrob Agents Chemother 2007;51:423–8.
172 Markowitz N, Quinn EL, Saravolatz LD. Trimethoprim–sulfamethoxazole compared with vancomycin for the treatment of *Staphylococcus aureus* infection. Ann Intern Med 1992; 117:390–8.
173 Szumowski JD, Cohen DE, Kanaya F, Mayer KH. Treatment and outcomes of methicillin-resistant *Staphylococcus aureus* MRSA infections at an ambulatory clinic. Antimicrob Agents Chemother 2007;51:423–8.
174 Kerry DW, Hamilton-Miller JM, Brumfitt W. Trimethoprim and rifampicin: in vitro activities separately and in combination. J Antimicrob Chemother 1975;1:417–27.
175 Libertin CR, Wold AD, Washington JA II. Effects of trimethoprim–sulfamethoxazole and incubation atmosphere on isolation of group A streptococci. J Clin Microbiol 1983;18:680–2.
176 Kunin CM, Brandt D, Wood H. Bacteriologic studies of rifampin, a new semisynthetic antibiotic. J Infect Dis 1969;119: 132–7.
177 Baddour LM, Wilson WR, Bayer AS *et al.* Infective endocarditis: diagnosis, antimicrobial therapy, and management of complications: a statement for healthcare professionals from the Committee on Rheumatic Fever, Endocarditis, and Kawasaki Disease, Council on Cardiovascular Disease in the Young, and the Councils on Clinical Cardiology, Stroke, and Cardiovascular Surgery and Anesthesia, American Heart Association: endorsed by the Infectious Diseases Society of America. Circulation 2005;111:e394–e434.
178 Zimmerli W, Widmer AF, Blatter M, Frei R, Ochsner PE. Role of rifampin for treatment of orthopedic implant-related staphylococcal infections: a randomized controlled trial. Foreign-Body Infection (FBI) Study Group. JAMA 1998;279:1537–41.
179 Levine DP, Fromm BS, Reddy BR. Slow response to vancomycin or vancomycin plus rifampin in methicillin-resistant *Staphylococcus aureus* endocarditis. Ann Intern Med 1991;115: 674–80.
180 Le J, Lieberman JM. Management of community-associated methicillin-resistant *Staphylococcus aureus* infections in children. Pharmacotherapy 2006;26:1758–70.
181 Segreti J, Gvazdinskas LC, Trenholme GM. In vitro activity of minocycline and rifampin against staphylococci. Diagn Microbiol Infect Dis 1989;12:253–5.
182 Kang SL, Rybak MJ, McGrath BJ, Kaatz GW, Seo SM. Pharmacodynamics of levofloxacin, ofloxacin, and ciprofloxacin, alone and in combination with rifampin, against methicillin-susceptible and -resistant *Staphylococcus aureus* in an in vitro infection model. Antimicrob Agents Chemother 1994;38:2702–9.
183 Piercy EA, Barbaro D, Luby JP, Mackowiak PA. Ciprofloxacin for methicillin-resistant *Staphylococcus aureus* infections. Antimicrob Agents Chemother 1989;33:128–30.
184 Blumberg HM, Rimland D, Carroll DJ, Terry P, Wachsmuth IK. Rapid development of ciprofloxacin resistance in methicillin-susceptible and -resistant *Staphylococcus aureus*. J Infect Dis 1991;163:1279–85.
185 Stevens DL, Herr D, Lampiris H, Hunt JL, Batts DH, Hafkin B. Linezolid versus vancomycin for the treatment of methicillin-resistant *Staphylococcus aureus* infections. Clin Infect Dis 2002; 34:1481–90.
186 Weigelt J, Itani K, Stevens D, Lau W, Dryden M, Knirsch C. Linezolid versus vancomycin in treatment of complicated skin and soft tissue infections. Antimicrob Agents Chemother 2005; 49:2260–6.
187 Lipsky BA, Itani K, Norden C. Treating foot infections in diabetic patients: a randomized, multicenter, open-label trial of linezolid versus ampicillin–sulbactam/amoxicillin–clavulanate. Clin Infect Dis 2004;38:17–24.
188 Wible K, Tregnaghi M, Bruss J, Fleishaker D, Naberhuis-Stehouwer S, Hilty M. Linezolid versus cefadroxil in the treatment of skin and skin structure infections in children. Pediatr Infect Dis J 2003;22:315–23.
189 Kaplan SL, Afghani B, Lopez P *et al.* Linezolid for the treatment of methicillin-resistant *Staphylococcus aureus* infections in children. Pediatr Infect Dis J 2003;22:S178–S185.
190 Peeters MJ, Sarria JC. Clinical characteristics of linezolid-resistant *Staphylococcus aureus* infections. Am J Med Sci 2005; 330:102–4.
191 Meka VG, Pillai SK, Sakoulas G *et al.* Linezolid resistance in sequential *Staphylococcus aureus* isolates associated with a T2500A mutation in the 23S rRNA gene and loss of a single copy of rRNA. J Infect Dis 2004;190:311–17.
192 Gerson SL, Kaplan SL, Bruss JB *et al.* Hematologic effects of linezolid: summary of clinical experience. Antimicrob Agents Chemother 2002;46:2723–6.
193 Apodaca AA, Rakita RM. Linezolid-induced lactic acidosis. N Engl J Med 2003;348:86–7.
194 De Vriese AS, Coster RV, Smet J *et al.* Linezolid-induced inhibition of mitochondrial protein synthesis. Clin Infect Dis 2006;42:1111–17.
195 Arbeit RD, Maki D, Tally FP, Campanaro E, Eisenstein BI. The safety and efficacy of daptomycin for the treatment of

complicated skin and skin-structure infections. Clin Infect Dis 2004;38:1673–81.

196 Ellis-Grosse EJ, Babinchak T, Dartois N, Rose G, Loh E. The efficacy and safety of tigecycline in the treatment of skin and skin-structure infections: results of 2 double-blind phase 3 comparison studies with vancomycin–aztreonam. Clin Infect Dis 2005;41(suppl 5):S341–S353.

197 Wang G, Hindler JF, Ward KW, Bruckner DA. Increased vancomycin MICs for *Staphylococcus aureus* clinical isolates from a university hospital during a 5-year period. J Clin Microbiol 2006;44:3883–6.

198 Steinkraus G, White R, Friedrich L. Vancomycin MIC creep in non-vancomycin-intermediate *Staphylococcus aureus* (VISA), vancomycin-susceptible clinical methicillin-resistant *S. aureus* (MRSA) blood isolates from 2001–05. J Antimicrob Chemother 2007;60:788–94.

199 Graber C, Wong M, Carleton HA, Perdreau-Remington F, Haller B, Chambers HF. Intermediate vancomycin susceptibility in a community-associated MRSA clone. Emerg Infect Dis 2007;13:491–3.

200 Ellis MW, Griffith ME, Dooley DP *et al.* Targeted intranasal mupirocin to prevent colonization and infection by community-associated methicillin-resistant *Staphylococcus aureus* strains in soldiers: a cluster randomized controlled trial. Antimicrob Agents Chemother 2007;51:3591–8.

201 Rahimian J, Khan R, LaScalea KA. Does nasal colonization or mupirocin treatment affect recurrence of methicillin-resistant *Staphylococcus aureus* skin and skin structure infections? Infect Control Hosp Epidemiol 2007;28:1415–16.

202 Yang ES. Body Site Colonization Prevalence in Patients with Community-Associated Methicillin-Resistant *Staphylococcus aureus* Infections. Infectious Diseases Society of America. San Diego, CA, October, 2007. Abstract 285.

203 Centers for Disease Control and Prevention. Methicillin-resistant *Staphylococcus aureus* infections among competitive sports participants: Colorado, Indiana, Pennsylvania, and Los Angeles County, 2000–2003. MMWR 2003;52:793–5.

204 Charlebois ED, Bangsberg DR, Moss NJ *et al.* Population-based community prevalence of methicillin-resistant *Staphylococcus aureus* in the urban poor of San Francisco. Clin Infect Dis 2002; 34:425–33.

205 Centers for Disease Control and Prevention. Severe methicillin-resistant *Staphylococcus aureus* community-acquired pneumonia associated with influenza: Louisiana and Georgia, December 2006 to January 2007. MMWR 2007;56:325–9.

206 Tsigrelis C, Armstrong MD, Vlahakis NE, Batsis JA, Baddour LM. Infective endocarditis due to community-associated methicillin-resistant *Staphylococcus aureus* in injection drug users may be associated with Panton–Valentine leukocidin-negative strains. Scand J Infect Dis 2007;39:299–302.

207 Borer A, Gilad J, Yagupsky P *et al.* Community-acquired methicillin-resistant *Staphylococcus aureus* in institutionalized adults with developmental disabilities. Emerg Infect Dis 2002;8:966–70.

208 Centers for Disease Control and Prevention. Methicillin-resistant *Staphylococcus aureus* skin infections among tattoo recipients: Ohio, Kentucky, and Vermont, 2004–2005. MMWR 2006;55: 677–9.

209 Baggett HC, Hennessy TW, Leman R *et al.* An outbreak of community-onset methicillin-resistant *Staphylococcus aureus* skin infections in southwestern Alaska. Infect Control Hosp Epidemiol 2003;24:397–402.

210 Saiman L, O'Keefe M, Graham PL III *et al.* Hospital transmission of community-acquired methicillin-resistant *Staphylococcus aureus* among postpartum women. Clin Infect Dis 2003;37: 1313–19.

211 Centers for Disease Control and Prevention. Community-associated methicillin-resistant *Staphylococcus aureus* infections in Pacific Islanders: Hawaii, 2001–2003. MMWR 2004;53:767–70.

Section IV
Prevention and Treatment of Staphylococcal Infections

Chapter 30
Elimination of *Staphylococcus aureus* Carriage: Importance and Strategies

Loreen A. Herwaldt[1] *and John M. Boyce*[2]

[1] University of Iowa Carver College of Medicine and University of Iowa College of Public Health, and University of Iowa Hospitals and Clinics, Iowa City, Iowa, USA

[2] Hospital of Saint Raphael and Yale University School of Medicine, New Haven, Connecticut, USA

Introduction

Staphylococcus aureus frequently causes serious infections such as endocarditis, pneumonia, osteomyelitis, and bloodstream infections [1,2]. Before antimicrobial therapy was introduced, the mortality rate attributed to *S. aureus* bacteremia was over 80% [3], but even with appropriate therapy the attributable mortality rate remains above 20% [4,5]. Investigators in the early twentieth century recognized that *S. aureus* carriage was a risk factor for subsequent infections and investigators continue to confirm these observations [6–10]. For example, 14 of 1278 patients with *S. aureus* nasal colonization subsequently acquired *S. aureus* bacteremia [10]. Of 14 nares isolates, 12 (86%) were identical to the isolates obtained from blood. Because carriage of *S. aureus* increases the risk of subsequent infections and because most infections are caused by isolates carried by the patient, many clinicians and investigators have tried to prevent infections by decolonizing persons who carry this organism [10–13].

Recently, investigators have tested decolonization strategies primarily among persons colonized or infected with methicillin-resistant *S. aureus* (MRSA) rather than those with methicillin-susceptible *S. aureus* (MSSA). Glycopeptide-resistant strains of *S. aureus* provide added incentive for clinicians and infection control staff to prevent these infections. Specific reasons to decolonize persons who carry *S. aureus* include:

- preventing infections in vulnerable patients, particularly those undergoing invasive procedures such as dialysis or operations;
- terminating outbreaks of *S. aureus* colonization or infection;
- reducing endemic rates of MRSA colonization or infection;
- decreasing use of systemic antimicrobials by preventing infections.

The perfect decolonizing agent would be a topical agent that is cheap, nontoxic, unrelated to systemic antimicrobials, and effective (i.e., decolonizes and prevents recolonization). It would also have a low risk of selecting resistant *S. aureus* isolates. Unfortunately, all currently available agents are imperfect. This chapter reviews data on decolonization of persons who carry *S. aureus*, the agents that have been tested, and the patient populations or situations in which decolonization protocols have been evaluated.

Efforts to eradicate *S. aureus* colonization

For over 60 years, investigators have assessed whether antimicrobial agents and other substances decolonize *S. aureus* carriers. In 1941, Delafield and Straker [14] developed snuffs containing either proflavine, penicillin, or sulphathiazole with menthol and lycopodium (moss) spores. Carriers applied the snuffs to the backs of their hands and inhaled this material into each nostril. Colony counts of *S. aureus* decreased during therapy but staphylococci often returned after therapy was stopped. Twenty years later, Elek and Fleming [15] sprayed methicillin into the air of a hospital nursery. The frequency of *S. aureus* nasal colonization among infants decreased but infants became colonized with methicillin-resistant strains of coagulase-negative staphylococci, which may explain why this procedure never became popular.

Investigators have used many other approaches to eradicate *S. aureus* nasal colonization over the last 60 years. Boyce [16], Chow and Yu [17], and Friedel and Climo [18] reviewed the literature and described many early decolonization efforts. Investigators have tested numerous oral agents, nebulized solutions, and topical preparations. Clinicians have not adopted nebulized regimens because they were not very effective. Of the systemic agents evaluated, some agents with activity against *S. aureus* (e.g.,

Staphylococci in Human Disease, 2nd edition. Edited by Kent B. Crossley, Kimberly K. Jefferson, Gordon Archer, Vance G. Fowler, Jr.
 ISBN 978-14051-6332-3.

gentamicin, vancomycin) did not decolonize the nares effectively and others (e.g., cefalexin and erythromycin) decolonized the nares for brief periods but *S. aureus* carriage rapidly returned after treatment was completed [17]. Oral quinolones decolonized the nares, but MRSA quickly became resistant to these agents [19–21]. Lipsky *et al.* [19] demonstrated that clindamycin eliminated nasal carriage of *S. aureus* and that patients remained decolonized for at least 3 weeks. Trimethoprim–sulfamethoxazole plus rifampin and minocycline plus rifampin are two regimens that have eliminated MRSA nasal colonization effectively [22]. However, even these regimens have significant failure rates. Also, many MRSA strains, particularly those that are healthcare-associated, are resistant to trimethoprim–sulfamethoxazole and some strains are resistant to rifampin. Of note, Keene *et al.* [6] found that parenteral antimicrobial agents did not clear nasal colonization.

Early trials with intranasal antimicrobial therapy were disappointing. Mupirocin, which inhibits bacterial protein synthesis by binding to the bacterial isoleucyl-tRNA-synthetase, was introduced in the late 1980s. Mupirocin eliminated nasal colonization among healthy participants in several clinical trials [23,24]. For example, Doebbeling *et al.* [23] analyzed six double-blind independently randomized studies assessing the efficacy of mupirocin ointment for eliminating *S. aureus* colonization. At 2–3 days after treatment with intranasal nasal mupirocin (twice daily for 5 days), 13% of the persons who received mupirocin still carried *S. aureus* compared with 93% of those who received placebo. The results were similar 4 weeks after treatment (18% carriers in the mupirocin group vs. 88% carriers in the placebo group). Among the subjects who were followed for 6 months and for 1 year after treatment, *S. aureus* nasal colonization rates were 48–53% (mupirocin group) and 72–76% (placebo group). Fernandez *et al.* [24] found similar results in a randomized, double-blind, placebo-controlled study of 2% intranasal mupirocin (twice daily for 5 days) among 68 healthcare workers. At the end of treatment, 86.7% of healthcare workers in the treatment group were decolonized; 57%, 44%, and 33% remained free of nasal carriage at 1 month, 2–4 months, and 6 months after treatment, respectively.

Parras *et al.* [25] compared the efficacy of intranasal 2% mupirocin (three times daily) and chlorhexidine baths with that of intranasal 2% sodium fusidate (three times daily), trimethoprim–sulfamethoxazole 160 mg/800 mg daily (administered orally or by nasogastric tube), and chlorhexidine bathing for 5 days. All patients in both groups had negative nares cultures 1 week after treatment. At 3 months after treatment, 78% of the mupirocin group and 71% of the sodium fusidate and trimethoprim–sulfamethoxazole groups did not carry *S. aureus*.

When *S. aureus* nasal colonization is eliminated, other areas (e.g., hands) are often decolonized as well [25–28]. However, eliminating carriage is difficult in patients with disorders that interrupt the keratinized squamous epithelium of the skin and in patients who carry the organism at extranasal sites [29]. Such sites can serve as sources from which the nares can become recolonized. For example, Laterre [30] used intranasal mupirocin (5 days), chlorhexidine baths, and chlorhexidine rinses for the oropharynx to treat 25 consecutive intubated patients who had *S. aureus* colonization, often involving multiple body sites. This protocol eliminated nasal colonization from only one of 25 patients. In contrast, other investigators claim that intensive regimens including systemic antimicrobials can eliminate carriage. Buehlmann *et al.* [31] reported that a combination of intranasal mupirocin ointment, chlorhexidine mouth rinses and full-body wash, oral vancomycin (for patients with gastrointestinal colonization), and trimethoprim–sulfamethoxazole (for patients with positive urine cultures) successfully decolonized 85% of patients (intent-to-treat analysis) colonized with MRSA. These investigators obtained cultures from six or more body sites to document the extent of colonization and the efficacy of the decolonization regimen.

Several investigators have used intensive regimens to decolonize the respiratory tract. Wenisch *et al.* [32] treated 21 intubated patients who had MRSA pneumonia with intravenous linezolid (600 mg twice daily), intravenous rifampin (600 mg twice daily), endotracheal vancomycin (100 mg four times daily), 1% chlorhexidine mouth and throat washes (three times daily), intranasal mupirocin (three times daily), and 4% chlorhexidine baths and hair washes for 7 days. If appropriate, they treated tracheostomy wounds with povidone-iodine. All 14 evaluable patients were free of MRSA for 2 months after treatment. Macfarlane *et al.* [33] used an intensive regimen to decolonize pediatric cystic fibrosis patients whose sputum cultures were positive for MRSA. After 5 days of treatment with intranasal 2% mupirocin (twice daily), rifampin (20 mg/kg daily), and fusidic acid (50 mg/kg daily), 8 of 17 patients (47%) no longer had positive cultures after one course. Four more patients (24%) had negative cultures after a second course; four of five remaining patients had negative cultures after they were treated with intravenous teicoplanin (5–7.5 mg/kg every 12 hours for three doses and then 10–15 mg/kg daily for 9–13 days). Ultimately, these investigators decolonized 16 of 17 (94.1%) patients (at least three negative cultures over 1 year).

Decolonizing patients and healthcare workers to terminate outbreaks

Efficacy of decolonization efforts for terminating MRSA outbreaks

Infection control personnel have treated colonized or infected patients and epidemiologically implicated healthcare workers to control *S. aureus* (usually, but not always,

MRSA) outbreaks. In many instances, this intervention has been associated with control of the outbreak [34–50]. For example, Redhead *et al.* [40] assessed whether mupirocin (two to three times daily for 3–8 days) decolonized inpatients, outpatients, and healthcare workers during outbreaks of MRSA at 102 hospitals in the UK. Of the 766 assessable subjects, 628 were colonized with MRSA, of whom 97.8% were decolonized; 138 people were colonized with MSSA, 97.8% of whom were decolonized. These investigators did not address whether use of mupirocin appeared to terminate the outbreaks.

Meier *et al.* [35] terminated an outbreak of MRSA in a burn/trauma unit after they treated three healthcare workers who carried the epidemic stain in their nares. One of the healthcare workers, a surgical resident, helped with skin graft procedures for 6 of 10 patients before they acquired MRSA. A colonized nurse cared for five of these 10 patients and the investigators could not determine whether a colonized nursing assistant cared for affected patients. Rashid *et al.* [47] terminated an MRSA outbreak, which affected 18 patients [12 had the epidemic (E)MRSA-15 strain] and nine staff members on a burn/plastic surgery unit (five had EMRSA-15), with a more complex intervention. The investigators placed the colonized healthcare workers on leave and treated them with intranasal mupirocin (three times daily for 5 days) and triclosan body washes (daily for 1 week). They allowed all healthcare workers to return to work after their follow-up cultures (on day 9) were negative. The investigators noted that the index case could not be decolonized but did not report whether other patients were decolonized. In addition, the investigators closed, refurbished, and decontaminated the unit.

Hitomi *et al.* [45] reported that standard infection control measures did not stop spread of MRSA in their neonatal intensive care unit (NICU). They treated all MRSA carriers with intranasal mupirocin three times daily for 3 days and then three times weekly. These investigators also prescribed intranasal mupirocin three times weekly for all noncarriers and all patients who were admitted to the unit (prophylactic treatment). After 1 month, only one intubated patient remained colonized. These investigators did not identify mupirocin-resistant isolates or adverse reactions to mupirocin.

Similary, Rodriguez *et al.* [48] reported that they could not terminate an MRSA outbreak in a 12-bed surgical recovery unit despite:

- culturing patients and healthcare workers to identify the entire reservoir;
- isolating carriers and discharging them as rapidly as possible;
- enforcing hygiene, especially hand-washing, among healthcare workers;
- treating infected patients with intravenous vancomycin;
- treating colonized patients with intranasal mupirocin, chlorhexidine mouthwashes, and chlorhexidine bathing.

They reported that the outbreak was terminated only after they began treating patients who did not carry MRSA on admission to the unit with prophylactic mupirocin (three times daily for 1 week).

Several groups have used mupirocin as one component of aggressive interventions to terminate outbreaks in NICUs [41–43,46,51]. The interventions also included contact precautions, cohorting, and active surveillance for colonized patients [38–40,43]. Khoury *et al.* [43] used active surveillance, aggressive implementation of contact isolation, cohorting, and decolonization to eradicate MRSA from the NICU for 2.5 years following an outbreak. They treated colonized patients with mupirocin ointment twice daily to the anterior nares and umbilical area for 7 days. Healthcare workers who carried MRSA took a hexachlorophene shower daily and received rifampin 600 mg and one double-strength tablet of trimethoprim–sulfamethoxazole twice daily for 1 week. Nambiar *et al.* [41] also cultured healthcare workers, treated those who were colonized, and closed the unit to new admissions. Lally *et al.* [46] treated all staff with intranasal mupirocin, regardless of their nasal carriage status, and treated neonates with this agent after their nares cultures were obtained but before the results were available.

Some investigators have used mupirocin in conjunction with systemic antimicrobial agents to terminate MRSA outbreaks [52,53]. For example, Embil *et al.* [52] successfully decolonized four of six patients on a plastic surgery and burn unit and all three patients in a second hospital with a combination of trimethoprim–sulfamethoxazole (160 mg/800 mg orally twice daily), rifampin (600 mg orally each day for 14 days), and mupirocin 2% ointment (applied to the nares and all open colonized skin lesions three times daily for 5 days). Of the four patients who were decolonized on the plastic surgery and burn unit, three required more than one course of treatment.

During an outbreak of MRSA on a urology unit, Maraha *et al.* [53] treated 35 colonized patients with a 5-day course of oral vancomycin (120 mL at 83.3 mg/mL) every 6 hours, intranasal mupirocin every 8 hours, and daily baths with povidone-iodine shampoo. The 35 patients received 55 courses of decolonization therapy (1.6/patient, SD 0.9). All patients had negative cultures 5 and 14 days after treatment. Six (17%) patients were switched to other oral antimicrobial agents because they did not tolerate vancomycin and 21 (60%) of the patients had diarrhea during therapy.

Several outbreaks have been caused by healthcare workers who were chronically infected or colonized with MRSA. Two outbreaks of MRSA were associated with healthcare workers who had chronic MRSA sinusitis [34,54]. Boyce *et al.* [34] used mupirocin as part of their strategy to terminate a hospital-wide MRSA outbreak but they could not terminate the outbreak until an implicated respiratory therapist underwent a sinus operation and was treated with systemic antimicrobial agents. Recently, Faibis *et al.* [54] identified seven surgical patients who became infected after being exposed to an employee in the operating room who had chronic sinusitis. After the healthcare worker was removed from the operating room, the investigators did not identify further cases. The healthcare worker was treated with intranasal mupirocin (three times daily) and body washes with povidone-iodine soap and then transferred to another ward. Cultures after two nasal treatments were negative but the healthcare worker and a family member carried the outbreak strain 10 months later.

Two outbreaks in NICUs were associated with healthcare workers who had MRSA cultured from their ears [51,55]. Bertin *et al.* [55] described a prolonged outbreak (August 2003 to July 2004) related to a newly hired employee who had chronic external otitis. Intensive interventions, including mupirocin treatment (nares and umbilicus three times daily for 10 days) for infants colonized or infected with MRSA, did not terminate the outbreak. The outbreak ended when the staff member was removed from the NICU. Mean *et al.* [51] linked an outbreak to a neonatal practitioner who had seven recurrent episodes of MRSA colonization (nose and ears). The healthcare worker did not have external otitis but the isolate became resistant to mupirocin after 11 monthly treatment courses. The outbreak ended when the neonatal practitioner left the hospital.

The outbreaks described by Boyce *et al.* [34], Faibis *et al.* [54], Mean *et al.* [51], and Bertin *et al.* [55] illustrate that decolonization alone may not terminate outbreaks related to persons with chronic infections or chronic colonization of sites like the ear. Additional measures, particularly removing the implicated healthcare worker from the unit, may be necessary to stop transmission. In some cases, treating underlying defects surgically, using intensive decolonization regimens, decolonizing close contacts, or decontaminating the home may facilitate decolonization of the implicated carrier so that he or she may return to work. Healthcare workers who cannot be decolonized may need to work in areas where they do not pose a risk to patients.

Irish *et al.* [50] investigated an outbreak of EMRSA-3 affecting a healthcare district in the UK. These investigators followed the government's guidelines for terminating outbreaks, including using intranasal mupirocin to eliminate nasal carriage and to protect patients and healthcare workers who were not carriers. However, the epidemic strain became resistant to mupirocin and the mupirocin-resistant EMRSA-3 (Mu-MRSA) affected 14 persons: 12 patients and two healthcare workers. The investigators treated patients with:

- 1% chlorhexidine obstetric cream (in the nares and on lesions);
- 2% triclosan concentrate on the hair and skin;
- 1% silver sulfadiazine on pressure sores and other lesions;
- 2% triclosan skin cleanser;
- topical bacitracin and fusidic acid creams (replaced chlorhexidine nasal cream).

After this regimen failed, the investigators treated five patients (all of whom had Mu-MRSA in their throats) for 21 days and two healthcare workers for 10 days with ciprofloxacin (500 mg twice daily) and rifampin (600 mg once daily). The two staff members and two of the five patients were decolonized; three patients died before they could be evaluated further. In addition, the investigators closed the unit to new admissions and cleaned the unit extensively. In subsequent years, they did not identify new cases. However, the investigators could not determine whether decolonization or closing and cleaning the unit was more important in terminating the outbreak.

Black *et al.* [56] introduced intensive microbiological surveillance, cohorting, and contact precautions to control spread of MRSA in their NICU. They cultured healthcare workers, changed their hand-washing soap from 0.5% PCMX to 2% chlorhexidine gluconate, treated all infants with mupirocin (nares and umbilicus twice daily for 5 days), treated parents of colonized infants with intranasal mupirocin (5 days), and treated healthcare workers caring for colonized infants with intranasal mupirocin (5 days). Mupirocin temporarily suppressed MRSA in five of six colonized infants but eradicated carriage from only one patient. The investigators implemented intensive microbiological surveillance again when they identified new cases. They terminated the second outbreak in 2 weeks. On the basis of their results, the investigators concluded that intensive microbiological surveillance and isolation precautions terminated the outbreak and that mupirocin did not eradicate MRSA from their patients.

The outbreak investigated by Sax *et al.* [42] is particularly interesting because it was caused by a community-associated (CA)-MRSA strain [ST5, SCC*mec* type VI, Panton–Valentine leukocidin (PVL)-positive]. This outbreak affected five neonates, two mothers, and a sibling. The authors improved hygiene measures in the unit, used barrier precautions, and applied mupirocin to the nares and umbilicus of all MRSA carriers (five neonates with the outbreak strain and two neonates with another MRSA strain) and they bathed infants aged over 32 weeks' gestational age with chlorhexidine. Four neonates were decolonized, two were lost to follow-up, and one remained colonized. The authors attributed their success in terminating the outbreak to the combination of interventions.

At present, we have very little data on the efficacy of decolonization efforts among persons colonized with CA-MRSA strains. Longtin *et al.* [57] followed 45 patients who were infected or colonized with PVL-positive CA-MRSA and who were treated with intranasal mupirocin and chlorhexidine showers. Of these patients, 39 had no clinical relapses and were MRSA-negative at their last follow-up visit. Five of the six who remained colonized were from a family cluster. In contrast, Rihn *et al.* [58] reported that prescribing mupirocin for high-school football players did not help them control an outbreak of CA-MRSA infections. However, only 36% of the players used mupirocin as prescribed.

Efficacy of decolonization efforts for terminating MSSA outbreaks

Weber *et al.* [44] used mupirocin to terminate an outbreak of MSSA among children who had undergone cardiothoracic surgical procedures. In this instance, numerous staff caring for these children, not just the two staff members implicated by the epidemiological study, carried the epidemic strain. These investigators treated all carriers with intranasal mupirocin (twice daily for 5 days) and required those who also carried the epidemic strain on their hands to wash their hands with chlorhexidine. The investigators did not allow the implicated surgeon to operate until two consecutive hand cultures were negative. Six months later, the investigators obtained nares cultures from 22 of 31 treated healthcare workers; 13 (60%) had negative nares cultures, six (27.3%) were recolonized with the epidemic strain, and three (13.6%) had acquired new *S. aureus* strains. Active surveillance did not identify additional cases.

Martorell *et al.* [59] tracked rates of *S. aureus* surgical-site infection after cardiac operations. During an 11-year period, they identified three clusters of *S. aureus* surgical-site infections. MSSA caused 11 of 14 infections (78.6%). One cluster was related to a colonized healthcare worker. This cluster was terminated after the investigators improved "traffic flow" and treated the carrier (they did not describe the treatment regimen). Two other clusters were associated with carriage among healthcare workers. In these instances, the investigators removed the carriers from direct patient care for 72 hours and treated them with mupirocin (twice daily for 5 days), rifampin (600 mg daily for 14 days), dicloxacillin (500 mg four times daily for 14 days), and chlorhexidine showers (daily for 5 days). The investigators also treated all patients who were scheduled to undergo cardiac operations with intranasal mupirocin for 3 days preoperatively and chlorhexidine showers. Subsequently, the overall surgical-site infection rate decreased from 4.1% to 2.6% ($P < 0.05$) and the proportion of surgical-site infections caused by *S. aureus* decreased from 57.9% to 25.0%.

Decolonizing patients with furunculosis

Raz *et al.* [60] studied 34 patients with recurrent staphylococcal nasal colonization and infection. They treated all patients with intranasal mupirocin for 5 days. For the next year, they treated 17 patients with a 5-day course of mupirocin every month and treated the other 17 with placebo. The total number of positive cultures (22 vs. 83) and the number of skin infections (26 vs. 62) were significantly lower in the treatment group. Only 1 of 10 patients who were no longer colonized acquired an infection compared with 24 of 24 patients who remained colonized ($P < 0.01$).

Recently, Wiese-Posselt *et al.* [61] investigated an outbreak of furunculosis caused by MSSA (*lukS-lukF*-positive). The outbreak affected 42 persons in one village, 27 of whom had 59 relapses. The investigators obtained cultures from 140 of 144 village residents; 51 persons were colonized with *S. aureus*, nine of whom had *lukS-lukF*-positive MSSA strains. To control this village-wide outbreak, the investigators treated carriers with intranasal mupirocin (three times daily for 5 days), an alcohol-based antibacterial hand sanitizer (after applying mupirocin), octenidin-based wash solution for the body and hair (daily), and 0.1% chlorhexidine for gargling (three times daily). In addition to these treatments, the investigators instructed the carriers to increase their hand hygiene, to disinfect personal items (e.g., combs, razors, glasses, jewelry), to clean their bathtubs or shower floors with an alcohol-based antimicrobial cleanser, and to wash their clothing, towels and bedlinen daily at 60°C. Subsequently, one new case was identified and three persons in two families had relapses. Persons with recurrent furuncles were treated by their own physicians and these patients repeated the decolonization protocol. Passive surveillance did not detect subsequent furuncles caused by *lukS-lukF*-positive MSSA in the following year.

Decolonizing surgical patients

Rationale

Investigators determined in the late 1950s that nasal carriage of *S. aureus* was a risk factor for autoinfection of surgical wounds. In the 1960s, White and Smith suggested a possible mechanism by which *S. aureus* in the nares could affect surgical sites [62,63]. These investigators demonstrated that the proportion of patients with *S. aureus* on their skin increased as the number of colony-forming units of this organism in their nares increased [62]. White also documented that the incidence of *S. aureus* surgical-site infections increased as the density of nasal colonization increased [63]. Recent studies have confirmed that the risk of acquiring *S. aureus* surgical-site infections is 4.5–9.6 times higher for carriers than noncarriers [13,64,65].

Studies using historical controls

Several studies have compared patients who received mupirocin with historical controls to assess whether mupirocin prevents *S. aureus* surgical-site infections [59,65–74]. Most of these studies found significantly decreased rates of *S. aureus* surgical-site infections in the treatment groups (Table 30.1). Several groups have conducted controlled

Table 30.1 Studies assessing the efficacy of mupriocin for preventing *S. aureus* infections in surgical patients.

Reference	Study designs	Patients studied	Agents studied	Decolonization rates	Infections evaluated	Infection rates			
						Treatment group	Control group	Historical period	Statistical significance
Kluytmans *et al.* [74]	Historical controls	Patients undergoing cardiothoracic surgery	Intranasal mupirocin for 5 days, beginning 1 day before the operation	93% of treated patients	Surgical-site infections	2%	7.8% among patients who did not receive mupirocin as planned during the treatment period	7%	$P = 0.02$
					S. aureus surgical-site infections	0.9%	1.7% among patients who did not receive mupirocin as planned during the treatment period	2.9%	
Yangco *et al.* [68]	Historical controls	Open heart surgical procedures	Intranasal mupirocin twice daily for 5 days; mupirocin was stopped if the nasal culture was negative	Not specified	Surgical site infections	1.4%		1.4%	
					S. aureus sternal wound infections	0%		0.7%	$P = 0.005$
Coskun *et al.* [70]	Historical controls (1999–2000)	All patients undergoing cardiovascular procedures 1999–2004	Intranasal mupirocin three times daily for 3 days before surgical procedure (2001–2004)	Not specified	Surgical-site infections	2.9% → 0.8%		1.4–1.5%	$P < 0.001$
					S. aureus surgical-site infections	0.9% → 0.1%		0.3–0.8%	$P < 0.001$
					MRSA surgical-site infections	0.6% → 0%		0.1–0.5%	$P < 0.001$
Nicholson & Huesman [66]	Historical control group	All patients undergoing cardiac surgical procedures	Intranasal mupirocin preoperatively for all patients; carriers continued mupirocin postoperatively until they received a total of 7 days	Not specified	Surgical-site infections	1.1%		1.9%	NS
					S. aureus surgical-site infections	0.37%		1.7%	$P < 0.006$
					S. aureus deep sternal infections	0.09%		1.0%	$P < 0.009$

Cimochowski *et al.* [72]	Historical control group (1/1/1995 to 10/31/1996)	All patients undergoing open heart surgical procedures 1/1/1995 to 3/31/1999	Intranasal mupirocin; two doses preoperatively and twice daily for 5 days postoperatively (12/1/1997 to 3/31/1999)	Not specified	Surgical-site infections	0.9%		2.7%	$P = 0.005$
					Deep surgical-site infections	0.4%		1.2%	$P = 0.04$
					Superficial surgical-site infections	0.6%		1.5%	$P = 0.05$
Konvalinka *et al.* [76]	RBPCS	*S. aureus* carriers having cardiac surgical procedures	Intranasal mupirocin ($N = 130$) or placebo ($N = 127$) twice daily for 7 days before the operation	81.5% of the treatment group and 46.5% of the placebo group	Surgical-site infections	13.8%	8.6%		OR 1.61, 95% CI 0.69–3.75
					S. aureus surgical-site infections	3.8%	3.2%		OR 1.23, 95% CI 0.32–4.68
Gernaat-van der Sluis *et al.* [71]	Historical control group	All patients undergoing orthopedic procedures	Intranasal mupirocin, three doses before the operation	Not defined	Surgical-site infections	1.3%		2.7%	$P = 0.02$
					S. aureus surgical-site infections	0.7%		1.1%	NS
Wilcox *et al.* [67]	Historical control group	Patients undergoing orthopedic procedures involving implantation of metal prostheses and/or fixation	Intranasal mupirocin and 2% triclosan showers or baths	Not specified	MRSA surgical-site infections	3.3–4 per 1000 operations		23 per 1000 operations	$P < 0.001$
Coskun *et al.* [69]	Historical controls	All patients undergoing elective orthopedic procedures	Intranasal mupirocin three times daily for 3 days before the procedure	Not specified	Surgical-site infections	1.4% → 1.0%		2.2–3.6%	$P < 0.001$
					S. aureus surgical-site infections	0.4% → 0.1%		1.3–1.6%	$P < 0.001$
					MRSA surgical-site infections	0.3% → 0.1%		1.3–0.9%	$P < 0.001$
Kalmeijer *et al.* [77]	RBPCS	All patients undergoing orthopedic operations	Intranasal mupirocin ($N = 315$) or placebo ($N = 299$) twice daily; ≥ 2 doses were given before the operation	84.2% of the treatment group, 29.1% of the placebo group	Surgical-site infections	3.8%	4.7%		RR 0.81, 95% CI 0.38–1.73
					S. aureus surgical-site infections	1.6%	2.7%		RR 0.59, 95% CI 0.20–1.79
					Endogenous *S. aureus* infections	0.3%	1.7%		RR 0.19, 95% CI 0.02–1.62

Table 30.1 (*cont'd*)

Reference	Study designs	Patients studied	Agents studied	Decolonization rates	Infections evaluated	Infection rates			
						Treatment group	Control group	Historical period	Statistical significance
Yano *et al.* [73][1]	Historical control group	Consecutive patients undergoing upper gastrointestinal surgical procedures	Intranasal mupirocin three times daily for 3 days preoperatively	Not specified	Postoperative infections	23.4%		28.1%	NS
					Staphylococcal infections	0.71%		11.7%	$P < 0.001$
					MRSA infections	0%		7.0%	$P = 0.001$
					MSSA infections	0.71%		4.7%	$P = 0.056$
Horiuchi *et al.* [75]	Prospective	72 patients who had percutaneous endoscopic gastrostomy tubes placed	Intranasal mupirocin alone (three times daily) for 5 days; followed by inhaled arebakacin (twice daily) if mupirocin was ineffective; inhaled arbekacin, and oral TMP–SMX (800/160 mg twice daily); each treatment was repeated once if the first was not effective	Mupirocin alone 25% Mupirocin + arebakacin 29.2% Mupirocin + arebakacin + TMP–SMX 45.8%	Peristomal infections	0% (0/24) of the decolonized patients 0% (0/24) of the patients who were not colonized	100% (24/24) of the patients who were colonized but not treated		$P < 0.0001$
Perl *et al.* [13]	RBPCS	4030 patients who underwent cardiothoracic, general, gynecological, or neurosurgical procedures	Intranasal mupirocin ($N = 444$) twice daily for up to 5 days vs. placebo ointment ($N = 447$)	83.4% of the treatment group, 24.7% of the placebo group	*S. aureus* surgical-site infections (primary end point)	2.3%	2.4%		NS
					S. aureus nosocomial infections among nasal carriers	4.0%	7.7%		$P = 0.02$ (OR 0.49, 95% CI 0.25–0.92)
Suzuki *et al.* [78]	Randomized and prospective	395 consecutive patients undergoing major digestive operations	Intranasal mupirocin ($N = 193$) three times daily for 3 days before the operation vs. no treatment ($N = 202$)	Not specified	All postoperative infections	2.1% Gram-positive infections	2.5% Gram-positive infections		NS

[1] In the study by Yano *et al.*, the rate of streptococcal infections was significantly increased during the treatment period compared with the historical period.
NS, not significant; OR, odds ratio; RBPCS, randomized, blinded, placebo-controlled study; RR, relative risk; TMP–SMX, trimethoprim–sulfamethoxazole.

trials of mupirocin [13,75–77]. Unlike the results of studies using historical controls, the primary end points for most of the controlled trials were not different between the treatment and control groups [13,76,77]. For example, in the randomized, double-blind, placebo-controlled study of mupirocin conducted by Perl *et al.* [13], the rate of *S. aureus* surgical-site infections, the primary end point, was the same among the mupirocin and placebo recipients but the rate of *S. aureus* nosocomial infections among patients who carried *S. aureus* in their nares was significantly lower for those who received mupirocin (4.0%) than for those who received placebo (7.7%) [odds ratio 0.49, 95% confidence interval (CI) 0.25–0.92; $P = 0.02$]. There are several possible reasons why the incidence of *S. aureus* surgical-site infections did not decrease significantly. First, the rate of these infections was lower than expected. Second, only 47.2% of patients with *S. aureus* surgical-site infections carried this organism preoperatively, which was lower than the a priori estimate. Thus, the study may not have been large enough to detect a significant difference. Third, molecular typing suggested that several *S. aureus* strains may have been transmitted among the patients. Intranasal mupirocin might not prevent transmission of *S. aureus* from healthcare workers to patients and thus might not prevent such infections.

Similarly, in the randomized, double-blind, placebo-controlled study conducted by Kalmeijer *et al.* [77] among orthopedic surgery patients, nasal carriage of *S. aureus* was eliminated from 83.5% of the mupirocin group but from only 27.8% of the placebo group. However, mupirocin prophylaxis did not reduce the rate of surgical-site infections (primary end point), the rate of *S. aureus* surgical-site infections, or the length of hospital stay (Table 30.1). However, the rate of endogenous *S. aureus* infections was five times lower in the treatment group than in the control group. The rate of surgical-site infections also decreased in the placebo group, in part because the investigators implemented intensive surveillance during the clinical trial. The investigators felt that the "unexpected decrease in the [surgical-site infection] rate observed in the placebo group resulted in insufficient power" and they therefore felt they could not draw conclusions about the efficacy of mupirocin.

Konvalinka *et al.* [76] conducted a randomized, double-blind, placebo-controlled trial of intranasal mupirocin in *S. aureus* carriers undergoing cardiac surgical procedures. The rate of surgical-site infections was higher in the mupirocin group than in the placebo group but this difference did not reach statistical significance (Table 30.1). The rate of *S. aureus* surgical-site infections was nearly identical in both groups. The investigators had done a priori power calculations but they concluded that the rates of *S. aureus* surgical-site infections were probably too low to allow them to demonstrate a significant difference between the two groups. In addition, the investigators were surprised that 46% of the patients in the placebo group were no longer colonized with *S. aureus* in the postoperative period. The investigators wondered whether some of the patients in the placebo group purchased mupirocin over the counter and used it instead of placebo.

Kallen *et al.* [79] included three randomized and four before–after trials [13,71–74,77,78] in a metaanalysis of studies that assessed perioperative use of mupirocin to prevent surgical-site infections. (The clinical trial performed by Konvalinka *et al.* [76] was published after the metaanalysis was published.) Kallen *et al.* found that the rate of surgical-site infections was not decreased in the randomized general surgery trials [summary estimates: 8.4% in the mupirocin group and 8.1% in the control group; relative risk (RR) 1.04, 95% CI 0.81–1.33]. In the randomized trials on surgical services other than general surgery, the summary estimates were 6.0% in the mupirocin group and 7.6% in the control group (RR 0.80, 95% CI 0.58–1.10). Summary estimates for the before–after trials were much stronger than those for the randomized trials: 1.7% in the mupirocin group and 4.1% in the control group (RR 0.40, 95% CI 0.29–0.56). Kallen *et al.* noted that the randomized trials conducted by Perl *et al.* [13] and Kalmeijer *et al.* [77] both found 20% reductions in the rate of surgical-site infections among patients who underwent nongeneral surgical procedures. Kallen *et al.* suggested that these studies were affected by type 2 statistical errors because 14 000 patients would be needed to detect a 20% decrease in surgical-site infections given a baseline rate of 5% [79]. They also noted that the before–after studies were done well and that bias was unlikely to account for the entire difference between the treatment and control groups.

Decolonizing hospitalized patients

A number of investigators have attempted to decolonize hospitalized patients. For example, Sandri *et al.* [80] carried out active surveillance in their ICU for patients colonized with MRSA. They treated all carriers with intranasal mupirocin three times daily for 5 days and daily baths with 2% chlorhexidine for 3 days. Over the study period, the proportion of patients who acquired nosocomial MRSA infections decreased from 8.2% in 1999 to 6.3% in 2000, 4.3% in 2001, 3.6% in 2002, and 2.8% in 2003. The overall downward trend did not meet statistical significance but the authors stated that "there was a significant decrease in 2003 ($P = 0.001$)." The percentage of nasal swab cultures positive for *S. aureus* or for MRSA both decreased significantly ($P < 0.001$ and $P = 0.006$, respectively). However, these investigators did not report the rates of colonization and infection before they began their intervention and they did not use time-series analysis to assess the significance of the changes they observed.

Wertheim *et al.* [29] conducted a randomized, double-blind, placebo-controlled study to assess whether mupirocin prevented *S. aureus* infections among adult patients who did not have an operative procedure. The investigators randomized patients whose nasal cultures at the time of admission were positive for *S. aureus* to receive either mupirocin ointment ($N = 793$) or placebo ointment ($N = 809$) twice daily for 5 days. The rates of *S. aureus* infections did not differ significantly between the mupirocin group (2.6%) and the placebo group (2.8%) but the time to occurrence of *S. aureus* infections was increased significantly, from 13 days in the placebo group to 32 days in the mupirocin group ($P = 0.02$). The authors subsequently suggested that one course of mupirocin might not be adequate to prevent infections among patients with prolonged hospitalizations [81]. In addition, this study had two major limitations. First, the decolonization process did not start until after the nasal culture results were available (up to 3 days after admission). Thus, the investigators might have begun treatment with mupirocin too late to prevent infections. Second, the rate of *S. aureus* nasal colonization was lower than the investigators predicted, which may have decreased the study's power.

Rumbak and Cancio [82] evaluated the effect of intranasal mupirocin ointment and bathing with chlorhexidine (both twice weekly) among patients on long-term acute-care mechanical ventilation. The investigators retrospectively reviewed medical records for 180 patients who were ventilated mechanically for a median of 18 ± 17 months between April 1990 and March 1991 and for 332 patients who were ventilated mechanically for a median of 17 ± 15 months between April 1991 and March 1993. The latter patients received prophylactic treatment regardless of whether they carried *S. aureus*. During the historical control period, 0.2% episodes of *S. aureus* ventilator-associated pneumonia occurred per ventilator-day compared with 0.026% episodes per ventilator-day during the treatment period ($P < 0.001$) for a relative risk reduction of 87% and an absolute risk reduction of 6.

Paterson *et al.* [83] studied the effect of mupirocin prophylaxis on liver transplant candidates and recipients who carried *S. aureus* in their nares. They observed that 87% were decolonized but 37% of these patients became recolonized. Overall, 23% of the patients acquired *S. aureus* infections during the study period. On the basis of these results, the authors concluded that mupirocin was ineffective. Subsequently, the same group compared 47 patients who underwent liver transplants during 1996–1999 with 97 patients who underwent these procedures during 2000–2004 after active surveillance for *S. aureus* was introduced [84]. The investigators cohorted patients who had nasal or rectal colonization, placed them in contact precautions, and treated them with intranasal mupirocin (twice daily for 5 days). The rate of *S. aureus* acquisition after transplantation decreased from 45.6% to 9.9% ($P < 0.001$) as did the rate of *S. aureus* infections (from 40.4% to 4.1%; $P < 0.001$) and the rate of bacteremia (from 25.5% to 4.1%; $P < 0.001$).

Dupeyron *et al.* [85] successfully used intranasal mupirocin (three times daily for 5 days) to decolonize 85 of 86 (98.8%) stable nasal MRSA carriers hospitalized on a gastroenterology unit. However, 25.9% became recolonized and stool carriage was an independent risk for recolonization. However, the prevalence of MRSA infections did not change after mupirocin prophylaxis was introduced. The authors subsequently began treating colonized patients with intranasal mupirocin (three times daily for 5 days) and 4% chlorhexidine (showers and hair-washing every other day) [86]. Over several years, the proportion of patients who acquired MRSA decreased from 14.3% to 10.2% and the incidence of MRSA infection decreased from 1.41 to 0.59 per 1000 patient-days ($P = 0.002$). However, the investigators did not use time-series analysis techniques to assess the significance of the changes over time.

Shitrit *et al.* [87] obtained cultures for MRSA from all patients at high risk of acquiring MRSA bacteremia. They placed MRSA carriers in contact precautions and treated them with one 5-day course of intranasal mupirocin (three times daily) and 4% chlorhexidine showers (once daily). The number of surveillance cultures and the percent surveillance cultures positive for MRSA increased significantly from the historical control period to the intervention period, while the incidence of MRSA bacteremia decreased significantly from 3.6 to 1.8 cases per month. Of note, the authors concluded that surveillance cultures "are important for identifying hidden reservoirs" and that "contact isolation can prevent new colonization and infection" with MRSA but they did not comment on the usefulness of intranasal mupirocin. In addition, they did not use time-series methods to analyze their data.

Muller *et al.* [88] observed rates of MRSA colonization and infection in a medical ICU. During the first 2 years, they treated colonized patients with intranasal mupirocin for 5 days; during the subsequent 2 years they did not treat carriers. Compared with the prior treatment period, the mean length of stay was significantly shorter (9.73 vs. 11.44 days; $P = 0.02$) and the decolonization rate among patients hospitalized more than 14 days was significantly worse during the nontreatment period (86.4% vs. 46.4%; $P = 0.002$). The number of MRSA infections did not change but the number of endogenous MRSA infections increased from 1 to 11 ($P = 0.006$) after mupirocin treatment was stopped. Of note, Wertheim and Vos put the results of this study in perspective when they commented in an accompanying editorial that the study design was subject to many biases [89].

Decolonizing residents of long-term care facilities

MRSA is endemic in many long-term care facilities and infections with MRSA in this setting increase costs more than those caused by MSSA [90]. Several groups have assessed decolonization efforts in this setting [91–95].

Kaufman *et al.* [92] applied mupirocin ointment to the anterior nares of colonized residents for 7 months and subsequently to their nares and wounds for 5 months. The investigators treated the residents' nares daily for 1 week and wounds daily for 2 weeks. They then treated the residents' nares and wounds three days per week for 3 weeks and once per week for a minimum of 3 months after all cultures were negative for MRSA. Overall, carriage recurred at least once in 33% of the residents and most recurrences involved the nares. The proportion of colonized residents decreased from 22.7 ± 2.1% to 11.5 ± 1.8% but the rate of transmission from room-mate to room-mate and the rate of MRSA infections did not decrease. Moreover, 10.8% of the residents acquired mupirocin-resistant isolates of MRSA. On the basis of their results, the investigators concluded that mupirocin should be saved for use in outbreak situations and should not be used for prolonged periods in facilities with endemic MRSA colonization.

Subsequently, Mody *et al.* [93] conducted a randomized, double-blind, placebo-controlled trial among persistent *S. aureus* carriers who resided in two long-term care facilities. Residents were treated with either mupirocin or placebo for 2 weeks and followed for 6 months. Immediately after treatment, 93% of the residents in the treatment arm and 15% of those in the placebo arm were no longer colonized ($P < 0.001$). At 90 days after entry into the study, 61% of the residents in the treatment group remained decolonized. Of the 14 residents who became recolonized, 13 (86%) were recolonized with their pretreatment strains. *Staphylococus aureus* infections occurred in 5% of residents treated with mupirocin and 15% of those who received placebo ($P = 0.10$). Three of four patients who were not decolonized after mupirocin treatment had mupirocin-resistant isolates.

Kotilainen *et al.* [94] described an outbreak of MRSA affecting eight patients in a 40-bed long-term ward of a healthcare center and 4 of 59 (6.8%) residents of a long-term care facility in Finland. Because they felt the outbreak was a "serious threat to the entire healthcare district," the investigators used contact precautions and screened patients and residents for asymptomatic carriage. Healthcare workers applied mupirocin to sites colonized with MRSA three times daily for 5–7 days and bathed colonized patients and residents daily with 4% chlorhexidine. The investigators treated patients who were colonized in the throat or other deep sites with two systemic agents for about 2 weeks. They successfully decolonized all but one resident and terminated the outbreak.

Jaqua-Stewart *et al.* [95] implemented a similar regimen on the extended-care unit and in the long-term care facility at the Sioux Falls Veterans Administration Medical Center to control an outbreak of MRSA. These investigators implemented contact isolation, bathed patients with chlorhexidine, treated nasal carriers with mupirocin, and treated patients with systemic antimicrobial agents if they were colonized at other sites or were infected. Subsequently, MRSA colonization and infection rates decreased from 52% to 2% and from 8.5% to 1.4%, respectively. Jaqua-Stewart *et al.* estimated that they prevented 93 infections, saving $429 500 [85]. The intervention cost $35 500 and the investigators assumed that each infection cost $5000. However, if one uses Capitano *et al.*'s more conservative approximation of $2607 [90], then one would estimate that Jaqua-Stewart *et al.* may have saved $206 951 if they prevented 93 infections.

Bradley [96] and McNeil *et al.* [97] do not recommend routinely decolonizing residents of long-term care facilities who carry MRSA. However, McNeil *et al.* [97] suggested that healthcare workers linked to transmission within long-term care facilities should be removed from work and that infection control staff should consider treating them with intranasal mupirocin.

Decolonizing patients treated with hemodialysis and peritoneal dialysis

Rationale

Staphylococcus aureus is the most common bacterium causing infections in patients treated with hemodialysis [98]. It causes 67–90% of vascular access site infections and these infections often cause bacteremia [17,99–103], which frequently causes metastatic infections of numerous sites including heart valves, bones, joints, and eyes [104–106]. Between 32 and 82% of patients treated with hemodialysis carry *S. aureus* in their nares [99,107–114]. The rate of bloodstream infection among *S. aureus* carriers is four times that of noncarriers [99], and 80–90% of *S. aureus* infections in hemodialysis patients are caused by endogenous strains [11,99,115]. Similarly, *S. aureus* causes 25–85% of exit-site infections and 9–40% of peritonitis episodes in patients treated with peritoneal dialysis [116]. Rates of *S. aureus* nasal carriage range from 17 to 67% in these patients [11,12,115,117–128]. Compared with noncarriers, carriers have higher rates of exit-site infection (1.1–13.6 times), peritonitis (2.5–8.5 times), and catheter loss (2.4 times) [12,122,123,125]. Between 50 and 86% of exit-site infections and peritonitis episodes are caused by endogenous strains [12,118,120,129].

Effect of treatment on nasal carriage and rates of *S. aureus* infection among dialysis patients

Hemodialysis

Yu *et al.* [99] demonstrated in 1986 that rifampin significantly reduced the *S. aureus* infection rate among hemodialysis patients (Table 30.2). Most nephrologists did not implement rifampin prophylaxis [116] because this agent has several substantial disadvantages: it turns secretions orange, can cause adverse reactions, is a systemic

Table 30.2 Studies assessing the efficacy of rifampin, mupirocin, and povidone-iodine for prevention of *S. aureus* infections in hemodialysis patients.[1]

Reference	Date[2]	Study design	Patients studied	Definition of carriage	Agents studied	Infections evaluated	Infection rates			*P* value
							Treatment group	Control group	Historical period	
Yu *et al.* [99]	1986 (1980–1983)	Prospective, randomized	*S. aureus* nasal carriers	One positive nares culture	Rifampin 600 mg twice daily for 5 days plus intranasal bacitracin four times daily for 7 days; repeated every 3 months for patients whose nares cultures were positive or no treatment	All *S. aureus* infections	2/18 (11%)	12/26 (46%)	NA	0.02
Boelaert *et al.* [111]	1989 (NS)	Prospective, randomized, double-blind, placebo-controlled	*S. aureus* nasal carriers	NS	Intranasal mupirocin three times daily for 2 weeks, then three times weekly	All *S. aureus* infections	0.12/ patient-year	0.49/ patient-year	NA	≤ 0.05
Boelaert *et al.* [112]	1993 (10/1/1989 to 9/30/1991)	Prospective, open trial	*S. aureus* nasal carriers	Two nares cultures taken 1 week apart were positive	Intranasal mupirocin three times weekly (10/1/1989 to 3/31/1990), then once weekly (4/1/1990 to 9/30/1991)	*S. aureus* bacteremia	0.024/ patient-year	NA	0.097/ patient-year	0.008
Kluytmans *et al.* [110]	1996 (2/1/1992 to 11/1/1993)	Prospective, open trial	*S. aureus* nasal carriers	One positive nares culture	Intranasal mupirocin once per week	*S. aureus* bacteremia	0.04/ patient-year	NA	0.25/ patient-year	< 0.001
Fong [113]	1993 (not specified)	Prospective, randomized, open trial	Patients who were dialyzed through subclavian catheters, regardless of nasal carriage status	Not specified	Povidone-iodine at the exit site and sterile dressing with each dressing change or sterile dressing alone	Bacteremia ESI CTI	0/14 (0%) 0/14 (0%) 2/17 (12%)	6/21 (29%) 5/21 (24%) 11/26 (42%)	NA	All < 0.05
Sesso *et al.* [131]	1998 (6/1994 to 12/1996)	Randomized, prospective trial	Patients with end-stage renal disease who had not had a central venous catheter within 1 month of the study	Not specified	Compared skin disinfection alone with skin disinfection followed by mupirocin at the catheter exit site	*S. aureus* skin infection *S. aureus* bacteremia	4.3% 0.71/1000 patient-days	23.9% 8.92/1000 patient-days	NA	0.001 < 0.001
Johnson *et al.* [132]	2002 (8/1/1999 to 5/31/2001)	Open-label, randomized controlled trial	All adult patients with acute or chronic renal failure who were dialyzed through a newly inserted tunneled, cuffed central venous catheter	Not specified	Mupirocin at the hemodialysis catheter exit site (three times weekly) compared with standard catheter care; all catheters were cuffed tunneled catheters	Catheter-related bacteremia Median time to first bacteremia Median duration of catheter survival	7% 108 days 108 days	35% 55 days 31 days	NA	< 0.01 < 0.01 < 0.05

[1] Table updated from Herwaldt [116].
[2] The year outside parentheses is the year in which the study was published; the year within parentheses is the year in which the study was done.
CTI, catheter-tip infection; ESI, exit-site infection; NA, not applicable; NS, not specified.

antimicrobial agent, is used to treat serious infections, and selects resistance quickly. Therefore, when mupirocin became available, numerous investigators began to evaluate this agent's effect on *S. aureus* nasal carriage and infection. Several research groups evaluated the effect of one course of intranasal mupirocin on *S. aureus* nasal carriage among hemodialysis patients, using various regimens: three times daily for 5 days [107]; three times daily for 10 days [108]; two times daily for 7 days plus chlorhexidine body scrubs for 3 days [109]. Immediately after one course of intranasal mupirocin, carriage rates decreased from 100% to 17–27% [107–109]. Three months after treatment, 58–77% of patients who received one course of mupirocin alone [107,108] carried *S. aureus* compared with only 31% of those who were treated with mupirocin and chlorhexidine body scrubs [109].

Pena *et al.* [130] have found that intranasal mupirocin (three times daily for 5 days) eliminated *S. aureus* from the nares of 88.5% of patients on hemodialysis but 43.5% subsequently had positive nares cultures. Of the recurrences, 70% were relapses and 30% were recolonizations with different strains. Boelaert *et al.* [28] and Kluytmans *et al.* [110] treated hemodialysis patients with intranasal mupirocin once weekly over prolonged time periods and found that 6–15% of these patients carried *S. aureus* in their nares at any one time despite prophylactic treatment.

Several investigators postulated that intranasal mupirocin may prevent *S. aureus* infections in hemodialysis patients because it eliminates the reservoir from which this organism colonizes other sites. Indeed, Bommer *et al.* [108] demonstrated that, compared with a placebo ointment, one course (10 days) of intranasal mupirocin reduced the rate of *S. aureus* skin carriage among hemodialysis patients from 91% to 33%, although the proportion of patients carrying *S. aureus* on their skin subsequently increased to 61% over the 3-month observation period as nasal carriage increased. The proportion of patients in the placebo group who carried *S. aureus* on their skin fluctuated from 70 to 90% during the study period.

Boelaert *et al.* [28] studied 20 hemodialysis patients who carried *S. aureus* in their nares and 20 patients who did not carry this organism. When the study began, 15 of 20 (75%) nasal carriers also had *S. aureus* on their hands compared with only 2 of 20 (10%) patients who did not carry this organism in their nares. Patients who carried *S. aureus* at the onset of the study were treated with one dose of intranasal mupirocin each week. Patients who did not carry *S. aureus* at study onset were not treated. Over 6 months, the rate of nasal carriage and hand carriage in the mupirocin group ranged from 11 to 15% and from 12 to 24%, respectively. Among patients who did not carry *S. aureus* in their nares initially, rates of nasal and hand carriage ranged from 0 to 24% and from 10 to 22%, respectively. These investigators concluded that patients who carry *S. aureus* in their nares often contaminate their hands with this organism. When patients touch their vascular access sites, they may contaminate these sites with *S. aureus*. Alternatively, organisms in the patients' nares might directly contaminate their access sites. These data help explain how an intervention limited to the nares could prevent *S. aureus* bloodstream infection in hemodialysis patients [28].

Boelaert *et al.* [111] have conducted the only randomized, double-blind, placebo-controlled clinical trial of intranasal mupirocin for prevention of *S. aureus* infections in hemodialysis patients (see Table 30.2). One bloodstream infection occurred in the mupirocin group compared with six infections in the placebo group, which the investigators reported as a significant difference. However, one of us (L.A.H.) has used a 1-tail binomial distribution to assess the statistical significance of these results and obtained a P-value of 0.14, suggesting that mupirocin decreased the incidence of *S. aureus* infection but the study was not large enough to detect a statistically significant difference. Subsequently, Boelaert's group [112] and Kluytmans' group [110] used historical control groups in studies of mupirocin prophylaxis among hemodialysis patients who carried *S. aureus* in their nares (see Table 30.2). Both studies found significantly lower rates of *S. aureus* bacteremia during the treatment period than during the historical control periods.

Sesso *et al.* [131] and Johnson *et al.* [132] have conducted prospective randomized trials of mupirocin at the hemodialysis catheter exit site. In the study by Sesso *et al.* [131], patients treated with pericatheter mupirocin had significantly lower rates of skin infection and bacteremia caused by *S. aureus*. In the study by Johnson *et al.* [132], the rate of exit-site infections and the rate of catheter-related bacteremia decreased in the treatment group compared with the control group, while the time to first exit-site infection, the time to first bacteremia, and the median duration of catheter survival increased significantly. *Staphylococcus aureus* caused half of the bacteremias in the controls and none among the treatment group. The investigators estimated that one would need to treat 3.7 patients to prevent one episode of bacteremia.

Peritoneal dialysis

Effect of mupirocin on rates of S. aureus *infections in patients treated with peritoneal dialysis*

Several groups have used historical controls in studies of intranasal mupirocin [125,126,133] or pericatheter mupirocin [124,134] for preventing infections among patients on continuous ambulatory peritoneal dialysis (CAPD). All these studies found lower rates of infection during the intervention periods. In a study conducted by Perez-Fontan *et al.* [125,126], the proportion of exit-site infections and peritonitis episodes caused by *S. aureus* decreased significantly during the mupirocin treatment period but the proportion of peritonitis episodes caused by Gram-negative organisms increased significantly (Table 30.3). Of the 24 patients treated by Mylotte *et al.* [133], 15 had no further positive

Table 30.3 Studies assessing the efficacy of rifampin and mupirocin for prevention of *S. aureus* infections in peritoneal dialysis patients.[1]

Reference	Date[2]	Study design	Patients studied	Definition of carriage	Agents studied	Infections evaluated	Infection rates: Treatment group	Infection rates: Control group	Infection rates: Historical period	*P* value
Zimmerman *et al.* [135]	1991 (9/1987 to 5/1989)	Prospective, randomized	Patients who had completed more than 6 months of CAPD, regardless of nasal carriage status	NA	Rifampin (300 mg twice daily for 5 days every 3 months) or no treatment	*S. aureus* CI	0.22/patient-year	0.65/patient-year	NA	< 0.05
						S. aureus peritonitis	0.11/patient-year	0.16/patient-year		NS
Perez-Fontan *et al.* [125]	1993 (9/1990 to 8/1992)	Prospective, randomized, placebo-controlled during first 9 months; then prospective open trial	Patients treated with CAPD who carried *S. aureus* in their nares	One of three cultures done at monthly intervals was positive	During first 9 months, intranasal mupirocin or intranasal 0.1% neomycin three times daily for 7 days, repeated every month if patient still carried *S. aureus*; next 15 months all carriers treated with mupirocin	*S. aureus* ESI	0.02/patient-year		0.22/patient-year	
						Proportion of ESI caused by *S. aureus*	44%		90%	< 0.01
						S. aureus peritonitis	0.09/patient-year		0.21/patient-year	
						Proportion of peritonitis episodes caused by *S. aureus*	2.9%		23.7%	< 0.001
						Proportion of peritonitis episodes caused by Gram-negative organisms	23.1%		9.2%	< 0.05
						Rate of peritonitis episodes caused by Gram-negative organisms	0.17		0.08	?
Bernadini *et al.* [124]	1996 (8/1992 to 9/1994)	Randomized prospective comparison of two treatments, compared with historical period	All patients on PD were randomized, controlling for nasal carriage, to one of two treatment groups	One or more nares cultures positive for *S. aureus*	Mupirocin at exit site daily or rifampin 300 mg for 5 days every 3 months	*S. aureus* CI and peritonitis	**Mupirocin** *S. aureus* CI: 0.13/patient-year*‡ *S. aureus* peritonitis: 0.04/patient-year†§ **Rifampin** *S. aureus* CI: 0.15/patient-year* *S. aureus* peritonitis: 0.02/patient-year†	NA	**No treatment** *S. aureus* CI: 0.46/year‡ *S. aureus* peritonitis: 0.16/year§	* NS † NS ‡ < 0.001 § < 0.02

Mupirocin Study Group [128]	1996 (not specified)	Randomized, double-blind, placebo-controlled, multicenter	*S. aureus* nasal carriers who were treated with CAPD in nine European countries	Two of three nasal cultures positive for *S. aureus*	Mupirocin or placebo twice daily for 5 days every 4 weeks	*S. aureus* ESI	0.12/patient-year	0.43/patient-year	NA	0.006
						S. aureus peritonitis	0.15/patient-year	0.22/patient-year		NS
						Tunnel infection	0.078/patient-year	0.097		NS
Mylotte *et al.* [133]	1999 (1/1995 to 5/1998)	Noncomparative, nonblinded study (4/1996 to 5/1998) with historical controls (1/1995 to 3/1996)	24 patients on CAPD who carried *S. aureus*	Two consecutive cultures positive (4/1996 to 6/1997); one positive culture (7/1997 to 5/1998)	Intranasal mupirocin twice daily for 5 days and then two times per month	All peritonitis	12.1 ± 4.3 (1997), 14.3 ± 6.7 (1998)	NA	9.6 ± 2.6 (1995), 9.4 ± 4.3 (1996)	NS
						S. aureus peritonitis	5.6 ± 3.5 (1997), 4.1 ± 3.1 (1998)		3.7 ± 1.7 (1995), 3.6 ± 1.6 (1996)	NS
						All ESI	3.4 ± 3.3 (1997), 4.0 ± 3.2 (1998)		8.8 ± 3.9 (1995), 7.4 ± 4.4 (1996)	0.008
						S. aureus ESI	2.5 ± 2.4 (1997), 0.9 ± 1.7 (1998)		5.6 ± 3.5 (1995), 4.9 ± 3.6 (1996)	0.03
Thodis *et al.* [134]	1998 (11/1/1995 to 10/31/1997)	Quasi-experimental study in which the same group of patients served as the intervention group (11/1/1996 to 10/31/1997) and the comparison group (11/1/1996 to 10/31/1996)	181 patients on CAPD regardless of carrier status	Not defined	Pericatheter mupirocin either daily or three times weekly for 1 year	*S. aureus* exit-site infections	0.01 episodes/ patient/year	NA	0.11 episodes/ patient/year	< 0.01
						S. aureus peritonitis	0.06 episodes/ patient/year		0.19 episodes/ patient/year	< 0.05
						Peritonitis caused by other organisms	0.37 episodes/ patient/year		0.68 episodes/ patient/year	< 0.05

[1] Table updated from Herwaldt [116].
[2] The year outside parentheses is the year in which the study was published; the year within parentheses is the year in which the study was done.
CAPD, continuous ambulatory peritoneal dialysis; CI, catheter infection; ESI, exit-site infection; NA, not applicable; NS, not significant; PD, peritoneal dialysis.

cultures and eight had only one positive culture during the follow-up period (median 8.5 months). The rates of all peritonitis cases and of *S. aureus* peritonitis cases did not change significantly after mupirocin was introduced but the rates of all exit-site infections and *S. aureus* exit-site infections decreased significantly. Bernardini *et al.* [124] prospectively compared the effect of oral rifampin with mupirocin applied to the exit site. Over 1 year, 12% of the patients treated with rifampin and none of those treated with mupirocin stopped treatment because of side effects. Rates of catheter-associated infections, peritonitis, and catheter loss caused by *S. aureus* were not significantly different in the rifampin and mupirocin groups but these rates were significantly lower than the rates during a historical comparison period. Thodis *et al.* [134] treated 181 patients on CAPD with pericatheter mupirocin. Compared with the rates among this same group of patients the previous year, the rates of exit-site infections and peritonitis caused by *S. aureus* decreased significantly during the intervention period as did the rate of peritonitis caused by other organisms.

The Mupirocin Study Group [128] have published the only randomized, double-blind, placebo-controlled trial of mupirocin in CAPD patients who carried *S. aureus* in their nares. The rate of *S. aureus* exit-site infection was significantly lower in the mupirocin group than in the placebo group. However, the overall rate of exit-site infection and the rates of tunnel infections, *S. aureus* peritonitis, all peritonitis, and catheter loss related to *S. aureus* infections were not significantly different in the two groups.

Effect of other agents on rates of S. aureus *infections in patients treated with peritoneal dialysis*

Zimmerman *et al.* [135] randomized 64 patients on peritoneal dialysis to no treatment or to rifampin. The rate of nasal carriage and the rate of peritonitis were not significantly different in the two groups but the rate of catheter infections caused by *S. aureus* decreased significantly in the treatment group (see Table 30.2). These investigators subsequently assessed 169 patients treated with peritoneal dialysis [122]. Age less than 20 years ($P = 0.008$) and *S. aureus* nasal carriage ($P = 0.06$) significantly increased the risk of new peritonitis; the ULTRA Set exchange system ($P = 0.001$) and intermittent prophylactic rifampin ($P = 0.001$) significantly decreased the risk of new peritonitis. However, rifampin did not decrease the risk of new catheter-related infections.

Blowey *et al.* [136] randomized seven children on peritoneal dialysis who carried *S. aureus* in their nares to receive rifampin (20 mg/kg daily in two doses for 5 days) and intranasal bacitracin (two times daily for 7 days) and eight children to no treatment. None of the seven treated children acquired *S. aureus* infection in the month after treatment but four of four untreated patients acquired infections ($P < 0.05$). Hanevold *et al.* [137] treated six children on peritoneal dialysis who carried *S. aureus* in their nares with rifampin (600 mg daily) and cloxacillin (500 mg four times daily) for 7 days. All six patients' nares were decolonized but four patients' nares became recolonized and exit-site colonization was eliminated in only three of five (60%) patients.

Sesso *et al.* [138] randomized nine patients on peritoneal dialysis who carried *S. aureus* in their nares and/or at their catheter exit sites to treatment with intranasal 2% sodium fusidate (twice daily for 5 days). They randomized nine patients to receive oral ofloxacin (200 mg every 48 hours for 5 days) and 13 patients served as a no-treatment control group. The rates of decolonization of the nares (33–43%), rates of decolonization of the exit site (11–43%), and rates of *S. aureus* infection (1.14–1.25 episodes/patient-year) were not significantly different among the three groups.

Summary of studies evaluating whether decolonizing dialysis patients decreases *S. aureus* infection rates

Tacconelli *et al.* [139] conducted a metaanalysis of mupirocin prophylaxis in dialysis patients. The pooled estimates of 10 studies and 9 papers [110–112,125,128, 131,134,140,141] suggested significant risk reductions for *S. aureus* infections among patients undergoing hemodialysis (80%, 95% CI 65–89). The risk reduction among peritoneal dialysis patients was also significant (63%, 95% CI 50–73); the incidence of exit-site infections and peritonitis were reduced 62% and 66%, respectively.

Currently available data suggest that decolonizing the nares prevents *S. aureus* infection in dialysis patients. However, we need additional studies to define the optimal prophylactic regimens, define the role of chlorhexidine in prophylactic regimens, and evaluate whether povidone-iodine or other topical agents decolonize the nares and prevent infection among dialysis patients.

If povidone-iodine or other topical agents are efficacious (see section below on alternative agents), investigators should assess whether alternating mupirocin and another agent reduces infection rates and also prevents selection of resistant *S. aureus* isolates. Staff in dialysis centers that routinely decolonize patients must monitor *S. aureus* susceptibility patterns continuously for resistance to mupirocin or to other agents used in the center to assess whether this practice selects resistant isolates.

Mupirocin resistance

Early studies found few mupirocin-resistant *S. aureus* isolates when this agent was used for limited periods of time [40]. Similarly, in the clinical trial by Perl *et al.* [13] among surgical patients treated prophylactically with mupirocin, only 0.6% of the isolates tested were resistant to mupirocin. Boelaert *et al.* [111] found one high-level mupirocin-resistant isolate among hemodialysis patients who were treated with intranasal mupirocin during 168 person-years of follow-up. Thus, in some patient populations, mupirocin prophylaxis does not appear to increase the incidence of mupirocin-resistant *S. aureus* isolates. In addition, several large studies have found mupirocin-resistance rates of only 1–5.6% [142–144].

Unfortunately, the incidence of mupirocin-resistant MRSA isolates increased when the agent was used extensively for prolonged time periods in endemic settings and when it was applied repeatedly to chronic nonhealing wounds [92,145–150]. For example, Miller *et al.* [145] used mupirocin extensively to decolonize patients during 1990–1993. For 2.5 years, these investigators treated all patients who had positive cultures for MRSA with intranasal mupirocin three times daily and with chlorhexidine showers or baths twice weekly during their entire hospital stay and for 6 months all patients were treated. During this time, the incidence of mupirocin-resistant MRSA increased from 2.7 to 65%.

Vasquez *et al.* [147] used mupirocin as part of a program to reduce endemic MRSA in a Veterans Administration Medical Center and its accompanying long-term-care facility. During 1993–1995, the incidence of high-level mupirocin-resistant MRSA [minimum inhibitory concentration (MIC) ≥ 512 μg/mL] increased significantly but the incidence of low-level mupirocin-resistant MRSA (MIC 4–256 μg/mL) did not change. Patients with decubitus ulcers were at higher risk of high-level mupirocin-resistant MRSA than those without this problem. Exposure to mupirocin was not a risk factor for high-level or low-level mupirocin resistance. Pulsed-field gel electrophoresis patterns of susceptible and resistant strains were similar, suggesting that the endemic MRSA clone acquired the plasmid that carries mupirocin resistance and that the plasmid-carrying strain was spread nosocomially. The authors concluded that mupirocin should not be used extensively in settings where MRSA is endemic.

Perez-Roth *et al.* [151] studied 375 MRSA isolates obtained from patients hospitalized between 1998 and 2002 at a university hospital in the Canary Islands; 48 (12.8%) isolates manifested high-level mupirocin resistance and the proportion of resistant isolates increased from 0% in 1998 to 15.6% in 2002 ($P < 0.001$). These investigators demonstrated that nine different plasmids carrying the *ileS2* locus spread mupirocin resistance among pandemic MRSA lineages from four clonal complexes (CC5, CC8, CC22, CC30), including the clone ST36-II, which replaced ST247-IA (the Iberian clone) as the predominant clone in this area.

In contrast, Caierão *et al.* [152] observed decreasing rates of high-level mupirocin-resistant MRSA and increasing rates of low-level resistance when they used intranasal mupirocin (three times daily for 5 days) and daily baths with 2% chlorhexidine to decolonize MRSA carriers in their ICU. Between May 2000 and April 2003, 5.1–6.7% of the patients in the ICU had MRSA. During the same time period, the proportion of MRSA isolates that had high-level resistance to mupirocin decreased from 13.0% to 0% ($P = 0.02$) and the proportion that had low-level resistance increased from 6.5 to 13.3% ($P = 0.01$). The investigators postulated that the incidence of high-level resistance decreased partly because the resistance determinant was on a mobile plasmid that was lost. However, five of eight patients who had these resistant isolates died within the first year after their isolates were identified and the other three patients were not readmitted during the study period.

The risk of selecting mupirocin-resistant *S. aureus* may be particularly high among patients on CAPD who use mupirocin at their catheter-exit sites. For example, Annigeri *et al.* [117] found that 15% of *S. aureus* isolates obtained from patients who applied mupirocin daily to the exit sites of their peritoneal dialysis catheters were resistant to this agent. Similarly, Perez-Fontan *et al.* [153] noted that the incidence of high-level mupirocin-resistant *S. aureus* increased significantly from 0% (1990–1996) to 12.4% (1999–2000) after patients began using mupirocin at peritoneal dialysis catheter-exit sites. Moreover, patients who carried the mupirocin-resistant isolates had a higher cumulative incidence of exit-site infection than did those with susceptible isolates (32.3% vs. 14.5%; $P = 0.03$).

Fortunately when facilities have strictly controlled the use of mupirocin, resistance to mupirocin has decreased. For example, Walker *et al.* [154] reported that the proportion of high-level mupirocin-resistant *S. aureus* isolates decreased from 31% to 4% after the use of mupirocin was restricted in their hospital. Similarly, Vivoni *et al.* [150] noted that the proportion of MRSA infections caused by mupirocin-resistant isolates decreased from 65% to 15% after mupirocin use was restricted to patients colonized with MRSA who were not infected and who did not have skin lesions. The amount of mupirocin purchased by the hospital also decreased from 10.7 to 3.5 g per 1000 admissions ($P < 0.001$).

Mupirocin resistance has extended into the community. In New Zealand, the incidence of mupirocin-resistant *S. aureus* increased significantly during the 1990s. Upton *et al.* [155] attributed the high rate of resistance (28%) to the fact that mupirocin was available over the counter.

Alternative agents for decolonizing *S. aureus* carriers

Mupirocin is currently the most effective agent for decolonizing persons who carry *S. aureus*. However, investigators are motivated to find other effective agents because a substantial proportion of patients are not decolonized by mupirocin and because resistance to mupirocin is increasing [156]. *In vitro* experiments on some agents have had promising results, including allicin (a garlic extract) [157], indolmycin (discovered in 1960 but not developed because it was active against a limited number of organisms) [158], and lauric acid monoesters [156]. A few studies have assessed the *in vitro* or *in vivo* efficacy of agents such as honey [159–161], gentian violet [162,163], silver sulfadiazine and cerium nitrate [164], tea tree oil [165–167], and extracts of green tea [168].

Probiotics and bacterial interference may also play a role in the future but at present their use is purely experimental. Investigators have attempted to eradicate MRSA colonization by applying "nonpathogenic" bacteria to the anterior nares of colonized persons (bacterial interference) [169]. However, these nonpathogenic strains of *S. aureus* can cause serious complications, including sepsis [170], that may limit use of this approach.

Numerous groups have evaluated whether chlorhexidine bathing alone or in combination with other agents can eliminate *S. aureus* carriage and decrease infections caused by this organism (see following section) [25,30,32,42,48, 59,80,82,87,94,95,109,152,171–179]. Several investigators have used chlorhexidine at other sites [30,32,48,50,61]. For example, Segers *et al.* [180] conducted a double-blind placebo-controlled clinical trial of nasal ointment and mouth wash containing 0.12% chlorhexidine gluconate compared with placebo in patients undergoing elective cardiac surgical procedures. *Staphylococcus aureus* nasal carriage decreased 57.5% in the chlorhexidine group compared with 18.1% in the placebo group ($P < 0.001$). Moreover, the rates of nosocomial infections were 19.8% and 26.2% in the treatment and placebo groups, respectively, for an absolute risk reduction of 6.4% (95% CI 2.3–10.7; $P = 0.002$).

Lysostaphin is a glycylglycine endopeptidase that specifically cleaves the cross-linking pentaglycine bridges of *S. aureus*. Investigators evaluated lysostaphin in the 1960s and 1970s and found that it was active *in vitro* against MRSA [167,181]. Recently, Kokai-Kun *et al.* [182] found that one dose of lysostaphin more effectively eradicates *S. aureus* in a cotton rat model than does mupirocin. Lysostaphin is active *in vitro* against both methicillin-resistant and vancomycin-intermediate resistant strains of *S. aureus* [183]. Some *S. aureus* isolates are resistant to lysostaphin; however, administering lysostaphin and β-lactam antimicrobials together can suppress resistance *in vitro* [184].

Povidone-iodine rapidly kills MRSA and MSSA *in vitro*. Masano *et al.* [185] demonstrated that povidone-iodine can decrease nasal carriage among healthcare workers. Fong [113] randomized 129 patients to receive either a sterile dressing alone or povidone-iodine ointment and a sterile dressing at the exit sites of their hemodialysis catheters; 14 of 63 (22%) patients in the treatment group and 21 of 66 (32%) patients in the control group carried *S. aureus* in their nares. Rates of bacteremia (0% vs. 29%), exit-site infections (0% vs. 24%), and catheter-tip infections (12% vs. 42%) were significantly lower in the treatment group than in the control group ($P < 0.05$). Several groups have assessed whether applying povidone-iodine and other topical antiseptic agents to catheter exit sites can prevent *S. aureus* infections among patients treated with peritoneal dialysis. However, the results of these studies have conflicted.

Fung *et al.* [186] assessed whether polysporin ointment (bacitracin, polymyxin B, and gramicidin; formulation not available in the USA) and bed baths with 4% chlorhexidine could decolonize 11 medical patients who carried MRSA. Prior mupirocin treatment had not decolonized 10 of these patients and five patients had mupirocin-resistant isolates. Nine patients were successfully decolonized, including all six patients who had mupirocin-susceptible isolates and three of five patients who had resistant isolates. However, the authors noted that "concomitant use of oral antibiotics during decolonization with [polysporin] may have confounded the results for four patients in this series." The investigators did not describe the oral regimens received by these patients. In contrast, Soto *et al.* [187] conducted a blinded, randomized, controlled trial of bacitracin and mupirocin among healthcare workers who were *S. aureus* nasal carriers and found that mupirocin was significantly more effective at 72–96 hours (94% vs. 44%) and at 30 days (80% vs. 23%) after treatment.

Some investigators have compared novel agents with agents used commonly in decolonization protocols. For example, Johnson *et al.* [161] compared Medihoney with mupirocin at the catheter exit site for patients dialyzed through intravascular catheters. The incidence of catheter-associated bloodstream infections was similar in the Medihoney group (0.97/1000 catheter-days) and mupirocin group (0.85/1000 catheter-days) (*P* not significant). Other investigators have assessed novel antimicrobial agents in the pleuromutilin family, particularly retapamulin [188, 189,190–196]. The latter agent has good activity against *S. aureus*, including MRSA [191] and is as effective for treating impetigo as 2% sodium fusidate ointment [192].

Bathing with antiseptic solutions

Numerous investigators have used an antimicrobial soap alone or in combination with other agents to decolonize patients [25,30–32,42,48,59,80,82,87,94,95,109,152,171–179, 197–202]. Various groups have used triclosan [173,197], octenidine dihydrochloride [61,200], 0.1% octenidine dihydrochloride and 2% phenoxyethanol [198], and chlorhexidine [18,25,30,32,42,48,59,80,82,87,94,95,109,152,171–179, 200–202] for this purpose.

After the prevalence of patients with MRSA carriage or infection increased on their cardiothoracic surgery ward, Brady *et al.* [197] introduced preoperative and postoperative bathing with 1% triclosan and they decreased the duration of prophylactic cephalothin. The prevalence of MRSA (colonization and infection) was 3.9% before the intervention and 1.8% after the intervention. The prevalence of MRSA infection decreased from 1.0–1.38% in the 3 years before the intervention to 0.15% in the first year after the intervention and increased to 0.71% in the subsequent 6 months. These investigators concluded that their intervention was successful. However, their results could be explained by regression to the mean because they intervened when the rates were high and they did not use time-series methods to analyze the data.

Rengelshausen *et al.* [198] treated five patients who carried MRSA in their nares and at other sites with intranasal mupirocin (three times daily) and 0.1% octenidine dihydrochloride and 2% phenoxyethanol bathing (every other day) and mouth washes (twice daily) for 25 ± 13 days. This regimen decolonized only one of five patients. Rohr *et al.* [199] treated 32 hospitalized MRSA carriers (100% of whom had skin colonization) with intranasal mupirocin and octenidine dihydrochloride body washes for 5 days. The investigators obtained quantitative cultures from the patients' foreheads and necks and semiquantitative cultures from their noses, axillae, and groins. The investigators obtained follow-up cultures 24–48 hours (time II) and 7–9 days (time III) after treatment. All sites were decolonized for 53% of the patients at time II and for 64% at time III. The decolonization rate was 89% for the nares and 56–68% for skin sites at times II and III, respectively.

Simor *et al.* [178] randomized (3 : 1) patients colonized with MRSA to receive either intranasal mupirocin, 2% chlorhexidine baths, and oral rifampin and doxycycline for 7 days or no treatment. Of the 146 patients, 112 were followed for 3 months; 64 of 87 (74%) patients in the treatment arm and 8 of 25 (32%) patients in the no-treatment arm were no longer colonized (RR 1.55, 95% CI 1.17–2.04; $P = 0.0003$). Survival analysis confirmed that treated patients were significantly less likely than patients in the no-treatment group to have MRSA recovered from their cultures ($P < 0.0001$ by log-rank test).

Ridenour *et al.* [200] recently studied whether daily baths with chlorhexidine and selective use of intranasal mupirocin would decrease acquisition of MRSA among patients hospitalized in ICUs. After daily bathing with chlorhexidine was introduced, incident cases of MRSA decreased 52%, from 8.45 to 4.05 cases per 1000 patient-days ($P = 0.48$). Climo *et al.* [201] subsequently studied whether chlorhexidine bathing alone would decrease acquisition of MRSA and vancomycin-resistant enterococci (VRE) and bloodstream infection rates among patients hospitalized in ICUs at four academic medical centers. After daily bathing with chlorhexidine was introduced, acquisition of MRSA decreased 32%, from 5.04 to 3.44 cases per 1000 patient-days. The rate of bloodstream infections also decreased significantly because bloodstream infections caused by Gram-positive organisms (primarily VRE) decreased. The abstract did not report the rate of decolonization.

Girou *et al.* [176] implemented the following MRSA control strategy in their 26-bed medical ICU: (i) active screening, (ii) barrier precautions, (iii) bathing with chlorhexidine for patients who carried MRSA, and (iv) intranasal mupirocin for patients who carried MRSA in their nares. The incidence of all ICU-acquired MRSA cases (5.8% vs. 2.6%; $P = 0.002$) and of acquired MRSA colonization or infection (5.6% vs. 1.4%; $P < 0.001$) decreased after they introduced the control measures but the incidence of imported cases remained stable at 3.8–4.3% ($P = 0.8$). Of note, these authors did not use time-series methods to analyze their data.

In contrast, Harbarth *et al.* [177] randomized 102 hospitalized patients, many of whom were colonized with MRSA at several body sites, to one of two treatment arms: intranasal mupirocin plus chlorhexidine baths or placebo plus chlorhexidine baths. One-quarter of patients who were treated with both intranasal mupirocin and chlorhexidine baths and 8% of those treated with placebo plus chlorhexidine baths were decolonized. The investigators concluded that intranasal mupirocin therapy was only marginally effective for eradicating MRSA carriage from patients who are colonized at several sites and who are treated in facilities where MRSA is endemic.

Wendt *et al.* [202] have conducted the only placebo-controlled trial of bathing with 4% chlorhexidine. They randomized 114 patients to the treatment group ($N = 56$) and to the placebo group ($N = 58$). The placebo was water with 0.1% polysorbate 20 (Tween 20), which looked and smelled similar to chlorhexidine. All patients received intranasal mupirocin ointment three times daily and rinsed their mouths with 2% chlorhexidine solution twice daily. The patients' bedlinen, towels, and clothes were changed daily and their environment was disinfected. Four patients in the treatment group and seven in the placebo group were MRSA-free 30 days after treatment ($P = 0.47$). The only independent predictor of "total eradication" was a small number of colonized sites. The odds of treatment failure was 10 times higher for patients who had more than one colonized site than for patients who only had one colonized site.

Watanakunakorn *et al.* [174] randomized MRSA carriers residing in a long-term care facility to receive either intranasal mupirocin (5 days) and chlorhexidine baths (3 days) or intranasal mupirocin alone. Both treatments temporarily eliminated intranasal colonization in most residents, but 24% of residents who were treated with only intranasal mupirocin and 15% of residents who were treated with mupirocin and chlorhexidine baths became recolonized within 12 weeks. The difference in rates of eradication was not statistically significant.

Failure to decolonize carriers or recolonization of carriers

Troche *et al.* [203] treated 69 MRSA carriers in their ICU with mupirocin (twice daily for 5 days). Only 16 (23%)

were decolonized. Unfortunately, this is not an isolated report. As noted previously, patients whose wounds or other extranasal body sites are colonized with MRSA [39,85,93,177,180,199] and those who have colonized foreign bodies (e.g., tracheostomy tubes, gastrostomy tubes, dentures [204]) are particularly difficult to decolonize. Vasquez *et al.* [147] determined that decubitus ulcers were independent risk factors for mupirocin-resistant MRSA. Several investigators have demonstrated that mupirocin resistance may cause MRSA decolonization efforts to fail [85,159,178]. Simor *et al.* [178] found that patients colonized with mupirocin-resistant MRSA isolates and treated with intranasal mupirocin, chlorhexidine baths, and oral rifampin and doxycycline were less likely to be decolonized than patients colonized with mupirocin-susceptible MRSA isolates.

Hurdle *et al.* [205] have described a patient who was persistently colonized with MRSA and who was not decolonized by treatment with mupirocin. The patient's MRSA isolate was initially susceptible to mupirocin but became resistant during therapy. The investigators identified a mupirocin-resistant *Staphylococcus epidermidis* in the patient's nares. This isolate and the mupirocin-resistant MRSA isolate both harbored a conjugative plasmid that carried the *mupA* determinant. The investigators postulated that the *S. epidermidis* isolate transferred its plasmid to the MRSA isolate while the patient was treated with mupirocin, conferring high-level mupirocin resistance on the MRSA isolate and preventing decolonization. Moreover, Rocha Ferreira *et al.* [206] documented that 16 of 112 coagulase-negative staphylococci (most were *S. epidermidis*) from Brazilian hospitals carried the *ileS-2* gene for mupirocin resistance.

In addition, decolonization may fail if family members, pets, or farm animals carry *S. aureus* [207–210] or if the home environment is contaminated [211]. Decolonization may also fail if patients carry *S. aureus* in their gastrointestinal tracts [85,212–215] or if patients pick their noses [216]. Marschall and Mühlemann [217] found that patients who still carried MRSA after treatment for 5 days with intranasal mupirocin, 4% chlorhexidine baths, and 0.1% chlorhexidine gargles had significantly more risk factors for MRSA carriage than did the patients who were decolonized (mean number of risk factors 1.3 ± 1.37 vs. 0.39 ± 0.65; $P = 0.01$). Harbarth *et al.* [177] and Wendt *et al.* [203] found that patients who have more body sites colonized were more likely to fail decolonization than those who had fewer colonized sites.

Thus, there are several reasons why decolonization regimens may fail to eliminate *S. aureus* carriage. Clinicians who are seeing patients with persistent *S. aureus* carriage that does not respond to decolonization treatment should determine whether *S. aureus* carriage substantially increases the patients' risk for infection and whether the patients have risk factors for persistent carriage. If patients are at increased risk of infection and have remediable risk factors for carriage, clinicians should consider eliminating or ameliorating the risk factors and then attempt again to decolonize the patients.

Cost-effectiveness of nasal decolonization

Boelaert *et al.* [111] reported that the time patients on hemodialysis were hospitalized with *S. aureus* bacteremia decreased from 434 to 74 days after mupirocin prophylaxis was implemented. Moreover, the cost per patient-year for treating bacteremia decreased from $896 to $231. Bloom *et al.* [218] performed a theoretical decision analysis to evaluate the cost-effectiveness of mupirocin prophylaxis. This indicated that mupirocin prophylaxis would save $784 000–1 117 000 per 1000 hemodialysis patient-years.

Davey *et al.* [219] used data from the clinical trial of mupirocin among peritoneal dialysis patients [128] to assess the cost-effectiveness of mupirocin decolonization in this patient population. Compared with patients in the placebo group, patients in the mupirocin group with exit-site infections had lower costs for antimicrobial agents ($P = 0.02$) and hospitalization ($P = 0.065$) but overall antimicrobial costs for treating all infections combined were significantly higher in the mupirocin group ($P = 0.02$). Mupirocin prophylaxis would have been cost neutral if the exit-site infection rate in the placebo group was greater than 75%, if the cost of screening was £3 not £15, or if the cost of treatment was £40 not £93.

However, even if mupirocin or other agents do not decrease the cost of treating infections in patients on CAPD, prophylaxis could be beneficial. For example, mupirocin prophylaxis decreases the incidence of exit-site infections. Thus, the total use of systemic antimicrobial agents including vancomycin may decrease, which in turn could decrease the risk of selecting resistant organisms, including VRE. In addition, individual patients might experience less morbidity and might be able to continue on CAPD longer if they were treated prophylactically.

VandenBergh *et al.* [220] used data from a quasi-experimental study of mupirocin prophylaxsis among patients undergoing cardiothoracic operation. The cost of mupirocin was $11 per patient and the saving per surgical-site infection prevented was $16 633. Their sensitivity analysis demonstrated that the cost of surgical-site infections was the only factor that influenced the model substantially.

Young and Winston [221] conducted a theoretical cost-effectiveness analysis of preoperative use of mupirocin to prevent *S. aureus* healthcare-associated infections. They found that the screen-and-treat strategy (saving $102/patient treated) and the treat-all strategy (saving $88/patient treated) were cost-saving. A one-way sensitivity analysis revealed that the model was robust over the ranges the investigators evaluated for all parameters except the efficacy of mupirocin treatment. If mupirocin's efficacy was less than 16.1%, then the screen-and-treat strategy would incur costs. Young and Winston concluded that use of mupirocin preoperatively would save money primarily because healthcare-associated infections are very expensive.

Summary and conclusions

Clinicians and investigators have long thought that eradicating *S. aureus* (including MRSA) colonization, and thereby preventing infections and spread of the organism, would be simple. We just needed to find the perfect decolonizing agent, the magic bullet, and all our problems with staphylococcal infections and with transmission of this organism would be eliminated. This search has been much like the search for the Holy Grail or the fountain of youth. Despite all our hard work, we have not found what we were looking for.

Not only have we failed to find the one perfect agent, but studies have produced conflicting data. Investigators have used very different methodologies. They have assessed different decolonization regimens, different doses and treatment periods, different follow-up periods, and different primary end points. Moreover, numerous papers describe complex interventions in which several agents were used simultaneously or sequentially. Furthermore, most studies have been quasi-experimental or have used historical controls and most investigators have not used time-series analysis to assess the significance of their findings. Some well-designed studies have shown a benefit for decolonization, while others have not. Thus, clinicians and epidemiologists have had difficulty determining whether any single agent or combination of agents effectively decolonizes patients, preventing *S. aureus* infections, interrupting nosocomial outbreaks, or significantly reducing nosocomial transmission of *S. aureus* in endemic settings. Even the conclusions from the various systematic reviews and metaanalyses differ.

The issue of whether to attempt decolonization is particularly important given that some states have passed laws requiring that hospitals screen patients for MRSA. An early version of a bill in Illinois required that the "hospital must so inform the patient and offer treatment to the patient" [222]. Such a mandate would not be supported by the literature and could, as discussed previously, select MRSA isolates that are also resistant to the agents used commonly for decolonization.

We believe the data on the efficacy of decolonization is strongest for patients on hemodialysis or peritoneal dialysis. The randomized, placebo-controlled, clinical trials and the studies using historical controls produced similar results and essentially all the studies support decolonization. In contrast, the results of studies assessing the efficacy of decolonization to prevent surgical-site infections have been less consistent. Six studies that used historical controls reported reduced rates of *S. aureus* surgical-site infections among mupirocin recipients, with reductions ranging from 36.4 to 88% [66,67,69–72,74]. Most of these studies did not establish the extent to which decolonization reduced *S. aureus* surgical infection rates among patients who were carriers. In addition, we cannot exclude other temporal factors that may have helped reduce *S. aureus* surgical-site infection reported in these studies. A recent Cochrane review of randomized controlled trials of mupirocin decolonization concluded that use of this drug was associated with a significant reduction in *S. aureus* infections [223].

Prospective randomized trials have yielded less convincing reductions in the rate of *S. aureus* surgical-site infection. The large trial by Perl *et al.* [13] found a 50% lower rate of *S. aureus* surgical-site infection among carriers who received mupirocin than among those who received placebo. However, this difference did not reach statistical significance. The incidence of *S. aureus* healthcare-associated infections among carriers who received perioperative mupirocin was significantly lower in the treatment group than in the placebo group. In the trial by Kalmeijer *et al.* [77], perioperative mupirocin treatment did not reduce *S. aureus* surgical-site infection rates significantly but the rate of endogenous *S. aureus* infections among patients who received mupirocin was five times lower than in the placebo group. Similarly, in the trial by Konvalinka *et al.* [76], perioperative mupirocin treatment did not reduce the overall incidence of *S. aureus* surgical-site infections significantly. However, the investigators did not confirm a number of the surgical-site infections in the mupirocin group and the etiological agents were not documented by clinical cultures. Segers *et al.* [180] reported that using chlorhexidine to decolonize the nares and pharynx significantly reduced the overall incidence of postoperative healthcare-associated infections. The incidence of *S. aureus* surgical-site infections was 24.2% lower among those patients who were decolonized than those who were not decolonized, but the difference was not statistically significant.

Given these findings, we believe further studies of *S. aureus* decolonization are warranted, particularly among surgical patients. A large multicenter trial among patients who carry *S. aureus* (the only patients likely to benefit) will be needed to achieve the power necessary to determine whether decolonization prevents *S. aureus* surgical-site infections. Future investigators must consider the duration of preoperative and postoperative mupirocin treatment and whether patients will use antimicrobial soap for their preoperative showers or baths in addition to an agent to decolonize their nares.

Finally, we would like to make several general observations based on our review of the literature and on our clinical experience.

1 Decolonizing patients who carry *S. aureus* in their nares only is relatively easy. Some of these patients may remain free of this organism while others become recolonized with their original strain or with new strains.
2 Patients who carry *S. aureus* at multiple sites are very difficult to decolonize even for brief periods. Several investigators have reported success with complex combinations, which have varied considerably from study to study. Large multicenter trials will be necessary to determine which combinations are most useful and whether such regimens cause significant adverse events or increase resistance.
3 Some patients who initially remain colonized can be decolonized if specific obstacles to decolonization (e.g., colonized family members or contaminated environmental surfaces) are identified and remediated.
4 If healthcare providers continue to use single agents long term in endemic situations or to treat patients with colonized wounds, *S. aureus* strains will become more resistant and the efficacy of current agents will decrease.
5 Investigators must study agents with novel mechanisms. Such agents are unlikely to be the silver bullets we have been seeking but they might improve our ability to eliminate *S. aureus* carriage, decrease infection rates, and decrease transmission, which is certainly a worthy goal.

References

1 Diekema DJ, Pfaller MA, Schmitz FJ *et al.* Survey of infections due to *Staphylococcus* species: frequency of occurrence and antimicrobial susceptibility of isolates collected in the United States, Canada, Latin America, Europe, and the Western Pacific region for the SENTRY Antimicrobial Surveillance Program, 1997–1999. Clin Infect Dis 2001;32(suppl 2):S114–S132.

2 Lowy FD. *Staphylococcus aureus* infections. N Engl J Med 1998; 339:520–32.

3 Skinner D, Keefer CS. Significance of bacteremia caused by *Staphylococcus aureus*. Arch Intern Med 1941;68:851–75.

4 Diekema DJ, Beekmann SE, Chapin KC *et al.* Epidemiology and outcome of nosocomial and community-onset bloodstream infection. J Clin Microbiol 2003;41:3655–60.

5 Blot SI, Vandewoude KH, Hoste EA, Colardyn FA. Outcome and attributable mortality in critically ill patients with bacteremia involving methicillin-susceptible and methicillin-resistant *Staphylococcus aureus*. Arch Intern Med 2002;162:2229–35.

6 Keene A, Vavagiakis P, Lee MH *et al. Staphylococcus aureus* colonization and the risk of infection in critically ill patients. Infect Control Hosp Epidemiol 2005;26:622–8.

7 Campbell W, Hendrix E, Schwalbe R, Farrom A, Edelman R. Head-injured patients who are nasal carriers of *Staphylococcus aureus* are at high risk for *Staphylococcus aureus* pneumonia. Crit Care Med 1999;27:798–801.

8 Mest DR, Wong DH, Shimoda KJ, Mulligan ME, Wilson SE. Nasal colonization with methicillin-resistant *Staphylococcus aureus* on admission to the surgical intensive care unit increases the risk of infection. Anesth Analg 1994;78:644–50.

9 Pujol M, Pena C, Pallares R *et al.* Nosocomial *Staphylococcus aureus* bacteremia among nasal carriers of methicillin-resistant and methicillin-susceptible strains. Am J Med 1996;100:509–16.

10 von Eiff C, Becker K, Machka K, Stammer H, Peters G. Nasal carriage as a source of *Staphylococcus aureus* bacteremia. N Engl J Med 2001;344:11–16.

11 Ena J, Boelaert JR, Boyken LD *et al.* Epidemiology of *Staphylococcus aureus* infections in patients on hemodialysis. Infect Control Hosp Epidemiol 1994;15:78–81.

12 Luzar MA, Coles GA, Faller B *et al. Staphylococcus aureus* nasal carriage and infection in patients on continuous ambulatory peritoneal dialysis. N Engl J Med 1990;322:505–9.

13 Perl TM, Cullen JJ, Wenzel RP *et al.* Intranasal mupirocin to prevent postoperative *Staphylococcus aureus* infections. N Engl J Med 2002;346:1871–7.

14 Delafield ME, Straker D. Antiseptic snuffs. BMJ 1941;1:145–50.

15 Elek SD, Fleming PC. A new technique for the control of hospital cross-infection. Lancet 1960;ii:569–72.

16 Boyce JM. MRSA patients: proven methods to treat colonization and infection. J Hosp Infect 2004;48:S9–S14.

17 Chow JW, Yu VL. *Staphylococcus aureus* nasal carriage in hemodialysis patients: its role in infection and approaches to prophylaxis. Arch Intern Med 1989;149:1258–62.

18 Friedel D, Climo M. Nasal colonization with methicillin-resistant *Staphylococcus aureus*: clinical implications and treatment. Curr Infect Dis Rep 2007;9:201–7.

19 Lipsky BA, Pecoraro RE, Hanley ME. Immediate and long-term efficacy of ofloxacin and other antibiotics for eradication of *Staphylococcus aureus* nasal colonization [Abstract]. In: International Congress for Infectious Diseases, Rio de Janeiro, April 17–21, 1988. New York: International Society for Infectious Diseases, 1988:105.

20 Mulligan ME, Ruane PJ, Johnson L *et al.* Ciprofloxacin for eradication of methicillin-resistant *Staphylococcus aureus* colonization. Am J Med 1987;82(suppl 4A):215–19.

21 Mulligan ME, Citron DM, Kwok YY. Ciprofloxacin resistance during therapy for oxacillin-resistant *Staphylococcus aureus* colonization. In: Program and Abstracts of the 27th Interscience Conference on Antimicrobial Agents and Chemotherapy, New York, 1987, Abstract 277.

22 Mulligan M, Murray-Leisure KA, Ribner BS *et al.* Methicillin-resistant *Staphylococcus aureus*: a consensus review of the microbiology, pathogenesis, and epidemiology with implications for prevention and management. Am J Med 1993;94:313–28.

23 Doebbeling BD, Breneman DL, Neu HC *et al.* Elimination of *Staphylococcus aureus* nasal carriage in health care workers: analysis of six clinical trials with calcium mupirocin ointment. Clin Infect Dis 1993;17:466–74.

24 Fernandez C, Gaspar C, Torrellas A, Vindel A. A double-blind, randomized, placebo-controlled clinical trial to evaluate the safety and efficacy of mupirocin calcium ointment for eliminating nasal carriage of *Staphylococcus aureus* among hospital personnel. J Antimicrob Chemother 1995;35:399–408.

25 Parras F, Guerrero MC, Bouza E *et al.* Comparative study of mupirocin and oral co-trimoxazole plus topical fusidic acid in eradication of nasal carriage of methicillin-resistant *Staphylococcus aureus*. Antimicrob Agents Chemother 1995;39:175–9.

26 Reagan DR, Doebbeling BN, Pfaller MA *et al.* Elimination of coincident *Staphylococcus aureus* nasal and hand carriage with

intranasal application of mupirocin calcium ointment. Ann Intern Med 1991;114:101–6.
27 Moss B, Squire JR, Topley E, Johnston CM. Nose and skin carriage of *Staphylococcus aureus* in patients receiving penicillin. Lancet 1948;i:320–5.
28 Boelaert JR, Van Landuyt HW, Gordts BZ *et al.* Nasal and cutaneous carriage of *Staphylococcus aureus* in hemodialysis patients: the effect of nasal mupirocin. Infect Control Hosp Epidemiol 1996;17:809–11.
29 Wertheim HFL, Vos MC, Ott A. Mupirocin prophylaxis against nosocomial *Staphylococcus aureus* infections in nonsurgical patients: a randomized study. Ann Intern Med 2004;140:419–25.
30 Laterre PR. Failure of mupirocin and chlorhexidine to eradicate methicillin-resistant *Staphylococcus aureus* carriage in an intensive care unit. In: Program and Abstracts of the 39th Interscience Conference on Antimicrobial Agents and Chemotherapy, San Francisco, 1999, Abstract 1702.
31 Buehlmann M, Dangel M, Frei R *et al.* Highly effective regimen for decolonization of methicillin-resistant *S. aureus* (MRSA) carriers. In: Program and Abstracts of the 47th Interscience Conference on Antimicrobial Agents and Chemotherapy, Chicago, 2007, Abstract K-461.
32 Wenisch C, Laferl H, Szell M *et al.* A holistic approach to MRSA eradication in critically ill patients with MRSA pneumonia. Infection 2006;34:148–54.
33 Mcfarlane M, Leavy A, McCaughan J, Fair R, Reid AJM. Successful decolonization of meticillin-resistant *Staphylococcus aureus* in paediatric patients with cystic fibrosis (CF) using a three-step protocol. J Hosp Infect 2006;65:231–6.
34 Boyce JM, Opal SM, Potter-Bynoe G, Medeiros AA. Spread of methicillin-resistant *Staphylococcus aureus* in a hospital after exposure to a health care worker with chronic sinusitis. Clin Infect Dis 1993;17:496–504.
35 Meier PA, Carter CD, Wallace SE *et al.* A prolonged outbreak of methicillin-resistant *Staphylococcus aureus* in the burn unit of a tertiary medical center. Infect Control Hosp Epidemiol 1996; 17:798–802.
36 Sheretz RJ, Reagan DR, Hampton KD *et al.* A cloud adult: the *Staphylococcus aureus*–virus interaction revisited. Ann Intern Med 1996;124:539–47.
37 Casewell MW. New threats to the control of methicillin-resistant *Staphylococcus aureus*. Hosp Infect 1995;30(suppl):465–71.
38 Cookson BD. The emergence of mupirocin resistance: a challenge to infection control and antibiotic prescribing practice. J Antimicrob Chemother 1998;41:11–18.
39 Hill RL, Duckworth GJ, Casewell MW. Elimination of nasal carriage of methicillin-resistant *Staphylococcus aureus* with mupirocin during a hospital outbreak. Antimicrob Agents Chemother 1988;22:377–84.
40 Redhead RJ, Lamb YJ, Rowsel RB. The efficacy of calcium mupirocin in the eradication of nasal *Staphylococcus aureus* carriage. Br J Clin Pract 1991;45:252–4.
41 Nambiar S, Herwaldt LA, Singh N. Outbreak of invasive disease caused by methicillin-resistant *Staphylococcus aureus* in neonates and prevalence in the neonatal intensive care unit. Pediatr Crit Care Med 2003;4:220–6.
42 Sax H, Posfay-Barbe K, Harbarth S *et al.* Control of a cluster of community-associated methicillin-resistant *Staphylococcus aureus* in neonatology. J Hosp Infect 2006;63:93–100.
43 Khoury J, Jones M, Grim A, Dunne WM Jr, Fraser V. Eradication of methicillin-resistant *Staphylococcus aureus* from a neonatal intensive care unit by active surveillance and aggressive infection control measures. Infect Control Hosp Epidemiol 2005;26:616–21.
44 Weber S, Herwaldt LA, McNutt LA *et al.* An outbreak of *Staphylococcus aureus* in a pediatric cardiothoracic surgery unit. Infect Control Hosp Epidemiol 2002;23:77–81.
45 Hitomi S, Kubota M, Mori N *et al.* Control of a methicillin-resistant *Staphylococcus aureus* outbreak in a neonatal intensive care unit by unselective use of nasal mupirocin ointment. J Hosp Infect 2000;46:123–9.
46 Lally RT, Lanz E, Schrock CG. Rapid control of an outbreak of *Staphylococcus aureus* on a neonatal intensive care department using standard infection control practices and nasal mupirocin. Am J Infect Control 2004;32:44–7.
47 Rashid A, Solomon LK, Lewis HG, Khan K. Outbreak of epidemic methicillin-resistant *Staphylococcus aureus* in a regional burns unit: management and implications. Burns 2006;32: 452–7.
48 Rodriguez G, Gaspar MC, Mariano A *et al.* Management of an outbreak of methicillin-resistant *Staphylococcus aureus* in a risk area with empirical intranasal mupirocin. J Hosp Infect 1997; 36:155–61.
49 Mayall B, Martin R, Keenan AM *et al.* Blanket use of intranasal mupirocin for outbreak control and long-term prophylaxis of endemic methicillin-resistant *Staphylococcus aureus* in an open ward. J Hosp Infect 1996;32:257–66.
50 Irish D, Eltringham I, Teall A *et al.* Control of an outbreak of an epidemic methicillin-resistant *Staphylococcus aureus* also resistant to mupirocin. J Hosp Infect 1998;39:19–26.
51 Mean M, Mallaret MR, Andrini P *et al.* A neonatal specialist with recurrent methicillin-resistant *Staphylococcus aureus* (MRSA) carriage implicated in the transmission of MRSA to newborns. Infect Control Hosp Epidemiol 2007;28:625–8.
52 Embil JM, McLeod JA, Al-Barrak AM *et al.* An outbreak of methicillin resistant *Staphylococcus aureus* on a burn unit: potential role of contaminated hydrotherapy equipment. Burns 2001;27:681–8.
53 Maraha B, van Halteren J, Verzijl JM, Wintermans RGF, Buiting AGM. Decolonization of methicillin-resistant *Staphylococcus aureus* using oral vancomycin and topical mupirocin. Clin Microbiol Infect 2001;8:671–5.
54 Faibis F, Laporte C, Fiacre A *et al.* An outbreak of methicillin-resistant *Staphylococcus aureus* surgical-site infections initiated by a healthcare worker with chronic sinusitis. Infect Control Hosp Epidemiol 2005;26:213–15.
55 Bertin ML, Vinski J, Schmitt S *et al.* Outbreak of methicillin-resistant *Staphylococcus aureus* colonization and infection in a neonatal intensive care unit epidemiologically linked to a healthcare worker with chronic otitis. Infect Control Hosp Epidemiol 2006;27:581–5.
56 Black NA, Linnemann CC, Staneck JL, Kotagal UR. Control of methicillin-resistant *Staphylococcus aureus* in a neonatal intensive-care unit: use of intensive microbiologic surveillance and mupirocin. Infect Control Hosp Epidemiol 1996;17:227–31.
57 Longtin Y, Schrenzel J, Francois P, Pittet D, Harbarth S. Long-term follow-up of patients colonized or infected with Panton–Valentine-Leucocidin (PVL)-positive, community-acquired methicillin-resistant *Staphylococcus aureus*. In Program

and Abstracts of the 47th Interscience Conference on Antimicrobial Agents and Chemotherapy, Chicago, 2007, Abstract L-1137.

58 Rihn JA, Posfay-Barbe K, Harner CD *et al.* Community-acquired methicillin-resistant *Staphylococcus aureus* outbreak in a local high school football team: unsuccessful interventions. Pediatr Infect Dis J 2005;24:841–3.

59 Martorell C, Engelman R, Corl A, Brown RB. Surgical site infections in cardiac surgery: an 11-year perspective. Am J Infect Control 2004;32:63–8.

60 Raz R, Miron D, Colodner R *et al.* A one year trial of nasal mupirocin in the prevention of recurrent staphylococcal nasal colonization and skin infection. Arch Intern Med 1996;156: 1109–12.

61 Wiese-Posselt M, Heuck D, Draeger A *et al.* Successful termination of a furunculosis outbreak due to lukS-lukF-positive, methicillin-susceptible *Staphylococcus aureus* in a German village by stringent decolonization, 2002–2005. Clin Infect Dis 2007; 44:e88–e95.

62 White A, Smith J. Nasal reservoir as the source of extranasal staphylococci. Antimicrob Agents Chemother 1963;161:679–83.

63 White A. Increased infection rates in heavy nasal carriers of coagulase-positive staphylococci. Antimicrob Agents Chemother 1963;161:667–70.

64 Kalmeijer MD, van Nieuwland-Bollen E, Bogaers-Hofman D, de Baere GAJ, Kluytmans JAJW. Nasal carriage of *Staphylococcus aureus* is a major risk factor for surgical-site infections in orthopedic surgery. Infect Control Hosp Epidemiol 2000;21: 319–23.

65 Kluytmans JAJW, Mouton JW, Ijzerman EP. Nasal carriage of *Staphylococcus aureus* as a major risk factor for wound infection after cardiac surgery. J Infect Dis 1995;171:216–19.

66 Nicholson MR, Huesman LA. Controlling the usage of intranasal mupirocin does impact the rate of *Staphylococcus aureus* deep sternal wound infections in cardiac surgery patients. Am J Infect Control 2006;34:44–8.

67 Wilcox MH, Hall J, Pike H *et al.* Use of perioperative mupirocin to prevent methicillin-resistant *Staphylococcus aureus* (MRSA) orthopaedic surgical site infections. J Hosp Infect 2003;54: 196–201.

68 Yangco BG, Chandler S, Fisher T, Lauretta J, Pentella M. Reduction of postoperative *Staphylococcus aureus* infections in open heart surgery by intranasal mupirocin. In: Program and Abstracts of the 39th ICAAC, San Francisco, 1999, Abstract 512.

69 Coskun D, Aytac J. Decrease in *Staphylococcus aureus* surgical-site infection rates after orthopaedic surgery after intranasal mupirocin ointment. J Hosp Infect 2004;58:90–1.

70 Coskun D, Aytac J. Decrease in *Staphylococcus aureus* surgical-site infections following cardiovascular surgery. J Hosp Infect 2005;58:287–289.

71 Gernaat-van der Sluis AJ, Hoogenboom-Verdegaal AMM, Edixhoven PJ, Spies-van Rooijen NH. Prophylactic mupirocin could reduce orthopedic wound infections: 1044 patients treated with mupirocin compared with 1260 historical controls. Acta Orthop Scand 1998;69:412–14.

72 Cimochowski GE, Harostock MD, Brown R *et al.* Intranasal mupirocin reduces sternal wound infection after open heart surgery in diabetics and nondiabetics. Ann Thorac Surg 2001; 71:1572–9.

73 Yano J, Doki Y, Inoue M *et al.* Preoperative intranasal mupirocin ointment significantly reduces postoperative infection with *Staphylococcus aureus* in patients undergoing upper gastrointestinal surgery. Surg Today 2000;30:16–21.

74 Kluytmans JAJW, Mouton JW, VandenBergh MFQ *et al.* Reduction of surgical-site infections in cardiothoracic surgery by elimination of nasal carriage of *Staphylococcus aureus*. Infect Control Hosp Epidemiol 1996;17:780–5.

75 Horiuchi A, Nakayama Y, Kajiyama M, Fujii H, Tanaka N. Nasopharyngeal decolonization of methicillin-resistant *Staphylococcus aureus* can reduce PEG peristomal wound infection. Am J Gastroeneterol 2006;101:274–7.

76 Konvalinka A, Errett L, Fong IW. Impact of treating *Staphylococcus aureus* nasal carriers on wound infections in cardiac surgery. J Hosp Infect 2006;64:162–8.

77 Kalmeijer MD, Coertjens H, van Nieuwland-Bollen PM *et al.* Surgical site infections in orthopedic surgery: the effect of mupirocin nasal ointment in a double-blind, randomized, placebo-controlled study. Clin Infect Dis 2002;35:353–8.

78 Suzuki Y, Kamigaki T, Fujino Y *et al.* Randomized clinical trial of preoperative intranasal mupirocin to reduce surgical-site infection after digestive surgery. Br J Surg 2003;90:1072–5.

79 Kallen AJ, Wilson CT, Larson RJ. Perioperative intranasal mupirocin for the prevention of surgical-site infections: systematic review of the literature and meta-analysis. Infect Control Hosp Epidemiol 2005;26:916–22.

80 Sandri AM, Dalarosa MG, de Alcântara LR, Elias LD, Zavascki AP. Reduction in the incidence of nosocomial methicillin-resistant *Staphylococcus aureus* (MRSA) infection in an intensive care unit: role of treatment with mupirocin ointment and chlorhexidine baths for nasal carriers of MRSA. Infect Control Hosp Epidemiol 2006;27:185–7.

81 Kluytmans JAJW, Wertheim HFL. Nasal carriage of *Staphylococcus aureus* and prevention of nosocomial infections. Infection 2005;33:3–8.

82 Rumbak MF, Cancio MR. Significant reduction in methicillin-resistant *Staphylococcus aureus* ventilator-associated pneumonia associated with the institution of a prevention protocol. Crit Care Med 1995;23:1200–3.

83 Paterson DL, Rihs JD, Squier C *et al.* Lack of efficacy of mupirocin in the prevention of infections with *Staphylococcus aureus* in liver transplant recipients and candidates. Transplantation 2003;75:194–8.

84 Singh N, Squier C, Wannstedt C *et al.* Impact of an aggressive infection control strategy on endemic *Staphylococcus aureus* infection in liver transplant recipients. Infect Control Hosp Epidemiol 2006;27:122–6.

85 Dupeyron C, Campillo B, Bordes M *et al.* A clinical trial of mupirocin in the eradication of methicillin-resistant *Staphylococcus aureus* nasal carriage in a digestive disease unit. J Hosp Infect 2002;52:281–7.

86 Dupeyron C, Campillo B, Richardet J-P, Soussy C-J. Long-term efficacy of mupirocin in the prevention of infections with meticillin-resistant *Staphylococcus aureus* in a gastroenterology unit. J Hosp Infect 2006;63:385–92.

87 Shitrit P, Gottesman B-S, Katzir M *et al.* Active surveillance for methicillin-resistant *Staphylococcus aureus* (MRSA) decreases the incidence of MRSA bacteremia. Infect Control Hosp Epidemiol 2006;27:1004–8.

88 Muller A, Talon D, Potier A *et al*. Use of intranasal mupirocin to prevent methicillin-resistant *Staphylococcus aureus* infection in intensive care units. Crit Care 2005;9:R246–R250.

89 Wertheim HFL, Vos MC. Can mupirocin prevent methicillin-resistant *Staphylococcus aureus* infections? Crit Care 2005;9: 257–8.

90 Capitano B, Leshem, OA, Nightingale CH, Nicolau DP. Cost effect of managing methicillin-resistant *Staphylococcus aureus* in a long-term care facility. J Am Geriatr Soc 2003;51:10–16.

91 Cederna JE, Terpenning MS, Ensberg M, Bradley SF, Kauffman CA. *Staphylococcus aureus* nasal colonization in a nursing home: eradication with mupirocin. Infect Control Hosp Epidemiol 1990;11:13–16.

92 Kauffman CA, Terpenning MS, He X *et al*. Attempts to eradicate methicillin-resistant *Staphylococcus aureus* from a long-term-care facility with the use of mupirocin ointment. Am J Med 1993;94: 371–8.

93 Mody L, Kauffman CA, McNeil SA, Galecki AT, Bradley SF. Mupirocin-based decolonization of *Staphylococcus aureus* carriers in residents of two long-term care facilities: a randomized, double-blind, placebo-controlled trial. Clin Infect Dis 2003;37: 1467–74.

94 Kotilainen P, Routamaa M, Peltonen R *et al*. Eradication of methicillin-resistant *Staphylococcus aureus* from a health center ward and associated nursing home. Arch Intern Med 2001;161: 859–63.

95 Jaqua-Stewart MJ, Tjaden J, Humphreys DW *et al*. Reduction in methicillin-resistant *Staphylococcus aureus* infection rate in a nursing home by aggressive containment strategies. S D J Med 1999;52:241–7.

96 Bradley SF. Methicillin-resistant *Staphylococcus aureus*: long-term care concerns. Am J Med 1999;106:2S–10S.

97 McNeil SA, Mody L, Bradley SF. Methicillin-resistant *Staphylococcus aureus*: management of asymptomatic colonization and outbreaks of infection in long-term care. Geriatrics 2002;57: 16–27.

98 Nsouli KA, Lazarus M, Schoenbaum SC *et al*. Bacteremic infection in hemodialysis. Arch Intern Med 1979;139:1255–8.

99 Yu VL, Goetz A, Wagener M *et al*. *Staphylococcus aureus* nasal carriage and infection in patients on hemodialysis: efficacy of antibiotic prophylaxis. N Engl J Med 1986;315:91–6.

100 Quarles LD, Rutsky EA, Rostand SG. *Staphylococcus aureus* bacteremia in patients on chronic hemodialysis. Am J Kidney Dis 1985;6:412–19.

101 Barcenas CG, Fuller TJ, Elms J, Cohen R, White MG. Staphylococcal sepsis in patients on chronic hemodialysis regimens: intravenous treatment with vancomycin given once weekly. Arch Intern Med 1976;136:1131–4.

102 Mennes PA, Gilula LA, Anderson CB *et al*. Complications associated with arteriovenous fistulas in patients undergoing chronic hemodialysis. Arch Intern Med 1978;138:1117–21.

103 Kaplowitz LG, Comstock JA, Landwehr DM, Dalton HP, Mayhall CG. A prospective study of infections in hemodialysis patients: patient hygiene and other risk factors for infection. Infect Control Hosp Epidemiol 1988;9:534–41.

104 Francioli P, Masur H. Complications of *Staphylococcus aureus* bacteremia: occurrence in patients undergoing long-term hemodialysis. Arch Intern Med 1982;142:1655–8.

105 Mathews M, Shen F-H, Lindner A, Sherrard DJ. Septic arthritis in hemodialysis patients. Nephron 1980;25:87–91.

106 Moxley GF, Moffatt TL, Falls WF Jr. Hemodialysis-related osteomyelitis. South Med J 1980;73:376–9.

107 Holton DL, Nicolle LE, Diley D, Bernstein K. Efficacy of mupirocin nasal ointment in eradicating *Staphylococcus aureus* nasal carriage in chronic haemodialysis patients. J Hosp Infect 1991;17:133–7.

108 Bommer J, Vergetis W, Andrassy K *et al*. Elimination of *Staphylococcus aureus* in hemodialysis patients. ASAIO J 1995; 41:127–31.

109 Watanakunakorn C, Brandt J, Durkin P *et al*. The efficacy of mupirocin ointment and chlorhexidine body scrubs in the eradication of nasal carriage of *Staphylococcus aureus* among patients undergoing long-term hemodialysis. Am J Infect Control 1992;20:138–41.

110 Kluytmans JAJW, Manders M-J, van Bommel E, Verbrugh H. Elimination of nasal carriage of *Staphylococcus aureus* in hemodialysis patients. Infect Control Hosp Epidemiol 1996;17: 793–7.

111 Boelaert JR, De Smedt RA, De Baere YA *et al*. The influence of calcium mupirocin nasal ointment on the incidence of *Staphylococcus aureus* infections in haemodialysis patients. Nephrol Dial Transplant 1989;4:278–81.

112 Boelaert JR, Van Landuyt HW, Godard CA *et al*. Nasal mupirocin ointment decreases the incidence of *Staphylococcus aureus* bacteraemias in haemodialysis patients. Nephrol Dial Transplant 1993;8:235–9.

113 Fong IW. Prevention of haemodialysis and peritoneal dialysis catheter related infection by topical povidone-iodine. Postgrad Med J 1993;69:S15–S17.

114 Kirmani N, Tuazon CU, Murray HW, Parrish AE, Sheagren JN. *Staphylococcus aureus* carriage rate of patients receiving long-term hemodialysis. Arch Intern Med 1978;138:1657–9.

115 Martin AM, Clunie GJA, Tonkin RW, Robson JS. The aetiology and management of shunt infections in patients on intermittent haemodialysis. Proc Eur Dial Transplant Assoc 1967;4:67–72.

116 Herwaldt LA. Reduction of *Staphylococcus aureus* nasal carriage and infection in dialysis patients. J Hosp Infect 1998;40:S13–S23.

117 Annigeri R, Conly J, Vas SI *et al*. Emergence of mupirocin-resistant *Staphylococcus aureus* in chronic peritoneal dialysis patients using mupirocin prophylaxis to prevent exit-site infection. Perit Dial Int 2001;21:554–9.

118 Davies SJ, Ogg CS, Cameron JS, Poston S, Noble WC. *Staphylococcus aureus* nasal carriage, exit-site infection and catheter loss in patients treated with continuous ambulatory peritoneal dialysis (CAPD). Perit Dial Int 1989;9:61–4.

119 Sewell CM, Clarridge J, Lacke C, Weinman EJ, Young EJ. *Staphylococcal* nasal carriage and subsequent infection in peritoneal dialysis patients. JAMA 1982;248:1493–5.

120 Sesso R, Draibe S, Castelo A. *Staphylococcus aureus* skin carriage and development of peritonitis in patients on continuous ambulatory peritoneal dialysis. Clin Nephrol 1989;31:264–8.

121 Wanten GJA, van Oost P, Schneeberger PM, Koolen MI. Nasal carriage and peritonitis by *Staphylococcus aureus* in patients on continuous ambulatory peritoneal dialysis: a prospective study. Perit Dial Int 1996;16:352–6.

122 Oxton LL, Zimmerman SW, Roecker EB, Wakeen M. Risk factors for peritoneal dialysis-related infections. Perit Dial Int 1994;14:137–44.

123 Piraino B, Perlmutter JA, Holley JL, Bernardini J. *Staphylococcus aureus* peritonitis is associated with *Staphylococcus aureus* nasal

carriage in peritoneal dialysis patients. Perit Dial Int 1992;13: S332–S334.
124 Bernardini J, Piraino B, Holley J, Johnston JR, Lutes R. A randomized trial of *Staphylococcus aureus* prophylaxis in peritoneal dialysis patients: mupirocin calcium ointment 2% applied to the exit site versus cyclic oral rifampin. Am J Kidney Dis 1996; 27:695–700.
125 Perez-Fontan M, Garcia-Falcon T, Rosales M *et al.* Treatment of *Staphylococcus aureus* nasal carriers in continuous ambulatory peritoneal dialysis with mupirocin: long-term results. Am J Kidney Dis 1993;22:708–12.
126 Perez-Fontan M, Rosales M, Rodriguez-Carmona A *et al.* Treatment of *Staphylococcus aureus* nasal carriers in CAPD with mupirocin. Adv Perit Dial 1992;8:242–5.
127 Lye WC, Leong SO, van der Straaten J, Lee EJC. *Staphylococcus aureus* CAPD-related infections are associated with nasal carriage. Adv Perit Dial 1994;10:163–5.
128 Mupirocin Study Group. Nasal mupriocin prevents *Staphylococcus aureus* exit-site infection during peritoneal dialysis. J Am Soc Nephrol 1996;7:2403–8.
129 Pignatari A, Pfaller M, Hollis R *et al. Staphylococcus aureus* colonization and infection in patients on continuous ambulatory peritoneal dialysis. J Clin Microbiol 1990;28:1898–902.
130 Pena C, Fernandez-Sabe N, Dominguez MA *et al. Staphylococcus aureus* nasal carriage in patients on haemodialysis: role of cutaneous colonization. J Hosp Infect 2004;58:20–7.
131 Sesso R, Barbosa D, Leme IL *et al. Staphylococcus aureus* prophylaxis in hemodialysis patients using central venous catheter: effect of mupirocin ointment. J Am Soc Nephrol 1998;9: 1085–92.
132 Johnson DW, MacGinley R, Kay TD *et al.* A randomized controlled trial of topical exit site mupirocin application in patients with tunneled, cuffed haemodialysis catheters. Nephrol Dial Transplant 2002;17:1802–7.
133 Mylotte JM, Kahler L, Jackson E. "Pulse" nasal mupirocin maintenance regimen in patients undergoing continuous ambulatory peritoneal dialysis. Infect Control Hosp Epidemol 1999;20:741–5.
134 Thodis E, Bhaskaran S, Pasadakis P *et al.* Decrease in *Staphylococcus aureus* exit-site infections and peritonitis in CAPD patients by local application of mupirocin ointment at the catheter exit site. Perit Dial Int 1998;18:261–70.
135 Zimmerman SW, Ahrens E, Johnson CA *et al.* Randomized controlled trial of prophylactic rifampin for peritoneal dialysis-related infections. Am J Kidney Dis 1991;18:225–31.
136 Blowey DL, Warady BA, McFarland KS. The treatment of *Staphylococcus aureus* nasal carriage in pediatric peritoneal dialysis patients. Adv Perit Dial 1994;10:297–9.
137 Hanevold CD, Fisher MC, Waltz R, Bartosh S, Baluarte HJ. Effect of rifampin on *Staphylococcus aureus* colonization in children on chronic peritoneal dialysis. Pediatr Nephrol 1995;9:609–11.
138 Sesso R, Parisio K, Dalboni A *et al.* Effect of sodium fusidate and ofloxacin on *Staphylococcus aureus* colonization and infection in patients on continuous ambulatory peritoneal dialysis. Clin Nephrol 1994;41:370–6.
139 Tacconelli E, Carmeli Y, Aizer A *et al.* Mupirocin prophylaxis to prevent *Staphylococcus aureus* infection in patients undergoing dialysis: a meta-analysis. Clin Infect Dis 2003;37:1629–38.
140 Casey M, Taylor J, Clinard P *et al.* Application of mupirocin cream at the catheter exit site reduces exit-site infections and peritonitis in peritoneal dialysis patients. Perit Dial Int 2000;20: 566–8.
141 Crabtree JH, Hadnott LL, Burchette RJ, Siddiqi RA. Outcome and clinical implications of a surveillance and treatment program for *Staphylococcus aureus* nasal carriage in peritoneal dialysis patients. Adv Perit Dial 2000;16:271–5.
142 Bischoff WE, Wallis ML, Tucker KB, Reboussin BA, Sherertz RJ. *Staphylococcus aureus* nasal carriage in a student community: prevalence, clonal relationships, and risk factors. Infect Control Hosp Epidemiol 2004;25:485–91.
143 Schmitz F-J, Lindenlauf E, Hofmann B *et al.* The prevalence of low- and high-level mupirocin resistance in *staphylococci* from 19 European hospitals. J Antimicrob Chemother 1998;42:489–95.
144 Deshpanda LM, Fix AM, Pfaller MA, Jones RN. Emerging elevated mupirocin resistance rates among staphylococcal isolates in the SENTRY Antimicrobial Surveillance Program (2000): correlations of results from disk diffusion, Etest and reference dilution methods. Diagn Microbiol Infect Dis 2002;42: 283–90.
145 Miller MA, Dascal A, Portnoy J, Mendelson J. Development of mupirocin resistance among methicillin-resistant *Staphylococcus aureus* (MRSA) after widespread use of nasal mupirocin ointment. Infect Control Hosp Epidemiol 1996;17:811–13.
146 Netto dos Santos KR, Fonseca LD, Filhe PPG. Emergence of high-level mupirocin resistance in methicillin-resistant *Staphylococcus aureus* isolated from Brazilian university hospitals. Infect Control Hosp Epidemiol 1996;17:813–16.
147 Vasquez JE, Walker ES, Franzus BW *et al.* The epidemiology of mupirocin resistance among methicillin-resistant *Staphylococcus aureus* at a Veterans' Affairs hospital. Infect Control Hosp Epidemiol 2000;21:459–64.
148 Cookson BD. The emergence of mupirocin resistance: a challenge to infection control and antibiotic prescribing practice. J Antimicrob Chemother 1998;41:11–18.
149 Rahman M, Noble WC, Cookson B. Transmissible mupirocin resistance in *Staphylococcus aureus*. Epidemiol Infect 1989;102: 261–70.
150 Vivoni AM, Santos KRN, de-Oliveira MP *et al.* Mupirocin for control of methicillin-resistant *Staphylococcus aureus*: lessons from a decade of use at a university hospital. Infect Control Hosp Epidemiol 2005;26:662–7.
151 Perez-Roth E, Lopez-Aguilar C, Alcoba-Florez J, Mendez-Alvarez S. High-level mupirocin resistance within methicillin-resistant *Staphylococcus aureus* pandemic lineages. Antimicrob Agents Chemother 2006;50:3207–11.
152 Caierão J, Berquó L, Cicero D, d'Azevedo PA. Decrease in the incidence of mupirocin resistance among methicillin-resistant *Staphylococcus aureus* in carriers from an intensive care unit. Am J Infect Control 2006;34:6–9.
153. Perez-Fontan M, Rosales M, Rodríguez-Carmona A, Falcón TG, Valdés F. Mupirocin resistance after long-term use for *Staphylococcus aureus* colonization in patients undergoing chronic peritoneal dialysis. Am J Kidney Dis 2002;39:337–41.
154 Walker ES, Vasquez JE, Dula R, Bullock H, Sarubbi FA. A decline in mupirocin resistance in methicillin-resistant *Staphylococcus aureus* accompanied administrative control of prescriptions. J Clin Microbiol 2004;42:2792–5.
155 Upton A, Lang S, Heffernan H. Mupirocin and *Staphylococcus aureus*: a recent paradigm of emerging antibiotic resistance. J Antimicrob Chemother 2003;51:613–17.

156 Rouse MS, Rotger M, Piper KE *et al.* In vitro and in vivo evaluation of the activities of lauric acid monoester formulations against *Staphylococcus aureus*. Antimicrob Agents Chemother 2005;49:3187–91.
157 Cutler RR, Wilson P. Antibacterial activity of a new, stable, aqueous extract of allicin against methicillin-resistant *Staphylococcus aureus*. Br J Biomed Sci 2004;61:71–4.
158 Hurdle JG, O'Neill AJ, Chopra I. Anti-staphylococcal activity of indolmycin, a potential topical agent for control of staphylococcal infections. J Antimicrob Chemother 2004;54:549–52.
159 Natarajan S, Williamson D, Grey J, Harding KG, Cooper RA. Healing of an MRSA-colonized, hydroxyurea-induced leg ulcer with honey. J Dermatol Treat 2001;12:33–6.
160 Miorin PL, Levy NC Jr, Custodio AR, Bretz WA, Marcucci MC. Antibacterial activity of honey and propolis from *Apis mellifera* and *Tetragonisca angustula* against *Staphylococcus aureus*. J Appl Microbiol 2003;95:913–20.
161 Johnson DW, van Eps C, Mudge DW *et al.* Randomized, controlled trial of topical exit-site application of honey (Medihoney) versus mupirocin for the prevention of catheter-associated infections in hemodialysis patients. J Am Soc Nephrol 2005;16: 1456–62.
162 Okano M, Noguchi S, Tabata K, Matsumoto Y. Topical gentian violet for cutaneous infection and nasal carriage with MRSA. Int J Dermatol 2000;39:942–4.
163 Saji M, Taguchi S, Uchiyama K *et al.* Efficacy of gentian violet in the eradication of methicillin-resistant *Staphylococcus aureus* from skin lesions. J Hosp Infect 1995;31:225–8.
164 Schuenck RP, Dadalti P, Silva MG, Fonseca LS, Santos KRN. Oxacillin- and mupirocin-resistant *Staphylococcus aureus*: in vitro activity of silver sulphadiazine and cerium nitrate in hospital strains. Chemotherapy 2004;16:453–8.
165 Dryden MS, Dailly S, Crouch M. A randomized, controlled trial of tea tree topical preparations versus a standard topical regimen for the clearance of MRSA colonization. J Hosp Infect 2004;56:283–6.
166 Caelli M, Porteous J, Carson CF, Heller R. Tea tree oil as an alternative topical decolonization agent for methicillin-resistant *Staphylococcus aureus*. J Hosp Infect 2000;46:236–7.
167 LaPlante KL. In vitro activity of lysostaphin, mupirocin, and tea tree oil against clinical methicillin-resistant *Staphylococcus aureus*. Diagn Microbiol Infect Dis 2007;57:413–18.
168 Matsumura T, Saito T, Nozaki S, Miyai I, Kang J. MRSA infection control in the wards for progressive muscular dystrophy: the effects of encouraged hand-washing. Rinsho Shinkeigaku 2000;40:8–13.
169 Uehara Y, Nakama H, Agematsu K, Uchida M. Bacterial interference among nasal inhabitants: eradication of *Staphylococcus aureus* from nasal cavities by artificial implantation of *Corynebacterium* sp. Hosp Infect 2000;44:127–33.
170 Houck PW, Nelson JD, Kay JL. Fatal septicemia due to *Staphylococcus aureus* 502A. Report of a case and review of the infectious complications of bacterial interference programs. Am J Dis Child 1972;123:45–8.
171 Bartzokas CA, Paton JH, Gibson MF *et al.* Control and eradication of methicillin-resistant *Staphylococcus aureus* on a surgical unit. N Engl J Med 1984;311:1422–5.
172 Tyzack R. The management of methicillin-resistant *Staphylococcus aureus* in a major hospital. Hosp Infect 1985;6:195–9.
173 Zafar AB, Butler RC, Reese DJ, Gaydos LA, Mennonna PA. Use of 0.3% triclosan (Bacti-Stat*) to eradicate an outbreak of methicillin-resistant *Staphylococcus aureus* in a neonatal nursery. Am J Infect Control 1995;23:200–8.
174 Watanakunakorn C, Axelson C, Bota B, Stahl C. Mupirocin ointment with and without chlorhexidine baths in the eradication of *Staphylococcus aureus* nasal carriage in nursing home residents. Am J Infect Control 1995;23:306–9.
175 Sloot N, Siebert J, Hoffler U. Eradication of MRSA from carriers by means of whole-body washing with an antiseptic in combination with mupirocin nasal ointment. Zentralbl Hyg Umweltmed 1999;202:513–23.
176 Girou E, Pujade G, Legrand P, Cizeau F, Brun-Buisson C. Selective screening of carriers for control of methicillin-resistant *Staphylococcus aureus* (MRSA) in high-risk hospital areas with a high level of endemic MRSA. Clin Infect Dis 1998; 27:543–50.
177 Harbarth S, Dharan S, Liassine N *et al.* Randomized, placebo-controlled, double-blind trial to evaluate the efficacy of mupirocin for eradicating carriage of methicillin-resistant *Staphylococcus aureus*. Antimicrob Agents Chemother 1999;43: 1412–16.
178 Simor AE, Phillips E, McGeer A. Randomized controlled trial of chlorhexidine gluconate for washing, intranasal mupirocin, and rifampin and doxycycline versus no treatment for the eradication of methicillin-resistant *Staphylococcus aureus* colonization. Clin Infect Dis 2007;44:178–85.
179 Semret M, Miller MA. Topical mupirocin for eradication of MRSA colonization with mupirocin-resistant strains. Infect Control Hosp Epidemiol 2001;22:578–80.
180 Segers P, Speekenbrink RGH, Ubbink DT, van Ogtrop ML, de Mol BA. Prevention of nosocomial infection in cardiac surgery by decontamination of the nasopharynx and oropharynx with chlorhexidine gluconate. A randomized trial. JAMA 2006;296: 2460–6.
181 Quickel KE Jr, Selden R, Caldwell JR, Nora NF, Schaffner W. Efficacy and safety of topical lysostaphin treatment of persistent nasal carriage of *Staphylococcus aureus*. Appl Microbiol 1971;22:446–50.
182 Kokai-Kun JF, Walsh SM, Chanturiya T, Mond JJ. Lysostaphin cream eradicates *Staphylococcus aureus* nasal colonization in a cotton rat model. Antimicrob Agents Chemother 2003;47:1589–97.
183 von Eiff C, Kokai-Kun JF, Becker K, Peters G. In vitro activity of recombinant lysostaphin against *Staphylococcus aureus* isolates from anterior nares and blood. Antimicrob Agents Chemother 2003;47:3613–15.
184 Climo MW, Ehlert K, Archer GL. Mechanism and suppression of lysostaphin resistance in oxacillin-resistant *Staphylococcus aureus*. Antimicrob Agents Chemother 2001;45:1431–7.
185 Masano H, Fukuchi K, Wakuta R, Tanaka Y. Efficacy of intranasal application of povidone-iodine cream in eradicating nasal methicillin-resistant *Staphylococcus aureus* in neonatal intensive care unit (NICU) staff. Postgrad Med J 1993;69:S122–S125.
186 Fung S, O'Grady S, Kennedy C *et al.* The utility of polysporin ointment in the eradication of methicillin-resistant *Staphylococcus aureus* colonization: a pilot study. Infect Control Hosp Epidemiol 2000;21:653–5.
187 Soto NE, Vaghijimal A, Stahl-Avicolli A *et al.* Bacitracin versus mupirocin for *Staphylococcus aureus* nasal colonization. Infect Control Hosp Epidemiol 1999;20:351–3.

188 Brooks G, Burgess W, Colthurst D *et al.* Pleuromutilins. Part 1. The identification of novel mutilin 14-carbamates. Bioorg Med Chem 2001;9:1221–31.
189 Champney WS, Rodgers WK. Retapamulin inhibition of translation and 50S ribosomal subunit formation in *Staphylococcus aureus* cells. Antimicrob Agents Chemother 2007;51:3385–7.
190 Pankuch GA, Lin G, Hoellman DB *et al.* Activity of retapamulin against *Streptococcus pyogenes* and *Staphylococcus aureus* evaluated by agar dilution, microdilution, E-test, and disk diffusion methodologies. Antimicrob Agents Chemother 2006;50:1727–30.
191 Jones RN, Fritsche TR, Sader HS, Ross JE. Activity of retapamulin (SB-275833), a novel pleuromutilin, against selected resistant Gram-positive cocci. Antimicrob Agents Chemother 2006;50:2583–6.
192 Oranje AP, Chosidow O, Sacchidanand S *et al.* Topical retapamulin ointment, 1%, versus sodium fusidate ointment, 2%, for impetigo: a randomized, observer-blinded, noninferiority study. Dermatology 2007;215:331–40.
193 Bitar CM, Mayhall CG, Lamb VA *et al.* Outbreak due to methicillin- and rifampin-resistant *Staphylococcus aureus*: epidemiology and eradication of the resistant strain from the hospital. Infect Control 1987;8:15–23.
194 Bryan CS, Wilson RS, Meade P, Sill LG. Topical antibiotic ointments for staphylococcal nasal carriers: survey of current practices and comparison of bacitracin and vancomycin ointments. Infect Control 1980;1:153–6.
195 Weathers L, Riggs D, Santeiro M, Weibley RE. Aerosolized vancomycin for treatment of airway colonization by methicillin-resistant *Staphylococcus aureus*. Pediatr Infect Dis J 1990; 9:220–1.
196 Gradon JD, Wu EH, Lutwick LI. Aerosolized vancomycin therapy facilitating nursing home placement. Ann Pharmacother 1992;26:209–10.
197 Brady LM, Thomson M, Palmer MA, Harkness JL. Successful control of endemic MRSA in a cardiothoracic surgical unit. Med J Aust 1990;152:240–5.
198 Rengelshausen J, Nürnberger J, Philipp T, Kribben A. Decolonization of methicillin-resistant *Staphylococcus aureus* by disinfection of the skin. JAMA 2000;108:685–6.
199 Rohr U, Mueller C, Wilhelm M, Muhr G, Gatermann S. Methicillin-resistant *Staphylococcus aureus* whole-body decolonization among hospitalized patients with variable site colonization by using mupirocin in combination with octenidine dihydrochloride. J Hosp Infect 2003;54:305–9.
200 Ridenour G, Lampen R, Federspiel J *et al.* Selective use of intranasal mupirocin and chlorhexidine bathing and the incidence of methicillin-resistant *Staphylococcus aureus* colonization and infection among intensive care unit patients. Infect Control Hosp Epidemiol 2007;28:1155–61.
201 Climo MW, Bush A, Fraser VJ *et al.* Daily bathing with chlorhexidine reduces the incidence of methicillin resistant *Staphylococcus aureus* (MRSA), vancomycin-resistant enterococci (VRE), and healthcare-associated bloodstream infections (HABSI): results of a multicenter trial. In: Program and Abstracts of the 17th Annual Meeting of the Society for Healthcare Epidemiology in America, Baltimore, 2007, Abstract 297.
202 Wendt C, Schinke S, Wurttemberger M *et al.* Value of whole-body washing with chlorhexidine for the eradication of methicillin-resistant *Staphylococcus aureus*: a randomized, placebo-controlled, double-blind clinical trial. Infect Control Hosp Epidemiol 2007;28:1036–43.
203 Troche G, Joly L-M, Guibert M, Zazzo J-F. Detection and treatment of antibiotic-resistant bacterial carriage in a surgical intensive care unit: a 6-year prospective survey. Infect Control Hosp Epidemiol 2005;26:161–5.
204 Rossi T, Peltonen R, Laine J *et al.* Eradication of the long-term carriage of methicillin-resistant *Staphylococcus aureus* in patients wearing dentures: a follow-up of 10 patients. J Hosp Infect 1996;34:311–20.
205 Hurdle JG, O'Neill AJ, Mody L, Chopra I, Bradley SF. *In vivo* transfer of high-level mupirocin resistance from *Staphylococcus epidermidis* to methicillin-resistant *Staphylococcus aureus* associated with failure of mupirocin prophylaxis. J Antimicrob Chemother 2005;26:1166–8.
206 Rocha Ferreira BR, Nunes APF, Kokis VM. Simultaneous detection of the *mecA* and *ileS-2* genes in coagulase-negative staphylococci isolated from Brazilian hospitals by multiplex PCR. Diagn Microbiol Infect Dis 2002;42:205–12.
207 Hollis R, Barr J, Doebbeling B, Pfaller M, Wenzel R. Familial carriage of methicillin-resistant *Staphylococcus aureus* and subsequent infection in a premature neonate. Clin Infect Dis 1995;21:328–32.
208 Widmer AF, Doebbeling BN, Costigan M *et al.* Source of recolonization following elimination of *Staphylococcus aureus* nasal carriage from chronic carriers [Abstract]. In: Program and Abstracts of the 32nd annual meeting of the Interscience Conference on Antimicrobial Agents and Chemotherapy, Anaheim, 1992.
209 Voss A, Loeffen F, Bakker J, Klaassen C, Wulf M. Methicillin-resistant *Staphylococcus aureus* in pig farming. Emerg Infect Dis 2005;11:1965–6.
210 Manian FA. Asymptomatic nasal carriage of mupirocin-resistant, methicillin-resistant *Staphylococcus aureus* (MRSA) in a pet dog associated with MRSA infection in household contacts. Clin Infect Dis 2003:36:26–8.
211 de Boer HE, van Elzelingen-Dekker CM, van Rheenen-Verberg CM, Spanjaard L. Use of gaseous ozone for eradication of methicillin-resistant *Staphylococcus aureus* from the home environment of a colonized hospital employee. Infect Control Hosp Epidemiol 2006;27:1120–2.
212 Bhalla A, Aron DC, Donskey CJ. *Staphylococcus aureus* intestinal colonization is associated with increased frequency of *S. aureus* on skin of hospitalized patients. BMC Infect Dis 2007;7:105.
213 Boyce JM, Havill NL, Maria B. Frequency and possible infection control implications of gastrointestinal colonization with methicillin-resistant *Staphylococcus aureus*. J Clin Microbiol 2005;43:5992–5.
214 Klotz M, Zimmermann S, Opper S, Heeg K, Mutters R. Possible risk for re-colonization with methicillin-resistant *Staphylococcus aureus* (MRSA) by faecal transmission. Int J Hyg Environ Health 2005;208:401–5.
215 Squire C, Rihs JD, Risa KJ *et al.* *Staphylococcus aureus* rectal carriage and its association with infections in patiens in a surgical intensive care unit and a liver transplant unit. Infect Control Hosp Epidemiol 2002;23:495–501.
216 Wertheim HFL, van Kleef M, Vos MC *et al.* Nose picking and nasal carriage of *Staphylococcus aureus*. Infect Control Hosp Epidemiol 2006;27:863–7.

217 Marschall J, Mühlemann K. Duration of methicillin-resistant *Staphylococcus aureus* carriage according to risk factors for acquisition. Infect Control Hosp Epidemiol 2006;27:1206–12.

218 Bloom BS, Fendrick AM, Chernew ME, Patel P. Clinical and economic effects of mupirocin calcium on preventing *Staphylococcus aureus* infection in hemodialysis patients: a decision analysis. Am J Kidney Dis 1996;27:687–94.

219 Davey P, Craig A-M, Hau C, Malek M. Cost-effectiveness of prophylactic nasal mupirocin in patients undergoing peritoneal dialysis based on a randomized placebo-controlled trial. J Antimicrob Chemother 1999;43:105–12.

220 VandenBergh MFQ, Kluytmans JAJW, van Hout BA *et al*. Cost-effectiveness of perioperative mupirocin nasal ointment in cardiothoracic surgery. Infect Control Hosp Epidemol 1996;17:786–92.

221 Young LS, Winston LG. Perioperative use of mupirocin for the prevention of healthcare-associated *Staphylococcus aureus* infections: a cost-effective analysis. Infect Control Hosp Epidemiol 2006;27:1304–12.

222 http://www.ilga.gov/legislation/94/SB/09400SB2771.htm. Accessed 12/4/06.

223 van Rijen M, Bonten M, Wenzel R, Kluytmans J. Mupirocin ointment for preventing *Staphylococcus aureus* infections in nasal carriers. Cochrane Database Syst Rev 2008;4:CD006216.

Chapter 31
Treatment of Staphylococcal Infection

Kent B. Crossley[1] *and Joseph John*[2]

[1] Department Veterans Affairs Medical Center and University of Minnesota Medical School, Minneapolis, Minnesota, USA
[2] Ralph H. Johnson Department of Veterans Affairs Medical Center, and Medical University of South Carolina, Charleston, South Carolina, USA

Introduction

Staphylococcal infections have been an inherent part of human suffering for millennia. There is clear evidence that pyogenic infections with the characteristics of those caused by *Staphylococcus aureus* existed in the Neolithic period some 5000 years ago [1,2]. As hospitals developed in the Middle Ages, infections almost certainly caused by *S. aureus* became a major cause of debility and death in those institutions [3]. For centuries, staphylococci have been not only important community pathogens but also a menace to the hospitalized patient.

Evidence of the treatment of staphylococcal infection by surgical drainage dates back as far as Neolithic times. In contrast, effective drug therapy for these infections has been available for less than 70 years. The modern treatment of staphylococcal disease has been a continuous challenge because of the severity of the infections, the facility with which these organisms acquire new pathogenic mechanisms, and the development of antimicrobial resistance. Penicillin-resistant strains, emerging in the mid-twentieth century, were treated first with vancomycin and soon thereafter with new effective nontoxic antistaphylococcal antibiotics [4,5]. Over the last 50 years progressively more resistant staphylococci have emerged [6]. Relatively few new antibiotics active against these organisms have been introduced. Mortality associated with infections caused by resistant *S. aureus* has remained very significant over time (Figure 31.1).

Although the multiresistant staphylococci collectively grouped as "methicillin resistant" arose primarily as nosocomial pathogens [7–10], even the lay public is now very well aware of the risks associated with methicillin-resistant *S. aureus* (MRSA) infection in the hospital and the community [11,12]. The treatment of these infections has relied on older antibiotics, such as vancomycin and trimethoprim–sulfamethoxazole (TMP–SMX) that are less than optimal in efficacy, safety, and cost. Several new agents, designed to be effective against MRSA and to address the shortcomings of the older agents, will be introduced in the next several years [13].

Each of the clinical chapters in this book includes discussion about specific aspects of therapy. This chapter is intended to recommend an approach to the antibiotic management of staphylococcal infection and to offer information about the drugs commonly used to treat staphylococcal infection.

Approach to the management of staphylococcal infection

An approach to a seriously ill patient with staphylococcal infection is outlined in the algorithm in Figure 31.2. *Staphylococcus aureus* must be considered a possible cause in any patient with evidence of acute life-threatening infection. Unless there is clear indication of another etiology (e.g., symptoms and signs of urinary tract infection with Gram-negative bacteria evident in the urine), antibiotic coverage for staphylococci should be included in the initial treatment of a seriously ill febrile patient. Management of coagulase-negative staphylococcal infection should follow the same process as described here for *S. aureus*. These organisms are very often methicillin resistant. While the discussion of *Staphylococcus epidermidis* infections in Chapter 15 contains additional detail, discussion of these organisms is included here as appropriate.

Although untrue in certain parts of Europe, in much of the world MRSA accounts for a substantial portion of cases of *S. aureus* infection in both hospital and community settings. For this reason, initial treatment of presumed or documented staphylococcal infections before susceptibility information is available requires therapy effective against both MRSA and methicillin-sensitive *S. aureus* (MSSA). In practical terms, this means the initiation of treatment with vancomycin for patients who require intravenous therapy or who are hospitalized.

At the same time as therapy is initiated, studies need to be done to determine the primary focus of the infection

Staphylococci in Human Disease, 2nd edition. Edited by Kent B. Crossley, Kimberly K. Jefferson, Gordon Archer, Vance G. Fowler, Jr.
 ISBN 978-14051-6332-3.

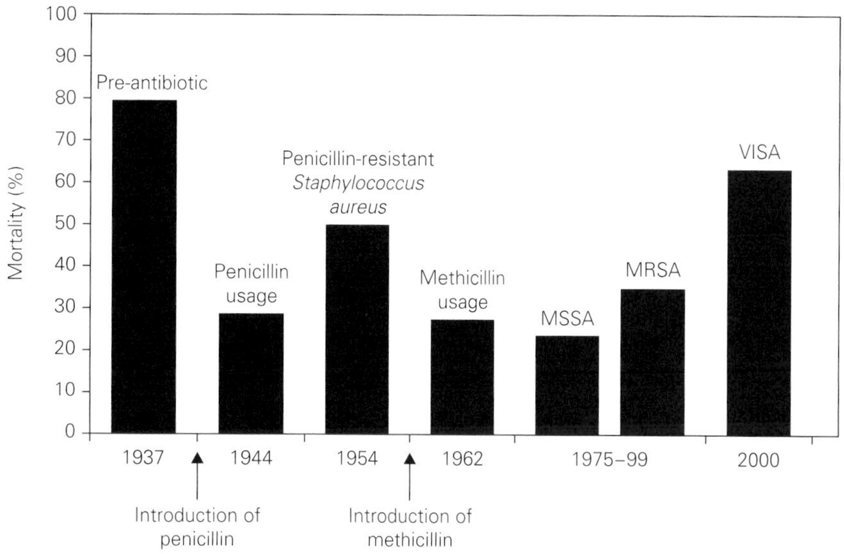

Figure 31.1 Mortality rates of antibiotic-resistant staphylococcal bacteremia over time. Data are from three US studies of mortality. VISA, vancomycin-intermediate *S. aureus*. (From Dancer [7] with permission).

if one is not evident (Figure 31.2). This requires a careful physical examination (including a digital rectal examination to exclude a prostatic abscess), chest radiography, and abdominal and pelvic imaging if there is a history of recent surgery or evidence of intraabdominal pathology (e.g., organomegaly and/or tenderness on physical examination). In large recent series of staphylococcal bacteremia, the most common sites of infection include intravascular devices, skin and soft tissue, bone, and heart valves [14,15]. These should be thoroughly evaluated for evidence of infection. Intravascular catheters are especially important and need to be carefully assessed and usually removed (see Chapter 18 for details).

Once antibiotic susceptibilities are available, decisions about therapy can be made. If the organism is MRSA or methicillin-resistant *S. epidermidis* (MRSE), vancomycin needs to be continued for a full course of treatment or until an oral agent is considered appropriate. Vancomycin serum levels are usually measured and dosing is adjusted to yield desired trough levels [16,17]. This is done primarily in an attempt to increase effectiveness, rather than minimize toxicity. There is limited evidence that this is useful, although recent studies suggest increased toxicity at the higher serum levels recommended especially for staphylococcal pneumonia [18,19].

Although another glycopeptide (teicoplanin) is available in many countries and other possible therapies might be considered (e.g., linezolid or daptomycin), there is little evidence to suggest that initiating therapy with, or changing to, these drugs is likely to be beneficial. There is some controversial evidence to suggest that linezolid may possibly be more effective in treating *S. aureus* pneumonia than vancomycin (see Chapter 23 for a discussion of the issues). As additional comparative trials are done in future years, vancomycin may be replaced by newer agents (discussed at the end of this chapter) as the most appropriate empirical therapy for *S. aureus* bacteremia. A summary of parenteral agents that may be used for treatment of MRSA bacteremia is presented in Table 31.1.

If the staphylococcal isolate is found to be methicillin susceptible, treatment should be changed to a β-lactam antibiotic (usually oxacillin, nafcillin or cefazolin). This is an important step because the antibiotics that are appropriate for methicillin-resistant staphylococci are not necessarily optimal for treatment of methicillin-susceptible strains. While there are scant data about outcomes of MSSA infection when treated with linezolid or daptomycin, the evidence of vancomycin's inferiority is extensive. Vancomycin is less effective than β-lactam antibiotics in the management of pneumonia caused by MSSA [19]. In another trial, use of vancomycin for treatment of methicillin-susceptible staphylococcal bacteremia in dialysis patients was less effective than cefazolin [20]. A recently published study of MSSA bacteremia found that mortality rates were more than three times higher among patients who received vancomycin than among those who were given a β-lactam [21]. This confirms findings of an earlier study [14]. Vancomycin is also associated with significantly more side effects than the β-lactam antibiotics [22].

If the patient's signs of infection do not promptly resolve, it is necessary to search for untreated infected foci that may require drainage or surgical management. Additional blood cultures should be collected in patients with ongoing symptoms of infection such as fever, leukocytosis, or rigors. With both MRSA and MSSA, localized infection needs to be identified (usually by imaging studies) and purulent material drained. Examples of common staphylococcal infections that may need drainage include soft tissue and renal abscesses and deep postoperative infections. In one recent study, 39% of patients with

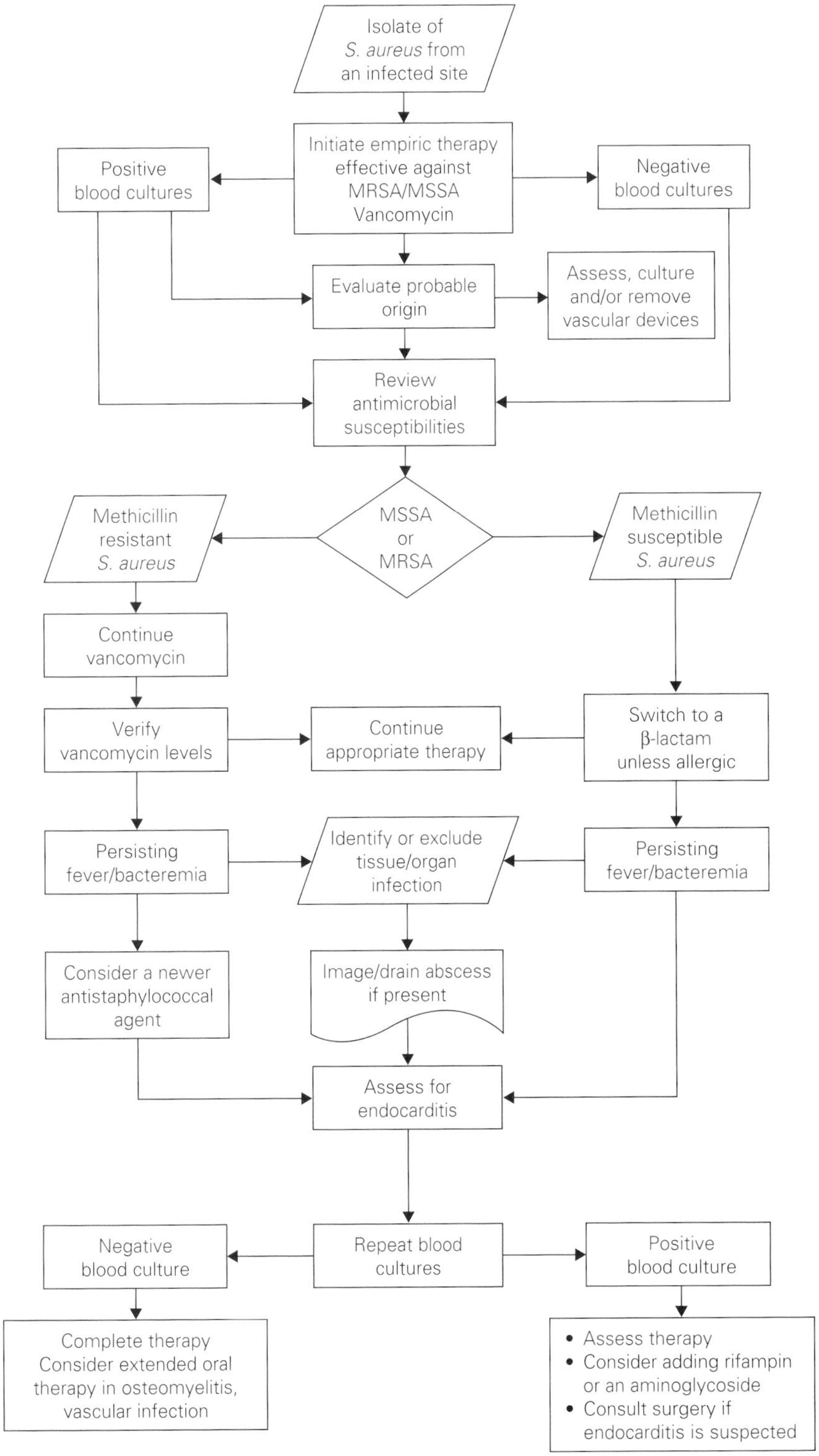

Figure 31.2 Algorithmic approach to the management of serious staphylococcal infection. See text for details.

S. aureus bacteremia had "complicating infectious foci." One-third of these had no associated signs or symptoms and 10% were detected initially at autopsy. Mortality was significantly higher in patients with these foci of infection than in those without [23].

Management of coagulase-negative staphylococcal bacteremia is similar. While abscesses are uncommonly caused by *S. epidermidis*, biofilm on prosthetic surfaces (such as heart valves and artificial joints) that contain these organisms is often the focus for coagulase-negative staphylococcal bacteremia. Some species of coagulase-negative staphylococci (notably *S. haemolyticus* and *S. lugdunensis*) may cause local infections, endocarditis, and bacteremia that are clinically similar in many ways to those caused by *S. aureus*.

Table 31.1 Parenteral agents for use in treatment of methicillin-resistant *S. aureus* infections. (Modified from Moellering [26] with permission.)

Drug	Usual adult dose	Cost[1]	Adverse effects	Comments
Proven efficacy				
Vancomycin	1 g every 12 hours	193	Neutropenia, "red man" syndrome	Treatment failures frequent
Daptomycin	4 mg/kg every 24 hours	1625	Elevated muscle enzymes	Resistance has developed during therapy. Not for pneumonia
Other agents with limited data regarding efficacy				
Linezolid	600 mg every 24 hours	2277	Thrombocytopenia, neuropathy	Treatment failures reported
Quinupristin–dalfopristin	7.5 mg/kg every 12 hours	5120	Myalgias, reactions at infusion site	Reasonable efficacy in one clinical trial
Trimethoprim–sulfamethoxazole	10–15 mg/kg daily in 2–3 divided doses	350	Rash and other allergic reactions	Effective when compared with vancomycin in one clinical trial

[1] Average wholesale price for 10 days' treatment in US dollars.

Endocarditis always needs to be considered when there is clinical evidence of ongoing infection. Seemingly trivial skin or soft tissue infection may result in *S. aureus* bacteremia and endocarditis. Unless another endovascular focus is recognized, transesophageal echocardiography is usually a key part of the evaluation of a patient with persisting bacteremia [24]. Patients with evidence of endocarditis (or other endovascular infection) need to be evaluated for surgical intervention as part of their therapy. Addition of an aminoglycoside and/or rifampin is also commonly recommended for treatment of endocarditis caused by either MRSA or MRSE [25].

If there is no evidence of endovascular infection, treatment should be continued for an appropriate period based on the probable focus of the infection. Duration of therapy is discussed in the chapters that deal with specific clinical conditions. In general, however, there has been a trend in the past decade to extend duration of therapy (e.g., to 6–8 weeks) and to use long-term follow-up treatment with oral agents in both vascular infections and osteomyelitis.

In patients who are not severely ill and not thought to be bacteremic, oral antibiotic therapy may be used as initial treatment (or as follow-up treatment after intravenous antibiotics). Selection of oral agents for MRSA infection is based on relatively limited data. Linezolid is effective against MRSA and is available as an oral antibiotic. However, because of cost and potential side effects, it is generally used only for serious documented methicillin-resistant staphylococcal infection. Many community-acquired MRSA infections are caused by isolates that remain susceptible to TMP–SMX, the tetracyclines, and clindamycin. There is only modest evidence of the efficacy of any of these agents against MRSA infection [26]. A summary of information about oral antibiotics used in the treatment of MRSA is provided in Table 31.2.

Specific agents for the treatment of staphylococcal infection

Although sulfonamides, the first widely available antimicrobials, were effective against *S. aureus*, isolates rapidly became resistant by over producing para-aminobenzoic acid [27]. The advent of effective therapy for *S. aureus* infection began with the availability of penicillin in the early 1940s. While the action of penicillin had been discovered by Fleming a number of years earlier in 1928, it was the development of novel methods for the production and concentration of this antibiotic that made it available for clinical use [28].

Most staphylococci were penicillin susceptible until the mid-1950s. In that decade, penicillin-resistant isolates of *S. aureus* began to be widely seen in hospitals in the USA. Vancomycin, introduced in 1955, was the first effective therapy for infection caused by these penicillin-resistant isolates [17]. Penicillinase-resistant penicillins, introduced several years later, soon became the mainstay of therapy because they were cheaper and less toxic than vancomycin. A variety of other antibacterials, including macrolides, tetracyclines, and cephalosporins that were also effective against many isolates of *S. aureus*, were introduced at about the same time.

The β-lactam antibiotics

Penicillins

Nearly all isolates of *S. aureus* and *S. epidermidis* produce β-lactamase and are resistant to benzylpenicillin. However, this antibiotic remains useful for treatment of infection

Table 31.2 Oral agents for treatment of methicillin-resistant *S. aureus* infections. (Modified from Proctor [176] with permission.)

Drug	Usual adult dose	Cost[1]	Adverse effects	Comments
TMP–SMX	1–2 double-strength tablets every 12 hours	9.40 (generic) 39.40 (Bactrim DS)	Rash and other allergic reactions	No adequate controlled trials to prove efficacy. May not provide adequate coverage for *Streptococcus pyogenes*
Doxycycline	100 mg every 12 hours	22.00 (generic) 100.00 (Vibramycin)	Allergic reactions, nausea, anorexia	Good *in vitro* activity against staphylococci and streptococci but recent emergence of resistance among CA-MRSA in California and Boston
Minocycline	100 mg every 12 hours	50.80 (generic) 77.00 (Minocin)	Vertigo, headache, photosensitivity	See comments for doxycycline
Rifampin	600 mg/day	38.00 (generic)	Flu-like syndrome, thrombocytopenia	Rapid emergence of resistance if used alone. May be added to TMP–SMX or tetracycline regimens. No clinical evidence of benefit
Clindamycin	300–600 mg every 6–8 hours	95.10 (generic)	Diarrhea, anaphylaxis, thrombocytopenia	Possibility of emergence of resistance when used against organisms with MLS_B resistance
Linezolid	600 mg every 12 hours	1286.80	Thrombocytopenia, neuropathy	Expensive. Efficacy against MRSA demonstrated in controlled trials

[1] Cost for 10 days' treatment in US dollars.

CA-MRSA, community-acquired methicillin-resistant *S. aureus*; MLS_B, macrolide lincosamide streptogramin B; TMP–SMX, trimethoprim–sulfamethoxazole.

caused by susceptible staphylococcal isolates. It is several fold more active against these organisms than other penicillins [29]. The short half-life of the drug (approximately 30 min) requires frequent dosing and it may only be given by the intravenous route. For these reasons and because almost all *S. aureus* isolates are resistant, benzylpenicillin is rarely used at present to treat staphylococcal infection.

The so-called "semisynthetic" penicillins are a group of related antibiotics with a molecular structure designed to resist hydrolysis by staphylococcal β-lactamase [30] (Figure 31.3). Oxacillin, cloxacillin, and dicloxacillin are isoxazolyl penicillins; nafcillin is structurally different from these compounds. These antibiotics (as is true of other β-lactams) have several different mechanisms of action against staphylococci, the most important of which is interfering with cross-linking of the cell wall. These drugs are rapidly bactericidal against susceptible staphylococci at relatively low concentrations (i.e., ≤ 8 μg/mL).

Methicillin, the initial representative of this class of drugs, is no longer available in the USA because it was more frequently associated with interstitial nephritis than similar drugs. The most commonly used semisynthetic penicillins are oxacillin and nafcillin. Although structurally different, these drugs are both highly effective against staphylococcal infections, achieve high serum concentrations, and have limited toxicity. Dosing is similar for both agents (e.g., 4–12 g/day in four to six divided doses). Nafcillin is more extensively eliminated via the biliary route than oxacillin and some physicians prefer to use this drug in patients with changing or impaired renal function as no modification in dosing is needed. In contrast, renal dosing is often recommended for oxacillin [31].

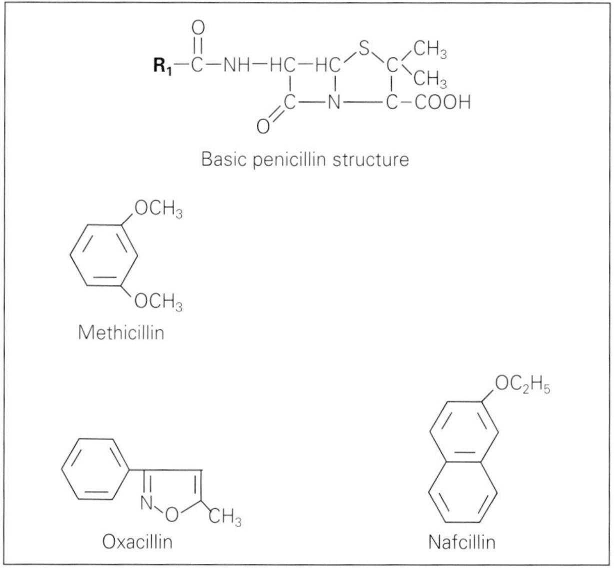

Figure 31.3 Structure of the semisynthetic penicillinase-resistant penicillins. Note that nafcillin has a different chemical structure from methicillin and oxacillin.

In animal models of infective endocarditis, both oxacillin and nafcillin are highly effective [32]. Because this is a particularly difficult infection to treat, data from endocarditis studies are often used as a proxy for overall efficacy. Animal experiments and clinical studies both indicate that these drugs are more effective than vancomycin against MSSA infections [21,33].

Because of the experimental evidence, extensive clinical experience, and limited toxicity, nafcillin and oxacillin continue to be the drugs of choice for the parenteral treatment of methicillin-susceptible staphylococcal infections. There are limited data to position one of these drugs over the other. Maraqa *et al.* [34] compared adverse reactions to nafcillin and oxacillin and found that hepatotoxicity and rash were more common with oxacillin than with nafcillin in a group of 222 children treated with outpatient parenteral antimicrobial therapy.

Nafcillin and oxacillin are not suitable for oral administration because of limited and erratic absorption. Cloxacillin and dicloxacillin are isoxazolyl penicillins given by mouth that are resistant to the action of gastric acid and absorbed in a reliable fashion. Both of these drugs are well absorbed if there is food present in the stomach. They are very highly protein bound and share a relatively short half-life. Because cloxacillin and dicloxacillin were introduced before extensive clinical trials were the norm, published data about the efficacy of these drugs are limited. For this reason and because they have remained expensive, many experienced clinicians prefer a cephalosporin (e.g., cephalexin) for the oral therapy of staphylococcal infection.

Side effects with the antistaphylococcal penicillins are relatively infrequent. Significant allergic reactions are uncommon. It should be assumed that a patient who has had a reaction to one penicillin would have a similar reaction to other drugs in the same class [35]. Because of the greater efficacy of penicillins in serious MSSA infection, desensitization should be considered in penicillin-allergic patients with infections such as MSSA endocarditis. Desensitization is not without risk and consultation with an allergist is strongly recommended if this procedure is considered.

Oxacillin and nafcillin may occasionally be associated with development of interstitial nephritis [36,37]. The process is thought to be the result of activation of drug-specific T cells that secrete cytokines responsible for the renal damage [38]. It is often associated with presence of eosinophils in the urine. On occasion, nafcillin and oxacillin (as well as cloxacillin and dicloxacillin) may cause cholestatic hepatitis [39–43]. The orally administered antistaphylococcal penicillins may be associated with development of diarrhea and *Clostridium difficile* infection [44], but the risk is relatively low with these compounds (Figure 31.4).

There is extensive clinical experience with these penicillins in pregnancy but no well-controlled studies in pregnant women. These drugs (as well as other penicillins and cephalosporins) are therefore placed in Pregnancy Category B by the Food and Drug Administration (FDA). A recent review of antibiotics commonly used in pregnancy concluded that there was no teratogenic potential with benzylpenicillin and phenoxymethylpenicillin [45].

Combinations of β-lactam and β-lactamase inhibitor

The combinations of amoxicillin or ticarcillin with clavulanic acid, piperacillin with tazobactam, and ampicillin with sulbactam are all effective against methicillin-susceptible staphylococci. The β-lactamase inhibitor lowers the minimal inhibitory concentration (MIC) for the penicillin when tested against MSSA. These agents are not generally used as first-line therapy for staphylococcal infection because they are more appropriate for treatment of Gram-negative organisms and have a broader than needed spectrum. They are also more often associated with *C. difficile* colitis

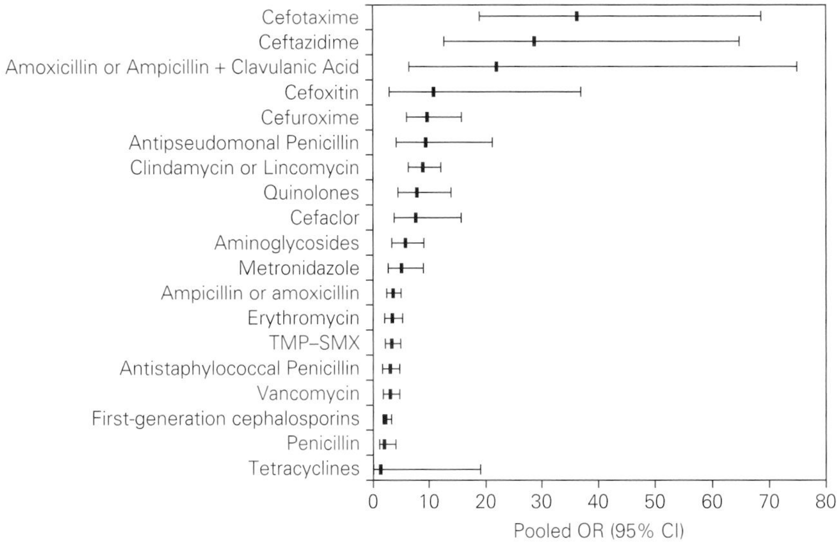

Figure 31.4 Risk of *Clostridium difficile* colitis as a function of oral antibiotic selection. Note that the antistaphylococcal penicillins are relatively uncommon causes of *C. difficile* colitis. CI, confidence interval; OR, odds ratio; TMP–SMX, trimethoprim–sulfamethoxazole. (From Owens *et al.* [44] with permission.)

than the antistaphylococcal penicillins [44]. Amoxicillin–clavulanic acid tends to be associated with more gastrointestinal side effects than dicloxacillin. When these combination drugs are selected as treatment for patients with mixed infection or as empirical therapy, they are effective against MSSA infection [46,47].

Cephalosporins

The cephalosporin antibiotics are another group of β-lactam antibiotics useful in the treatment of staphylococcal infections. Though most of the cephalosporins are very effective against staphylococci, some variation in activity among members of this family exists. As is true of the penicillins, marketed drugs in this class are only useful for treatment of methicillin-susceptible staphylococcal infection. A new broad-spectrum cephalosporin (ceftobiprole) with activity against MRSA is presently in late-stage clinical trials [48,49].

Of the parenteral cephalosporins, cefazolin is probably most often used for the treatment of MSSA infection. The drug has a relatively narrow spectrum of activity. Although there are few data, use of this antibiotic is assumed to be associated with less suprainfection and colonization with resistant organisms than broader-spectrum cephalosporins [50]. The drug's half-life (1.5–2 hours) allows it to be dosed every 8 hours. Because of reduced administration costs and apparent comparable efficacy in most situations, cefazolin has largely replaced the parenteral semisynthetic penicillins for outpatient parenteral antistaphylococcal therapy. With the exception of cefipime, most other cephalosporins are somewhat less active against staphylococci than cefazolin. Ceftazidime, ceftriaxone, ceftizoxime, and cefoxitin are less active than cefuroxime and cefotaxime [51].

These are some data to suggest that the cephalosporins are less effective than the semisynthetic penicillins in serious staphylococcal infection. In an animal model of endocarditis, cefazolin, ceftizoxime, ceftriaxone, cefotaxime, cefoperazone, and cefuroxime were all less effective than nafcillin [52]. In another study, methicillin was significantly more active than cefazolin or cephalothin in reducing numbers of *S. aureus* in cardiac vegetations [53]. In general, because of these and similar data, antistaphylococcal penicillins are preferable to cephalosporins in serious staphylococcal infections such as endocarditis.

Controversy surrounds the clinical importance of type A β-lactamase, a more effective inactivator of cefazolin than other β-lactamases [54]. There are occasional reports of clinical failure with cefazolin therapy in some patients with staphylococcal endocarditis [54,55]. Lack of association between the presence of type A β-lactamase and failure in treatment of joint infection with cefazolin has been documented [56].

There are a number of oral cephalosporins available that may be useful in treating staphylococcal infection. As is true of the marketed parenteral agents, broader-spectrum oral cephalosporins are generally less active against staphylococci than older agents such as cephalexin. Agents that are clinically useful against staphylococci when administered by mouth would include cephalexin and cefuroxime axetil. The antistaphylococcal activity of cefpodoxime is limited. Orally administered cephalosporins are well absorbed; however, cefuroxime axetil has the lowest bioavailability and its absorption may be increased significantly by administration with food. Most oral cephalosporins are not significantly metabolized but rather eliminated unchanged by renal excretion [51].

The cephalosporin antibiotics share a side-effect profile very similar to the penicillins. Allergic reactions are most frequent in patients who have had a reaction to a penicillin; there is a 5–10% probability of a cross-reaction when these individuals are given a cephalosporin [57]. In patients with immediate allergic reactions to the penicillins (i.e., urticaria or bronchospasm), a cephalosporin antibiotic should be avoided. Cephalosporins may be used in a patient who has had a nonurticarial rash or other benign allergic reaction to a penicillin. A recent paper suggests that cross-reactivity is primarily an issue with the first-generation cephalosporins and that more recently introduced agents are uncommonly associated with cross-reactions in penicillin-allergic patients [58].

Other side effects of this group of drugs include nausea, vomiting, and diarrhea. Diarrhea may be a significant problem with larger oral doses of cephalexin. As with the oral penicillins, these drugs are believed to be safe for use in pregnancy [45].

Macrolides and lincosamides

Both the macrolides and the lincosamides, primarily clindamycin, have a long track record in the treatment of staphylococcal infection. These drugs, along with the streptogramins, everninomycins, and oxazolidinones, block the 30S and 50S subunits of the bacterial ribosome [59]. Erythromycin and the expanded 14-membered macrolide antibiotics like clarithromycin all bind at the entrance to the 50S polypeptide exit tunnel. At that site there is a build-up of t-RNA, eventually leading to termination of elongation of the polypeptide.

The newer macrolides are more stable in the acid pH of the stomach and have less gastrointestinal toxicity. They also have better tissue penetration and longer half-lives, which allow dosing once or twice a day. Azithromycin has gained widespread acceptance due to its low toxicity and the option for both parenteral and oral dosing. MSSA isolates are often susceptible to macrolides but multiresistant nosocomial isolates of *S. aureus* tend to exhibit high-level resistance to all the macrolides. Some community-acquired isolates of MRSA remain susceptible to the macrolides but this varies by geography [60,61]. Telithromycin is a third-generation macrolide that has extended activity against staphylococci but it has been indicted for occasional severe hepatic toxicity and thus has to be used with extreme caution, particularly for long-term treatment.

Clindamycin has the most appeal in this class of drugs for therapy of staphylococcal infection. It has extraordinary penetration into tissue, including bone, and many clinicians have become very comfortable with the agent even though it is expensive and needs to be given at least three times daily (in doses of 150–300 mg). While macrolide therapy is appropriate only for mild to moderate staphylococcal infection, over the last 20 years clindamycin has been increasingly used for therapy of severe staphylococcal infection, including acute and chronic osteomyelitis and pulmonary and abdominal infection. The drug can be given parenterally or orally, has excellent oral bioavailability, and is generally well tolerated.

Increased rates of resistance have been recently reported in staphylococci recovered from patients with cystic fibrosis [62]. Strains of both hospital-acquired and community-associated MRSA may be resistant to clindamycin or demonstrate inducible clindamycin resistance when tested by special microbiological assays [63,64]. In some locations (e.g., Bogota, Colombia), there are high rates of both erythromycin (58%) and clindamycin (57%) resistance [61]. With susceptible strains, one advantage of clindamycin therapy is that it can be used for prolonged periods of time (e.g., for chronic vertebral osteomyelitis) without the problems of bone marrow suppression or peripheral neuropathy that may be seen with TMP–SMX [65]. The risk of *C. difficile* diarrhea is a concern with long-term oral clindamycin usage [44]. Although clindamycin remains a common cause of *C. difficile*-associated diarrhea, many other classes of antibiotics besides the lincomycins are implicated (see Figure 31.4).

Tetracyclines

The tetracyclines have variable activity against staphylococci and historically have not been considered ideal agents for treating staphylococcal infection. Resistance determinants, specifically tetM and tetK, render many staphylococci resistant to tetracycline, minocycline, and doxycycline. These and other tetracycline-resistance determinants are commonly found in nosocomial strains of *S. aureus*. The tetracyclines are generally effective against community-associated strains of MRSA and have been used with success in mild to moderately severe infections during the US epidemic. Tetracyclines are highly bioavailable and congeners like doxycycline can be dosed once or twice a day depending on the severity of the infection.

A novel glycylcycline, tigecycline, a derivative of minocycline, has excellent activity against staphylococci including MRSA [66]. Almost all staphylococci originally studied were inhibited by 2 μg/mL or less of tigecycline. Subsequently, over 90% of community-acquired MRSA from the USA were found to be susceptible [67,68]. Studies in Taiwan found 40% of MRSA strains (and all MSSA strains) to be tigecycline tolerant (i.e., the drug lacked bactericidal activity against these isolates) [69]. Peak serum concentrations approach 30 μg/mL so the mean MIC can be easily exceeded. Levels in colonic epithelial lining may be variable as predicted by Monte Carlo simulation and could explain some clinical failures in the therapy of abdominal infection [70]. Early clinical trials in patients with skin and skin-structure infection and with intraabdominal infection were very encouraging [71]. Tigecycline was marketed in 2006 but there is limited postmarketing information on the compound [72].

Glycopeptides

Vancomycin

Despite its imperfections, vancomycin remains the most important single antimicrobial for the treatment of methicillin-resistant staphylococcal infection [18]. It is remarkable that an agent introduced more than 50 years ago continues to be the drug of choice for the treatment of methicillin-resistant staphylococci. The drug also remains the first-choice alternate for the treatment of methicillin-susceptible staphylococcal infection in individuals with a history of serious reactions to the β-lactam antibiotics.

Vancomycin was first available in the late 1950s at a time when penicillin-resistant *S. aureus* was the major nosocomial pathogen in the USA [73]. The drug was introduced before the semisynthetic β-lactamase-resistant penicillins (e.g., methicillin, oxacillin, and nafcillin) and was widely used until those drugs were available. It was intended to "vanquish" staphylococcal infection, hence its name (R.S. Griffith, personal communication).

Vancomycin's use as a first-line agent for staphylococcal infection was largely limited to penicillin-allergic patients after the introduction of the semisynthetic penicillins and cephalosporins. However, with the resurgence of MRSA infections, it again became widely used throughout the world [74].

Activity

Vancomycin inhibits cell wall synthesis and is active against many Gram-positive organisms. Against staphylococci its activity is nearly universal. Some strains that are heteroresistant (i.e., a strain that produces a subclone at a frequency of $> 10^{-6}$ colonies with a vancomycin MIC of ≥ 8 μg/mL, with the stability of the strain persisting beyond 9 days in an antibiotic-free medium) have been recognized for years but are of unknown significance. Falagas *et al.* [75] recently reviewed the relevant studies and concluded that it was unclear if emergence of heteroresistance during treatment was of clinical importance.

A small number of *S. aureus* strains have been described that are of intermediate vancomycin susceptibility (VISA) or resistant to vancomycin (VRSA). VISA was first reported in 1996 and resistant isolates some 6 years later. These strains do not appear to be "epidemiologically virulent" and they have not spread widely in the years since they were first identified [76–78]. Only a half dozen isolates of vancomycin-resistant staphylococci have been recovered from clinical specimens [79]. The mechanisms of resistance are complex and discussed in detail in Chapter 9.

Among other species of staphylococci, some isolates of *S. epidermidis* and *S. haemolyticus* are vancomycin heteroresistant [80–82]. Tolerance (defined as the ability to survive but not grow in the presence of a normally lethal dose of an antibiotic) to vancomycin has been documented in *S. lugdunensis* but only infrequently in other coagulase-negative staphylococci when tested by the killing curve method [83].

There has been speculation that the vancomycin MICs for MRSA have increased over the last decade. Although this remains controversial, a recent comprehensive review found no evidence for this [84] nor did a study in a single medical center in Texas that examined isolates for the years 1999–2006 [85]. A recent analysis of data from 2002–2006 in a hospital in Madrid reached the same conclusion [86]. However, considerable evidence suggests that vancomycin is less effective against *S. aureus* now than in the past [87].

In the individual patient, higher MICs appear to predict a greater probability of treatment failure. Sakoulas *et al.* [88] reported that a lower vancomycin MIC was associated with a higher probability of treatment success. A more recent study reported that patients treated with vancomycin for bacteremic *S. aureus* infection caused by an isolate with an MIC above 1 μg/mL have significantly higher mortality than patients infected with strains with lower MICs [89].

Pharmacology

Vancomycin is poorly absorbed when given by mouth and cannot be administered by the intramuscular route. The drug is modestly bound to plasma proteins and has an elimination half-life of about 6 hours. A 1-g dose given by slow intravenous infusion yields concentrations of 20–30 μg/mL after 1 hour. The drug is eliminated by the renal route. Since nearly all of a dose is renally excreted, it is possible to maintain therapeutic concentrations in patents who are hemodialyzed by administering the drug every 5–7 days.

Vancomycin is distributed to many body fluids including pleural, pericardial, ascitic, and synovial fluids. It achieves significant concentrations in the cerebrospinal fluid (CSF) in the presence of inflamed meninges. The levels following a single intravenous dose in children with suspected shunt infection varied considerably, with penetration ranging from 0.77 to 18% [90]. In children without suspected infection who received the drug for prophylaxis, 40% had undetectable levels. A recent French study reported that patients with pneumococcal meningitis treated with cefotaxime, vancomycin, and dexamethasone had substantial CSF vancomycin levels. The drug was administered as a continuous intravenous infusion; mean serum concentration was 25.2 mg/L and CSF concentration 7.2 mg/L [91]. A case report of a neonate with staphylococcal ventriculitis also noted significant CSF vancomycin levels after parenteral administration and much higher levels following intraventricular administration that were not associated with apparent toxicity [92].

Serum levels are often monitored in patients receiving vancomycin. A recent consensus statement about monitoring has been published [93]. Because the drug appears to cause limited toxicity, measurement is done primarily to assure that therapeutic concentrations are achieved. This is important in obese subjects because of the risk of underdosing [94]. It may also be important in diabetic patients. In a recent study of patients undergoing cardiac surgery, tissue levels in diabetic and nondiabetic patients were compared. In six diabetic subjects, soft tissue concentrations of vancomycin were about one-third of the level noted in controls (3.7 vs. 11.9 mg/L) [95].

Although usually administered by intermittent infusion, Vuagnat *et al.* [96] found that continuous infusion of an identical dose of vancomycin yielded higher mean serum levels than did intermittent dosing [96].

Indications

By default, vancomycin is the preferred drug for initial therapy in any patient who needs empirical treatment for *S. aureus* infection. In the unusual parts of the world where MRSA is uncommon (e.g., the Netherlands), it would be possible to begin treatment for presumed *S. aureus* infection with a semisynthetic penicillin. In most other countries, the prevalence of methicillin-resistant staphylococci requires use of vancomycin. The other major indication for this drug is treatment of methicillin-sensitive staphylococcal infection in patients with a serious β-lactam allergy.

Vancomycin has been associated with significant failure rates in serious staphylococcal infection. One recent study noted that there is a need for careful prospective studies of the frequency of treatment failure with vancomycin [97]. These same authors reported failure rates of 46% in osteomyelitis in a retrospective study of vancomycin treatment of MRSA infections [97]. Given failure rates in MSSA endocarditis of 30–50% [98,99] and failure in a significant proportion of other bacteremic infections [15], desensitization should be considered in a penicillin-allergic patient with serious MSSA infection.

Because MRSA has become a common cause of postoperative infection, vancomycin has been increasingly used for prophylaxis in patients undergoing cardiac surgery [100]. In one study, optimal serum levels and a corresponding reduction in surgical wound infection were found to occur when the drug was given between 16 and 60 min before the first surgical incision [101]. It has been suggested that a dose of 15 mg/kg (as opposed to a standard

1-g dose for any patient) may be most appropriate [102]. A recent analysis of a large population of patients undergoing cardiac surgery showed that vancomycin was more effective than cefuroxime in the prevention of staphylococcal postoperative infections [103].

Side effects

Vancomycin has been associated with a variety of side effects. The drug, when initially manufactured, was less pure than later formulations and initial reports of frequent renal toxicity and ototoxicity have not been confirmed in more recent studies [104]. Most contemporary studies suggest that these side effects are relatively uncommon. Although the incidence of ototoxicity is not well studied, a recent report noted high-frequency hearing loss in 19% of older patients [105].

There is no general agreement on the magnitude of the nephrotoxicity of this agent when administered alone or on the importance of serum level measurements in determining dosages [106]. The study by Lodise *et al.* [18] of a group of 246 patients who received vancomycin found that nephrotoxicity was significantly more common among patients who received 4 g/day or more. Patients who received less than 4 g/day did not have nephrotoxicity more often than a cohort of patients who received linezolid (Figure 31.5).

There is good evidence that when vancomycin is administered with an aminoglycoside the combination is more toxic than either agent alone. A metaanalysis completed 15 years ago reported that nephrotoxicity was 13.3 ± 3.1% more common in patients receiving vancomycin and an aminoglycoside than in those receiving vancomycin as a single agent [107]. This same observation was also made in a recent study of toxicity factors associated with continuous infusion of vancomycin [108]. There have been reports of acute renal failure following use of cement impregnated with vancomycin and an aminoglycoside [109].

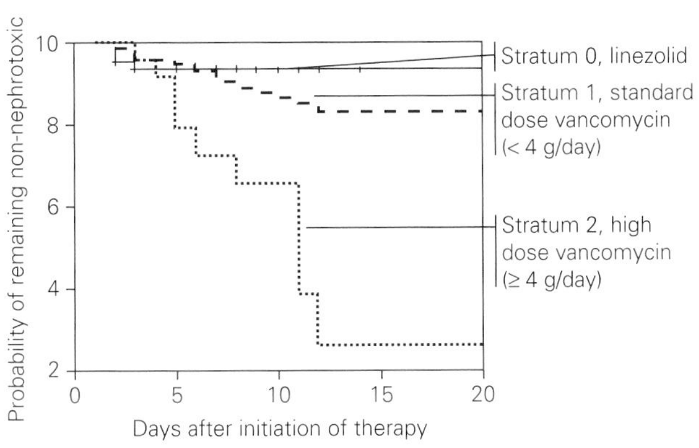

Figure 31.5 Probability of development of nephrotoxicity while being treated with vancomycin. The likelihood of nephrotoxicity is much higher at higher vancomycin doses. (Redrawn from Lodise *et al.* [18] with permission.)

A useful paper that examines the spectrum of vancomycin-associated toxicity reported the complications associated with this drug in 742 cancer patients treated over a 3-month period a decade ago [104]. Phlebitis occurred in 3% of patients and rashes developed in 11% (although all but four of these patients were receiving β-lactams as well). Ototoxicity was documented in 3% of the patients not receiving other ototoxic drugs. Nephrotoxicity (defined as a 20% or greater decline in renal function) occurred in 17% of cases.

The best-known complication of vancomycin is "red man" syndrome, a side effect associated with rapid infusion of the drug [110]. It occurs in 3.7–47% of infected patients (and in up to 90% of normal volunteers) [110–113]. The reaction is manifest by sudden onset of pruritis and erythema involving the face, chest, and neck shortly after an infusion of vancomycin. Patients are often alarmed and complain of diffuse burning and itching. The syndrome results from histamine release triggered by vancomycin. It may be prevented or managed with diphenhydramine and its severity controlled by pretreatment with hydroxyzine. Some patients may also have significant hemodynamic compromise with vancomycin infusion. Bertolissi *et al.* [114] suggested that onset of pruritus correlated with a decline in systemic vascular resistance and arterial oxygen tension and that a beta-blocker could protect against these changes.

Some 50 years after its introduction, vancomycin continues to be the mainstay of therapy against MRSA. It is not a perfect antibiotic and its lower efficacy against MSSA compared with nafcillin or oxacillin means it should not be used in infections caused by these organisms unless there is a significant allergic issue [74,115].

Teicoplanin

Teicoplanin, which is not marketed in the USA, is the only other glycopeptide antibiotic currently available. Other drugs in this class (e.g., oritavancin) are likely to be marked in the near future.

Teicoplanin is twofold to fourfold more active than vancomycin against most staphylococci. The major exception to this is *S. haemolyticus*, against which its activity is considerably less. Recent evidence suggests that resistance among *S. epidermidis* has increased in recent years [116]. *Staphylococcus lugdunensis* has also been found to be relatively resistant to the killing effect of this antibiotic (and of vancomycin) [83].

In contrast to vancomycin, teicoplanin may be given by either the intravenous or intramuscular route. Very little of the drug is metabolized and it is eliminated by glomerular filtration. Teicoplanin has a long half-life (about 30 hours) and after a loading dose it is given as a single daily dose. Use of a loading dose is needed to achieve a therapeutic serum concentration promptly [117].

The drug is associated with fewer side effects than vancomycin [118]. It does not cause histamine release and "red man" syndrome occurs rarely, if ever, after teicoplanin. Ototoxicity and nephrotoxicity are also both uncommon and are not dose related. Fever and skin rash are infrequent but more common at higher doses. One recent study in febrile neutropenic patients noted that the combination of teicoplanin and amphotericin was significantly less nephrotoxic than vancomycin and amphotericin [119].

There are few comparative trials of teicoplanin but those that are published indicated that the drug appears comparable in efficacy to vancomycin. A recent retrospective study reported that teicoplanin and vancomycin were equivalent in the treatment of MRSA endocarditis [120]. The agent can be given by the intramuscular route on a daily basis and, for that reason, has been extensively used for outpatient therapy [121].

Daptomycin

Daptomycin is a cyclic lipopeptide with a novel mechanism of action at the level of the bacterial cell membrane. It displays activity against a wide range of Gram-positive cocci including the staphylococci. Given at a dose of 6 mg/kg intravenously, it reaches peak levels of 10–16 μg/mL. The drug is highly active against *S. aureus* and the coagulase-negative staphylococci, with an MIC_{90} at or below 1.0 μg/mL [122]. It is bactericidal against *S. aureus*. Early studies showed that resistance developed slowly *in vitro* but recent studies have reported that *S. aureus* MICs in some patients increase sharply after 5–15 days of treatment and clinical failure may result [123]. Nevertheless, many patients have been successfully treated, often in closely followed clinical trials.

In two international randomized studies of complicated skin and skin-structure infections that analyzed 902 clinically evaluable patients, penicillinase-resistant penicillins and vancomycin were the comparative agents. Almost 70% of these patients had infections due to *S. aureus* [124]. Rates of success were about 84% in both groups, although the daptomycin group required fewer days of therapy. A follow-up study of a South African subset of 326 patients from these two registrational studies was performed [125]. *Staphylococcus aureus* was the responsible pathogen in about 45% of both the daptomycin- and the comparator-treated groups. A detailed analysis of symptoms and signs (including erythema, tenderness, edema ulceration and drainage) showed that patients receiving daptomycin required a shorter length of therapy (7.0 vs. 8.0 days; $P < 0.001$) but there was no organism-specific breakdown of the data. A prospective open-label study of skin and skin-structure infections in 51 patients, 27 of whom had MRSA, compared daptomycin with a historical control group of 212 patients treated with vancomycin [126]. Half of the study patients had *S. aureus* infections. For all patients, resolution of the infections at 3 or 5 days was 90% and 98% respectively in the daptomycin group; these results were significantly different from the vancomycin group.

In a randomized study of patients with endocarditis or bacteremia caused by *S. aureus*, rates of cure were much lower [127]. In this landmark study, 44.2% of patients in the daptomycin group compared with 41.7% of patients who received standard therapy were cured. A later analysis of the patients who had MRSA infection found that daptomycin was as effective as vancomycin/gentamicin in both endocarditis and bacteremia [128]. In a retrospective study of a daptomycin registry for endocarditis through 2004, rates of cure were better than for the randomized study, although the trial included patients infected with coagulase-negative staphylococci and enterococci in addition to *S. aureus* [129]. Daptomycin was successful in 12 of 14 evaluable patients with *S. aureus* endocarditis.

The dosage of daptomycin has emerged as an important factor in success. In a registry review of the treatment of osteomyelitis with daptomycin (in which MRSA was the most common pathogen), success rates were 88% with a daily dose in excess of 4 mg/kg compared with only 65% with a daily dose of 4 mg/kg or less [130]. A study of septic arthritis, most often caused by *S. aureus*, showed cure in 41% and improvement in 50%, with a median final dose of 5 mg/kg and median duration of 22 days [131]. All the patients in this study received an antibiotic before daptomycin, which itself was combined with another antibiotic in two-thirds of the patients.

Studies in children are much less common. Of 15 children treated for invasive staphylococcal disease in Dallas, 14 were improved at the time they were discharged [132]. Daptomycin was added to failing regimens for persistent bacteremia and resulted in cure of six of seven of these children.

There was early concern that adverse effects on muscle would be a limiting factor in the use of daptomycin. Randomized studies, in particular, have shown that the rate of muscle enzyme elevation is very small and frank myositis rare [124]. Rates of renal toxicity in all reported studies are extremely low. Resistance to daptomycin in primary staphylococcal isolates is rare but resistance due to complex mechanisms of membrane alteration has been described in some well-studied isolates [133].

Aminoglycosides

Aminoglycosides have been used for years, usually in combination with other agents, for the therapy of staphylococcal infections. It was believed two decades ago that the addition of an aminoglycoside to standard regimens of penicillinase-resistant penicillins would clear bacteremia faster or reduce mortality but most studies did not support this bias. Moreover, over this time, the gene *aac(6')-aph(2")* (which specifies a bifunctional aminoglycoside-modifying enzyme that reduces the antibacterial activity of these agents) became prevalent, adding to the spectrum of multiple drug resistance in MRSA and reducing the potential for aminoglycoside addition or synergy with other agents. However, some recent work from France suggests that the incidence of septic shock itself, but not mortality, may be reduced when aminoglycoside antibiotic combinations are used to treat *S. aureus* bacteremia [134].

Persistent *S. aureus* bacteremia is a special clinical situation [135]. In the setting of persistent bacteremia, aminoglycosides are added occasionally to other regimens, particularly vancomycin, even though the combination poses an increased risk of nephrotoxicity or ototoxicity. When *S. aureus* bacteremia is due to prosthetic valve endocarditis, because of the historic high mortality, aminoglycosides are used in double- and occasionally triple-drug regimens. A Mayo Clinic study reported that 71% of 55 patients with *S. aureus* prosthetic valve endocarditis had an aminoglycoside added to their regimen [136]. Of 23 patients treated medically, 52% survived and no patients under 50 years of age died. Use of an aminoglycoside in addition to a β-lactam with or without rifampin will likely remain the regimen of choice in prosthetic valve endocarditis [25]. Therefore, in the USA today, while aminoglycosides are considered to play a minor role in the therapy of staphylococcal infection, there may be situations when their addition to an antibiotic regimen may be the best therapeutic option. There are only limited evidence-based data for use of these drugs in *S. aureus* infection.

There are other clinical settings in which aminoglycosides are used for the therapy for staphylococcal infection. Some nephrologists utilize vancomycin and gentamicin combinations for the therapy of hemodialysis catheter-related bacteremia or its prevention [137]. Gentamicin plus ampicillin is one combination that has been compared with chloramphenicol for therapy of severe pneumonia in children in developing countries including Pakistan [138].

Gentamicin or tobramycin enmeshed in plastic beads is still routinely utilized in prevention and treatment of orthopedic infections [139,140]. Few studies are available to evaluate their efficacy in orthopedic device infections compared with systemic antimicrobials used alone. Tobramycin beads seem to quicken healing when used with debridement in treatment of adult osteomyelitis [140].

Oxazolidinones

Linezolid has made a profound impact on the therapy of staphylococcal infections since its introduction in 2000 [141]. It is a synthetic drug that interacts with the 50S ribosome at a unique site within the V domain of the 23S peptidyltransferase core of the 50S unit. When linezolid binds to the peptidyltransferase, it likely interferes with processing of the tRNA by the ribosome. In turn, the 70S initiation complex does not form properly and protein synthesis is interrupted.

The kinetics of oral linezolid and intravenous linezolid are the same, a 600-mg dose by either route yielding peak serum levels of around 20 μg/mL. Tissue penetration, including muscle, fat and bone, are excellent. Bone concentrations approach 50% of serum concentrations and thus exceed the MIC for most pathogens that cause osteomyelitis [142]. Linezolid has a broad spectrum of activity against most Gram-positive cocci, including the staphylococci, with an MIC_{90} of 2–3 μg/mL for MSSA and MRSA [141]. Toxicity centers around bone marrow suppression, seen mostly in depression of platelet and red cell production, an effect usually associated with chronic administration.

In order to evaluate the efficacy of linezolid, there have been multiple randomized controlled trials to determine if it is superior or equivalent to glycopeptides or β-lactams. A metaanalysis of 14 appropriate randomized controlled trials selected from 44 papers ultimately analyzed 12. Of the 12 studies, which included 2661 patients, the overall odds ratio was 1.41 with a 95% confidence interval (CI) of 1.11–1.81 [143]. When *S. aureus* eradication was considered, the total odds ratio was 1.81 (95% CI 1.40–2.34); for MRSA the odds ratio was 1.69 (95% CI 0.84–3.41). Adverse effects showed no difference from the comparative antibiotic. No new resistance to linezolid was reported. The rates of *S. aureus* bacteremia were so low that the effectiveness of linezolid versus comparators could not be determined. Comparison in pneumonia was possible and linezolid showed equivalence for patients with MRSA pneumonia and equivalence for nosocomial pneumonia due to other Gram-positive cocci.

The randomized controlled trial that enrolled the most patients also did a subanalysis of patients with MSSA (29%) and MRSA (42%) [144]. For MRSA, for both evaluable and for the modified intent-to-treat patient populations, linezolid was superior to vancomycin. For the MSSA populations, the higher rates of cure in the linezolid group did not reach statistical significance. Regarding adverse reactions, nausea, diarrhea and thrombocytopenia were more common in the linezolid group, as was phlebitis in the vancomycin group.

Resistance to linezolid has been rare in *S. aureus*. It is conferred by mutations in domain V of the 23sRNA gene, in particular G2447, T2500A, and G2576 [145]. For a G2576 mutation in one isolate, increasing gene dosage contributes to an increasing, to a relatively stable resistance phenotype with an MIC increasing to 128 μg/L. The good news is that the increasing gene dose of the resistance mutation is associated with decreased fitness, as shown by a reduced rate of growth.

Quinolones

The quinolones are a diverse group of antibiotics that play a relatively minor role in the treatment of staphylococcal infections. Those quinolones in current clinical use are both well absorbed after oral dosing and widely distributed in the body. Elimination route varies with the compound. Ciprofloxacin, levofloxacin, and gatifloxacin are renally eliminated. Moxifloxacin is eliminated by both hepatic and renal mechanisms, although impaired renal or hepatic function does not require changes in dosing with this drug. Adverse events are similar for all the quinolones. Most are gastrointestinal; about 5% of patients experience nausea, diarrhea, or anorexia [146].

Quinolones are not indicated for staphylococcal infection because (i) resistance to all the currently marketed drugs in this class has been seen in staphylococci; (ii) multidrug resistance in staphylococci appears to parallel the frequency of quinolone use in an institution; and (iii) these drugs are no more effective than other compounds against staphylococci and tend to be associated with more side effects than other agents.

Resistance

Following the introduction of the fluoroquinolones to clinical medicine in the mid-1980s, staphylococci were found to rapidly develop resistance to these drugs. The number of nosocomial infections caused by quinolone-resistant isolates of *S. aureus* increased dramatically over a period of several years [147]. Interestingly, quinolone resistance was much more frequent in MRSA than MSSA isolates [148].

Recently introduced agents (e.g., moxifloxacin) have significantly greater activity against *S. aureus* in comparison with older quinolones (e.g., ciprofloxacin). A variety of structural modifications (alkylation, addition of a piperazine group at C-7 and of a fluorine group at C-6) in the newer quinolone compounds have resulted in improved activity against staphylococci. Representative MICs for *S. aureus* are as follows: ciprofloxacin 0.25–1.0 μg/mL, levofloxacin 0.25 μg/mL, gatifloxacin 0.125 μg/mL, and moxifloxacin 0.06 μg/mL. Mutations that result in resistance to all these drugs have been described in *S. aureus* [149]. Because of significantly greater activity against staphylococci, some authors have suggested that the C-8 modified quinolones (e.g., moxifloxacin) might be an appropriate option for treatment of community-acquired MRSA [150]. In a rabbit experimental arthritis model, moxifloxacin was found to be as effective as cloxacillin or vancomycin [151].

Rapid one-step resistance has developed in MRSA when evaluated in experimental models of infection [152]. In clinical MRSA infection as well, treatment has often been ineffective and associated with emergence of quinolone-resistant strains [153].

Prevalence of resistance and quinolone usage

Several studies have found a relationship between the extent of use of the quinolones and the frequency of MRSA isolation in hospitals. In a study using data from 47 French hospitals, Rogues *et al.* [154] found that the incidence of MRSA increased as the use of ciprofloxacin and levofloxacin increased. Ciprofloxacin use was associated with increased MRSA isolation in a group of German intensive care units [155]. In a study conducted in a group of 17 US hospitals, total fluoroquinolone use in a hospital was significantly associated with the proportion of staphylococcal isolates that were MRSA [156]. In another study, fluoroquinolone use was markedly limited in one French hospital for 1 year. Monthly rates of MRSA isolation in this hospital dropped significantly compared with control institutions [157]. In an *in vitro* experiment, duration of drug use was found to be an important determinant of development of resistance [158].

Clinical effectiveness

Ruotsalainen *et al.* [159] conducted a randomized study to determine if levofloxacin, added to standard therapy, would improve outcomes in *S. aureus* bacteremia. In 381 patients with *S. aureus* isolates that were fluoroquinolone and methicillin susceptible, there was no difference in complication rate, time to defervescence, or mortality when a quinolone was added to usual treatment regimens. A recent metaanalysis assessed the role of fluoroquinolones versus β-lactam antibiotics in the empirical therapy of immunocompetent patients with skin and soft tissue infection [160]. Overall, the quinolones were as effective as the comparator antibiotics but associated with more frequent side effects.

Although there are only infrequent appropriate uses for quinolones in staphylococcal infection, the drugs continue to be used with some success in two situations. Quinolones are used in prevention and management of ocular infection, although the increasing incidence of resistance in *S. aureus* has limited this use (see Chapter 21 for additional information) [161]. The quinolones are also used in combination with other antibiotics in "suppressive therapy" in patients with prosthetic joint infection in whom the prosthesis is not removed. In one study of 60 patients who received levofloxacin and rifampin, significant failure rates occurred (35%) with higher failure rates in patients with MRSA infections [162]. A recent study found *in vivo* antagonism between these two agents [163].

Fusidic acid

Fusidic acid is a unique compound with activity directed only against Gram-positive cocci. It is most active against staphylococci and MICs are typically less than 0.1 mg/L. The drug is bactericidal at high concentrations.

Resistance, mediated by chromosomal mutation or plasmid-mediated genetic transfer, has been relatively uncommon, even with extensive topical use of this drug. A resistant clone emerged among children with bullous impetigo in Sweden in the late 1990s [164]. Nearly half of fusidic acid-resistant isolates in one study were from patients who had received the same drug topically in the prior 6 months [165]. Because of the drug's unique role in treatment of multiply resistant *S. aureus*, strong arguments have been made to eliminate topical use of this agent [166].

Resistance occurs more commonly in coagulase-negative staphylococci. Isolates of *S. saprophyticus* carry a gene (FusD) different from that usually seen in *S. aureus*, while resistant isolates of *S. lugdunensis* have a gene (FusB) that is common in *S. aureus* [167,168]. A recent study found that 46% of 50 strains of *S. epidermidis* were fusidic acid resistant; most carried FusB [169].

Fusidic acid may be used topically or administered by the intravenous or oral route. It is very well absorbed after oral administration. The drug has a half-life of about 9 hours. It is widely distributed in the body and penetrates most tissues excluding the CSF. Fusidic acid is metabolized in the liver, with only a very small amount eliminated in the urine.

The drug has relatively few side effects. Those which are documented include uncommon episodes of gastrointestinal irritation, dermatitis, and sideroblastic anemia [170]. Uncommonly, hepatitis may occur after intravenous administration. For this reason, it is recommended that fusidic acid be avoided in patients with liver impairment.

Clinical use of fusidic acid is largely limited to patients with osteomyelitis or other severe infection, or patients with staphylococcal infections requiring long-term oral therapy. In both cases, the drug is usually given with another antibiotic because of the possibility that resistance may develop when fusidic acid is given alone [168,171]. Although of proven effectiveness in staphylococcal bacteremia, there are only limited data (despite four decades of use) to support this drug as appropriate treatment for endocarditis [172].

Orally administered fusidic acid is not effective in eliminating MRSA nasal colonization. In several cases in one study, organisms isolated from the nares appeared to develop resistance during treatment [173]. Fusidic acid has been given by mouth in combination with rifampin for managing prosthetic joint infection. In one such trial, after 1 year of treatment, the risk of failure was about 10% [174].

Along with clindamycin, rifampin, and linezolid, fusidic acid inhibits release of Panton–Valentine leukocidin [175]. The clinical importance of this is not clear. Although the drug is used throughout the world, it has never been commercially available in the USA.

Trimethoprim–sulfamethoxazole

TMP–SMX has retained considerable utility over the years since its introduction. It is of interest in the treatment of staphylococcal infection because many MRSA isolates (73–98% in one study) are susceptible [176]. The drug consists of two agents (one part trimethoprim to five parts sulfamethoxazole) that act sequentially to inhibit folate synthesis. Both drugs are widely distributed in the body. Since trimethoprim and sulfamethoxazole are both eliminated by renal excretion, dosages need to be adjusted in renal failure. Adverse reactions are usually related to the sulfamethoxazole component.

In vitro, TMP–SMX is rapidly lethal to staphylococci. When compared with rifampin, linezolid, clindamycin, moxifloxacin, and minocycline, it was the most rapidly bactericidal of this group of drugs [177]. In a single animal study, TMP–SMX did not appear to be effective for treatment of MRSA or MSSA endocarditis [178]. These authors cautioned that use of TMP–SMX in infections with high numbers of organisms was potentially problematic.

Although TMP–SMX has been widely recommended for treatment of minor community-acquired MRSA infection, clinical data about the effectiveness of this drug in staphylococcal infection are very limited [179]. A retrospective review of treatment of MRSA skin and soft tissue infections in a Boston clinic found TMP–SMX resistance to be uncommon (< 1%), the drug to be clinically effective, and side effects to be infrequent. Therapy was stopped in 5.3% of cases treated with this drug because of side effects. Interestingly, about half of MRSA isolates from this clinic were clindamycin resistant [180].

A recent study compared oral doxycycline (100 mg b.i.d.) to TMP–SMX (160/800 mg b.i.d.) in patients with skin and soft tissue infection that required incision, drainage, and wound packing. There were three treatment failures and all occurred among the 14 patients treated with TMP–SMX. Two of these were in patients from whom MRSA was recovered; one was a patient with a *Streptococcus milleri* infection [181]. While there was no statistically significant difference between the treatment groups, the authors noted a need for additional prospective studies. In addition to skin and soft tissue infection, oral TMP–SMX has been used for long-term treatment of prosthetic implants infected with staphylococci [182].

Only a single clinical study has evaluated use of TMP–SMX in serious staphylococcal infection. This trial was a randomized double-blind study of vancomycin versus TMP–SMX in the treatment of serious *S. aureus* infection in intravenous drug users [183]. The authors found that duration of bacteremia was higher and cure rates lower in the group that received TMP–SMX. They also reported that side effects (largely nausea and vomiting) were more frequent in this group. Interestingly, although nearly half of infections were caused by MRSA, all the treatment failures were in the MSSA-infected group. The authors concluded that TMP–SMX may be useful for selected MRSA infections. While this drug does appear to be appropriate for skin and soft tissue infections caused by MRSA, the data that support its use for other types of staphylococcal infection are very limited.

There are at least two potential concerns about use of TMP–SMX for staphylococcal infection. Firstly, it is unclear if resistance will develop in isolates of MRSA as this drug continues to be used for these infections. Resistance has been associated with increased exposure to this drug. Among HIV-infected patients receiving TMP–SMX for *Pneumocystis* prophylaxis, the rates of resistance in *S. aureus* increased from 0 to 48% between 1988 and 1995 [184]. Secondly, as Proctor [176] noted recently, the presence of thymidine in tissues and purulent material can allow staphylococci to bypass the action of TMP–SMX [176].

Quinupristin–dalfopristin

Quinupristin–dalfopristin is a combination of two streptogramin antibiotics derived from pristinomycin [185]. This agent (marketed as Synercid) is active against multiresistant Gram-positive aerobes and many Gram-positive anaerobes. The two related components are synergistic against many organisms. Even though the components are bacteriostatic, the combination is reported to often be bactericidal [186]. Fuchs *et al.* [187] found that of 516 strains of *S. aureus*, 97.1% were susceptible to this drug. They noted that clindamycin- and macrolide-resistant strains were not killed by quinupristin–dalfopristin. Although active against MRSA, the drug is not approved for treatment of these infections in the USA.

A survey of the sensitivity of 2132 clinically significant staphylococcal isolates to quinupristin–dalfopristin was reported in 2000 [188]. This study examined organisms collected from Europe, Africa, and the Middle East. Most (68%) of the isolates were *S. aureus*. Of all isolates, 97.6% had MICs of 1 mg/L or less. Tested isolates of VISA have been susceptible to this agent [189].

Quinupristin–dalfopristin was assessed in two randomized open-label trials in patients with skin and soft tissue infection [190]. The drug was found to be as effective as the comparative agents (cefazolin, oxacillin, and vancomycin). In a multicenter European study of patients with Gram-positive nosocomial pneumonia, quinupristin–dalfopristin was compared with vancomycin [191]. The clinical response rates, including those when analyzed by pathogen, were the same for both drugs.

The primary side effect of quinupristin–dalfopristin in these studies was vein irritation. Myalgias and arthralgias have also been reported in a significant number of patients (7–50%) in other trials [192,193]. Quinupristin–dalfopristin also interacts with the cytochrome P450 system and significant drug interactions are a concern [185].

Because of its broad-spectrum activity against Gram-positive organisms (excluding some enterococci), quinupristin–dalfopristin has been suggested as an alternative agent to glycopeptides in patients with multiply-resistant Gram-positive infections [194].

Rifampin

Rifampin is a bactericidal antibiotic with impressive activity against Gram-positive cocci and Mycobacteria. It is not as highly active against most Gram-negative organisms. The major advantages of rifampin in treating staphylococcal infection are its potent activity and ability to penetrate virtually all the tissues and cells in the body.

The drug is virtually always used in combination with other antimicrobials because of the ease with which resistance develops. In a recent study in three Japanese hospitals, 88–94% of isolates of MRSA from tuberculosis wards were found to be resistant to rifampin; no isolates from other wards were resistant [195]. All the resistant isolates had mutations in the *rpoB* gene. Changes in this gene responsible for resistance are usually, but not always, associated with compromised biological fitness [196].

Although there is an intravenous formulation, rifampin is well absorbed after oral administration. It is primarily excreted in the bile and half-life is not affected by renal function. The drug is associated with several notable side effects, including skin reactions, gastrointestinal side effects (e.g., nausea), and abnormalities of liver function. All are relatively uncommon [197]. Rifampin is a potent inducer of cytochrome P450 and therefore modifies the metabolism of a number of drugs, including warfarin, hypoglycemic agents, oral contraceptives, and digoxin.

Rifampin has three primary uses in treating staphylococcal infection: (i) as part of a regimen for decolonization; (ii) as an agent in the long-term treatment of prosthetic joint infection; and (iii) as an adjunct to other antibiotics in patients with serious staphylococcal infections (e.g., endocarditis). Use of rifampin as part of a decolonization regimen was recently reviewed by Falagas *et al.* [198]. These authors noted that in nine comparative trials, rifampin-containing regimens appeared to be more effective than single agents including cloxacillin, ciprofloxacin, minocycline, and vancomycin. The most effective combination was rifampin and minocycline given for 14 days. Resistance to rifampin developed during treatment in 17% of the subjects in the comparative trials. Use of rifampin in prevention of dialysis-associated infection was examined in a recent metaanalysis of the four published randomized controlled trials. The authors found that prophylaxis with rifampin was no more effective than use of mupirocin ointment at the access site for any studied outcome measure [199].

Rifampin has been used in combination with other agents such as quinolones in the treatment of prosthetic joint infection. In one report, rifampin and levofloxacin were used together; overall failure occurred in 35% of subjects, with higher rates in those patients with methicillin-resistant organisms, knee infections, and a longer duration of symptoms [162]. In another trial, rifampin was used with fusidic acid [174]. Treatment failure occurred in 10% of patients after 1 year. In an animal model of prosthetic knee joint infection, rifampin combined with quinupristin–dalfopristin or vancomycin was significantly more effective than either vancomycin or quinupristin–dalfopristin alone [200].

Rifampin has been used for many years as an adjunct to other antistaphylococcal therapies. Bliziotis *et al.* [201] have reviewed results of the published randomized controlled trials assessing rifampin as part of a treatment regimen for staphylococci. These authors noted that there was no significant difference in mortality in any of the trials. Another more recent review concluded there is need for larger, more powerful trials [202]. In one of the five clinical studies comparing regimens including rifampin and those excluding rifampin, the authors concluded that clinical cures were significantly more common in the rifampin arm than in those patients who did not receive this drug [203]. The same study was discontinued prematurely because all of the failures were in the nonrifampin arm of the trial. In another study, statistical significance was reached only by pooling the improved and cured patient groups [204] (Table 31.3).

Although rifampin is recommended by the American Heart Association for treatment of staphylococcal (both coagulase-negative staphylococci and *S. aureus*) prosthetic valve endocarditis, the authors of these quidelines note that published data are limited [25]. The paper cites an animal study noting the unique ability of rifampin to sterilize foreign bodies infected with *S. aureus* [208]. Rifampin is not recommended for routine treatment of patients with native valve endocarditis but may be considered for patients who do not respond to conventional therapy. Significant issues with toxicity and emergence of resistant isolates of *S. aureus* were recently documented in a retrospective study of patients who received rifampin as part of therapy for endocarditis [209].

Rifampin is also commonly used in treatment of patients with vascular graft infections. A recent review noted the benefit of systemic antibiotic prophylaxis in preventing infection in peripheral arterial reconstruction. The same paper examined the role of rifampin bonded to Dacron grafts in two published trials with 2 years of follow-up and concluded that there was no evidence that rates of infection were reduced at either 1 month or 2 years [210].

New antistaphylococcal agents

Many factors have driven the need for new agents to treat staphylococcal infections, including the decline of infections due to Gram-negative bacilli over the last 20 years, continued emergence of antimicrobial resistance in staphylococci, the relatively high mortality and morbidity of invasive infection due to *S. aureus*, the propensity of staphylococci to form recalcitrant biofilm-related infections, and the increasing percentage of isolates that display heteroresistance to older agents like vancomycin. Additional phenotypic variation among the genus (e.g., the ability to form small-colony variants with associated increased resistance) has likely reduced the efficacy of standard antimicrobial regimens [211]. In response to the growing importance and resistance of staphylococcal infection, pharmaceutical companies and other laboratories involved with basic research have unveiled a series of new compounds that show promise in the therapy of staphylococcal infection.

New glycopeptides are always attractive because of the track record of vancomycin over many years, although there are major questions now as to the efficacy of this drug [115]. Several promising new glycopeptides have surfaced, each with slightly different pharmacokinetic characteristics. Dalbavancin is related to teicoplanin, an agent that has been used widely in Europe over the last two decades [13,212]. It is substantially more active than vancomycin against staphylococci [213]. This drug has a half-life of about 7 days, allowing weekly dosing, a novel concept for treating acute Gram-positive infections. Several clinical trials have shown efficacy in skin and skin-structure infections.

Telavancin is another glycopeptide, a derivative of vancomycin with increased activity against *S. aureus* [214]. The drug is equal in efficacy to vancomycin in therapy of skin and soft tissue infection [215,216]. The agent also functioned well in a murine model of MRSA pneumonia [217] and other animal models [13]. One advantage of telavancin may be its sustained antibacterial activity in biofilm models [218].

Oritavancin is derived from chloroeremomycin, a vancomycin-like natural fermentation product of *Amycolatopsis orientalis*. No *S. aureus* strains resistant to this drug are known and the MICs are lower than those of vancomycin [219]. The drug was as effective as vancomycin in a rabbit model of MRSA endocarditis [220]. Oritavancin has some of the advantages of telavancin including penetration into biofilm and would likely be dosed once daily [221].

New antistaphylococcal agents in the rifamycin and dihydrofolate reductase classes of antimicrobials have also been developed [222]. One new diaminopyrimidine dihydrofolate reductase inhibitor, iclaprim, has good antistaphylococcal activity and is particularly promising, advancing through phase II and phase III trials [223]. A new rifamycin derivative, ABI-0043, unlike other rifampicins, is actually bactericidal with excellent antistaphylococcal activity [224]. Given alone, resistance develops rapidly but when administered in combination with levofloxacin, it was very effective in a foreign-body model of infection.

Probably the most unexpected new antistaphylococcal agents are in the β-lactam class. Activity against MRSA is surprising because the production of aberrant penicillin-binding proteins is the basis of methicillin resistance. Ceftobiprole and ceftaroline are two agents that actually bind to PBP2′ (the penicillin-binding protein present in MRSA) and thus are active against these organisms. More

Table 31.3 Randomized controlled trials of antistaphylococcal therapy with or without rifampin.[1] (Modified from Bliziotis *et al.* [201] with permission.)

Reference	Number of patients		Type of infection	Causative pathogen	Regimen	Cure		Mortality	
	Regimen	Regimen + rifampin				Regimen	Regimen + rifampin	Regimen	Regimen + rifampin
Zimmerli *et al.* [203]	15	18	Staphylococcal infection associated with stable orthopedic implants	*S. aureus* (26/33) *S. epidermidis* (7/33)	Flucloxacillin 2 g i.v. every 6 hours or vancomycin 1 g i.v. every 12 hours for 2 weeks, then ciprofloxacin 750 mg p.o. every 12 hours	7/12 (58%)	12/12 (100%)	0/12 (0%)	0/12 (0%)
Levine *et al.* [205]	22	20	Endocarditis	MRSA	Vancomycin 1 g i.v. every 12 hours	15/19 (79%)	16/18 (89%)	2/22 (9%)	1/20 (5%)
Norden *et al.* [206]	8	10	Chronic osteomyelitis	*Staphylococcus aureus*	Nafcillin (or cephalothin or cephapirin) 20 mg/kg i.v. every 4 hours (maximum 12 g/day)	4/8 (50%)	8/10 (80%)	0/8 (0%)	0/10 (0%)
Van der Auwera *et al.* [207]	32	33	Staphylococcal infections	*Staphylococcus aureus*	Oxacillin 3 g every 6 hours or vancomycin 1 g i.v. every 12 hours	18/32 (56.2%)	20/33 (60.6%)	Due to infection 2/32 (6.25%) All-cause 2/32 (6.25%)	Due to infection 1/33 (3%) All-cause 2/33 (6%)
Van Der Auwera *et al.* [204]	29	27	Staphylococcal infections	*Staphylococcus aureus*	Oxacillin 3 g every 6 hours or vancomycin 1 g i.v. every 12 hours	12/29 (41%)	18/27 (67%)	Due to infection 4/29 (14%) All-cause 4/29 (14%)	Due to infection 1/27 (4%) All-cause 3/27 (11%)

[1] In each study, rifampin 600–1200 mg/day was added to the regimen noted. There was no difference in mortality between the regimen and regimen plus rifampin in any of the studies.

clinical work has been done with ceftobiprole. Ceftobiprole demonstrates time-dependent killing and has a spectrum of activity against Gram-negative bacilli similar to that of cefipime. The drug is more active than cefipime against *Pseudomonas* [225]. The cure rate of MRSA skin and skin-structure infections in two human clinical trials approached or exceeded 90%, while adverse reactions were no higher than in the comparator arms [48,49].

Agents are also being developed to exploit virulence factors of staphylococci. Specific monoclonal antibodies against microbial surface factors that determine adhesion have been studied in clinical trials. Tefibazumab is one such agent that inhibits staphylococcal clumping factor and was thought to be additive to the effects of antimicrobials in the therapy of staphylococcal bacteremia [226]. Other agents that inhibit the so-called quorum-sensing mechanism have been very successful in treatment of infections in animal models [227].

Because staphylococci usually colonize human skin and mucous membranes before producing disease, topical agents have had some success in limiting colonizing strains from producing disease and in treating active skin infections (see Chapter 30 for a detailed discussion). Mupirocin is one topical agent that has had an extremely successful run in this regard. A related agent, retapamulin, has recently been marketed for the treatment of staphylococcal skin infection [228]. Even more novel agents, like copper silicate, may eventually find use in topical application or limitation of environmental spread based on the bactericidal activity of copper [229]. It is likely that the next decade of antistaphylococcal chemotherapy will witness emergence of agents that attack staphylococci at many sites of the pathogenicity cycle [230].

References

1 Lagier R, Baud CA, Kramer C. Brodie's abscess in a tibia dating from the Neolithic period. Pathol Anat 1983;401:153–7.

2 Lagier R, Baud CA, Arnaud G *et al.* Lesions characteristic of infection or malignant tumor in Paleo-Eskimo skulls. Pathol Anat 1982;395:237–43.

3 Ayliffe GAJ, English MP. Hospital Infection: From Miasma to MRSA. Cambridge: Cambridge University Press, 2003.

4 Jevons MP. Celbenin-resistant staphylococci. BMJ 1961;1:124–5.

5 Casey AL, Lambert PA, Elliott TS. Staphylococci. Int J Antimicrob Agents 2007;3:S23–S32.

6 Pope SD, Roecker AM. Vancomycin for treatment of invasive, multi-drug resistant *Staphylococcus aureus* infections. Expert Opin Pharmacother 2007;8:1245–61.

7 Dancer SJ. The effect of antibiotics on methicillin-resistant *Staphylococcus aureus*. J Antimicrob Chemother 2008;61:246–53.

8 Crossley K, Landesman B, Zaske D. An outbreak of infections caused by strains of *Staphylococcus aureus* resistant to methicillin and aminoglycosides. II. Epidemiologic studies. J Infect Dis 1979;139:280–7.

9 Duckworth GJ, Lothian JL, Williams JD. Methicillin-resistant *Staphylococcus aureus*: report of an outbreak in a London teaching hospital. J Hosp Infect 1988;11:1–15.

10 Boucher HW, Corey GR. Epidemiology of methicillin-resistant *Staphylococcus aureus*. Clin Infect Dis 2008;46(suppl 5):S344–S349.

11 Adler J, Interlandi J, Philips M *et al.* Caution: killing germs may be hazardous to your health. Newsweek 2007;150:44–8.

12 Gorman C. Surviving the new killer bug. Time 2006;167:52–3.

13 Aksoy DY, Unal S. New antimicrobial agents for the treatment of Gram-positive bacterial infections. Clin Microbiol Infect 2008;14:411–20.

14 Chang FY, Peacock JE, Musher DM *et al. Staphylococcus aureus* bacteremia: recurrence and the impact of antibiotic treatment in a prospective multicenter study. Medicine 2003;82:333–9.

15 Jensen AG. *Staphylococcus aureus* bacteremia. Dan Med Bull 2003;50:423–38.

16 Cantu TG, Yamanaka-Yuen NA, Lietman PS. Serum vancomycin concentrations: reappraisal of their clinical value. Clin Infect Dis 1994;18:533–43.

17 Cunha BA. Vancomycin revisited: a reappraisal of clinical use. Crit Care Clin 2008;24:393–420.

18 Lodise TP, Lomaestro B, Graves J *et al.* Larger vancomycin doses (at least four grams per day) are associated with an increased incidence of nephrotoxicity. Antimicrob Agents Chemother 2008;52:1330–6.

19 Gonzalez C, Rubio M, Romero-Vivas J *et al.* Bacteraemic pneumonia due to *Staphylococcus aureus*: a comparison of disease caused by methicillin-resistant and methicillin-susceptible organisms. Clin Infect Dis 1999;29:1171–7.

20 Stryjewski ME, Szczech LA, Benjamin DK Jr *et al.* Use of vancomycin or first-generation cephalosporins for the treatment of hemodialysis-dependent patients with methicillin-susceptible *Staphylococcus aureus* bacteremia. Clin Infect Dis 2007;44:190–6.

21 Kim SH, Kim KH, Kim HB *et al.* Outcome of vancomycin treatment in patients with methicillin-susceptible *Staphylococcus aureus* bacteremia. Antimicrob Agents Chemother 2008;52: 192–7.

22 Wynn M, Dalovisio JR, Tice AD *et al.* Evaluation of the efficacy and safety of outpatient parenteral antimicrobial therapy for infections with methicillin-sensitive *Staphylococcus aureus*. South Med J 2005;98:590–5.

23 Cuijpers ML, Vos FJ, Bleeker-Rovers CP *et al.* Complicating infectious foci in patients with *Staphylococcus aureus* or *Streptococcus* species bacteraemia. Eur J Clin Microbiol Infect Dis 2007;26:105–13.

24 Mugge A, Daniel WG. Echocardiographic assessment of vegetations in patients with infective endocarditis: prognostic implications. Echocardiography 1995;12:651–61.

25 Baddour LM, Wilson WR, Bayer AS *et al.* Infective endocarditis: diagnosis, antimicrobial therapy, and management of complications. A statement for healthcare professionals from the Committee on Rheumatic Fever, Endocarditis, and Kawasaki Disease, Council on Cardiovascular Disease in the Young, and the Councils on Clinical Cardiology, Stroke, and Cardiovascular Surgery and Anesthesia, American Heart Association: endorsed by the Infectious Diseases Society of America. Circulation 2005;111:e394–e434.

26 Moellering RC Jr. Current treatment options for community-acquired methicillin-resistant *Staphylococcus aureus* infection. Clin Infect Dis 2008;46:1032–7.

27 Landy M, Larkum NW, Oswald EJ *et al.* Increased synthesis of *p*-aminobenzoic acid associated with the development of sulfonamide resistance in *Staphylococcus aureus*. Science 1943; 97:265–7.
28 Bud R. Penicillin: Triumph and Tragedy. Oxford: Oxford University Press, 2007.
29 Petri WA Jr. Penicillins, cephalosporins, and other β-lactam antibiotics. In: Brunton LL, Lazo JS, Parker KL, eds. Goodman and Gilman's The Pharmacological Basis of Therapeutics, 11th edn. New York: McGraw-Hill, 2006:1127–54.
30 Bush K. β-Lactam antibiotics: penicillins. In: Finch RG, Greenwood D, Norrby SR, Whitley RJ, eds. Antibiotic and Chemotherapy, 8th edn. Edinburgh: Churchill Livingstone, 2003: 224–58.
31 Diaz CR, Kane JG, Parker RH *et al.* Pharmacokinetics of nafcillin in patients with renal failure. Antimicrob Agents Chemother 1977;12:98–101.
32 Watanakunakorn C. A general survey of antibiotic treatment of staphylococcal septicaemia and endocarditis. Scand J Infect Dis Suppl 1983;41:151–7.
33 Apellaniz G, Valdes M, Perez R *et al.* Comparison of the effectiveness of various antibiotics in the treatment of methicillin-susceptible *Staphylococcus aureus* experimental infective endocarditis. J Chemother 1991;3:91–7.
34 Maraqa NF, Gomes MM, Rathore MH, Alvarez AM. Higher occurrence of hepatotoxicity and rash in patients treated with oxacillin, compared with those treated with nafcillin and other commonly used antimicrobials. Clin Infect Dis 2002;34:50–4.
35 Gruchalla RS, Pirmohamed M. Antibiotic allergy. N Engl J Med 2006;354:601–9.
36 Hoppes T, Prikis M, Segal A. Four cases of nafcillin-associated acute interstitial nephritis in one institution. Nat Clin Pract Nephrol 2007;3:456–61.
37 Tillman DB, Oill PA, Guze LB. Oxacillin nephritis. Arch Intern Med 1980;140:1552.
38 Spanou Z, Keller M, Britschgi M *et al.* Involvement of drug-specific T cells in acute drug-induced interstitial nephritis. J Am Soc Nephrol 2006;17:2919–27.
39 Goland S, Malnick SD, Gratz R *et al.* Severe cholestatic hepatitis following cloxacillin treatment. Postgrad Med J 1998;74:59–60.
40 Al Homaidhi H, Abdel-Haq NM, El-Baba M *et al.* Severe hepatitis associated with oxacillin therapy. South Med J 2002; 95:650–2.
41 Kleinman MS, Presberg JE. Cholestatic hepatitis after dicloxacillin-sodium therapy. J Clin Gastroenterol 1986;8:77–8.
42 Mazuryk H, Kastenberg D, Rubin R *et al.* Cholestatic hepatitis associated with the use of nafcillin. Am J Gastroenterol 1993; 88:1960–2.
43 Siegmund JB, Tarshis AM. Prolonged jaundice after dicloxacillin therapy. Am J Gastroenterol 1993;88:1299–300.
44 Owens RC Jr, Donskey CJ, Gaynes RP *et al.* Antimicrobial-associated risk factors for *Clostridium difficile* infection. Clin Infect Dis 2008;46(suppl 1):S19–S31.
45 Nahum GG, Uhl K, Kennedy DL. Antibiotic use in pregnancy and lactation: what is and is not known about teratogenic and toxic risks. Obstet Gynecol 2006;107:1120–38.
46 Philpott-Howard J, Burroughs A, Fisher N *et al.* Piperacillin–tazobactam versus ciprofloxacin plus amoxicillin in the treatment of infective episodes after liver transplantation. J Antimicrob Chemother 2003;52:993–1000.
47 Davey PG, Main J, Scott AC. An open study of timentin for the initial treatment of serious infections. J Antimicrob Chemother 1986;17(suppl C):161–8.
48 Noel GJ, Bush K, Bagchi P *et al.* A randomized, double-blind trial comparing ceftobiprole medocaril with vancomycin plus ceftazidime for the treatment of patients with complicated skin and skin-structure infections. Clin Infect Dis 2008;46:647–55.
49 Noel GJ, Strauss RS, Amsler K *et al.* Results of a double-blind, randomized trial of ceftobiprole treatment of complicated skin and skin structure infections caused by Gram-positive bacteria. Antimicrob Agents Chemother 2008;52:37–44.
50 Neu HC, Duma RJ, Jones RN *et al.* Therapeutic and epidemiologic recommendations to reduce the spread of type-1-beta-lactamase resistance. Diagn Microbiol Infect Dis 1992;15 (2 suppl):49S–52S.
51 Marshall WF, Blair JE. The cephalosporins. Mayo Clin Proc 1999;74:187–95.
52 Steckelberg JM, Rouse MS, Tallan BM *et al.* Relative efficacies of broad-spectrum cephalosporins for treatment of methicillin-susceptible *Staphylococcus aureus* experimental infective endocarditis. Antimicrob Agents Chemother 1993;37:554–8.
53 Carrizosa J, Santoro J, Kaye D. Treatment of experimental *Staphylococcus aureus* endocarditis: comparison of cephalothin, cefazolin, and methicillin. Antimicrob Agents Chemother 1978;13:74–7.
54 Nannini EC, Singh KV, Murray BE. Relapse of type A beta-lactamase-producing *Staphylococcus aureus* native valve endocarditis during cefazolin therapy: revisiting the issue. Clin Infect Dis 2003;37:1194–8.
55 Bryant RE, Alford RH. Unsuccessful treatment of staphylococcal endocarditis with cefazolin. JAMA 1977;237:569–70.
56 Shuford JA, Piper KE, Hein M *et al.* Lack of association of *Staphylococcus aureus* type A beta-lactamase with cefazolin combined with antimicrobial spacer placement prosthetic joint infection treatment failure. Diagn Microbiol Infect Dis 2006; 54:189–92.
57 Romano A, Guéant-Rodriguez RM, Viola M *et al.* Cross-reactivity and tolerability of cephalosporins in patients with immediate hypersensitivity to penicillins. Ann Intern Med 2004;141:16–22.
58 Pichichero ME. Use of selected cephalosporins in penicillin-allergic patients: a paradigm shift. Diagn Microbiol Infect Dis 2007;57(3 suppl):13S–18S.
59 Walsh C. Antibiotics: Actions, Origins, Resistance. Washington, DC: ASM Press, 2003.
60 Kaplan SL. Community-acquired methicillin-resistant *Staphylococcus aureus* infections in children. Semin Pediatr Infect Dis 2006;17:113–19.
61 Reyes J, Hidalgo M, Diaz L *et al.* Characterization of macrolide resistance in Gram-positive cocci from Colombian hospitals: a countrywide surveillance. Int J Infect Dis 2007;11:329–36.
62 Moore ZS, Jerris RC, Hilinski JA. High prevalence of inducible clindamycin resistance among *Staphylococcus aureus* isolates from patients with cystic fibrosis. J Cyst Fibros 2008;7:206–9.
63 Yilmaz G, Avdin K, Iskender S *et al.* Detection and prevalence of inducible clindamycin resistance in staphylococci. J Med Microbiol 2007;56:342–5.
64 Daurel C, Huet C, Dhalluin A *et al.* Differences in potential for selection of clindamycin-resistant mutants between inducible erm(A) and erm(C) *Staphylococcus aureus* genes. J Clin Microbiol 2008;46:546–50.

65 Martinez-Aguilar G, Hammerman WA, Mason EO Jr *et al.* Clindamycin treatment of invasive infections caused by community-acquired, methicillin-resistant and methicillin-susceptible *Staphylococcus aureus* in children. Pediatr Infect Dis J 2003;22:593–8.
66 Gales AC, Sader HS, Fritsche TR. Tigecycline activity tested against 11808 bacterial pathogens recently collected from US medical centers. Diagn Microbiol Infect Dis 2008;60:421–7.
67 Mendes RE, Sader HS, Deshpande L *et al.* Antimicrobial activity of tigecycline against community-acquired methicillin-resistant *Staphylococcus aureus* isolates recovered from North American medical centers. Diagn Microbiol Infect Dis 2008; 60:433–6.
68 Goff DA, Dowzicky MJ. Prevalence and regional variation in methicillin-resistant *Staphylococcus aureus* (MRSA) in the USA and comparative in vitro activity of tigecycline, a glycylcycline antimicrobial. J Med Microbiol 2007;56:1189–93.
69 Huang YT, Liao CH, Teng LJ *et al.* Comparative bactericidal activities of daptomycin, glycopeptides, linezolid and tigecycline against blood isolates of Gram-positive bacteria in Taiwan. Clin Microbiol Infect 2008;14:124–9.
70 Rubino CM, Ma L, Bhavnani SM *et al.* Evaluation of tigecycline penetration into colon wall tissue and epithelial lining fluid using a population pharmacokinetic model and Monte Carlo simulation. Antimicrob Agents Chemother 2007;51:4085–9.
71 Garrison MW, Neumiller JJ, Setter SM. Tigecycline: an investigational glycycycline antimicrobial with activity against resistant Gram-positive organisms. Clin Ther 2005;27:12–22.
72 Grolman DC. Therapeutic applications of tigecycline in the management of complicated skin and skin structure infections. Int J Infect Dis 2007;11(suppl 1):S7–S15.
73 Levine DP. Vancomycin: a history. Clin Infect Dis 2006; 42(suppl 1):S5–S12.
74 Levine DP. Vancomycin: understanding its past and preserving its future. South Med J 2008;10:284–91.
75 Falagas ME, Makris GC, Dimopoulos G *et al.* Heteroresistance: a concern of increasing clinical significance. Clin Microbiol Infect 2008;14:101–4.
76 Courvalin P. Vancomycin resistance in Gram-positive cocci. Clin Infect Dis 2006;42(suppl 1):S25–S34.
77 Sievert DM, Rudrile JT, Patel JB *et al.* Vancomycin-resistant *Staphylococcus aureus* in the United States, 2002–2006. Clin Infect Dis 2008;46:668–74.
78 Appelbaum PC, Bozdogan B. Vancomycin resistance in *Staphylococcus aureus*. Clin Lab Med 2004;24:381–402.
79 Tenover FC, McDonald LC. Vancomycin-resistant staphylococci and enterococci: epidemiology and control. Curr Opin Infect Dis 2005;18:300–5.
80 Chiew YF, Charles M, Johnstone MC *et al.* Detection of vancomycin heteroresistant *Staphylococcus haemolyticus* and vancomycin intermediate resistant *Staphylococcus epidermidis* by means of vancomycin screening agar. Pathology 2007;39:375–7.
81 Nunes AP, Teixeira LM, Iorio NL *et al.* Heterogeneous resistance to vancomycin in *Staphylococcus epidermidis*, *Staphylococcus haemolyticus* and *Staphylococcus warneri* clinical strains: characterization of glycopeptides susceptibility profiles and cell wall thickening. Int J Antimicrob Agents 2006;27:307–15.
82 Biavasco F, Vignaroli C, Lazzarini R *et al.* Glycopeptide susceptibility profiles of *Staphylococcus haemolyticus* bloodstream isolates. Antimicrob Agents Chemother 2000;44:3122–6.
83 Bourgeois I, Pestel-Caron M, Lemeland JF *et al.* Tolerance to the glycopeptides vancomycin and teicoplanin in coagulase-negative staphylococci. Antimicrob Agents Chemother 2007;51: 740–3.
84 Jones RN. Microbiological features of vancomycin in the 21st century: minimum inhibitory concentration creep, bactericidal/static activity, and applied breakpoints to predict clinical outcomes or detect resistant strains. Clin Infect Dis 2006;42(suppl 1):S13–S24.
85 Holmes RL, Jorgensen JH. Inhibitory activities of 11 antimicrobial agents and bactericidal activities of vancomycin and daptomycin against invasive methicillin-resistant *Staphylococcus aureus* isolates obtained from 1999 through 2006. Antimicrob Agents Chemother 2008;52:757–60.
86 Alós JI, Garcia-Cañas A, Garcia-Hierro P *et al.* Vancomycin MICs did not creep in *Staphylococcus aureus* isolates from 2002 to 2006 in a setting with low vancomycin usage. J Antimicrob Chemother 2008;62:773–5.
87 Sakoulas G, Moellering RC Jr. Increasing antibiotic resistance among methicillin-resistant *Staphylococcus aureus* strains. Clin Infect Dis 2008;46(suppl 5):S360–S367.
88 Sakoulas G, Moise-Broder PA, Schentag J *et al.* Relationship of MIC and bactericidal activity to efficacy of vancomycin for treatment of methicillin-resistant *Staphylococcus aureus* bacteremia. J Clin Microbiol 2004;42:2398–402.
89 Soriano A, Marco F, Martinez JA *et al.* Influence of vancomycin minimum inhibitory concentrations on the treatment of methicillin-resistant *Staphylococcus aureus* bacteremia. Clin Infect Dis 2008;46:193–200.
90 Jorgenson L, Reiter PD, Freeman JE *et al.* Vancomycin disposition and penetration into ventricular fluid of the central nervous system following intravenous therapy in patients with cerebrospinal devices. Pediatr Neurosurg 2007;43:449–55.
91 Ricard JD, Wolff M, Lacherade JC *et al.* Levels of vancomycin in cerebrospinal fluid of adult patients receiving adjunctive corticosteriods to treat pneumococcal meningitis: a prospective multicenter observational study. Clin Infect Dis 2007;44:250–5.
92 Nava-Ocampo AA, Mojica-Madera JA, Villanueva-Garcia D *et al.* Antimicrobial therapy and local toxicity of intraventricular administration of vancomycin in a neonate with ventriculitis. Ther Drug Monit 2006;28:474–6.
93 Rybak M, Lomaestro B, Rotschafer JC. Therapeutic monitoring of vancomycin in adult patients: a consensus review of the American Society of Health-System Pharmacists, the Infectious Diseases Society of America, and the Society of Infectious Diseases Pharmacists. Am J Health Syst Pharm 2009;66:82–98.
94 Bauer LA, Black DJ, Lill JS. Vancomycin dosing in morbidly obese patients. Eur J Clin Pharmacol 1998;54:621–5.
95 Skhirtladze K, Hutschala D, Fleck T *et al.* Impaired target site penetration of vancomycin in diabetic patients following cardiac surgery. Antimicrob Agents Chemother 2006;50:1372–5.
96 Vuagnat A, Stern R, Lotthe A *et al.* High dose vancomycin for osteomyelitis: continuous vs. intermittent infusion. J Clin Pharm Ther 2004;29:351–7.
97 Dombrowski JC, Winston LG. Clinical failures of appropriately-treated methicillin-resistant *Staphylococcus aureus* infection. J Infect 2008;57:110–15.
98 Small PM, Chambers HF. Vancomycin for *Staphylococcus aureus* endocarditis in intravenous drug users. Antimicrob Agents Chemother 1990;34:1227–31.

99 Gentry CA, Rodvold KA, Novak RM *et al.* Retrospective evaluation of therapies for *Staphylococcus aureus* endocarditis. Pharmacotherapy 1997;17:990–7.

100 Maki DG, Bohn MJ, Stolz SM *et al.* Comparative study of cefazolin, cefamandole, and vancomycin for surgical prophylaxis in cardiac and vascular operations. A double-blind randomized trial. J Thorac Cardiovasc Surg 1992;104:1423–34.

101 Garey KW, Dao T, Chen H *et al.* Timing of vancomycin prophylaxis for cardiac surgery patients and the risk of surgical site infections. J Antimicrob Chemother 2006;58:645–50.

102 Movahed MR, Kasravi B, Bryan CS. Prophylactic use of vancomycin in adult cardiology and cardiac surgery. J Cardiovasc Pharmacol Ther 2004;9:13–20.

103 Garey KW, Lai D, Dao-Tran TK *et al.* Interrupted time series analysis of vancomycin compared to cefuroxime for surgical prophylaxis in patients undergoing cardiac surgery. Antimicrob Agents Chemother 2008;52:446–51.

104 Elting LS, Rubenstein EB, Kurtin D *et al.* Mississippi mud in the 1990s: risks and outcomes of vancomycin-associated toxicity in general oncology practice. Cancer 1998;83:2597–607.

105 Forouzesh A, Moise PA, Sakoulas G. Vancomycin ototoxicity: a re-evaluation in an era of increasing doses. Antimicrob Agents Chemother 2009;53:483–6.

106 Cunha BA, Mohan SS, Hamid N *et al.* Cost-ineffectiveness of serum vancomycin levels. Eur J Clin Microbiol Infect Dis 2007;26:509–11.

107 Goetz MB, Sayers J. Nephrotoxicity of vancomycin and aminoglycoside therapy separately and in combination. J Antimicrob Chemother 1993;32:325–34.

108 Ingram PR, Lye DC, Tambyah PA *et al.* Risk factors for nephrotoxicity associated with continuous vancomycin infusion in outpatient parenteral antibiotic therapy. J Antimicrob Chemother 2008;62:168–71.

109 Dovas S, Liakopoulos V, Papatheodorou L *et al.* Acute renal failure after antibiotic-impregnated bone cement treatment of an infected total knee arthroplasty. Clin Nephrol 2008;69:207–11.

110 Sivagnanam S, Deleu D. Red man syndrome. Crit Care 2003;7:119–20.

111 Polk RE, Healy DP, Schwartz LB *et al.* Vancomycin and the red-man syndrome: pharmacodynamics of histamine release. J Infect Dis 1988;157:502–7.

112 Wallace MR, Mascola JR, Oldfied EC. Red man syndrome: incidence, etiology, and prophlaxis. J Infect Dis 1991;164: 1180–5.

113 Sorrell TC, Collignon PJ. A prospective study of adverse reactions associated with vancomycin therapy. J Antimicrob Chemother 1985;16:235–41.

114 Bertolissi M, Bassi F, Cecotti R *et al.* Pruritus: a useful sign for predicting the haemodynamic changes that occur following administration of vancomycin. Crit Care 2002;6:234–9.

115 Deresinski S. Counterpoint: vancomycin and *Staphylococcus aureus*: an antibiotic enters obsolescence. Clin Infect Dis 2007; 44:1543–8.

116 Trueba F, Garrabe E, Hadef R *et al.* High prevalence of teicoplanin resistance among *Staphylococcus epidermidis* strains in a 5-year retrospective study. J Clin Microbiol 2006;44:1922–3.

117 Pea F, Brollo L, Viale P *et al.* Teicoplanin therapeutic drug monitoring in critically ill patients: a retrospective study emphasizing the importance of a loading dose. J Antimicrob Chemother 2003;51:971–5.

118 Finch RG, Eliopoulos GM. Safety and efficacy of glycopeptide antibiotics. J Antimicrob Chemother 2005;55(suppl S2):ii5–ii13.

119 Hahn-Ast C, Glasmacher A, Arns A *et al.* An audit of efficacy and toxicity of teicoplanin versus vancomycin in febrile neutropenia: is the different toxicity profile clinically relevant? Infection 2008;36:54–8.

120 Huang JH, Hsu RB. Treatment of infective endocarditis caused by methicillin-resistant *Staphylococcus aureus*: teicoplanin versus vancomycin in a retrospective study. Scand J Infect Dis 2008; 40:462–7.

121 Brogden RN, Peters DH. Teicoplanin: a reappraisal of its antimicrobial activity, pharmacokinetic properties and therapeutic efficacy. Drugs 1994;47:823–54.

122 Castanheira M, Jones RN, Sader HS. Update of the *in vitro* activity of daptomycin tested against 6710 Gram-positive cocci isolated in North America (2006). Diagn Microbiol Infect Dis 2008;61:235–9.

123 Sharma M, Riederer K, Chase P *et al.* High rate of decreasing daptomycin susceptibility during the treatment of persistent *Staphylococcus aureus* bacteremia. Eur J Clin Microbiol Infect Dis 2008;27:433–7.

124 Arbeit RD, Maki D, Tally FP *et al.* The safety and efficacy of daptomycin for the treatment of complicated skin and skin-structure infections. Clin Infect Dis 2004;38:1673–81.

125 Krige JE, Lindfield K, Friedrich L *et al.* Effectiveness and duration of daptomycin therapy in resolving clinical symptoms in the treatment of complicated skin and skin structure infections. Curr Med Res Opin 2007;23:2147–56.

126 Davis SL, McKinnon PS, Hall LM *et al.* Daptomycin versus vancomycin for complicated skin and skin structure infections: clinical and economic outcomes. Pharmacotherapy 2007;27: 1611–18.

127 Fowler VG Jr, Boucher HW, Corey GR *et al.* Daptomycin versus standard therapy for bacteremia and endocarditis caused by *Staphylococcus aureus*. N Engl J Med 2006;355:653–65.

128 Rehm SJ, Boucher H, Levine D *et al.* Daptomycin versus vancomycin plus gentamicin for treatment of bacteraemia and endocarditis due to *Staphylococcus aureus*: subset analysis of patients infected with methicillin-resistant isolates. J Antimicrob Chemother 2008;62:1413–21.

129 Levine DP, Lamp KC. Daptomycin in the treatment of patients with infective endocarditis: experience from a registry. Am J Med 2007;120(10 suppl 1):S28–S33.

130 Lamp KC, Friedrich LV, Mendez-Vigo L *et al.* Clinical experience with daptomycin for the treatment of patients with osteomyelitis. Am J Med 2007;120:S13–S20.

131 Forrest GN, Donovan BJ, Lamp KC *et al.* Clinical experience with daptomycin for the treatment of patients with documented Gram-positive septic arthritis. Ann Pharmacother 2008;42:213–17.

132 Ardura MI, Mejias A, Katz KS *et al.* Daptomycin therapy for invasive Gram-positive bacterial infections in children. Pediatr Infect Dis J 2007;26:1128–32.

133 Jones T, Yeaman MR, Sakoulas G *et al.* Failures in clinical treatment of *Staphylococcus aureus* infection with daptomycin are associated with alterations in surface charge, membrane phospholipid asymmetry and drug binding. Antimicrob Agents Chemother 2008;52:269–78.

134 Lesens O, Brannigan E, Bergin C *et al.* Impact of the use of aminoglycosides in combination antibiotic therapy on septic

shock and mortality due to *Staphylococcus aureus* bacteremia. Eur J Intern Med 2006;17:276–80.
135 Hawkins C, Huang J, Jin N *et al.* Persistent *Staphylococcus aureus* bacteremia: analysis of risk factors and outcomes. Arch Intern Med 2007;167:1861–7.
136 Sohail MR, Martin KR, Wilson WR *et al.* Medical versus surgical management of *Staphylococcus aureus* prosthetic valve endocarditis. Am J Med 2006;119:147–54.
137 Araya CE, Fennell RS, Neiberger RE *et al.* Hemodialysis catheter-related bacteremia in children: increasing antibiotic resistance and changing bacteriological profile. Am J Kidney Dis 2007;50:119–23.
138 Asghar R, Banajeh S, Egas J *et al.* Chloramphenicol versus ampicillin plus gentamicin for community acquired very severe pneumonia among children aged 2–59 months in low resource settings: multicentre randomized controlled trial (SPEAR study). BMJ 2008;336:80–4.
139 Kent ME, Rapp RP, Smith KM. Antibiotic beads and osteomyelitis: here today, what's coming tomorrow? Orthopedics 2006;29:599–603.
140 Chang W, Colangeli M, Colangeli S *et al.* Adult osteomyelitis: debridement plus Osteoset T pellets. Acta Orthop Belg 2007; 73:238–43.
141 Norrby R. Linezolid: a review of the first oxazolidinone. Expert Opin Pharmacother 2001;2:293–302.
142 Falagas ME, Siempos II, Papagelopoulos PJ *et al.* Linezolid for the treatment of adults with bone and joint infections. Int J Antimicrob Agents 2007;29:233–9.
143 Falagas ME, Siempos II, Vardakas KZ. Linezolid versus glycopeptides or beta-lactam for treatment of Gram-positive bacterial infections: meta-analysis of randomized controlled trials. Lancet Infect Dis 2008;8:53–66.
144 Weigelt J, Itani K, Stevens D *et al.* Linezolid versus vancomycin in treatment of complicated skin and soft tissue infections. Antimicrob Agents Chemother 2005;49:2260–6.
145 Besier S, Ludwig A, Zander J *et al.* Linezolid resistance in *Staphylococcus aureus*: gene dosage effect, stability, fitness costs, and cross-resistances. Antimicrob Agents Chemother 2008;52:1570–2.
146 Andriole VT. Quinolones. In: Finch RG, Greenwood D, Norrby SR, Whitley RJ, eds. Antibiotic and Chemotherapy. Anti-infective Agents and Their Use in Therapy, 8th edn. Edinburgh: Churchill Livingstone, 2003:349–73.
147 Daum TE, Schaberg DR, Terpenning MS. Increasing resistance of *Staphylococcus aureus* to ciprofloxacin. Antimicrob Agents Chemother 1990;34:1862–3.
148 Aldridge KE, Gelfand MS, Schiro DD *et al.* The rapid emergence of fluoroquinolone-methicillin-resistant *Staphylococcus aureus* infections in a community hospital. An in vitro look at alternative antimicrobial agents. Diagn Microbiol Infect Dis 1992;15:601–8.
149 Schmitz FJ, Higgins PG, Mayer S *et al.* Activity of quinolones against Gram-positive cocci: mechanisms of drug action and bacterial resistance. Eur J Clin Microbiol Infect Dis 2002;21: 647–59.
150 Shopsin B, Zhao X, Kreiswirth BN. Are the new quinolones appropriate treatment for community-acquired methicillin-resistant *Staphylococcus aureus*? Int J Antimicrob Agents 2004; 24:32–4.
151 Grossi O, Caillon J, Arvieux C *et al.* In vivo efficacy of moxifloxacin compared with cloxacillin and vancomycin in a *Staphylococcus aureus* rabbit arthritis experimental model. Antimicrob Agents Chemother 2007;51:3401–3.
152 Kaatz GW, Seo SM, Barriere SL *et al.* Development of resistance to fleroxacin during therapy of experimental methicillin-susceptible *Staphylococcus aureus* endocarditis. Antimicrob Agents Chemother 1991;35:1547–50.
153 Hooper DC. Fluoroquinolone resistance among Gram-positive cocci. Lancet Infect Dis 2002;2:530–8.
154 Rogues AM, Dumartin C, Amadeo B *et al.* Relationship between rates of antimicrobial consumption and the incidence of antimicrobial resistance in *Staphylococcus aureus* and *Pseudomonas aeruginosa* isolates from 47 French hospitals. Infect Control Hosp Epidemiol 2007;28:1389–95.
155 Meyer E, Schwab F, Gastmeier P *et al.* Methicillin-resistant *Staphylococcus aureus* in German intensive care units during 2000–2003: data from project SARI (Surveillance of Antimicrobial Use and Antimicrobial Resistance in Intensive Care Units). Infect Control Hosp Epidemiol 2006;27:146–54.
156 MacDougall C, Powell JP, Johnson CK *et al.* Hospital and community fluoroquinolone use and resistance in *Staphylococcus aureus* and *Escherichia coli* in 17 US hospitals. Clin Infect Dis 2005;41:435–40.
157 Charbonneau P, Parienti JJ, Thibon P *et al.* Fluoroquinolone use and methicillin-resistant *Staphylococcus aureus* isolation rates in hospitalized patients: a quasi experimental study. Clin Infect Dis 2006;42:778–84.
158 Tam VH, Louie A, Fritsche TR *et al.* Impact of drug-exposure intensity and duration of therapy on the emergence of *Staphylococcus aureus* resistance to a quinolone antimicrobial. J Infect Dis 2007;195:1818–27.
159 Ruotsalainen E, Jarvinen A, Koivula I *et al.* Levofloxacin does not decrease mortality in *Staphylococcus aureus* bacteremia when added to the standard treatment: a prospective and randomized clinical trial of 381 patients. J Intern Med 2006; 259:179–90.
160 Falagas ME, Matthaiou DK, Vardakas KZ. Fluoroquinolones vs. beta-lactams for empirical treatment of immunocompetent patients with skin and soft tissue infections: a meta-analysis of randomized controlled trials. Mayo Clin Proc 2006;81: 1553–66.
161 Moshirfar M, Feiz V, Vitale AT *et al.* Endophthalmitis after uncomplicated cataract surgery with the use of fourth-generation fluoroquinolones: a retrospective observational case series. Ophthalmology 2007;114:686–91.
162 Barberan J, Aguilar L, Carroquino G *et al.* Conservative treatment of staphylococcal prosthetic joint infections in elderly patients. Am J Med 2006;119:993 e7–10.
163 Murillo O, Pachón ME, Euba G *et al.* Antagonistic effect of rifampin on the efficacy of high-dose levofloxacin in staphylococcal experimental foreign-body infection. Antimicrob Agents Chemother 2008;52:3681–6.
164 Osterlund A, Kahlmeter G, Haeggman S *et al.* On fusidic acid resistant *S. aureus*. *Staphylococcus aureus* resistant to fusidic acid among Swedish children: a follow-up study. Scand J Infect Dis 2006;38:334–4.
165 Ravenscroft JC, Layton A, Barnham M. Observations on high levels of fusidic acid resistant *Staphylococcus aureus* in Harrogate, North Yorkshire, UK. Clin Exp Dermatol 2000;25:327–30.
166 Howden BP, Grayson ML. Dumb and dumber: the potential waste of a useful antistaphylococcal agent: emerging fusidic

acid resistance in *Staphylococcus aureus*. Clin Infect Dis 2006; 42:394–400.
167 O'Neill AJ, McLaws F, Kahlmeter G *et al*. Genetic basis of resistance to fusidic acid in staphylococci. Antimicrob Agents Chemother 2007;51:1737–40.
168 Brown EM, Thomas P. Fusidic acid resistance in *Staphylococcus aureus* isolates. Lancet 2002;359:803.
169 McLaws F, Chopra I, O'Neill AJ. High prevalence of resistance to fusidic acid in clinical isolates of *Staphylococcus epidermidis*. J Antimicrob Chemother 2008;61:1040–3.
170 Christiansen K. Fusidic acid adverse drug reactions. Int J Antimicrob Agents 1991;12(suppl 2):S3–S9.
171 Falagas ME, Kopterides P. Old antibiotics for infections in critically ill patients. Curr Opin Crit Care 2007;13:592–7.
172 Whitby M. Fusidic acid in septicaemia and endocarditis. Int J Antimicrob Agents 1999;12(suppl 2):S17–S22.
173 Chang SC, Hsieh SM, Chen ML *et al*. Oral fusidic acid fails to eradicate methicillin-resistant *Staphylococcus aureus* colonization and results in emergence of fusidic acid-resistant strains. Diagn Microbiol Infect Dis 2000;36:131–6.
174 Aboltins CA, Page MA, Buising KL *et al*. Treatment of staphylococcal prosthetic joint infections with debridement, prosthesis retention and oral rifampicin and fusidic acid. Clin Microbiol Infect 2007;13:586–91.
175 Dumitrescu O, Badiou C, Bes M *et al*. Effect of antibiotics, alone and in combination, on Panton–Valentine leukocidin production by a *Staphylococcus aureus* reference strain. Clin Microbiol Infect 2008;14:384–8.
176 Proctor RA. Role of folate antagonists in the treatment of methicillin-resistant *Staphylococcus aureus* infection. Clin Infect Dis 2008;46:584–93.
177 Kaka AS, Rueda AM, Shelburne SA III *et al*. Bactericidal activity of orally available agents against methicillin-resistant *Staphylococcus aureus*. J Antimicrob Chemother 2006;58:680–3.
178 deGorgolas M, Aviles P, Verdejo C *et al*. Treatment of experimental endocarditis due to methicillin-susceptible or methicillin-resistant *Staphylococcus aureus* with trimethoprim–sulfamethoxazole and antibiotics that inhibit cell wall synthesis. Antimicrob Agents Chemother 1995;39:953–7.
179 Moellering RC Jr. A 39-year-old man with a skin infection. JAMA 2008;299:79–87.
180 Szumowski JD, Cohen DE, Kanaya F *et al*. Treatment and outcomes of infections by methicillin-resistant *Staphylococcus aureus* at an ambulatory clinic. Antimicrob Agents Chemother 2007;51:423–8.
181 Cenizal MJ, Skiest D, Luber S *et al*. Prospective randomized trial of empiric therapy with trimethoprim–sulfamethoxazole or doxycycline for outpatient skin and soft tissue infections in an area of high prevalence of methicillin-resistant *Staphylococcus aureus*. Antimicrob Agents Chemother 2007;51:2628–30.
182 Stein A, Bataille JF, Drancourt M *et al*. Ambulatory treatment of multidrug-resistant *Staphylococcus*-infected orthopedic implants with high-dose oral co-trimoxazole (trimethoprim–sulfamethoxazole). Antimicrob Agents Chemother 1998;42: 3086–91.
183 Markowitz N, Quinn EL, Saravolatz LD. Trimethoprim–sulfamethoxazole compared with vancomycin for the treatment of *Staphylococcus aureus* infection. Ann Intern Med 1992; 117:390–8.
184 Martin JN, Rose DA, Hadley WK *et al*. Emergence of trimethoprim–sulfamethoxazole resistance in the AIDS era. J Infect Dis 1999;180:1809–18.
185 Lamb HM, Figgitt DP, Faulds D. Quinupristin/dalfopristin: a review of its use in the management of serious Gram-positive infections. Drugs 1999;58:1061–97.
186 Eliopoulos GM. Quinupristin–dalfopristin and linezolid: evidence and opinion. Clin Infect Dis 2003;36:473–81.
187 Fuchs PC, Barry AL, Brown SD. Bactericidal activity of quinupristin–dalfopristin against *Staphylococcus aureus*: clindamycin susceptibility as a surrogate indicator. Antimicrob Agents Chemother 2000;44:2880–2.
188 Auckenthaler R, Courvalin P, Feger C *et al*. International study working group. In vitro activity of quinupristin/dalfopristin in comparison with five antibiotics against worldwide clinical isolates of staphylococci. Clin Microbiol Infect 2000;6:608–12.
189 Cohen MA, Huband MD. Activity of clinafloxacin, trovafloxacin, quinupristin/dalfopristin, and other antimicrobial agents versus *Staphylococcus aureus* isolates with reduced susceptibility to vancomycin. Diagn Microbiol Infect Dis 1999;33:43–6.
190 Nichols RL, Graham DR, Barriere SL *et al*. Treatment of hospitalized patients with complicated Gram-positive skin and skin structure infections: two randomized, multicentre studies of quinupristin/dalfopristin versus cefazolin, oxacillin, or vancomycin. Synercid Skin and Skin Structure Infection Group. J Antimicrob Chemother 1999;44:263–73.
191 Fagon JY, Patrick H, Haas DW *et al*. Treatment of Gram-positive nosocomial pneumonia. Prospective randomized comparison of quinupristin/dalfoprisin versus vancomycin. Am J Respir Crit Care Med 2000;161:753–62.
192 Rubinstein E, Prokocimer P, Talbot GH. Safety and tolerability of quinupristin/dalfopristin: administration guidelines. J Antimicrob Chemother 1999;44(suppl A):37–46.
193 Olsen KM, Rebuck JA, Rupp ME. Arthralgias and myalgias related to quinupristin–dalfopristin administration. Clin Infect Dis 2001;32:e83–e86.
194 Klastersky J. Role of quinupristin/dalfopristin in the treatment of Gram-positive nosocomial infections in haematological or oncological patients. Cancer Treat Rev 2003;29:431–40.
195 Sekiguchi J, Fujino T, Araake M *et al*. Emergence of rifampicin resistance in methicillin-resistant *Staphylococcus aureus* in tuberculosis wards. J Infect Chemother 2006;12:47–50.
196 Wichelhaus TA, Boddinghaus B, Besier S. Biological cost of rifampin resistance from the perspective of *Staphylococcus aureus*. Antimicrob Agents Chemother 2002;46:3381–5.
197 Parenti F, Lancini G. Rifamycins. In: Finch RG, Greenwood D, Norrby SR, Whitley RJ, eds. Antibiotic and Chemotherapy. Anti-infective Agents and Their Use in Therapy, 8th edn. Edinburgh: Churchill Livingstone, 2003:374–81.
198 Falagas ME, Bliziotis IA, Fragoulis KN. Oral rifampin for eradication of *Staphylococcus aureus* carriage from healthy and sick populations: a systematic review of the evidence from comparative trials. Am J Infect Control 2007;35:106–14.
199 Falagas ME, Fragoulis KN, Bliziotis IA. Oral rifampin for prevention of *S. aureus* carriage-related infections in patients with renal failure: a meta-analysis of randomized controlled trials. Nephrol Dial Transplant 2006;21:2536–42.
200 Saleh-Mghir A, Ameur N, Muller-Serieys C *et al*. Combination of quinupristin–dalfopristin (Synercid) and rifampin is highly synergistic in experimental *Staphylococcus aureus* joint

prosthesis infection. Antimicrob Agents Chemother 2002;46: 1122–4.

201 Bliziotis IA, Ntziora F, Lawrence KR *et al.* Rifampin as adjuvant treatment of Gram-positive bacterial infections: a systematic review of comparative clinical trials. Eur J Clin Microbiol Infect Dis 2007;26:849–56.

202 Periroth J, Kuo M, Tan J *et al.* Adjunctive use of rifampin for the treatment of *Staphylococcus aureus* infections: a systematic review of the literature. Arch Intern Med 2008;168:805–19.

203 Zimmerli W, Widmer AF, Blatter M *et al.* Role of rifampin for treatment of orthopaedic implant-related staphylococcal infections. A randomized controlled trial. JAMA 1998;279: 1537–41.

204 Van der Auwera P, Meunier-Carpentier F, Klastersky J. Clinical study of combination therapy with oxacillin and rifampin for staphylococcal infections. Rev Infect Dis 1983;5(suppl 3): 515–22.

205 Levine DP, Fromm BS, Reddy BR. Slow response to vancomycin or vancomycin plus rifampin in methicillin-resistant *Staphylococcus aureus* endocarditis. Ann Intern Med 1991;115: 674–80.

206 Norden CW, Bryant R, Palmer D *et al.* Chronic osteomyelitis caused by *Staphylococcus aureus*: controlled clinical trial of nafcillin therapy and nafcillin–rifampin therapy. South Med J 1986;79:947–51.

207 Van der Auwera P, Klastersky J, Thys JP *et al.* Double-blind, placebo-controlled study of oxacillin combined with rifampin in the treatment of staphylococcal infections. Antimicrob Agents Chemother 1985;28:467–72.

208 Chuard C, Herrmann M, Vaudaux P *et al.* Successful therapy of experimental chronic foreign-body infection due to methicillin-resistant *Staphylococcus aureus* by antimicrobial combinations. Antimicrob Agents Chemother 1991;35:2611–16.

209 Riedel DJ, Weekes E, Forrest GN. Addition of rifampin to standard therapy for treatment of native valve infective endocarditis caused by *Staphylococcus aureus*. Antimicrob Agents Chemother 2008;52:2463–7.

210 Stewart AH, Eyers PS, Earnshaw JJ. Prevention of infection in peripheral arterial reconstruction: a systematic review and meta-analysis. J Vasc Surg 2007;46:148–55.

211 Proctor RA, von Eiff C, Kahl BC *et al.* Small colony variants: a pathogenic form of bacteria that facilitates persistent and recurrent infections. Nat Rev Microbiol 2006;4:295–305.

212 Anderson VR, Keating GM. Dalbavancin. Drugs 2008;68:639–48.

213 Biedenbach DJ, Bell JM, Sader HS, Turnidge JD, Jones RN. Activity of dalbavancin tested against a worldwide collection of 81,673 Gram-positive bacterial isolates. Antimicrob Agents Chemother 2009;53:1260–3.

214 Laohavaleeson S, Kuti JL, Nicolau DP. Telavancin: a novel lipoglycopeptide for serious Gram-positive infections. Expert Opin Investig Drugs 2007;16:347–57.

215 Stryjewski ME, Chu VH, O'Riordan WD *et al.* Telavancin versus standard therapy for treatment of complicated skin and skin structure infections caused by Gram-positive bacteria: FAST 2 study. Antimicrob Agents Chemother 2006;50:862–7.

216 Stryjewski ME, Graham DR, Wilson SE *et al.* Telavancin versus vancomycin for the treatment of complicated skin and skin-structure infections caused by Gram-positive organisms. Clin Infect Dis 2008;46:1683–93.

217 Reyes N, Skinner R, Kaniga K *et al.* Efficacy of telavancin (TD-6424), a rapidly bactericidal lipoglycopeptide with multiple mechanisms of action, in a murine model of pneumonia induced by methicillin-resistant *Staphylococcus aureus*. Antimicrob Agents Chemother 2005;49:4344–6.

218 Gander S, Kinnaird A, Finch R. Telavancin: in vitro activity against staphylococci in a biofilm model. J Antimicrob Chemother 2005;56:337–43.

219 Lentino JR, Narita M, Yu VL. New antimicrobial agents as therapy for resistant Gram-positive cocci. Eur J Clin Microbiol Infect Dis 2008;27:3–15.

220 Kaatz GW, Seo SM, Aeschlimann JR *et al.* Efficacy of LY333328 against experimental methicillin-resistant *Staphylococcus aureus* endocarditis. Antimicrob Agents Chemother 1998;42:981–3.

221 Poulakou G, Giamarellou H. Oritavancin: a new promising agent in the treatment of infections due to Gram-positive pathogens. Expert Opin Investig Drugs 2008;17:225–43.

222 Murphy CK, Karginova E, Sahm D *et al.* In vitro activity of novel rifamycins against Gram-positive clinical isolates. J Antibiot 2007;60:572–6.

223 Peppard WJ, Schuenke CD. Iclaprim, a diaminopyrimidine dihydrofolate reductase inhibitor for the potential treatment of antibiotic-resistant staphylococcal infections. Curr Opin Investig Drugs 2008;9:210–25.

224 Trampuz A, Murphy CK, Rothstein DM *et al.* Efficacy of a novel rifamycin derivative, ABI-0043, against *Staphylococcus aureus* in an experimental model of foreign-body infection. Antimicrob Agents Chemother 2007;51:2540–5.

225 Fritsche TR, Sader HS, Jones RN. Antimicrobial activity of ceftobiprole, a novel anti-methicillin-resistant *Staphylococcus aureus* cephalosporin, tested against contemporary pathogens: results from the SENTRY Antimicrobial Surveillance Program (2005–2006). Diagn Microbiol Infect Dis 2008;61:86–95.

226 John JF Jr. Drug evaluation. Tefibazumab: a monoclonal antibody against staphylococcal infection. Curr Opin Mol Ther 2006;8:455–60.

227 Balaban N, Cirioni O, Giacometti A *et al.* Treatment of *Staphylococcus aureus* biofilm infection by the quorum sensing inhibitor RIP. Antimicrob Agents Chemother 2007;51:2226–9.

228 Champney WS, Rodgers WK. Retapamulin inhibition of translation and 50S ribosomal subunit formation in *Staphylococcus aureus* cells. Antimicrob Agents Chemother 2007;51:3385–7.

229 Carson KC, Bartlett JG, Tan TJ *et al.* In vitro susceptibility of methicillin-resistant *Staphylococcus aureus* and methicillin-susceptible *Staphylococcus aureus* to a new antimicrobial, copper silicate. Antimicrob Agents Chemother 2007;51:4504–7.

230 Foster TJ. The *Staphylococcus aureus* "superbug". J Clin Invest 2004;114:1693–6.

Chapter 32
Vaccine-based Strategies for Prevention of *Staphylococcus aureus* Infection

Adam C. Schaffer and Jean C. Lee
Department of Medicine, Brigham and Women's Hospital and Harvard Medical School, Boston, Massachusetts, USA

Introduction

Staphylococcus aureus is an important bacterial pathogen that causes a variety of human infections, some of them life-threatening [1,2]. It is a well-established pathogen in the hospital, where it causes a variety of infections, especially in immunocompromised hosts, surgical patients, and those with indwelling medical devices. Methicillin-resistant *S. aureus* (MRSA) strains are responsible for 40–60% of nosocomial staphylococcal infections in the USA, and many of these isolates are multidrug resistant [2]. Under the influence of antibiotic pressure, *S. aureus* may cause outbreaks among patients in intensive care units [3] and nurseries [4].

The emergence of community-associated MRSA infections has heightened concern about this microbe [5–7] and has led to redoubled efforts among academic researchers and pharmaceutical companies to develop new treatment and prevention strategies. Although new antimicrobial agents are under investigation, there is little doubt that *S. aureus* will ultimately devise resistance mechanisms to circumvent the effectiveness of antibiotics [8]. Not only has resistance to methicillin among *S. aureus* isolates become markedly more common [2], but MRSA strains with reduced susceptibility to vancomycin have also been reported [9]. Furthermore, 9 MRSA clinical isolates that carry the *vanA* resistance gene and which are fully resistant to vancomycin have been isolated [10–12]. Because *S. aureus* cannot always be controlled by commonly used antibiotics and because MRSA isolates are becoming increasingly prevalent in the community, additional control strategies are sorely needed.

An *S. aureus* vaccine offers a mechanism to boost the immune system so that effector molecules are elicited by the host to contain and eradicate the infecting microbe. Because many of the individuals most susceptible to staphylococcal infections are the least competent to mount an effective immune response, passive as well as active immunization strategies must be explored. This chapter emphasizes accomplishments over the past 10 years, since numerous other reviews [13–16] have adequately summarized earlier work.

Is an effective *S. aureus* vaccine feasible?

Controversy has existed for years over the feasibility of designing and producing an *S. aureus* vaccine. Successful vaccine design relies on an understanding of how the pathogen relates to the host. Although our understanding of *S. aureus* pathogenesis has increased exponentially over the last 10 years, the protean clinical manifestations of staphylococcal infections still leave many gaps in our understanding of the interactions between the host and this versatile microbial pathogen. Importantly, little evidence supports the premise that immunity to *S. aureus* infection exists, at least for the unimmunized host. With the recent increase in community-associated staphylococcal infections, *S. aureus* is commonly isolated from skin and soft tissue infections of individuals without predisposing risk factors. Recovery from an *S. aureus* infection does not appear to confer immunity against subsequent infections. Does resistance to staphylococcal infection correlate with the presence of antibodies to specific staphylococcal antigens? Dryla *et al.* [17] reported that healthy individuals have higher antibody levels to *S. aureus* proteins than patients with staphylococcal infections. Although *S. aureus* nasal carriage is a risk factor for *S. aureus* infection [18,19], epidemiological evidence suggests that colonized hosts are less likely to die as a result of staphylococcal infection than individuals who are noncarriers [20]. This fact suggests that some degree of immunity induced by colonization protects *S. aureus* carriers from lethal infection. Our poor understanding of the relationship between protection and specific immune responses can be partially attributed to the limitations of rodent models of staphylococcal infection. In the absence of a foreign body, very large inocula

Staphylococci in Human Disease, 2nd edition. Edited by Kent B. Crossley, Kimberly K. Jefferson, Gordon Archer, Vance G. Fowler, Jr.
 ISBN 978-14051-6332-3.

Table 32.1 Target populations for an *S. aureus* vaccine.

Active immunization	Passive immunization
Hemodialysis patients	Patients undergoing emergency surgery
Residents of nursing homes and other long-term care facilities	Patients implanted with intravascular or prosthetic devices
Men who have sex with men	Trauma victims
Military personnel	Immunocompromised individuals
Prisoners	Low-birthweight neonates
Patients undergoing elective surgery	Patients in intensive care units
Diabetics	
Intravenous drug users	
Heathcare providers	
Athletes	
School children	

($> 10^6$ cfu) are needed to produce experimental infections in rats and mice. An understanding of the *in vitro* correlates that predict enhanced immunity to staphylococcal infections are sorely needed for rational vaccine design.

Bacteria are, in general, less likely to develop resistance to a vaccine than to an antibiotic. Although some microbes undergo antigenic variation to escape vaccine-induced immunity, this is not a trait that is characteristic of *S. aureus*. Instead, this organism produces a large array of molecules with redundant functions, such that if one is eliminated (or targeted by a vaccine), other staphylococcal products may compensate for that loss of function. Other challenges to vaccine development include the diverse strategies that *S. aureus* has developed to avoid human innate immunity [21], as well as its ability to persist in biofilms [22,23] and as small-colony variants [24,25].

Target populations

A crucial question that one faces in promoting a vaccine to prevent staphylococcal infections is who would constitute the target population for such a vaccine. There are certain groups, listed in Table 32.1, that are obvious candidates for vaccination against staphylococcal disease. Hemodialysis patients are at elevated risk for *S. aureus* infection because their vascular compartment is frequently accessed, they spend many hours a week in healthcare facilities, they have numerous comorbidities, and the uremia accompanying their renal failure itself may suppress the immune system [26]. Similarly, peritoneal dialysis patients, military personnel, soldiers, firefighters, police officers, and individuals undergoing elective major surgery are prime vaccine candidates. Other groups, such as healthcare providers, intravenous drug abusers, and men who have sex with men, might also benefit from an *S. aureus* vaccine.

Passive immunoprophylaxis against staphylococcal infections is indicated for persons who are unable to respond to active immunization because they are immunocompromised (Table 32.1). This group would include patients undergoing chemotherapy and patients with immune disorders. Likewise, passive immunotherapy would be appropriate for individuals who are at immediate risk of infection and for whom time constraints prohibit an active immunization approach. Patients undergoing emergency surgery and premature neonates are examples of populations that would benefit from passive immunotherapy. Among very-low-birthweight infants (< 1500 g), the rate of late-onset (> 3 days after birth) sepsis is approximately 20%, with the majority of cases caused by Gram-positive organisms, most commonly coagulase-negative staphylococci followed by *S. aureus* [27]. Factors predisposing these neonates to sepsis include hypogammaglobulinemia (given that transplacental transfer of maternal antibodies occurs after 32–35 weeks' gestation), an immature oxidative burst from neutrophils, and indwelling catheters [28,29]. The expense of making antibody preparations for passive immunotherapy requires that discussions of appropriate target populations consider cost–benefit analyses. However, the high costs of *S. aureus* infections [30,31] make it likely that there will be populations for whom the cost–benefit balance indicates that immunotherapy is more favorable than treatment with antibiotics alone.

Active immunization approaches in clinical trials (Table 32.2)

StaphVAX

Most *S. aureus* strains are encapsulated, and strains producing either capsular polysaccharide serotype 5 (CP5) or serotype 8 (CP8) (Figure 32.1) are the most prevalent among clinical isolates [32]. Capsular antigens were obvious targets for vaccine development, since capsule-based vaccines directed against other encapsulated bacterial pathogens have shown high success rates. Capsular polysaccharides from *Haemophilus influenzae* [33,34], *Neisseria meningitidis* [35,36], and *Streptococcus pneumoniae* [37,38] have been purified, conjugated to protein, and used as

Table 32.2 *Staphylococcus aureus* vaccines in clinical trials.

Product	Corporate sponsor	Composition	Status
Active immunization			
StaphVAX	Nabi	CP5 and CP8	Phase III failed
V710	Merck	IsdB	Phase II in progress
SA75	Vaccine Research International	Killed *S. aureus*	Phase I completed
Passive immunization			
INH-A21 (Veronate)	Inhibitex	ClfA (selected IVIG)	Phase III failed
Tefibazumab (Aurexis)	Inhibitex	ClfA (monoclonal antibody)	Phase II completed
AltaStaph	Nabi	CP5 and CP8	Phase II completed
Aurograb	NeuTec	ABC transporter	Phase III completed
Pagibaximab (BSYX-A110)	Biosynexus	Lipoteichoic acid	Phase II completed

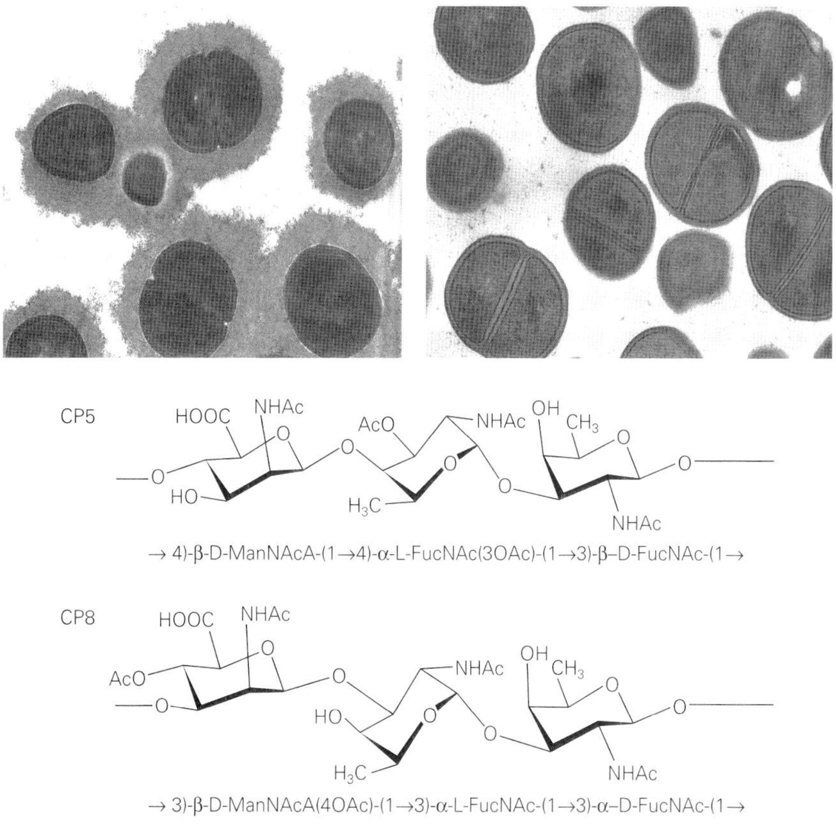

Figure 32.1 Transmission electron micrographs of stationary-phase *S. aureus* cells. Prior to fixation, the bacteria were incubated with CP5-specific antibodies to stabilize and visualize the capsule: (*left*) CP5-producing strain Reynolds; (*right*) acapsular *S. aureus* mutant. (*Bottom*) Structural composition of *S. aureus* CP5 and CP8. ManNAcA, 2-acetamido-2-deoxy-mannuronic acid; FucNAc, 2-acetamido-2,6-dideoxygalactose. (Adapted from O'Riordan & Lee [32] with permission.)

effective immunogens to elicit protective anticapsular antibodies.

Fattom *et al.* [39] were the first to conjugate CP5 and CP8 to protein (recombinant *Pseudomonas aeruginosa* exoprotein A or rEPA). The conjugate vaccines were highly immunogenic in mice and humans, and antibodies elicited by immunization opsonized encapsulated *S. aureus* for phagocytosis [39,40]. Passive immunization with antibodies to CP5 was protective in a mouse model of *S. aureus* lethality and disseminated infection [41]. Similarly, administration of antibodies to the *S. aureus* CP5 conjugate vaccine protected rats against infection in a catheter-induced model of staphylococcal endocarditis, if the animals were challenged by the intraperitoneal route [42].

Nabi Biopharmaceuticals combined the CP5 and CP8 conjugate vaccines into a bivalent vaccine called StaphVAX for immunization of humans at elevated risk for *S. aureus* infection. The vaccine was composed of *S. aureus* CP5 and CP8 (100 μg of each type) conjugated to an equal weight of rEPA. The phase III clinical trial of the vaccine, conducted between April 1998 and April 2000, enrolled 1804 end-stage renal disease patients on hemodialysis [43]. Subjects were randomized to receive either a single intramuscular injection of the vaccine or a placebo injection.

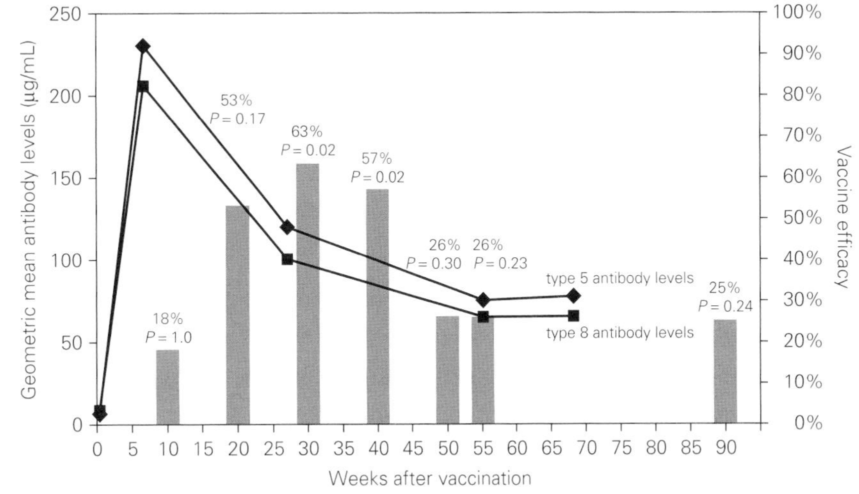

Figure 32.2 Results of Nabi's first phase III clinical trial of StaphVAX in hemodialysis patients. The graph depicts the temporal relationship between vaccine efficacy and serum antibody levels to CP5 and CP8. Vaccine efficacy was evaluated at weeks 10, 20, 30, 40, 50, 54, and 91. A significant reduction in bacteremia was observed between 3–40 weeks after immunization, but not at the later time points. The outcome of the second phase III trial of StaphVax did not confirm these results (unpublished data). (From Shinefield *et al.* [43] with permission.)

Randomization was stratified by type of vascular access (fistula or graft) and *S. aureus* nasal carriage status (carrier or noncarrier).

The primary hypothesis of the study was that the vaccine would prevent *S. aureus* bacteremia during the period from week 3 to week 54 after immunization. However, at week 54 the cumulative reduction in episodes of *S. aureus* bacteremia was only 26%, which was not statistically significant (Figure 32.2). When earlier time intervals were analyzed, the vaccine was found to significantly reduce the incidence of *S. aureus* bacteremia between weeks 3 and 40. During this period, *S. aureus* bacteremia occurred among 11 of 892 patients who received the vaccine, compared with 26 of 906 control patients. The reduction in the incidence of *S. aureus* bacteremia occurring up to 40 weeks after immunization was 57% ($P = 0.02$).

The study authors concluded that the mean antibody level necessary for protection was 80 μg/mL, an estimate based on the antibody levels found in study patients 40 weeks after immunization. This level of antibody response was achieved in approximately 75% of vaccine recipients. Levels of antibodies peaked 8 weeks after vaccination, at which time the geometric mean level of CP5 antibodies was 230 μg/mL and the geometric mean level of CP8 antibodies was 208 μg/mL; these levels fell to 78.1 and 65.8 μg/mL, respectively, by week 67 (Figure 32.2).

A confirmatory phase III clinical trial involved 3600 hemodialysis patients who were evaluated for bacteremia from 3 to 35 weeks after receipt of StaphVAX. Following a booster dose of StaphVAX, the patients were followed for an additional 6 months. Results from the second trial, announced in November 2005 (but not yet published), showed that StaphVAX offered no significant protection against bacteremia over the placebo control, and thus Nabi halted further development of StaphVAX (http://www.nabi.com/pipeline/clinicaltrials.php; accessed February 6, 2008). Although Nabi attributed the clinical failure of the vaccine to the immunocompromised status of the patients in the trial and a manufacturing problem in vaccine production, these data suggest that a conjugate vaccine that targets *S. aureus* CPs alone is insufficient to protect against staphylococcal bacteremia. Nabi has plans to develop a "next-generation" vaccine that will contain CP5, CP8, 336 antigen (wall teichoic acid), α-toxin, and Panton–Valentine leukocidin (PVL) (http://www.nabi. com/pipeline/pipeline.php?id=1, accessed February 29, 2008). However, the Nabi program is apparently on hold pending partnership or external funding.

Why, then, is a CP-conjugate vaccine protective against pathogens like *H. influenzae* type b and *Strep. pneumoniae*, but not *S. aureus*? Indeed, antibodies to CP5 and CP8 have been shown to opsonize *S. aureus* for phagocytic killing by human neutrophils [44]. However, differences become apparent when one considers experimental animal studies that have examined the effect of CP production on bacterial virulence. The CPs elaborated by *Strep. pneumoniae* and *H. influenzae* type b play critical roles in the virulence of these invasive pathogens, i.e., the bacteria are rendered avirulent in the absence of CP production. In contrast, *S. aureus* shows only a modest reduction in virulence in animal models of abscess formation, arthritis, wound infection, and bacteremia in the absence of CP expression [32]. Moreover, capsule-negative mutants are more virulent than the parental isolates in the catheter-induced endocarditis infection model [45]. Only 75–80% of *S. aureus* clinical isolates are encapsulated by CP5 or CP8; the remaining strains produce no CP due to mutations in the *cap5(8)* locus or in genes that regulate CP expression [46]. Importantly, serotype 5 and 8 *S. aureus* elaborate CPs *in vitro* only during the stationary growth phase; thus actively replicating staphylococci are acapsular [32,47].

Vaccine V710 (IsdB)

In an effort to identify *in vivo* expressed staphylococcal vaccine candidate antigens, Etz *et al.* [48] prepared *S. aureus* peptide expression libraries in *Escherichia coli.*

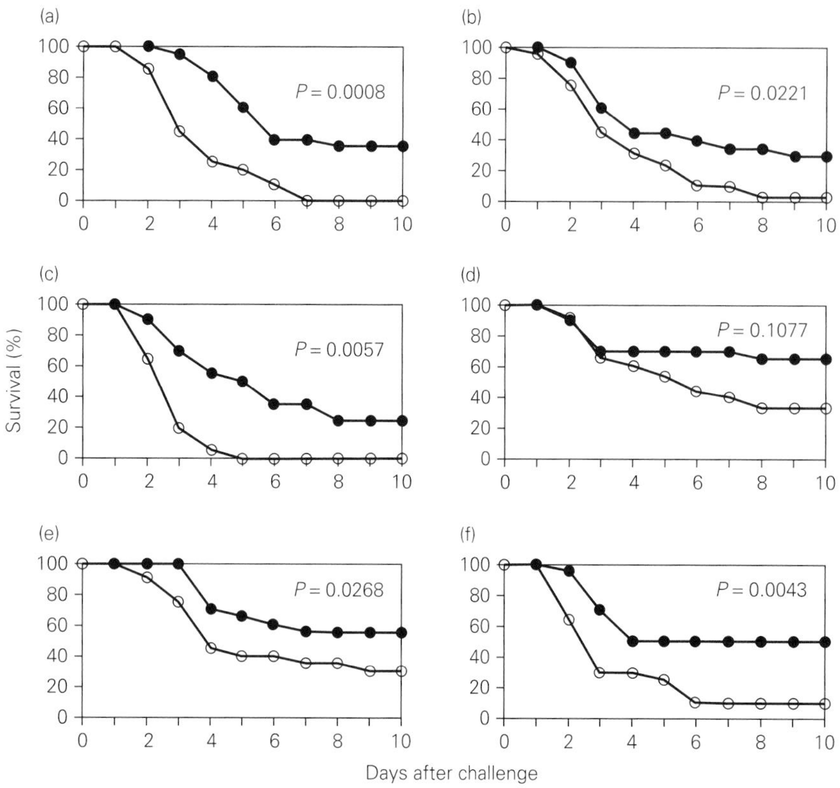

Figure 32.3 Survival of mice immunized with three doses of recombinant IsdB and challenged with diverse clinical isolates of *S. aureus*: (a) *S. aureus* ME60; (b) *S. aureus* MCL8538; (c) *S. aureus* ME27; (d) *S. aureus* ME31; (e) *S. aureus* ME11; (f) *S. aureus* Becker. Closed circles indicate survival of mice immunized with IsdB plus adjuvant; open circles indicate survival of mice immunized with adjuvant alone. (Adapted from Kuklin *et al.* [49] with permission.)

The recombinant polypeptides fused to *E. coli* surface proteins were then probed with sera from patients and sera from healthy donors with high levels of antibodies to *S. aureus*. The cell wall-anchored IsdB protein reacted with convalescent-phase serum from patients who recovered from *S. aureus* infections [49], and it has been targeted by Merck, Intercell, and Vaxgen as a candidate antigen for staphylococcal vaccine development. The iron-regulated IsdB protein was originally described and characterized by Mazmanian *et al.* [50]. IsdB, expressed only under conditions of limiting iron, binds to hemoglobin, and this interaction plays a role in the acquisition of heme iron by *S. aureus*. This surface-associated protein is conserved among diverse clinical isolates of *S. aureus*, and it was immunogenic in mice and rhesus monkeys. Compared with sham-immunized animals, mice immunized by the intramuscular route three times with 20 μg of recombinant IsdB showed improved survival following intravenous challenge with five of six clinical strains of *S. aureus* (Figure 32.3). Protection against lethality was not observed when the immunized animals were challenged with an IsdB mutant strain, which demonstrated the specificity of the protective response [49].

Merck's V710 vaccine (previously designated 0657nl) completed phase I testing and is currently being tested in a phase II clinical trial. The first trial is designed to assess the efficacy, immunogencity, and safety of a single preoperative dose of V710 for the prevention of serious *S. aureus* infection in 8044 patients undergoing cardiothoracic surgery involving a median sternotomy (http://clinicaltrials.gov/ct2/show/NCT00518687; accessed February 28, 2008). A second phase II trial will evaluate the safety and immunogenicity of the V710 vaccine in 198 patients with end-stage renal disease on chronic hemodialysis (http://www.clinicaltrials.gov/ct2/show/NCT00572910, accessed February 28, 2008).

Vaccine SA75

Vaccine Research International (UK) has conducted a phase I clinical trial of its chloroform-inactivated *S. aureus* vaccine [51]. A double-blind placebo-controlled phase I clinical trial was conducted in 2005 to test safety and immunogenicity of the vaccine. Three dosage groups (0.15–0.45 mg/dose) of 16 males were evaluated, wherein 12 subjects received vaccine (four immunizations given at 2-week intervals) and 4 subjects received placebo in each group. Significant adverse reactions were observed only at the high vaccine dose. The majority of the vaccinees produced antibodies to the homologous bacterium and to collagen-binding protein. However, there were minimal antibody responses to clumping factor (Clf)A, fibronectin-binding protein, or the *S. aureus* extracellular adherence protein. The company hopes to embark on additional clinical trials aimed at proving efficacy of the vaccine in preventing staphylococcal infections among vulnerable patient groups (http://www.vri.org.uk, http://www.vri.org.uk/PhaseITrial.pdf; accessed February 28, 2008).

Passive immunization approaches in clinical trials (Table 32.2)

Staphylococcus aureus ClfA-based products

Staphylococcus aureus adheres to host molecules such as fibrinogen, fibronectin, collagen, and IgG through surface protein adhesins, also referred to as microbial surface components recognizing adhesive matrix molecules (MSCRAMMs) [52,53]. ClfA is an adhesin that mediates *S. aureus* binding to fibrinogen [54] and promotes the attachment of *S. aureus* to biomaterial surfaces [55], blood clots [56], and damaged endothelial surfaces [56]. The fibrinogen-binding domain of ClfA is located within region A of the full-length protein [57]. ClfA plays an important role in *S. aureus* binding to platelets, an interaction that is critical in animal models of catheter-induced staphylococcal endocarditis [58].

Preclinical studies by scientists at Inhibitex revealed that mice immunized with a recombinant form of the binding region A of ClfA showed reductions in arthritis and lethality induced by *S. aureus*, but protection was strain-dependent [59]. Passive immunization experiments were performed in rabbits given a human polyclonal immunoglobulin preparation that contained elevated levels of antibodies specific for ClfA [60]. In rabbits with catheter-induced *S. aureus* endocarditis, the combination therapy resulted in better bacterial clearance from the blood than that induced by vancomycin. However, the bacterial burdens in the kidneys and endocardial vegetations of the infected animals were not significantly reduced.

A related Inhibitex product, INH-A21 (Veronate), is a pooled human immunoglobulin preparation from donors selected for high antibody titers against staphylococcal adhesins that bind fibrinogen and fibrin (*S. aureus* ClfA and *S. epidermidis* SdrG). This product, at a dose of 1000 mg/kg, protected neonatal rats from *S. epidermidis* infection compared with normal IgG for intravenous injection (IVIG). Protection studies in suckling rats challenged with *S. aureus* were not reported. However, pretreatment of rabbits with INH-A21 significantly deceased the infection rates of both *S. aureus* and *S. epidermidis* in a catheter-induced endocarditis infection model [61].

A human trial enrolling 512 subjects conducted from 2002 to 2003 studied escalating doses of INH-A21 in infants 3–7 days old with birthweights between 500 and 1250 g [62]. Subjects received four infusions of placebo or 250, 500, or 750 mg/kg of INH-A21. The rate of *S. aureus* infections in the highest-dose INH-A21 group (2.5%) was lower than the rate of *S. aureus* infections in the placebo group (7.0%), but this decrease did not achieve statistical significance ($P = 0.14$). The infants who received up to four doses of INH-A21 (750 mg/kg) also showed trends toward fewer episodes of candidemia and lower mortality than the placebo-treated cohort.

These findings prompted a phase III, double-blind, placebo-controlled study of INH-A21 in 1983 infants who received either placebo or INH-A21 750 mg/kg [63]. The primary outcome measure was the rate of late-onset sepsis caused by *S. aureus*, and in this measure there was no significant difference between the 6% rate in the INH-A21 group and the 5% rate in the placebo group ($P = 0.34$) (Table 32.3). Similarly, there were no differences between the two groups in mortality or in the rates of late-onset sepsis caused by coagulase-negative staphylococci or *Candida* species. This failure of INH-A21 is striking since the outcome of the infants who were given INH-A21 was compared with that of infants who received placebo rather than an IVIG preparation lacking elevated levels of antibodies to ClfA and SdrG. The results were particularly disappointing since, in effect, the INH-A21 product, although selected for its antibodies to ClfA and SdrG, likely contained antibodies to many other staphylococcal antigens. Thus, the product could loosely be considered a "multi-component" passive immunotherapy. However, the INH-A21 product was not elicited by immunization but by natural exposure to staphylococci, and so the antibodies might have recognized the wrong ClfA epitopes or may have been of low affinity or avidity toward their target antigens. Moreover, low-birthweight premature neonates may require additional immune stimulators, such as cytokines (e.g., G-CSF or GM-CSF) to boost neutrophil function [64,65], as well as effective antibiotics and antibodies to staphylococcal antigens, in order to fend off staphylococcal infections.

Table 32.3 Incidence of late-onset bloodstream infection in premature infants infused with placebo or INH-A21. (Data adapted from DeJonge *et al.* [63] with permission.)

Outcome	Placebo no. of patients (%)	INH-A21 no. of patients (%)
S. aureus	50 (5%)	60 (6%)
Coagulase-negative staphylococci	227 (23%)	247 (25%)
Candida spp.	30 (3%)	33 (3%)
Mortality	73 (7%)	57 (6%)

Another Inhibitex product in the pipeline is the murine monoclonal antibody 12-9 that binds ClfA and inhibits fibrinogen binding to ClfA. In preclinical studies, 12-9 given by the intraperitoneal route protected mice in a lethal sepsis model [66]. A humanized version of 12-9, known as tefibazumab (Aurexis), was produced by Inhibitex. In a rabbit model of endocarditis, two doses of tefibazumab (30 mg/kg) in combination with vancomycin resulted in fewer animals with bacteremia and significantly fewer bacteria in the spleens and kidneys than in animals given vancomycin alone [67].

A phase II study of tefibazumab enrolled hospitalized patients with documented *S. aureus* bacteremia [68]. Subjects were randomized to receive either a single tefibazumab dose of 20 mg/kg plus standard therapy, or standard therapy alone. To evaluate efficacy, a composite clinical end point was used that consisted of relapse of *S. aureus* bacteremia, a complication related to *S. aureus* bacteremia (such as endocarditis), or death. In the tefibazumab group, 2 of 30 patients (6.7%) reached the composite clinical end point compared with 4 of 30 (13.3%) in the placebo group ($P = 0.455$). Although preliminary clinical trials of tefibazumab in hemodialysis patients [69] and cystic fibrosis patients have been performed, Inhibitex is seeking a partner to support further efforts before proceeding with additional clinical trials to address the dosing range and efficacy of tefibazumab.

AltaStaph

AltaStaph, produced by Nabi, is a hyperimmune polyclonal antibody preparation derived from healthy volunteers immunized with the bivalent StaphVAX preparation. The product contains high levels of vaccine-induced antibodies to *S. aureus* CP5 and CP8 and is intended for intravenous administration. In a phase II study designed primarily to assess the safety of AltaStaph, 206 neonates, weighing 500–1500 g, were given an initial 1000 mg/kg dose of AltaStaph or placebo [28]. A second dose was given 14 days later. No significant difference was seen in the rate of adverse events between the two arms. Though not specifically powered to look for differences in the rates of *S. aureus* bacteremia, this was a secondary end point of the study, and the rates of *S. aureus* bacteremia were nearly identical in both groups (about 3%).

Another phase II trial looking at AltaStaph enrolled patients with documented *S. aureus* bacteremia, as well as persistent fever [70]. Five of 21 patients (24%) who received AltaStaph died, compared with 2 of 18 patients (11%) in the placebo group ($P = 0.42$). There was a trend toward quicker resolution of fever and a shorter length of hospital stay in the AltaStaph group. Nonetheless, these results provide additional support for the premise that vaccine-induced antibodies to CP5 and CP8 are insufficient to significantly reduce *S. aureus* bacteremia in at-risk populations.

Aurograb

NeuTec Pharma has identified an *S. aureus* ATP-binding cassette (ABC) transporter as a novel target for passive immunization therapies against staphylococcal infection [71]. This 61-kDa protein was reported to elicit an antibody response in patients who recovered from septicemia and wound infections caused by an epidemic MRSA strain [72]. A significant correlation was reported between patient survival and serum IgG reactive with this immunodominant protein. Epitope mapping of a recombinant form of the protein identified peptides that reacted with sera from patients infected with *S. aureus*. The peptides were synthesized and used to isolate recombinant human antibodies from a phage antibody display library. Hyperimmune rabbit serum or recombinant antibodies reactive with certain epitopes of the ABC transporter were used to treat mice that had been challenged intravenously with 2×0^7 cfu of the epidemic MRSA strain. Treated animals showed an approximately 1-log lower bacterial burden recovered from the liver, kidney, and spleen after 24–48 hours compared with control mice. Based on these findings, NeuTec developed Aurograb, which is a single-chain variable antibody fragment against the *S. aureus* ABC transporter. In June 2006 the company completed a double-blind, placebo-controlled, phase III clinical trial (http://clinicaltrial.gov/ct2/show/NCT00217841; accessed February 10, 2008). The study was performed in six European countries and involved the recruitment of 161 adult hospitalized patients with deep-seated staphylococcal infections. The trial compared the effects of Aurograb (1 mg/kg i.v. twice daily) in combination with vancomycin versus vancomycin alone in the treatment of MRSA infections. The results of this trial have not been released, and in July 2006 NeuTec Pharma was taken over by Novartis but Novartis stopped development of Aurograb in 2008 after phase II clinical data showed lack of efficacy.

Pagibaximab

Lipoteichoic acid (LTA) is a plasma membrane-embedded glycolipid unique to Gram-positive bacteria [73]. Like its Gram-negative counterpart, lipopolysaccharide, purified LTA has immunostimulatory activity [74–76]. Biosynexus has developed a humanized mouse chimeric monoclonal antibody against LTA called pagibaximab (also known as BSYX-A110). The antibody is targeted at low-birthweight infants for the prevention of bloodstream infections by *S. aureus* and coagulase-negative staphylococci, the latter being the leading cause of bloodstream infections among premature neonates [27]. After a successful safety and pharmacokinetic phase I trial, the company embarked on a phase I/II clinical trial in which 55 low-birthweight neonates (≤ 1300 g) were randomized to receive two doses (10, 30, 60, or 90 mg/kg) of pagibaximab or placebo on days 0 and 14. The product was deemed safe and tolerable, although the clinical data indicated that more frequent administration of the highest dose should be pursued in future studies (77). Biosynexus is currently recruiting participants for a phase IIb/III trial to evaluate the safety and efficacy of pagibaximab in 1550 very low birth weight neonates for the prevention of staphylococcal sepsis.

Preclinical development

Surface-associated *S. aureus* antigens

Poly-*N*-acetylglucosamine

Poly-*N*-acetylglucosamine (PNAG), also known as polysaccharide intercellular adhesin [78], is a surface polymer produced by both *S. aureus* and *S. epidermidis*. PNAG promotes biofilm formation [79] and enhances staphylococcal virulence in mouse infection models [80]. PNAG is the product of the *icaADBC* genes of the intercellular adhesin (*ica*) locus in *S. epidermidis* [81] and *S. aureus* [79]. Consistent with the observation that the native form of PNAG is partially de-N-acetylated, the product of the *icaB* gene is an extracellular *N*-deacetylase that removes N-linked acetate groups from the PNAG polymer [82]. An *icaB* mutant produces only the fully acetylated PNAG, and this form of the antigen is not retained on the staphylococcal cell surface [80,82]. Kelly-Quintos *et al.* [83] postulated that antibodies to a deacetylated (backbone) form of PNAG (dPNAG) and the native acetylated form of PNAG might elicit functionally distinct antibodies. In fact, they demonstrated that only antibodies to dPNAG were opsonic, i.e., mediated antibody-dependent opsonophagocytic killing of *S. aureus* by human neutrophils. In a follow-up study, the investigators immunized mice, rabbits, and goats with either native PNAG or dPNAG conjugated to diphtheria toxoid [84]. Mice were passively immunized intraperitoneally with immune or nonimmune serum and challenged intravenously with *S. aureus* 48 hours later. Quantitative blood cultures performed 2 hours after bacterial challenge revealed that mice given dPNAG antibodies had 54–91% fewer *S. aureus* in their blood than mice given normal rabbit serum. Antibodies to the native (acetylated) PNAG conjugate were ineffective in clearing the bacteremia in mice.

These data indicate that antibodies to dPNAG (but not native PNAG) are opsonic and provide significant protection against experimental *S. aureus* infections in mice. Because dPNAG is preferentially retained on the bacterial cell surface, antibodies to dPNAG may be more effective in achieving protection than PNAG antibodies [80]. Moreover, in human sera, levels of antibodies to dPNAG correlated with levels of *in vitro* opsonophagocytic killing [83].

Collagen-binding protein/fibronectin-binding protein fusion protein

A review of the recent literature revealed few reports of multicomponent vaccine approaches against *S. aureus*. Zhou *et al.* [85] engineered a collagen-binding protein (Cna)–fibronectin-binding protein (Fnb) fusion protein by combining the genes for these two *S. aureus* adhesins and expressing them in *E. coli*. Mice were immunized three times over a 28-day interval with phosphate-buffered saline (PBS), Cna, Fnb, or the Cna–Fnb fusion protein, and then they were challenged intraperitoneally with 5×10^7 cfu of *S. aureus* in 5% hog mucin. Although 75% of the mice given the fusion protein survived compared with 17% of the animals given PBS, immunization with the Cna–Fnb fusion protein did not prove superior to immunization with either Cna or Fnb alone.

Multicomponent *S. aureus* adhesin vaccine

An elegant study by Stranger-Jones *et al.* [86] systematically evaluated 19 cell wall-anchored *S. aureus* protein adhesins for their vaccine potential in mice. The animals were immunized twice via the intramuscular route with 100 μg of each protein with adjuvant. The mice were challenged retroorbitally on day 21 with *S. aureus* Newman, and the bacterial burden in the kidneys was evaluated 4 days later. The authors identified four antigens (SdrE, IsdA, SdrD, and IsdB) that were conserved among *S. aureus* isolates and showed the best protection in the renal infection model. IsdB was previously identified by Merck scientists as a protective staphylococcal antigen [49]. IsdA, a heme-binding surface protein, is also involved in heme iron uptake [87]. SdrD and SdrE are surface proteins that are structurally similar to ClfA, but their molecular functions remain unknown.

Rabbit antiserum raised to each of the proteins (together with rabbit complement) was opsonic in an *in vitro* opsonophagocytic killing assay against a protein A-negative mutant of *S. aureus* Newman. The opsonic activity of rabbit complement in the absence of antibodies was not reported. A mixture of antibodies to the four recombinant proteins showed higher opsonic activity than any of the individual sera. Animals immunized with the combination of all four surface components and then challenged intraperitoneally with 2×10^{10} cfu of strain Newman had 100% survival at 7 days (Figure 32.4). In comparison, animals immunized with either PBS or one of the individual components had survival rates of 50–70%. Immunization with the multivalent vaccine significantly reduced *S. aureus*-induced mortality in mice compared with PBS for four of five *S. aureus* clinical isolates [86].

Heteropolymers

A novel heteropolymer technology is being developed by Elusys Therapeutics to combat *S. aureus* bacteremias. The product (ETI-211) consists of a monoclonal antibody to *S. aureus* protein A linked to another monoclonal antibody directed against the human complement receptor 1 (CR1) [88,89]. The concept promoted by Elusys is that blood-borne *S. aureus*, bridged by the bispecific monoclonal

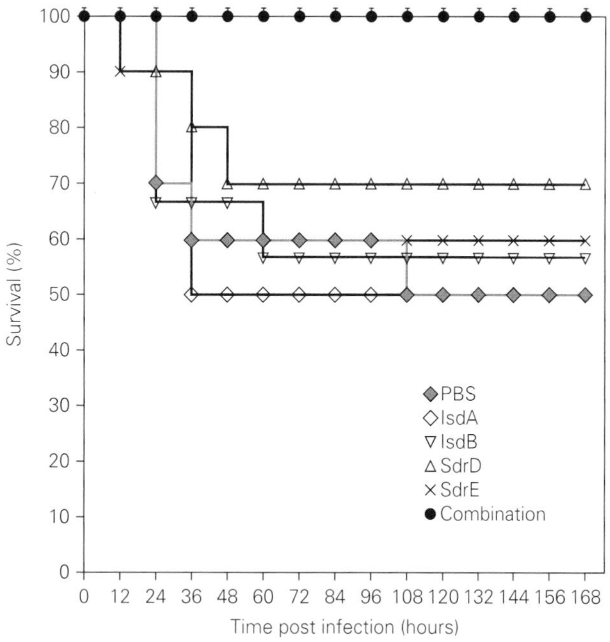

Figure 32.4 Mice immunized with a combination protein adhesin vaccine survived challenge with an intraperitoneal lethal dose of *S. aureus* Newman. Animals immunized with individual surface-protein antigens (IsdA, IsdB, SdrD, or SdrE) or with PBS showed survival rates of 50–70%. (Data from Stranger-Jones *et al.* [86] with permission.)

antibody complex, binds to CR1 on erythrocytes, and that this complex is taken up and destroyed by tissue macrophages in the liver and spleen [88–90]. Preclinical studies to demonstrate efficacy utilized transgenic mice expressing human CR1 on red blood cells. Mice pretreated with the heteropolymers survived a lethal *S. aureus* challenge dose, in contrast to mice pretreated with the protein A monoclonal antibody alone. Therapeutic administration of the heteropolymer to infected mice resulted in more efficient clearance of bacteria from the liver, kidneys, and spleen than in control mice given PBS. Preliminary data suggest that mice treated with the heteropolymer develop protective immunity against subsequent challenge with *S. aureus*, implying that the heteropolymer has adjuvant-like properties. Elusys now has a research and license agreement with Pfizer to evaluate heteropolymers targeting *S. aureus*, and so the research community awaits publication of further research and clinical trials. Questions about the specificity of the response and whether the adjuvant effects of the heteropolymer persist after the innate immune response wanes will need to be resolved.

Extracellular fibrinogen-binding protein

Extracellular fibrinogen-binding protein (Efb), a secreted staphylococcal protein thought to contribute to virulence in a rat wound infection model [91], has been investigated for its potential as a vaccine target [92]. Mice were immunized four times via the subcutaneous route with 10 μg Efb or PBS in adjuvant. The animals were challenged by application of 10^2 cfu of *S. aureus* Newman to a small piece of cotton inserted into a neck incision. Clinical signs of wound infection 10 days after bacterial inoculation were scored by a blinded investigator as mild or severe. The proportion of mice with severe infections was higher among the control mice (73%) than among mice given Efb (17%), but there was no difference in weight loss in the infected mice or the bacterial burden recovered from the wounded tissue.

Exotoxin vaccines

α-Hemolysin

α-Hemolysin (also known as α-toxin) is a secreted *S. aureus* protein that can cause pore formation within eukaryotic cells [93] and interfere with *S. aureus* adhesion to epithelial cells [94]. Adlam *et al.* [95] first reported that immunization with a toxoid prepared from α-toxin-protected rabbits against the lethal gangrenous form of *S. aureus* mastitis but did not prevent abscess formation. Similarly, in an experimental model of *S. aureus* keratitis, rabbits actively immunized with an α-hemolysin toxoid showed less corneal pathology and epithelial erosion than rabbits immunized with adjuvant alone [96]. However, there was no difference in the number of bacteria recovered from the infected corneas of immunized or control rabbits. Menzies and Kernodle [97] created a nontoxic and nonhemolytic α-hemolysin mutant toxin (H35L) by site-directed mutagenesis. Passive immunization with rabbit anti-H35L serum protected mice from lethal challenge with native α-hemolysin and against acute lethal challenge with a high-α-hemolysin-producing *S. aureus* strain.

In a recent study, the severity of staphylococcal lung infection in mice was shown to correlate with the levels of α-hemolysin produced by different *S. aureus* isolates [98]. α-Hemolysin is critical in the pathogenesis of community-associated MRSA pneumonia caused by USA300 strains [99]. Wardenburg and Schneewind [98] used the H35L α-hemolysin mutant protein to immunize mice and evaluate protection against *S. aureus* in a murine pneumonia model. Mice immunized with the H35L protein and then challenged intranasally with *S. aureus* showed significantly less lethality attributable to three different *S. aureus* isolates than animals immunized with PBS (Figure 32.5). Vaccine-induced protection correlated with reduced inflammation and destruction of lung tissue, as well as an approximately 1-log decrease in bacterial counts in the lung tissue of infected animals. Similarly, in passive immunization experiments, antibodies to the H35L protein administered intraperitoneally protected mice against lethality after intranasal challenge with either methicillin-resistant or -sensitive *S. aureus* strains. Mice given antibodies to α-hemolysin showed an approximately 1-log

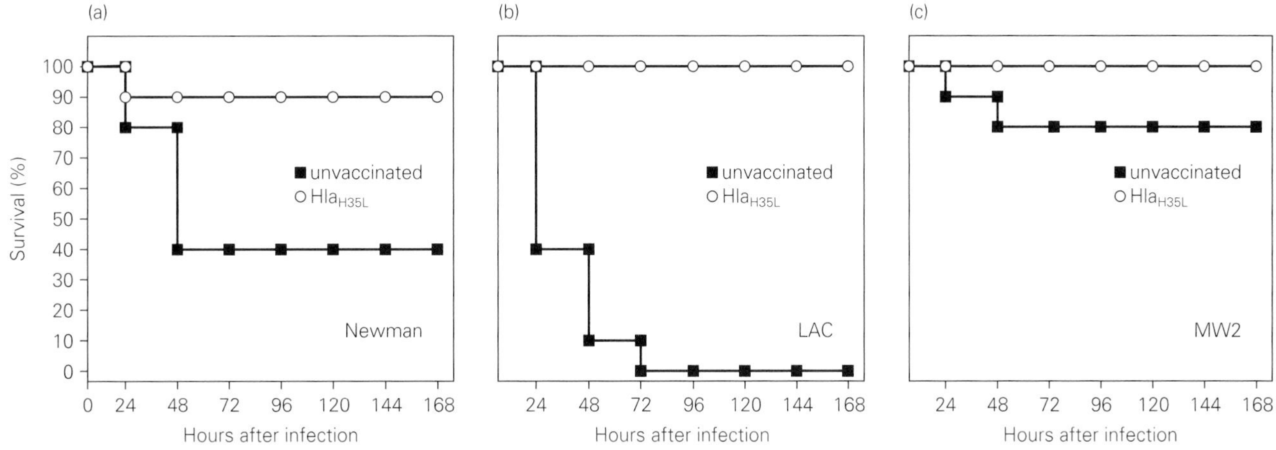

Figure 32.5 Survival curves of mice immunized with α-hemolysin H35L compared with unimmunized mice. The animals were challenged intranasally with *S. aureus* strain Newman (a), LAC (b), or MW2 (c). Survival in the control mice showed an inverse correlation with the amount of α-hemolysin produced by each strain. (Data from Wardenburg & Schneewind [98] with permission.)

decrease in *S. aureus* counts in the lungs compared with control mice given normal rabbit serum. Antibodies to α-hemolysin clearly play a role in neutralizing the lethal effects induced by this toxin; their efficacy in modulating other types of staphylococcal infections remains to be determined.

Superantigens

Staphylococcus aureus can secrete a wide variety of superantigen exoproteins, including toxic shock syndrome toxin (TSST)-1 and approximately 15 different enterotoxins. The genes encoding the superantigens are carried on mobile genetic elements, such as bacteriophages and pathogenicity islands; thus, clinical isolates vary markedly in their production of these proteins. Superantigens act as potent oligoclonal T-cell activators, stimulating massive release of proinflammatory cytokines [100,101]. Aerosol exposure of nonhuman primates to staphylococcal enterotoxin B (SEB) results in gastrointestinal symptoms, lethargy, shock, and death. Early studies, reviewed previously [13], indicate that mutant forms of the superantigenic proteins that are devoid of their biological properties can be used as vaccines to elicit antibodies that neutralize the native toxin molecules. Importantly, when monkeys were actively immunized with a proteasome-SEB toxoid vaccine, all the animals were protected against severe symptoms and death due to aerosolized SEB intoxication [102]. Passive immunization with antibodies to SEB before or 4 hours after aerosol exposure to SEB provided similar protection to rhesus monkeys [103]. Likewise, rabbits immunized with nontoxic recombinant TSST-1 were protected against death induced by lethal doses of native TSST-1 administered with lipopolysaccharide [104]. Nontoxic derivatives of the staphylococcal superantigens may be useful vaccine candidates for either active or passive protection strategies against toxic shock syndrome or against the potential use of aerosolized superantigens in biological warfare.

Several recent reports have claimed that immunization with site-directed mutants of TSST-1 or staphylococcal enterotoxins can protect mice against *S. aureus*-induced lethality or infection [105–109]. Mice were immunized via the subcutaneous or intranasal route with 10–20 μg of the mutant toxins mixed with adjuvant or adjuvant alone. Following intravenous challenge with about 5×10^7 cfu of a superantigen-producing *S. aureus* strain, there was greater survival of the toxoid-vaccinated mice than control mice. Some of the reports demonstrated that active immunization reduced the numbers of staphylococci in the spleens and livers of vaccinated mice by approximately 1-log cfu [105,106,108,109]. A specificity control lacking in all the infection studies was the inclusion of an experiment wherein the immunized animals were inoculated with an *S. aureus* strain lacking the targeted superantigen.

Antibodies to block *S. aureus* virulence

To circumvent *S. aureus* multiple-antibiotic resistance, some investigators have proposed targeting bacterial virulence rather than genes essential for bacterial viability. Such a strategy could debilitate the microbe so that the host immune system could more easily eradicate it. The major global regulator of virulence in *S. aureus* is the accessory gene regulator (*agr*), which modulates bacterial physiology and virulence factor expression through quorum sensing mediated by the secretion of small cyclic autoinducing peptides (AIPs) [110,111]. Strains of *S. aureus* can be classified into four *agr* groups, depending on the amino acid

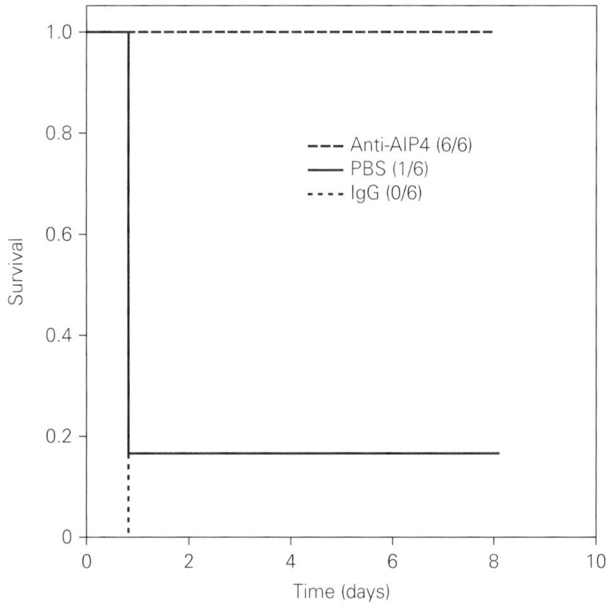

Figure 32.6 Mice passively immunized intraperitoneally with 1 mg of a monoclonal antibody to AIP-4 survived a lethal intraperitoneal inoculum of *S. aureus* RN4850, whereas mice given PBS or an isotype-matched monoclonal antibody succumbed to the infection. (Data from Park *et al.* [112] with permission.)

sequence of the exported AIP, and AIPs from the different groups inhibit *agr* expression by members of the heterologous groups. A recent elegant study by Park *et al.* [112] described the preparation of a monoclonal antibody to AIP-4 that inhibits *agr* function, i.e., the monoclonal antibody reduced the expression of RNAIII (the effector molecule of the *agr* locus) and α-toxin, and it increased protein A expression and biofilm formation in an AIP subgroup-specific manner. The monoclonal antibody to AIP-4 did not affect bacterial growth *in vitro*. Importantly, mice passively immunized intaperitoneally with 1 mg of the AIP-4 monoclonal antibody were protected from a lethal dose of *S. aureus* administered by the intraperitoneal route; mice given an isotype-matched monoclonal antibody were not protected (Figure 32.6). Likewise, mice challenged with *S. aureus* mixed with cytodex beads and 0.6 mg of the AIP-4 monoclonal antibody (but not the control monoclonal antibody) were protected from subcutaneous abscess formation.

Whether disruption of quorum-sensing signaling will be beneficial against other *S. aureus* strains and other AIP groups will likely be addressed in future studies. Since *agr* negatively regulates staphylococcal biofilm formation and the production of many surface adhesins, it is questionable whether antibodies to AIPs will be beneficial against all manifestations of *S. aureus* disease. For example, inhibition of *agr* might enhance staphylococcal infections that are initiated by adherence to traumatized tissue or prosthetic devices and promote chronic infection. Nonetheless, this conceptual approach of targeting *S. aureus* virulence factors is intriguing and has potential to aid in the control of acute infections caused by multidrug-resistant staphylococcal strains.

DNA vaccines

DNA vaccination is an approach whereby a mammalian expression vector carrying one or more genes encoding vaccine antigens is administered to a host, usually via the intramuscular route. Gene expression within the muscle cells of the host results in an immune response to the expressed antigen [113,114]. DNA vaccines stimulate both a T-cell response and a serum antibody response in mice, and they typically induce a higher proportion of the mouse IgG2a isotype, which enhances the opsonic antibody titer in the immunized host, than of IgG1. One of the earliest approaches to an *S. aureus* DNA vaccine utilized a plasmid encoding the fibrinogen-binding region A of ClfA [115]. In this study, the authors vaccinated mice intramuscularly with 100 μg of the ClfA plasmid or the empty expression plasmid at 3-week intervals for a total of three immunizations. Animals injected with the ClfA plasmid produced an elevated ClfA antibody response, and serum from the immunized mice inhibited *S. aureus* binding *in vitro* to immobilized fibrinogen. Nonetheless, the ClfA DNA vaccine afforded no protection over the vector control when the immunized mice were challenged intraperitoneally with *S. aureus*; the bacterial burden in the liver, kidneys, and peritoneal washings was similar in both groups. Analogous (negative) results were obtained when the same group vaccinated mice with a recombinant plasmid encoding Cna [116]. Actively immunized mice showed high titers of antibodies to Cna, but they showed no protection against staphylococcal infection. Moreover, mice challenged with *S. aureus* that were pre-opsonized with Cna antiserum from vaccinated mice actually had a higher *S. aureus* burden in the kidneys and livers than mice challenged with *S. aureus* pre-opsonized with normal serum.

In an effort to develop a multigene DNA vaccine against *S. aureus*, Gaudreau *et al.* [117] engineered a plasmid that expressed a single fusion polyprotein that contained ClfA, fibronectin-binding protein A, and sortase A. Fibronectin-binding protein A is a cell wall-anchored protein adhesin that allows *S. aureus* to bind to and invade eukaryotic cells, and sortase is an enzyme involved in covalently linking 19 different surface proteins of *S. aureus* to the bacterial cell wall [118]. The combined DNA vaccine effectively elicited an antibody response to each of the component antigens, and the antiserum partially blocked *S. aureus* binding to fibrinogen but not fibronectin. Compared with mice given the vector alone, mice immunized with the multigene DNA vaccine showed enhanced survival 21 days after intravenous challenge with *S. aureus* (55% vs. 15%). Whether this protection was greater than that afforded by the individual antigens is an important question that was not addressed in this study. Moreover, the multigene DNA vaccine provided no protection against arthritis. Because of its documented role in arthritis, inclusion of the *cna* gene may have enhanced the protective efficacy of a multigene vaccine against septic arthritis.

In an attempt to target MRSA specifically, two different groups have prepared DNA vaccines based on the *S. aureus mecA* gene, which encodes the altered penicillin-binding protein PBP2a that confers resistance to methicillin and other β-lactam antibiotics. In the first study [119], immunization with a *mecA* plasmid resulted in an antibody response to PBP2a that promoted the uptake of *S. aureus* by mouse peritoneal macrophages. However, when immunized mice were challenged intravenously with MRSA, the animals immunized with the *mecA*-expressing plasmid showed only a 0.32-log reduction in *S. aureus* numbers recovered from the kidneys, compared with animals immunized with the vector alone. In the second study, mice were immunized with a plasmid containing an internal fragment (transpeptidase domain) of the *mecA* gene or the vector alone [120]. The mice were challenged with a sublethal dose of MRSA administered intraperitoneally. Mice immunized with *mecA* had fewer *S. aureus* in their kidneys than mice given the vector alone. One clinical application of this approach would be to generate anti-PBP2a antibodies that could be used for passive immunization of hosts infected with multidrug-resistant MRSA strains [121].

Vaccine to prevent nasal colonization

The primary niche for *S. aureus* in humans is the nares, and nasal carriage is a documented risk factor for staphylococcal infection [18,19]. The source of about 80% of *S. aureus* bacteremias is endogenous since infecting bacteria have been shown by genotypic analysis to be identical to organisms recovered from the nasal mucosa [20,122]. These observations support an approach in which systemic *S. aureus* infections are prevented by eliminating or reducing nasal carriage. Although topical treatment with mupirocin is usually effective in decolonizing nasal carriers [123], the emergence of mupirocin resistance in *S. aureus* potentially limits the effectiveness of this approach [124]. Moreover, recolonization of mupirocin-sensitive strains often occurs from extranasal carriage sites. A mouse model of nasal colonization was used to demonstrate that *S. aureus* mutants that lack ClfA, Cna, fibronectin-binding proteins A and B, PNAG, or the accessory gene regulator colonized as well as wild-type strains [125]. In contrast, mutants deficient in sortase A or ClfB showed reduced nasal colonization. Mice immunized intranasally with killed *S. aureus* cells showed less nasal colonization than control animals. Likewise, mice that were immunized systemically or intranasally with a recombinant vaccine composed of domain A of ClfB demonstrated lower levels of colonization than control animals. A ClfB monoclonal antibody inhibited *S. aureus* binding to mouse cytokeratin 10. Passive immunization of mice with the monoclonal antibody resulted in less nasal colonization than with an isotype-matched control antibody.

Clarke *et al.* [126] took a different approach to development of a vaccine to eradicate nasal colonization by probing *S. aureus* expression libraries with sera from infected and uninfected patients to identify immunogenic proteins. Eleven proteins identified in their screen were further investigated by measuring antibodies reactive with the recombinant proteins in serum from healthy individuals (*S. aureus* nasal carriers and noncarriers), as well as patient serum. Antibodies to IsdA and IsdH were higher among noncarriers, and so the investigators immunized cotton rats with the recombinant proteins. The animals responded with high serum antibody titers to the proteins. Rats immunized with IsdA or IsdH and inoculated with *S. aureus* showed less nasal colonization than control rats.

Another antigen that merits investigation as an *S. aureus* vaccine component to prevent nasal colonization is wall teichoic acid. These ribitol phosphate polymers are produced by all *S. aureus* strains and are critical for nasal colonization [127], biofilm formation [128], and staphylococcal adherence to human endothelial cells under high-flow conditions [129].

The feasibility of reducing nasal colonization is based on clinical studies that have documented decreased nasopharyngeal carriage of *H. influenzae* and *Strep. pneumoniae* vaccine serotypes following immunization with relevant capsule conjugate vaccines [130–133]. Secretory IgA responses are best achieved by mucosal immunization [134], which offers the added advantage of eliciting a more Th1-like antibody subclass pattern of response than immunization by the systemic route [135]. Nonetheless, the relative importance of IgG versus IgA antibodies in preventing *S. aureus* colonization is not known. The mucosal immunization route has been shown to stimulate both mucosal and systemic immunity and thus might offer immune protection against both invasive disease and nasal carriage [125,136,137].

Conclusions and considerations

Despite the progress made over the past 10 years in developing an *S. aureus* vaccine, unresolved issues and unanswered questions remain (Table 32.4). There are lessons to be learned from the initial promising results and ultimate failures of the StaphVAX [43] and Veronate [62,63] phase III clinical trials, and these lessons are broadly applicable to the development of a vaccine against *S. aureus*. First, a multicomponent vaccine will no doubt

Table 32.4 Unresolved issues in *S. aureus* vaccine development.

Can *S. aureus* infections be prevented by vaccination?
Who should receive the *S. aureus* vaccine?
What are the measurable correlates of protective immunity?
What are the appropriate antigens for inclusion in a multicomponent staphylococcal vaccine?
Can a multicomponent vaccine address the protean clinical manifestations of *S. aureus* disease?
Can one expect a vaccine to protect against an infection involving a prosthetic device?
Do the animal models chosen for preclinical studies reflect the pathogenesis of human disease?
Will a vaccine that reduces *S. aureus* nasal colonization reduce staphylococcal infections?

be essential. It is not surprising that a vaccine based only on a single *S. aureus* virulence determinant would be unsuccessful, given the multifactorial nature of the pathogenesis of staphylococcal infections. Neutralizing one of the myriad staphylococcal virulence factors is not sufficient to protect a susceptible human host.

The second lesson we learned from the Nabi and Inhibitex trials focuses on the vaccine target population. The patients in most need of a staphylococcal vaccine comprise a population whose immune systems may not adequately respond to immunization. For example, hemodialysis patients are at persistently elevated risk for *S. aureus* bacteremia, and they are an obvious target population for active immunization. However, the immune response to vaccination may be suboptimal in this cohort, as was seen with StaphVAX [138], hepatitis B [139], and influenza [140] vaccine administration to hemodialysis patients [141]. Likewise, about 20% of low-birthweight neonates develop late-onset sepsis and could benefit from passive immunization against staphylococcal infection. However, antibodies alone may be insufficient to protect these premature babies with poorly developed innate immunity. Targeting otherwise healthy individuals, such as those undergoing elective surgical procedures, may be the best way to demonstrate vaccine efficacy in clinical trials. Such trials may be essential in order to demonstrate proof of principle, i.e., a protective *S. aureus* vaccine can be formulated. However, such a trial will not solve the greater problem of protecting compromised hosts from life-threatening *S. aureus* infections.

Choosing appropriate antigens to include in a multicomponent vaccine is a major challenge in the development of a staphylococcal vaccine. Candidate antigens should be surface exposed, be expressed by the majority of clinical *S. aureus* isolates belonging to diverse lineages, and show minimal serological variability among strains. At least some of the candidate antigens should elicit antibodies that promote opsonophagocytic killing *in vitro* by human neutrophils. In addition, an ideal vaccine would include antigens that elicit antibodies to block staphylococcal adherence and/or biofilm formation and neutralize toxic *S. aureus* exoproteins. Vaccine efficacy would need to be tested in diverse models of *S. aureus* infection, such as endocarditis, bacteremia, pneumonia, and lethal sepsis.

The accessibility of *S. aureus* surface antigens has important implications for vaccine development since optimal targets for immunization should be surface exposed. This does not necessarily translate into recognition by antibodies to the antigen on *S. aureus* cells evaluated in flow cytometry experiments, since antibodies to surface proteins can penetrate the *S. aureus* CP layer and bind to proteins that are masked by capsule [142]. For example, ClfA and CP are both expressed by *S. aureus* in postexponential growth, but CP production at least partially masks cell wall-associated ClfA and prevents it from binding to fibrinogen [143]. If an antibody to a surface antigen is masked by CP, it will not retain functionality (mediating opsonization or blocking attachment).

Evaluation of the results of the clinical and preclinical studies summarized herein suggests several good candidate vaccine antigens: CP5, CP8, PNAG, cell wall-anchored proteins (ClfA and IsdB), and α-hemolysin H135A. These candidates are under investigation by academicians and researchers in various industrial settings. We would argue for development of a multicomponent staphylococcal vaccine that includes at least one surface antigen (such a fibronectin-binding protein A or IsdB) that is expressed during the exponential phase of bacterial growth. Antigen expression *in vivo* and under different growth conditions and media should also be explored.

Ultimately, it is likely that an *S. aureus* vaccine will form only part of our antistaphylococcal armamentarium. In developing an *S. aureus* vaccine, both active and passive approaches should be pursued, as these are not mutually exclusive and may very well turn out to be complementary. For severe *S. aureus* infections such as endocarditis, passive antistaphylococcal immunization could be used as an adjunct to antibiotics (as was studied with Aurograb and Aurexis). Eradication of nasal carriage by treatment with mupirocin, followed by administration of a vaccine that would prevent reacquisition of *S. aureus* nasal colonization, might reduce serious staphylococcal infections in certain at-risk populations. Ten years ago, there was much skepticism about the pursuit of a vaccine against *S. aureus*. Today, there is considerably more optimism, as the array of recently discovered proteins and polysaccharides that may be critical targets for protective immunity against *S. aureus* raise the prospect that an effective vaccine could be developed. However, our expectations need to be tempered, as developing an *S. aureus* vaccine that provides the levels of protection offered by other bacterial vaccines will be a formidable challenge.

Acknowledgment

This work is supported by NIH Grant AI29040.

References

1 Lowy FD. *Staphylococcus aureus* infections. N Engl J Med 1998; 339:520–32.
2 Klein E, Smith DL, Laxminarayan R. Hospitalizations and deaths caused by methicillin-resistant *Staphylococcus aureus*, United States, 1999–2005. Emerg Infect Dis 2007;13:1840–6.
3 de Lassence A, Hidri N, Timsit J-F *et al*. Control and outcome of a large outbreak of colonization and infection with glycopeptide-intermediate *Staphylococcus aureus* in an intensive care unit. Clin Infect Dis 2006;42:170–8.
4 McDonald JR, Carriker CM, Pien BC *et al*. Methicillin-resistant *Staphylococcus aureus* outbreak in an intensive care nursery: potential for interinstitutional spread. Pediatr Infect Dis J 2007;26:678–83.
5 Chambers HF. The changing epidemiology of *Staphylococcus aureus*? Emerg Infect Dis 2001;7:178–82.
6 Shastry L, Rahimian J, Lascher S. Community-associated methicillin-resistant *Staphylococcus aureus* skin and soft tissue infections in men who have sex with men in New York City. Arch Intern Med 2007;167:854–7.
7 Daum RS. Clinical practice. Skin and soft-tissue infections caused by methicillin-resistant *Staphylococcus aureus*. N Engl J Med 2007;357:380–90.
8 de Lencastre H, Oliveira D, Tomasz A. Antibiotic resistant *Staphylococcus aureus*: a paradigm of adaptive power. Curr Opin Microbiol 2007;10:428–35.
9 Graber CJ, Wong MK, Carleton HA *et al*. Intermediate vancomycin susceptibility in a community-associated MRSA clone. Emerg Infect Dis 2007;13:491–3.
10 Chang S, Sievert DM, Hageman JC *et al*. Infection with vancomycin-resistant *Staphylococcus aureus* containing the *vanA* resistance gene. N Engl J Med 2003;348:1342–7.
11 Centers for Disease Control and Prevention. Vancomycin-resistant *Staphylococcus aureus*: New York, 2004. MMWR 2004; 53:322–3.
12 Centers for Disease Control and Prevention. *Staphylococcus aureus* resistant to vancomycin: United States, 2002. MMWR 2002;51: 565–7.
13 Lee JC. *Staphylococcus aureus* vaccine. In: Ellis RW, Brodeur BR, eds. New Bacterial Vaccines. New York: Kluwer Academic/ Plenum Publishers, 2003:283–93.
14 Deresinski S. Antistaphylococcal vaccines and immunoglobulins: current status and future prospects. Drugs 2006;66:1797–806.
15 Projan SJ, Nesin M, Dunman PM, Projan SJ, Nesin M, Dunman PM. Staphylococcal vaccines and immunotherapy: to dream the impossible dream? Curr Opin Pharmacol 2006;6:473–9.
16 Otto M. Targeted immunotherapy for staphylococcal infections: focus on anti-MSCRAMM antibodies. BioDrugs 2008;22: 27–36.
17 Dryla A, Prustomersky S, Gelbmann D *et al*. Comparison of antibody repertoires against *Staphylococcus aureus* in healthy individuals and in acutely infected patients. Clin Diagn Lab Immunol 2005;12:387–98.
18 Kluytmans J, van Belkum A, Verbrugh H. Nasal carriage of *Staphylococcus aureus*: epidemiology, underlying mechanisms, and associated risks. Clin Microbiol Rev 1997;10:505–20.
19 Wertheim HFL, Melles DC, Vos MC *et al*. The role of nasal carriage in *Staphylococcus aureus* infections. Lancet Infect Dis 2005; 5:751–62.
20 Wertheim HF, Vos MC, Ott A *et al*. Risk and outcome of nosocomial *Staphylococcus aureus* bacteraemia in nasal carriers versus non-carriers. Lancet 2004;364:703–5.
21 Foster TJ. Immune evasion by staphylococci. Nat Rev Microbiol 2005;3:948–58.
22 Yarwood JM, Paquette KM, Tikh IB, Volper EM, Greenberg EP. Generation of virulence factor variants in *Staphylococcus aureus* biofilms. J Bacteriol 2007;189:7961–7.
23 Gotz F. *Staphylococcus* and biofilms. Mol Microbiol 2002;43: 1367–78.
24 Vaudaux P, Kelley WL, Lew DP. *Staphylococcus aureus* small colony variants: difficult to diagnose and difficult to treat. Clin Infect Dis 2006;43:968–70.
25 Sendi P, Rohrbach M, Graber P *et al*. *Staphylococcus aureus* small colony variants in prosthetic joint infection. Clin Infect Dis 2006;43:961–7.
26 Minnaganti VR, Cunha BA. Infections associated with uremia and dialysis. Infect Dis Clin North Am 2001;15:385–406.
27 Stoll BJ, Hansen N, Fanaroff AA *et al*. Late-onset sepsis in very low birth weight neonates: the experience of the NICHD neonatal research network. Pediatrics 2002;110:285–91.
28 Benjamin DK, Schelonka R, White R *et al*. A blinded, randomized, multicenter study of an intravenous *Staphylococcus aureus* immune globulin. J Perinatol 2006;26:290–5.
29 Kaufman D, Fairchild KD. Clinical microbiology of bacterial and fungal sepsis in very-low-birth-weight infants. Clin Microbiol Rev 2004;17:638–80.
30 Shorr AF. Epidemiology and economic impact of meticillin-resistant *Staphylococcus aureus*: review and analysis of the literature. Pharmacoeconomics 2007;25:751–68.
31 Cosgrove SE, Qi Y, Kaye KS, Harbarth S, Karchmer AW, Carmeli Y. The impact of methicillin resistance in *Staphylococcus aureus* bacteremia on patient outcomes: mortality, length of stay, and hospital charges. Infect Control Hosp Epidemiol 2005;26:166–74.
32 O'Riordan K, Lee JC. *Staphylococcus aureus* capsular polysaccharides. Clin Microbiol Rev 2004;17:218–34.
33 Eskola J, Kayhty H, Takala AK *et al*. A randomized, prospective field trial of a conjugate vaccine in the protection of infants and young children against invasive *Haemophilus influenzae* type b disease. N Engl J Med 1990;323:1381–7.
34 Swingler G, Fransman D, Hussey G. Conjugate vaccines for preventing *Haemophilus influenzae* type b infections. Cochrane Database of Systematic Reviews 2007;2:CD001729.
35 Gardner P. Clinical practice. Prevention of meningococcal disease. N Engl J Med 2006;355:1466–73.
36 Maiden MCJ, Stuart JM. Carriage of serogroup C meningococci 1 year after meningococcal C conjugate polysaccharide vaccination. Lancet 2002;359:1829–31.
37 Rennels MB, Edwards KM, Keyserling HL *et al*. Safety and immunogenicity of heptavalent pneumococcal vaccine conjugated to CRM197 in United States infants. Pediatrics 1998; 101:604–11.
38 Black SB, Shinefield HR, Ling S *et al*. Effectiveness of heptavalent pneumococcal conjugate vaccine in children younger than

five years of age for prevention of pneumonia. Pediatr Infect Dis J 2002;21:810–15.

39 Fattom A, Schneerson R, Szu SC *et al.* Synthesis and immunologic properties in mice of vaccines composed of *Staphylococcus aureus* type 5 and type 8 capsular polysaccharides conjugated to *Pseudomonas aeruginosa* exotoxin A. Infect Immun 1990;58: 2367–74.

40 Fattom A, Schneerson R, Watson DC *et al.* Laboratory and clinical evaluation of conjugate vaccines composed of *Staphylococcus aureus* type 5 and type 8 capsular polysaccharides bound to *Pseudomonas aeruginosa* recombinant exoprotein A. Infect Immun 1993;61:1023–32.

41 Fattom AI, Sarwar J, Ortiz A, Naso R. A *Staphylococcus aureus* capsular polysaccharide (CP) vaccine and CP-specific antibodies protect mice against bacterial challenge. Infect Immun 1996;64:1659–65.

42 Lee JC, Park JS, Shepherd SE, Carey V, Fattom A. Protective efficacy of antibodies to the *Staphylococcus aureus* type 5 capsular polysaccharide in a modified model of endocarditis in rats. Infect Immun 1997;65:4146–51.

43 Shinefield H, Black S, Fattom A *et al.* Use of a *Staphylococcus aureus* conjugate vaccine in patients receiving hemodialysis. N Engl J Med 2002;346:491–6.

44 Karakawa WW, Sutton A, Schneerson R, Karpas A, Vann WF. Capsular antibodies induce type-specific phagocytosis of capsulated *Staphylococcus aureus* by human polymorphonuclear leukocytes. Infect Immun 1988;56:1090–5.

45 Baddour LM, Tayidi MM, Walker E, McDevitt D, Foster TJ. Virulence of coagulase-deficient mutants of *Staphylococcus aureus* in experimental endocarditis. J Med Microbiol 1994;41:259–63.

46 Cocchiaro JL, Gomez MI, Risley A, Solinga R, Sordelli DO, Lee JC. Molecular characterization of the capsule locus from non-typeable *Staphylococcus aureus*. Mol Microbiol 2006;59: 948–60.

47 Pohlmann-Dietze P, Ulrich M, Kiser KB *et al.* Adherence of *Staphylococcus aureus* to endothelial cells: influence of capsular polysaccharide, global regulator *agr*, and bacterial growth phase. Infect Immun 2000;68:4865–71.

48 Etz H, Minh DB, Henics T *et al.* Identification of in vivo expressed vaccine candidate antigens from *Staphylococcus aureus*. Proc Natl Acad Sci USA 2002;99:6573–8.

49 Kuklin NA, Clark DJ, Secore S *et al.* A novel *Staphylococcus aureus* vaccine: iron surface determinant b induces rapid antibody responses in rhesus macaques and specific increased survival in a murine *S. aureus* sepsis model. Infect Immun 2006;74:2215–23.

50 Mazmanian SK, Ton-That H, Su K, Schneewind O. An iron-regulated sortase anchors a class of surface protein during *Staphylococcus aureus* pathogenesis. Proc Natl Acad Sci USA 2002;99:2293–8.

51 Ahmad A, Davies JA, Ravenhill KL, Skinner GRB. Development of a vaccine against staphylococcal infections. In 12th International Symposium on Staphylococci and Staphylococcal Infections, Maastricht, The Netherlands, 2006, Abstract p-091.

52 Foster TJ, Hook M. Surface protein adhesins of *Staphylococcus aureus*. Trends Microbiol 1998;6:484–8.

53 Clarke SR, Foster SJ. Surface adhesins of *Staphylococcus aureus*. Adv Microb Physiol 2006;51:187–224.

54 McDevitt D, Francois P, Vaudaux P, Foster TJ. Molecular characterization of the clumping factor (fibrinogen receptor) of *Staphylococcus aureus*. Mol Microbiol 1994;11:237–48.

55 Vaudaux PE, Francois P, Proctor RA *et al.* Use of adhesion-defective mutants of *Staphylococcus aureus* to define the role of specific plasma proteins in promoting bacterial adhesion to canine arteriovenous shunts. Infect Immun 1995;63:585–90.

56 Moreillon P, Entenza JM, Francioli P *et al.* Role of *Staphylococcus aureus* coagulase and clumping factor in pathogenesis of experimental endocarditis. Infect Immun 1995;63:4738–43.

57 McDevitt D, Francois P, Vaudaux P, Foster TJ. Identification of the ligand-binding domain of the surface-located fibrinogen receptor (clumping factor) of *Staphylococcus aureus*. Mol Microbiol 1995;16:895–907.

58 Sullam PM, Bayer AS, Foss WM, Cheung AL. Diminished platelet binding in vitro by *Staphylococcus aureus* is associated with reduced virulence in a rabbit model of infective endocarditis. Infect Immun 1996;64:4915–21.

59 Josefsson E, Hartford O, O'Brien L, Patti JM, Foster T. Protection against experimental *Staphylococcus aureus* arthritis by vaccination with clumping factor A, a novel virulence determinant. J Infect Dis 2001;184:1572–80.

60 Vernachio J, Bayer AS, Le T *et al.* Anti-clumping factor A immunoglobulin reduces the duration of methicillin-resistant *Staphylococcus aureus* bacteremia in an experimental model of infective endocarditis. Antimicrob Agents Chemother 2003;47: 3400–6.

61 Vernachio JH, Bayer AS, Ames B *et al.* Human immunoglobulin G recognizing fibrinogen-binding surface proteins is protective against both *Staphylococcus aureus* and *Staphylococcus epidermidis* infections in vivo. Antimicrob Agents Chemother 2006;50:511–18.

62 Bloom B, Schelonka R, Kueser T *et al.* Multicenter study to assess safety and efficacy of INH-A21, a donor-selected human staphylococcal immunoglobulin, for prevention of nosocomial infections in very low birth weight infants. Pediatr Infect Dis J 2005;24:858–66.

63 DeJonge M, Burchfield D, Bloom B *et al.* Clinical trial of safety and efficacy of INH-A21 for the prevention of nosocomial staphylococcal bloodstream infection in premature infants. J Pediatr 2007;151:260–5.

64 Banerjea MC, Speer CP. The current role of colony-stimulating factors in prevention and treatment of neonatal sepsis. Semin Neonatol 2002;7:335–49.

65 Carr R, Modi N, Dore C. G-CSF and GM-CSF for treating or preventing neonatal infections. Cochrane Database of Systematic Reviews 2003;3:CD003066.

66 Hall AE, Domanski PJ, Patel PR *et al.* Characterization of a protective monoclonal antibody recognizing *Staphylococcus aureus* MSCRAMM protein clumping factor A. Infect Immun 2003;71:6864–70.

67 Patti JM. A humanized monoclonal antibody targeting *Staphylococcus aureus*. Vaccine 2004;22(suppl 1):S39–S43.

68 Weems JJ Jr, Steinberg JP, Filler S *et al.* Phase II, randomized, double-blind, multicenter study comparing the safety and pharmacokinetics of tefibazumab to placebo for treatment of *Staphylococcus aureus* bacteremia. Antimicrob Agents Chemother 2006;50:2751–5.

69 Hetherington S, Texter M, Wenzel E *et al.* Phase I dose escalation study to evaluate the safety and pharmacokinetic profile

of tefibazumab in subjects with end-stage renal disease requiring hemodialysis. Antimicrob Agents Chemother 2006;50: 3499–500.

70 Rupp ME, Holley HP Jr, Lutz J *et al.* Phase II, randomized, multicenter, double-blind, placebo-controlled trial of a polyclonal anti-*Staphylococcus aureus* capsular polysaccharide immune globulin in treatment of *Staphylococcus aureus* bacteremia. Antimicrob Agents Chemother 2007;51:4249–54.

71 Garmory HS, Titball RW. ATP-binding cassette transporters are targets for the development of antibacterial vaccines and therapies. Infect Immun 2004;72:6757–63.

72 Burnie JP, Matthews RC, Carter T *et al.* Identification of an immunodominant ABC transporter in methicillin-resistant *Staphylococcus aureus* infections. Infect Immun 2000;68:3200–9.

73 Ruhland GJ, Fiedler F. Occurrence and structure of lipoteichoic acids in the genus *Staphylococcus*. Arch Microbiol 1990;154: 375–9.

74 von Aulock S, Morath S, Hareng L *et al.* Lipoteichoic acid from *Staphylococcus aureus* is a potent stimulus for neutrophil recruitment. Immunobiology 2003;208:413–22.

75 Morath S, Geyer A, Hartung T. Structure–function relationship of cytokine induction by lipoteichoic acid from *Staphylococcus aureus*. J Exp Med 2001;193:393–7.

76 Morath S, Stadelmaier A, Geyer A, Schmidt RR, Hartung T. Synthetic lipoteichoic acid from *Staphylococcus aureus* is a potent stimulus of cytokine release. J Exp Med 2002;195:1635–40.

77 Weisman LE, Thackray HM, Garcia-Prats JA *et al.* A phase 1/2 double blind, placebo-controlled, dose escalation, safety, and pharmo kinetic study in very low birth weight neonates of pagibaximab (BSYX-ALLO), an anti-staphylococcal monodonal antibody for the prevention of staphylococcal bloodstream infections. Antimicrob Agents Chemother 2009 Apr 20 (Epub ahead of print).

78 Maira-Litran T, Kropec A, Joyce J, Mark G III, Goldmann DA, Pier GB. Immunochemical properties of the staphylococcal poly-N-acetylglucosamine surface polysaccharide. Infect Immun 2002;70:4433–40.

79 Cramton SE, Gerke C, Schnell NF, Nichols WW, Gotz F. The intercellular adhesion (*ica*) locus is present in *Staphylococcus aureus* and is required for biofilm formation. Infect Immun 1999;67:5427–33.

80 Cerca N, Jefferson KK, Maira-Litran T *et al.* Molecular basis for preferential protective efficacy of antibodies directed to the poorly acetylated form of staphylococcal poly-N-acetyl-beta-(1-6)-glucosamine. Infect Immun 2007;75:3406–13.

81 Heilmann C, Schweitzer O, Gerke C, Vanittanakom N, Mack D, Gotz F. Molecular basis of intercellular adhesion in the biofilm-forming *Staphylococcus epidermidis*. Mol Microbiol 1996;20:1083–91.

82 Vuong C, Kocianova S, Voyich JM *et al.* A crucial role for exopolysaccharide modification in bacterial biofilm formation, immune evasion, and virulence. J Biol Chem 2004;279: 54881–6.

83 Kelly-Quintos C, Kropec A, Briggs S, Ordonez CL, Goldmann DA, Pier GB. The role of epitope specificity in the human opsonic antibody response to the staphylococcal surface polysaccharide poly N-acetyl glucosamine. J Infect Dis 2005;192: 2012–19.

84 Maira-Litran T, Kropec A, Goldmann DA, Pier GB. Comparative opsonic and protective activities of *Staphylococcus aureus* conjugate vaccines containing native or deacetylated staphylococcal poly-N-acetyl-beta-(1-6)-glucosamine. Infect Immun 2005;73:6752–62.

85 Zhou H, Xiong ZY, Li HP *et al.* An immunogenicity study of a newly fusion protein Cna–FnBP vaccinated against *Staphylococcus aureus* infections in a mice model. Vaccine 2006;24: 4830–7.

86 Stranger-Jones YK, Bae T, Schneewind O. Vaccine assembly from surface proteins of *Staphylococcus aureus*. Proc Natl Acad Sci USA 2006;103:16942–7.

87 Mazmanian SK, Skaar EP, Gaspar AH *et al.* Passage of heme-iron across the envelope of *Staphylococcus aureus*. Science 2003; 299:906–9.

88 Gyimesi E, Bankovich AJ, Schuman TA, Goldberg JB, Lindorfer MA, Taylor RP. *Staphylococcus aureus* bound to complement receptor 1 on human erythrocytes by bispecific monoclonal antibodies is phagocytosed by acceptor macrophages. Immunol Lett 2004;95:185–92.

89 Mohamed N, Jones SM, Casey LS, Pincus SE, Spitalny GL. Heteropolymers: a novel technology against blood-borne infections. Curr Opin Mol Ther 2005;7:144–50.

90 Lindorfer MA, Hahn CS, Foley PL, Taylor RP. Heteropolymer-mediated clearance of immune complexes via erythrocyte CR1: mechanisms and applications. Immunol Rev 2001;183: 10–24.

91 Palma M, Nozohoor S, Schennings T, Heimdahl A, Flock JI. Lack of the extracellular 19-kilodalton fibrinogen-binding protein from *Staphylococcus aureus* decreases virulence in experimental wound infection. Infect Immun 1996;64:5284–9.

92 Shannon O, Uekotter A, Flock JI. The neutralizing effects of hyperimmune antibodies against extracellular fibrinogen-binding protein, Efb, from *Staphylococcus aureus*. Scand J Immunol 2006;63:184–90.

93 Song L, Hobaugh MR, Shustak C, Cheley S, Bayley H, Gouaux JE. Structure of staphylococcal alpha-hemolysin, a heptameric transmembrane pore. Science 1996;274:1859–66.

94 Liang X, Ji Y, Liang X, Ji Y. Alpha-toxin interferes with integrin-mediated adhesion and internalization of *Staphylococcus aureus* by epithelial cells. Cell Microbiol 2006;8:1656–68.

95 Adlam C, Ward PD, McCartney AC, Arbuthnott JP, Thorley CM. Effect of immunization with highly purified alpha- and beta-toxins on staphylococcal mastitis in rabbits. Infect Immun 1977;17:250–6.

96 Hume EB, Dajcs JJ, Moreau JM, O'Callaghan RJ. Immunization with alpha-toxin toxoid protects the cornea against tissue damage during experimental *Staphylococcus aureus* keratitis. Infect Immun 2000;68:6052–5.

97 Menzies BE, Kernodle DS. Passive immunization with antiserum to a nontoxic alpha-toxin mutant from *Staphylococcus aureus* is protective in a murine model. Infect Immun 1996;64: 1839–41.

98 Wardenburg JB, Schneewind O. Vaccine protection against *Staphylococcus aureus* pneumonia. J Exp Med 2008;205:287–94.

99 Wardenburg JB, Bae T, Otto M *et al.* Poring over pores: alpha-hemolysin and Panton–Valentine leukocidin in *Staphylococcus aureus* pneumonia. Nature Med 2007;13:1405–6.

100 Dinges MM, Orwin PM, Schlievert PM. Exotoxins of *Staphylococcus aureus*. Clin Microbiol Rev 2000;13:16–34.

101 Murray RJ. Recognition and management of *Staphylococcus aureus* toxin-mediated disease. Intern Med J 2005;35(suppl 2): S106–S119.

102 Lowell GH, Colleton C, Frost D *et al.* Immunogenicity and efficacy against lethal aerosol staphylococcal enterotoxin B challenge in monkeys by intramuscular and respiratory delivery of proteosome-toxoid vaccines. Infect Immun 1996;64:4686–93.

103 LeClaire RD, Hunt RE, Bavari S, LeClaire RD, Hunt RE, Bavari S. Protection against bacterial superantigen staphylococcal enterotoxin B by passive vaccination. Infect Immun 2002;70: 2278–81.

104 Gampfer J, Thon V, Gulle H, Wolf HM, Eibl MM. Double mutant and formaldehyde inactivated TSST-1 as vaccine candidates for TSST-1-induced toxic shock syndrome. Vaccine 2002;20:1354–64.

105 Cui JC, Hu DL, Lin YC, Qian AD, Nakane A. Immunization with glutathione S-transferase and mutant toxic shock syndrome toxin 1 fusion protein protects against *Staphylococcus aureus* infection. FEMS Immunol Med Microbiol 2005;45:45–51.

106 Hu D-L, Cui J-C, Omoe K *et al.* A mutant of staphylococcal enterotoxin C devoid of bacterial superantigenic activity elicits a Th2 immune response for protection against *Staphylococcus aureus* infection. Infect Immun 2005;73:174–80.

107 Nilsson IM, Verdrengh M, Ulrich RG, Bavari S, Tarkowski A. Protection against *Staphylococcus aureus* sepsis by vaccination with recombinant staphylococcal enterotoxin A devoid of superantigenicity. J Infect Dis 1999;180:1370–3.

108 Hu DL, Omoe K, Sasaki S *et al.* Vaccination with nontoxic mutant toxic shock syndrome toxin 1 protects against *Staphylococcus aureus* infection. J Infect Dis 2003;188:743–52.

109 Hu D-L, Omoe K, Narita K, Cui J-C, Shinagawa K, Nakane A. Intranasal vaccination with a double mutant of staphylococcal enterotoxin C provides protection against *Staphylococcus aureus* infection. Microbes Infect 2006;8:2841–8.

110 George EA, Muir TW. Molecular mechanisms of *agr* quorum sensing in virulent staphylococci. ChemBioChem 2007;8:847–55.

111 Goerke C, Wolz C. Regulatory and genomic plasticity of *Staphylococcus aureus* during persistent colonization and infection. Int J Med Microbiol 2004;294:195–202.

112 Park J, Jagasia R, Kaufmann GF *et al.* Infection control by antibody disruption of bacterial quorum sensing signaling. Chem Biol 2007;14:1119–27.

113 Donnelly JJ, Wahren B, Liu MA. DNA vaccines: progress and challenges. J Immunol 2005;175:633–9.

114 Srivastava IK, Liu MA. Gene vaccines. Ann Intern Med 2003; 138:550–9.

115 Brouillette E, Lacasse P, Shkreta L *et al.* DNA immunization against the clumping factor A (ClfA) of *Staphylococcus aureus.* Vaccine 2002;20:2348–57.

116 Therrien R, Lacasse P, Grondin G, Talbot BG. Lack of protection of mice against *Staphylococcus aureus* despite a significant immune response to immunization with a DNA vaccine encoding collagen-binding protein. Vaccine 2007;25:5053–61.

117 Gaudreau M-C, Lacasse P, Talbot BG. Protective immune responses to a multi-gene DNA vaccine against *Staphylococcus aureus.* Vaccine 2007;25:814–24.

118 Cossart P, Jonquieres R. Sortase, a universal target for therapeutic agents against Gram-positive bacteria? Proc Natl Acad Sci USA 2000;97:5013–15.

119 Ohwada A, Sekiya M, Hanaki H *et al.* DNA vaccination by *mecA* sequence evokes an antibacterial immune response against methicillin-resistant *Staphylococcus aureus.* J Antimicrob Chemother 1999;44:767–74.

120 Senna JPM, Roth DM, Oliveira JS, Machado DC, Santos DS. Protective immune response against methicillin resistant *Staphylococcus aureus* in a murine model using a DNA vaccine approach. Vaccine 2003;21:2661–6.

121 Roth DM, Senna JPM, Machado DC. Evaluation of the humoral immune response in Balb/C mice immunized with a naked DNA vaccine anti-methicillin-resistant *Staphylococcus aureus.* Genet Mol Res 2006;5:503–12.

122 von Eiff C, Becker K, Machka K, Stammer H, Peters G. Nasal carriage as a source of *Staphylococcus aureus* bacteremia. N Engl J Med 2001;344:11–16.

123 Kluytmans JA, Wertheim HF. Nasal carriage of *Staphylococcus aureus* and prevention of nosocomial infections. Infection 2005; 33:3–8.

124 Jones JC, Rogers TJ, Brookmeyer P *et al.* Mupirocin resistance in patients colonized with methicillin-resistant *Staphylococcus aureus* in a surgical intensive care unit. Clin Infect Dis 2007; 45:541–7.

125 Schaffer AC, Solinga RM, Cocchiaro J *et al.* Immunization with *Staphylococcus aureus* clumping factor B, a major determinant in nasal carriage, reduces nasal colonization in a murine model. Infect Immun 2006;74:2145–53.

126 Clarke SR, Brummell KJ, Horsburgh MJ *et al.* Identification of in vivo-expressed antigens of *Staphylococcus aureus* and their use in vaccinations for protection against nasal carriage. J Infect Dis 2006;193:1098–108.

127 Weidenmaier C, Kokai-Kun JF, Kristian SA *et al.* Role of teichoic acids in *Staphylococcus aureus* nasal colonization, a major risk factor in nosocomial infections. Nature Med 2004; 10:243–5.

128 Vinogradov E, Sadovskaya I, Li J, Jabbouri S. Structural elucidation of the extracellular and cell-wall teichoic acids of *Staphylococcus aureus* MN8m, a biofilm forming strain. Carbohydr Res 2006;341:738–43.

129 Weidenmaier C, Peschel A, Xiong YQ *et al.* Lack of wall teichoic acids in *Staphylococcus aureus* leads to reduced interactions with endothelial cells and to attenuated virulence in a rabbit model of endocarditis. J Infect Dis 2005;191:1771–7.

130 Kauppi M, Saarinen L, Kayhty H. Anti-capsular polysaccharide antibodies reduce nasopharyngeal colonization by *Haemophilus influenzae* type b in infant rats. J Infect Dis 1993;167: 365–71.

131 Barbour ML, Mayon-White RT, Coles C, Crook DW, Moxon ER. The impact of conjugate vaccine on carriage of *Haemophilus influenzae* type b. J Infect Dis 1995;171:93–8.

132 Pelton SI, Loughlin AM, Marchant CD. Seven valent pneumococcal conjugate vaccine immunization in two Boston communities: changes in serotypes and antimicrobial susceptibility among *Streptococcus pneumoniae* isolates. Pediatr Infect Dis J 2004;23:1015–22.

133 Ghaffar F, Barton T, Lozano J *et al.* Effect of the 7-valent pneumococcal conjugate vaccine on nasopharyngeal colonization by *Streptococcus pneumoniae* in the first 2 years of life. Clin Infect Dis 2004;39:930–8.

134 Brandtzaeg P. Role of secretory antibodies in the defense against infections. Int J Med Microbiol 2003;293:3–15.

135 Hanniffy SB, Carter AT, Hitchin E, Wells JM. Mucosal delivery of a pneumococcal vaccine using *Lactococcus lactis* affords protection against respiratory infection. J Infect Dis 2007;195: 185–93.

136 Stiles BG, Garza AR, Ulrich RG, Boles JW. Mucosal vaccination with recombinantly attenuated staphylococcal enterotoxin B and protection in a murine model. Infect Immun 2001;69:2031–6.

137 Castagliuolo I, Piccinini R, Beggiao E *et al.* Mucosal genetic immunization against four adhesins protects against *Staphylococcus aureus*-induced mastitis in mice. Vaccine 2006;24:4393–402.

138 Welch PG, Fattom A, Moore J Jr *et al.* Safety and immunogenicity of *Staphylococcus aureus* type 5 capsular polysaccharide–*Pseudomonas aeruginosa* recombinant exoprotein A conjugate vaccine in patients on hemodialysis. J Am Soc Nephrol 1996; 7:247–53.

139 Davis JP. Experience with hepatitis A and B vaccines. Am J Med 2005;118(suppl 10A):7S–15S.

140 Tanzi E, Amendola A, Pariani E *et al.* Lack of effect of a booster dose of influenza vaccine in hemodialysis patients. J Med Virol 2007;79:1176–9.

141 Johnson DW, Fleming SJ. The use of vaccines in renal failure. Clin Pharmacokinet 1992;22:434–46.

142 Watts A, Ke D, Wang Q, Pillay A, Nicholson-Weller A, Lee JC. *Staphylococcus aureus* strains that express serotype 5 or serotype 8 capsular polysaccharides differ in virulence. Infect Immun 2005;73:3502–11.

143 Risley AL, Loughman A, Cywes-Bentley C, Foster TJ, Lee JC. Capsular polysaccharide masks clumping factor A-mediated adherence of *Staphylococcus aureus* to fibrinogen and platelets. J Infect Dis 2007;196:919–27.

Index

Page numbers in **bold** represent tables, those in *italics* represent figures.

As most of the text applies to *S. aureus*, entries under that heading have been kept to a minimum, and readers should look for more specific topics.